D1758575

Foundations of Anesthesia Basic and Clinical Sciences

Hugh C Hemmings Jr BS MD PhD
Associate Professor of Pharmacology and Anesthesiology
Vice Chairman of Research in Anesthesiology
Weill Medical College of Cornell University, and
Attending Anesthesiologist, New York Presbyterian Hospital
New York
USA

Philip M Hopkins MB BS MD FRCA
Senior Lecturer in Anaesthesia, University of Leeds, and
Honorary Consultant in Anaesthesia, Leeds Teaching Hospitals Trust
Academic Unit of Anaesthesia
St James's University Hospital
Leeds
UK

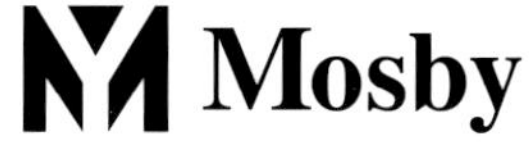

London Edinburgh Philadelphia St Louis Sydney Toronto 2000

MOSBY
An imprint of Harcourt Publishers Limited

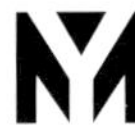

First published 2000

ISBN 0–7234–27879

British Library Cataloguing in Publication Data
A catalogue record for this book is available from the British Library

Library of Congress Cataloging in Publication Data
A catalog record for this book is available from the Library of Congress

Drug Notice
The contributors, the editors, and the publishers have made every effort to ensure the accuracy and appropriateness of the drug dosages presented in this textbook. The medications described do not necessarily have specific approval by drug regulatory authorities in all countries for use in the diseases and dosages for which they are recommended. The package insert for each drug should be consulted for use and dosage as approved by the relevant drug regulatory authority. Because standards for usage change, it is advisable to keep abreast of revised recommendations, particularly those concerning new drugs.

Medical Editor	Maria Khan
Development Editor	Maria Stewart
Project Manager	Philip Dauncey
Illustration Manager	Mick Ruddy
Senior Designer	Ian Spick
Production Manager	Mark Sanderson

Printed in Spain

Foreword

Drs Hemmings and Hopkins have assembled seventy chapters written by well-recognized authorities from both sides of the Atlantic. Though the sea of knowledge is never full, they have completed an extraordinary and successful labor in producing a significant tidal surge that will be regarded as the high water mark to be noted by generations of anesthesiologists yet unborn.

Essential to the understanding of this text is the editor's 'conviction that the successful practice of the art of anesthesia requires a sound understanding of the underlying scientific principles'. This quotation from the invitational letter to each contributor summarizes the philosophy which underlies the entire work. The seventy chapters are grouped under eight major headings (General Principles, Neurosciences, Cardiovascular system, Respiratory system, Pathological sciences, Renal system, Gastrointestinal system and metabolism, and Adaptive physiology). Within each section of the book, there are chapters that cover the essential basic science information necessary for the understanding of the section's utility in clinical practice.

The amount of basic science information has grown tremendously during my half century in medicine. When I started my training, I was initially taught clinical anesthesia by very skillful nurse anesthetists who were far more concerned with the art of anesthesia. Scientific information was scarce. John Snow's classic monograph on the inhalation of the vapor of ether was one of the first publications to provide a scientific basis for the practice of our art. In 1924, Howard Haggard published five classic papers in the *Journal of Biological Chemistry* on the uptake and elimination of diethyl ether, attributing his failure to effect quantitative recovery to the volatility of ether rather than to the possibility of its metabolism by the body. The importance of water solubility on the speed of anesthetic action was soon elucidated by Seymour Kety. And so opened a new era in the scientific understanding of what had previously been largely a clinical art.

When Dr Hemmings honored me by asking me to write this piece, I asked myself not only what to say, but also who might have said it very well in the past. The answer rose immediately to mind: more than 30 years ago, John Severinghaus wrote the foreword for the first edition of John Nunn's classic book on respiratory physiology – a book which, like this one, combined and correlated basic science with clinical practice. He chose the title 'A Flame for Hypnos', and illustrated it with a photograph of a lighted candle before the statue of the god of sleep. No one has ever said it so well. Never have I read a more beautiful foreword and append a part of it here with the permission of Dr Severinghaus (who himself has contributed a chapter to this book). So from the work of many minds and hands this book goes forth, that we too, by understanding the process, may better the art.

Alan Van Poznak, M.D.
New York City
1999

The world will little note nor long remember what I say here, but it can never forget what we did here.

Abraham Lincoln, Gettysburg, November 19, 1863

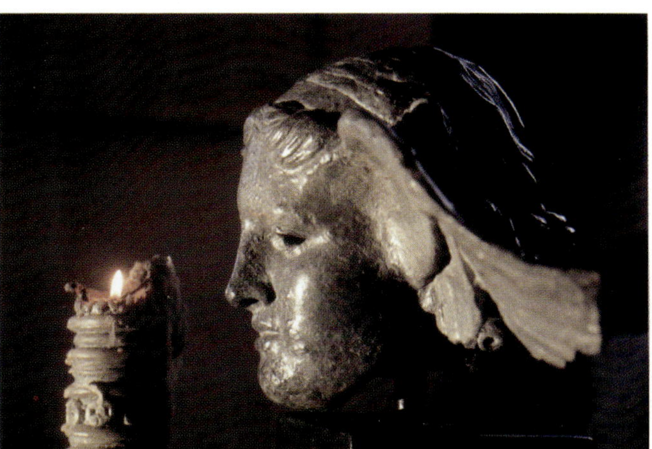

Excerpted from the foreword to the first edition (1969) of *Applied Respiratory Physiology* by John F. Nunn, reprinted with the permission of Butterworth-Heinemann:

The lighted candle respires and we call it flame. The body respires and we call it life. Neither flame nor life is substance, but process. The flame is as different from the wick and wax as life from the body, as gravitation from the falling apple, or love from a hormone. Newton taught science to have faith in processes as well as substances – to compute, predict and depend upon an irrational attraction. Caught up in enlightenment, man began to regard himself as a part of nature, a subject for investigation. The web of self-knowledge, woven so slowly between process and substance, still weaves physiology, the process, and anatomy, the substance, into the whole cloth of clinical medicine. Within this multihued fabric, the warp fibres of process shine most clearly in the newest patterns, among which must be numbered anaesthesiology.

And what of the god of sleep, patron of anaesthesia? The centuries themselves number more than 21 since Hypnos wrapped his cloak of sleep over Hellas. Now before Hypnos, the artisan, is set the respiring flame – that he may, by knowing the process, better the art.

John W. Severinghaus
San Francisco

Preface

The successful practice of the art of anesthesia and critical care demands a sound understanding of underlying scientific concepts. This is recognized in the postgraduate examinations in anesthesia in North America, Europe and Australasia, for which a thorough understanding of the relevant basic sciences is required. There is no single currently available text that presents basic scientific principles relevant to the practice of anesthesia. Furthermore, many trainees in anesthesia come to view learning the basic sciences to the required depth as a necessary chore. This is disappointing to those of us who find the scientific basis for our clinical practice to be a constant source of interest, fascination and, indeed, sometimes excitement. Part of the problem is that basic science texts directed towards anesthetists tend to be fact, rather than concept-oriented, and therefore difficult to read and to learn from.

Foundations of Anesthesia: Basic and Clinical Sciences emphasizes the principles and clinical applications of the four major areas of basic science that are relevant to anesthesia practice: molecular and cell biology, physiology, pharmacology, and physics and measurement. The approach is integrated and systems oriented, avoiding the artificial boundaries between the basic sciences. Recognizing that no single author possesses the breadth and depth of understanding of all relevant subjects, each chapter is authored by an expert in that area. These authorities represent many of the finest institutions of North America and the United Kingdom. This allows an international presentation of current anesthesia science presented by relevant experts at the cutting edge of anesthesia research and education.

Each chapter stresses the scientific principles necessary to understand and manage various situations encountered in anesthesia. Detailed explanations of techniques are avoided since this information is available in many subspecialty anesthesia texts. Nor is this book intended to provide a detailed review of specialized research areas for the scientist. Rather, the fundamental information necessary to understand "why" and "how" is stressed, and basic concepts are related to relevant anesthesia situations. The style stresses a conceptual approach to learning, using factual information to illustrate the concepts. Chapters are self-contained with minimal repetition, and include a short list of Key References and suggestions for Further Reading. This style and approach is modeled after the ground-breaking text *Scientific Foundations of Anesthesia*, edited by Cyril Scurr and Stanley Feldman, updated to cover the revolutionary developments in modern molecular biology and physiology. Recognizing that graphics are the most expressive way of conveying concepts, full-color illustrations facilitate use of the book as a learning aid and make it enjoyable to read.

Hugh C Hemmings Jr
Philip M Hopkins
1999

Acknowledgements

We would like to acknowledge our mentors and students, who have taught us and from whom we continue to learn.

Dedication

To our wives Katherine Albert and Carmel Hopkins, whose countless contributions and support were vital.

Contents

Section 3 Cardiovascular system

Section 4 Respiratory system

Section 5 Pathological sciences

Section 6 Renal system

Section 7 Gastrointestinal system and metabolism

Section 8 Adaptive physiology

Contributors

James Arden, MD PhD
Assistant Professor of Anesthesiology, Department of Anesthesiology, Weill Cornell Medical College of Cornell University, New York, New York, USA

Solomon Aronson, MD
Department of Anesthesiology and Critical Care Medicine, University of Chicago School of Medicine, Chicago, Illinois, USA

John L Atlee, MD FACA FACC
Professor of Anesthesiology, Department of Anesthesiology, Medical College of Wisconsin, Milwaukee, Wisconsin, USA

Jeffrey R Balser, MD PhD
Associate Professor of Anesthesiology and Pharmacology, The James Taloe Gwathmey Chair, Vanderbilt University School of Medicine, Nashville, Tennessee, USA

Paul R Barach, MD BSc MPH
Instructor, Harvard Medical School, Massachusetts General Hospital, Boston, Massachusetts, USA

Paul C W Beatty, PhD
ISBE, University of Manchester, Manchester, UK

Mark C Bellamy, MA MB BS FRCA
Consultant, Intensive Care Unit, St James's University Hospital, Leeds, West Yorkshire, UK

Heith H Berge, MD
Instructor of Anesthesiology, Mayo Medical School, Rochester, Minnesota, USA

Thomas J J Blanck, MD PhD
Director of Anesthesiology, Hospital for Special Surgery, Professor of Anesthesiology, Physiology and Biophysics, Weill Cornell Medical College of Cornell University, New York, New York, USA

Andrew R Bodenham, MBBS FRCA
Director of Intensive Care and Consultant Anaesthetist, Leeds General Infirmary, Leeds, West Yorkshire, UK

Simon Christopher Body, MB ChB FANZCA
Assistant Professor, Department of Anesthesia, Perioperative and Pain Medicine, Brigham and Women's Hospital, Boston, Massachusetts, USA

John V Booth, MB ChB FRCA
Assistant Professor of Anesthesiology, Department of Anesthesiology, Duke University Medical Center, Durham, North Carolina, USA

Emery N Brown, MD PhD
Assistant Professor of Anesthesia, Harvard Medical School, Department of Anesthesia and Critical Care, Massachusetts General Hospital, Boston, Massachusetts, USA

John Butterworth, MD
Professor and Head, Section of Cardiothoracic Anesthesia, Department of Anesthesia, Wake Forest University School of Medicine, Winston-Salem, North Carolina, USA

Iain T Campbell, FRCA
Reader, University Department of Anaesthesia, University Hospitals of South Manchester, Withenston Hospital, Manchester, UK

Andrew T Cohen, MB ChB FRCA
Consultant in Anaesthesia and Intensive Care, Intensive Care Unit, St James's University Hospital, Leeds, West Yorkshire, UK

Alan Davey-Quinn, MB ChB FRCA
Specialist Registrar, Intensive Care Unit, St James's University Hospital, Leeds, West Yorkshire, UK

Joan P Desborough, MD FRCA
Consultant Anaesthetist, Epsom County Hospital, Epsom, Surrey, UK

Thomas J Ebert, MD PhD
Professor of Anesthesiology; Adjunct Professor of Physiology, VA Medical Center, Milwaukee, Wisconsin, USA

Simon M Enright, MB ChB FRCA
Consultant Anaesthetist and Director of Intensive Care, Intensive Care Unit, Pinderfields Hospital, Wakefield, West Yorkshire, UK

John Feiner, MD
Department of Anesthesiology, University of California at San Francisco School of Medicine, San Francisco, California, USA

Pierre Foëx, DPhil FRCA FANZCA FMedSci
Professor, Nuffield Department of Anaesthetics, Radcliffe Infirmary, Oxford, Oxfordshire, UK

Patricia Fogarty Mack, MD
Assistant Professor of Anesthesiology, Department of Anesthesiology, Weill Medical College of Cornell University, New York, New York, USA

Steven M. Frank, MD
Associate Professor, Department of Anesthesiology and Critical Care Medicine, Johns Hopkins Hospital, Baltimore, Maryland, USA

Helen F Galley PhD FIMLS
Lecturer in Anaesthesia and Intensive Care, Academic Unit of Anaesthesia and Intensive Care, University of Aberdeen, Aberdeen, UK

Susan Garwood, MB ChB BSc FRCA
Assistant Professor of Anesthesiology, Department of Anesthesiology, Yale University, New Haven, Connecticut, USA

Kevin J Gingrich, MD
Associate Professor of Anesthesiology, Department of Anesthesiology, University of Rochester Medical Center, Rochester, New York, USA

Nikolaus Gravenstein, MD BCA
Professor and Chairman of Anesthesiology, Department of Anesthesiology, University of Florida College of Medicine, Gainesville, Florida, USA

Roger Hainsworth, MB ChB PhD DSc
Professor of Applied Physiology, Institute for Cardiovascular Research, University of Leeds, Leeds, West Yorkshire, UK

Philip Meade Hartigan, MD
Instructor in Anesthesia, Department of Anesthesia, Perioperative and Pain Medicine, Brigham and Women's Hospital, Boston, Massachusetts, USA

Paul M Heerdt, MD
Associate Professor of Anesthesiology and Pharmacology, Department of Anesthesiology, Weill Medical College of Cornell University, New York, New York, USA

Norman L Herman, MD PhD
Assistant Professor of Anesthesiology; Director, Obstetric Anesthesia, Department of Anesthesiology, Weill Medical College of Cornell University, New York, New York, USA

Andrew T Hindle, MB BCh DA BSc FRCA
Consultant Anaesthetist, Department of Anaesthesia, Warrington Hospital, Warrington, Lancashire, UK

Kirk Hogan, MD
Associate Professor of Anesthesiology, Department of Anesthesiology, University of Wisconsin Medical School, Madison, Wisconsin, USA

Simon Howell, MSc MBBS MRCP FRCA
Consultant Senior Lecturer in Anaesthesia, Sir Humphrey Davy Department of Anaesthesia, Bristol Royal Infirmary, Bristol, UK

Michael J Hudspith, MBBS BSc PhD FRCA
Consultant Anaesthesia and Pain Relief, Norfolk and Norwich Hospital, Norwich, Norfolk, UK

Christopher J Hull, MB BS FRCA
Emeritus Professor of Anaesthesia, University of Newcastle-upon-Tyne, Newcastle-upon-Tyne, UK

Uday Jain, MD PhD
Clinical Associate Professor, Department of Anesthesia, Stanford University School of Medicine, Stanford, California, USA

E Heidi Jerome, MD
Associate Professor of Anesthesiology and Pediatrics, College of Physicians and Surgeons of Columbia University, New York, New York, USA

David C Leach, MD
Associate Professor of Internal Medicine, Loyola University School of Medicine, Executive Director of the ACGME, Chicago, Illinois, USA

David L Lee, MD
Assistant Professor of Anesthesiology, Weill Medical College of Cornell University; Attending Anesthesiologist, Hospital for Special Surgery, New York, New York, USA

Jerrold Lerman, MD BASc FRPC FANZCA
Professor of Anaesthesia, Department of Anaesthesia, Hospital for Sick Children, Toronto, Ontario, Canada

Cynthia A Lien, MD
Associate Professor of Anesthesiology, Department of Anesthesiology, Weill Medical College of Cornell University, New York, New York, USA

Emilio B Lobato, MD BCA BCIM
Associate Professor in Anesthesiology, University of Florida College of Medicine, Gainesville, Florida, USA

Martin J London, MD
Professor in Residence – Anesthesia, VA Medical Center, San Francisco, California, USA

Louise Lynch, MB ChB FRCA
Specialist Registrar in Anaesthesia, St James's Hospital, Leeds, West Yorkshire, UK

Ken Mackie, MD
Associate Professor, Department of Anesthesiology, University of Washington, Seattle, Washington, USA

Abhraim Mallick, MB BS FRCA FFARCSI
Consultant in Anaesthesia and Intensive Care, Huddersfield Royal Infirmary, Huddersfield, UK

Harold M Marsh, MB BS BSc FANZCA FCCP FACA
Professor and Chair of Anesthesiology, Wayne State University, Specialist-in-Chief, Department of Anesthesiology, Detroit Medical Center, Detroit, Michigan, USA

Iain G Marshall, BSc PhD
Emeritus Professor, Department of Physiology and Pharmacology, University of Strathclyde, Glasgow, UK

Henry J McQuay, DM FRCA
Professor of Pain Relief, Pain Research, University of Oxford, Churchill Hospital, Oxford, Oxfordshire, UK

Jose Melendez, MD
Memorial Sloan–Kettering Cancer Center, New York, New York, USA

Eric J Moody, MD
Associate Professor of Anesthesia and Critical Care Medicine, Johns Hopkins Hospital, Baltimore, Maryland, USA

R Andrew Moore, DSc
Consultant Biochemist, Pain Research, University of Oxford, Churchill Hospital, Oxford, Oxfordshire, UK

Salim Mujais, MD
Medical Director, Renal Division, Baxter Healthcare Corporation, Deerfield, Illinois, USA

Rajesh Munglani
Senior Lecturer in Anaesthesia and Pain Relief, University of Cambridge, Addenbrooke's Hospital, Cambridge, UK

Paul G Murphy, MA MB ChB FRCA
Consultant Anaesthetist, Department of Anaesthesia, The General Infirmary at Leeds, Leeds, West Yorkshire, UK

Daniel Nyhan, MD
Department of Anesthesia and Critical Care Medicine, Johns Hopkins Medical Hospital, Baltimore, Maryland, USA

Hugh A O'Beirne, MB BAO BCh FFARCSI
Consultant in Anaesthesia and Intensive Care, Intensive Care Unit, Pinderfields Hospital, Wakefield, West Yorkshire, UK

Peter J Papadakos, MD FCCM FCCP
Associate Professor of Anesthesiolgy, University of Rochester, Professor of Respiratory Care, State University of New York, Department of Anesthesiology, University of Rochester, New York, USA

Gavril W Pasternak, MD PhD
Member and Attending Neurologist, Memorial Sloan–Kettering Cancer Center, New York, New York, USA

Alison J Pittard, MD FRCA
Consultant in Anaesthesia and Intensive Care, The General Infirmary at Leeds, Leeds, West Yorkshire, UK

Christopher B Prior, BSc PhD
Department of Physiology and Pharmacology, University of Strathclyde, Glasgow, UK

David J Rowbotham, MB ChB FRCA MRCP
Professor of Anaesthesia and Pain Management, Leicester University, Leicester, UK

Keith J Ruskin, MD
Associate Professor of Anesthesiology, Yale University School of Medicine, New Haven, Connecticut, USA

John J Savarese, MD
Professor and Chairman, Department of Anesthesiology, Weill Medical College of Cornell University, New York, New York, USA

Debra A Schwinn, MD
Professor of Anesthesiology, Pharmacology, Cancer Biology and Surgery, Department of Anesthesiology, Duke University Medical Center, Durham, North Carolina, USA

John Severinghaus, MD
Professor Emeritus, Department of Anesthesiology, University of California at San Francisco School of Medicine, San Francisco, California, USA

Nitin Shah, MD
Associate Clinical Professor, Department of Anesthesiology, VAMC, Long Beach, California, USA

Philip J Siddall FRCA
University of Cambridge, Addenbrookes Hospital, Cambridge, UK

Jeffrey H Silverstein, MD
Department of Anesthesia, Mount Sinai Medical Center, New York, New York, USA

Brett A Simon, MD PhD
Associate Professor, Anesthesiology and Critical Care Medicine, Johns Hopkins Hospital, Baltimore, Maryland, USA

Karen H Simpson, MB ChB FRCA
Consultant in Anaesthesia and Pain Management, St James's University Hospital, Leeds, West Yorkshire, UK

Tod B Sloan, MD PhD
Professor of Anesthesiology, Department of Anesthesiology, University of Texas Health Science Center, San Antonio, Texas, USA

Robert E Study, MD PhD
Staff Anesthesiologist, Department of Anesthesia, Faulkner Hospital, Jamaica Plain, Massachusetts, USA

Richard Teplick, MD
Vice Chairman, Department of Anesthesia, Brigham Women's Hospital, and Associate Professor of Anesthesia, Harvard Medical School, Boston, Massachusetts, USA

Stephen J Thomas, MD
Professor and Vice Chair, Department of Anesthesiology, Weill Medical College of Cornell University, New York, New York, USA

Howard M Thompson FRCA
Consultant in Anaesthesia and Pain Management , Pilgrim Hospital, Boston, UK

Robert A Veselis, MD
Director, Neuroanesthesiology Research Laboratory, Department of Anesthesiology, Weill Medical College of Cornell University, New York, NY, USA

Mladen Vidovich, MD
Anesthesia Department, Northwestern University, Chicago, Illinois, USA

H Ronald Vinik, MD
Professor of Anesthesia, Eye Foundation Hospital, Birmingham, Alabama, USA

David O Warner, MD
Professor of Anesthesiology, Mayo Medical School, Rochester, Minnesota, USA

Lisa Warren, MD
Department of Anesthesiology, Weill Medical College of Cornell University, New York, New York, USA

Nigel R Webster, BSc MB ChB PhD FRCA FRCP
Professor in Anaesthesia and Intensive Care, Academic Unit of Anaesthesia and Intensive Care, University of Aberdeen, Aberdeen, UK

Ian G Wilson, MB ChB FRCA
Consultant Anaesthetist, Department of Anaesthesia, St James's University Hospital, Leeds, West Yorkshire, UK

William Winlow, PhD
Professor of Neuroscience; Head, Department of Biological Sciences, University of Central Lancashire, Preston, UK

Jacques Ya Deau, MD PhD
Assistant Professor of Anesthesiology, Weill Medical College of Cornell University, Hospital for Special Surgery, New York, New York, USA

Jay Yang, MD PhD
Associate Professor of Anesthesiology and Pharmacology/Physiology, University of Rochester Medical Center, Rochester, New York, New York, USA

William L Young, MD BCA
Professor of Anesthesiology (in Neurological Surgery and Radiology), College of Physicians and Surgeons of Columbia University, New York, New York, USA

Michael Zaugg, MD
Department of Anesthesia, Mount Sinai Medical Center, New York, New York, USA

Michael Zwillman, MD
Department of Medicine, Huntington Hospital, New York, New York, USA

Chapter 1 Molecular structure and biochemistry

James Arden

Topics covered in this chapter

Molecular structure
Biochemistry
Solution chemistry
Molecular interactions

In this chapter fundamental ideas of molecular structure and principles of biochemistry, pharmacology, and physiology relevant to anesthesiology are introduced.

MOLECULAR STRUCTURE

Atoms

An atom consists of *elementary particles*, protons, neutrons, and electrons, and approximately 20 *subatomic particles* (mesons, bosons, etc.). The mass of the atom is provided principally by the *protons* and the slightly larger *neutrons*. *Electron*s are much smaller, with a mass approximately 0.05% that of a proton. The number of protons (and electrons in an uncharged atom) is the *atomic number* (6, 7, and 8 for carbon, nitrogen, and oxygen, respectively), and the total mass of the protons plus neutrons is the *atomic mass* or *mass number* (12, 14, and 16 for carbon, nitrogen, and oxygen, respectively). Mass numbers are indicated by superscripts before the element symbol (e.g. ^{12}C, ^{14}N, ^{16}O). *Isotopes* are atoms with the same atomic numbers but with different atomic masses. Naturally occurring elements are found as mixtures of isotopes. For hydrogen, the hydrogen atom of atomic number 1 and atomic mass 1 (^{1}H) is about 5000 times more common than its stable isotope, deuterium (^{2}H) which has one neutron (atomic number 1, atomic mass 2). The atomic mass of an element is actually the weighted average of the masses of the isotopes of that element. A *mole* of a substance contains as many atoms or molecules as there are atoms in exactly 12g of ^{12}C (6.022×10^{23}). By analogy to atomic mass, the *molecular mass* of a molecule is described in reference to the mass of ^{12}C, and hence the term 'relative' molecular mass.

Bonding: the basis of structure

Atoms interact to form molecules by chemical bonds, which are described by two theories. The *valence bond theory* concentrates on the transfer (ionic bond) or sharing (covalent bond) of electrons and is the basis for traditional organic chemistry. *Molecular orbital theory* considers bonding as a coalescence of electron orbitals (probabilistic electron density maps) of two atoms to create a new orbital that spreads over the entire molecule. To describe electron orbitals mathematically, electrons are described as waves, rather than as negatively charged points. Like light waves, sound waves, or sine waves, an electron wave is defined by a formula. Since an electron moves in three dimensions, its formula has x-, y-, and z-components; changes along the three axes are described by partial derivatives. Since it is hard to freeze electrons in time and space, their location is defined as a probability (ψ). For example, $\partial^2\psi/\partial x^2$ is the derivative of ψ calculated in the x-dimension with the y- and z-dimensions held constant. An electron has a small mass (m) that is included in energy calculations and, depending on its position, it also has potential energy (V). Adding constants to balance the function mathematically (h), electron energy (E) is defined in probability terms ($E\psi$) by Equation 1.1, the Schrödinger equation.

Equation 1.1

$$E\psi = V\psi + [(\partial^2\psi/\partial x^2) + (\partial^2\psi/\partial y^2) + (\partial^2\psi/\partial z^2)]\,(h/2m)$$

The solutions to this differential equation for a single particle are simple equations that can be plotted on a graph to give mathematical pictures of electron densities, called *orbitals*. The orbitals of molecules can be defined by combining the equations for the electron orbitals of individual atoms, which defines three types of molecular orbitals (Fig. 1.1):

- those with a high probability of finding electrons (*bonding orbital*, σ or π);
- those with a low probability of finding electrons (*antibonding orbital*, σ^* or π^*); or
- those of lower energy, inner shell electrons that do not participate in bonding (*nonbonding*).

'Antibonding' does not refer to a repulsive interaction, but rather an electron distribution determined from the wave equation that shows a low probability of finding an electron between the nuclei of the bonded atoms.

Special arrangements of electrons

Radicals

Certain electron configurations are of special interest to physicians. *Radicals* (sometimes called free radicals) are molecules or atoms that contain one or more unpaired electrons. 'Pairing' of electrons refers to the orientation ($+\frac{1}{2}$ or $-\frac{1}{2}$) of the electron 'spin', which is an intrinsic property of electrons (like mass) rather than a spinning movement. Atoms like Cl and Na (not the ions Na^+ and Cl^-) have unpaired electrons and are radicals. *Nitric oxide* ($NO^\bullet$) has an unpaired electron, and is thus a radical. It is composed of N (nitrogen), which has seven electrons,

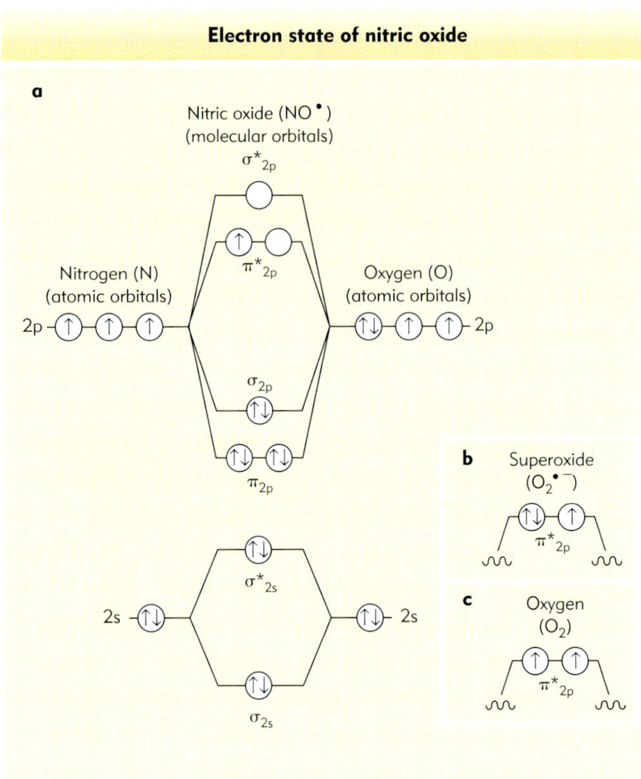

Figure 1.1 Electron diagram of nitric oxide. (a) Oxygen (eight electrons, 8e⁻) and nitrogen (7e⁻) are the components of nitric oxide. Electrons in the inner shells are not depicted. The remaining 11 electrons are shown for nitrogen (left) and oxygen (right). The molecular orbital model distributes these electrons into bonding and antibonding orbitals in order of increasing energy level: two into σ_{2s}, two into σ^*_{2s}, four into π_{2p}, two into σ_{2p}, and one into π^*_{2p}. The electron in a π^*_{2p} orbital remains unpaired, which defines $NO^•$ as a radical. (b) An electron diagram for superoxide ($O_2^{•-}$) distributes 16 electrons from the two oxygen atoms similarly, except that 3e⁻ are in the π^*_{2p} orbital. (c) Ground state oxygen (O_2) is also formally a radical and has one electron in each π^*_{2p} orbital with spins unpaired.

and O (oxygen), which has eight electrons (see Fig. 1.1). The radical $NO^•$ has received considerable attention as a diffusible modulator of cell signaling via the cyclic guanosine monophosphate pathway (Chapter 3) and as a direct vasodilator (Chapter 33). Another radical of physiologic interest is the *superoxide radical* ($O_2^{•-}$), generated by the addition of an electron to molecular oxygen (O_2). Excessive production of superoxide produces *oxidative stress* and ultimately cell death. Superoxide is converted into less reactive products (hydrogen peroxide and oxygen) by the enzyme *superoxide dismutase*.

Dipoles

Since molecules consist of combinations of charged atoms, an uneven distribution of charge over the molecule can exist when atoms with different atomic numbers are combined. Most biomolecules, which combine N, C, O, H, and a few other atoms, have a complex distribution of charge. The charge of a molecule may also be distorted by an externally applied electric field, which need only be as large as a neighboring molecule with its own uneven charge distribution. When charges on a molecule are separated by a distance, they constitute an *electric dipole*. The dipole is represented by a vector (which has magnitude and direction), which points by convention from the negative toward the positive charge, and is called the *dipole moment* [the unit is a Debye, or coulomb meter (Cm) in SI units, i.e. charge × distance). Some molecules are polar and have an *intrinsic* dipole moment. Nonpolar molecules, when placed in an externally applied electric field, can have an *induced* dipole. The dipole moment determines in part the solubility of molecules. A polar molecule with a large dipole moment is difficult to integrate into a nonpolar medium, such as the interior of the plasma membrane of a cell, which results in a slow transfer into the cell interior (Chapter 7).

Molecular magnetism

A moving charge generates a magnetic field. For molecules, the *electron spin* and *orbital motion* of electrons around the nucleus of each atom result in a molecular *magnetic moment*. When an external magnetic field is applied, molecules become oriented in the field according to their magnetic moment. Three types of interaction occur between the external field and the molecular magnetic moment – *diamagnetism*, *paramagnetism*, and *ferromagnetism*. If the molecular field opposes the external magnetic field, the material is referred to as *diamagnetic*. Diamagnetic molecules (such as N_2) have paired electron spins in the outer shell. If the molecular field augments the applied magnetic field, the molecule is termed *paramagnetic*. Paramagnetic molecules (such as O_2) have unpaired electron spins in the outer shell. In *ferromagnetic* materials, electron spins align in parallel and greatly augment an external magnetic field (by as much as 10^5). Magnetic interactions are the physical basis for oxygen analyzers (paramagnetism) and magnetic resonance imaging (ferromagnetism). Nuclear magnetic resonance manipulates molecular magnetism to define molecular structure.

Stereochemistry

Stuctural isomers are molecules that have the same molecular formula, but with the atoms arranged differently in space; for example, glucose, galactose, and mannose (all $C_6H_{12}O_6$) or isoflurane and enflurane ($C_3H_2OF_5Cl$) are structural isomers with distinct structures and properties. In *stereoisomers*, molecules have identical structures, except for the arrangement of substituents around one atom (the *stereocenter*) so that the two molecules are not superimposable on one another (e.g. pseudoephedrine is a stereoisomer of ephedrine). Stereoisomers have identical structures except for the configuration or spatial arrangement of atoms at the stereocenter. If this difference in configuration produces a mirror image of the original structure, the compounds are *chiral* and are called *enantiomers*.

Stereochemistry can be described according to three different systems – *optical activity*, *'relative' configuration*, and the *Cahn–Ingold–Prelog system*.

Optical activity is a property of molecules which can rotate plane polarized light. *Dextrorotary* molecules have a positive (+) angle of rotation and rotate plane polarized light to the right (or clockwise, as viewed when looking into the beam). *Levorotary* molecules have a negative (–) angle of rotation and rotate plane polarized light counterclockwise. Molecules that can rotate plane polarized light have a *chiral* (handed) center, are *not superimposable* on their mirror images, and are known as *enantiomers*. Enantiomeric pairs have identical chemical and physical properties (e.g. boiling point, density, solubility, spectrum), but each enantiomer rotates plane polarized light in the opposite direction. A mixture of equal amounts of enantiomers of a molecule is a *racemic* mixture, which is optically *inactive*. Racemic epinephrine (adrenaline) contains equal amounts of the two enantiomers of epinephrine.

Relative configuration defines the structure of a molecule as either the D- or L-form by relating it to the two forms of a standard molecule, glutaraldehyde. Most naturally occurring sugars are of the D-configuration [e.g. D-(+)-glucose]. The optical rotation of a molecule, (+) or (–), is independent of its relative configuration. These two nomenclatures are sometimes confused by the use of the lower case *d*- and *l*- to denote optical rotation. Thus, *l*-epinephrine (optical rotation) and L-epinephrine (configuration) are not the same enantiomer; only *l*-epinephrine (the D-configuration) is biologically active.

The *Cahn–Ingold–Prelog* system can only be applied if the absolute stereochemistry is known. This system defines the *absolute configuration* based on the atomic mass of the four substituents attached to a chiral carbon center. The three highest mass number substituents at the chiral center are projected onto a triangle (the lowest mass substituent is projected backward behind the triangle) and ranked in order of decreasing mass number, starting with the highest mass at the top of the triangle. If the mass numbers of the substituents follow a clockwise direction from the top, the molecule is in the (*R*)-configuration; if it is counterclockwise, it is in the (*S*)-configuration. The stereochemical standard molecule is (*R*)-glyceraldehyde, which, coincidentally, is the same as D-(+)-glyceraldehyde. *Conformation* refers to the arrangements of a molecule that are achieved by rotation of substituents at a bond (the molecules are superimposable if correctly rotated), while the *configuration* (e.g. 'absolute configuration') of a molecule cannot be converted by bond rotation.

About 60% of drugs used in anesthesia are chiral. Chirality influences the actions of intravenous hypnotics – etomidate is administered as a single enantiomer, and the enantiomers of ketamine and thiopental have small differences in pharmacodynamic and pharmacokinetic effects. The volatile anesthetics in current use are racemic mixtures, except sevoflurane, which is achiral (Chapter 24). Many new drugs will be introduced as the single safest and most efficacious enantiomer.

Amino acid classification and abbreviations

Nonpolar		
Aspartate	A	Asp
Cysteine	C	Cys
Phenylalanine	F	Phe
Glycine	G	Gly
Isoleucine	I	Ile
Leucine	L	Leu
Methionine	M	Met
Proline	P	Pro
Valine	V	Val
Tryptophan	W	Trp
Polar uncharged		
Asparagine	N	Asp
Glutamine	Q	Gln
Serine	S	Ser
Threonine	T	Thr
Tyrosine	Y	Tyr
Acidic		
Aspartic Acid	D	Asp
Glutamic Acid	E	Glu
Basic		
Histidine	H	His
Lysine	K	Lys
Arginine	R	Arg

Figure 1.2 Amino acid classification and abbreviations.

Biomolecular structure: amino acids and proteins

The 20 common amino acids (Fig. 1.2) are distinguished by the side chains attached to the α-carbon. The side chains are chemically distinct, and are classified as nonpolar, polar uncharged, acidic, or basic. At neutral pH, amino acids and proteins are mostly in a form with both positive and negative charges (*zwitterions*). Amino acids are almost always of the L-form. Glycine, the simplest amino acid, is the only amino acid that is not chiral, since it has two hydrogens on the α-carbon. Amino acids can have other functions in addition to being components of proteins (e.g. glutamate and glycine are excitatory and inhibitory neurotransmitters, respectively).

Peptides are short chains of amino acids joined by *peptide bonds* (Fig. 1.3), and proteins are longer *polypeptides* (as long as 8000 amino acids). Both peptides and proteins are broken down by the addition of water (*hydrolysis*), which is catalyzed by enzymes called *proteases*. Proteins contain successive levels of organization, which endows them with complex three-dimensional structures (Fig. 1.4a). The *primary structure* is the sequence of amino acids. Certain *motifs*, or short segments of amino acids, are associated with cellular functions [e.g. NPXY for internalization of the low-density lipoprotein (LDL) receptor where X is any amino acid] or identified as sites of enzyme action (e.g. RRXS is a consensus site for phosphorylation by cyclic adenosine monophosphate-dependent protein kinase). Certain amino acids can be modified by the addition of a phosphoryl group (on Y, S, or T), carbohydrate chains (on O or N), or lipids (on S or N), thus affecting activity or subcellular location (Chapter 2).

Secondary structure incorporates more information into the protein by organizing some sections along the chain into regular conformations such as the right-handed α-helix (10–15 amino acids) and the β-sheet (3–10 amino acids). In the α-helix the polypeptide backbone is closely packed with hydrogen bonds at every fourth residue of the helix. All the side chains project outward into the surrounding solution. Many α-helices are *amphipathic*, i.e. they have nonpolar amino acids along one face and polar residues around the rest of the helix, which can stabilize helix–helix interactions in lipid environments like the interior of the cell membrane. At a higher level of organization, sequences of approximately 70–100 amino acids are organized into *domains*, which are loosely defined organizational units that do not have distinct structures.

Tertiary structure is the overall pattern of folding or topology. Unlike secondary structure, which consists of repeating patterns, tertiary structure is diverse and results from interaction of the side chains that project from the peptide backbone. Through a variety of interactions, including hydrogen, electrostatic, hydrophobic and disulfide bonds (between the sulfur

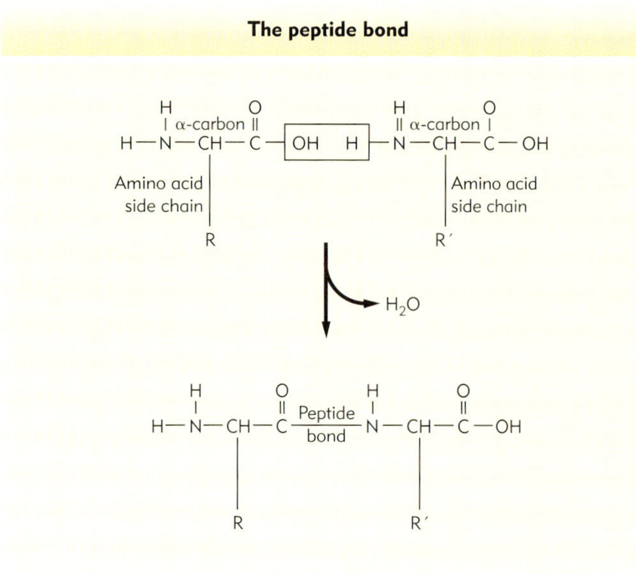

Figure 1.3 The peptide bond. The peptide bond of the polypeptide backbone is an amide bond formed by the condensation of amino acids. This bond has some double-bond character and acts as a rigid, planar unit. R and R′ are linked to the α-carbon and denote the side-chain groups specific to each amino acid. The amino terminus is on the left, and the carboxy terminus is on the right.

atoms on cysteine), a complex, energetically favorable conformation is generated. The tertiary structures of most soluble (i.e. not membrane-bound or transmembrane) proteins are tightly packed, water excluding, and stable. Tertiary structure is not static since conformational changes are essential to protein functions such as catalysis, ligand binding, and signal transduction. The tertiary structures of more than five thousand proteins are known at the atomic level, and have been described by several methods, including *X-ray and electron diffraction* of protein crystals (Fig. 1.4b), and *mass spectrometry* and *nuclear magnetic resonance* of small proteins in solution. For example, structural studies of proteins have direct applications in medicine. X-ray diffraction analysis and molecular dynamic calculations of the structure of human immunodeficiency virus (HIV) protease have contributed to the development of HIV-1 protease inhibitors, which have dramatically altered the therapy of HIV infection.

Quarternary structure refers to the grouping of two or more proteins by noncovalent bonds. A well-known example is hemoglobin, which consists of two pairs of subunits (2α, 2β), each with its own tertiary structure. The interaction of the subunits alters their affinity for oxygen through conformational changes.

Membrane structure: lipids

The lipids of cell membranes are amphipathic; they have a *nonpolar* (or *hydrophobic*) *hydrocarbon tail* and a *polar* (or *hydrophilic*) *head group*. In the cell membrane lipid bilayer (Chapter 2), the tails are clustered in the interior and the head groups face the aqueous environments. Thus, the cell membrane is dynamic, and the lipids and proteins embedded in the membrane are able to move laterally within it (the fluid mosaic model of cell membrane structure), although specific membrane proteins can be immobilized to particular domains by anchoring proteins.

The head groups of *phospholipids* are small, charged molecules (e.g. serine, ethanolamine, choline) linked by a phosphate group to the hydrocarbon tail (Fig. 1.5). The hydrocarbon tail usually consists of two long-chain *fatty acids* linked by glycerol. The tail molecules may be of different lengths (14–24 carbons), and may be saturated ($-CH_2-CH_2-$) or unsaturated ($-C=C-$). Saturated tails are straighter and more flexible than kinked, unsaturated tails. A simple fatty acid, palmitic acid, has a carboxyl (COO^-) head and a straight tail of 15 methylene groups. Myristic acid has 14 carbons in a similar arrangement. The hydrocarbon tail is poorly soluble in water and the exclusion of water by collections of hydrocarbon chains allows an energetically more favorable arrangement of the water molecules, which stabilizes the hydrocarbon cluster. This is called the 'hydrophobic' effect, although the arrangement is more a property of water packing than of hydrocarbons excluding water. This water–hydrocarbon separation is the basis for the formation of the lipid bilayer of the cell plasma membrane.

The cell membrane is not symmetric, instead the inner and outer leaflets of the cell membrane contain different phospholipids. The inner leaflet contains more phosphatidylserine and phosphatidylethanolamine and the outer leaflet contains more phosphatidylcholine and sphingosine. Cholesterol, a planar steroid molecule, is a major component (about 20%) of mammalian plasma membranes. The rigidity of cholesterol helps to 'stiffen' the plasma membrane.

Lipids have functions in addition to membrane structure. *Phosphatidylinositol bisphosphate*, a phospholipid, is involved in G protein-coupled transmembrane signaling cascades (Chapter 3). LDL, a large complex of phospholipids and cholesterol packed together and bound to a protein, is a cholesterol storage and transport molecule, the regulation of which is critical in atherogenesis.

BIOCHEMISTRY AND SOLUTION CHEMISTRY

Carbohydrates

Sugars have carbons arranged in a straight chain or ring form with the general formula $(CH_2O)_n$, where $n = 3$ (triose), 5 (pentose, e.g. ribose), or 6 (hexose, e.g. glucose). Sugars are generally depicted in their closed ring form (Fig. 1.6). Chains of sugars may be linked together in pairs (e.g. sucrose = glucose–fructose, lactose = galactose–glucose). Longer chains, including branched chains, are *polysaccharides*, and shorter chains are *oligosaccharides*. A number of biologically important molecules are branched chain polysaccharides, including red cell surface antigens and heparin.

The vast majority of glucose synthesis (*gluconeogenesis*) occurs in the liver, from which it is secreted into the blood and transported to other tissues (Chapter 62). Gluconeogenesis involves the conversion of pyruvate to glucose (Equation 1.2).

Equation 1.2

$$\underset{\text{pyruvate}}{C_3H_3O_3} \rightarrow \underset{\text{glucose}}{C_6H_{12}O_6}$$

Some amino acids and glycerol (derived from fats) can enter the synthetic pathway as pyruvate when they are broken down. Gluconeogenesis and glucose breakdown (*glycolysis*) are not simply reversals of the same reactions. Rather, each pathway has its own energetically favorable reactions, mediated by different sets of enzymes.

The addition of an electron (and a negative charge) is called *reduction* and removal of an electron is called *oxidation*. In the

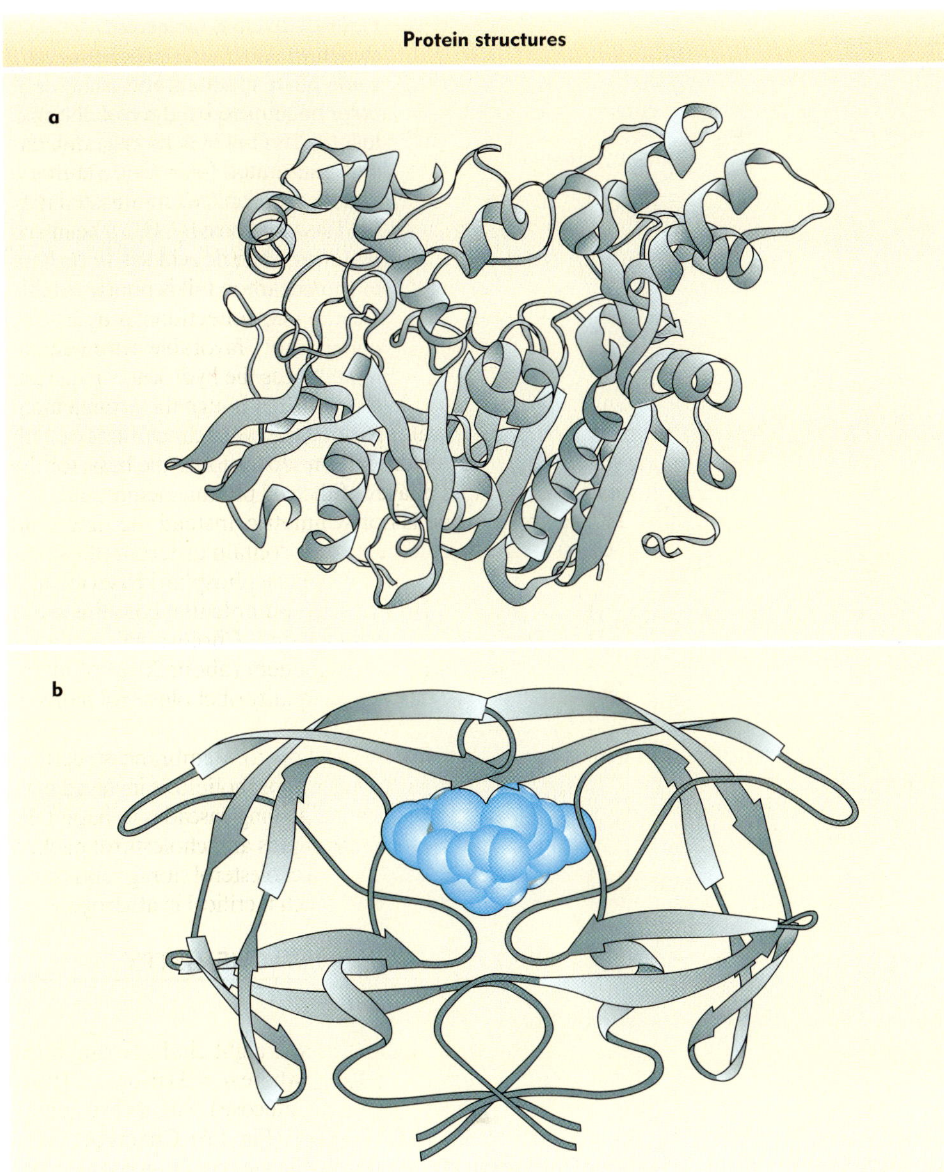

Figure 1.4 Protein structures. (a) In X-ray diffraction, X-rays (wavelength 1.5Å) are scattered by the electrons of the protein crystal. The regular, repeating arrangement, called a *crystal lattice*, acts like a *diffraction grating* and the X-rays are scattered in a pattern that is the reciprocal of the crystal lattice pattern. The structure of the molecule is calculated mathematically from this diffraction pattern by *Fourier transformation*. Here, a ribbon diagram of acetylcholinesterase from coordinates stored in the Brookhaven Protein Data Bank was generated using RasMol software. The binding site is within the open area slightly above center. (See: Sussman JL, Harel M, Frolow F, *et al*. Atomic structure of acetylcholinesterase from *Torpedo californica*: a prototypic acetylcholine-binding protein. Science. 1991;253:872–79.) (b) Human immunodeficiency virus (HIV) protease complexed with an inhibitor. The protease dimer is shown in ribbon form. The inhibitor molecule is colored blue. The two fold axis of symmetry of the dimer is vertical, in the plane of the figure. (See Silva AM, Cachau RE, Sham HL, Erickson JW. Inhibition and catalytic mechanism of HIV-1 aspartic protease. J Mol Biol. 1996;255;321–46.)

oxidative breakdown of glucose, nicotinamide adenine dinucleotide (NAD^+) receives an electron and proton and is converted into NADH. The breakdown of sugar can be summarized as in Equation 1.3. Electrons and protons are removed from glucose, which is oxidized and released as CO_2. The transfer of electrons is converted into energy by oxidative phosphorylation (Chapter 62).

Equation 1.3

$$\underset{\text{glucose}}{C_6H_{12}O_6} \rightarrow \underset{\text{pyruvate}}{C_3H_3O_3} \rightarrow CO_2 + H_2O + \text{energy}$$

Transport of glucose across membranes of most animal cells is via *carrier* molecules (uniporters) which move glucose passively down its concentration gradient. A family of transport proteins with 12 membrane-spanning helices has been identified. The transporters GLUT1, GLUT3, and GLUT5 transport glucose into the brain. The heart, which normally uses fatty acids as an energy source, transports glucose via the GLUT1 and GLUT4 uniporters. During myocardial ischemia, manipulation of these energy sources may be critical, since fatty acids appear to be detrimental. In some cells (intestine and kidney) in which glucose must be transported from lower luminal to higher cytosolic concentrations against its concentration gradient, transporters (synporters) are coupled to Na^+ transport in the same direction.

Carbohydrates have other cellular functions in addition to storing and releasing metabolic energy. Inositol (Fig. 1.6) is phosphorylated to different degrees with 1–4 phosphates and is an intracellular signaling molecule (Chapter 3). A variety of cellular proteins and lipids are also modified by oligosaccharides, the function of which is unclear.

SOLUTION CHEMISTRY

A *solution* is a mixture of two or more components to make a homogenous dispersion in a single phase. As the particle size in the solvent increases, a solution is referred to as a *colloidal dispersion* (particle diameter about 10nm) and as a *coarse dispersion* (particle diameter about 100nm). The component in the greater amount is the *solvent* and that in the lesser is the

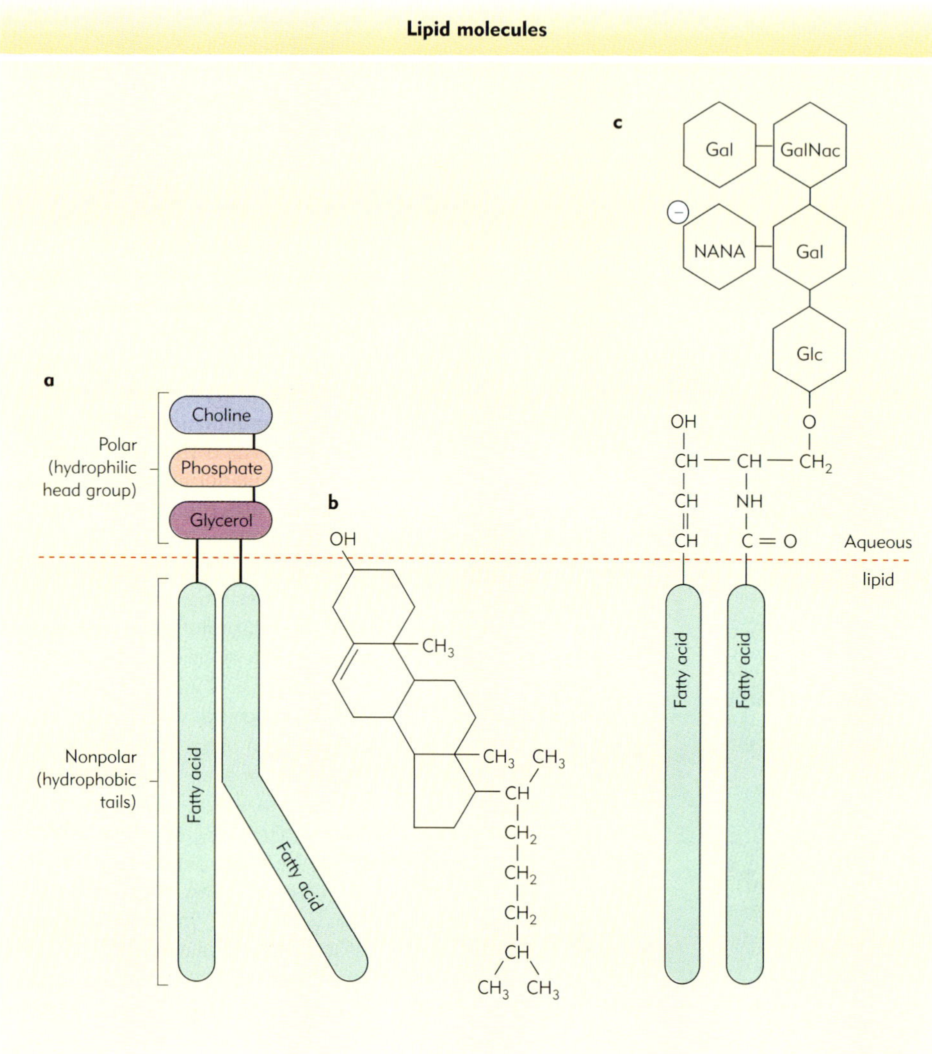

Figure 1.5 Lipid molecules structure. Lipid molecules have the same basic structure, consisting of a polar *head group* and a hydrophobic *tail*. (a) The tail may be extended as in the saturated fatty acid or bent if double bonds (–C=C–) are present. (b) The head group may be small and the hydrocarbon tail compact as in cholesterol or (c) the head group may be large and complex as in ganglioside GM_1, which contains multiple sugars. The overall structural elements are the same for each lipid. (Gal, galactose; Glc, glucose; GalNAc, *N*-acetylgalactosamine; NANA, *N*-acetylneuraminic acid.

solute. Since there are three states of components (solid, liquid, and gas), nine solute–solvent combinations are possible. Anesthesia involves solid–liquid, gas–gas, and gas–liquid solutions, which are the usual drug delivery and disposition combinations. Note that a vapor refers to the gaseous form of any substance that is either liquid or solid under normal conditions of temperature and pressure (e.g. isoflurane). The *colligative properties* of a solution depend primarily on the number of solute particles, and include osmotic pressure, vapor pressure lowering, freezing point lowering, and boiling point elevation.

Concentrations of a solution are defined in several ways. *Molarity* is moles of solute per liter of solution (mol/L). Note that the denominator is for the total solution, not the volume of solvent. Molarity is temperature dependent, since the solvent expands or contracts as temperature changes. *Molality* is defined as moles of solute per kilogram (mol/kg) of solvent. Note that the denominator is mass. Molality has experimental advantages because it is not temperature dependent and is useful in examining colligative properties. The *mole fraction* (X_A) is used to calculate partial pressures of gases and in working with vapor pressures, and is defined as '(moles of component A)/(moles of all components)'. As a result of solute interactions, the properties of a solution are not simply the additive sum of the properties of each component.

Nonelectrolytes

Nonelectrolytes do not form ions when placed in water solution. Solutions of nonelectrolytes are defined as either ideal or real. In an ideal solution, made by mixing components with similar properties, no change in component properties (e.g. vapor pressure, refraction of light, viscosity, surface tension) occurs on mixing the components. This implies an absence of attractive forces (for gas mixtures) or a complete uniformity of attractive forces among liquid molecules. The properties of an ideal solution are equal to the property for an individual component multiplied by the mole fraction of that component. As an example, consider vapor pressure, that is the tendency of molecules of a liquid to escape from the liquid phase into the vapor phase. If the vapor pressure of component A over a solution (p_A) is proportional to the vapor pressure of the pure component (p^*_A) times its mole fraction (X_A), that is if $p_A = X_A\, p^*_A$, the solution obeys Raoult's Law and is said to be an ideal solution.

Most solutions, however, are *real* or *nonideal*. When intermolecular forces between molecules of the different components are stronger (or weaker) than the attraction between like

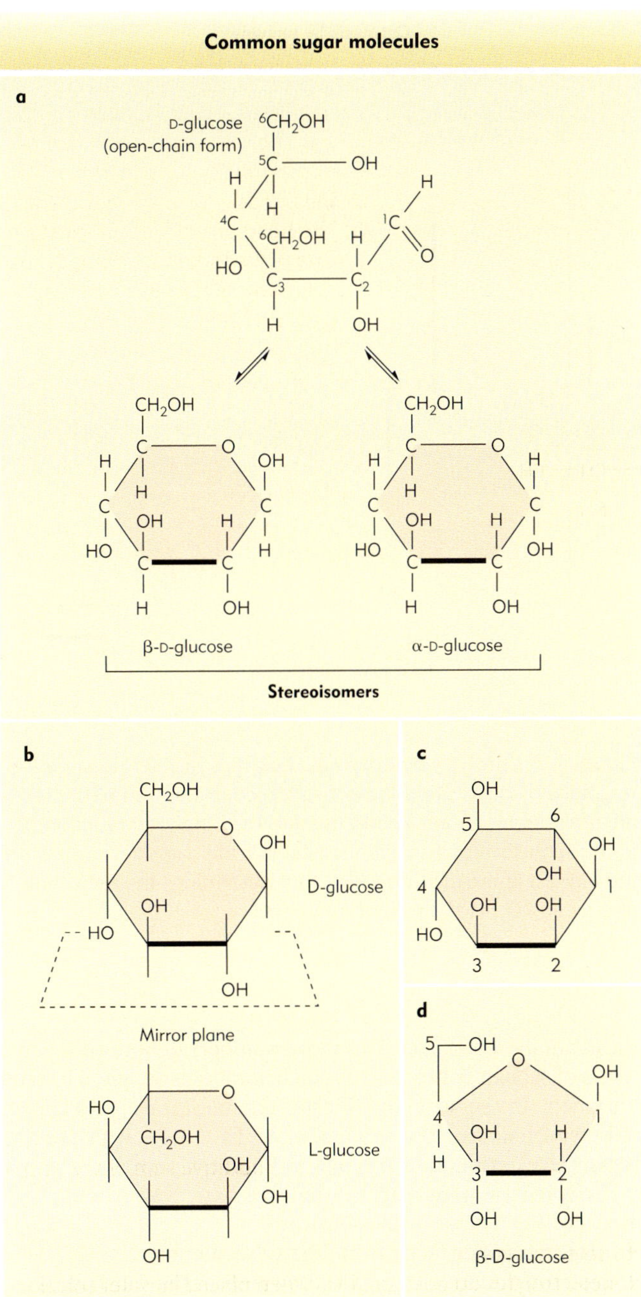

Figure 1.6 Common sugar molecules. (a) Opening the glucose ring and closing it during bonding can result in reconfiguration of the OH group at C1 into an α- or β- linkage. (b) The two enantiomers of glucose. (c) Inositol, with phosphates (PO_4) at the 1, 4, and 5 positions, is an intracellular signaling molecule (inositol trisphosphate). (d) In RNA, the phosphate backbone of ribose is attached at the 3- and 5-positions.

molecules, Raoult's Law is not obeyed. Instead, the solute makes its contribution to solution vapor pressure based on a proportionality constant specific to the solute (K_{solute}), rather than on the vapor pressure of the pure solute (p^*_{solute}); that is $p_{solute} = X_{solute}K_{solute}$. This is Henry's Law, which is usually applied to very low concentrations of gases in liquid solutions. Henry's Law states that the solubility of a gas in a solution increases in direct proportion to the partial pressure of the gas. Thus, nitrogen, which is in solution in a diver's blood at depth, becomes less soluble as pressure decreases, and can form bubbles in the blood.

Electrolytes

Electrolytes form ions when dissolved in water, conduct electric current, and have exaggerated (compared with nonelectrolytes) freezing point depression and boiling point elevation (colligative properties). Electrolytes are classified as strong (e.g. NaCl, HCl) or weak (e.g. acetic acid, ammonium hydroxide). Strong electrolytes are highly dissociated in water solution, but the large number of positive and negative charges results in electrostatic attractions between ions in moderately concentrated solutions. One result of electrostatic attraction is that the ions sometimes form *ion pairs*, rather than being free ions. The net result of these attractions between ions is that the 'effective' concentration of ions is lower than the actual concentration, which gives rise to the use of *activity*, rather than concentration, to describe ionic solutions.

Transport processes

Diffusion is the transport by random motion of particles down a concentration gradient, *electrical conduction* is the transport of charge down a potential gradient, and *thermal conduction* is the transport of energy (thermal motion) down a temperature gradient. Somewhat less intuitive than these processes is *viscosity*, which involves the transport of momentum. To approach viscosity, the idea of *flux* must be examined. Flux is a *rate* of movement and is dependent on a *gradient* of the property that is moving. The flux (J) of a particle is its rate of diffusion (in one direction) along its concentration gradient (in the same direction). If C is the concentration along a gradient, $J = -D(\partial C/\partial x)$, where x is a distance along the gradient and D is the diffusion coefficient (the minus sign indicates that movement is toward decreasing concentration). This is Fick's First Law of Diffusion. The usual model for viscosity is a series of liquid plates stacked together and moving along the x-axis. As the top plate moves, it drags the plates beneath it. Successively lower plates are accelerated to a lesser extent, so a *gradient* occurs in the velocity of the plates down the z-direction. The rate of movement in the x-direction (flux, J_x) is proportional to the gradient in velocity down the plates in the z-direction, $J \propto \partial v/\partial z$. If a constant is substituted for the proportionality sign, $J_x = \eta(\partial v/\partial z)$, where η is the *viscosity coefficient*, which describes the ammount of drag between the plates. Viscosity is a determinant of gas and liquid flow through a tube, which is described by *Poiseuille's Law* for laminar flow through a cylinder, $\partial V/\partial t = [(P_a - P_b)\pi r^4]/(8\eta l)$, where V is the volume of gas or liquid, P_a and P_b are the pressures at each end, l is the length, and r is the radius.

Electrochemistry, pH, and buffers

Acid–base chemistry is intimately tied to electrochemistry – the movement of protons (H^+) is the movement of positive charge and results in ionization. The pH of a solution is determined by measuring the *electromotive force*, the potential difference in a reversible electrochemical cell when no current flows. More commonly, pH is defined as the negative logarithm of the proton concentration, $pH = -\log_{10}[H^+]$. The measurement of pH relative to the pH of water (pH = 7.0) leads to the definition of an *acid* as a proton donor, $HA \rightarrow H^+ + A^-$, where A^- is the *conjugate base* of acid HA. A *base* is a proton acceptor, $B^- + H^+ \rightarrow BH$, and BH is the *conjugate acid*. More general definitions also exist – a Lewis acid is an electron-pair acceptor and a Lewis base is an electron-pair donor. The extent of dissociation of the acid HA is quantified by the dissociation constant $K_a = [H^+][A^-]/[HA]$. Separating the proton concentration and taking the negative $\log_{10}$ of both sides gives Equation 1.4, the Henderson–Hasselbach equation.

Equation 1.4

$$pH = pK_a + \log \frac{[A^-]}{[HA]}$$

The pK_a is the pH at which the concentrations of A^- and HA are equal. The pH may be calculated from this equation if the ratio of $[A^-]/[HA]$ is known, but it is only accurate between pH 3 and 11 (beyond this range water ionization must be included).

A *buffer* can be made to attenuate pH changes by combining a weak acid and its conjugate base (i.e. salt of its conjugate base). Combining a weak base and its conjugate acid also makes a buffer. The *buffering capacity* is the quantity of acid (or base) that may be added to a buffer to change the pH by one unit. Buffers are most effective (permit the smallest pH change) in the region of their pK_a. Bicarbonate ($pK_a = 6.1$) is the principle buffer in blood.

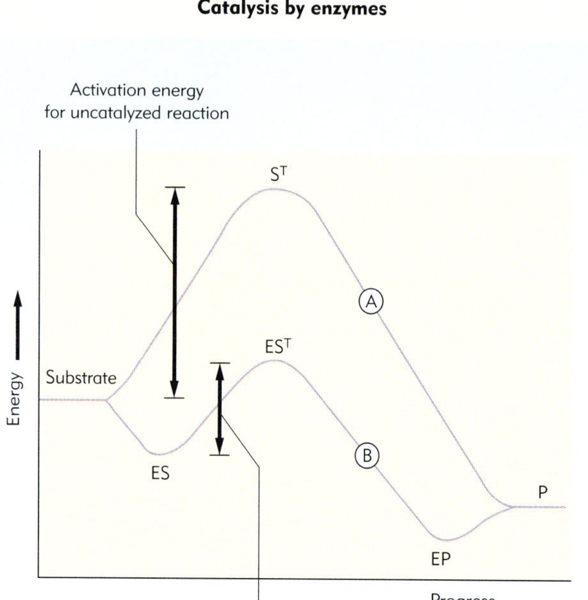

Figure 1.7 Catalysis by enzymes. Enzymes accelerate chemical reactions by decreasing the activation energy. Often both the uncatalyzed reaction (A) and the enzyme-catalyzed reaction (B) go through several transition states. It is the transition state with the highest energy (S^T and ES^T) that determines the activation energy and limits the rate of the reaction.

MOLECULAR INTERACTIONS

Surface interactions

The surface at which a phase interaction (gas–liquid, solid–liquid, etc.) occurs is an *interface*. If a liquid forms an interface with a gas, the cohesive force of the molecules of liquid holds the liquid together. A small attractive force also occurs between the liquid and gas. The work that must be done (or the energy expended) by the liquid to counteract this attraction at the interface is the *surface tension*. Surface tension is a critical factor in defining the relationship between the pressure inside a cavity and the cavity curvature (the *Laplace relation*, $P_{in} = P_{out} + 2\gamma/r$, where γ is the surface tension and r is the radius of curvature). Extensions of this relationship to the ventricle and the alveolus are important in cardiac and pulmonary physiology. The units of surface tension are those of energy/area ($ergs/cm^2$) or force/distance (dyne/cm). *Adsorption* refers to the movement of molecules in solution to an interface, which results in an interface concentration higher than that of the solution. Molecules and ions that are adsorbed at interfaces are called *surfactants* (surface-active agents), which are essential to pulmonary alveolar function (Chapter 42).

Enzymes

Enzymes *catalyze* chemical reactions, that is, they lower the *activation energy barrier* between products and reactants or substrates (Fig. 1.7). Enzymes are proteins, though ribonucleotides can catalyze reactions of RNA. Enzymes can increase the *rate* of a reaction by as much as a billion times over the rate of the spontaneous reaction, but they do not change the equilibrium (ratio of products to reactants) of a reaction, and cannot by themselves drive an energetically unfavorable reaction. A cell has thousands of enzymes. Some enzymes catalyze specific reactions, while others facilitate reactions of several related substrates. The large number of enzymes has required the development of an enzyme classification (EC) system. An enzyme is classified as (1) oxidoreductase, (2) transferase, (3) hydrolase, (4) lyase, (5) isomerase, or (6) ligase. Starting with these numbered classes, two more numbers denote successive levels of subcategories, and a fourth number is assigned to each enzyme in the subcategory. Plasma cholinesterase, also known as butyrylcholinesterase, is a hydrolase, EC 3.1.1.8, which breaks down the ester bond of succinylcholine.

Enzymes catalyze reactions in three basic ways:

- distorting a bond of the substrate;
- proton transfer to, or from, the substrate; or
- electron donation to or withdrawal from the substrate.

In each case the few amino acid residues involved are positioned together from separate parts of the polypeptide chain by precise protein folding to create an *active site* (see Fig. 1.4). The active site usually contains amino acids such as C, H, S, D, E, and K, which have available protons or electrons or can bind with a substrate. Prosthetic groups are also located at active sites, which, as described by X-ray diffraction studies, are actually pockets or grooves in enzymes where the substrate binds. Most naturally occurring amino acids are of the L-configuration, and it is consistent that enzymes are *stereospecific* in their choice of substrates.

The rate of an enzyme-catalyzed reaction increases with increasing substrate concentration. At high substrate concentrations, the increase in reaction rate attained by increasing the substrate concentration reaches a limit (i.e. the reaction is *saturable*), which is reflected by the hyperbolic shape of the plot of reaction velocity (v) versus substrate concentration [S] (Fig. 1.8a). This curve is described by Equation

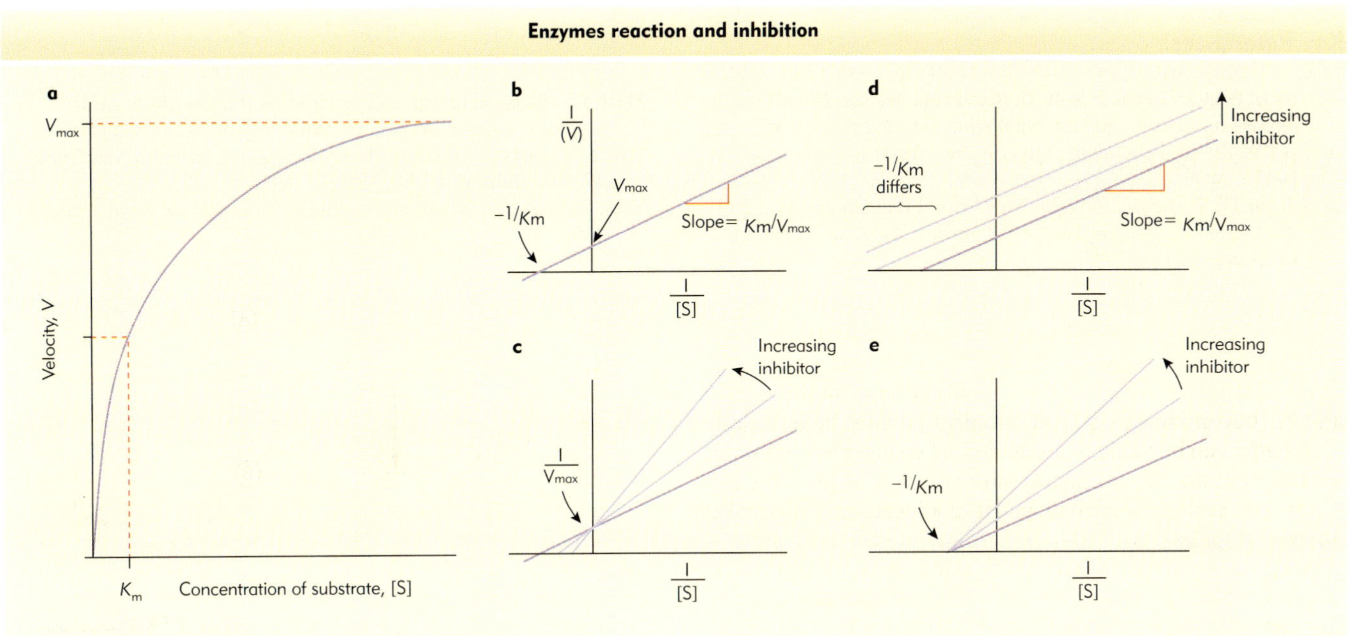

Figure 1.8 Enzyme reaction and inhibition. (a) Enzyme reaction velocity is described by a plot of velocity (V) versus substrate concentration [S]. (b-e) Different types of enzyme inhibition are described by *double reciprocal plots* of 1/V versus 1/[S] – the values of the normal plot (b) are shown in dark blue in each plot. (c) In competitive inhibition, all lines intersect the y-axis at $1/V_{max}$. (d) In uncompetitive inhibition, the slopes (K_m/V_{max}) are parallel. (e) In noncompetitive inhibition, lines intersect the x-axis (1/[S]) at $-1/K_m$.

1.5, the *Michaelis–Menten equation*, in which V_{max} is the maximal rate at saturating substrate concentration, and K_m is a combination of rate constants that is also equal to the substrate concentration at which the reaction velocity is one half of V_{max} ($v = V_{max}/2$).

■ Equation 1.5

$$v = \frac{(V_{max}[S])}{(K_m + [S])}$$

The curve of Equation 1.5 is based on a two-step model in which enzyme and substrate join initially to form an enzyme–substrate (ES) complex in a reversible equilibrium, followed by the formation of the product (P) (Equation 1.6).

■ Equation 1.6

$$E + S \underset{k_{-1}}{\overset{k_1}{\rightleftharpoons}} ES \overset{k_{cat}}{\rightarrow} E + P$$

The term k_{cat} describes the maximum number of substrate molecules converted into product per active site per unit time, or how often the enzyme 'turns over'. The k_{cat}/K_m value is a measure of an enzyme's *efficiency* as a catalyst: if $k_{cat}/K_m = k_1$ the enzyme is 100% efficient, and catalyzes a reaction every time it encounters a substrate molecule. In this case, the reaction is *diffusion rate limited*, that is the reaction proceeds as quickly as substrate and enzyme make contact and product leaves. Acetylcholinesterase is an example of a nearly perfectly efficient enzyme in these terms.

Replotting the velocity–substrate concentration plot as the reciprocals gives a linear plot of 1/[S] versus $1/v$ (Fig. 1.8b). These plots are valuable to describe different enzyme inhibitors (Figs 1.8c–e). In *competitive inhibition*, substrate and inhibitor compete for the substrate binding site on the enzyme. In *uncompetitive* inhibition, the inhibitor binds to the enzyme–substrate complex, but not to the free enzyme. In *noncompetitive inhibition*, the inhibitor binds the enzyme at a site that inhibits both catalysis and substrate binding.

Enzyme action may also be modulated by *allosteric regulation*. A modulator or *regulator* binds to the enzyme at a distinct site and either enhances or inhibits the binding of the substrate with the enzyme or its catalytic efficiency. Many enzymes that are allosterically regulated are composed of two or more protein subunits bound together – one subunit binds the regulator (*regulatory subunit*) and the other contains the active site (*catalytic subunit*). These functions may also be achieved by separate domains of the same protein.

Key References

Alberts B, Bray D, Lewis J, Raff M, Roberts K, Watson JD. Molecular biology of the cell, 3rd edn. New York: Garland Press; 1994.
Atkins PW. Physical chemistry, 6th edn. New York: Freeman and Co.; 1997.
Creighton TE. Proteins, 2nd edn. New York: Freeman and Co.; 1993.
Ferscht A. Enzyme structure and mechanisms, 2nd edn. New York: Freeman and Co.; 1985.
Martin A. Physical pharmacy principles in the pharmaceutical sciences, 4th edn. New York: Williams and Wilkins; 1993.
Tipler PA. Physics for scientists and engineers, 3rd edn. New York: Worth Publishers; 1991.
Voex D, Voex JG. Biochemistry, 2nd edn. New York: John Wiley; 1995.

Further Reading

Bonner FT. Nitric oxide, Part A: nitric oxide gas. Meth Enzymol. 1996;268:50–7.
Calvey TN. Isomerism and anaesthetic drugs. Acta Anaesth Scand. 1995;39:83–90.
Egan TD. Stereochemistry and anesthetic pharmacology: joining hands with the medicinal chemists. Anesth Analg. 1996;83:447–50.
Feynman RP, Leighton RB, Sands M. Polarization. In: The Feynman Lectures on Physics. Reading: Addison-Wesley, 1963.
Halliwell B, Gutteridge MC. Oxygen radicals in biological systems, Part B: role of free radicals and catalytic metal ions in human disease: an overview. Meth Enzymol. 1990;186:1–85.

Chapter 2 Cell structure and function

Jacques Ya Deau

Topics covered in this chapter

Plasma membrane: structure and transport mechanisms
Mitosis and the cell cycle
Protein folding,degradation, and post-translational modification
The cytoskeleton
Intracellular transport, protein trafficking, and secretion

PLASMA MEMBRANE: STRUCTURE AND TRANSPORT MECHANISMS

The plasma membrane, a thin (5nm) bilayer of lipids and proteins, delineates the cell, confines cellular organelles and proteins, and allows ion gradients to exist across the membrane (Figs 2.1 & 2.2). The lipids of the plasma membrane are chemically diverse, but phospholipids are the most common. Phospholipid molecules are amphipathic and spontaneously form bilayers in water. The plasma membrane also contains cholesterol. Cholesterol helps to maintain membrane fluidity by inhibiting crystallization of the hydrocarbon chains of other lipids. As long as the membrane remains fluid, lipid molecules generally diffuse freely laterally within the bilayer. Lipid bilayers, in the absence of proteins, allow hydrophobic and small uncharged polar molecules (such as water and urea) to pass through them but largely block the diffusion of ions and larger polar molecules (e.g. sugars). Cholesterol hinders the passage of hydrophilic compounds through the plasma membrane.

Biologic membranes contain two major types of membrane transport protein; these facilitate the passage of molecules across membranes. Carrier proteins have at least two different conformational states. They bind a solute on one side of the membrane and release it on the other side. Channel proteins span the membrane and allow the passage of molecules across the membrane. Channel proteins allow more rapid transfer than can occur with carrier proteins, but they can only facilitate diffusion of certain molecules down electrochemical gradients. Most channel proteins are not simple pores but are highly selective for particular molecules or ions. In general, channels are not constantly open but act as gated pores and open in response to a particular stimulus. Carrier proteins, by comparison, can actively transport compounds; they are often pumps driven by the energy derived from ATP hydrolysis or by the energy stored in ion gradients.

The two sides (faces) of the lipid bilayer have different lipid compositions. For example, inositol phospholipids tend to be concentrated on the cytoplasmic face of the plasma membrane. This is significant because inositol phospholipids are substrates for enzymes that create second messengers such as inositol trisphosphate (Chapter 3). Glycolipids (i.e. lipids with sugars attached to their head groups) are found on the extracellular face of the plasma membrane. Glycolipids are particularly prominent in the myelin membrane that sheaths the axons of many nerves.

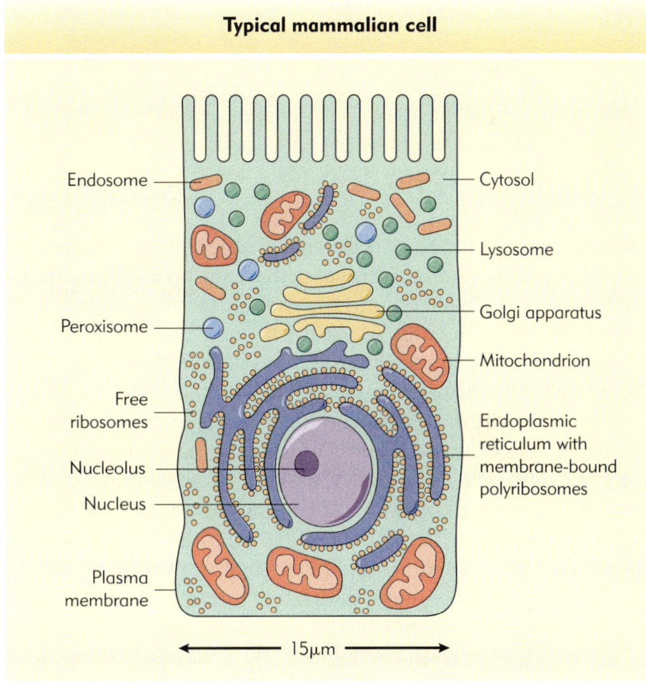

Figure 2.1 Typical mammalian cell. The membrane-bound compartments typical of a mammalian cell are indicated.

Membranes and membrane proteins are of particular interest to anesthesiologists with an interest in mechanisms of anesthesia. It is still controversial how volatile anesthetics cause anesthesia, but current theories focus on membrane proteins as targets (Chapter 22 & 24).

Mitochondria

Mitochondria are membrane-delimited organelles that oxidize organic compounds, generate an electrochemical proton gradient across the mitochondrial membrane, and synthesize adenosine triphosphate (ATP) from adenosine diphosphate (ADP) and phosphate ions. Glycolysis, the conversion of glucose to

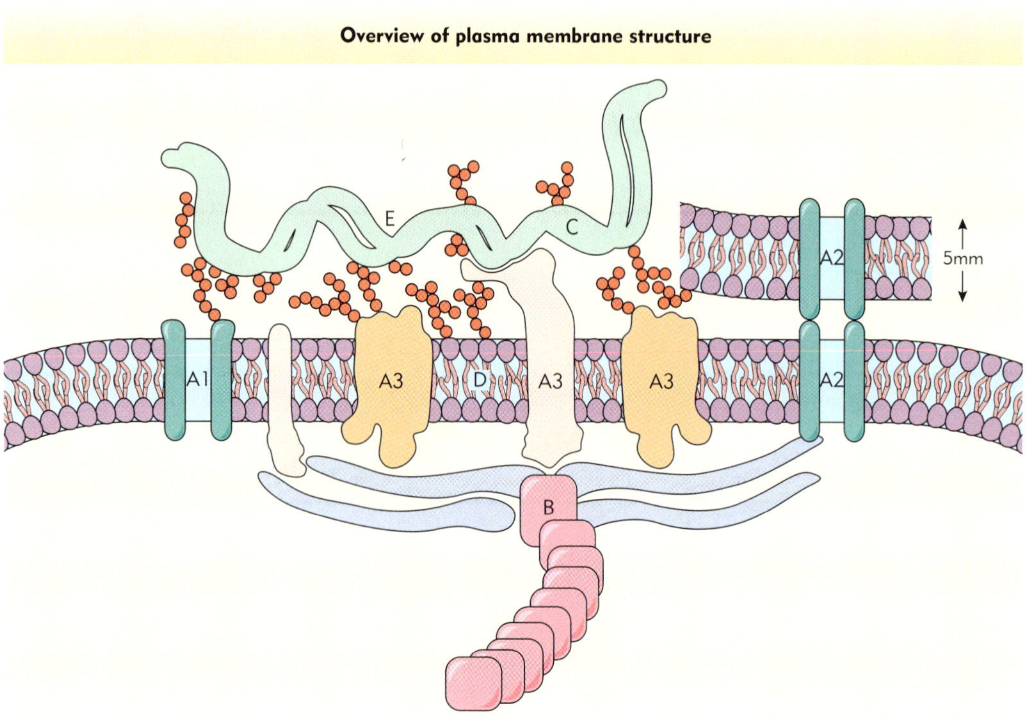

Figure 2.2 Overview of plasma membrane structure. Plasma membranes are distinguishable from other cellular membranes by the presence of both glycolipids and glycoproteins on their outer surfaces and the attachment of cytoskeletal proteins to their cytoplasmic surfaces. Proteins that are inserted through the lipid bilayer (A1–A3), termed 'integral' membrane proteins, are often glycosylated (dark orange circles), as are some bilayer lipids (D) and many components of the extracellular matrix (E) Certain integral membrane proteins can interact with intracellular proteins (B), with extracellular components (C) and to form specific junctions with other cells (A2). (Modified with permission from Albers, 1999.)

pyruvate, occurs in the cytoplasm and generates two molecules of ATP. Pyruvate then undergoes active transport into the mitochondria and is oxidized into water and carbon dioxide, yielding up to 30 molecules of ATP for each glucose molecule (Chapter 62). The intracellular location of mitochondria is influenced by their coassociation with microtubules.

The two membranes of the mitochondria are very different. The outer membrane contains large channels composed of porin protein, which renders the outer membrane permeable to solutes of less than 5kDa. The inner membrane is a convoluted membrane with a large surface area that surrounds the mitochondrial matrix. Most solutes, such as protons, hydroxyl ions, and other ions, cannot pass freely through the inner mitochondrial membrane, but carrier proteins facilitate movement of metabolites across the membrane. Proteins of the respiratory chain, located in the inner membrane, oxidize metabolic substrates and establish an electrochemical proton gradient across the inner membrane. Protons are pumped across the inner membrane out of the matrix. Adenosine triphosphate synthase, a large protein complex, uses the proton gradient to synthesize ATP as the protons return into the matrix. The inner matrix contains enzymes used in breaking down nutrients; it also contains the mitochondrial DNA, mitochondrial transfer RNAs, and ribosomes for translation of mitochondrial proteins. Enzymes located in the matrix include proteins that catalyze the tricarboxylic acid cycle (also known as the Krebs cycle or the citric acid cycle), which catalyzes the breakdown of acetyl coenzyme A (CoA) to produce high-energy electrons (NADH) used by the respiratory chain to pump protons out of the matrix.

Evolutionarily, mitochondria are probably derived from endosymbiotic prokaryotic organisms. Like bacteria, they reproduce by fission. The number of mitochondria per cell is not fixed, and repeated exercise of muscles leads to a large increase in mitochondrial number. The bacterial origin of mitochondria explains the existence of mitochondrial DNA, which encodes some of the mitochondrial proteins. The mitochondrial DNA is circular, and each mitochondrion has multiple copies of the molecule. However, most mitochondrial proteins are derived from nuclear genes.

Mitochondrial inheritance is non-Mendelian in nature. Unlike the precise segregation of nuclear genes during meiosis, mitochondrial inheritance is the result of random separation of mitochondria. The ovum has much more cytoplasm than the sperm, and the zygotic mitochondria are descended from maternal mitochondria. Therefore inheritance of mitochondrial DNA follows the maternal line.

The nucleus

The double nuclear membrane physically segregates DNA from the cytoplasm. This may serve two functions. First, separation of gene transcription in the nucleus from messenger RNA translation in the cytoplasm may facilitate RNA processing. Second, the nuclear membrane and its associated cytoskeleton may protect chromosomes from physical stress. Cytoplasmic intermediate filaments surround the outer membrane, and nuclear filaments known as lamins form a mesh underneath the inner nuclear membrane. The two nuclear membranes are bridged by nuclear pores, which are large protein complexes that regulate movement of molecules into and out of the nucleus. Proteins synthesized in the cytosol that contain nuclear localization signals bind to the nuclear pore and are actively transported into the nucleus. Ribosomes are assembled in a specialized portion of the nucleus, the nucleolus, and exported to the cytosol through nuclear pores.

Chromosomes

Most of the DNA in mammals does not encode proteins; some is used to encode RNA, some is regulatory, but most has no known function (Chapter 4). Chromosomes are linear molecules of DNA, extensively bound to proteins. Histones are proteins that facilitate packing of the DNA into condensed loops of DNA, which are called nucleosomes. Nucleosomes pack together to form fibers, which in turn form higher order structures such as loops. Certain gene regulatory proteins can decondense the chromosomes, unwind the loops, and create nucleosome-free regions. Genes being transcribed are found in decondensed portions of chromosomes, which are termed active chromatin. All chromatin becomes tightly condensed as a prelude to mitosis. As a result of condensation, mitotic chromosomes can be stained to reveal the distinct banding patterns (karyotyping).

MITOSIS AND THE CELL CYCLE

The cell division cycle is a co-ordinated process of duplicating the cell and dividing the contents into two daughter cells. Division of the nucleus occurs during mitosis, which is also referred to as the M phase. The rest of the cycle is termed interphase. Deoxyribonucleic acid is synthesized during the S phase of the cell cycle. The period between the end of the M phase and the beginning of the S phase is termed G_1 (for gap), and the time from the end of S phase to the beginning of M phase is termed G_2 (Fig. 2.3).

Certain cells, such as endothelial cells, divide rapidly. For other cells, such as hepatocytes in an adult human, the cell cycle may last a year. Mature neurons do not progress through the cell cycle at all. In tissue culture, the cell cycle for many cell lines lasts about 24 hours. Under these conditions, the total protein content of the cell increases throughout the cycle. Progression through the cycle is tightly regulated and depends upon checkpoints of the cell-cycle control system. Progression through the cycle will stop at a checkpoint if the cell is not ready to proceed. Checkpoints occur in G_1, G_2, and metaphase. The most studied of these is the G_2 checkpoint, which regulates entry into M phase. However, in many cells the most critical checkpoint occurs at G_1, where the cell cycle pauses to allow for growth of the cell.

Cyclins are proteins that regulate progression through the cell cycle. Mitotic cyclins build up during interphase and are broken down as the cell progresses from metaphase to anaphase. When sufficient levels of mitotic cyclins have accumulated, they bind cyclin-dependent protein kinases (Cdks), forming a complex termed M-phase promoting factor (MPF). Once MPF is activated via an autocatalytic positive-feedback system, the cell passes through the G_2 checkpoint and enters mitosis. The MPF protein kinase phosphorylates many proteins, including microtubule-associated proteins and lamins. Progression through the G_1 checkpoint similarly requires accumulation of sufficient G_1 cyclins to bind Cdk to form the Start kinase complex.

Chromosomal replication defines the S phase, or DNA synthesis phase, of the cell cycle. Duplicated chromosomes are linked together at their centromeres, which are the sites of attachment of chromosomes to the mitotic spindle. Mammalian chromosomes are too long to duplicate efficiently by beginning replication at one end of the chromosome and traversing to the other. Instead, there are many replication origins. During S phase, different portions of the chromosomes replicate at different times. Active chromatin is replicated first, while condensed chromatin is replicated late in S phase. Histones are synthesized in S phase, and the new DNA is assembled into nucleosomes. Once a stretch of chromatin has replicated, further DNA synthesis from that portion cannot occur until the nuclear envelope dissociates. This rereplication block limits replication to once per cell cycle.

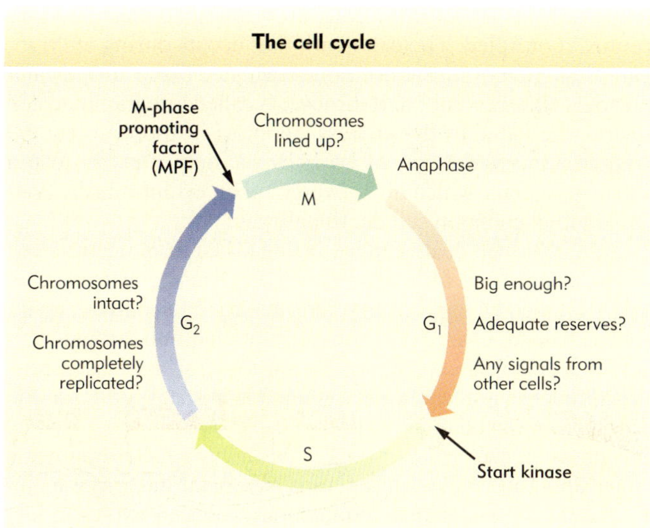

Figure 2.3 The cell cycle. Dividing cells progress through the phases of the cell cycle. Checkpoints (some of which are listed in the figure) act to ensure that the cell is ready to proceed to the next phase. (Modified with permission from Hunt, 1991.)

Deoxyribonucleic acid polymerase synthesizes DNA from the 5′ end to the 3′ end. Because of the directional nature of DNA polymerase, the ends of a chromosome cannot be fully replicated by DNA polymerase. If uncorrected, over time this would lead to progressively shorter chromosomes, with loss of genetic information. This problem is addressed by sequences at the ends of chromosomes termed telomeres. The enzyme telomerase binds to these sequences and synthesizes further tandem repeats of the telomeric sequence. Deoxyribonucleic acid polymerase can then complete the replication of the complementary sequence. The number of repeated telomeric sequences varies between cells and with cell age (Chapter 4).

Mitotic division of the nucleus, along with cytoplasmic division or cytokinesis, defines the M phase of the cell cycle. The first step, prophase, is marked by compaction of the duplicated chromosomes into chromatids (pairs of chromosomes attached at their centromeres) and formation of the mitotic spindle in the cytoplasm. At prometaphase the nuclear envelope disintegrates into vesicles, and the chromatids attach to the microtubules of the mitotic spindle. Kinetochores are protein complexes that link centromeres to microtubules. During metaphase, the chromatids line up in the metaphase plate. The chromatids separate during anaphase and move towards the spindle poles. When the chromosomes reach the poles, the cell enters telophase. The nuclear envelope coalesces around the chromosomes, and the nucleolus reappears as RNA synthesis resumes. After mitosis is complete, the cytoplasm separates into two cells. The cell divides at the site of the metaphase plate. If division is asymmetric, this is initiated by asymmetric location of the mitotic ring. The first sign of cell division is the formation of a cleavage furrow, which is powered by an actomyosin contractile ring that assembles in anaphase.

APOPTOSIS

Cell proliferation is a highly regulated process with numerous checks and balances. Cell death is also a highly regulated process. Throughout life, and particularly during development, many surplus or harmful cells are generated that must be removed or killed. The cell death that occurs during embryogenesis, metamorphosis, hormone-regulated tissue atrophy and normal cell senescence and turnover is called ìprogrammed cell deathî, mediated by the process ìapoptosisî. Apoptosis can be triggered in a variety of cell types by a variety of extrinsic and intrinsic signals, which all converge on an evolutionarily conserved final common cell death pathway.

Apoptotic cell death can be distinguished from necrotic cell death, a pathologic form of acute cell death resulting from acute injury typified by rapid cell swelling and lysis. In contrast, apoptotic cell death involves a controlled autodigestion through activation of endogenous proteases leading to cytoskeletal disruption, cell shrinkage, mitochondrial dysfunction, nuclear condensation and membrane blebbing. Apoptotic cells are phagocytosed by neighboring phagocytes or broken down into smaller fragments called apoptotic bodies while plasma membrane integrity is maintained. This maintenance of membrane integrity avoids induction of an inflammatory response, a hallmark of apoptosis, in contrast to necrotic cell death, which results in early leakage of cell contents and induction of inflammation. Cell survival usually depends on the constant presence of survival signals such that removal of extracellular signals leads to apoptosis, which may be viewed as a default pathway. In other cells, apoptosis may be induced and requires new protein synthesis.

Cell accumulation can result from increased proliferation, or from failure to undergo apoptosis. The latter is increasingly recognized as an important mechanism in diseases of cell accumulation such as cancer and autoimmune disease. Many malignant cells have a reduced ability to undergo apoptosis in response to physiologic stimuli. Most chemotherapeutic agents and radiation induce cell death by deranging cellular physiology, usually by initiating DNA damage, which leads to induction of apoptosis. Myocardial infarction and stroke are common disorders resulting from acute loss of blood flow producing a central area of ischemia characterized by necrotic cell death and a peripheral area (penumbra) which undergoes apoptosis upon reperfusion.

The morphologic similarities of different cell types undergoing apoptosis first suggested the existence of a central apoptotic pathway. A family of genes related to Bcl-2 and Bcl-XL have been identified which have both positive and negative effects on apoptosis by unclear mechanisms. This pathway results in cytochrome c release from mitochondria, followed by the activation of procaspases by proteolytic processing to form an active aspartyl protease, which in turn triggers a proteolytic cascade of caspase family members. The signalling pathways regulating apoptosis have been studied most extensively in lymphocytes, which express a variety of cell surface receptors that inhibit or activate apoptosis. The tumor necrosis factor receptor (TNFR) family is the largest group of receptors that regulate apoptosis in lymphocytes. Apoptosis-inducing receptors such as TNFR1 and Fas share an intracellular death domain, along with several cytoplasmic proteins, which can heterodimerize with these receptors to recruit and activate caspases. Apoptosis inhibiting receptors interact with the TRAF proteins, but their role in apoptotic signalling remains to be defined. These complex signaling pathways integrate a variety of signals to regulate apoptosis and ultimately determine cell fate.

MEIOSIS

Meiosis produces haploid gametes from a diploid cell. A cell with two homologous copies of each chromosome (except the XY pair in males) divides twice to form four cells, each with a single copy of each chromosome. Chromosomal crossing-over occurs during prophase of the first meiotic division, termed meiosis I. The pairs of homologous condensed chromosomes become physically connected as they exchange DNA; this genetic recombination increases the diversity of the gametes. Protein complexes called recombination nodules carry out recombination. The crossover sites, known as chiasmata, hold the homologous chromosomes together during meiotic division I, until they separate during anaphase I. During mitosis, chromosomes duplicate to form sister chromatids linked by centromeres; segregation during anaphase ensures that each sister chromatid goes to a different cell. In contrast, during meiosis I, each daughter cell receives a pair of sister chromatids derived from either the maternal or the paternal homolog. Deoxyribonucleic acid replication does not occur during meiosis II, the second meiotic division. The sister chromatids are separated forming four haploid gametes.

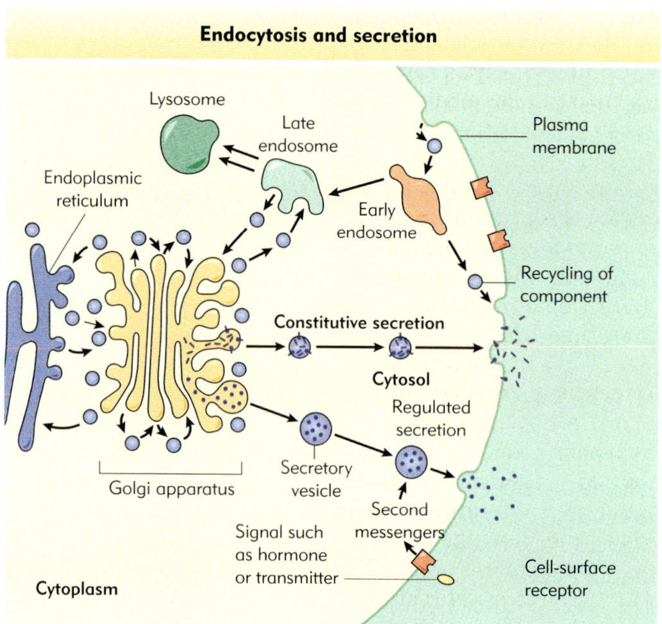

Figure 2.4 Endocytosis and secretion. Transport vesicles shuttle materials between the various intracellular compartments and the exterior of the cell. Endocytosis begins with invagination of a coated pit and formation of an early endosome. Some of the components of the endosome (such as membrane proteins) are recycled to the cell surface. Others progress to the late endosome and the lysosome for degradation. Protein secretion begins with protein synthesis in the endoplasmic reticulum. Proteins are modified as they pass through the Golgi apparatus and are packaged into vesicles. All cells have constitutive secretion of proteins. Cells such as neurons and secretory cells also have regulated section. Secretory vesicles are formed and stored until a signal triggers their release.

THE ENDOPLASMIC RETICULUM

The endoplasmic reticulum (ER) is an extensive web of membranes that courses throughout the cytoplasm of eukaryotic cells. In a typical cell, the ER makes up about half of the total cellular membrane and encloses about one-tenth of the cell volume. Ribosomes associated with the rough ER synthesize cellular proteins. The ER also synthesizes much of the cellular lipid and plays a role in Ca^{2+} homeostasis. The ER is the beginning of the secretory pathway. Proteins synthesized on the rough ER pass through the Golgi en route to their final destination, which could be lysosomes, endosomes, secretory vesicles, or the plasma membrane (Fig. 2.4). Topologically, the ER lumen is equivalent to the exterior of the cell. The rough ER is continuous with the outer nuclear membrane.

Smooth ER appears smooth by electron microscopy because there are no ribosomes bound to it. Most cells have relatively little smooth ER. Hepatocytes, however, have abundant smooth ER containing many membrane-bound enzymes. The hepatic cytochrome P450 system, located in smooth ER, metabolizes many drugs including volatile anesthetics (in particular halothane and methoxyflurane) (see Chapter 7). Chronic ingestion of certain drugs that are metabolized by smooth ER induces proliferation of hepatic smooth ER. Barbiturates, phenytoin, and ethanol are well-known hepatic P450 enzyme inducers. Synthesis of steroid hormones is another cellular function that necessitates an abundance of smooth ER. The sarcoplasmic reticulum of muscle cells is actually smooth ER that is specialized for efficient Ca^{2+} sequestration.

The cytosolic face of the rough ER is studded with ribosomes. As free (cytoplasmic) ribosomes synthesize a secretory protein, the N-terminal signal sequence emerges from the ribosome and is bound by a signal-recognition particle. The signal-recognition particle receptor on the rough ER binds the complex of ribosome, nascent protein, and signal-recognition particle. Protein synthesis continues as the nascent protein is translocated into the lumen of the ER. Recent evidence indicates that polypeptides pass through a protein-conducting channel, not through the membrane itself. The signal sequence is often removed by signal peptidase. Transmembrane proteins and proteins for many cellular organelles follow the same pathway. Transmembrane proteins contain hydrophobic sequences that remain embedded in the membrane. Proteins imported into mitochondria or peroxisomes are synthesized in the cytosol and have signal sequences that are different from the signal sequences that mediate translocation into the ER.

Synthesis of cell membrane lipids occurs on the outer, cytoplasmic side of the ER. Movement of lipids to the other face of the membrane is catalyzed by phospholipid translocators that flip lipids from one side of the membrane to the other. Membrane lipids are transported along the secretory pathway by transport vesicles to the Golgi apparatus and then to the plasma membrane, endosomes, or lysosomes. Many lipids undergo further modification in the Golgi. However, mitochondria and peroxisomes are not part of the secretory pathway, and cytosolic phospholipid transfer proteins shuttle lipids from the secretory pathway to these other membrane-bound organelles.

Transport vesicles ferry proteins between membrane-bound compartments. After passing through the ER, proteins and lipids are carried to the Golgi apparatus. The Golgi is a stack of flattened plate-like membranes and is involved in maturation of proteins and lipids, including attachment or modification of polysaccharides.

PROTEIN FOLDING, DEGRADATION, AND POST-TRANSLATIONAL MODIFICATION

Rapid folding of proteins into secondary structures (e.g. α-helices, β-sheets, and random coils) occurs during and shortly after synthesis. Then the slower process of searching for the final correct protein conformation occurs. For some proteins, this state is reached spontaneously. Others require assistance to fold to their final shape. Chaperonin proteins are ATPases that bind nascent or incorrectly folded proteins to promote correct folding and block unwanted aggregation. Despite these safeguards, some proteins become irreversibly misfolded and are destroyed. Abnormal protein folding can cause diseases; some mutations cause loss of function through abnormal folding of the final protein. 'Mad cow disease', or bovine spongiform encephalopathy, and Creutzfeld–Jacob disease are diseases of protein folding. It appears that in these diseases, known as prion diseases, a normal cellular protein adopts a pathologic, contagious state through abnormal folding. This then causes neurologic deterioration and death.

Protein degradation can occur in the cytosol, in lysosomes, or in the ER. Reasons for selective degradation of proteins include misfolding, damage, overproduction, or targeted

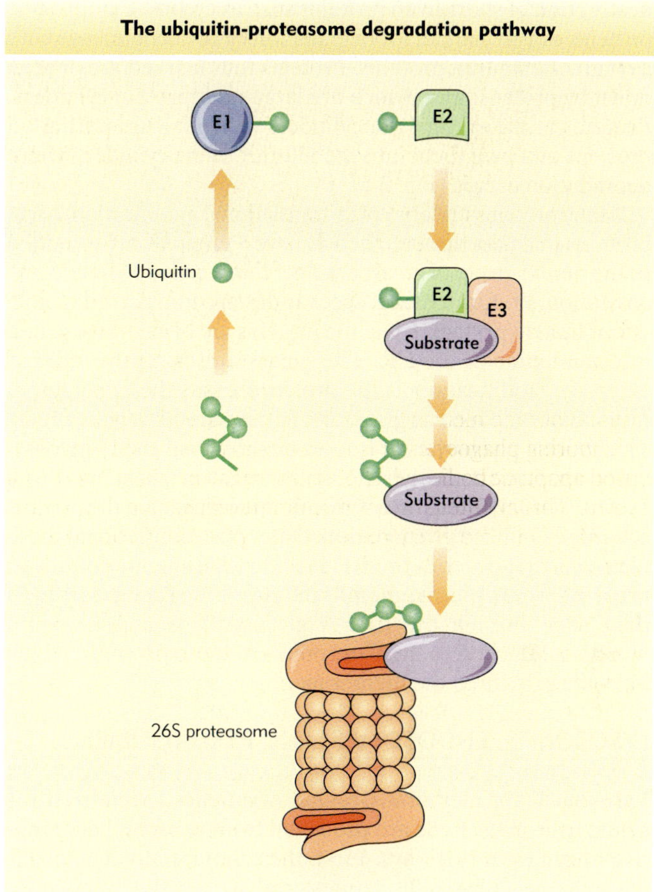

Figure 2.5 The ubiquitin–proteasome degradation pathway. The ubiquitin-activating enzyme E1 forms a thioester linkage with ubiquitin using its C-terminus. The activated ubiquitin is transferred to the active cysteine group on the ubiquitin-conjugating enzyme E2. E2, sometimes with the help of ubiquitin ligase E3, transfers ubiquitin to lysine residues on other proteins. Repeated conjugation leads to the formation of multiubiquitin chains. Proteasomes recognize proteins with ubiquitin chains and degrade the labeled proteins. Multi-ubiquitin chains are released and recycled. (Modified with permission from Hilt and Wolf, 1996.)

destruction of short-lived proteins such as cyclins. Cytoplasmic proteins can be marked for degradation by covalent linkage with a chain of ubiquitin proteins. Proteins thus marked are broken down by proteosomes, which are large multiprotein cylinders. Proteins at the ends of the cylinders recognize ubiquitinated proteins and pass them into the interior of the cylinder, where degradation occurs (Fig. 2.5).

Many proteins undergo post-translational modification. Most proteins that pass through the ER have a group of sugars added to the amino group of an asparagine; this is called N-linked glycosylation. Preformed oligosaccharides are transferred from a donor lipid to proteins while the proteins are being translocated into the lumen of the ER. The sugars subsequently undergo extensive modification as the protein transits the Golgi apparatus. Glycosylation can also occur in the cytosol or in the Golgi. This type of glycosylation is less common than the N-glycosylation that occurs in the ER. If the sugar is transferred to a hydroxyl (–OH) group on a serine or threonine, then the process is termed O-linked glycosylation. Other post-translational modifications that occur in the ER include attachment of lipids to proteins. Some plasma membrane proteins receive a lipid as they pass through the ER. A glycosylphosphatidylinositol moiety is attached to the C-terminus of these proteins, which links the protein to the membrane.

LYSOSOMES, ENDOSOMES, AND PEROXISOMES

Lysosomes are membrane-bound organelles specialized for acidic hydrolysis. Cells are protected from lysosomal degradative enzymes in two ways. First, these potentially dangerous enzymes are physically sequestered within the lysosomes. Second, the enzymes are optimally active at acid pH, but the pH of the cytosol is neutral. The pH inside lysosomes is kept at about 5 (versus the cytosolic pH of 7.2) by a H^+-ATPase that pumps protons into the lysosome.

Molecules can follow several pathways to the lysosome. Lysosomal enzymes receive a specific marker (mannose-6-phosphate) in the Golgi apparatus. Proteins that carry this modification bind to mannose-6-phosphate receptor proteins, which mediate movement of lysosomal enzymes through transport vesicles to lysosomes. Proteins, other solutes, and fluids are taken up by cells by endocytosis and enter vesicles called early endosomes. This continuous process is termed pinocytosis and results in the formation of small vesicles. Pinocytosis occurs at invaginated portions of the plasma membrane. The cytosolic face is coated with clathrin, a protein that mediates pinching off of the clathrin-coated pit into clathrin-coated vesicles. Specific proteins are taken up during pinocytosis by inclusion of receptors in clathrin-coated pits. Many cells have another type of invagination termed caveolae or plasmalemmal vesicles, which may function in transcytosis and as subcellular compartments to store and concentrate various signaling molecules. Some endosomes undergo maturation into late endosomes, and the internal pH begins to drop. Transport vesicles containing lysosomal enzymes fuse with the late endosomes, creating lysosomes. Other proteins contained in early endosomes, such as cell-surface receptors, do not go to lysosomes but are recycled to the plasma membrane.

Specialized cells, such as macrophages or neutrophils, engulf large particles or micro-organisms by phagocytosis, creating a large vesicle known as a phagosome. Phagocytosis is triggered after a particle binds to a specific receptor, such as the Fc receptor, which recognizes antibodies. Phagosomes fuse with lysosomes, which degrade the engulfed object. Organelles no longer needed by the cell, such as aged mitochondria, are surrounded by membranes derived from the ER to form an autophagosome. The autophagosome fuses with lysosomes, and the contents are broken down.

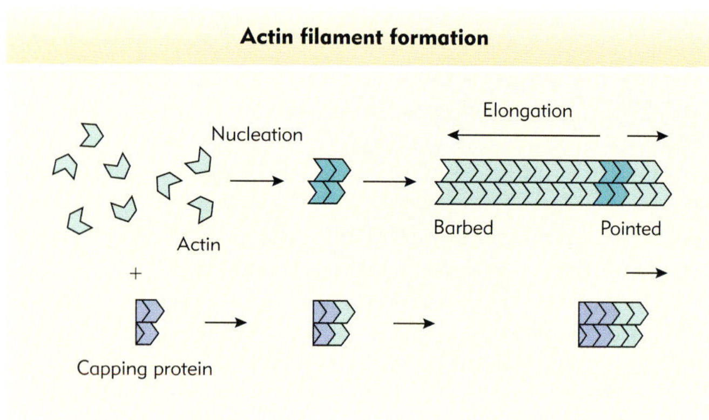

Figure 2.6 Actin filament formation. Actin filaments are unstable in the absence of actin-binding proteins. Capping protein binds the fast-growing, or plus, end of actin filaments. It blocks further addition or loss of actin monomers from that end. Similarly, other proteins can block the minus end. Capping protein also binds small actin oligomers and thereby promotes nucleation of new filaments.

Peroxisomes are membrane-bounded organelles that produce hydrogen peroxide by enzymatically oxidizing an organic compound (indicated as R):

$$RH_2 + O_2 \rightarrow R + H_2O_2$$

The hydrogen peroxide is transformed to less toxic compounds by the enzyme catalase:

$$H_2O_2 + R'H_2 \rightarrow R' + 2H_2O$$

The substrates of this reaction include toxins such as ethanol, which is converted to acetaldehyde by catalase. Oxidation of fatty acids into acetyl CoA occurs both in peroxisomes and mitochondria.

Peroxisomes are present in all eukaryotic cells. Structurally, peroxisomes have only one membrane (unlike the double membrane surrounding mitochondria and nuclei). They do not have a genome; therefore, all peroxisomal proteins are imported. Proteins destined for the peroxisome are synthesized in the cytosol with a specific C-terminal signal sequence that triggers uptake of proteins into the peroxisome. New peroxisomes are formed by fission of pre-existing peroxisomes.

THE CYTOSKELETON

The cytoskeleton is a cytoplasmic web of filamentous proteins. It provides structure to the cell, allows for movement of organelles, and generates force for movement of the cell. Components of the cytoskeleton include microtubules (polymerized tubulin), intermediate filaments (polymers of tissue-specific proteins, such as vimentin), and actin filaments. All eukaryotic cells have microtubules and actin; intermediate filaments are present in most cells from multicellular eukaryotes. The nucleus also has a filamentous protein structure, the nuclear lamina, composed of intermediate filament proteins termed lamins.

Actin

Actin is the most abundant protein in many cells. Actin filaments are flexible double-stranded helices with a diameter of 5–9nm. Actin cross-linking proteins dictate the structure of actin filaments. The cell cortex is an actin-containing gel located beneath the cell membrane. The network of actin polymers is cross-linked by actin-binding proteins such as filamin. Other cross-linking proteins, such as α-actinin, promote formation of parallel bundles of actin filaments. Alpha-actinin is found in stress fibers, which are loosely packed bundles that span large distances in cells. Stress fibers also contain myosin, which produces tension in the fibers. Transmembrane proteins, such as integrins, anchor stress fibers to the extracellular substrate of the cell (see Fig. 2.2).

Pure actin filaments are unstable. An actin filament is a polar structure; the plus end has a high affinity for free actin molecules while the minus end has a lower affinity. Actin filaments can simultaneously grow by net addition of actin subunits at the plus end and shrink by loss of subunits from the minus end (Fig. 2.6). Free actin subunits bind ATP, which is hydrolyzed after they are incorporated into actin filaments. At steady state, the filaments undergo treadmilling: the average length of the filaments remains constant but subunits progress through the filaments by binding to the plus end and passing along the length of the filament until they reach the minus end and dissociate from the filament. Energetically, treadmilling is driven by the hydrolysis of bound ATP. Normal functions of cells depend upon the instability of actin. If actin filaments are stabilized by toxins (such as the mushroom toxin phalloidin) cell structure is grossly distorted and the cell may die. Toxins that block actin polymerization also disrupt cellular function.

Actin-binding proteins control the polymerization and depolymerization of actin filaments. Some of these proteins bind actin monomers and sequester them from polymerizing. Others, such as tropomyosin, stabilize and strengthen actin filaments. Capping protein binds the plus end of the filament and blocks elongation from that end (Fig. 2.6). Gelsolin is an example of an actin-severing protein; it cuts filaments and binds to the plus end, thereby generating shorter filaments that are less likely to extend in length. Gelsolin is activated by Ca^{2+}. By shortening filaments, gelsolin can liquify the cell cortex. Localized transformation of the cell cortex from a gel to a solution plays a role in cell movement and release of the contents of secretory vesicles.

Actin is released into the bloodstream following massive cell death, as occurs in fulminant hepatic necrosis and septic shock. In normal circumstances, circulating actin is depolymerized and bound by gelsolin and G_c protein in the plasma. If this actin-scavenging system is saturated by excessive amounts of actin, free G_c protein is depleted. Clinically, this is associated with a fatal outcome. Intravenous injection into rats of large amounts of actin causes pulmonary lesions similar to those found in the lungs of patients who have adult respiratory distress syndrome (ARDS). This suggests that excessive actin in the blood may play a role in pathogenesis of ARDS (Chapter 49).

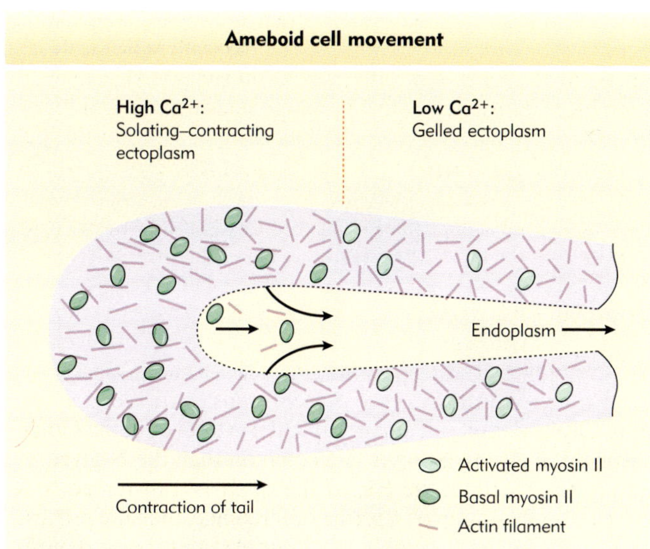

Figure 2.7 Ameboid cell movement. The ectoplasm, or the cortical gel layer, consists of actin filaments cross-linked by actin binding proteins and myosin II motor proteins. It is hypothesized that local increases in Ca^{2+} induces partial solation of the cortical gel. Ca^{2+} activates proteins that shorten actin filaments, decreases the extent of cross-linking of filaments, and activates myosin (causing local contraction). The combination of solation and contraction generates hydrostatic pressure, and the contracting tail is pulled forward. (Modified with permission from Janson and Taylor, 1993.)

Myosin

Myosin generates force by ATP-driven sliding of myosin filaments past actin filaments. Skeletal muscle cells are giant multinucleated syncytia that contain actin and myosin filaments tightly organized into sarcomeres (Chapter 30). Cardiac muscle cells are also highly organized, but each cell is smaller and has only one nucleus. Cardiac cells are physically tightly linked via binding of actin filaments to desmosomes and are electrically linked by gap junctions (Chapter 34). Smooth muscle cells are much less organized. The cells have individual nuclei, and lack sarcomeres. The loose organization of actin and myosin filaments in smooth muscle cells allows only slow contractions, but permits the cells to stretch or contract through a broad range of lengths (Chapter 33). Myosin and actin also have many important functions in cells other than muscle cells. Myosin generates force for division of cells, movement of cells, alteration of cell shape, and intracellular movement of some organelles. Stable actin filaments are found in microvilli, small extensions that greatly increase the surface area of intestinal epithelial cells. Other actin filaments exhibit rapid turnover and reorganization. Changes in actin filaments can alter cell shape by inducing formation of spikes, invaginations, or sheet-like extension of the cell. Ameboid movement of cells such as leukocytes is mediated by actin filaments (Fig. 2.7).

Microtubules

Microtubules are large, relatively rigid cylinders with a diameter of approximately 25nm. They are heterodimeric polymers of α- and β-tubulin. Like actin filaments, microtubules are polar structures. One end of a microtubule is often attached to the centrosome, also called the microtubule-organizing center.

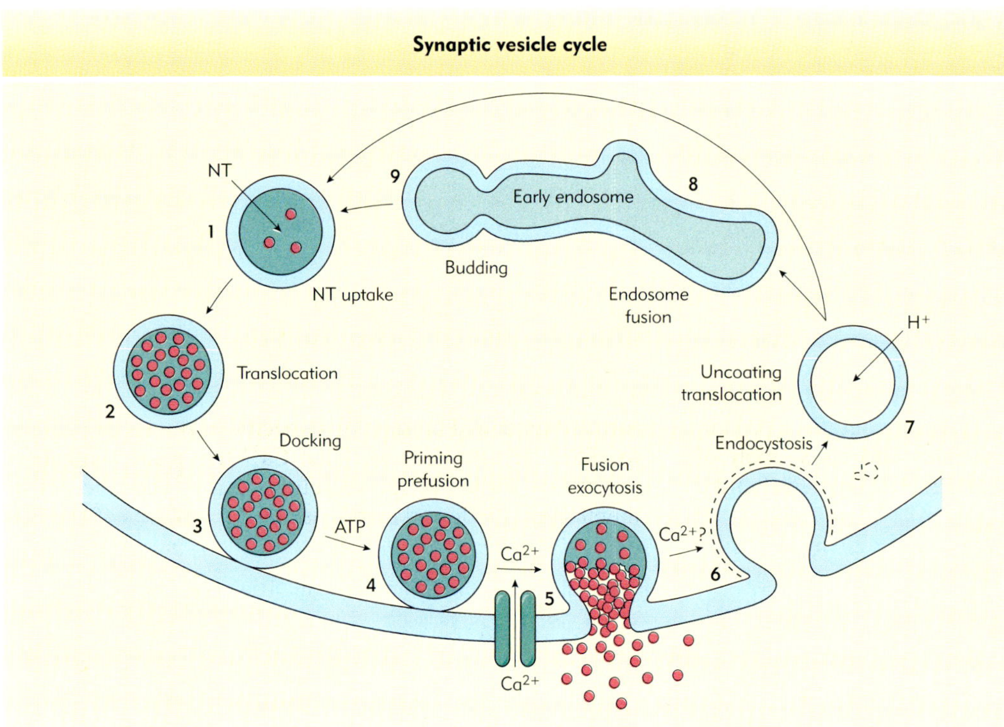

Figure 2.8 The synaptic vesicle cycle. (1) Empty synaptic vesicles take up neurotransmitters (NT) by active transport into their lumen using an electrochemical gradient that is established by a proton pump activity. (2) Filled synaptic vesicles are translocated to the active zone. (3) Synaptic vesicles attach to the active zone of the presynaptic plasma membrane but, to no other component of the presynaptic plasma membrane, in a targeted reaction (docking). (4) Synaptic vesicles are primed for fusion in order to be able to respond rapidly to a Ca^{2+} signal later. (5) Ca^{2+} influx through voltage-gated channels triggers neurotransmitter release in less than 1 msec. Ca^{2+} stimulates completion of a partial fusion reaction initiated during priming. (6) Empty synaptic vesicles are coated by clathrin and associated proteins in preparation for endocytosis. Ca^{2+} may be involved in this process. (7) Empty synaptic vesicles shed their clathrin coat, acidify via proton pump activity and retranslocate into the backfield of the nerve terminal. (8) Synaptic vesicles fuse with early endosomes as an intermediate sorting compartment to eliminate aged or mis-sorted proteins. (9) Synaptic vesicles are freshly generated by budding from endosomes. Although some synaptic vesicles may recycle via endosomes (steps 8 and 9), it is likely that the endosomal intermediate is not obligatory for recycling and that synaptic vesicles can go directly from step 7 to step 1. Multiple molecular chaperones are involved at each step. (Modified with permission from Südhof, 1999.)

As the name implies, the centrosome is often located near the center of the cell. The end of the microtubules attached to the centrosome is the minus end (i.e. the end of the filament with lower affinity for binding of free tubulin). Free filaments tend to lose subunits from the minus end and tend to add subunits at the plus end.

About half of the tubulin in a typical cell is polymerized into microtubules, and half exists as free tubulin. The tubulin heterodimer is the structural subunit of microtubules. Microtubule arrays grow and shrink rapidly; this dynamic instability is crucial for microtubule function in intracellular transport and cell division.The tubulin subunits can dissociate from a microtubule only after the bound GTP is hydrolyzed to GDP. Hydrolysis of the tubulin-bound GTP does not occur immediately upon polymerization but requires passage of a 'lag time'. A rapidly growing microtubule has a GTP cap on its growing end composed of tubulin bound to GTP. The GTP cap is stable and tends to elongate. If a microtubule starts to disassemble and loses its GTP cap, further disassembly will be favored by the weaker coassociation of subunits bound to GDP. A filament that has lost its GTP cap is unstable and is likely to dissociate completely. Certain drugs alter the stability of microtubules. Paclitaxel (Taxol), a tumor chemotherapeutic agent, stabilizes microtubules and favors the assembly of tubulin into microtubules. Paclitaxel causes mitotic arrest in dividing cells. Colchicine (used for gout), and vinblastine and vincristine (used for cancer chemotherapy) all bind tubulin monomers and cause dissassembly of microtubules.

Microtubule-associated proteins (MAPs) stabilize assemblies of microtubules and link microtubules to other cellular components. Organelles are often associated with microtubules and are propelled along microtubules to other parts of the cell by the action of microtubule-dependent motor proteins such as kinesins or dyneins. Axons of nerve cells contain microtubules. All of the microtubules of an axon have the same polarity; the plus end points towards the synapse. This unipolar organization has functional importance, as secretory vesicles use motor proteins to move along microtubules towards the plus end, where the contents are released. The shorter microtubules of dendrites have a mixed polarity. Motor proteins also play essential roles in cell division and motion of cilia and flagella.

Intermediate filaments

Intermediate filaments are polymers with a diameter of approximately 10nm. Intermediate filament proteins are diverse and vary by cell type. Pathologists can use intermediate filament subtype to determine the tissue of origin of tumors. The fibrous subunits of intermediate filaments are structurally different from the globular subunits of actin and tubulin.

Intermediate filaments play a major role in distributing mechanical forces within and across cells. Keratin filaments are intermediate filaments found in epidermal cells. Desmosomes, which link cells together, and hemidesmosomes, which fix cells to their substrate, are attached to keratin filaments. The keratin filaments distribute stress between and within cells. The disease epidermosa bullosa simplex is the result of a mutation in the keratin protein. It is characterized by a fragile epidermis that is easily ruptured by mechanical stress.

INTRACELLULAR TRANSPORT, PROTEIN TRAFFICKING, AND SECRETION

Constitutive exocytosis of proteins is a nonregulated process that occurs in all cells. It is a continuation of the default pathway of secretion, which begins in the ER and passes through the Golgi to the plasma membrane. Transport vesicles involved in the default pathway of secretion have a cytosolic coat of the protein coatamer. A GTPase regulates assembly and disassembly of coatamer-coated vesicles. The coatamer coat is removed after the vesicle reaches its destination.

Many cells, such as neurons, hormone-secreting cells, and other specialized secretory cells, have a regulated secretory system. Secretory vesicles are stored for subsequent release. Proteins and other compounds stored in secretory vesicles are sorted into clathrin-coated vesicles as they leave the Golgi apparatus. As the secretory vesicles mature, they lose the clathrin coat and the contents of the vesicle become concentrated. Further processing of secretory proteins, such as proteolytic cleavage of proopiomelanocortin into β-endorphin and adrenocorticotropic hormone, occurs as the secretory vesicle matures. Transport vesicles contain surface proteins that mediate binding to the correct destination. The fidelity of binding is ensured by GTPases known as Rab proteins. Different Rab proteins are associated with different membrane systems.

In neuronal cells, protein-containing secretory vesicles are synthesized in the cell body and then transported along microtubules of the nerve axon until they reach the axonal terminus. The vesicles accumulate, and some of them undergo a modification known as priming that readies them for release of their contents (Fig 2.8). The next step in release is docking, the close association of vesicles with the plasma membrane. Actual release of vesicular contents occurs after protein-mediated fusion of the two membranes. In nerve cells, an action potential leads to depolarization of the axonal terminal, which causes influx of Ca^{2+} through Ca^{2+} channels and subsequent secretion (Chapter 18). In other cells regulated secretion is often receptor mediated, and binding of a specific hormone can cause a localized increase in intracellular Ca^{2+} that leads to regulated exocytosis. Fusion of the secretory vesicles with the plasma membrane is followed by release of the contents of the vesicle, and rapid recycling of the secretory vesicle membrane proteins by endocytosis.

Neurons are best known for their secretion of small neurotransmitters such as acetylcholine or γ-aminobutyric acid. The 'classical' neurotransmitters are synthesized near the synapse. They are contained in the morphologically and functionally distinct small synaptic vesicles. After release of the contents of small synaptic vesicles, the associated membrane proteins undergo endocytosis and are reconstituted into synaptic vesicles. Neurotransmitter carrier proteins in the synaptic vesicle membrane load neurotransmitters into the vesicles and rapidly restore the vesicle's contents.

Key References

Blobel G. Intracellular protein topogenesis. Proc Natl Acad Sci USA. 1980;77:1496–500.

Hilt W, Wolf DH. Proteasomes: destruction as a programme. Trend Biochem Sci. 1996;21:96–102.

Schafer DA, Cooper JA. Control of actin assembly at filament ends. Annu Rev Cell Dev Biol. 1995;11:497–518.

Singer, SJ, Nicolson,GL. The fluid mosaic model of the structure of cell membranes. Science. 1972;175:720–31.

Further Reading

Alberts B, Bray D, Lewis J, et al., eds. Molecular biology of the cell. New York: Garland; 1994.

Alberts RW. Cell membrane structures and functions. In: Basic Neurochemistry: molecular, cellular and medical aspects. 6th edn. Philadelphia, PA: Lippincott-Raven; 1999:31–46.

Blobel G. Unidirectional and bidirectional protein traffic across membranes. In: Cold Spring Harbor Symposia in Quantitative Biology, Vol. LX. Protein kinesis: the dynamics of protein trafficking and stability. Cold Spring Harbor, NY: Cold Spring Harbor Laboratory Press; 1995:1–10.

Burns ME, Beushausen SA, Chin GJ, et al. Proteins involved in synaptic vessel docking and fusion. In: Cold Spring Harbor Symposia in Quantitative Biology, Vol. LX. Protein kinesis: the dynamics of protein trafficking and stability. Cold Spring Harbor, NY: Cold Spring Harbor Laboratory Press; 1995:337–48.

Dragovitch T, Rudin CM, Thompson CB. Signal transduction pathways that regulate cell survival and cell death. Oncogene. 1998;17:3207–13.

Hunt T. In: Cold Spring Harbor Symposia in Quantitative Biology, Vol. LVI. Summary: put out more flags. Cold Spring Harbor, NY: Cold Spring Harbor Laboratory Press; 1991:757–69.

Janson LW, Taylor DL. In vitro models of tail contraction and cytoplasmic streaming in amoeboid cells. J Cell Biol. 1993;123: 345–56.

Lee WM, Galbraith RM. The extracellular actin-scavenging system and actin toxicity. N Engl J Med. 1992;326:1335–41.

Matthews G. Neurotransmitter release. Annu Rev Neurosci. 1996;19:219–33.

Südhof TC. Intracellular trafficking. In: Basic Neurochemistry: molecular, cellular and medical aspects. 6th edn. Philadelphia, PA: Lippincott-Raven; 1999:175–90.

Thomas PJ, Qu BH, Pedersen PL. Defective protein folding as a basis of human disease. Trend Biochem Sci. 1995;20:456–9.

Chapter 3 Cell signaling

Hugh C Hemmings, Jr

Topics covered in this chapter

Extracellular signals
Cell-surface receptors: structure and function
Second messengers and protein phosphorylation
Anesthetic effects on cell signaling mechanisms

Functional coordination in multicellular organisms requires intercellular communication between individual cells in various tissues and organs. Adjacent cells can communicate directly by specialized plasma membrane junctions (gap junctions). Long range cell-to-cell communication is possible through the involvement of extracellular signaling molecules (such as hormones and neurotransmitters) that are synthesized and released by specific cells, diffuse or circulate to target cells, and elicit specific responses in target cells that express receptors for the particular extracellular signal. The responses to the extracellular signal are generated by diverse signal transduction mechanisms that frequently involve intracellular signals (second messengers) that transmit signals from activated receptors to the cell interior. These intercellular and intracellular signaling pathways are essential to the growth, differentiation, metabolic regulation and behaviour of the organism. Cell signaling pathways are involved in the pathophysiology of many diseases and in the mechanism of action of many drugs, including local and general anesthetics. Knowledge of basic cell signaling mechanisms is therefore essential for understanding many pathophysiologic and pharmacologic mechanisms. Recently, specific signal transduction mechanisms have become important targets for new drug development.

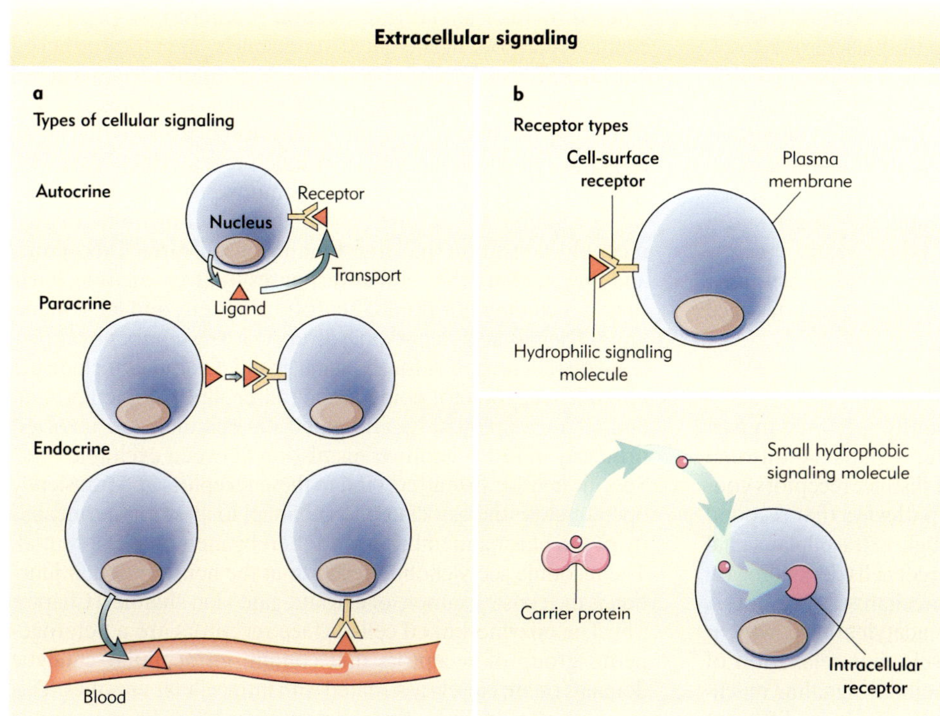

Figure 3.1 Extracellular signaling. (a) In autocrine signaling the hormone signal acts back on the cell of origin or adjacent cells. In paracrine signaling the hormone signal is carried to an adjacent target cell over short distances via the interstitial fluid. In endocrine signaling the signal is carried to a distant target via the bloodstream. (From Brody et al., 1994, with permission.) (b) Receptor types for extracellular signaling molecules. Most signaling molecules are hydrophilic and are therefore unable to cross the plasma membrane. They bind to cell-surface receptors, which in turn generate one or more signals (second messengers) inside the target cell, or activate a protein kinase or ion channel. Some hydrophobic signaling molecules, by contrast, diffuse across the plasma membrane and bind to receptors inside the target cell, either in the cytosol (as shown) or in the nucleus. Many of these small signaling molecules are nearly insoluble in aqueous solutions; they are therefore transported in extracellular fluids bound to carrier proteins, from which they dissociate before entering the target cell. (Modified from Alberts et al., 1994, with permission.)

EXTRACELLULAR SIGNALS

Communication by extracellular signaling is usually classified on the basis of the distance over which the signal acts (Fig. 3.1a). In *autocrine* signaling, the signaling cell is its own target. This situation occurs with many growth factors which are released by cells to stimulate their own growth. *Paracrine* signaling involves the release of extracellular signals that affect target cells in close proximity to the signaling cell, as occurs via neurotransmitters in neuromuscular transmission and synaptic transmission. *Endocrine* signaling involves the release of hormones, which are extracellular signals that usually act on distant target cells after being transported by the circulatory system from their sites of release. This classification is not strict in that many signals function in more than one manner, as both a neurotransmitter and a hormone, for example.

The cellular response to an extracellular signal requires binding of the signal to a specific receptor (Fig. 3.1b), which is then coupled to changes in the functional properties of the target cell. The particular receptors expressed by the target cell determine its sensitivity to various signals and are responsible for the specificity involved in cellular responses to various signals. Receptors can be classified by their cellular localization (Fig. 3.2). Most signaling molecules are hydrophilic and interact with cell-surface receptors that are directly or indirectly coupled to various effector molecules. Water-soluble (hydrophilic) signaling molecules that interact with cell-surface receptors include the majority of hormones and neurotransmitters, such as peptides, catecholamines, amino acids, and their derivatives. Prostaglandins are the major class of lipid-soluble signaling molecules that interact with cell-surface receptors. A number of lipid-soluble (hydrophobic) signaling molecules diffuse across the plasma membrane and interact with intracellular receptors. Steroid hormones, retinoids, vitamin D, and thyroxine are transported in the blood bound to specific transporter proteins, from which they dissociate and diffuse across cell membranes to bind to specific receptors in the nucleus or cytosol. The hormone-receptor complex then acts as a ligand-regulated transcription factor to modulate gene expression by binding to cis-acting regulatory DNA sequences in target genes that alter their transcription and thereby regulate target cell function. Nitric oxide (NO), and possibly carbon monoxide (CO), are members of a new class of gaseous signaling molecules that readily diffuse across cell membranes to affect neighboring cells. Nitric oxide, which is unstable and has a short half-life (5–10 seconds), acts as a paracrine signal since it is able to diffuse only a short distance before breaking down.

Receptors

Diverse cellular functions are independently regulated in part by the existence of distinct extracellular signals. Additional specificity is imparted by the existence of distinct receptors coupled to different intracellular signaling pathways that respond to the same extracellular signal. Thus a single extracellular signal can elicit different effects on different target cells depending on the receptor subtype and the signaling mechanisms present. A good example is the neurotransmitter acetylcholine, which stimulates contraction of skeletal muscle, but relaxation of smooth muscle. Differences in the intracellular signaling mechanisms also allow the same receptor to produce different responses in different target cells.

The intracellular receptors are all structurally related and act by directly regulating the transcription of specific genes. In contrast, there are three known classes of cell-surface receptors, defined by their signal transduction mechanisms: G protein-coupled receptors, ligand-gated ion channels, and receptor-linked enzymes (Fig. 3.3). These cell-surface receptor proteins act as signal transducers by binding the extracellular signal molecule and converting this information into an intracellular signal that alters target cell function. G protein-coupled receptors interact with specific G proteins in the plasma membrane, which in turn activate or inhibit an enzyme or ion channel. G protein-coupled receptors constitute the largest family of cell-surface receptors, and they mediate the cellular responses to diverse extracellular signals including hormones, neurotransmitters, and local mediators. There is also remarkable diversity in the number of G protein-coupled receptors for the same ligand. Examples include the multiple receptors for epinephrine (adrenaline), dopamine, and endogenous opioids. Ligand-gated ion channels are involved primarily in fast synaptic transmission between excitable cells. Specific neurotransmitters bind to these receptors and transiently open or close the associated ion channel to alter ion permeability of the plasma membrane and thereby membrane potential. The nicotinic acetylcholine receptor at the neuromuscular junction is the classic example of a ligand-gated ion channel (Chapter 31). The enzyme-linked cell-surface receptors are a heterogeneous group of receptors that contain intracellular catalytic domains or are closely associated with intracellular enzymes. This receptor class includes the receptor guanylyl cyclases, receptor tyrosine kinases, tyrosine-kinase-associated receptors, receptor tyrosine phosphatases, and receptor serine/threonine kinases, in which ligand binding to the receptor activates intrinsic catalytic

Receptor classification

Cell-surface receptors

G protein-coupled – receptors for hormones, neurotransmitters (biogenic amines, amino acids) and neuropeptides.
- Activate adenylyl cyclase.
- Inhibit adenylyl cyclase.
- Activate phospholipase C.
- Modulate ion channels.

Ligand-gated ion channels – receptors for neurotransmitters (biogenic amines, amino acids, peptides).
- Mediate fast synaptic transmission.

Receptor guanylyl cyclases – receptors for atrial natriuretic peptide, *Escherichia coli* heat-stable enterotoxin.

Receptor serine/threonine kinases – receptors for activin, inhibin, transforming growth factor (TGF)-β, Müllerian inhibiting substance.

Receptor tyrosine kinases – receptors for peptide growth factors.

Tyrosine kinase-associated – receptors for cytokines, growth hormone, prolactin.

Receptor tyrosine phosphatases – ligands unknown in most cases

Intracellular receptors

Steroid receptor superfamily – receptors for steroids, sterols, thyroxine (T_3), retinoic acid, and vitamin D.

Figure 3.2 Receptor classification.

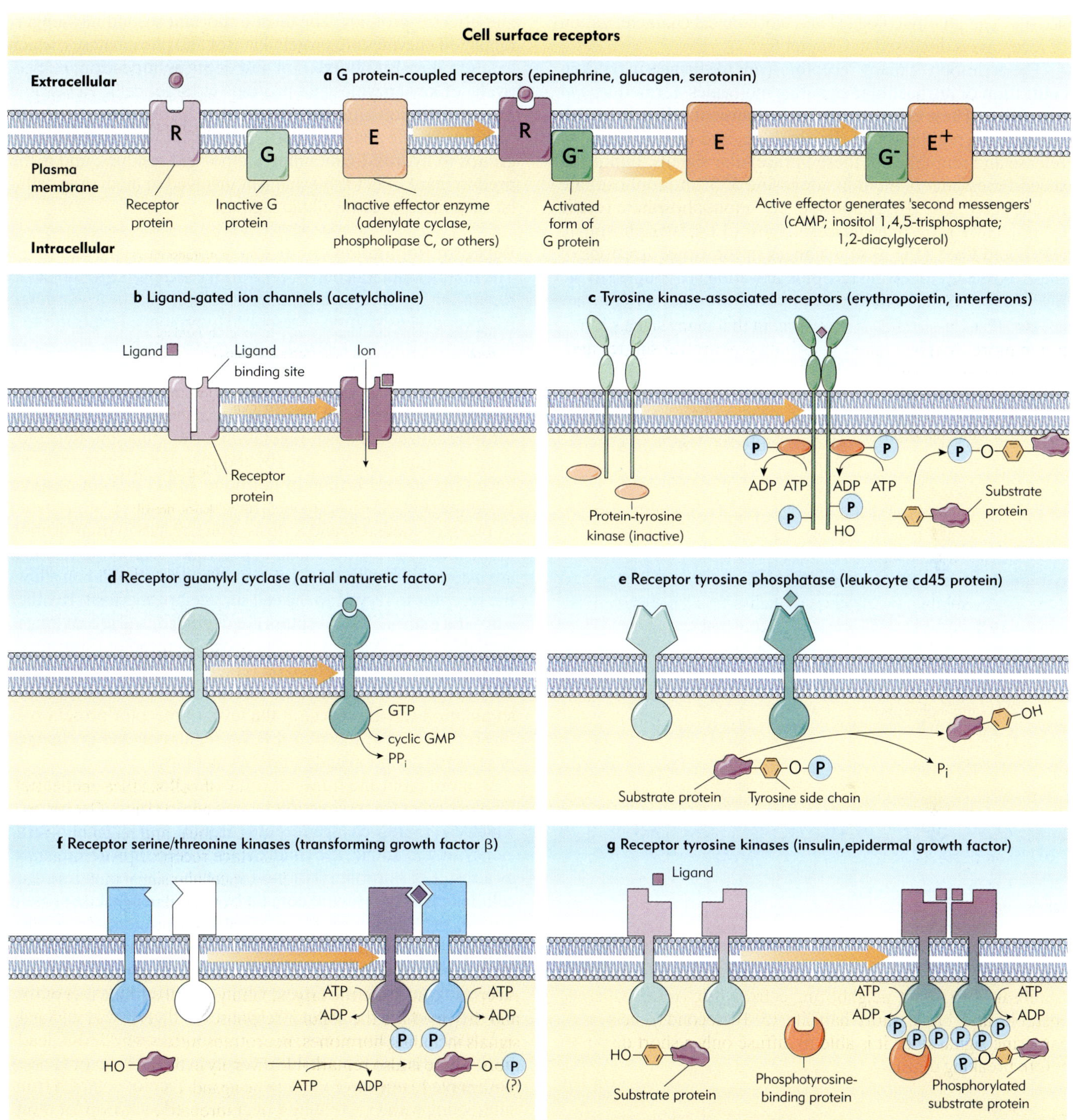

Figure 3.3 Cell-surface receptors. Common ligands for each receptor type are shown in parentheses. (a) G protein-coupled receptors. Ligand binding triggers activation of a G protein, which then binds to and activates an enzyme that catalyzes synthesis of a specific second messenger or regulates an ion channel. (b) Ligand-gated ion channels. A conformational change triggered by ligand binding opens the channel for ion flow. (c–g) Enzyme-linked cell-surface receptors: (c) Tyrosine kinase-associated receptors. Ligand binding causes formation of a homodimer or heterodimer, triggering the binding and activation of a cytosolic protein tyrosine kinase. The activated kinase phosphorylates tyrosines in the receptor and autophosphorylates; substrate proteins then bind to these phosphotyrosine residues and are phosphorylated. (d) Some activated receptors are monomers with guanylyl cyclase activity that generate the second messenger cGMP. (e) Ligand binding to other receptors activates intrinsic tyrosine phosphatase activity; these receptors can remove phosphate groups from phosphotyrosine residues in substrate proteins, thereby modifying their activity. (f–g) The receptors for many growth factors have intrinsic protein kinase activity. Ligand binding to these receptors causes either identical or nonidentical receptor monomers to dimerize and activates their enzymatic activity. Activated receptors with serine/threonine kinase activity are heterodimers (f), whereas those with tyrosine kinase activity are heterodimers or homodimers (g). In both cases, the activated dimeric receptor phosphorylates several residues in its own cytosolic domain. (Modified from Lodish et al., 1995, with permission.)

activity. The pharmacological and biochemical characterization of receptors is discussed in Chapter 6.

The activation of many receptors leads to changes in the concentration of intracellular signaling molecules, termed *second messengers*. These changes are usually transient, which is a result of the tight regulation of the synthesis and degradation (or release and reuptake) of these intracellular signals. Important second messengers include adenosine 3′,5′-monophosphate (cyclic AMP; cAMP), guanosine 3′,5′-monophosphate (cyclic GMP; cGMP), 1,2-diacylglycerol, inositol 1,4,5-trisphosphate (IP_3), and Ca^{2+} (Fig. 3.4). Changes in the concentrations of these molecules following receptor activation are coupled to the modulation of the activities of important regulatory enzymes and effector proteins. The most important second messenger-regulated enzymes are protein kinases and phosphatases, which catalyze the phosphorylation and dephosphorylation, respectively, of key enzymes and proteins in target cells. Reversible phosphorylation alters the function or localization of specific proteins by the specific addition and removal of phosphoryl groups to hydroxyl-containing amino acid residues, and is the predominant effector mechanism involved in mediating cellular responses to extracellular signals.

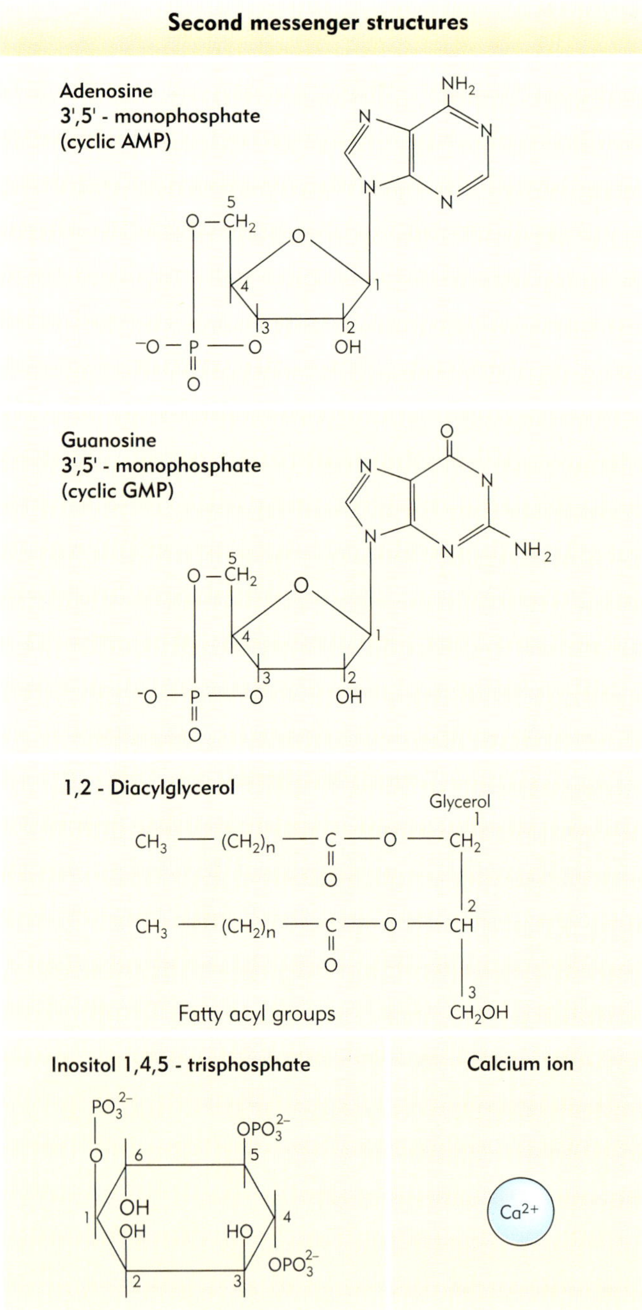

Figure 3.4. Second messengers. Structures of five common intracellular second messengers.

Receptor Regulation

The number and function of cell-surface receptors are subject to regulation by several mechanisms. Many receptors undergo receptor desensitization in response to prolonged exposure to a high concentration of ligand, a process by which the number or function of receptors is reduced, such that the physiological response to the ligand is attenuated (tachyphylaxis). Receptor desensitization can occur by several mechanisms, including receptor internalization, down-regulation, or modulation. Receptor internalization (sequestration) by endocytosis is a common mechanism for desensitization of hormone and G protein-coupled receptors (Fig. 3.5). The agonist-receptor complex is sequestered by receptor-mediated endocytosis, which results in translocation of the receptor to intracellular compartments (endosomes) that are inaccessible to ligand. Cessation of agonist stimulation allows the receptor to recycle to the cell surface by exocytosis. In other cases the internalized receptors are degraded, and are no longer available for recycling, a process known as receptor down-regulation. Receptors must then be replenished by protein synthesis. Receptor down-regulation in response to prolonged agonist stimulation can also occur at the level of receptor protein synthesis or at that of receptor mRNA regulation due to changes in gene transcription and/or mRNA stability.

A more rapid and transient form of receptor desensitization involves receptor modulation by phosphorylation (see below), which can rapidly change receptor affinity and/or signaling efficiency. For example, the β-adrenergic receptor is desensitized as a result of phosphorylation of a number of sites in its intracellular carboxy-terminal domain by cAMP-dependent protein kinase, protein kinase C, and β-adrenergic receptor kinase (βARK). The former kinase is activated as a result of β-receptor stimulation of adenylyl cyclase and results in homologous or heterologous desensitization, while the latter kinase is active only on β-receptor occupied by ligand and therefore results only in homologous desensitization. Phosphorylation by βARK leads to the binding of β-arrestin to the receptor. These processes both serve to uncouple the active ligand-receptor complex from interacting with G_s, creating a negative feedback loop for modulation of β-receptor activity. In other instances, receptor phosphorylation can affect ligand affinity or associated ion channel kinetics rather than G protein coupling.

CELL-SURFACE RECEPTORS: STRUCTURE AND FUNCTION

G Protein-coupled Receptors

A variety of signals, which include hormones, neurotransmitters, cytokines, pheromones, odorants, and photons, produce their intracellular actions by a pathway that involves interaction with receptors that activate heterotrimeric guanine nucleotide (GTP)-binding proteins (G proteins). G proteins act as molecular switches to relay information from activated receptors to the

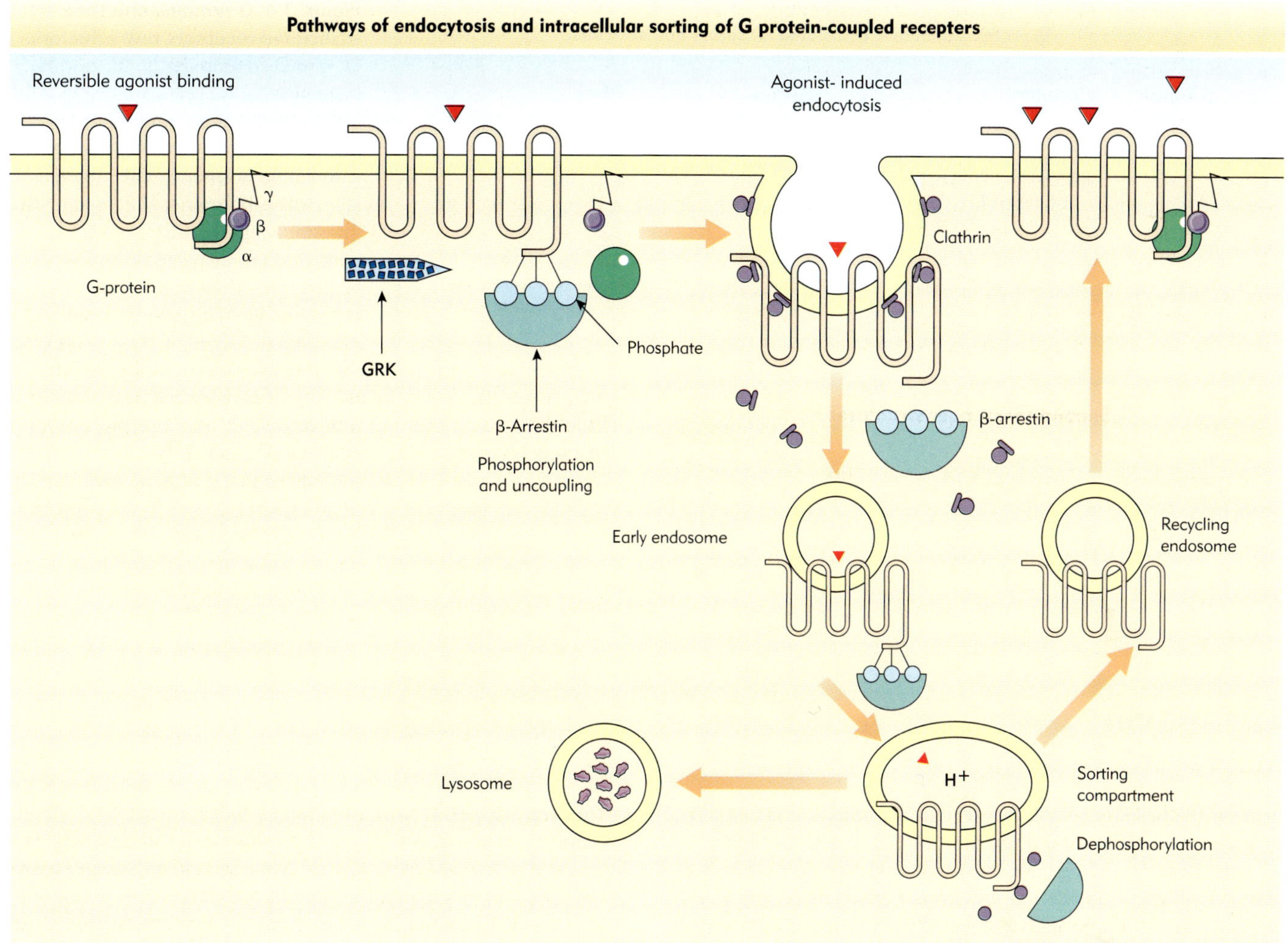

Figure 3.5 Pathways of endocytosis and intracellular sorting of G protein-coupled receptors. Typical pathway for a neurotransmitter receptor, exemplified by the NK1 receptor for substance P or the β_2 adrenergic receptor is shown. Agonist binding, which is reversible, is followed by receptor phosphorylation by G protein receptor kinases (GRKs). Interaction with β-arrestins and uncoupling from G proteins, mediates rapid desensitization. The ligand-receptor complex is internalized via clathrin-coated vesicles that soon shed their clathrin coat and become early endosomes. This may represent a second phase of desensitization. Ligand and receptor dissociate in an acidified perinuclear compartment. Endosomal phosphatases may dephosphorylate the receptor, allowing dissociation of β-arrestins. The ligand is degraded whereas the receptor is recycled to the plasma membrane, where it can interact with ligands with high affinity. Resensitization requires internalization, processing and recycling of receptor. Down-regulation occurs during prolonged exposure of cells to agonists, and may be mediated by increased degradation and diminished synthesis of receptors.

appropriate effectors. An agonist-stimulated receptor can activate several hundred G proteins, which in turn activate a variety of downstream effectors including enzymes and ion channels. G protein-coupled (or -linked) receptors form a large and functionally diverse receptor superfamily, of which over 100 members have been identified. The binding of extracellular signals to their specific receptors on the cell surface initiates a cycle of reactions that involves three major steps: (1) the signal (ligand) activates the *receptor* and induces a conformational change in the receptor; (2) the activated receptor turns on a heterotrimeric *G protein* in the cell membrane by forming a high-affinity ligand-receptor-G protein complex, which promotes guanine nucleotide exchange of GTP for GDP bound to the α subunit of the G protein, followed by dissociation of the α subunit and the βγ subunit dimer from the receptor and each other; (3) the appropriate *effector* protein(s) is then regulated by the dissociated G protein α or βγ (or both) subunits, which thereby transduces the signal. The dissociation of the G protein from the receptor reduces the affinity of the receptor for the agonist, and the system returns to its basal state as the GTP bound to the α subunit is hydrolyzed to GDP and the trimeric G protein complex reassociates and turns off the signal. A number of different isoforms of G protein α, β, and γ subunits have been identified which mediate the stimulation or inhibition of functionally diverse effector enzymes and ion channels (Fig. 3.6). Among the effector molecules regulated by G proteins are adenylyl cyclase, phospholipase C, phospholipase A_2, cGMP phosphodiesterase, and Ca^{2+} and K^+ channels. These effectors then produce changes in the concentrations of a variety of second messenger molecules or in the membrane potential of the target cell.

Despite the diversity in the extracellular signals that stimulate the various effector pathways activated by G protein-coupled

G proteins and their associated receptors and effectors

G Protein[a]	Receptors[b]	Effectors	Effect
G_s	β_1, β_2, β_3-adrenergic; D_1, D_5-dopamine ; H_1, H_2-histamine; glucagon; ACTH; LH; FSH; TSH; VIP; CRH; GHRH; GnRH; TRH; 5-HT_4 5-HT_6; prostacyclin	Adenylyl cyclase Ca^{2+} channels	Increased cAMP Increased Ca^{2+} influx
G_i	α_2-adrenergic; D_2; m_2, m_4-muscarinic; μ, δ, κ opioid; adenosine; 5-HT_{1A}; angiotensin; endothelin-1; thrombin; $GABA_B$; somatostatin	Adenylyl cyclase Phospholipase A_2 K^+ channels	Decreased cAMP Eicosanoid release Hyperpolarization
G_k	Atrial muscarinic	K^+ channel	Hyperpolarization
G_q	m_1, m_3-muscarinic; α_1-adrenergic; 5-HT_2	Phospholipase C β	Increased IP_3, DG, Ca^{2+}
G_{olf}	Odorants	Adenylyl cyclase	Increased cAMP (olfaction)
G_t	Photons	cGMP phosphodiesterase	Decreased cGMP (vision)
G_o	Not yet defined	Phospholipase C Ca^{2+} channels	Increased IP_3, DG, Ca^{2+} Decreased Ca^{2+} influx

[a] The G proteins are: Gs, stimulation; Gi, inhibition; Gk, potassium regulation; Gq, phospholipase C regulation; Golf, olfactory; Gt, transducin; Go, other.

Figure 3.6 G proteins and their associated receptors and effectors. D_1 and D_2 dopamine$_{1,2}$; H_1 and H_2, histamine$_{1,2}$; ACTH, adrenocorticotropic hormone; LH luteinizing hormone; FSH, follicle-stimulating hormone; TSH, thyroid-stimulating hormone; VIP, vasoactive intestinal peptide; CRH, corticotropin-releasing hormone; GHRH, growth hormone-releasing hormone; GnRH, gonadotropin-releasing hormone; TRH, thyrotropin-releasing hormone; GABA, γ-aminobutyric acid; cAMP, adenosine 3′,5′-monophosphate; cGMP, guanosine 3′,5′-monophosphate; IP_3, inositol trisphosphate; DG, 1,2-diacylglycerol. (Modified from Yost, 1993, with permission.)

receptors, these receptors are structurally homologous, which is consistent with their common mechanism of action. Molecular cloning and sequencing have shown that these receptors are characterized by seven hydrophobic transmembrane α helical segments of 20–25 amino acids connected by alternating intracellular and extracellular loops (Fig. 3.7). The structural domains of G protein-coupled receptors involved in ligand binding and in interactions with G proteins have been analyzed by deletion analysis, in which segments of the receptor are sequentially deleted, by site-directed mutagenesis, in which specific single amino acid residues are deleted or mutated, and by constructing chimeric receptor molecules, in which recombinant chimeras are formed by splicing together complementary segments of two related receptors. For example, the agonist isoproterenol binds among the seven transmembrane a helices of the β_2-adrenergic receptor near the extracellular surface of the membrane. The intracellular loop between α helices 5 and 6 and the C-terminal segment is important for specific G protein interactions.

Heterogeneity within the G protein-coupled receptor signaling pathway exists both at the level of the receptors and at the level of the G proteins. A single extracellular signal may have several closely related receptor subtypes (Chapters 6 and 19). For example, 6 genes for α-adrenergic receptors, 3 genes for β-adrenergic receptors and 5 genes for muscarinic cholinergic receptors have been identified. Likewise, G proteins consist of multiple subtypes. The 16 homologous a subunit genes are classified as G_s, G_i, G_k, G_q, etc., subtypes based on structural similarities, but their functional significance is incompletely understood. The significance of the structural diversity in β and γ subunits is also unclear since the functional importance of these subunits has been recognized only recently. Heterogeneity in effector pathways makes divergence possible within G protein-coupled receptor activated pathways. This effector heterogeneity can arise from two distinct mechanisms: (1) a single receptor can activate multiple G protein types, or (2) a single G protein type can activate more than one second messenger pathway. Thus, a single type of G protein-coupled receptor can activate several different effector pathways within a given cell, while the predominant pathway may vary between cell types.

The structure and function of the adrenergic receptors for epinephrine and norepinephrine (noradrenaline) and their

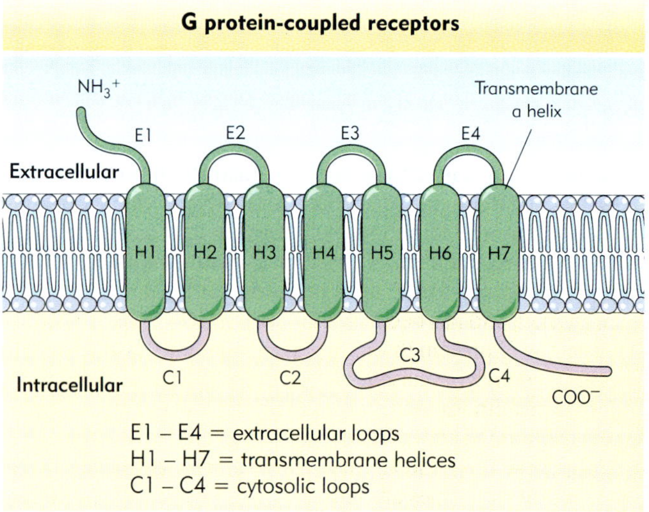

Figure 3.7 General structure of G protein-coupled receptors. Because all receptors of this type contain seven helical transmembrane loops, they also are called seven-transmembrane domain (or heptahelical) or serpentine receptors.

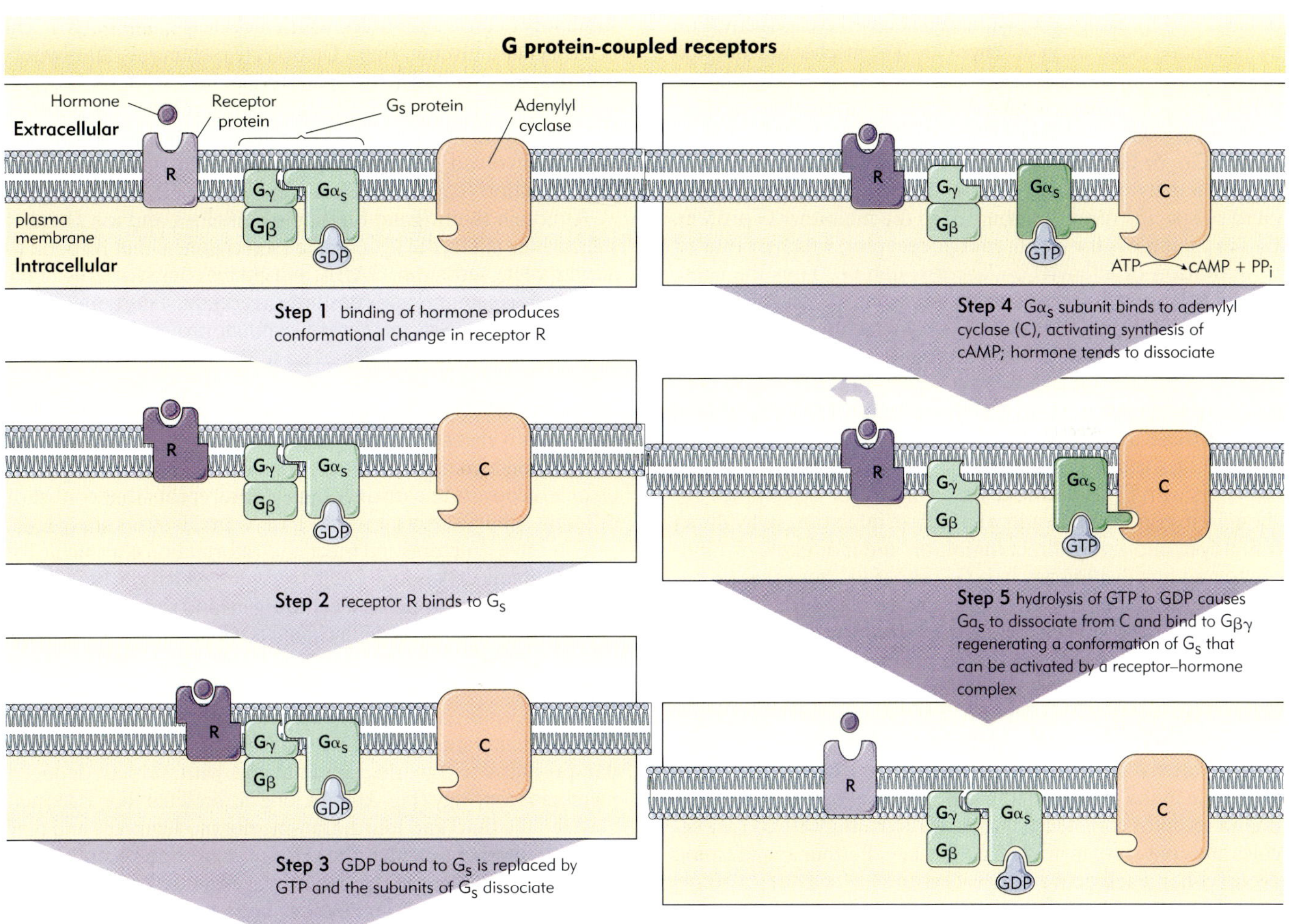

Figure 3.8 Activation of adenylyl cyclase following binding of an appropriate hormone to its receptor. The patch of cell membrane depicted contains two transmembrane proteins – a seven-transmembrane domain receptor (R; purple) and adenylyl cyclase (C; brown) – and the transducing protein G_s (green) on its cytosolic surface. The G_s protein relays the hormone signal to the effector protein, in this case adenylyl cyclase. $G\alpha_s$ cycles between an inactive form with bound GDP and active form with bound GTP. Dissociation of the active form yields the $G\alpha_s$-GTP complex, which directly activates adenylyl cyclase. Activation is short lived because GTP is rapidly hydrolyzed to GDP (step 5). This terminates the hormone signal and leads to reassembly on the inactive $G\alpha_s$-GDP complex, returning the system to its resting state. Binding of another hormone molecule causes repetition of the cycle. A similar scheme can be shown for inhibition of adenylyl cyclase by substituting $G\alpha_i$ for $G\alpha_s$. (Modified from Lodish et al., 1995, with permission.)

associated G proteins can be used to illustrate important principles of G protein-coupled receptors. β-Adrenergic receptors are coupled to the stimulation of adenylyl cyclase, a plasma membrane-associated enzyme that catalyzes the synthesis of the second messenger cAMP. cAMP was the first second messenger identified, and has been found to exist in all prokaryotes and animals. The G protein that couples β-adrenergic receptor stimulation to adenylyl cyclase activation is known as G_s, for stimulatory G protein. Epinephrine-stimulated cAMP synthesis can be reconstituted in phospholipid vesicles using purified β-adrenergic receptors, G_s, and adenylyl cyclase, which demonstrates that no other molecules are required for the initial steps of this signal transduction mechanism.

A current model of how G_s couples receptor stimulation to adenylyl cyclase activation is shown in Figure 3.8. In the resting state G_s exists as a heterotrimer consisting of $G\alpha_s$, β, and γ subunits with GDP bound to $G\alpha_s$. Agonist binding to the β-adrenergic receptor alters the conformation of the receptor and exposes a binding site for G_s. The agonist-activated receptor binds the GDP-G_s complex, and thereby reduces the affinity of $G\alpha_s$ for GDP, which dissociates, allowing GTP to bind. The $G\alpha_s$ subunit bound to GTP then dissociates from the G protein complex; this exposes a binding site for adenylyl cyclase, to which the GTP-$G\alpha_s$ complex binds, activating the cyclase. The affinity of the receptor for agonist is reduced following dissociation of the complex, leading to agonist dissociation and a return of the receptor to its inactive state. Activation of adenylyl cyclase is rapidly reversed following agonist dissociation from the receptor since the lifetime of active $G\alpha_s$ is limited by the intrinsic GTPase activity of $G\alpha_s$, which is stimulated by binding to adenylyl cyclase. The bound GTP is hydrolyzed to GDP, which returns the a subunit to its inactive conformation. The $G\alpha_s$ subunit then dissociates from adenylyl cyclase, which renders it inactive, and reassociates with βγ to reform G_s. Nonhydrolyzable analogues of GTP, such as GTPγS or GMPPNP, prolong agonist-induced adenylyl cyclase activation by preventing inactivation of active $G\alpha_s$. The mechanism of action of cholera toxin and pertussis toxin, which are ADP-ribosyltransferases, involves selective ADP ribosylation of $G\alpha_s$ or $G\alpha_i$ respectively, which inhibits GTPase activity and results in prolonged $G\alpha_s$ or $G\alpha_i$ activation.

The activity of adenylyl cyclase can also be negatively regulated by specific receptors coupled to the inhibitory G protein, G_i. An example is the α_2-adrenergic receptor, which is coupled to inhibition of adenylyl cyclase through G_i. Thus the same extracellular signal, epinephrine in this example, can either stimulate or inhibit the formation of the second messenger cAMP depending on the particular G protein that couples the receptor to the cyclase. G_i, like G_s, is a heterotrimeric protein consisting of an ai subunit and β and γ subunits, which can be the same as those in G_s. Activated α_2-receptors bind to G_i and lead to GDP dissociation, GTP binding, and complex dissociation, as occurs with G_s. Both the released ai and the bg complex are thought to contribute to adenylyl cyclase inhibition, α_i by direct inhibition, and βγ by direct inhibition and indirectly, by binding to and inactivating any free $G\alpha_s$ subunits. Activated G_i can also open K^+ channels, an example of how a single G protein can regulate multiple effector molecules. A similar G protein regulatory cycle applies to other G protein subtypes as well.

One of the hallmarks of signal transduction by G protein-coupled receptors, as well as other receptor/second messenger systems, is their ability to amplify the extracellular signal. Amplification is possible since the receptor and G protein are able to diffuse in the plasma membrane, which allows each agonist-bound receptor complex to interact with many inactive G_s molecules and convert them to their active state. Further amplification occurs when each active $G\alpha_s$-GTP complex activates a single adenylyl cyclase molecule, which then catalyzes the formation of many cAMP molecules in the period before the GTP is hydrolyzed, the complex dissociates, and adenylyl cyclase is inactivated.

Ligand-gated Ion Channels

Signals that utilize G protein-coupled receptors are involved in functions that operate with time courses of seconds to minutes, as occurs with slow synaptic transmission, in which receptor activation is coupled indirectly through a series of steps to a specific change in effector function. In contrast, signals that require rapid transduction, such as fast synaptic transmission, utilize ligand-gated ion channels, in which binding of the extracellular signal to the receptor directly causes an immediate conformational change in the receptor-ion channel complex that opens the associated ion channel and selectively changes its ion permeability independent of a second messenger. The ligand-binding site and the ion channel are part of the same molecule or macromolecular complex. Ion channel activation is dependent on the continued occupation of receptor by the ligand, and is rapidly reversible upon ligand dissociation. This allows ligand-gated ion channels to mediate rapid onset and rapidly reversible cell signaling.

Ligand-gated ion channels allow the direct conversion of extracellular chemical signals into electrical signals in excitable cells such as neurons and muscle. The ionic selectivity of the ion channel and the membrane potential of the target cell determine whether the ligand-gated ion channel has an excitatory or an inhibitory effect on neuronal excitability or synaptic transmission (Chapter 19). Excitatory neurotransmitters, which include acetylcholine and glutamate, open cation-selective channels that allow Na^+ influx, which depolarizes the membrane. Inhibitory neurotransmitters, which include γ-aminobutyric acid (GABA) and glycine, open Cl^--selective channels that hyperpolarize the membrane or prevent depolarization. A subclass of ligand-gated ion channels includes receptors for intracellular messengers that control Ca^{2+} channels on organelle membranes involved in the regulation of intracellular Ca^{2+} concentration (e.g. ryanodine receptors and IP_3 receptors).

Although their ligand binding specificities and ion channel selectivities differ, the ligand-gated ion channels that respond to acetylcholine, serotonin, GABA, and glycine consist of structurally homologous subunits and constitute a receptor superfamily. They are heteropentameric membrane-spanning proteins comprised of homologous subunits that interact to form a central transmembrane ion channel. Multiple isoforms of each subunit exist that interact in different combinations to form receptor-ion channel complexes with distinct ligand affinities, sensitivities to drugs, and channel conductance and kinetic properties. Glutamate-gated ion channels constitute a distinct family of receptors that consist of different subunits, but appear to have a similar structure overall.

Extensive structural and functional information is available for the nicotinic acetylcholine (ACh) receptor, which can be isolated in large quantities from fish electric organs and serves as an example for other ligand-gated ion channels (Chapter 31). This receptor contains four subunit types, which exist in the stoichiometry $\alpha_2\beta\gamma\delta$ (Fig. 3.9a). Each subunit of the nicotinic ACh receptor, GABA receptor, and glycine receptor contains four hydrophobic transmembrane domains in its carboxy-terminal region, in similar positions within the subunit, and with similar deduced membrane topology (Fig. 3.9b). A long intracellular loop is located between the third and fourth transmembrane segments and may mediate interactions with the cytoskeleton. The second transmembrane segment (M2) is the most hydrophilic of the four, and lines the aqueous ion channel. A large extracellular domain extends over the entire amino-terminal half of the subunit.

Molecular cloning techniques have identified a large number of isoforms of the five different subunit types that constitute the $GABA_A$ receptor (α_1–α_6; β_1–β_4; γ_1–γ_3; δ, and ρ subunits). Each isoform is homologous and has the general structure shown in Fig. 3.9b (Chapter 23). Experimental expression of specific subunit isoforms in cultured cells has identified pharmacologic differences produced by various subunit combinations. For example, benzodiazepine sensitivity can be altered depending on the specific α or γ subunit isoform present. Alternative splicing of subunit mRNA precursors has also been shown to generate a second isoform of each γ subunit, which may contain an additional phosphorylation site. The many alternative combinations of $GABA_A$ receptors have been shown to have a complex anatomical distribution within the CNS, which may have important functional and pharmacological implications.

The ligand-gated glutamate receptors are functionally divided into those activated by *N*-methyl-D-aspartate (NMDA) and the non-NMDA receptors, the latter of which can be distinguished by their sensitivities to α-amino-3-hydroxy-5-methylisoxazole-4-propionic acid (AMPA) and kainate (KA). Expression cloning was used to identify the first non-NMDA receptor subunit structure, from which a family of homologous non-NMDA receptor subunits has been identified (GluR1-GluR7 and KA1-KA2). These subunits have four deduced hydrophobic transmembrane domains, similar to $GABA_A$ receptor subunits, but the amino-terminal domains are significantly longer. More than one type of subunit is required to express glutamate-gated cation channel function, which suggests

Structure of the torpedo nicotinic acetylcholine receptor and transmembrane topography of the four subunits

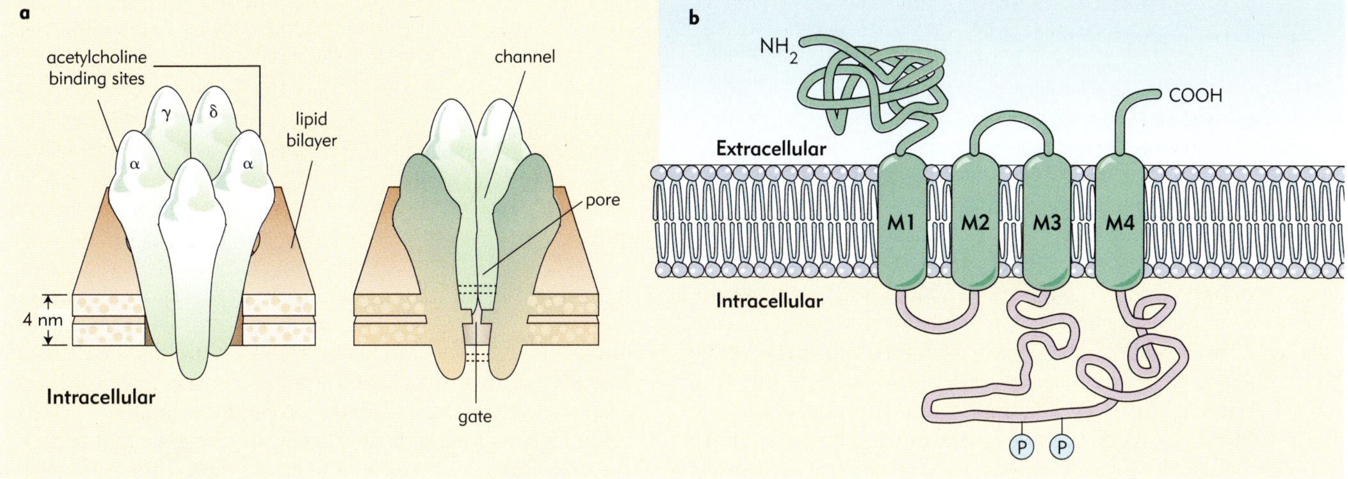

Figure 3.9 (a) Structure of the *Torpedo* nicotinic acetylcholine receptor. Five homologous subunits (α, α, β, γ, δ) combine to form a transmembrane aqueous pore. The pore is lined by a ring of five transmembrane a helices, one contributed by each subunit. The ring of a helices is probably surrounded by a continuous rim of transmembrane β sheet, made up of the other transmembrane segments of the five subunits. In its closed conformation the pore is thought to be occluded by the hydrophobic side chains of five leucine residues, one from each α helix, which form a gate near the middle of the lipid bilayer. The negatively charged side chains at either end of the pore (dotted lines) insure that only positively charged ions pass through the channel. Both of the α subunits contain an acetycholine binding site; when acetylcholine binds to both sites, the channel undergoes a conformational change that opens the gate, possibly by causing the leucine residues to move outward. (From Alberts et al., 1994, with permission.) **(b) Transmembrane topography of each of the four subunit types of the nicotinic acetylcholine receptor.** M1–M4 represent the four α-helical transmembrane domains of the receptor subunit. A region of the intracellular loop of each subunit is phosphorylated by cAMP-dependent protein kinase, protein kinase C, and a protein-tyrosine kinase. Phosphorylation of the receptor in this region increases its rate of rapid desensitization. The M2 domain of each subunit lines the ion pore. (Modified from Hemmings et al., 1989, with permission.)

that the functional form of the receptor exists as an oligomer. Alternative splicing results in additional subunit heterogeneity, as seen with the $GABA_A$ receptor. NMDA receptors possess many properties that are unique among ligand-gated ion channels; these include voltage sensitivity (in addition to glutamate sensitivity), the requirement of glycine as a co-agonist, slow kinetics, and blockade by Mg^{2+}. Identification of the structure of an NMDA receptor subunit by expression cloning (NR1) again revealed a topology consisting of four similar transmembrane domains (Chapter 23). Additional subunits have since been identified (NR2A-NR2C). Although NR1 can produce the above physiological properties in homomeric form, NR2A-NR2C are only functional in a heteromeric form with NR1. The NR2 subunits differ considerably from NR1 in amino acid sequence and subunit lengths due to variable carboxy-terminal extensions. While the various glutamate receptors show considerable sequence diversity overall, the similarities in their four transmembrane sequences justify their inclusion as a distinct subgroup within the ligand-gated ion channel superfamily.

Ligand-gated ion channels are important targets for drugs. Drug specificity is conferred in part by their specialized functions dictated by distinct combinations of receptor subtypes, their differing electrophysiological properties and pharmacological sensitivities, and their specialized anatomical localizations. Thus, the structural diversity of these receptors is reflected in a rich pharmacological diversity. Important examples include the actions of neuromuscular blocking drugs on nicotinic ACh receptors at the neuromuscular junction (Chapter 32), of barbiturates, benzodiazepines and volatile anesthetics on $GABA_A$ receptors, and of phencyclidine derivatives on NMDA receptors (Chapter 23).

Enzyme-linked Cell-Surface Receptors

Enzyme-linked receptors are transmembrane proteins that couple an extracellular ligand binding site with an intracellular enzyme activity. The enzyme activity is either contained within the intracellular domain of the receptor (intrinsic activity) or associated with the intracellular domain of the receptor (associated activity). Although this is a heterogeneous group of receptors, most possess a single transmembrane domain and are associated with the activation of protein kinase activity (see Fig. 3.3). The known enzyme-linked receptors can be divided into five classes: (1) receptor tyrosine kinases, (2) tyrosine kinase-associated receptors, (3) receptor tyrosine phosphatases, (4) receptor serine/threonine kinases, and (5) receptor guanylyl cyclases.

Receptor tyrosine kinases include the receptors for many peptide/protein growth factors, including epidermal growth factor (EGF), platelet-derived growth factor (PDGF), nerve growth factor (NGF), the fibroblast growth factors (FGFs), insulin, and insulin-like growth factor-1 (IGF-1). Signaling through receptor tyrosine kinases is central to many of the cell–cell interactions that regulate embryonic development, tissue maintenance, and repair. Ligand binding to the extracellular domain of most receptor tyrosine kinases induces dimerization and activation of the tyrosine kinase intrinsic to the intracellular domain, which catalyzes the phosphorylation of the receptor itself (autophosphorylation) and of specific intracellular proteins, which leads to specific physio-

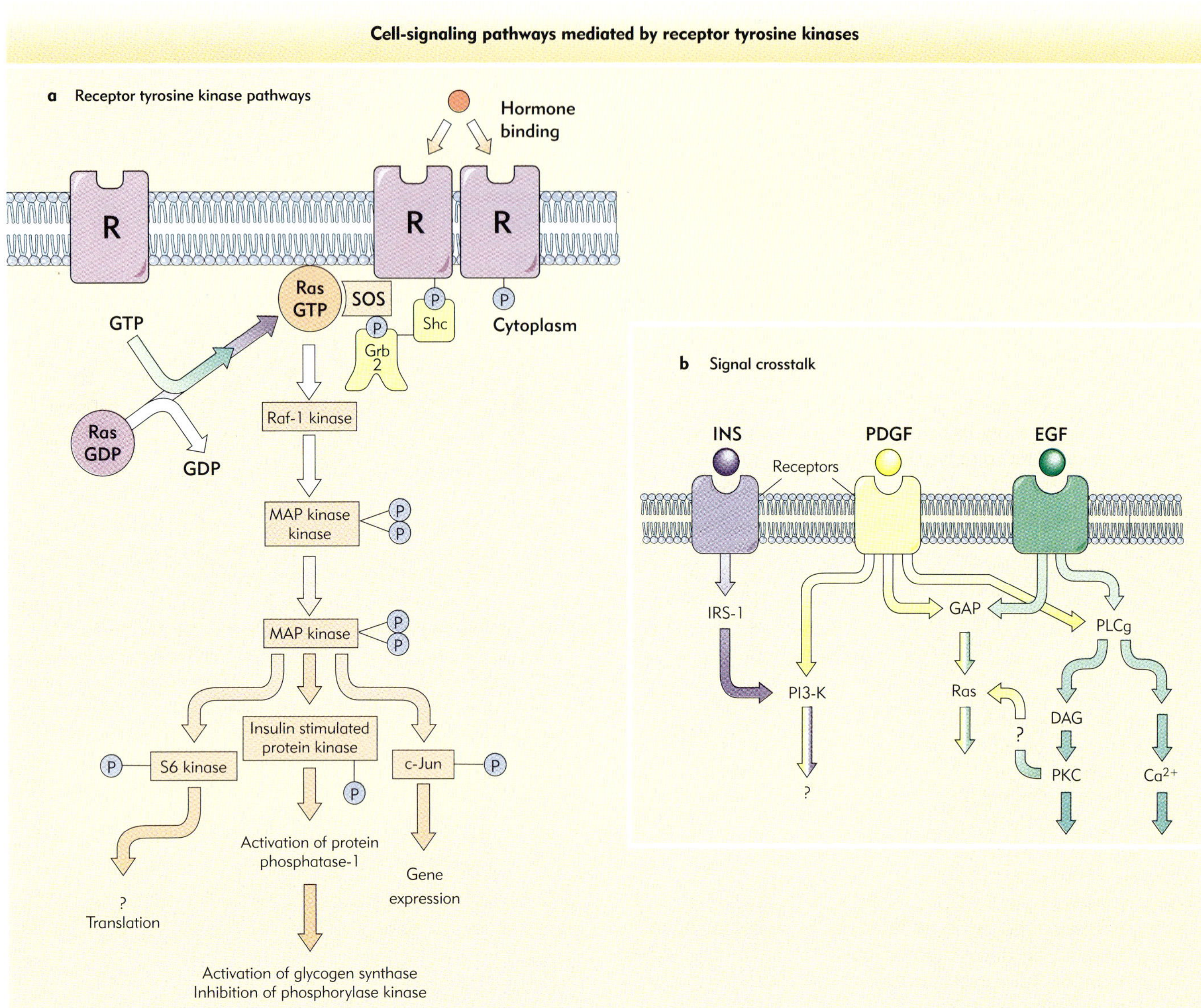

Figure 3.10 (a) Cell-signaling pathways mediated by receptor tyrosine kinases. Binding of a hormone such as insulin leads to receptor dimerization, autophosphorylation, and activation of receptor tyrosine kinase. On receptor stimulation, the adapter protein Shc binds to activated, tyrosine-phosphorylated receptors and becomes phosphorylated. Tyrosine-phosphorylated Shc subsequently interacts with the SH2 domain of Grb2, which binds by its SH3 domains to the guanine nucleotide exchange factor SOS, which activates Ras. SOS enhances GDP dissociation from Ras, promoting its activation by rebinding GTP; Ras then slowly hydrolyzes GTP to GDP and becomes inactive (note the similarity to the membrane-bound G proteins). Ras in turn activates Raf-1, a serine- threonine protein kinase. Raf-1 phosphorylates and activates MAP kinase kinase, a bifunctional protein tyrosine and protein threonine kinase (also called MEK, MAP, or extracellular signal-regulated kinase kinase). MAP kinase kinase activates MAP kinase by phosphorylation on both tyrosine and threonine residues. MAP kinase (also called ERK, extracellular signal-regulated kinase) itself phosphorylates and activates S6 kinase, which stimulates protein synthesis. MAP kinase also phosphorylates and activates the insulin-stimulated protein kinase p90rsk, which activates protein phosphatase-1. Glycogen synthase is activated and phosphorylase kinase inactivated by dephosphorylation by protein phosphatase-1. Nuclear gene expression is also activated by phosphorylation of transcription factors such as c-Jun. Thus three anabolic pathways are stimulated by insulin. **(b) Signaling mechanisms initiated by insulin (INS), PDGF, and EGF.** Insulin activates IRS-1 and PI3 kinase. PDGF activates PI3 kinase, the Ras-GAP sequence, and phospholipase Cγ (PLCγ). EGF activates the Ras-GAP sequence and PLCγ. Thus there is extensive cross-talk between these intracellular signaling pathways. (Modified from Brody et al., 1994, with permission.)

logical effects and changes in gene expression. Receptor dimerization is thought to play an important role in the activation of the intracellular tyrosine kinase activity since it allows cross-phosphorylation of the two intracellular domains. The autophosphorylated tyrosines on the receptors serve as high-affinity binding sites for specific intracellular signaling proteins in the target cell. Binding of these proteins frequently results in their phosphorylation on tyrosine and subsequent activation, or in their interaction with other signaling molecules. Receptor tyrosine autophosphorylation thereby triggers the assembly of a transient intracellular signaling complex that is involved in the signal transduction process (Fig. 3.10). Some of the proteins that interact with tyrosine phosphorylated receptors are phospholipase Cγ, GTPase activating proteins (GAPs), c-Src-like nonreceptor tyrosine kinases, and phosphatidylinositol 3-kinase. These proteins usually contain Src homology domains (SH2 or SH3 domains), which recognize phosphorylated tyrosine residues in the receptor.

Ras proteins are small GTPase proteins involved in transducing mitogenic signals from activated receptor tyrosine kinases to the nucleus to stimulate cell growth and differentiation (Fig. 3.10). Ras activation by receptor tyrosine kinases requires the adapter proteins Shc, Grb2, and SOS, which couple receptor activation to Ras activation. An SH2 domain in Grb2 specifically interacts with a phosphotyrosine residue on the intracellular portion of the activated receptor tyrosine kinase (e.g. EGF receptor) or on the adapter protein Shc. Grb2 then binds and activates SOS through two SH3 domains on SOS, thereby linking the receptor with SOS, a guanine nucleotide exchange protein that activates Ras by stimulating release of GDP and subsequent GTP binding. The active GTP-bound form of Ras then associates with several potential downstream signaling molecules including the Raf-1 protein kinase that initiates a serine/threonine protein kinase cascade that activates MAP-kinase (mitogen-activated protein kinase), which relays the signal downstream by phosphorylating various effector molecules involved in gene regulation. The MAP-kinase pathway is a highly conserved eukaryotic signaling pathway that couples various receptor signals to cell proliferation, differentiation, and metabolic regulation. Activated GTP-Ras is slowly converted to the inactive, GDP-bound form by its intrinsic GTPase activity, which can be accelerated by GAPs.

Tyrosine kinase-associated receptors are comparable to the receptor tyrosine kinases, but instead of activating an integral tyrosine kinase activity, they work through associated non-receptor tyrosine kinases. This diverse group of receptors includes those for some hormones (prolactin and growth hormone, for example), lymphocyte antigen receptors, and many cytokines. The associated tyrosine kinases belong to the c-Src family (e.g. Src, Fyn, Yes, and Lck) or the Janus family (e.g. JAK1 and JAK2) of nonreceptor tyrosine kinases. These receptors are thought to function like the receptor tyrosine kinases, except that the tyrosine kinase domain is a separate entity that attaches to the receptor noncovalently. As with the receptor tyrosine kinases, ligand binding usually induces receptor dimerization, tyrosine kinase activation, and phosphorylation of distinct sets of substrate proteins.

Receptor tyrosine phosphatases are a large and diverse group of membrane-bound enzymes that reverse the action of tyrosine kinases by catalyzing the dephosphorylation of specific phosphotyrosine residues. Receptor tyrosine phosphatases include an extracellular domain of variable length and composition, a single membrane-spanning domain, and one or two intracellular catalytic domains. CD45, the prototype of this family, has a single transmembrane domain and is activated by crosslinking with antibodies to the extracellular domain. The natural ligands for CD45, and for most other members of this family, are unknown.

Receptor serine/threonine kinases constitute a recently identified family of receptors for the transforming growth factor-β (TGF-β) family of signaling proteins. These receptors consist of a single transmembrane domain with an integral serine/threonine protein kinase domain within the intracellular portion of the receptor.

The receptor guanylyl cyclases are discussed below.

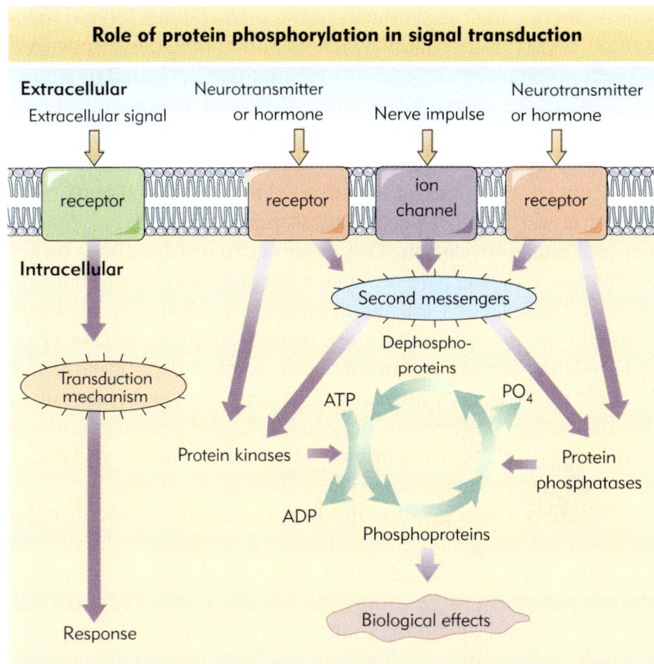

Figure 3.11 Schematic diagram of cellular regulation by extracellular signals acting through protein phosphorylation. A generalized scheme for cell-surface receptor-mediated signal transduction is shown on the left. Extracellular signals (first messengers), which include various neurotransmitters, hormones, and cytokines, produce specific biological effects in target cells via a series of intracellular signals. Cell membrane receptors for many extracellular signals are coupled to the activation of protein kinases, either directly by activating a protein kinase intimately associated with the receptor, or indirectly through changes in the intracellular levels of second messengers. Prominent second messengers involved in the regulation of protein kinases include cAMP, cGMP, Ca^{2+}, and 1,2-diacylglycerol. The activation of individual protein kinases causes the phosphorylation of specific substrate proteins (phosphoproteins) in target cells. In some cases these substrate proteins, or third messengers, appear to be the immediate effectors for the biological response, and in other cases they seem to produce the biological response indirectly, through additional intracellular messengers. Protein phosphatases are also subject to regulation by extracellular signals acting directly, or through second messengers acting on the protein phosphatases (e.g., Ca^{2+} on Ca^{2+}/calmodulin-dependent protein phosphatase-2B), or by the phosphorylation of specific protein phosphatase modulator proteins. Many, if not all, membrane receptors and ion channels are themselves regulated by phosphorylation/dephosphorylation. (Modified from Hemmings et al., 1989, with permission.)

SECOND MESSENGERS AND PROTEIN PHOSPHORYLATION

Work by Sutherland and colleagues in the late 1950s on the hormonal control of glycogen metabolism in the mammalian liver revealed that epinephrine and glucagon stimulated glycogenolysis by increasing the synthesis of the intracellular second messenger cAMP. Subsequently, Krebs and colleagues discovered a protein kinase in skeletal muscle that was activated by physiological increases in the levels of cAMP, and demonstrated that epinephrine stimulated glycogenolysis through activation of this protein kinase. Since this groundbreaking work, the mechanisms of action of a number of additional extracellular signals have been found to involve second messengers and/or regulation of protein phosphorylation. This process can involve either direct activation of a receptor-associated protein kinase or an alteration in the level of a second messenger, which then in turn regulates a specific protein kinase or protein phosphatase (Fig. 3.11). Thus, the regulation of the state of phosphorylation of specific substrates by a variety of protein kinases represents a final common pathway in the signal transduction mechanisms through which many hormones, neurotransmitters, and other extracellular signals produce their biological effects.

Protein phosphorylation involves the covalent modification of key substrate proteins by phosphoryl transfer, which in turn regulates their functional properties. All protein phosphorylation systems have three components in common: (1) a substrate protein (phosphoprotein) that can exist in either the dephospho- or phospho-form, (2) a protein kinase that catalyzes phosphoryl transfer from the terminal (γ) phosphate of ATP to a specific hydroxylated amino acid of the substrate protein (serine, threonine, or tyrosine), and (3) a protein phosphatase that catalyzes dephosphorylation of the phosphorylated substrate protein (Fig. 3.11). Several second messengers are involved in the control of protein phosphorylation by extracellular signals. These second messengers include cAMP, cGMP, Ca^{2+} (together with calmodulin), and 1,2-diacylglycerol, each of which is capable of activating one or more distinct protein kinases.

Protein kinases can be divided into two classes, protein-serine/threonine kinases and protein-tyrosine kinases. The protein-serine/threonine kinases can be further divided into those that are regulated by known second messengers (e.g. cAMP, cGMP, and Ca^{2+}) and those that are not (the Ca^{2+}-and cyclic nucleotide-independent protein kinases and the receptor serine/threonine protein kinases). Up to 1% of eukaryotic genes appear to encode protein kinases, most of which are protein-serine/threonine kinases.

Cyclic AMP

Cyclic AMP (cAMP), the first intracellular messenger identified, operates as a signaling molecule in all eukaryotic and prokaryotic cells. A variety of hormones and neurotransmitters have been found to regulate the levels of cAMP. Adenylyl cyclase, the membrane-bound enzyme which catalyzes the formation of cAMP, is controlled by receptor-mediated stimulation and inhibition. The rapid degradation of cAMP to adenosine 5′-monophosphate by one of several isoforms of cAMP phosphodiesterase provides the potential for rapid reversibility and responsiveness of this signaling mechanism. Most of the actions of cAMP are mediated through the activation of cAMP-dependent protein kinase (PKA) and the concomitant phosphorylation of substrate protein effectors on specific serine or threonine residues.

The widespread distribution of cAMP-dependent protein kinase throughout the animal kingdom led to the hypothesis that the diverse effects of cAMP on cell function are mediated through the activation of this enzyme, which has been shown to be the principal intracellular receptor for cAMP. Another known receptor for cAMP is a cAMP-sensitive ion channel in odorant-sensitive olfactory neurons. cAMP-dependent protein kinase exists as a tetramer composed of two types of dissimilar subunits, the regulatory (R) subunit and the catalytic (C) subunit. In the absence of cAMP, the inactive holoenzyme tetramer consists of two R subunits joined by disulfide bonds, bound to two C subunits (R_2C_2). The binding of cAMP to the R subunits of the inactive holoenzyme lowers their affinity for the C subunits and leads to the dissociation from the holoenzyme of the two free C subunits expressing phosphotransferase activity. Each R subunit contains two binding sites for cAMP, which activate the kinase synergistically and exhibit positively cooperative cAMP binding.

The phosphorylation of specific substrates brought about by cAMP-dependent protein kinase represents the next step in the molecular pathway by which cAMP produces its biological responses. Substrates for cAMP-dependent protein kinase are characterized by two or more basic amino acid residues on the amino-terminal side of the phosphorylated residue. The identification and characterization of the specific substrate(s) phosphorylated in response to cAMP are important goals in the study of agents whose actions are mediated by cAMP. The various substrates for cAMP-dependent protein kinase present in different cell types explain the diverse tissue-specific effects of cAMP.

Cyclic GMP/Nitric Oxide

Cyclic GMP (cGMP) is a key intracellular signaling molecule in virtually all cells. It plays a key role in signal transduction pathways activated by nitric oxide (NO) and the natriuretic peptides. Various tissues contain multiple forms of guanylyl cyclase and cGMP phosphodiesterase, the two enzymes that regulate the intracellular concentration of cGMP. Guanylyl cyclases exist in both soluble and particulate (cell-surface) forms. Soluble forms of the enzyme are activated by NO formed from L-arginine by activation of NO synthase or pharmacologically by exogenous nitroglycerin or nitroprusside which degrade to NO. Soluble guanylyl cyclase contains a heme moiety, which binds NO and other oxidants to stimulate enzyme activity. The family of NO synthases includes constitutive neuronal and endothelial forms and an inducible macrophage form. The endothelial and neuronal isoforms of NO synthase are dependent on Ca^{2+}/calmodulin for activation, while the inducible form is constitutive and Ca^{2+}-independent. Nitric oxide is thought to be the endogenous regulator of guanylyl cyclase activity that mediates the action of several vasodilators, including acetylcholine, bradykinin, and substance P (Fig. 3.12). These transmitters stimulate the production of a diffusable mediator known as endothelium-derived relaxing factor (EDRF), which has been identified as NO or a closely related molecule (Chapter 33). NO may also regulate the function of other proteins in addition to guanylyl cyclase by S-nitrosylation of specific protein thiols.

The NO/guanylyl cyclase signaling pathway has received considerable attention as the first example of a signaling system that involves a gaseous signaling molecule. Recent evidence suggests that carbon monoxide (CO) can also act as a signaling molecule to stimulate guanylyl cyclase. Because it readily diffuses within a restricted volume across cell membranes, NO formed in one cell is able to activate guanylyl cyclase in the same cell as a second messenger (autocrine effect) as well as in neighboring cells as a transmitter (paracrine effect), but its diffusion is limited by its chemical reactivity and short half-life. Nitric oxide is an important signaling molecule involved in the regulation of vascular tone and in host defense mechanisms. Nitric oxide donors, inhibitors of NO

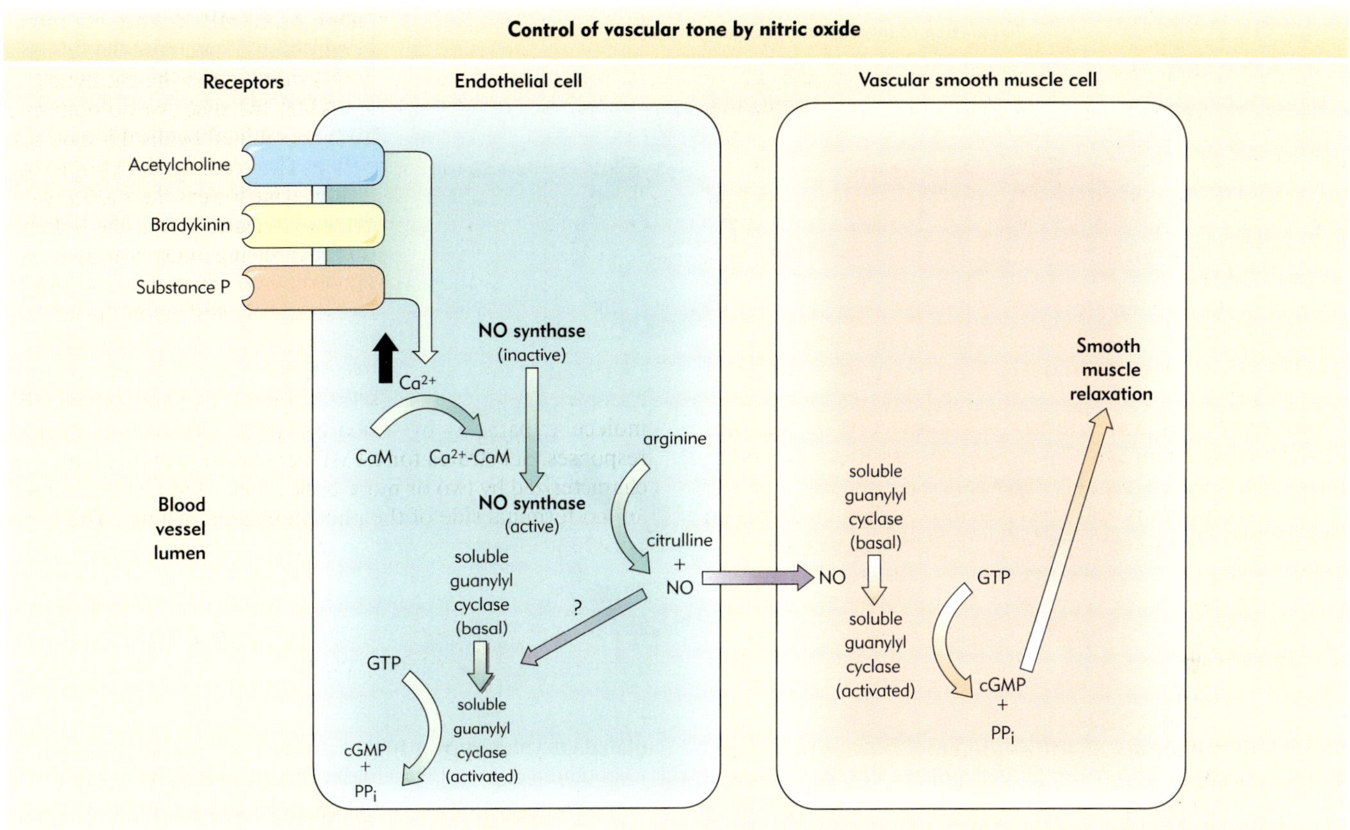

Figure 3.12 Control of vascular tone by nitric oxide. Model depicting the regulation of soluble guanylyl cyclase in a vascular smooth muscle cell by nitric oxide formed in an endothelial cell. Increases in intracellular Ca^{2+} concentration stimulate NO synthase activity through binding to calmodulin (CaM). Nitric oxide may also act on the soluble form of guanylyl cyclase within the same (endothelial) cell. (Modified from Schulz et al., 1991, with permission.)

synthase, and NO itself are providing new approaches to the management of a number of diseases, including sepsis, ARDS, pulmonary hypertension, ischemia, and degenerative diseases.

Particulate forms of guanylyl cyclase serve as cell-surface receptors for a variety of different peptide ligands, including the natriuretic peptides (e.g. atrial natriuretic peptide; ANP). These receptors contain a single transmembrane domain flanked by an extracellular peptide binding domain and intracellular guanylyl cyclase and protein kinase-like catalytic domains. Some forms of particulate guanylyl cyclase also appear to be sensitive to intracellular Ca^{2+}.

The cellular responses to cGMP are mediated in specific tissues by regulation of cGMP-regulated phosphodiesterase, cGMP-gated ion channels and cGMP-dependent protein kinase. cGMP-dependent protein kinase is a protein-serine/threonine kinase that is either a soluble dimer of identical subunits (type I) or a membrane-bound monomer (type II). cGMP-dependent protein kinase is activated by increases in intracellular cGMP, the formation of which is catalyzed by guanylyl cyclase. The primary mechanism of inactivation of cGMP-dependent protein kinase results from hydrolysis of cGMP by cyclic nucleotide phosphodiesterase, of which there is a form specific for cGMP. Each subunit of type I cGMP-dependent protein kinase contains a cGMP-binding domain and a catalytic domain, which is homologous to the cAMP-dependent protein kinase catalytic subunit. Upon binding of cGMP, a conformational change occurs in the enzyme, exposing the active catalytic domain; the mechanism of activation of the type II kinase has not been determined. In contrast to cAMP-dependent protein kinase, which is present in similar concentrations in most mammalian tissues, cGMP-dependent protein kinase has an uneven tissue distribution. Relatively high concentrations of the type I enzyme are found in lung, heart, smooth muscle, platelets, cerebellum, and intestine; the type II enzyme is widely distributed in the brain and intestine. *In vitro*, cGMP-dependent and cAMP-dependent protein kinases show similar substrate specificities. Although many physiological substrates for cAMP-dependent protein kinase have been identified, only a few specific physiological substrates for cGMP-dependent protein kinase have been found. Physiological roles for both kinases have been demonstrated in a number of tissues by microinjection into cells of the purified kinases or specific peptide inhibitors.

Calcium Ion and Inositol Trisphosphate

Along with cAMP, Ca^{2+} controls a wide variety of intracellular processes. Ca^{2+} entry through Ca^{2+} channels or its release from intracellular stores triggers hormone and neurotransmitter secretion, initiates muscle contraction, and activates many protein kinases and other enzymes. The concentration of free Ca^{2+} is maintained at a very low level in the cytosol of most cells ($<10^{-6}$ mol/L) compared to the extracellular fluid $\sim10^{-3}$ mol/L) by a number of homeostatic mechanisms. A Ca^{2+}-ATPase in the plasma membrane pumps Ca^{2+} from the cytosol to the cell exterior at the expense of ATP hydrolysis, a Ca^{2+}-ATPase in the

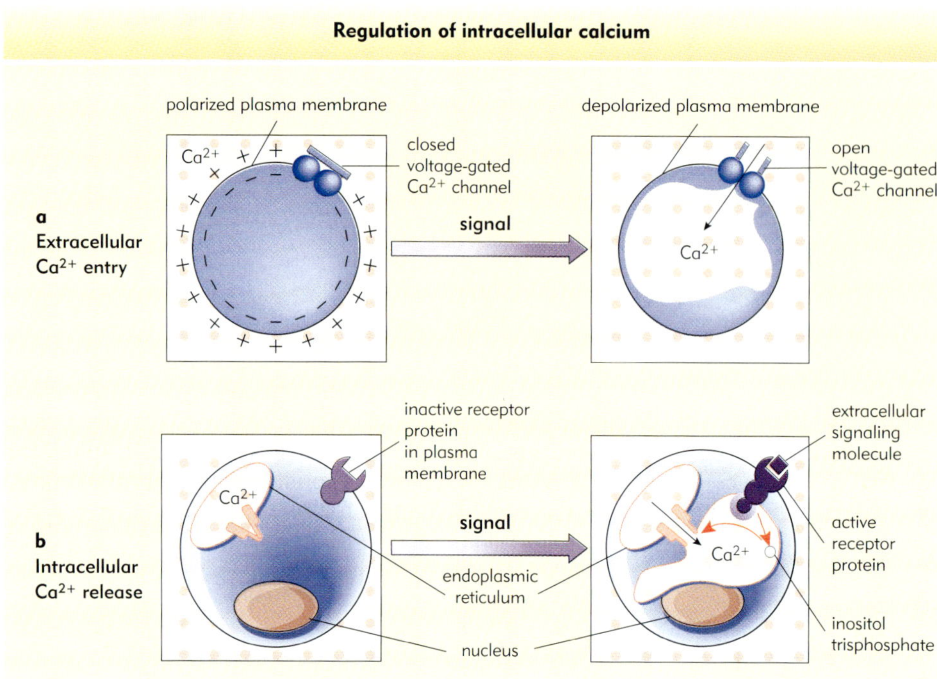

Figure 3.13 Two common pathways by which Ca^{2+} can enter the cytosol in response to extracellular signals. In (a) Ca^{2+} enters a nerve terminal from the extracellular fluid through voltage-gated Ca^{2+} channels when the nerve terminal membrane is depolarized by an action potential. In (b) the binding of an extracellular signaling molecule to a cell-surface receptor generates inositol trisphosphate, which stimulates the release of Ca^{2+} from the endoplasmic reticulum. (Modified from Alberts et al., 1994, with permission.)

endoplasmic and sarcoplasmic reticulum concentrates Ca^{2+} from the cytosol into intracellular storage organelles and a Na^+/Ca^{2+} exchanger, which is particularly active in excitable plasma membranes, couples the electrochemical potential of Na^+ influx to the efflux of Ca^{2+} (Na^+ driven Ca^{2+} antiport). Although mitochondria have the ability to take up and release Ca^{2+}, they are not widely felt to play a major role in cytosolic Ca^{2+} homeostasis under normal conditions.

Changes in intracellular free Ca^{2+} concentration can be induced directly by depolarization evoked Ca^{2+} entry through voltage-dependent Ca^{2+} channels (as in neurons and muscle) and by extracellular signals that activate Ca^{2+}-permeable ligand-gated ion channels (e.g. the NMDA receptor), or directly by extracellular signals coupled to the formation of IP_3 (Fig. 3.13). IP_3 is formed in response to a number of extracellular signals that interact with G protein-coupled cell-surface receptors (G_q) coupled to the activation of phospholipase C. Phospholipase C hydrolyzes phosphatidylinositol-4,5-bisphosphate to IP_3 and diacylglycerol; further degradation of diacylglycerol by phospholipase A_2 can result in the release of arachidonic acid. All three of these receptor-regulated metabolites are important second messengers. IP_3 increases intracellular Ca^{2+} by binding to specific IP_3 receptors on the endoplasmic reticulum, which are coupled to a Ca^{2+} channel that allows Ca^{2+} efflux into the cytosol. IP_3 receptors are similar to the Ca^{2+} release channels (ryanodine receptors) of muscle sarcoplasmic reticulum that release Ca^{2+} in response to excitation. Diacylglycerol remains in the plasma membrane where it activates protein kinase C, while arachidonic acid, in addition to its metabolism to biologically active prostaglandins and leukotrienes, can also activate protein kinase C. The Ca^{2+} signal is terminated by hydrolysis of IP_3 and by the rapid reuptake and extrusion of Ca^{2+}.

Ca^{2+} carries out it second messenger functions primarily after binding to intracellular Ca^{2+} binding proteins, of which *calmodulin* is the most important. Calmodulin is a ubiquitous multifunctional Ca^{2+} binding protein, highly conserved between species, that binds four atoms of Ca^{2+} with high affinity. Most calmodulin-regulated enzymes appear to be activated by a similar mechanism. Calmodulin does not bind to the enzyme in the absence of Ca^{2+}; however, in the presence of micromolar concentrations of Ca^{2+}, calmodulin undergoes a marked conformational change exposing hydrophobic binding sites. The exposed hydrophobic domain of the Ca^{2+}/calmodulin complex interacts with a calmodulin-binding domain present in a variety of effector proteins, including the Ca^{2+}/calmodulin-dependent protein kinases, which along with protein kinase C mediate most of the effects of Ca^{2+} in cells. Ca^{2+}/calmodulin-dependent activation of protein kinases was originally observed for phosphorylase kinase and myosin light chain kinase (Chapter 33). Subsequently Ca^{2+}/calmodulin-dependent protein phosphorylation was found to be widespread in various tissues. Ca^{2+}/calmodulin kinases I and II, myosin light chain kinase, and phosphorylase kinase appear to be responsible for most Ca^{2+}/calmodulin-dependent protein kinase activity.

Ca^{2+}/calmodulin kinase I has a widespread species and tissue distribution, and, like phosphorylase kinase or myosin light chain kinase, exhibits a limited substrate specificity. In contrast to other Ca^{2+}/calmodulin kinases, the isozymes of Ca^{2+}/calmodulin kinase II exhibit a relatively broad substrate specificity. This kinase is therefore referred to as the multifunctional Ca^{2+}/calmodulin-dependent protein kinase.

Protein kinase C was first purified from brain as a cyclic nucleotide-independent protein kinase which could be activated by a Ca^{2+}-dependent protease. The holoenzyme was subsequently found to be activated by the addition of Ca^{2+}, diacylglycerol, and membrane phospholipid. Protein kinase C has been shown to be the intracellular receptor for, and to be activated by, the tumor-promoting phorbol esters. The holoenzyme contains a hydrophobic regulatory domain which interacts with Ca^{2+}, phospholipid, and phorbol esters, and a hydrophilic catalytic domain, which can be cleaved from the holoenzyme by proteolysis to yield a fragment that is catalytically active in the absence of Ca^{2+}, diacylglycerol, and phospholipid. Protein kinase C has a broad substrate specificity, which differs from those of both cyclic nucleotide-dependent and Ca^{2+}/calmodulin-dependent protein kinases.

Protein kinase C is activated by micromolar concentrations of Ca^{2+} and membrane phospholipids of which phosphatidylserine is the most active. Addition of low concentrations of diacylglycerol increases its affinity for Ca^{2+}. Protein kinase C is activated in cells by an increase in the concentration of diacylglycerol produced by receptor-stimulated phosphatidylinositol turnover (Fig. 3.6). The activation of the kinase by diacylglycerol, although dependent on micromolar concentrations of Ca^{2+}, does not appear to be dependent on increases in intracellular Ca^{2+}. Tumor-promoting phorbol esters appear to substitute for diacylglycerol in the activation of protein kinase C. The hydrolysis of phosphatidylinositol 4,5-bisphosphate produces diacylglycerol and IP_3, and the latter compound mobilizes Ca^{2+} in cells. Activation of protein kinase C results from the synergistic actions of increases in the intracellular concentrations of both Ca^{2+} and diacylglycerol. The contributions of each second messenger may vary, however, depending on the cell type or receptor-mediated event. Activation of protein kinase C, which is predominantly a cytosolic enzyme, leads to its translocation to the plasma membrane, where it undergoes protease-mediated down-regulation in the presence of continuous stimulation. Translocation of PKC may be important in targeting the enzyme to specific substrates and cellular compartments.

Protein Phosphatases

The phosphorylation of specific sites on proteins is transient and regulated by protein phosphatases in addition to protein kinases. Rather than simply reversing the phosphorylation catalyzed by protein kinases, protein phosphatases exhibit distinct substrate specificities and are tightly regulated; regulation of both protein phosphorylation and dephosphorylation increases the complexity and flexibility of this regulatory mechanism. The protein phosphatases involved in the dephosphorylation of most of the known proteins phosphorylated on serine or threonine residues are principally accounted for by four enzymes: type 1 protein phosphatase (protein phosphatase-1) and type 2 protein phosphatases (protein phosphatases-2A, -2B, and -2C). Protein phosphatase-1 selectively dephosphorylates the β-subunit of phosphorylase kinase and is inhibited by nanomolar concentrations of phosphatase inhibitor-1, inhibitor-2, or DARPP-32, while type 2 protein phosphatases selectively dephosphorylate the α-subunit of phosphorylase kinase and are insensitive to these inhibitors. The type 2 protein phosphatases are further distinguished by their requirements for divalent cations. Protein phosphatases-1, -2A, and -2B share homologous catalytic subunits, and are complexed with one or more regulatory subunits. Protein phosphatase-2C is distinct and relatively minor in most tissues. Protein phosphatases-1, -2A, and -2C all exhibit relatively broad substrate specificities, while that of protein phosphatase-2B (also known as calcineurin) appears to be more restricted. Recently, multiple forms (>40 members) of both cytosolic and membrane-bound (receptor) phosphotyrosine-protein phosphatases have been demonstrated which are distinct from the phosphoserine/phosphothreonine-protein phosphatases.

Protein phosphatases, like protein kinases, are under tight physiological regulation. Protein phosphatase-2B, which is a prominent calmodulin-binding protein in brain, is activated by Ca^{2+} plus calmodulin. Protein phosphatase-1 is regulated indirectly by cAMP, which stimulates phosphorylation and activation of two potent and specific inhibitor proteins (DARPP-32 and phosphatase inhibitor-1). This provides a positive feedback mechanism for amplifying the effects of cAMP, and a mechanism for cAMP to modulate the phosphorylation state of substrate proteins for protein kinases other than cAMP-dependent protein kinases. Protein phosphatase-1 is also regulated by its interaction with phosphatase inhibitor-2. A complex of protein phosphatase-1 with phosphatase inhibitor-2 (together known as the Mg^{2+}-ATP-dependent protein phosphatase) is inactive, but is activated by incubation with glycogen synthase kinase-3 plus Mg^{2+}-ATP. Tissue-specific targeting subunits also serve to localize protein phosphatase-1 to important subcellular sites of action in muscle, liver, and brain.

ANESTHETIC EFFECTS ON CELL SIGNALING MECHANISMS

Cell signaling mechanisms are important targets for drug effects on many physiological systems. This is due in part to the fact that cell-surface receptors for hormones and neurotransmitters provide accessible targets for drug action. For example, a number of cardiovascular drugs interact with G protein-coupled receptors for epinephrine and/or norepinephrine (α1, α2, and β adrenergic receptors). Other components of cell signaling pathways are also affected by drugs that are relevant to the practice of anesthesiology, or are currently the focus of targeted drug development. Thus a thorough understanding of cell signaling mechanisms is essential to understanding the actions, interactions, and undesirable effects of many drugs.

The mechanisms of action of anesthetic agents is of particular relevance to anesthesiologists. This area of research has generated considerable controversy, and there is little agreement over how and where general anesthetics act at a cellular and molecular level. Most evidence implicates ligand-gated ion channels and voltage-dependent ion channels as important targets for anesthetic effects in the central nervous system; these topics are covered in more detail in Chapters 22–24. Other components of cell signaling pathways have also been implicated as potential anesthetic targets, and many of the effects of anesthetics may result from effects on transmembrane signaling mechanisms. In particular, intracellular second messenger systems are sensitive to general anesthetics in a variety of systems.

Considerable evidence suggests that general anesthetics have specific effects on the cAMP signaling system. The regulation of cAMP synthesis by neurotransmitters and hormones is involved in the control of neuronal excitability, myocardial contractility, smooth muscle contraction, and numerous other physiological processes. The results of experiments investigating the effects of anesthetics on these cell signaling mechanisms have been contradictory in many instances, a situation that is perhaps not surprising given the extreme complexity of the biochemical mechanisms involved. For example, barbiturates were found to inhibit adenylyl cyclase in a rat brain membrane preparation by disrupting the G_s-adenylyl cyclase interaction, while more recent studies have found that barbiturates stimulate adenylyl cyclase in an intact mouse lymphoma cell line by enhancing the interaction between $G\alpha_s$ and adenylyl cyclase. In contrast, halothane stimulated adenylyl cyclase activity in the same lymphoma cell line by a mechanism that was independent of $G\alpha_s$. In other experiments, volatile anesthetics were found to increase basal adenylyl cyclase activity in rat brain and heart membranes and liver homogenates, but to inhibit basal adenylyl cyclase in dog sarcolemmal membranes. Volatile anesthetics were also found to attenuate muscarinic inhibition of rat heart adenylyl cyclase by disrupting the muscarinic receptor-G_i protein interaction. Recent experiments have shown that halothane stimulates adenylyl cyclase activity in human heart membranes and in a mouse lymphoma cell line by interfering with the inhibitory effect of G_i on adenylyl cyclase. General anesthetic effects on the G protein pathway regulating phospholipase C have also been described. Barbiturates inhibit inositol phospholipid hydrolysis through an interaction with the G protein that couples antigen stimulation to histamine release in a rat leukemia cell line. This effect is thought to derive from an action of the barbiturates to block activation of G_q, a G protein coupled to phospholipase C stimulation. Anesthetic effects on lysophosphatidate signaling have been reported recently. Inhibition by propofol and halothane occurred at the level of the receptor or its G protein, since signaling through another G protein-coupled receptor was not affected. In summary, a number of studies indicate tissue-, species-, and anesthetic-specific effects of general anesthetics on G protein-mediated signal transduction pathways. This variability suggests the existence of specific effects depending on the particular receptor, G protein and/or adenylyl cyclase isoforms present, although this possibility has not been adequately investigated. The complexity of these systems makes generalization of anesthetic effects on the G protein-mediated signaling pathways difficult.

The NO/guanylyl cyclase signaling pathway has come under intense scrutiny as a possible target for anesthetic action. Although this system was originally identified as an important regulator of vascular tone, it is now recognized to exist in various tissues, including the central nervous system, in which it plays an important role in signal transduction. Volatile anesthetics attenuate NO-dependent vasodilation in the peripheral vasculature, and inhibit NO synthase activity and reduce cGMP levels in the brain. It is therefore generally accepted that volatile anesthetics inhibit the NO-guanylyl cyclase pathway. This effect is due to inhibition of receptor- or Ca^{2+}-stimulated NO formation, and not to inhibition of guanylyl cyclase activation, possibly due to direct inhibition of NO synthase activity. These findings implicate inhibition of the NO-guanylyl cyclase pathway as a mechanism for the anesthetic, analgesic and/or sedative effects of anesthetics, although studies to demonstrate such a role have been inconsistent. Administration of selective inhibitors of NO synthase has been reported to either reduce or not change the MAC of halothane in the rat. Furthermore, targeted deletion of the gene for neuronal NO synthase in mice did not alter their sensitivity to isoflurane anesthesia, although it did eliminate a MAC-sparing effect of NO synthase inhibition, which suggests the existence of compensatory nociceptive pathways in the mutant mice.

A variety of evidence has implicated protein kinase C-mediated protein phosphorylation as a target for general anesthetic effects in the central nervous system. Protein kinase C is involved in the regulation of a number of synaptic processes known to be affected by general anesthetics, including neurotransmitter release, ion channel function, and neurotransmitter receptor desensitization. Biochemical studies have demonstrated effects of general anesthetics on protein kinase C activation *in vitro*. However, the results of these studies have been contradictory in that halothane has been found to either stimulate or inhibit protein kinase C activity. More recently, halothane has been found to activate endogenous protein kinase C in synaptic membranes and in isolated nerve terminals. The protein kinase C signaling pathway is complicated by the existence of multiple protein kinase C isoforms and their regulation by subcellular translocation and down-regulation, factors that may affect the modulation of protein kinase C by anesthetics.

The role of intracellular Ca^{2+} as a second messenger in mediating anesthetic effects has been addressed in a number of studies. The considerable evidence for anesthetic inhibition of Ca^{2+} flux through both ligand-gated channels (e.g. the NMDA receptor) and voltage-dependent Ca^{2+} channels is discussed in Chapters 22–24. Further studies suggest that anesthetics may also affect Ca^{2+}-mediated signal transduction by interacting with the Ca^{2+}-binding protein calmodulin. The pharmacological significance of these effects in modulating the activity of the host of enzymes regulated by calmodulin remains to be determined.

It is now apparent that opioids and a2-adrenergic agents act by inhibition of adenylyl cyclase and presynaptic Ca^{2+} channels through receptor-mediated interactions with pertussis toxin-sensitive G proteins (G_i or G_o). These effects of opioids and α_2-adrenergic agents are described in more detail in Chapters 26 and 25, respectively.

Key References

Berridge MJ. Elementary and global aspects of calcium signalling. J Physiol. 1997;499:291–306.

Böhm SK, Grady EF, Bunnett NW. Regulatory mechanisms that modulate signalling by G protein-coupled receptors. J Biochem. 1997;322:1–18.

Cohen P. Signal integration at the level of protein kinases, protein phosphatases and their substrates. Trends Biochem Sci. 1992;17:408–13.

Hepler JR, Gilman AG. G proteins. Trends Biochem Sci. 1992;17:383–7.

Moncada S, Higgs A. The L-arginine-nitric oxide pathway. New Engl J Med. 1993;329:2002–12.

Further Reading

Alberts B et al. (eds). Cell signaling. In: Alberts B et al. (eds). Molecular Biology of the Cell, 3rd edn. New York: Garland Pub; 1994;721–85.

Hemmings HCJr, Nairn AC, McGuinness TL, Huganir RL, Greengard P. Role of protein phosphorylation in neuronal signal transduction. FASEB J. 1989;3:1583–92.

Jacobs SJ. Hormone receptors and signaling mechanisms, In: Brody TM (ed.). Human Pharmacology. St Louis, Mosby–Year Book, Inc., 1994:457–71.

Landers DF, Becker GL, Wong KC. Ca^{2+}, calmodulin and anesthesiology. Anesth Analg. 1989;69:100–12,.

Lodish H (ed). Cell-to-cell signaling: Hormones and receptors. In: Lodish H (ed.). Molecular Cell Biology, 3rd edn. New York: WH Freeman and Co.;1995;853–924.

Nishida E, Gotoh Y. The MAP kinase cascade is essential for diverse signal transduction pathways. Trends Biochem Sci. 1993;18:128–30.

Nishizuka T. Intracellular signaling by hydrolysis of phospholipids and activation of protein kinase C. Science. 1992;258:607–14.

Schulz S, Yuen PST, Garbers DL. The expanding family of guanylyl cyclases. Trends Pharmacol Sci. 1991;12:116–20.

Yost CS. G proteins: Basic characteristics and clinical potential for the practice of anesthesia. Anesth Analg. 1993;77:822–34.

Chapter 4 Principles and techniques of molecular biology

Kirk Hogan

Topics covered in this chapter

GENERAL PRINCIPLES

Deoxyribonucleic acid (DNA) and ribonucleic acid (RNA) comprise a cell-signaling system that defies the death of an organism, if not the extinction of a species. Not only are the nucleic acids responsible for coordinating the cellular mechanisms that underlie growth, development, disease, and senescence, but also their biochemical morphology enables successful adaptations to be communicated to an organism's progeny. To fulfill these diverse roles, nucleic acids are forever suspended in tension between the demands of error-free replication and those for the continuous variation required to fuel selection. Too much or too little stability in regions of an individual's DNA sequence that are unique, or in those that are shared with other individuals, entails identical lethal consequences.

It is now possible to measure with precision the extent of variation between creatures, from the identity of whole organism clones to that of phylogenetic ancestors long since extinct. Moreover, we have the capacity to introduce variation, to enable better understanding of the mysteries of anesthesia or to ameliorate pain. Described below are the fundamental concepts and tools of nucleic acid investigations (molecular biology). Inevitably, these principles and techniques will improve many areas of our practice, including pre-symptomatic diagnosis (malignant hyperthermia, plasma cholinesterase deficiency), anesthetic genotoxicology (compound A), workplace safety (nitrous oxide, viral pathogens), and therapeutic interventions (xenogenic organs, recombinant proteins). As nucleic acids are involved in virtually all cellular processes, the same set of tools can be used to address questions of outwardly unrelated origin. Although the vernacular of molecular biology is huge and daunting, the underlying notions are usually simple and concrete, reflecting the parsimony that unites nucleic acid structure with function.

CLASSICAL VERSUS MOLECULAR GENETICS

With the advent of contemporary molecular biology, the definition of a gene has shifted from abstract units of inheritance of specific traits to the correspondence of DNA sequence with expressed proteins and RNA. Nevertheless, an explicit distinction between the genotype and phenotype of an organism has been preserved. The genotype, or genetic constitution, of an organism can be described with extraordinary precision, and differences between species, populations, individuals, and even cells within the same individual can be compared. Conversely, the phenotype, or characteristics that result from the interaction of an organism's genotype and its environment, is much more indefinite. The perceived phenotype is largely a function of how well the investigator is able to observe (e.g. how accurate is the *in vitro* halothane contracture test used to phenotype malignant hyperthermia susceptibility?) and categorize biologic phenomena (e.g. how is the state of anesthesia defined?). The net result is that mapping phenotypic observations of interest on to concrete DNA sequences inevitably risks confusing biochemical with semantic logical domains.

With the exceptions of sex chromosomes and mitochondrial DNA (which is inherited only from the mother), the human genome is diploid with each gene present twice at a given chromosomal locus. Mitosis is the process of DNA replication in cell division that generates new diploid cells for development and replacement. Meiosis is DNA replication in the testis and ovary that results in the creation of haploid sperm and egg cells. The copy at one locus of a matched pair of chromosomes is inherited from the mother, and that of the other from the father. Each copy of a gene at a specific locus is called an allele. An organism that carries two unaltered, normal alleles is wild type. An altered allele is mutant. When a specific allele at a particular genetic locus is both necessary and sufficient for a trait to be expressed, given an otherwise normal genetic and environmental background, the trait (not gene) is said to be inherited in a mendelian fashion. Authentic mendelian traits are dominant if detectable in the heterozygote with a single copy of the allele, and recessive if two copies of the allele in the homozygote are needed for detection. Alleles at the level of the genotype (i.e. DNA sequence) are codominant, since both may be discerned unambiguously without reference to an expressed trait. In some conditions the heterozygote may have an intermediate phenotype, which is then referred to as semidominant. Roughly 10 000 pathologic and nonpathologic human mendelian characters, each with a six-digit call number, are recognized and cataloged in Online Mendelian Inheritance in Man (OMIM), with weekly updates on the Internet (http://www3.ncbi.nlm.nih.gov/Omim).

Mendelian traits are inherited in patterns (e.g. autosomal dominant) that may often represent more of an informed guess than an actual genetic mechanism. An outwardly identical trait may be caused by mutations in different genes (locus heterogeneity), or by distinct mutations in the same gene (allelic heterogeneity). Furthermore, different mutations in the same gene may give rise to apparently unrelated phenotypes. A basic mendelian pattern may be disguised by pleiotropic alleles (widespread and divergent effects of the genotype), the presence of phenocopies (phenotypes produced by environmental factors and masquerading as genetic traits), incomplete penetrance (the probability that an individual who has the genotype manifests the phenotype), and variable expressivity (the genotype gives rise to different phenotypes in related individuals). For a trait with high penetrance and variable expressivity, each affected individual manifests the genotype, but in different ways. A trait with reduced penetrance and limited expressivity is identical in all affected individuals, but some individuals who have the genotype may show no sign of the trait. Since the human genome is complex and outbred, and because environmental factors vary enormously between individuals, truly mendelian single-gene traits are the exception rather than the rule. Mutant alleles at several (oligogenic inheritance) or many (polygenic inheritance) loci, with greater or lesser contributions from genetic interactions (epistasis) and environmental factors (multifactorial inheritance), are required to account for most human characteristics.

DNA STRUCTURE, REPLICATION, AND REPAIR

Although Avery had established DNA as the carrier of genetic information by 1944, its structure was not elucidated until 1952. A further 10 years elapsed before the molecular mechanisms that underlie DNA self-replication and protein assembly were correlated with its structure. Both DNA and the family of RNAs are composed of linked sequences of nucleotides, each consisting of a nitrogenous base, a five-carbon sugar (pentose), and a phosphate group. Two classes of base are used: pyrimidines [cytosine (C), thymine (T) in DNA, and uracil (U), which substitutes for T in RNA] and purines [adenine (A) and guanine (G)] (Fig. 4.1). Covalent addition of a pentose to N_1 of a pyrimidine or N_9 of a purine creates the nucleosides (one base plus one sugar) cytidine, thymidine, uridine, adenosine, and guanosine. The difference between ribose (RNA) and deoxyribose (DNA) is the hydroxyl group at the 2´ position of the sugar (Chapter 1). A phosphate group is added to the 5´ position to form the cytidylic (C), thymidylic (T), uridylic (U), adenylic (A), and guanylic (G) acid nucleotides (one nucleoside plus one, two, or three phosphate groups), which constitute the basic repeat units of nucleic acids.

Nucleotides that form the nucleic acid chain are connected by a covalent phosphodiester bond between the 5´ and 3´ positions of adjacent sugar rings. Each nucleic acid chain begins with a free 5´ phosphate, and terminates with a free hydroxy group at the 3´ position. The designations 5´ (upstream) and 3´ (downstream) serve as a shorthand to orient relative position along the DNA and RNA linear sequence. Double-stranded DNA takes the shape of a helix of two polynucleotide chains. The abundant phosphate groups confer a net negative charge to the outside of the nucleic acid helix. Like the rungs of a ladder, the bases point inward and are enjoined such that the distance between the two phosphorylated sugar backbones remains constant. This results from the regular pairing of one purine with one pyrimidine, either A with T bound by two hydrogen bonds, or G with C linked by three hydrogen bonds. The capacity of noncovalent hydrogen bonds to break and reform under physiologic conditions is of crucial importance in nucleic acid function

The A–T and G–C dyads are referred to as base pairs (bps), and represent the basic unit of distance from point-to-point along the nucleic acid molecule [e.g. a kilobase (kb) equals 10^3 bps, a megabase (Mb) equals 10^6 bps]. Since a given purine only binds with a specific pyrimidine, one strand of DNA is complementary to the other, which permits reproduction of DNA, with one strand serving as a template for synthesis of its companion. Partner strands of the helix are oriented in an antiparallel direction, with the sense strand running from 5´ to 3´, and the complementary antisense strand from 3´ to 5´. Synthesis of new DNA molecules during replication proceeds in the 5´ to 3´ direction. The enzyme helicase first unwinds the double strand, which allows each single strand to serve as a template for the synthesis of an identical daughter strand catalyzed by DNA polymerase.

Each of the daughter DNA duplexes contains one parental strand and one newly synthesized strand. As the two parental strands are antiparallel in orientation only, the leading strand is continuously synthesized 5´ to 3´ from the origin of replication. The second lagging strand is assembled in small 5´ to 3´ fragments, which are covalently joined by DNA ligase. About 8 hours is required to complete the process of DNA replication in cultured human cells. Most errors that occur during DNA replication are corrected by DNA repair enzymes (glycosylase, phosphodiesterase, helicase), which continuously scan the DNA sequence to detect and replace damaged nucleotides. Two major repair pathways, single-base excision and polynucleotide excision (the latter for larger lesions up to 30bp), recognize and remove most changes in the DNA duplex. Alterations of fewer than 20bp/year arise in a mammalian germline cell with a genome size over 3000Mb.

RNA STRUCTURE, TRANSCRIPTION, TRANSCRIPTIONAL REGULATION, TRANSLATION, AND THE GENETIC CODE

The replacement of T with U and ribose for deoxyribose makes RNA chemically less stable than DNA. Its single-stranded polynucleotide chain is able to adopt secondary structures of functional significance. Three kinds of RNA, each synthesized by a different RNA polymerase, are present in the cell. The first step by which the genetic information encoded by DNA is converted to protein assembly is transcription, whereby a single strand of messenger RNA (mRNA) is assembled from 5´ to 3´ in the cell nucleus, to be identical in sequence with its sense DNA strand (Fig. 4.2).

In the subsequent step in the cytoplasm, translation, mRNA serves as a template for the synthesis of amino acids into proteins. Most (up to 99%) RNA in the cell is ribosomal (or rRNA), which does not code for proteins. Ribosomes that comprise rRNA and specific protein constituents are the active sites of translation, and contain binding sites for the interacting molecules necessary for initiation, elongation, and termination of peptide chains. Twenty distinct transfer RNA (tRNA) molecules in cloverleaf conformations participate in

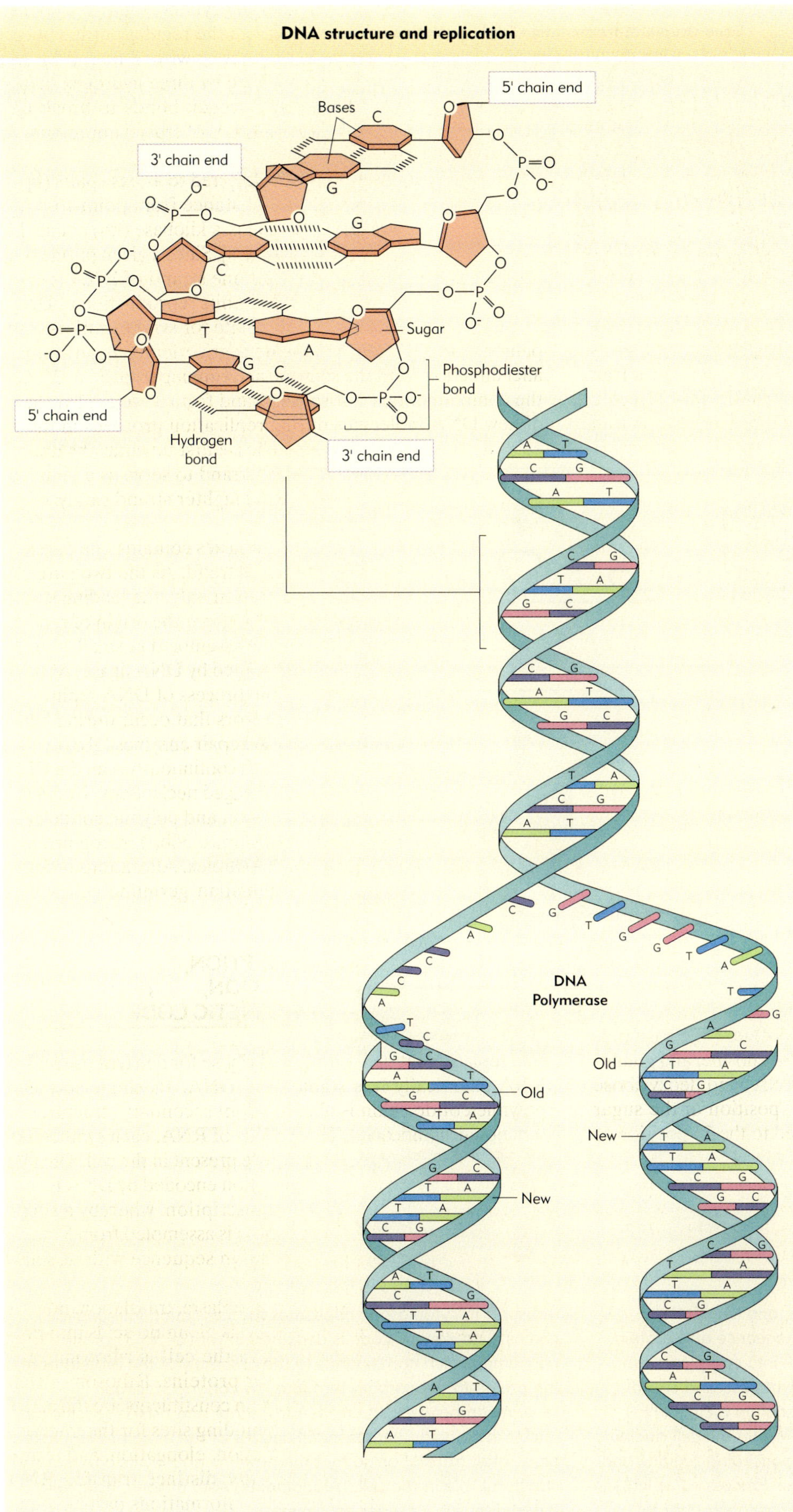

Figure 4.1 DNA structure and replication. The DNA strands in the 'double helix' consist of a deoxyribose sugar backbone held together by phosphodiester bonds. The two chains, which run in opposite (antiparallel) directions, are linked by either two (A–T) or three (G–C) hydrogen bonds between complementary purine and pyrimidine base pairs. During replication the strands unwind and separate such that each is able to serve as a template for the synthesis of a new complementary, antiparallel daughter strand using DNA polymerase. Each daughter duplex contains one parental and one new DNA strand that is identical in sequence and structure to the parental duplex.

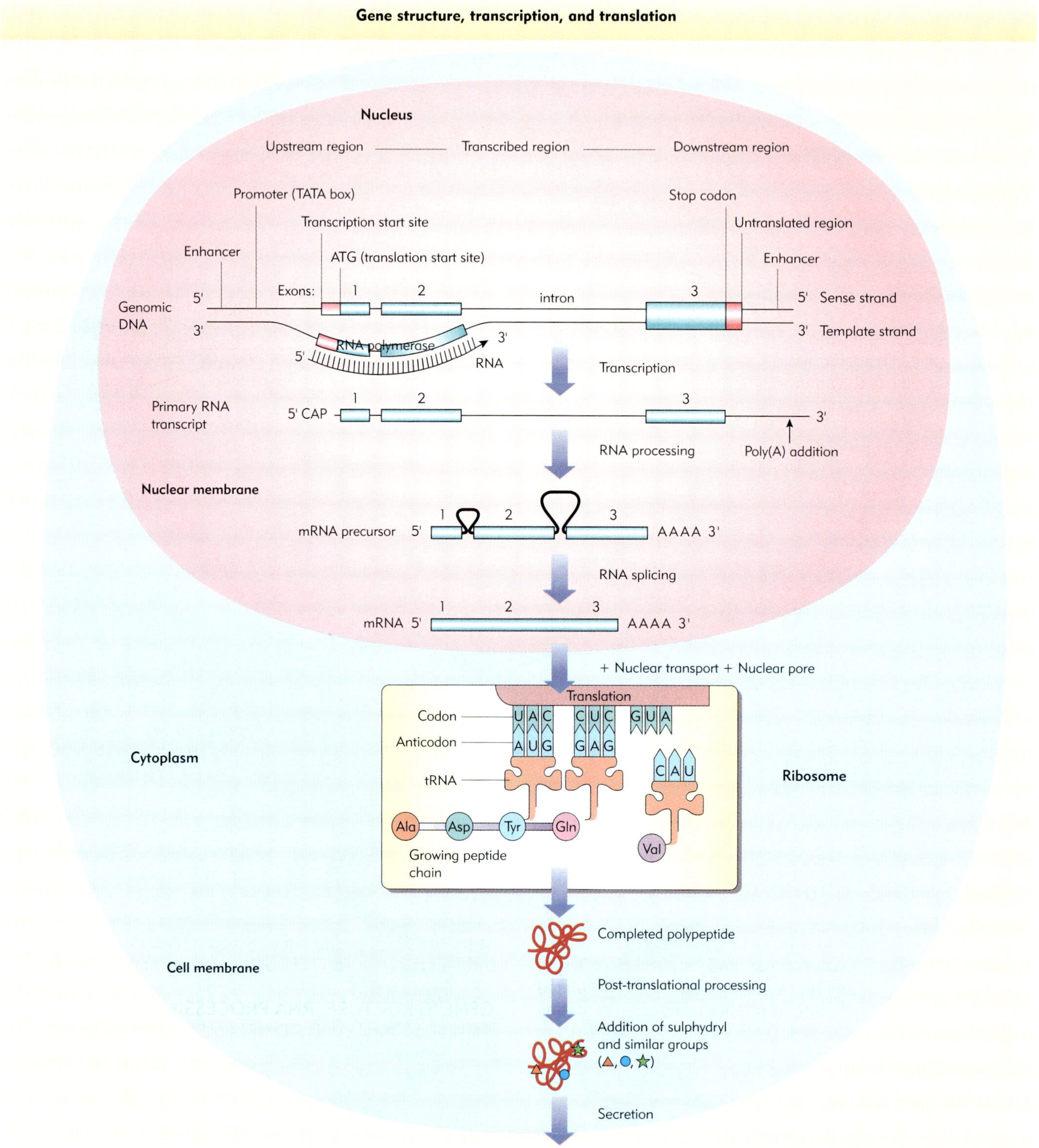

Gene structure, transcription, and translation

Figure 4.2 Gene structure, transcription, and translation. Information transfer between nucleotide sequence and protein synthesis begins with transcription of DNA into complementary mRNA. This step is catalyzed by RNA polymerase and coordinated by a variety of *cis*- and *trans*-acting transcription factors (TFs), which include enhancers and promoters. Within the cell nucleus, the mRNA transcript is edited to remove noncoding regions and splice exon segments (1–3 above) together. Processing of RNA is completed with 5´-capping and 3´-polyadenylation prior to transport to cytoplasmic ribosomes for translation into peptide chains. The genetic code is deciphered from 5´ to 3´ at the ribosome, which corresponds to the assembly of the protein from the amino to the carboxy terminus, by codon–anticodon recognition between the mRNA transcript and tRNAs specific for each amino acid. Further modifications of the gene product take place after translation so that the protein can play its enzymatic or structural role in the cell. (Ala, alanine; Asp, aspartic acid; Gln, glutamine; Tyr, tyrosine; Val, valine.)

translation by recognition and aminoacyl-tRNA synthetase-mediated covalent binding of a specific amino acid to an acceptor arm. Codons are mRNA triplets, each of which encodes a single amino acid (Fig. 4.3).

Of the 64 possible codons (4^3 combinations of nucleotides), 20 amino acids are designated. Thus, the genetic code is degenerate or redundant (i.e. several different codons may designate the same amino acid). A loop within another arm of each tRNA carries an anticodon nucleotide triplet complementary to an mRNA codon, which assures an orderly assembly of the nascent polypeptide chain in procession from the amino terminus to the carboxy terminus of the peptide corresponding to the 5´ to 3´ orientation of the DNA sequence. Successive amino acids are incorporated in the growing chain by peptide bonds created by a condensation reaction between the amino group of the incoming amino acid and the carboxyl group of the preceding amino acid (Chapter 1). Translation is begun at the initiation codon AUG, which encodes the amino acid methionine. Three codons (UAA, UAG, UGA) do not signify an amino acid, but are 'nonsense codons' that terminate translation at the 3´ end of the open reading frame. As a result of the triplet code, each stretch of DNA and corresponding transcribed RNA contain three potential translation frames. The open reading frame is that string of codons flanked on the 5´ side by an initiation codon, and on the 3´ side by a termination codon. It is therefore possible to infer DNA or RNA sequence one from the other, if either is known. Peptide translation products commonly undergo a variety of post-translational modifications that involve chemical (e.g. hydroxylation, phosphorylation) and side-chain (e.g. glycosylation) alterations, as well as cleavage of precursors to give mature proteins.

For biochemical purposes, a gene is defined as a segment of DNA responsible for the production of one or more related polypetide chains or structural RNA molecules. The gene or, more accurately, the transcription unit is a sequence of DNA that can be transcribed into a single mRNA, tRNA, or rRNA using a specific RNA polymerase. Included in the transcription unit are regions that precede (proximal promoter) and follow (distal terminator) the coding sequence. Upstream promoter sequences (e.g. a TATA box 25bp 5´ from a transcriptional start site) serve to bind various transcription factors (TFs), positioning and activating RNA polymerase to begin transcription. The TFs are referred to as *trans*-acting because they are synthesized by remotely located genes, and migrate to their specific *cis*-acting sites of action. Genes with expression regulated by external factors, including hormones or internal signaling molecules [e.g. cyclic adenosine monophosphate (cAMP)], are preceded by response elements capable of binding the signaling factor. Transcription is further stimulated by *cis*-acting elements (enhancers) for sequence-specific DNA-binding proteins that function independently of orientation and proximity to the coding sequence, and are responsible for tissue-specific and developmental regulation of the 30,000 genes per cell, which are differentially expressed along 40Mb of sequence.

Activation of gene expression is complex, and involves the state of DNA methylation (which represses transcription), modification of chromatin-associated histone proteins, and the state and stage of the cell in its cycle. The heteronuclear RNA transcript is processed shortly after transcription to mRNA with the addition of 5´ cap (guanosine), a substrate for methylation that contributes to the efficiency of mRNA transport to the cytoplasm, and splicing to facilitate translation. Most genes have 5´

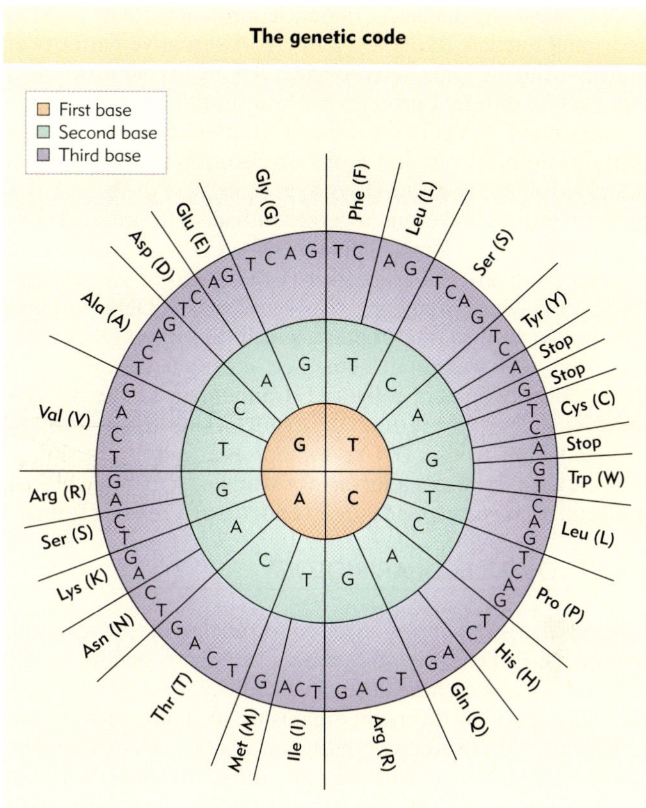

Figure 4.3 The genetic code. Codons composed of three nucleotides are translated into amino acids according to the rules shown, with the first, second, and third positions chosen from the inner to outermost circles, respectively. (Arg, arginine; Asn, asparagine; Cys, cysteine; Glu, glutamic acid; Gly, glycine; His, histidine; Ile, isoleucine; Lys, lysine; Met, methionine; Phe, phenylalanine; Pro, proline; Ser, serine; Thr, threonine; Trp, tryptophan.)

leader and 3´ trailer untranslated sequences added on after initiation of transcription. At the 3´ terminus, an untranslated poly(A) tail of 150–200 A nucleotides is added after an endonucleic cleavage of about 20 bases 3´ to an AAUAAA RNA sequence. The poly(A) tail may also stabilize the mRNA transcript in the cytoplasm, and assist transport and translation.

GENE STRUCTURE, RNA PROCESSING, AND GENOMIC AND COMPLEMENTARY DNA

The majority of mRNA transcripts are interrupted by large segments of intervening sequences, or introns, which are eventually edited out to leave only the coding sequences or exons linked together. Noncoding intron sequences, which contain defective copies of functional genes (pseudogenes and gene fragments) and repetitive noncoding DNA, are highly polymorphic since they are not subject to the same selective pressure as exons. On average, a polymorphic allele is detected once in 10^3bp of human exon sequence, and intron polymorphisms appear once in 10^2bp. The fuctional roles of introns are unclear, but it is speculated that they may act as TF binding sites and regions of spontaneous recombination. Splicing occurs at consensus sequences of splice donor and acceptor junctions, and results in the formation of a spliceosome, a large particulate complex made up of nuclear ribonucleoprotein particles (RNPs) and small nuclear RNPs, U1 and U2. Alternative patterns of splicing from the same heteronuclear RNA can lead to mRNAs that encode different proteins by exon shuffling.

Genomic DNA is DNA isolated from eukaryotic cells that contains both introns and exons. In addition to the elements described above, genomic DNA represents all of the boundaries between introns and exons, together with all of the internal non-coding sequences. Complementary DNA (cDNA) is synthesized *in vitro* from mRNA transcripts isolated from tissues that express the genes of interest. The synthesis of cDNA employs the enzyme reverse transcriptase, which (like other DNA polymerases) uses a template sequence, a primer {usually oligo deoxy-thymidylic acid [oligo(dT)] annealing to the mRNA poly(A) tail}, and the four deoxynucleotide tri-phosphates (dNTPs). Unlike other DNA polymerases, reverse transcriptase is able to use RNA as a template for synthesis, creating a cDNA molecule that corresponds to the edited open reading frame.

IN VITRO MOLECULAR BIOLOGY

The cellular mechanisms required for nucleotide segregation, lengthwise and end-to-end cleavage, sorting, recognition, editing, and replication have been elucidated by virtue of their conservation in widely divergent organisms, including prokaryotes (bacteria) and eukaryotes (yeast, mammalian cells). To detect variations in DNA sequence directly, and to correlate them with variations between cells, individuals, families, and species, tools were needed to reprise these processes *in vitro*. A revolution in human biology was heralded by the discovery and availability of restriction endonucleases (1962), DNA ligases (1967), vectors (1973), DNA sequencing (1977), and the polymerase chain reaction (PCR) (1984).

Chromosome sorting, nucleotide isolation, and cleavage

The complement of human chromosomes consists of 22 homologous pairs of autosomes numbered by convention from the largest (1) to the smallest (22), and one pair of sex chromosomes. Together, the human genome consists of 3×10exp9 base pairs (Fig. 4.4). During the mitotic interphase, chromosomes are decondensed and invisible to light microscopy. Use of agents such as colchicine to halt the cell cycle at metaphase permits the visualization of chromosomes, each of which reveals unique banding patterns when stained with appropriate reagents. Together with size and position of the centromere, chromosome banding enables accurate differentiation of the autosomes. The representation of the entire set of banded chromosomes is a karyogram. Alterations of chromosomal structure that arise during meiotic cross-over may result in duplications, deletions, or translocations up to 4Mb, which are apparent on the karyogram. These and other large abnormalities of genetic material [aberrations in chromosomal number (e.g. triploidy) or structure (e.g. chromosome rings, inversions)], when associated with specific clinical syndromes, may provide important clues to the sublocalization of genes.

The extraction of genomic DNA of high molecular weight from cells is incredibly easy. If of sufficient molecular weight, the DNA may be spooled on to a glass rod. In fact, the main difficulty in working with genomic DNA from eukaryotic cells in bulk is its viscosity and susceptibility to shearing forces. Much more challenging is the isolation of RNA. Ubiquitous tissue ribonucleases are amazingly hardy, and can even survive autoclaving.

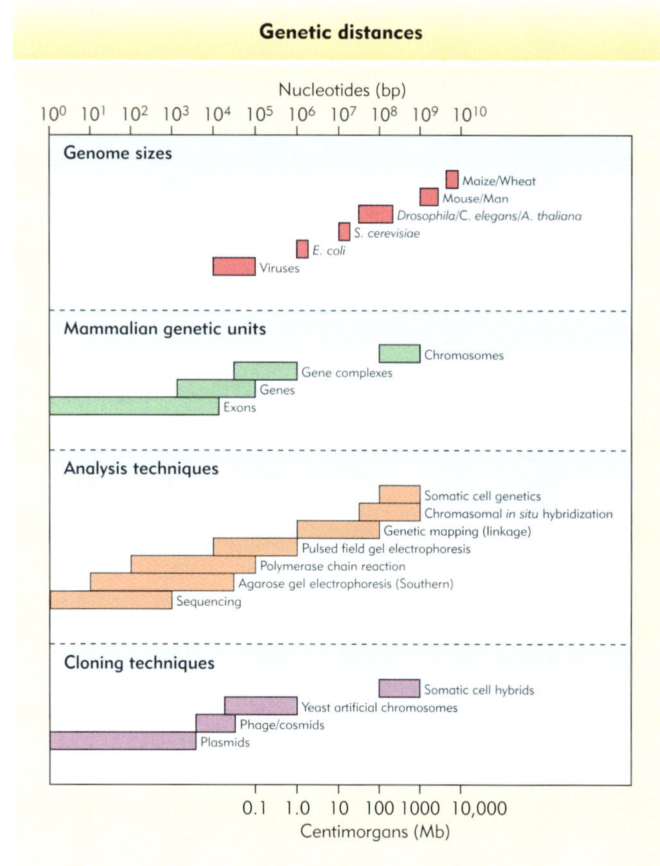

Figure 4.4 Genetic distances. (*E. coli*, *Escherichia coli*; *S. cerevisiae*, *Saccharomyces cerevisiae*; *C. elegans*, *Caenorhabditis elegans*; *A. thaliana*, *Arabidopsis thaliana*.)

Endonucleases are enzymes that cleave phosphodiester bonds within a nucleic acid chain. Restriction enzymes are a class of endonucleases that recognize short sequences of double-stranded DNA and cleave at or near a recognition sequence (Fig. 4.5). Selection from a catalog of restriction endonucleases, each with known recognition-specific sequences, enables segregation of DNA fragments by size based on the estimated frequency of the recognition site. Smaller fragments are generated by digestion with frequent cutters, whereas larger fragments are produced by rare cutters with longer and less frequently encountered recognition sites. The resultant fragments may have either blunt or sticky ends – the overhangs of the latter are especially useful for ligation of DNA from dissimilar sources. The number and arrangement of restriction sites can be assembled into a restriction map of a particular DNA sequence or even a whole genome.

Detection of restriction fragment length polymorphisms (RFLPs) was the first technique developed that used DNA sequence as a marker for the presence of mutant alleles in adjacent genes. Usually disclosed by Southern blotting (see below), an RFLP is a specific DNA fragment resulting from restriction endonuclease digestion of DNA, which differs in length between two alleles of the same gene in an individual, or between two individuals. The difference resides in the presence or absence of the specific cleavage site required by the enzyme, which may depend on a single bp change. In the presence of the site, two smaller fragments are generated after digestion. In its absence, only a single larger fragment results. The polymorphism is represented by the lengths of the fragments, which are easily measured.

Nucleotide separation

Fragments of DNA that arise from restriction endonuclease digestion are separated according to size on agarose or polyacrylamide gels. As a result of their phosphate groups, DNA fragments are negatively charged, and are therefore repelled from the negative electrode (cathode) toward the positive electrode (anode) as they sieve through a porous gel. Smaller fragments move faster. Agarose gel can separate DNA fragments that range in size from 100bp to 25kb. Pulse-field gel electrophoresis enables separation of very large fragments of DNA up to several Mbs using alternating current in two different directions.

Nucleotide visualization

Ethidium bromide binds DNA by intercalating between bps, which causes the DNA helix to partially unwind. Deoxyribonucleic acid bands in electrophoresis gels stained with ethidium are fluorescent upon exposure to ultraviolet light. Silver staining for small fragments in polyacrylamide gels and radiolabeling fragments prior to gel separation are alternative strategies for tracking the presence of a DNA sequence of interest. While these approaches can indicate the presence of DNA, none can disclose the bp composition of the DNA fragment that has been isolated. For this, probe-based tactics are necessary.

Nucleotide probes

A probe is any single-stranded nucleic acid that can be labeled with a marker, enabling identification and quantification, and hybridized (bound) to another nucleic acid on the basis of base complementarity. Labeled nucleic acid probes allow investigators to interrogate genetic material in solution, fixed on a filter, separated in an electrophoretic gel or on a histologic section. Nucleic acid probes can be used to detect a single nucleotide species from thousands of messages of varying abundance, and are easily prepared, stored, and handled. Such DNA probes may be 15–50bp oligonucleotides synthesized on the basis of prior knowledge of the DNA target, PCR (see below) products (<5kb), or full-length genomic or cDNA inserts (0.1–300kb) cloned from libraries and isolated by cell-based cloning (see below). When no DNA sequence is available, but the protein sequence is known, the DNA sequence can be deduced from the genetic code, and an array of degenerate synthetic oligomer nucleotides synthesized to represent all possible codon combinations. A variety of methods (nick translation, kinasing, random primer, RNA transcription) have been devised to incorporate nucleotide precursors with radionuclide (^{32}P, ^{3}H, or ^{35}S) tags. After hybridization to radiolabeled probes and washing, the filter is exposed to a film with autoradiographic emulsion. The resultant autoradiograph reveals the pattern of hybridization. Nonradioactive methods use nonisotopic adducts (biotin-labeled probes incubated with colorimetric streptavidin or fluorescent dyes).

In vitro hybridization, and Southern, Northern, and Western blotting

Sequences of DNA may be specifically identified by binding or molecular hybridization to a labeled, single-strand nucleotide of known composition. Hybridization is the formation of a duplex between two complementary nucleotide sequences. All nucleotide hybridization tests are based on the fact that two antiparallel, single-stranded nucleic acid molecules recognize one another and bind on the basis of hydrogen bonding (e.g. DNA:DNA, DNA:RNA, and RNA:RNA). The probability of hybridization depends on the free energy available for the formation of a particular structure, and is the sum of the individual base-pairing reactions involved. The total number of complementary bases in the two sequences is a major factor in determining the ability to form a stable hybrid, but the bp composition also plays a role. Multiple G–C pairings with three hydrogen bonds form a more stable duplex than A–T-rich (with two hydrogen bonds) structures.

The interaction between duplex strands of nucleic acid is strongly temperature dependent. Duplex stability is measured by the melting temperature, defined as the temperature that

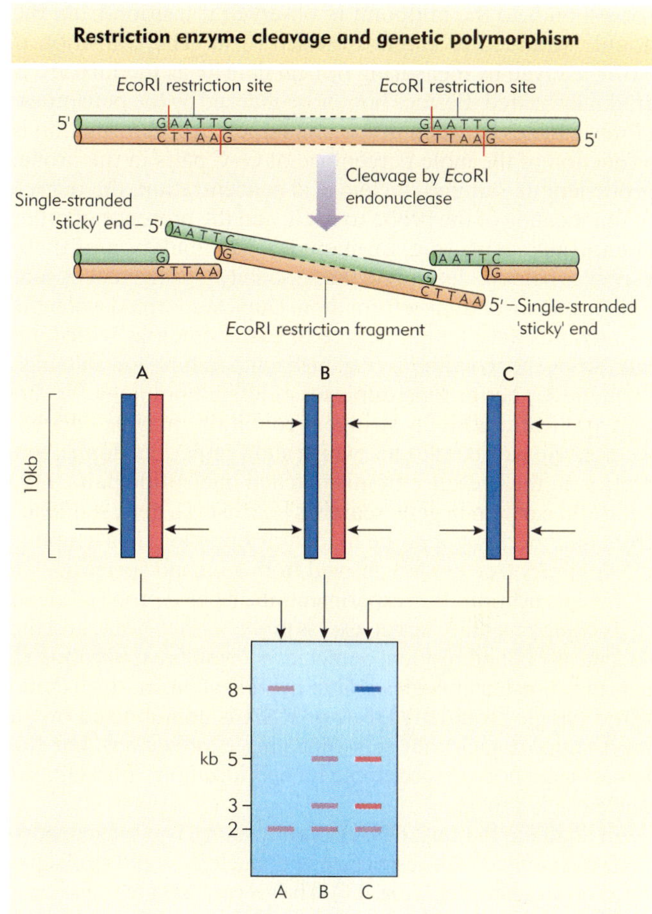

Figure 4.5 Restriction enzyme cleavage and genetic polymorphism. A molecule of DNA contains many short nucleotide sequences recognized by restriction endonucleases that bind and cut the DNA duplex at that site (e.g. the enzyme EcoRI cleaves wherever it encounters the sequence GAATTC, to leave staggered 'sticky' ends). Presence or absence of the recognition site can be inferred by the size of fragments separated by gel electrophoresis after enzymatic digestion. Unambiguous ordering of fragment sizes is used to discriminate chromosomal regions inherited from either parent (i.e. genetic 'markers'). In the example shown, a single digest of a 10kb fragment is sufficient to detect each homozygote (A and B) from the heterozygote in which all four possible configurations are represented.

corresponds to the midpoint in observed transition from the double-stranded to single-stranded form. The transition is easily assayed by measuring optical density as the mixture is gradually heated. Besides homology indexed by the percentage of mismatches between probe and target, hybrid formation is a function of the mole percentage of G–C pairs in the probe, probe length, salt and nucleic acid concentration, the degree of reannealing of the probe to itself, and the presence of other denaturing agents (e.g. formamide). Manipulation of these variables helps to determine the specificity (stringency) of conditions that favor duplex formation. Duplexes formed when the two strands have a high degree of base homology withstand high stringency conditions (e.g. high temperature, low salt, high formamide) better than duplexes of lesser homology. In certain applications highly stringent conditions may be desired, whereas relaxed conditions, which allow imperfect duplex formation in the presence of mismatched nucleotide pairs, may be useful early on in gene searches [e.g. using a gene sequence from one species as a probe to identify homologs in a genomic DNA library (see below) derived from a second species].

In most hybridization experiments the labeled probe is bound to its complementary target, excess probe washed away, and the specifically bound residual detected. A common application of hybridization technologies is filter hybridization, in which denatured (single-stranded) DNA or RNA is immobilized on an inert support such that self-annealing is prevented, but the bound sequences are accessible for hybridization with a labeled nucleic acid probe.

In Southern blotting, DNA from any source is extracted, purified, fragmented with restriction endonucleases, and size-separated on an agarose gel (Fig. 4.6). The gel contents are transferred or 'blotted' onto a solid support nitrocellulose or nylon filter. The flow of buffer by capillary action causes denatured DNA fragments to pass out of the gel onto the filter paper, with preservation of their relative positions. The DNA is hybridized with a complementary, labeled, single-stranded DNA nucleic acid probe and the nonspecifically bound excess probe is discarded. Thus, a restriction map of a particular DNA sequence is generated by digestion with a panel of restriction enzymes. Deoxyribonucleic acid fingerprinting using multilocus patterns that represent the summed contribution of two alleles at many variable loci throughout the genome enables unequivocal distinction between any two individuals who are not identical twins.

Laser scanning for evidence of hybridization of sample cDNAa to oligonucleotide probes representing thousands of genes fixed to glass chip microarrays enables simultaneous screening of thousands of alleles. This technology potentially identifies any genotype of interest to perioperative caregivers within several hours at low cost. Adaptation of these methods to ascertain patterns of gene expression by organ, cell, subcellular structure, or pathologic process yields insights into the components of complex events.

Northern blotting is the RNA counterpart of Southern blotting, and may be useful for the estimation of the steady-state level of specific mRNA transcription, or expression pattern, at the time of extraction from the tissue. It is also valuable in the detection of transcripts of differing size (alternate splice variants), and may indicate the presence of promoters, splice sites, or untranslated segments not apparent on Southern blotting of genomic DNA. Western blotting employs the same matrix and detection formats, but the targets are proteins and the labeled probes are antibodies.

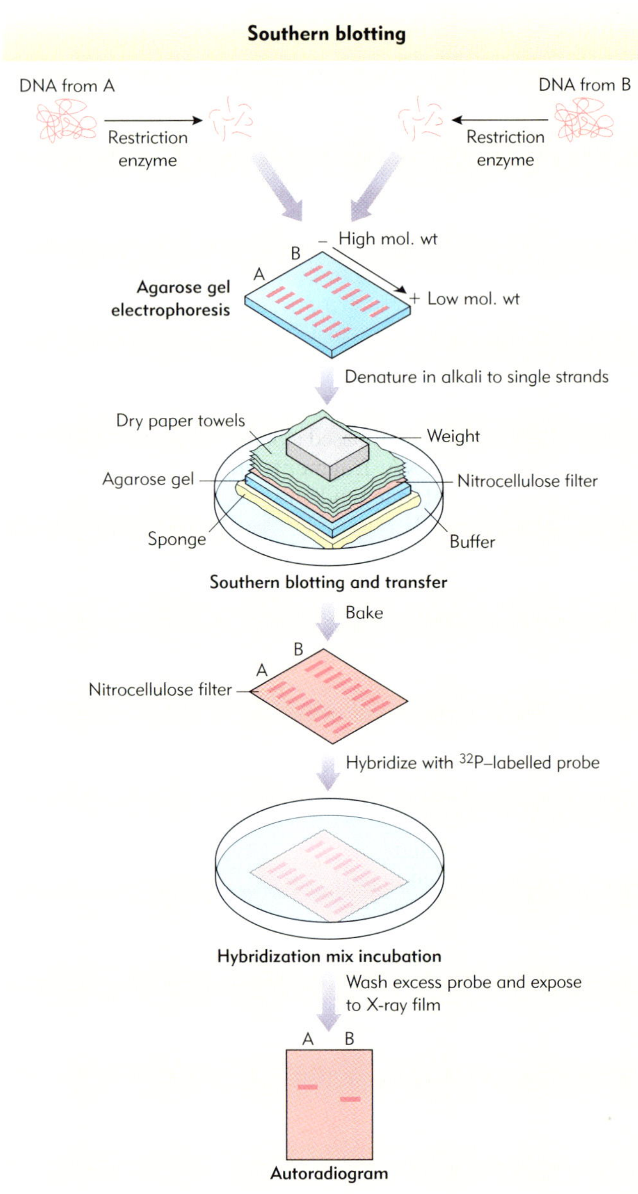

Figure 4.6 Southern blotting. Deoxyribnucleic acid samples are digested by a restriction endonuclease and fractionated by size on agarose gel by electrophoresis. The positions of DNA fragments complementary to the probe are detected as bands on the developed autoradiogram.

In situ hybridization

In situ hybridization, the technique of hybridization applied to cells, reveals the tissue or cellular distribution of nucleic acid sequences. Both the cellular localization of a specific DNA or RNA sequence (tissue *in situ* hybridization) and the chromosomal assignment (chromosomal *in situ* hybridization) of a probe can be established. Other than choosing between DNA and RNA targets, differences between *in situ* hybridization protocols center on maintaining tissue morphology while rendering the tissue permeable to the probe without losing the target. The sensitivity of *in situ* hybridization relies on the fraction of target in the tissue that is accessible for hybridization, the mass of probe relative to the target (saturation), and the specific activity of the probe. Noise in the hybridization reaction correlates with the extent to which the probe is able to bind non-specifically to the background. The specificity of hybridization is controlled by the sequence and stringency conditions, and can be measured using other probes [e.g. those that bind to the poly(A) tails of most mRNA species] as controls.

Nucleotide propagation: cell-based cloning, nucleotide libraries

Since a particular fragment of DNA may represent only a small fraction of the DNA in a cell, techniques are required to selectively amplify and purify the sequence of interest before its structure and function can be investigated (i.e. by sequencing or *in vitro* expression). Cell-based cloning is an *in vivo* technique in which foreign DNA fragments are attached to DNA sequences capable of independent replication, which are then propagated in suitable host cells. Recombinant DNA refers to novel hybrid DNA molecules constructed from DNA sources that cannot naturally occur. Vectors are DNA molecules capable of continuing a usual life cycle after insertion of foreign DNA. A vector with a foreign recombinant DNA insert capable of replication in bacteria represents a recombinant DNA clone. Cloning of recombinant DNA in bacteria allows the production of large amounts of the inserted fragment. The common property of all vectors is a site at which foreign DNA can be inserted without disrupting function. Plasmid vectors are autonomous circular DNAs capable of self-replication without incorporation into host-cell chromosomes. Most plasmid inserts are limited in size, usually <5kb (Fig. 4.7). Phages are viruses that infect bacteria and, unlike plasmids, are capable of extracellular existence. Up to 23kb DNA sequences can be stably packaged in phage particles. Cosmid vectors are plasmids with some phage sequences. Perpetuated in bacteria as plasmids, but retrieved by packaging *in vitro* into phages, cosmids carry inserts up to 45kb in length.

The ends of the DNA insert, whether cDNA or genomic DNA fragments, must be engineered to link with the vector at a specific locus. Any DNA fragment can be successfully cloned by generating sequences of the foreign DNA that are complementary to sequences of the vector and then selecting a unique restriction site in the vector to be used as the cloning site. The ends of the insert sequence are ligated to the complementary vector ends with DNA ligase. Often the restriction site is within a marker gene in the vector, so that interruption of the gene by the DNA insert can be used to select appropriate clones. If the interrupted gene confers antibiotic resistance (e.g. to ampicillin), the recombinant clones will be sensitive to the antibiotic. In other systems, inserts interrupt the β-galactosidase gene required to metabolize lactose. Recombinant clones are unable to cleave an artificial substrate (X-gal). Wild-type clones that lack the recombinant DNA inserts produce a blue color, while recombinant clones do not.

The recombinant plasmid molecule that consists of foreign DNA and vector-specific sequence is introduced into bacterial host cells, usually a strain of *Escherichia coli*, by the process of transformation. The host bacteria are made competent by pretreatment with calcium chloride, and exposed to heat in the presence of the plasmid. While only a small percentage of the competent cells take up foreign DNA, they can be selected and replicated many times. The transformed bacterial colonies are selected in antibiotic-containing media, and undergo secondary expansion to scale up large yields of cell clones, each with the desired insert. When the foreign DNA is ligated into phage DNA, the recombinant DNA is first packaged into the phage, which is allowed to infect the bacteria.

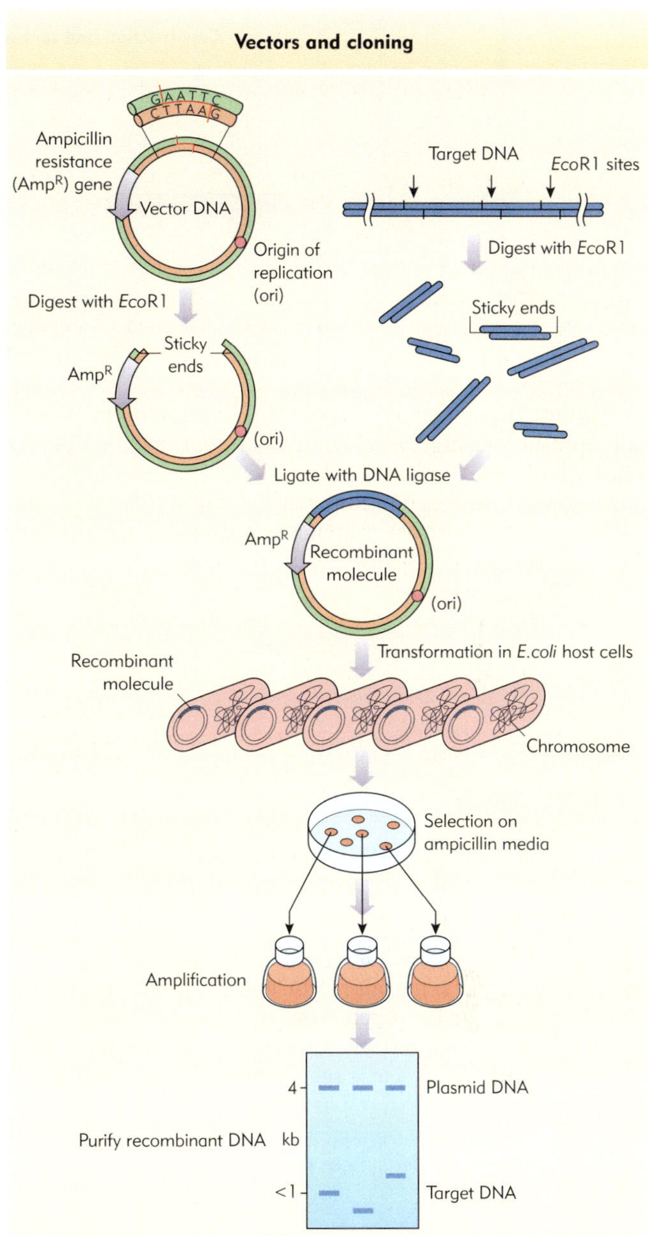

Figure 4.7 Vectors and cell-based cloning. Multiple copies of a DNA fragment of interest can be created by cell-based cloning. To clone DNA, a circular plasmid vector is linearized (cut) with a restriction endonuclease, to leave the vector and insert with compatible ends for ligation. The plasmids, which carry sequences for replication origin (ori) and antibiotic resistance (Amp^R), are introduced into *E. coli* host cells by transformation and replicate as drug-resistant elements. Bacterial colonies that contain the vector molecule are selected on antibiotic-containing media and amplified in culture. Bacterial and plasmid-vector DNA are discarded, and target recombinant DNA purified by electrophoresis.

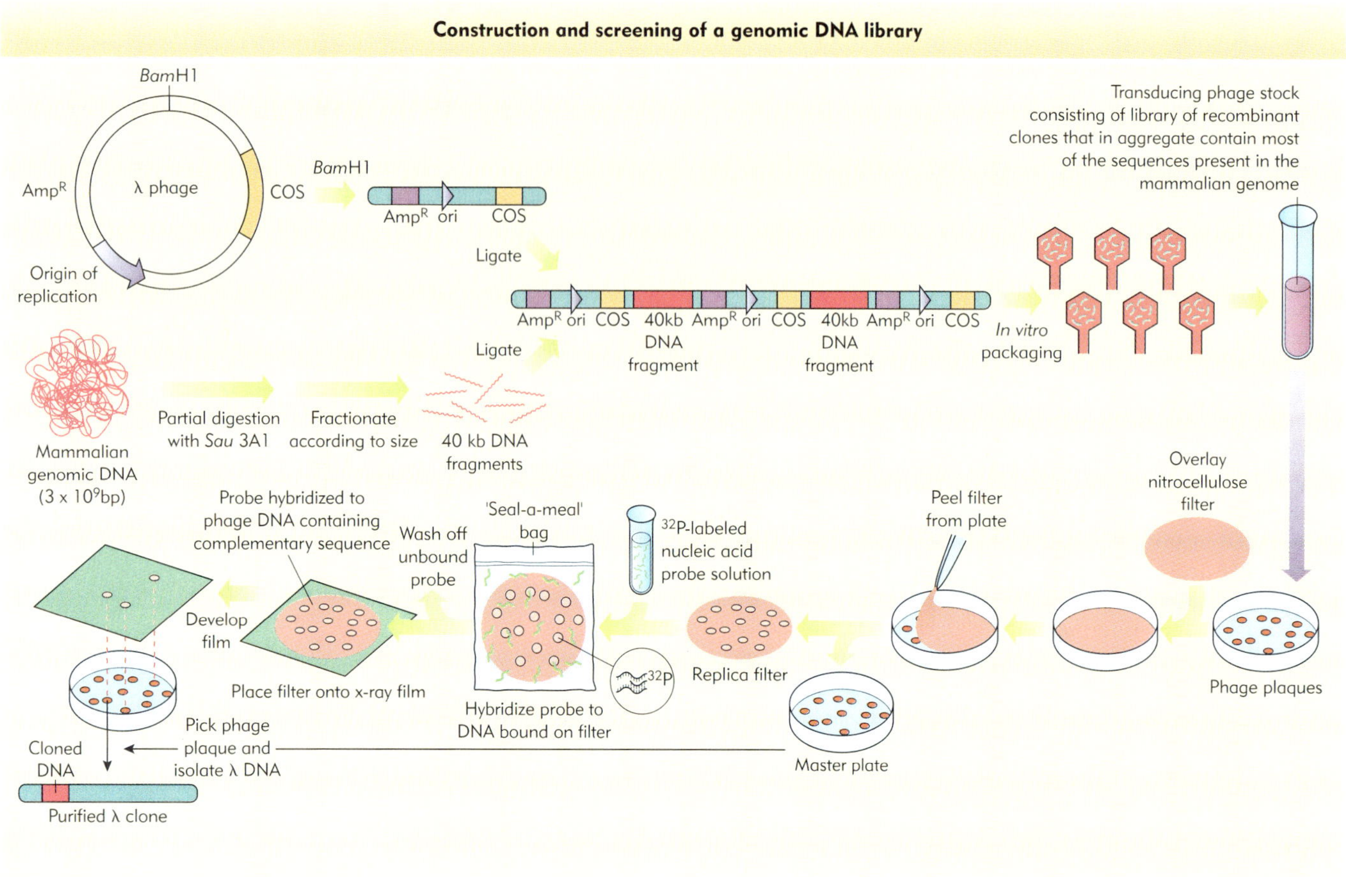

Figure 4.8 Construction and screening of a genomic DNA library. To construct a genomic DNA library, easily accessible cells (e.g. leukocytes) are harvested, lysed, and their DNA extracted. Partial digestion with a restriction endonuclease cleaves the DNA at a small number of available sites (with the pattern differing between molecules), which results in a near-random cleavage in aggregate. The series of overlapping restriction fragments that represents most of the sequences present in the genome is packaged in phage, and bacterial plaques are adsorbed from the master plate to overlaying filters. The filters are screened by hybridization to a radiolabeled probe and placed on radiographic film. Plaques that contain the recombinant fragment of interest appear as spots on the film, and can be picked from the master plate for amplification and purification. COS sequences are 12 bp sticky ends at either terminus of linear bacteriophage lamda (λ) DNA molecules

Preparation of the DNA insert and host vector with restriction endonucleases not only assures specific recombination, but permits later isolation and recovery of the cloned insert. To retrieve the cloned DNA the bacteria are lysed and the plasmid DNA extracted. Separation of the insert from its cloning vector is accomplished by restriction endonuclease digestion, followed by gel electrophoresis and visualization of the fragments with ethidium bromide staining. The gel band that contains the foreign DNA can be sliced out and eluted, and recombinant DNA molecules subcloned into a different vector molecule for structural or functional assays. Recently, new cloning vectors capable of accepting DNA inserts up to 3.0Mb have been developed. Bacterial artificial chromosomes were created to counteract the instability of large eukaryotic inserts (>300kb) cloned in bacterial hosts, but usually give only low yields of recombinant DNA. Cloning in yeast cells with the construction of yeast artificial chromosomes (YACs) enables the propagation of exogenous DNA fragments up to 2Mb, and has become essential for physical mapping of genomes. However, YACs are also hampered by relatively low yields of recombinant DNA.

Species-specific genomic DNA and tissue-specific cDNA fragments are available as libraries of clones supplied in plasmids, phage, and cosmids. Deoxyribonucleic acid sequences that are extremely rare in the starting population can be represented in a library of clones created by restriction endonuclease digestion, from which they can be selected and amplified. Hybridization is the most widely used method for screening a library to select individual clones of interest with DNA or RNA probes (Fig. 4.8). In colony hybridization with plasmid vectors or plaque hybridization with recombinant phage vectors, bacterial cells are used to propagate recombinants on an agar surface, which are transferred to a nitrocellulose or nylon membrane, denatured, and hybridized to a labeled probe. The position of positively hybridized probes identifies colonies that contain the cDNA sequence, which may be picked and expanded. Subsequent rounds of cloning and library rescreening (using one end of a newly identified clone to detect an overlapping clone) enables ever larger DNA fragments in the region of interest to be characterized by chromosome walking.

Interspecies somatic cell hybrids are created by radiation fragmentation of human cellular components. During fusion of rodent and human cells, hybrids that contain human, rodent, and recombinant human–rodent chromosomes are created. Hybrid cells randomly lose chromosomes in subsequent culture, which allows the selection of hybrid panels with one or a few remnant human chromosomes. Matching the presence or absence of a particular nucleic acid probe by hybridization on the panel with the presence or absence of known chromosome fragments leads to unambiguous identification of the chromosome that contains the gene from which the probe was derived.

Nucleotide propagation:cell-free cloning and the polymerase chain reaction

If the sequence of regions that flank both ends of a specific DNA fragment are known, it is possible to selectively amplify picogram (10^{-12}g) quantities of DNA using PCR. Defined as the *in vitro* enzymatic synthesis and amplification of specific DNA sequences, PCR is a simple and efficient technique to produce over 100 billion copies of a single molecule of DNA within several hours (Fig. 4.9). Its advantages are its capacity to use minute samples to produce a high yield of amplified target DNA, specificity of the reaction, flexibility of the methods, and rapidity and simplicity of the automated procedure. Owing to these attributes, PCR has been used to amplify degraded DNA successfully from Egyptian mummies, Neanderthal remains, and dyes used in Paleolithic cave art.

Major disadvantages compared with cell-based cloning include template contamination, the need for target-sequence information for primer assembly, short PCR product sizes (usually <3kb), and absence of proofreading mechanisms to correct copying errors. Since PCR may be successful in the presence of several DNA bases in the primer that are not complementary to the template DNA, it is possible to assemble amplified PCR fragments with modified restriction endonuclease recognition sites for use in subcloning, or to introduce site-directed mutations into amplified products of target DNA to investigate functional expression in host cells (see below). Knowledge of the intron–exon structure of a gene expressing pathogenic alleles allows exon-specific amplification by PCR using primers complementary to 5′ and 3′ boundary intron sequences. The resultant PCR products can then be analyzed for mutations by rapid screening methods or by direct sequencing. If primers are assembled to anneal with specific sequences that exhibit the pathogenic allele (allele-specific oligonucleotides) at the 3′ terminus of the primer, the presence of the mutant allele is inferred by the presence of the appropriately sized PCR product. Small deletions and insertions are readily detected by a change in the size of PCR products, or by a failure to produce any fragment if the primer is unable to anneal in the area of deletion.

DNA sequencing

The ultimate step in resolving the fine structure of DNA by direct sequencing was first attained in 1977. Subsequent refinements of the technique using novel cloning vectors and oligonucleotides led to the Sanger dideoxy sequencing method now in widespread use. The basic principle in sequencing methods is the assembly of a population of synthetic, single-stranded DNA molecules in which each base of a specimen is represented by DNA fragments of a length that conforms to the sample sequence that extends to that point,

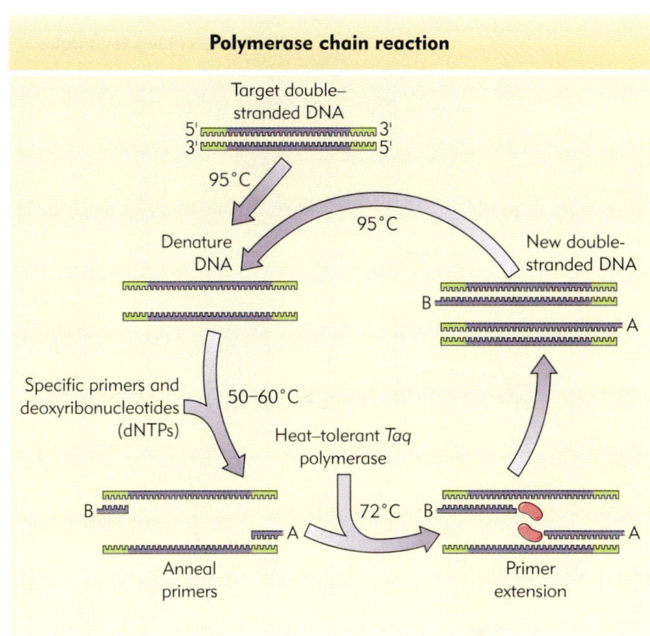

Figure 4.9 The polymerase chain reaction. In the first step of PCR, target double-stranded DNA is denatured at high temperature [e.g. 95°C (203°F)] for 1–2 minutes to give single-stranded DNA (denaturation step). Next, 20–30bp oligonucleotide primers specific for the flanking regions on opposite strands are annealed to the denatured DNA (annealing step) at 50–70°C (122–158°F). The primers are designed to be complementary to the opposite strands of DNA and not to one another, and bind at the 5′ ends of the cDNAs in a 5′ to 3′ orientation. Next, a heat-tolerant DNA polymerase uses the oligonucleotides as primers to synthesize cDNA with both strands as templates (primer extension step). *Taq* DNA polymerase, isolated from *Thermus aquaticus* bacteria living in the geysers of Yellowstone National Park, is active at temperatures used for extension [70–72°C (158–162°F)], and survives subsequent 95°C (203°F) denaturation steps. The strands are heat denatured, the cycle begun again, and the template amplified in a geometric expansion over 30–40 cycles. A programmable heating and cooling thermal cycler makes replication of DNA fragments rapid and cost-effective.

and not beyond (Fig. 4.10). Typically, several hundred bps of specimen sequence (up to 400bp) can be read with high fidelity. Synthesis of new oligonucleotide primers based on homology with this sequence enables ongoing sequencing using the same clone of template DNA. Novel sequencing methods now make it feasible to use double-stranded vectors such as plasmids and lambda phage, provided a short sequence of insert or vector is known to construct the priming oligonucleotides.

GENOME STRUCTURE, MUTATION, THE HUMAN GENOME PROJECT, AND BIOINFORMATICS

The human genome refers to the total DNA content in human cells, including the complex nuclear genome and a simple mitochondrial genome that specifies only a small proportion of mitochondrial functions in its 37 genes. The number of genes in the nuclear genome, estimated by genomic sequencing and random

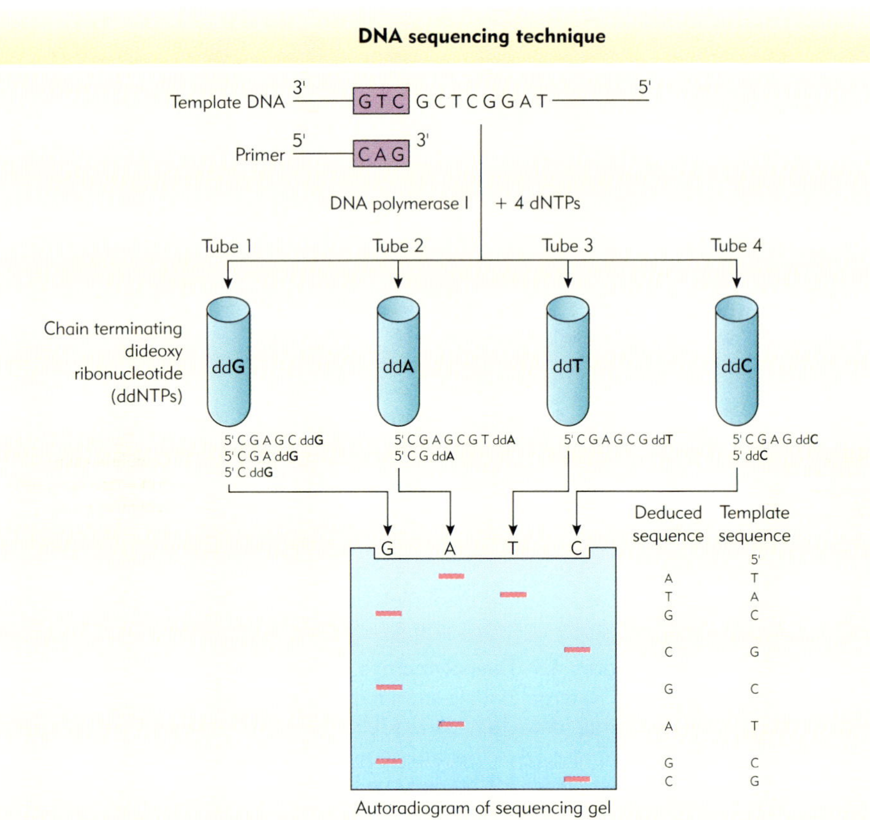

Figure 4.10 Sanger dideoxy DNA sequenci The DNA to be sequenced is inserted into a polycloning site of the M13 phage vector, w can produce single-stranded DNA as a template. A universal oligonucleotide prime annealed to the strand of sample DNA, and synthesis of new strands is initiated *in vitro* b addition of DNA polymerase I and dNTPs. Deoxyribonucleic acid polymerase I is able t incorporate the ddNTPs, but cannot add fur to the chain to form a new phosphodiester b with the next incoming nucleotide. Thus, a s of DNA molecules is constructed in each of reaction tubes; the series differ in length depending on the location of a particular ba relative to the 5′ end, as a result of 3′ chai termination by a specific ddNTP. The synthe strands are labeled by radionuclide or fluorescent markers linked either to the four bases individually, or to the primer itself. The four tubes of reaction products, which consi DNA fragments of the same sequence that in length by one base, are separated into fo parallel lanes of a polyacrylamide gel, one f each ddNTP. After autoradiography or laser detection, the sequence is read from one ba to the next according to the lanes in which t bands appear.

sequencing of partial cDNA clones, known as expressed sequence tags (ESTs), is estimated to be 60,000–100,000 genes, which are encoded by 3% or less of the 3000Mb genome. Human genes vary tremendously in size and internal organization. On average, a human gene consists of 10–20 boundaries between intron and exon sequences, 1–2kb of coding, and 10–30kb of genomic sequence. Genes as small as several hundred base pairs without introns and as large as the dystrophin gene, with 15kb of coding sequence and 60 introns that span an entire genomic sequence of 2.5Mb, are well-described. Overlapping genes, genes within genes, multiple copy numbers of the same gene, and gene families with homology between members have been identified. Intron sequence is characterized by microsatellite (1–4bp) and minisatellite (1–20kb) tandem repeats of high copy number and variable length, but of unknown functional significance.

Mutation, which produces heritable changes in DNA, includes both large changes (loss, duplication, or rearrangement of chromosome segments) and small point modifications (loss, duplication, or alteration of segments of DNA as small as a single bp). Based on estimates of gene frequency in a population and reproductive failure of a genotype because of natural selection, mutation rates for most organisms are 10^{-5}–10^{-7} per locus per generation. This low level of mutation represents a balance that allows occasional evolutionary novelty at the expense of disease or death of a proportion of members of a species. Methods available to detect human genes that carry novel mutant alleles are chosen based on the size of the defect. Visible chromosomal rearrangements that give rise to dysmorphic syndromes may represent contiguous gene defects disrupting a monogenic locus of interest. Animal models, traits associated with previously mapped loci, and candidate proteins in plausible pathways may indicate specific genes for direct sequencing. If there are no such shortcuts, investigators may resort to genetic maps of linked markers and positional candidate genes (see below). Once a mutation is identified, to screen individuals at risk is relatively simple using PCR-based approaches. Single bp alterations produce mismatches that modify the ability of a PCR product to form heteroduplexes with tagged RNA probes. More commonly, conformational changes in single-strand DNA fragments [single-strand conformation polymorphism (SSCP)] that differ at one bp are discriminated by gel electrophoresis to detect known mutations (Fig. 4.11).

A major goal of the Human Genome Project is to complete a composite cDNA and, ultimately, genomic DNA sequence (physical map) so that meaningful variations from normal can be compared with their respective phenotypes, and thereby improve the diagnosis and management of disease. The DNA sequence map will ultimately incorporate all the information obtained in the construction of earlier, lower resolution physical maps (e.g. cytogenetic maps, restriction maps, and EST maps; Fig. 4.12). To date, about 30,000 human genes have been mapped, designating approximately 1Mb of sequence, and 5000–10,000 of these genes represent full-length cDNA sequences. Roughly 8000 partial sequence cDNA ESTs are being added to this database per week. This superexponential explosion of sequence information generated from human and other model organism genome projects is made accessible worldwide using the Internet (http://compbio.ornl.gov/).

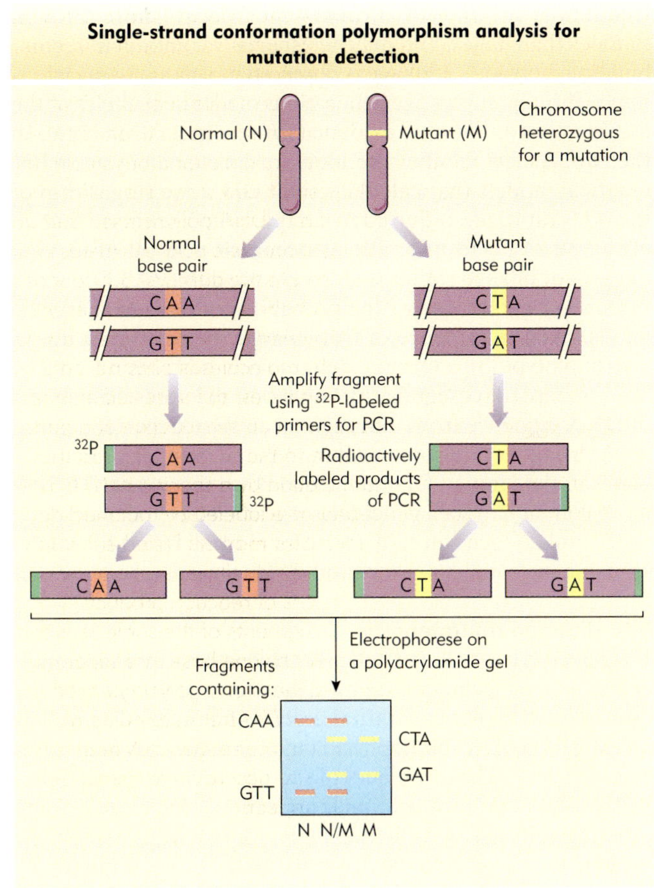

Figure 4.11 Single-strand conformation polymorphism analysis for mutation detection. Single-strand DNA forms complex structures stabilized by weak intermolecular bonds based on DNA composition that can be discriminated by altered electrophoretic mobility. Denatured PCR products tagged with radiolabeled primers are loaded on nondenaturing polyacrylamide gels – samples that differ by a single bp may be resolved. In the example shown, two bands are apparent from each of the homozygous normal (N) and mutant (M) strands, whereas all four bands are present in DNA from the heterozygote (N/M). Although SSCP is a sensitive technique with which to screen PCR products for mutations, it is limited to fragments of several hundred bps and cannot indicate the exact nature or position of the genetic alteration if this is not known *a priori*.

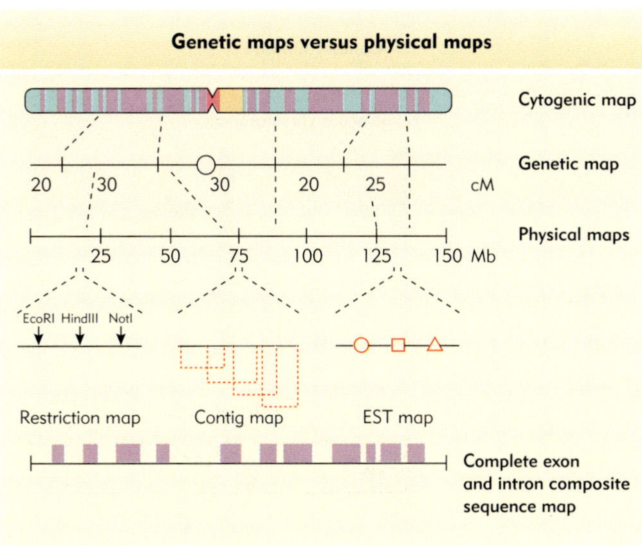

Figure 4.12 Genetic maps versus physical maps. Genetic maps represent the order of loci by the frequency of recombination events between two loci. Genetic loci in close approximation, <1 centimorgan (cM) apart, rarely dissociate in meiosis, while the greater the interval between loci, the greater is the likelihood that they sort independently. The genetic distance of 1cM corresponds loosely to the physical distance of 1Mb, but it is not constant throughout the genome (see text). When completed, the highest order human physical map of exon and intron sequence will encompass lower resolution cytogenetic, restriction, contig (contiguous overlapping DNA clones assembled by chromosome walking), and EST physical maps, and will incorporate chromosome-specific genetic maps.

Recombination, genetic maps, and genetic linkage

The basic principle in genetic mapping is to order loci using meiotic recombination to index the size of the intervening distance. Any phenotypic or genotypic character that is polymorphic and mendelian can be used as a marker for the presence of a genetic locus. In the simplest case of X-linked conditions, analysis of pedigrees using gender as a marker leads to many gene assignments to the X chromosome. For the remaining 22 autosomes, tremendous genetic variation arises during the first stage of meiosis, from independent assortment of maternal and paternal chromosomes to the gamete to recombination or crossing over (the exchange of chromosomal material between homologous chromosomes during meiosis). Taking advantage of the low probability of reassortment by crossing-over between genetic loci in close linear approximation, linkage analysis allows the detection of regions of the genome that contain genes associated with traits and diseases inherited in a mendelian single-gene manner. The strength of the approach is that no assumptions need to be made regarding the nature of the gene or its expressed product. Its weaknesses include the need for pedigrees of substantial size and specific character (multiple affected individuals in three generations, with both parents heterozygous for the marker), clear-cut phenotypic diagnosis, and assumptions about gene number, mechanisms of inheritance, expressivity, and penetrance that may or may not prevail.

Linkage refers to the co-inheritance of a marker and a region of DNA sequence thought to underlay a specific trait. Ideal markers are highly polymorphic (i.e. at least two or more alleles exist at the locus) and the least common allele has a frequency of at least 1% in the general population. Individuals are most likely to be heterozygous for markers that are highly polymorphic, which makes it possible to track inheritance of a particular marker-tagged chromosome within a family. In the simplest version of linkage analysis (Fig. 4.13), if a marker is mapped to a specific locus and a marker at a second locus is linked to the first, then the two loci must reside on the same chromosome. The map distance defined as a frequency of recombination between loci of 1% (theta = 0.01) is 1cM, which is estimated to represent about 1Mb, but genetic maps and physical maps are not isologous. Recombination is more

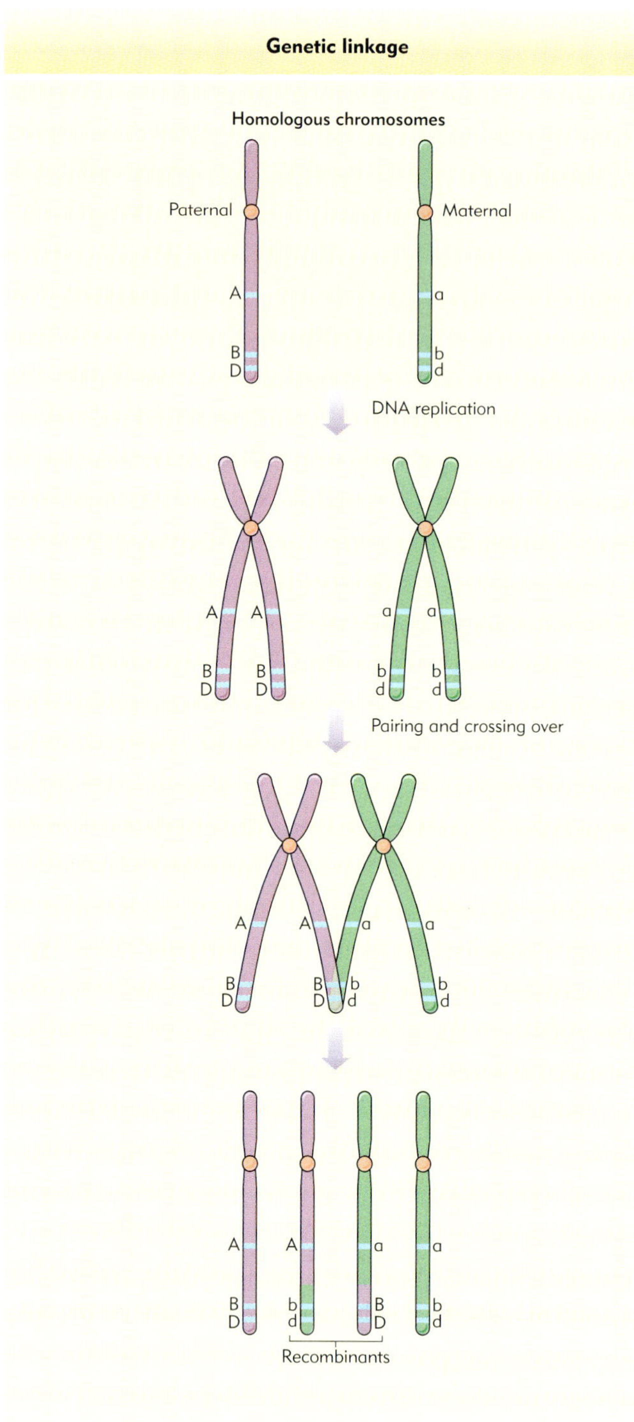

Figure 4.13 Genetic linkage. By isolating a series of polymorphic markers at loci linked to a locus associated with a specific trait or disease, it is possible to track the inheritance of specific chromosomal regions in families without knowledge of the function of the locus in question. If two loci are closely linked (e.g. Bb and Dd), their alleles are transmitted together to the gamete. Exchange of chromosomal material between homologous chromosomes during meiosis is a crossover event. The smaller the distance between two loci the less probable a crossover event (recombination) becomes between the two, and therefore the likelihood of recombinational events between two loci can be used to define genetic distances.

frequent at the ends of chromosomes, occurs more often in females than males, and may be especially common in recombination 'hotspots'. Linkage is observed by simultaneous inheritance through successive generations of identical alleles at the loci in question, with no evidence for recombination between the two. As few families are ideal for linkage analysis, mathematical models that calculate the LOD score (logarithm of the odds ratio) are required to compare the likelihood that an observed association of alleles occurs as a result of varying degrees of linkage rather than by chance alone. A LOD score of three or greater favors the probability of linkage at 1000:1, and is taken as evidence of true linkage. Once a set of markers (haplotype) in a chromosomal region have been found to be co-inherited (cosegregate) with a trait of interest, fragments of DNA sequence from that region can be searched for causal genes using chromosome walking. As the number of mapped genes in the Human Genome Project has increased, it is now more common to seek candidate genes that have been mapped to the linked locus already (positional candidates) for analysis using intragenic markers and direct mutation searches.

Site-directed mutagenesis

If a gene has been cloned and a suitable assay is available, molecular genetic techniques allow dissection and mapping of the operational elements within the gene and protein, as well as investigation of the pathophysiologic consequences of disease-causing alleles. The techniques of site-directed mutagenesis precisely alters one or more nucleotides in a DNA clone using either cell-based or cell-free PCR approaches. With PCR, primers are designed to be dissimilar to the target sequence by incorporating novel nucleotides in the PCR product, but not sufficiently different to inhibit amplification. Denatured PCR products of two reactions with partially overlapping sequences that contain the mutation of interest can then be combined to create a larger fragment with the mutation at midpoint in the sequence. In add-on mutagenesis, modified primers introduce a convenient restriction site, labeled group, promoter sequence, or other useful component to the 5′ end of the PCR product. Using the normal gene as a control, the mutant gene product may then be expressed in host cells and functional changes compared with the wild-type gene product.

Expression cloning

Most cloning efforts in the past have been aimed at acquisition and amplification of DNA to investigate its structure and function. More recently, the generation of bulk amounts of a specific protein, for therapy (insulin, growth hormone) or for direct studies of peptide function, has become feasible with the design of cloning systems that promote expression of eukaryotic genes in bacterial cells (expression cloning). An expression vector contains bacterial promoter sequences of DNA required to transcribe the cloned DNA insert and translate its mRNA into protein (i.e. sequences that position the mRNA on the ribosome and an initiation codon). The foreign DNA fragment may be cloned into a site within the coding region of a prokaryotic gene. Expression vectors are most appropriate for cDNA inserts, since bacteria lack mechanisms for intron splicing. They often include an inducible promoter, which overcomes the detrimental effects of foreign gene expression by switching on the foreign gene after the bacteria have been selected and propagated. Expression of eukaryotic proteins in bacterial cells may be useful in the identification and characterization of novel genes by antibody screening of a cDNA library in bacterial cells that express foreign proteins (phage display library). Clones that positively react for a specific antibody are isolated and used as probes for genomic library screens.

In the absence of many post-translational processing systems in bacterial prokaryotic cells, eukaryotic gene products may be unstable or reveal no biologic activity. Expression of eukaryotic genes in eukaryotic cells allows detection and quantification of a gene product, which might otherwise be impossible in bacteria. A crucial step in the development of DNA-mediated transfection techniques was the creation of mammalian expression vectors, which allow the transcription and translation of foreign genes in a wide variety of recipient cell types. Mammalian expression vectors contain a eukaryotic transcription unit, in addition to a prokaryotic plasmid region composed of a replication origin (ori) and an antibiotic resistance cistron (e.g. AmpR). To obtain a high level of expression in a broad range of host cell types, the transcription unit derived from a simian virus (SV40) that contains an early promoter is placed upstream (5´) from the insert coding region. The function of the SV40 transcription unit is to direct transcription, the processing and transport of the foreign mRNA to the host cell cytoplasm. An intervening intron sequence improves mRNA stability and transport to the cytoplasm, and a 3´ polyadenylation site prevents 'readthrough' to a prokaryotic plasmid sequence. Other modifications include restriction endonuclease sites for insertion of DNA sequences, or a eukaryotic DNA replication origin may be added for specific applications. To measure the function of exogenously introduced DNA, it is necessary to construct a foreign gene such that its expression can be distinguished from expression of the host cell gene. Foreign gene elements are marked by fusion with functional reporter genes expressing easily assayed proteins that are otherwise absent or expressed at low levels in mammalian cells (e.g. chloramphenicol acetyltransferase, *E. coli* β-galactosidase, and firefly luciferase).

Gene transfer

Despite the various mechanisms evolved by host cells to sequester and degrade foreign DNA, many physicochemical and viral techniques have been contrived to surmount obstacles to gene transfer. The major attribute of nonviral vectors is the absence of infectious and neoplastic hazards, whereas inefficient transfer is their greatest deficit. After physicochemical transfer, plasmid transgenes are maintained in the nucleus as episomal DNA, but as they are nonreplicating they may not be useful vectors in regenerating tissue. In the most fundamental method, plasmid DNA is delivered directly into the nucleus using microinjection. Although microinjection bypasses cytoplasmic and lysosomal degradation, only several hundred cells can be modified in a given experiment. Calcium phosphate–DNA coprecipitation to micron-size particles is a convenient and versatile technique for endocytosis-mediated gene transfer. It is effective with a wide range of cell types and can be used both with plasmid and high molecular weight genomic DNAs, although efficiency of transgene expression is below that required for most therapeutic applications. Electroporation, the technique used to create whole animal clones by nuclear transfer, generates pores in the cell membrane for DNA entry in the presence of transient, high-voltage pulses that result in stable transfectants. Upon cessation of the pulse, the pores close and entrap the transgene. Many cells do not survive the electric shock and, even under optimal conditions, most do not take up the foreign DNA. Particle bombardment with the 'gene gun' requires minimal manipulation of target cells, and is able to deliver controlled dosages of DNA that coat the heavy projectile beads. However, expression is transient with minimal stable integration of foreign DNA in the nuclei of treated cells. Artificial cationic liposomes that contain small plasmid DNAs are able to fuse to cells in tissue culture and deliver DNA into the mammalian host cell. In the past this technique was confined to low molecular weight DNA fragments, and yields of expression *in vivo* were low, but recent modifications of liposome composition and DNA packaging promise to make liposome-mediated gene transfer the method of choice, particularly in applications for which it is possible to select stable transfectants.

For long-term expression of large inserts *in vivo*, viral transfection vectors are preferred. The gene to be expressed is cloned into a site in the viral genome that replaces essential viral sequences and renders the recombinant host virus defective. The recombinant viral genome is then cotransfected into packaging cells in culture, and DNA from a second, defective helper virus carries functional genes that lack the recombinant viral genome. Cells that take up both the recombinant host virus and the helper virus express proteins required for replication of the introduced DNA. The DNA is packaged into infectious particles that are harvested to transfect cell targets for expression of protein from the cloned gene. Retroviral vectors capable of reverse transcriptase-mediated synthesis of cDNA are able to integrate into chromosomal DNA, accommodate large inserts (up to 7kb), and are highly efficient, easily manipulated, and propagate through daughter cells after mitosis. Chromosomal integration after viral transfection allows the transgene to be perpetuated by replication following cell division, which provides long-term stable expression at the risk of host cell death or undesired modification. Unfortunately, they do not readily transfect nondividing cells, may cause harmful insertional mutagenesis, and may be prone to rescue of the crippled helper virus by contamination with wild-type, replication-competent viruses. Adenoviral vectors enable gene delivery into differentiated post-mitotic cells, with limited risk of wild-type contamination. As adenoviral infection is ubiquitous in mammals, pre-existing immunity may account for unstable and depressed levels of expression. Other viral vectors are under investigation. A shared theme is that the qualities of a vector that promote gene transfer are closely entwined with properties that endanger the host.

Transgenic animals

Using transgenic animals, the consequences of discrete nucleotide alterations may be investigated in genetic backgrounds otherwise identical to those of the unmanipulated organism. Hence, a whole animal expression–cloning system is produced by transfection of exogenous DNA into cultured cells capable of differentiation into the cells of the adult animal. If the exogenous gene is found in only a proportion of cells, the animals are partially transgenic. If the foreign DNA is transferred into fertilized oocytes or embryonic stem (ES) cells that contribute to the development of the whole organism, the animals are fully transgenic and will transmit the modified genome to their offspring. Methods used in the assembly of transgenic animals include pronuclear microinjection of DNA into random chromosomal sites of individual oocytes, retroviral transfer into pre- or postimplantation embryos, and injection of modified ES

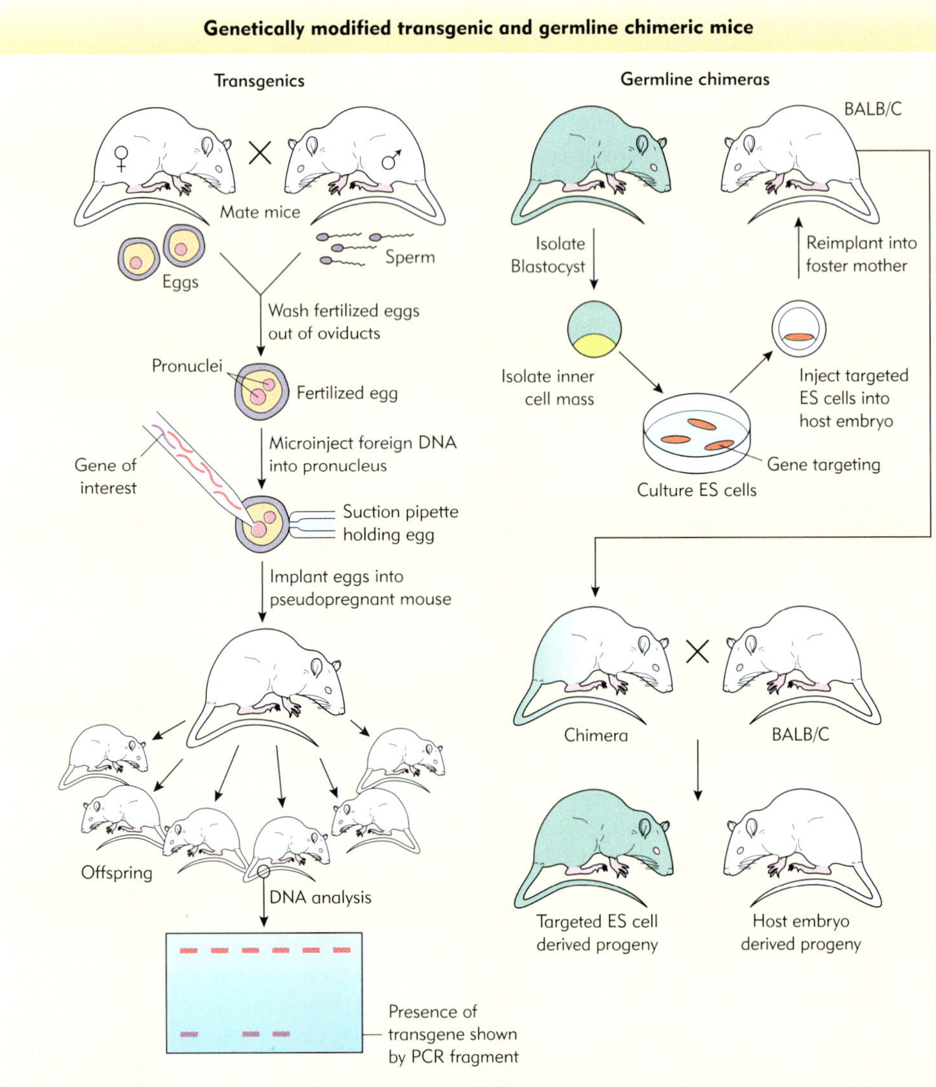

Figure 4.14 Genetically modified transgenic and germline chimeric animals. To create transgenic animals, fertilized eggs are transferred to pseudopregnant foster mothers after microinjection of the gene of interest into one of the pronuclei. Southern blotting of DNA from tail cells is used to screen the offspring for the presence of the transgene. To generate germline chimeras, ES cells isolated from the blastocyst are gene targeted for a mutation by homologous recombination in culture, injected into blastocysts from a different strain, and reimplanted into a pseudopregnant foster mother. Chimeric animals are bred to identify germline chimeras in which a proportion of the progeny arise from ES-derived gametes using coat color as a marker. Backcrossing and interbreeding of chimeras produces animals that are heterozygous or homozygous for the genetic modification. (BALB/C is a host mouse strain.)

cells into host blastocysts using coat color as a proxy to identify chimeras (organisms derived from more than a single zygote) that carry mutations for subsequent backcrossing (Fig. 4.14).

Gene knockouts

Introduction of a transgene into a preselected endogenous locus is a form of site-directed *in vivo* mutagenesis termed gene targeting. Gene targeting in ES cells leads to the creation of an animal in which all the nucleated cells carry a mutation at the gene of interest. This is usually accomplished by electroporation of a cloned gene that is closely related in sequence to an endogenous gene of an ES cell. Selected from the treated ES cells are those in which recombination between the introduced gene and its corresponding chromosomal homolog (homologous recombination) has occurred. The modified ES cells are injected into the blastocyst of a foster mother to produce an animal in which all of the nucleated cells have been mutated at the site of interest. If the mutagenesis results in the inactivation of gene expression, the mutation is termed a 'knockout' and the effect of the mutation on development and physiology is measured. Often the knockout mutation is lethal, but viable cells can be harvested for further investigation. On occasion little or no change may be detected in the phenotype of the animal, which indicates that other (redundant) genes are able to fulfill the required functions of the inactivated locus.

Gene therapy

In the broadest sense, gene therapy is the genetic modification of a patient's cells to enable disease treatment. This definition embraces many potential avenues for intervention, including transfer of whole or partial genes from identical or foreign genomes, synthetic genes, and antisense oligonucleotides to eliminate damaged cells or protect normal tissues from destruction. Originally envisaged as a method to correct human diseases that arise from single gene defects, gene therapy currently encompasses a much broader range of applications in acquired disorders, infectious disease, oncology, and symptom management. Due to profound ethical, legal, and social considerations, for the foreseeable future human gene therapy will be restricted to addressing disorders of somatic rather than germline cells.

Strategies that involve modification of somatic cells can be classified into *in vivo* 'direct' and *ex vivo* 'indirect' gene therapy (Fig. 4.15). *In vivo* methods, with transgene vectors directly introduced into the tissue space of a living organism, are limited by poor speci-

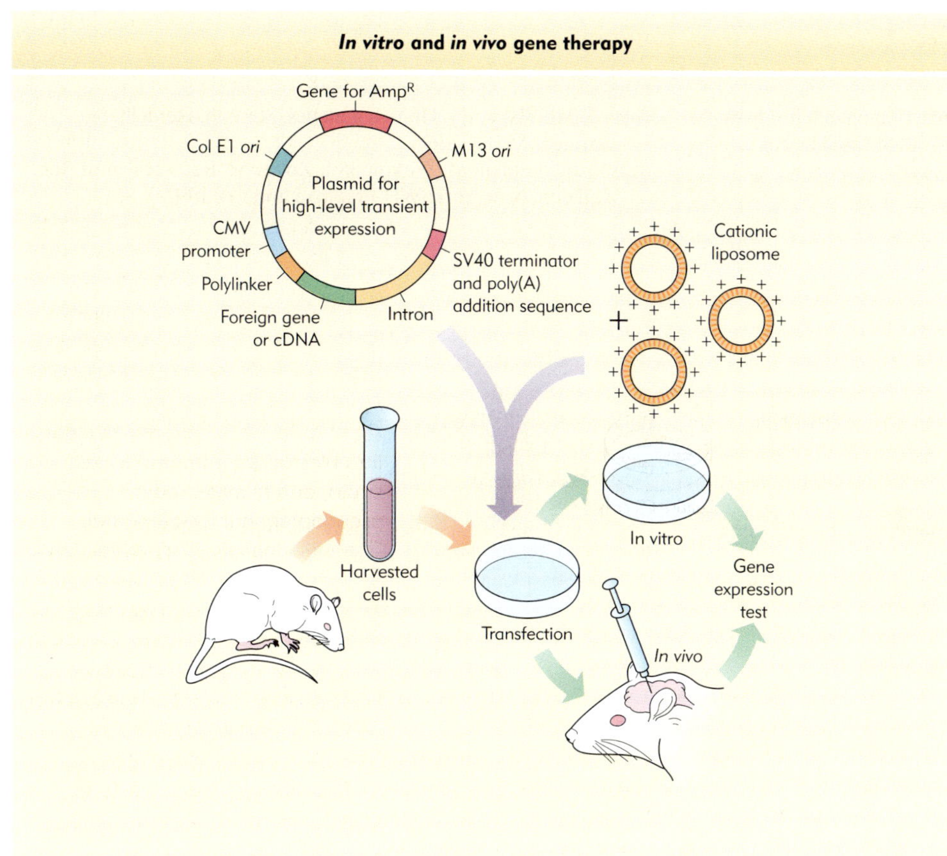

Figure 4.15. Gene therapy. Mammalian expression vectors contain prokaryotic regions required for replication (ori) and antibiotic resistance (Amp^R), together with promoter (CMV), polyadenylation, and intervening intron sequences to improve mRNA stability and transport. *Ex vivo* gene therapy entails modification of harvested primary cells by transfection, in this example with a plasmid DNA–cationic lipid complex, and reimplantation into the organism. Expression of the transgene is monitored *in vitro* and *in situ*. *In vivo* gene therapy refers to direct injection of viral or nonviral vectors into targeted host cells.

ficity and stability of gene transfer because of the inability to select and amplify transformed cells, which increases the need for repeated treatments that may engender immunogenicity. *Ex vivo* methods are based on grafting target cells that are transfected, selected, and expanded *in vitro* to deliver a required gene product fabricated in the host cell. Selectivity and specificity are expedited by physical removal and isolation of autogenic or allogenic target cells. To serve as *ex vivo* platforms for expression of transgenes, the host cells must be harvested, purified, and banked easily and safely. They must be tolerant to genetic manipulation by various means, survive transplantation without immunosuppression, and express the transgene for an appropriate interval with minimal oncogenic, infectious, and immunogenic potential.

Well-characterized genes and methods to transfer genes into appropriate target cells considered in earlier sections of this chapter are the first two prerequisites for gene therapy. Identification of conditions with well-defined phenotypes and clear-cut therapeutic end points to monitor efficacy is an additional significant barrier. For the ideal clinical target, the biochemical pathophysiology must be understood, a suitable animal model must be available or created using transgenic technologies, the human and appropriate model animal genes must have been cloned (e.g. genes that encode ligands, receptors, and metabolic enzymes), outcomes must be quantifiable and controlled (i.e. using identical vectors with nontherapeutic reporter genes replacing the gene of interest), and the shortcomings of competing approaches must be balanced by the magnitude of the clinical problem. Many of the conditions faced by anesthesiologists (e.g. cancer pain syndromes) meet these criteria, while knowledge of the fundamental pathophysiology of other disorders (e.g. complex regional pain syndromes) must be expanded before gene therapy will fulfill a management role.

Methods to regulate bioactivity of the gene product offer the prospect of temporal specificity to complement the topographic specificity realized by confining cell targets to discrete populations. These methods include control of transcription with administration of second drugs coupled to promoters (tetracycline, antiprogestins) or channeling gene products through alternative pathways of RNA splicing, post-translational modification, or pharmacokinetic transport and elimination. In this fashion, alterations engineered at the most fundamental molecular level of the cell may be placed directly under the will of the patient (i.e. patient-controlled gene therapy), while limiting toxicity and tolerance and maintaining bioactivity in reserve as needs dictate.

Key References

Sambrook J, Fritsch EF, Maniatis T. Molecular cloning: a laboratory manual, 2nd edn. Cold Spring Harbor: Cold Spring Harbor Laboratory Press; 1989.

Vogel F, Motulsky AG. Human genetics, 3rd edn. Heidelberg: Springer Verlag; 1996.

Watson JD, Gilman M, Witkowski J, Zoller M. Recombinant DNA, 2nd edn. New York: WH Freeman and Co; 1992.

Further Reading

Carlson EA. Defining the gene: an evolving concept. Am J Hum Genet. 1991;49:475–87.

Frankel WN, Schork NJ. Who's afraid of epistasis? Nature Genet. 1996;14:371–3.

Hogan K. To fire the train: the second malignant hyperthermia gene. Am J Hum Genet. 1997;60:1303–8.

Joyner AL (ed.). Gene Targeting: a Practical Approach. IRL Press, Oxford, 1993.

McPherson MJ, Taylor GR, Quirke P. PCR: a practical approach. Oxford: IRL Press; 1991.

Phimster B (ed.). The chipping forecast. Nature Genetics (Suppl). 1999;21:1–60.

Singer M, Berg P. Genes and genomes. Mill Way: University Science Books; 1991.

Wolff JA. Gene therapeutics. Boston: Birkhauser; 1994

Wolf U. The genetic contribution to the phenotype. Hum Genet. 1995;95:127–48.

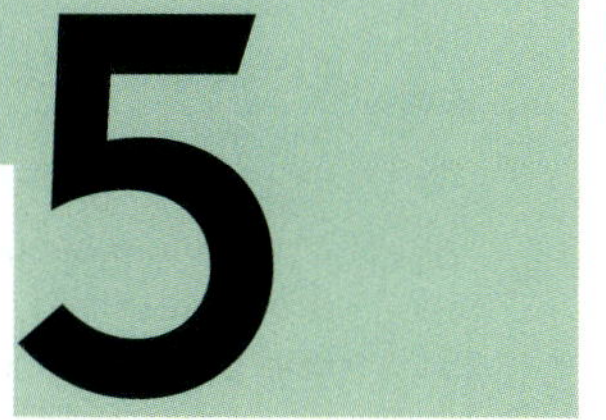

Chapter 5 Molecular physiology

Kevin Gingrich and Jay Yang

Topics covered in this chapter

Electrical principles
Gated ion channels
Membrane voltage
Carriers, pumps, and transporters
Current and voltage measurements
Measurement of ion concentrations
Relevance to anesthesia

Ion channels are specialized membrane proteins that mediate the rapid transmembrane ionic fluxes which are critical for the initiation and propagation of action potentials, synaptic transmission, and muscle contraction. Carriers, pumps, and transporters form another class of membrane proteins that carry ion fluxes essential to cellular homeostasis. In addition, they transport neurotransmitters and large organic molecules involved in metabolism. Electrophysiologic studies have identified the governing physiologic principles and provided functional characterization of these proteins. The techniques of molecular biology have advanced our knowledge of the molecular structural basis of their functions. The importance of ion channels and carrier proteins in normal cell function is self-evident, but some may also serve as targets for anesthetic agents and other therapeutic drugs. This chapter reviews the fundamental electrical principles that govern the behavior of all cells, the properties of ion channels and carrier proteins, and the methods used to study them.

ELECTRICAL PRINCIPLES

Potential, current, capacitance, and resistance

Ions range in size from small negatively charged electrons ($<10^{-14}$cm) to large organic molecules. Ion movement is determined by physical laws, which underlie the concepts of *electrical current*, *voltage*, *capacitance*, and *resistance* (Chapter 11).

To illustrate these concepts, consider two parallel plates composed of a conducting material that allows easy passage of ions (Fig. 5.1a). A nonconducting gas between the plates prohibits ion movement and electrically insulates one from the other. Overall, this configuration is a capacitive element which stores charge on parallel plates. Current (I) is defined (Fig 5.1a) as the flow of positive charge (Q) per unit time and has units of amperes (A). Current can also be carried by negatively charged ions (*anions*), where the direction of actual ion flow is opposite to that of current. Current delivered to the upper plate by the flow of positive ions (*cations*) leads to a net positive charge that electrostatically repels cations on the lower plate, driving them off and resulting in a net negative charge. Separated positive and negative charges create an electric field between the plates with a magnitude decribed by a *potential* or *voltage* (V) difference. The electric field exerts a force (F_v) on an ion with magnitude proportional to the voltage and in a direction towards the unlike charge. Therefore, voltage or potential differences drive current from positive to negative polarity.

Capacitance (C) is a measure of the ability to store charge. An electrical circuit equivalent of a capacitive element has two parallel lines representing parallel plates (Fig. 5.1b). Capacitance is expressed in terms of the amount of charge stored for the applied voltage and has units of Farads (F). A transient charging current is induced upon application of voltage that continues until the applied and capacitive voltages equalize.

Resistance (R) is the opposition to current flow and has units of ohms (Ω). As resistance increases, higher voltages are required to induce the same current through the element. Resistance is defined by the ratio of the applied voltage to the induced current (Fig. 5.1c). *Conductance* (G), the reciprocal of resistance, describes the ease with which ions are passed. The unit of conductance is the mho (the reverse spelling of ohm) or siemens (S).

Electrical properties of the cell membrane

The cell membrane separates the intracellular and extracellular environments (Chapter 2). Molecules energetically prefer surroundings with similar physicochemical properties (polarity, charge, etc.). The properties of aqueous environments are determined by the polar nature of water molecules. As a result, polar or charged molecules favor the company of water molecules and are called 'water loving' or *hydrophilic*. Long uncharged carbon chains prefer the absence of water molecules and are called 'water fearing' or *hydrophobic*. Since the extracellular and intracellular environs are aqueous they attract the polar hydrophilic phosphate heads of membrane phospholipids while repelling the nonpolar hydrocarbon tails; this favors formation of a phospholipid bilayer as molecules align in this manner (Fig. 5.1d). This bilayer allows passage of small nonpolar molecules but is impermeable to ions and large or polar molecules (e.g. sugars and amino acids), which must enter and exit the cell by means of ion channels and transporters. Since the membrane impedes ion flow, it electrically insulates the intracellular and extracellular solutions, which themselves are excellent conductors because of their high ion concentrations. This arrangement results in significant membrane

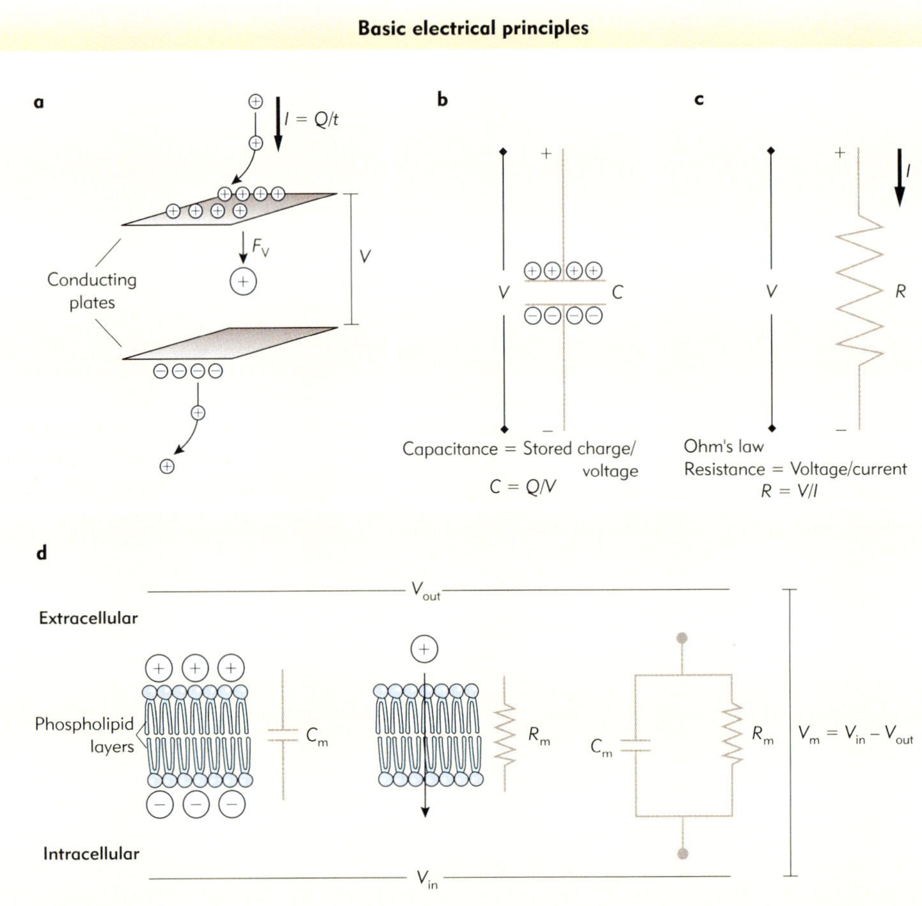

Figure 5.1 Basic electrical principles. (a) Two parallel conducting plates separated by a nonconducting gas constitute a capacitive element. Ions are represented by circles with minus and plus signs indicating polarity. Current (I) carried by cations is delivered to the upper plate. The voltage or potential difference (V) between the plates is indicated. A large cation placed between the plates experiences an electromotive force (F_V) arising from the electric field and the voltage difference. (b) The electrical circuit equivalent of a capacitive element. Charges are shown on each plate. (c) The electrical circuit equivalent for resistance (R). (d) The cell membrane is composed of a phospholipid bilayer; each molecule has a polar phosphate group and two nonpolar long-chain hydrocarbons. The cell membrane can store charges, demonstrating its capacitance (C_m). The membrane permits limited passage of cations, constituting a finite resistance (R_m). Alongside is the overall equivalent electrical circuit, which combines capacitive and resistive elements. The voltage difference is the transmembrane voltage (V_m).

capacitance (C_m). Ions, to a small degree, penetrate the bilayer, resulting in a finite but large membrane resistance (R_m). The electrical properties of the membrane can be represented by an equivalent circuit involving resistance and capacitance elements (Fig. 5.1d, right). The voltage across this circuit is the transmembrane voltage (V_m). Events that force V_m towards negative potentials are *polarizing* and those that drive V_m towards positive potentials are *depolarizing*. Thus the electrical properties of a cell can be represented by an electrical circuit made up of familiar electrical elements (resistors and capacitors).

GATED ION CHANNELS

Physiology

Ion channels are ion-selective macromolecular protein tunnels or pores that traverse the cell membrane and may, therefore, affect the membrane potential, which is critical to excitable cells. Ions are passed with high efficiency such that a few picoamperes (10^{-12}A) of current are generated by the ionic flow of a single open channel. This high efficiency means that relatively few channels, in the order of thousands, are needed in a particular cell to support its electrical function. The majority of ion channels fall into two broad categories: *voltage-gated* or *ligand-gated*. Gating is the progression of the channel through various conformational states, including a resting closed state and an open ion-conducting state. A triggering stimulus (membrane depolarization or ligand presentation) causes transition from resting to open through the process of activation. Permeation is the passage of ions through the channel. In this way, gating regulates ion permeation. Figure 5.2 shows a simple topologic model of a generic voltage-gated cation channel. Permeation occurs via the channel pore, which begins on the extracellular face as the outer vestibule and narrows to a selectivity filter responsible for ion discrimination. The pore then widens to an inner vestibule (in which there are binding sites for local anesthetics in Na^+ channels or antagonists in Ca^{2+} channels: Chapter 18). An activation gate is shown at the inner channel mouth, which is closed at rest and obstructs the pore. Membrane depolarization triggers activation by exerting force on a charged voltage sensor, leading to the open conformation. Persistent depolarization induces further gating that closes the channel by shutting an inactivation gate. Consequently, voltage-gated ion channels have three primary conformational states: resting and inactivated closed states, and an open conducting state. In contrast, ligand-gated ion channels are activated by ligand (such as neurotransmitters) binding to an extracellular receptor. Like voltage-gated channels, they manifest resting and open states. However, persistant ligand presence induces a closed desensitized state. Examples of common gated ion channels and their physiologic roles are given in Figure 5.3 (see also Chapter 19).

Molecular structure

Functional entities that define channel behavior (such as the selectivity filter, voltage sensor, etc.) have structural correlates. The molecular structure of an ion channel defines its properties. Channel proteins span the membrane and have

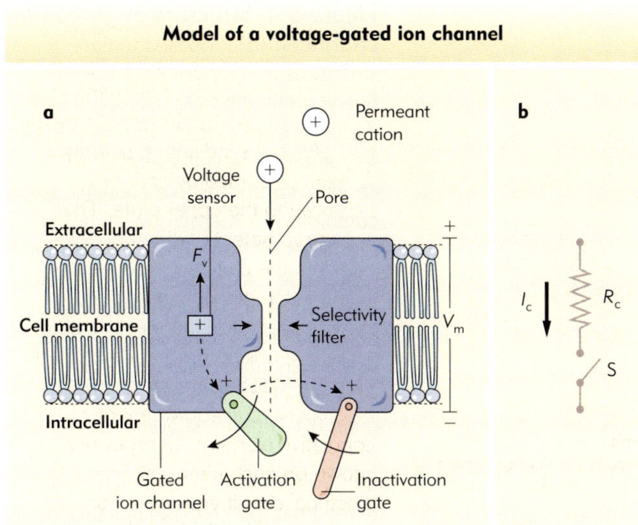

Figure 5.2 Model of a voltage-gated ion channel. (a) A simple general model of a voltage-gated ion channel residing within the cell membrane. A selectivity filter performs ion discrimination. An activation gate is shown at the intracellular mouth, which normally occludes the pore in the resting closed state and prevents permeation. Depolarization of the membrane voltage (V_m) exerts a force (F_V) on a positively charged voltage sensor, which triggers conformational changes leading to activation, gate opening, and ion permeation. Prolonged activation, caused by persistent depolarization, leads to closure of a normally open inactivation gate at the inner mouth. Negative V_m drives the permeant cation into the cell. (b) An electrical circuit can be drawn to describe a gated ion channel where the resistive element (R_c) is resistance to ion flow of the channel pore, I_c is the induced channel current, and the switch (S) represents the regulatory effect of channel gates on pore patency. When all gates are open, S is closed.

a hydrophobic exterior surface compatible with the hydrophobic environment of the lipid bilayer. The channel pore is lined with hydrophilic amino acids, providing a water-like environment for the ion to traverse the membrane. These pores are designed to pass ions of a particular kind, either anions or cations as determined by the selectivity filter. Cationic channels are somewhat more ion selective than the anionic channels. Many ligand-gated ion channels (e.g. the acetylcholine-gated channels that mediate the neuromuscular transmission or the glutamate-gated channels that are largely responsible for excitatory synaptic transmission) are permeable to several different cations.

Many ion channels have been cloned and their function directly assayed using oocytes harvested from South African toads (*Xenopus laevis*). These oocytes are large enough to be injected with messenger RNA (mRNA) from other species and are capable of synthesizing the encoded foreign protein (heterologous protein expression). Messenger RNA is derived from complementary DNA (cDNA) obtained from tissues rich in the channel of interest. Mutant cDNA clones with engineered alterations in the primary structure of the protein can be expressed and the properties of the mutated ion channel can be studied electrophysiologically to determine which regions of the protein are critical for a given channel function.

Most voltage-gated ion channel proteins are composed of subunits, with each subunit containing six α-helical hydrophobic transmembrane regions, S1 through S6. Voltage-gated K^+ channels (K_v; the subscript v indicates voltage gated) are composed of four separate subunits, (Fig. 5.4a,b). The subunits are assembled to form the central pore in a manner that also determines the basic properties of gating and permeation of the channel type. The peptide chain (H5 or P loop: permeation loop) between the membrane-spanning segments S5 and S6 projects into and lines the water-filled pore, as do portions of S6. The voltage sensor is composed of charged amino acid

Common gated ion channels

Voltage-gated channels	Abbreviation	Role
Na^+	I_{Na}	Rapid rising phase of action potential
K^+		
Delayed rectifier	I_K	Termination of action potential
Inward rectifier	I_{KIR}	Determines resting membrane potential
Ca^{2+}		
Low voltage activated or transient	LVAC or T-type	Automaticity in the heart, Ca^{2+} influx in nerve
High voltage activated (HVA)	HVAC	
Neuron	HVAC N-type	Synaptic transmission
Muscle	HVAC L-type	Ca^{2+} influx

Ligand-gated channels	Neurotransmitter	Primary permeable ion(s)	Role
$GABA_A$	GABA	Cl^-	Inhibition in CNS
Glycine	Glycine	Cl^-	Inhibition in spinal cord
Kainate	Glutamate	Na^+, K^+	Excitation in CNS
AMPA	Glutamate	Na^+, K^+	Excitation in CNS
NMDA	Glutamate	Na^+, Ca^{2+}	Excitation in CNS
Nicotinic acetylcholine	Acetylcholine	Na^+, K^+	Excitation in CNS and neuromuscular junction

Figure 5.3 Common gated ion channels. AMPA, 2-amino-3-hydroxy-5-methylisoxozole-4-propionic acid; GABA, γ-aminobutyric acid; NMDA, *N*-methyl-D-aspartate.

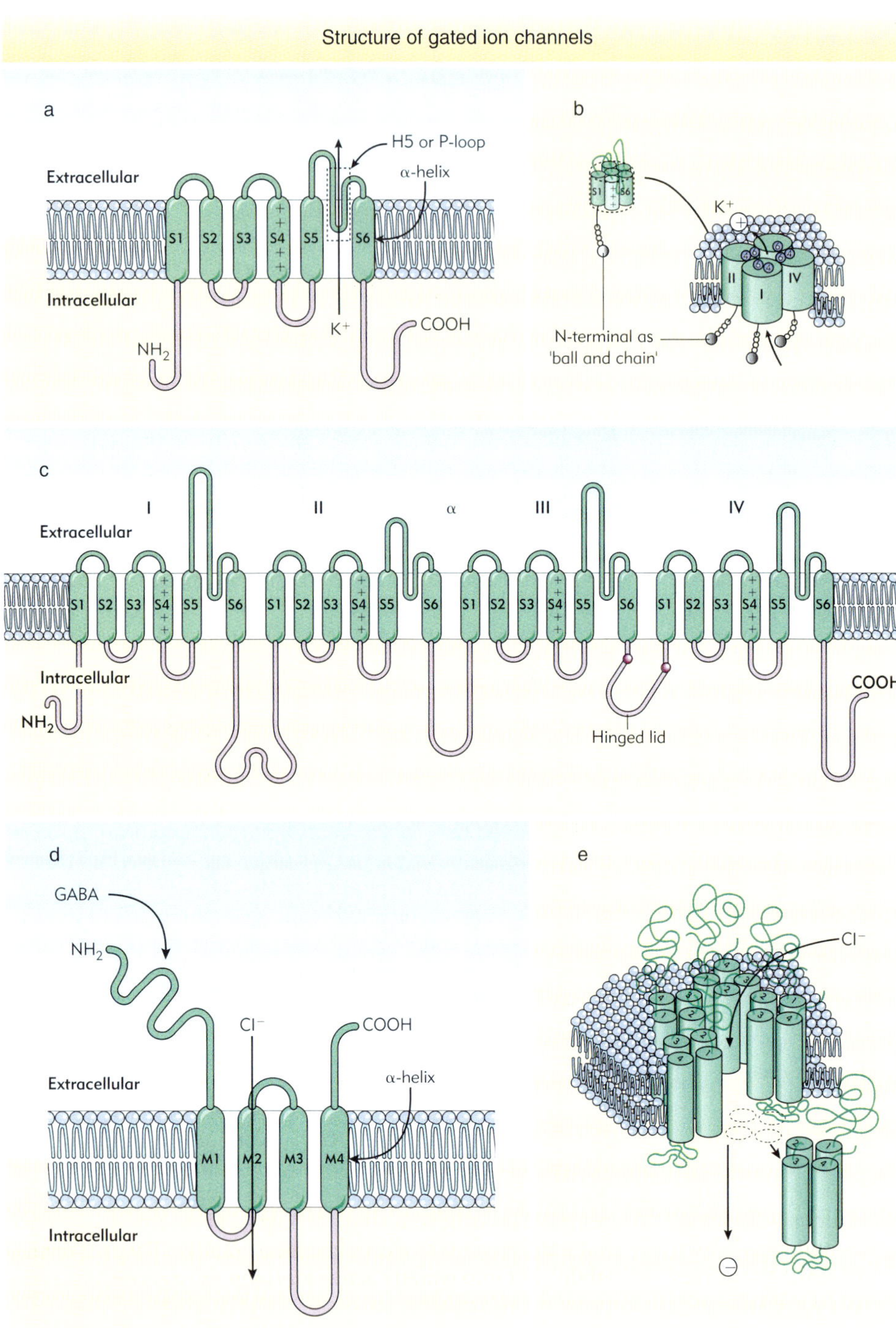

Figure 5.4 Structure of gated ion channels. (a) Proposed tertiary structures of a typical K^+ channel based on amino acid hydrophobicity deduced from cloned channel mRNA sequences. The voltage-gated K^+ channel comprises four subunits, each containing six membrane-spanning segments (S1–S6). Positively charged residues in S4 act as a voltage sensor. Residues of H5 (P-loop) line the pore and contribute to the selectivity filter, which is located between S5 and S6. S6 residues also contribute to the pore. (b) The four subunits assemble to form a K^+ channel in which the N terminus acts like a 'ball on a chain' to mediate fast (N-type) inactivation by occluding the permeation pathway at the inner mouth. (c) In Na^+ channels, the α-subunit comprises four repeats (domains I–IV) that are strikingly similar to a single K^+ channel subunit. The α-subunit alone forms the channel pore, although other auxillary subunits also exist (see Fig.18.10b). Voltage sensors are charged residues of S4 in each domain. All P-loops contribute to the pore, as well as portions of S6 in domain IV. The cytoplasmic loop between domains III and IV underlies fast inactivation and is considered a 'hinged lid'; it closes to occlude the pore. The structure of Ca^{2+} channels (not shown) is similar to that of the Na^+ channels. (d) The ligand-gated $GABA_A$ receptor has a subunit containing four membrane-spanning segments (M1–M4). M2 contributes to the pore and a chloride ion is shown traversing it. (e) Five subunits assemble to form a $GABA_A$ channel. This general structure also applies to several other ligand-gated ion channels (e.g. those for glycine, serotonin, nicotinic acetylcholine; see Chapter 19).

residues (lysine and arginine) on S4 that move outward during depolarization to trigger channel opening. Clones with K^+channels with varying numbers of positively charged amino acids in S4 show distinct voltage-dependent gating, supporting the idea that the S4 segment is a voltage sensor. Inactivation involves the movement of the N terminus into the inner mouth, thus obstructing the permeation pathway. The inactivation gate of Shaker channels, K^+ channels with a very rapid rate of inactivation, is the N terminus, which acts like a 'ball on a chain' to plug the inner mouth to prevent permeation. When the inside of the cell where the N terminus of the K^+ channel resides is treated with a proteolytic enzyme (digesting away the peptide), the inactivation disappears. Subsequently, if a synthetic polypeptide corresponding to the N-terminal amino acids of the ion channel is introduced to the cell, inactivation reappears, clearly supporting the notion that the structural basis for fast inactivation resides in the N terminus. The pore-forming α-subunit of Na^+ and Ca^{2+} channels contains four repeats of the six transmembrane-spanning motifs or domains (I–IV). These channels coassemble with accessory subunits that modulate channel gating but do not contribute to the pore. The structure of voltage-gated Na^+ and Ca^{2+} channels is fundamentally similar to that of K^+ channels (Fig. 5.4c).

Most ligand-gated ion channels comprise individual subunits or groups of subunits; however, in these, each subunit contains four hydrophobic transmembrane regions (Fig. 5.4). The subunits assemble in a pentameric fashion such that segment M2 from the five subunits forms the central pore and determines the permeation characteristics. Channel activation is triggered by ligand binding to site(s) on the extracellular segment of the polypeptide chain. The conformational change caused by ligand binding is 'transduced' by an undefined mechanism to open the channel pore. Molecular cloning has identified numerous isoforms of the subunits of ligand-gated ion-channel receptors (Chapter 19). The reason why so many receptor subunit isoforms exist in nature is unclear. The exact subunit composition of the γ-aminobutyric acid $(GABA)_A$ receptor may have significance for the action of general anesthetics.

MEMBRANE VOLTAGE

Many ions have different intracellular and extracellular concentrations, resulting in transmembrane concentration gradients. These gradients combined with ion-selective channels provide for the control of resting membrane potential that is critical to cell function. In addition, gated channels allow for modulaton of membrane voltage (Chapter 18). In the face of a concentration gradient representing a chemical potential, particles move by diffusion to give a net movement from the area of high concentration to that of the lower. As a simplification, the chemical potential gives rise to a diffusional force (F_D) pushing particles down the concentration gradient. The effects of diffusional forces and ion-selective or semipermeable channels on membrane voltage is shown in Figure 5.5. The permeant cation has a greater concentration inside than outside, similar to K^+ in actual cells. When the gated ion channel opens, F_D pushes the permeant cation through the channel pore to the outside solution. This charge movement constitutes an outward channel current. The permeant cation accumulates on the outer membrane surface because of electrostatic attraction from its partner anion, which itself is drawn to the inner surface. These charges, stored in the membrane capacitance, result in a negative membrane potential. In electrically quiescent cells, the resting membrane voltage is negative. Outward currents cause additional polarization or *hyperpolarization*. Conversely, inward currents drive the membrane voltage to more positive values and cause *depolarization*. The outward current continues until the forces owing to diffusion and the increasing membrane potential equalize. The Nernst equation describes the magnitude of the membrane voltage (Nernst potential) that exerts a force (F_V) that matches the diffusional force, thereby stopping ion flow through the channel. The equation for the Nernst potential of ion X is:

$$V_X = (RT/zF) \times \ln\frac{[X_{out}]}{[X_{in}]}$$

where R is the universal gas constant, T is temperature in Kelvin, F is the Faraday constant, and z is the valence of the ion. Applying the constants and converting to $\log_{10}$:

$$V_X = 61 \times \log\frac{[X_{out}]}{[X_{in}]} \text{ in mV at 37°C}$$

If we assume $[K^+_{out}] = 0.01$mol/L and $[K^+_{in}] = 0.1$mol/L, we obtain a Nernst potential for K^+ (V_K) of –61mV. Thus, when $V_m = -61$mV, K^+ will stop flowing through the channel. If there are only K^+ channels present, the voltage at which the measured current reaches zero and reverses polarity, the *reversal potential* (V_R), is equal to V_K. At equilibrium, the membrane potential is called the *resting membrane potential* and is equal to the reversal potential.

There are many ion-selective channels in cells, each with their own Nernst potential. The reversal potential will depend on all permeant ions. The Goldman, Hodgkin, and Katz equation is used to determine the reversal potential for two (X and Y) or more permeant ions:

$$V_{X,Y} = (RT/zF)\ \ln\left[\frac{(P_X \times [X_{out}]) + (P_Y \times [Y_{out}])}{(P_X \times [X_{in}]) + (P_Y \times [Y_{out}])}\right]$$

where the constants are the same and P is the permeability for each ion when its channel is open. Permeability represents the ease with which a concentration gradient induces a flow of ions and here reflects channel conductance summed over all channels present. The reversal potential is the voltage at which the net current through the membrane is zero. For two ions, this means that current carried by ion X is of equal magnitude and opposite polarity to that of Y.

CARRIERS, PUMPS, AND TRANSPORTERS

The cell membrane in preserving the intracellular milieu also excludes the free movement of larger and charged molecules in and out of cells. Substrate molecules required for cell metabolism, such as glucose and amino acids, metabolic end-products, and essentially all charged molecules must be transported. Carriers, pumps, and transporters are proteins that allow movement of these molecules across the cell membrane. Like voltage-gated ion channels, some protein carriers are highly selective, while others resemble neurotransmitter-gated ion channels in moving two or more molecules at the same time. Therefore, carrier proteins in many ways functionally resemble ion channels.

Carrier proteins are classified as active or passive depending on whether the translocated molecules are moved up or down their electrochemical gradients, respectively. Active carrier proteins expend energy through ATP hydrolysis to move molecules against the electrochemical gradient. They are further subdivided into *primary active transporters* or *secondary active transporters* depending on whether the transporter is directly or indirectly coupled to the energy-supplying process (Fig. 5.6). The best known primary active transporter is the Na^+/K^+-ATPase, which is present in all eukaryotic cells. This primary active transporter maintains the Na^+ and K^+ ionic gradients by translocating Na^+ outward and K^+ inward against their electrochemical gradients. The Ca^{2+}-ATPase, abundant in Ca^{2+} storage organelles such as skeletal muscle sarcoplasmic reticulum, moves Ca^{2+} against its electrochemical gradient. The ionic gradients established by these primary active transporters provide the potential energy necessary for the rapid membrane electrical events critical to the function of excitable membranes. Secondary active transporters lack endogenous ATPase activity and move molecules against their electrochemical gradient by coupling to an already established potential energy source. In most cases, movement of Na^+ and/or K^+ drives secondary active transport.

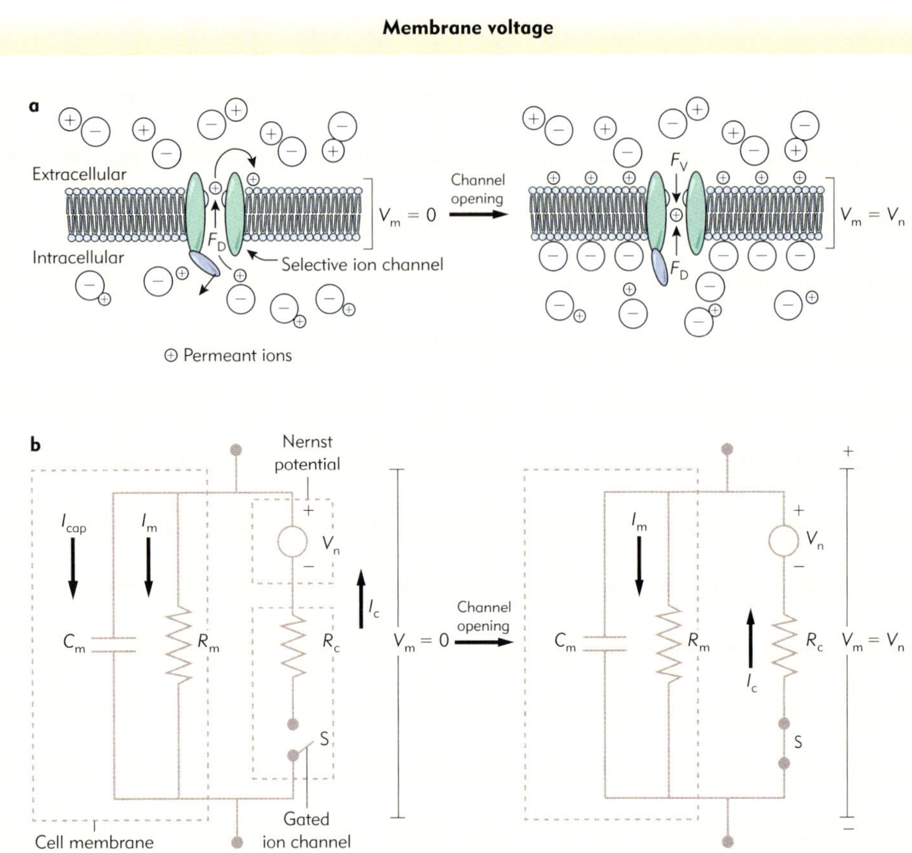

Figure 5.5 Membrane voltage. (a) Larger impermeant cations are at a high concentration outside and permeant ions are inside. Channel opening allows the diffusional force (F_D) to drive permeant cations through the channel where they collect on the outer surface as a result of electrostatic attraction with partner anions that move to the inner surface. In the new equilibrium condition, the diffusional force (F_D) is equal to the electromotive force (F_V) as a result of V_m. At this equilibrium, V_m is equal to the Nernst potential (V_n) for the permeant ion. (b) The Nernst potential is shown as a source of voltage that can induce an ion channel current. Initially V_m is zero. When the channel opens (closure of switch S) the channel current (I_c) is composed of capacitive charging current (I_{cap}) and transmembrane resistive current (I_m). At the new equilibrium I_c is equal to I_m. The current magnitude is such that the voltage induced in R_m (membrane resistance) is equal to V_n, assuming $R_m >> R_c$. Therefore, V_m equals V_n.

Examples include the Na^+/K^+-dependent glutamate transporters, Na^+/Cl^--dependent GABA transporter, Na^+–Ca^{2+} exchanger, and the Na^+–glucose cotransporters (SGLTs).

Passive transporters move molecules down their electrochemical gradient, which is sometimes referred to as *facilitated* or *carrier-mediated diffusion*. The carrier rate has a maximum, indicating a specific binding process. As the concentration gradient for the transported molecule is increased, a maximum transport velocity (V_{max}) is reached that depends only on the total binding sites available. The Na^+-independent amino acid and glucose transporters are examples of passive transporters. For an uncharged molecule, the electrochemical gradient is the concentration gradient. For charged molecules, transport depends on membrane potential as well. Transporters can translocate a single molecule in one direction (*uniport*) or two or more molecules in the same (*symport*) or opposite (*antiport*) directions (Fig. 5.6).

Transporters as a current source

The Na^+/K^+-ATPase couples the translocation of three Na^+ outward and two K^+ inward, both against their electrochemical gradients. Because of the unequal 3:2 coupling, there is a net movement of positive charge out of the cell. In electrical terms, the Na^+/K^+-ATPase is *electrogenic*, causing an outward current. An electrogenic pump has two major implications for cell function. First, its transmembrane current affects membrane potential. For the Na^+/K^+-ATPase, the outward current hyperpolarizes the membrane. Inhibition of this pump by drugs such as digoxin immediately depolarizes the cell membrane. Second, electrogenic pumps are influenced by membrane potential. Depolarization of the membrane enhances cation pumping. Therefore, during times of intense membrane depolarization, such as during skeletal muscle activity with exercise, ionic gradients can run down. Under these conditions, Na^+/K^+-ATPase activity is increased, enhancing gradient restoration.

Membrane potential also modulates electrogenic secondary active transporters such as the GABA and glutamate transporters. The GABA transporter is a symport carrier that couples the transport of two Na^+, one Cl^-, and one GABA molecule into the cell. Since GABA has no net charge, at physiologic pH this results in net transport of one positive charge into the cell for each cycle. The glutamate transporter is an antiport carrier that couples the inward translocation of two Na^+ and a glutamate anion, with outward transport of K^+ and OH^-. Glutamate is negatively charged at physiologic pH, resulting in net transport of one positive charge into the cell. Thus both GABA and glutamate transporters are electrogenic, causing a net inward current, and like the Na^+/K^+-ATPase, they are sensitive to membrane potential.

Transporter reversal

Neurotransmitter transporters are responsible for sequestering neurotransmitters released during synaptic transmission. The rapid sequestration of neurotransmitters away from postsynaptic receptors ensures rapid termination of the signal, which allows for high-speed information transfer. They may also serve as a nonvesicular source of neurotransmitter release during pathophysiologic conditions (e.g. ischemia). Under normal conditions, the GABA transporter removes the inhibitory neurotransmitter GABA from the extracellular space against its

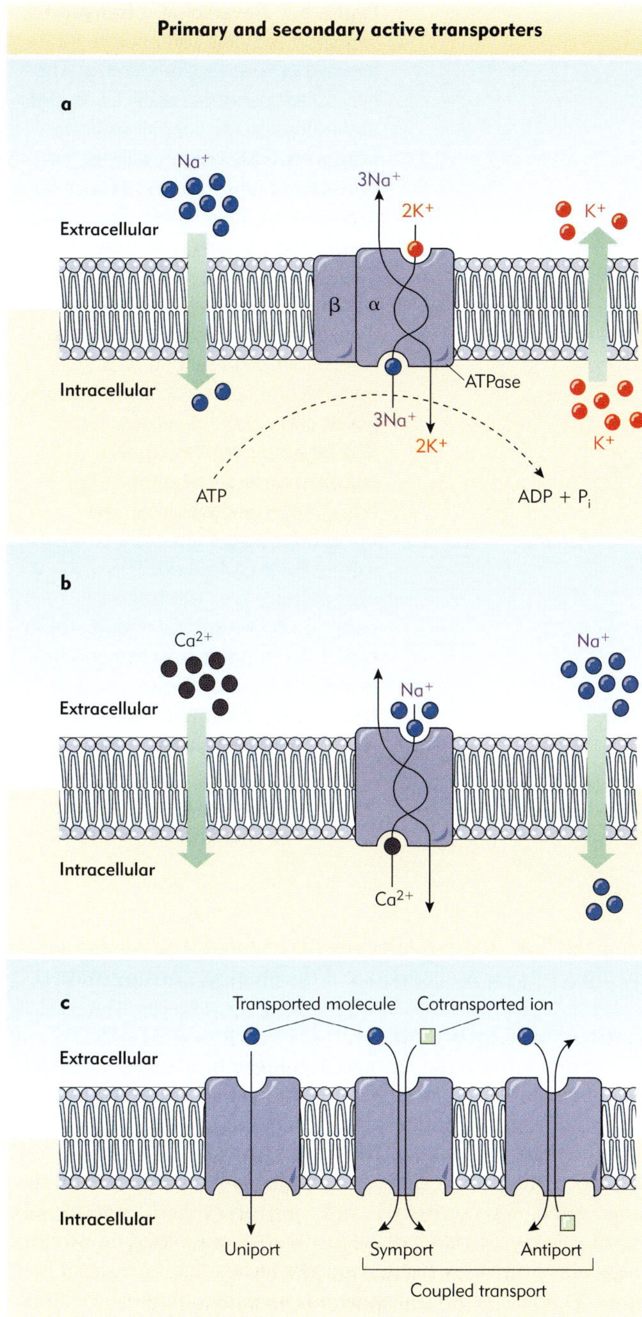

Figure 5.6 Primary and secondary active transporters. (a) The primary active transporter Na^+/K^+-ATPase has two binding sites for K^+ (red) facing the extracellular surface and three binding sites for Na^+ (blue) on the intracellular side. The movement of Na^+ outside and K^+ inside both against their respective concentration gradients (green arrows), is accomplished by energy derived from the hydrolysis of ATP. (b) The secondary active transporter Na^+–Ca^{2+} exchanger binds three Na^+ (blue) on the outside and one Ca^{2+} (black) inside. The translocation of Ca^{2+} against its concentration gradient is driven by the movement of Na^+. This carrier protein has 11 transmembrane domains; it does not hydrolyze ATP. (c) Three types of protein transporters exist depending on the coupling between the ions or molecules that they transport. Both active and passive transporters can function as uniporter, symporter, or antiporter. (Modified from Guyton, 1991; and Alberts et al., 1994.).

concentration gradient. With increased neuron excitability, such as during hypoxic–ischemic insult to the brain or seizure, the membrane depolarizes and the intracellular Na^+ concentration rises. Both factors oppose the normal inward electrogenic GABA transporter activity. In fact, under these conditions the GABA transporter may reverse, translocating Na^+, Cl^-, and GABA outward. γ-Aminobutyric acid can activate GABA receptors, inducing membrane hyperpolarization, and reducing electrical activity (Fig. 5.7a) such that reversal of the GABA transporter serves as a negative feedback mechanism, reducing neuronal excitability at times of greatest need.

In contrast, reversal of the glutamate transporter during neuronal hyperexcitability can result in greater glutamate release into the extracellular space, causing increased neuronal damage (Fig. 5.7b). During neuronal hyperexcitability, the increased intracellular Na^+ and extracellular K^+ concentrations and the depolarized membrane potential favor reversal of the glutamate transporter, resulting in the outward translocation of glutamate from the cytoplasmic pool. Released glutamate can activate its receptors leading to further neuronal excitation and ultimately to neuronal death ('excitotoxicity'). The *in vivo* significance of this positive feedback self-exacerbating mechanism may be limited by the effect of extracellular acidosis to block transporter function. Malfunction of the glutamate transporter may be important for the pathophysiology of a variety of neurodegenerative diseases.

CURRENT AND VOLTAGE MEASUREMENTS

A dramatic increase in our understanding of ion channels and carrier proteins has resulted largely from combining the powerful techniques of molecular biology (Chapter 4) and electrophysiology. This section provides an overview of selected electrophysiologic techniques that allow precise measurements of membrane currents and voltages.

Two-electrode voltage clamp

Channel currents are determined by the nature of channel opening, resistance or conductance, the Nernst potential, and membrane voltage. In order to study ion channel function, the essence of ion channel physiology, channel currents are precisely measured during the delivery of a triggering stimulus (for voltage-gated ion channels, a membrane voltage change).

The two-electrode voltage clamp technique yielded the first observations of currents through voltage-gated ion channels in the 1950s and remains an indispensable tool in ion channel physiology. This technique employs two electrodes to control or 'clamp' membrane voltage (V_m) (Fig. 5.8). The glass microelectrodes contain conducting solutions and communicate electrically with the cell cytosol. A voltage-sensing electrode in combination with a bath electrode provides measurement of V_m. When the gated channel opens, the resultant current (I_c) will drive V_m away from V_{ref} (see Fig. 5.8). This increases the error, causing an increase in I_a (current delivered by the amplifier) that exactly matches I_c to equalize V_m and V_{ref}. As a result, the change in I_a reports I_c under constant V_m. Two-electrode voltage clamp controls voltage of the entire cell membrane and, therefore, reports an average activity of all channels, which is known as *whole-cell* or *macroscopic* current. Two-electrode voltage clamp can only be used in cells large enough to tolerate puncture by two microelectrodes (e.g. cardiac Purkinje cells). As a result single-electrode voltage clamp techniques were developed, but the nature of currents through individual or *single channels* remained a mys-

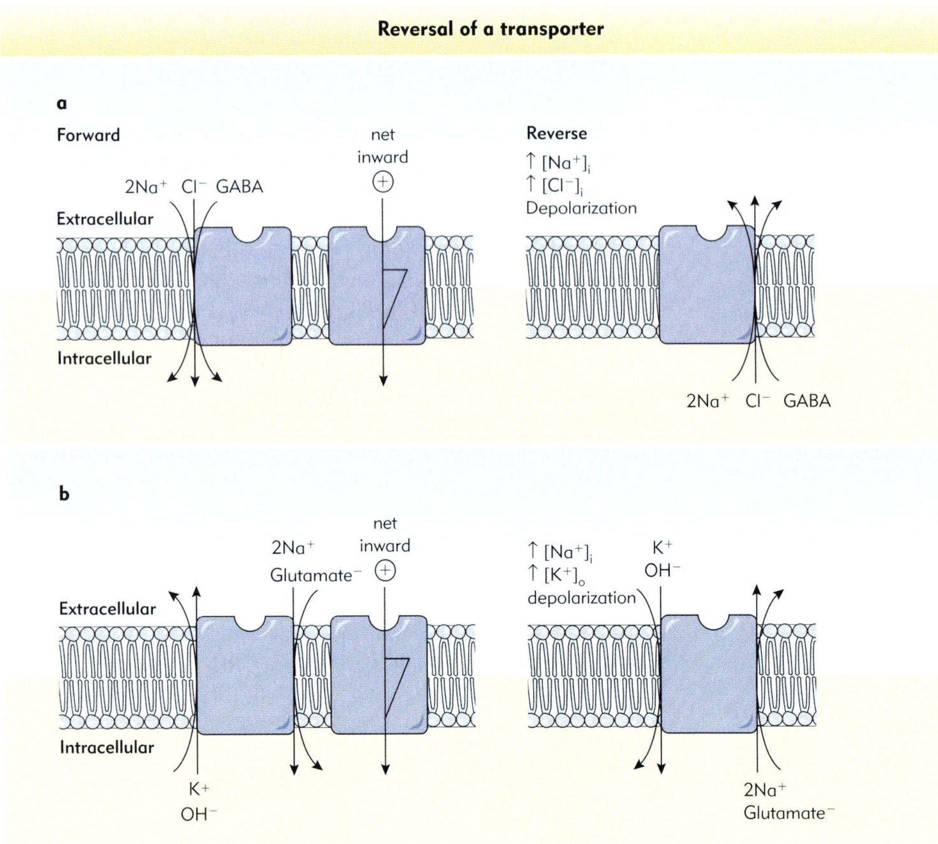

Figure 5.7 Reversal of a transporter. Transport proteins can operate in the forward or reverse direction. (a) The Na^+/Cl^--dependent GABA transporter under physiologic conditions (left) transports GABA along with the co-transported ions from the extracellular to the intracellular space. The net inward current flow is denoted as an inwardly directed current source. Under the conditions indicated (right), the transporter may operate in the reverse direction serving as a nonvesicular source of GABA release, which can act on its receptors to decrease neuronal excitability. (b) Normal forward operation of the Na^+/K^+-dependent glutamate transporter (left) sequesters extracellular glutamate. This transporter is also electrogenic causing an inwardly directed current. Under the conditions indicated (right), reversal of this transporter releases intracellular glutamate, exacerbating excitotoxicity of neurons.

tery until the 1970s when Neher and Sakmann developed the patch clamp technique, for which they received a Nobel Prize.

Patch clamp technique

The patch clamp technique provides voltage clamp of a membrane patch (hence the name). A single glass micropipette is pushed onto the cell membrane and negative pressure is carefully applied to form a 'tight seal' characterized by high resistance (giga-Ohm, >10exp12Ω). In essence, the electrode isolates and captures all the ions flowing through the $\sim 2\mu m^2$ membrane bounded by the micropipette. In this fashion, ionic current passing through a single channel in the membrane patch can be collected and measured. These *single-channel* or *microscopic currents* reflect closed or open conducting states (Fig. 5.9). Open channels conduct *unitary current,* which is determined by channel conductance, ionic conditions, and membrane potential. Single channel activity reports transitions among numerous possible conformational states; the analysis of these data requires probabilistic techniques such as histogram analysis. The patch clamp technique has a number of variations for the measurement of single channel currents that include cell-attached inside-out, cell-free inside-out and outside-out, as well as whole-cell formations.

Lipid bilayer technique

The lipid bilayer technique also allows the study of single channel activity. The recording chamber comprises two wells separated by a thin wall containing a 250μm hole, which is painted with lipid solution to form a lipid bilayer. Channel-containing vesicles are introduced in one well and fuse with the lipid covering the hole, thereby inserting the channel. The voltage across the lipid bilayer is clamped and the channel current studied.

Extracellular recording

While much has been learned about the fundamental properties of excitable membranes through voltage clamp techniques that require intracellular microelectrodes, essentially all clinical information is obtained through extracellular recording (e.g. electrocardiogram, electroencephalogram, and nerve conduction such as sensory- and motor-evoked potentials). Extracellular recording of electrical activity is based on two fundamental principles: excited membrane serves as a current generator, and current flowing between any two points on a tissue can be recorded as a resistive voltage difference.

The first principle is easy to understand based on the preceding discussions on gated ion channels. The net current flow across a short segment of axon or a membrane patch changes from zero at rest to net inward current at the peak of an action potential (inward Na^+ channels are fully open) to net outward current during the falling phase of an action potential (outward K^+ channels are fully open), and back to zero. These events sequentially cause the excitable membrane to be a current sink, then a current source, before returning to zero current. The charge flow that feeds the current sink or accepts the current source comes from the extracellular space surrounding the excitable membrane. When many membrane patches act as a time-dependent current generator, a corresponding extracellular current flow occurs. Quantitatively, the transmembrane current (i.e. the net current that flows across the cell membrane via the ion channels) is directly proportional to the first derivative of the extracellular

Two-electrode voltage clamp measurement of channel currents

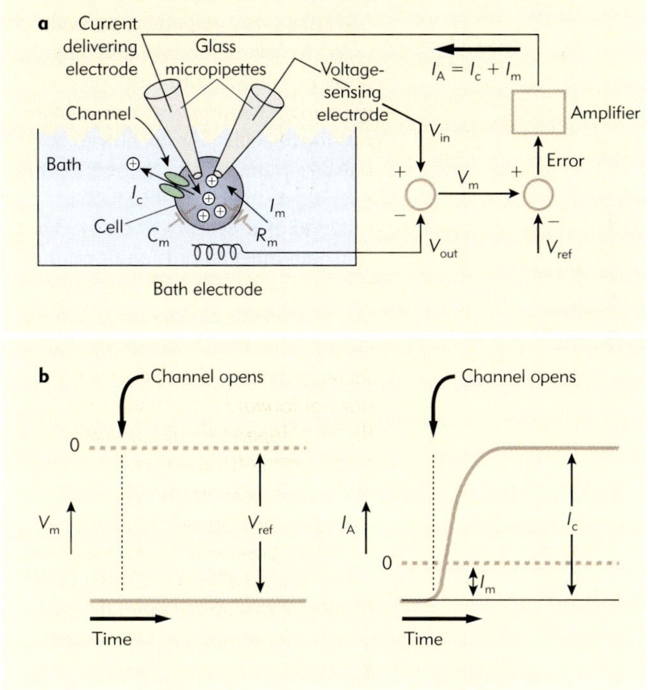

Figure 5.8 Two-electrode voltage clamp measurement of channel currents. (a) The method is illustrated for a single cell with a gated ion channel selective for an intracellular cation (circle with plus sign) that is concentrated in the cytosol. Electrical elements representing membrane capacitance (C_m) and resistance (R_m) are superimposed on the membrane. The intracellular voltage (V_{in}) is assayed by a glass micropipette (diameter 10^{-6}m) and voltage-sensing electrode. The transmembrane voltage (V_m) is determined by comparing V_{in} with the bath voltage (V_{out}) detected by the bath electrode (coiled wire); V_m is compared with its desired value (V_{ref}). The difference represents an error signal that is fed to an amplifier; this then generates a proportional current (I_A) that is delivered to the cell via a second electrode (current delivering). (b) Changes in V_m (left) and I_A (right) over time are also shown. Initially, when the gated channel is closed, I_A is equal to the negative resistive current (I_m) necessary to cause the voltage induced in R_m and, therefore, V_m to equal V_{ref} (< 0mV). Channel opening results in an outward hyperpolarizing current. The setup delivers additional current equal to I_c in order to maintain equality between V_m and V_{ref} (negative feedback control). This technique allows measurement of ion channel current at constant V_m.

action current. In experimental recording situations such as extracellular recording from a hippocampal slice preparation, this relationship is utilized and the first-derivative of the initial upstroke of the extracellular action current is used as an indirect measure of the transmembrane current indicative of the synaptic strength. In clinical situations when a fairly well-defined large amount of excitable tissue undergoes a more or less uniform change in its excitability (such as during the stimulation of a nerve bundle during a nerve conduction test) the total extracellular current flow resulting from these changes is recorded as the compound action potential. When billions of nerve cells all fire in a synchronous manner in the brain, all individually contributing a miniscule amount of extracellular current, the net aggregate extracellular current flow as recorded on the surface of the scalp is the *electroencephalogram* (EEG) (Chapter 13).

The second principle states that the final magnitude of the recording is a product of the actual current flow and the extracellular resistance between the two recording points. For a given amount of current flow, the ohmic voltage drop is proportional to the resistance. Therefore, a low-resistance contact provided by the electrocardiogram pads and the precise placement of the leads becomes essential for obtaining reproducible results (Chapter 12).

MEASUREMENT OF ION CONCENTRATIONS

Ion channels and protein carriers maintain the vital intracellular ion and substrate concentrations. Direct physicochemical techniques, such as radioisotopic tracer or ion-selective microelectrode methods, allow measurements of intracellular ion concentrations. Optical methods based on ion-selective indicators are now popular. Their principal advantages are that they are noninvasive and allow high spatial resolution of intracellular ion concentrations at the level of individual cells and organelles.

The physical principles underlying optical measurement of intracellular ions should be familiar to clinical anesthesiologists. The method is based on a concentration-dependent change in the absorbence/emission of light at a given wavelength, analogous to the principles underlying oxygen saturation determination by pulse oximetry (Chapter 15). Thus, determination of functional oxygen saturation of hemoglobin is accomplished by comparing light absorbence at 660 and 940nm. At 660nm, reduced hemoglobin (higher extinction coefficient) absorbs light better than oxyhemoglobin (lower extinction coefficient) while at 940nm the converse is true. Modern pulse oximeters take measurements of light absorption at these two wavelengths nearly 500 times a second and calculate the relative amounts of oxyhemoglobin and reduced hemoglobin and determine the hemoglobin oxygen saturation. Optical methods of determining ion concentrations follow the same principle. Binding of specific ions to their respective indicator molecule results in altered spectral properties. Unlike hemoglobin, many of the newly developed ion-selective indicators are fluorescent molecules. Light at shorter wavelength (excitation wavelength) is absorbed and lower energy light at a longer wavelength is given off (emission wavelength). Upon binding of a specific ion to its indicator, the emission and/or the excitation spectrum changes. For example, the commonly used Ca^{2+} indicator Fura-2 has a characteristic emission peak at 510nm. This molecule shows a Ca^{2+}-dependent increase in fluorescence with excitation at 340nm and concomitant decreases in fluorescence with excitation at 380nm. As the availability of free Ca^{2+} increases, the light intensity ratio measured at 510nm owing to excitation at 340nm compared with 380nm increases. Ion-selective indicators for other divalent ions (e.g. Mg^{2+}, Zn^{2+}, Cu^{2+}), for monovalent ions (e.g. Na^+, K^+, Cl^-), and for other inorganic ions are also available.

RELEVANCE TO ANESTHESIA

Voltage-gated ion channels not only are vital for normal cell function, but also may serve as important pharmacologic targets for anesthetic drugs. The Na^+ channels are clear targets of the local anesthetics, a vital class of drug used in major nerve conduction blockade (Chapter 28) and as cardiac antiarrythmics

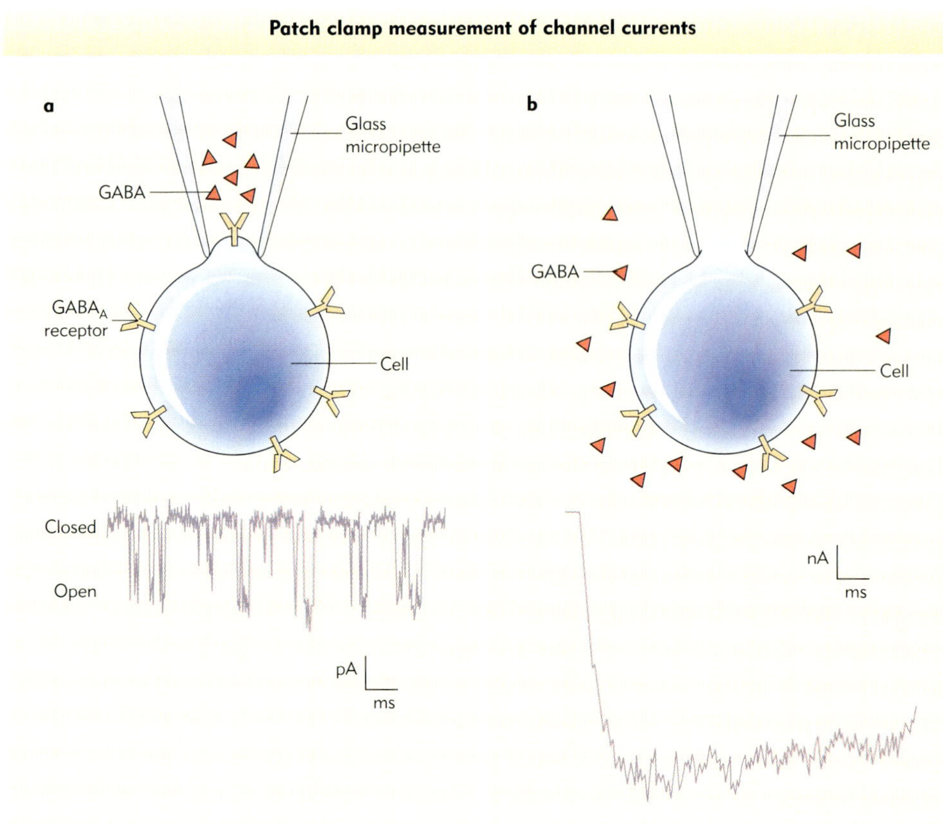

Figure 5.9 Patch clamp measurement of channel currents. In the 'membrane patch' arrangement (a) a glass micropipette is pushed onto the cell membrane and negative pressure is applied to the micropippette lumen to form a high-resistance seal. γ-Aminobutyric acid (GABA) in the pipette triggers the opening of the channel, which is reported as a Cl^- current below. These single-channel records demonstrate that individual channels open in a quantal fashion to conduct a unitary current. The membrane patch can be 'ripped' off the cell to achieve a cell-free inside-out configuration, (b) which allows the delivery of agents to the cytoplasmic side of the channel and membrane. In the 'whole-cell' configuration, transient negative pressure applied to the micropipette lumen disrupts the membrane patch, allowing the pipette lumen to communicate with the cell cytosol electrically. Delivery of GABA to the cell exterior triggers channel opening. The recorded current reflects the averaged activity of numerous channels in the entire membrane.

(Chapter 35). Recent evidence also suggests that Na^+ channels may be blocked by anesthetic agents and perhaps play a role in the mechanism of general anesthesia. The Ca^{2+} channels are blocked by volatile anesthetic agents, which may underly their cardiodepressant effects (see Chapters 24 and 34). Blockade of Ca^{2+} channels in the CNS may also play a role in the mechanism of general anesthesia. Experimental evidence indicates that the GABA$_A$ receptor is also a potential target for general anesthetics. Essentially all general anesthetics, both intravenous and inhalational, directly gate the GABA$_A$ channel and potentiate the action of GABA (Chapters 22–24). The idea that general anesthetics depress the brain by mimicking or potentiating the function of an inhibitory neurotransmitter is appealing. Recently, investigations have begun to identify the site(s) on the GABA$_A$ receptor where general anesthetics act. Use of techniques outlined in this chapter to define sites of general anesthetic action may allow the development of better agents devoid of side effects or of antagonists (i.e. general anesthetic reversal compounds).

Key References

Alberts B, Bray D, Lewis J, et al. Carrier proteins and active membrane transport. In: Lewis J, Rass M, Roberts K, Watson JD (eds). Molecular biology of the cell, 3rd edn. New York: Garland; 1994:512–22.

Amara SG, Arriza JL. Neurotransmitter transporters: three distinct gene families. Curr Opin Neurobiol. 1993;3:337–44.

Attwell D, Barbour B, Szatkowski M. Nonvesicular release of neurotransmitter. Neuron. 1993;11:401–7.

Catterall WA. Structure and function of voltage-gated ion channels. Trend Neurosci. 1993;16:500–4.

Hamill OP, Marty A, Neher E, Sakmann B, Sigworth FJ. Improved patch-clamp techniques for high-resolution current from cells and cell-free membrane patches. Pfluger Arch. 1981;391:85–100.

Rabow LE, Russek SJ, Farb DH. From ion current to genomic analysis: recent advances in GABA, receptor research. Synapse. 1995;21:189–274.

Richerson GB, Gaspary HL. Carrier-mediated GABA release: is there a functional role? Neuroscientist. 1997;3:151–7.

Further Reading

Yaksh TL, Lynch III C, Zapol WM, Maze M, Biebuyck JF, Saidman LJ. (eds). Anesthesia: biological foundations. Philadelphia, PA: Lippinincott-Raven; 1998.

Haugland RP (ed.). Handbook of fluorescent probes and research chemicals: molecular probes, 6th edn. Eugene, OR: Molecular Probes Inc; 1996.

Hille B (ed.). Ion channels of excitable membranes, 2nd edn. Sunderland, MA: Sinauer;1992.

Kandel ER, Schwartz JH, Jessel TM. (eds). Principles of neural science, 4th edn. Norwalk, CT: Appleton and Lange; 1996.

Sakmann B, Neher E (eds). Single-channel recording, 2nd edn. New York: Plenum; 1995.

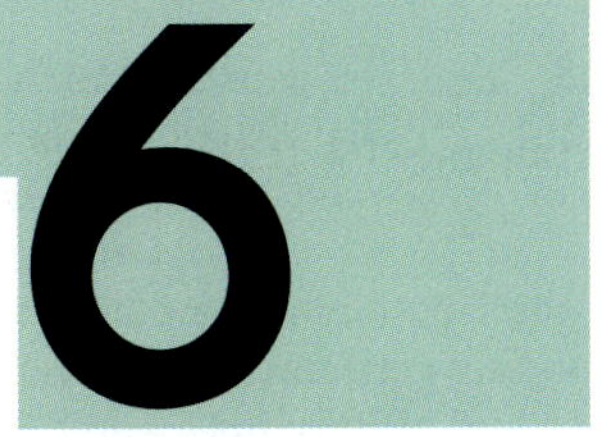

Chapter 6 Sites of drug action

John V Booth and Debra A Schwinn

Topics covered in this chapter

Nature of receptors
Receptor characterization
Receptor theories
Concentration–response relationships
Measurement of biological responses
Interactions of agonists with antagonists

NATURE OF RECEPTORS

A vast array of hormones, autocoids, neurotransmitters, toxins, and drugs transfer information to cells by interaction with specific membrane proteins known as receptors. The concept of specific sites residing on cell membranes with cognitive and transitive properties for drugs emerged at the turn of the century as a result of studies by Ehrlich (1854–1915), through his experiments with tissue stains, snake venoms, and bacterial toxins, and Langley (1852–1926), who studied the effects of pilocarpine and atropine on salivary secretion. The first axiom of a drug-initiated response is that the drug molecule and biological target must come together; they do not act at a distance. But mere interaction does not address selectivity. Therefore the second axiom is that the interaction must result in selective binding of drug to the biological target before a response occurs. This emphasizes the concept of *molecular level recognition.* Biological molecules which bind drugs must have locales both spatially and energetically favorable for binding of specific drug molecules. These locales are termed 'receptors' in a general sense.

Most drug binding sites discovered thus far are present on proteins, glycoproteins, or proteolipids (some drugs are capable of interacting with DNA directly). Proteins are folded to form unique three-dimensional structures, providing binding sites of the correct three-dimensional shape to accommodate drug molecules. Although receptors are present on cell membranes, in the cytoplasm, and in the nucleus, most receptors that bind water-soluble drugs and hormones are cell membrane proteins. The cell membrane consists of a phospholipid bilayer (Chapter 2). Phospholipid molecules are amphipathic; they contain two distinct regions, one nonpolar (consisting of tails of the fatty acyl chains), and the other polar (consisting of charged phosphate, choline, and ethanolamine head groups). Nonpolar regions tend to avoid contact with water by facing inward and self-associating, whereas polar headgroups tend to interact with water through hydrogen bonds. These interactions are optimized by the structure of the cell membrane (Fig. 6.1).

Proteins are important constituents of the cell membrane. Peripheral proteins are associated with external or internal surfaces of the lipid bilayer, while integral proteins are deeply embedded in the membrane. Membrane receptor proteins are integral transmembrane proteins, with extracellular portions binding water-soluble ligands, and intracellular portions capable of interacting with intracellular proteins in second messenger pathways (Chapter 3). Characteristically, transmembrane regions of receptors are formed by α helices composed of 19 to 24 predominantly lipophilic amino acids with nonpolar side groups. Several basic amino acids typically constitute the cytoplasmic end of the transmembrane sequence. These are believed to interact with phosphate headgroups of the bilayer and to anchor the receptor so that it cannot 'slip' from the bilayer.

Although movement of membrane receptors into and out of the bilayer is restricted by the amphipathic nature of the receptor, lateral diffusion of the receptor within the plane of the membrane occurs, unless specifically restrained by interaction with intracellular cytoskeletal elements. This lateral diffusion has been demonstrated experimentally by labeling receptors with fluorescently-tagged ligands and measuring rates of diffusion of the fluorescent tags into membrane areas rendered nonfluorescent by photobleaching. Lateral diffusion of receptors is an important concept because it means that membrane receptors can interact freely with other membrane proteins.

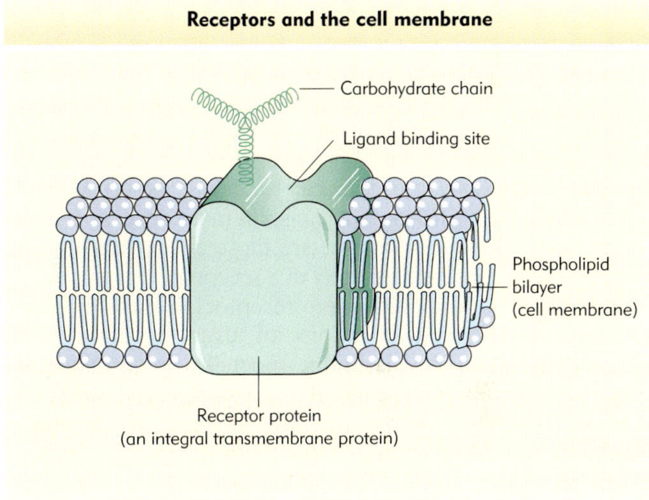

Figure 6.1. Receptors and the cell membrane.

Indeed, many receptors depend on such interactions to trigger a cellular response to receptor–ligand binding.

In summary, common properties of transmembrane receptors include those essential for all receptors, namely *recognition* of extracellular substances and *transduction* of information of these substances to the intracellular machinery. Models describing the interactions between receptors and ligands are useful in predicting drug effects. As modeling becomes more complex, aided by new discoveries at the molecular level, drugs can be designed with greater specificity and defined mechanisms to produce more refined effects.

RECEPTOR CHARACTERIZATION

Traditionally, drug receptors have been identified and classified primarily on the basis of the effects and relative potency of selective agonists and antagonists. For example, acetylcholine effects mimicked by the action of muscarine and selectively antagonized by atropine are classified as *muscarinic* effects. Other effects of acetylcholine mimicked by nicotine and not readily antagonized by atropine, but antagonized by other agents (e.g. d-tubocurare), are classified as *nicotinic* effects. These distinct actions of acetylcholine are said to result from an affinity for either *muscarinic* or *nicotinic* receptors. This means of pharmacological classification is convenient to use and generally consistent with clinical practice. However, once a receptor 'type' is classified, it is necessary to understand drug–receptor interactions or pharmacodynamics in more detail to explain drug effects. *Pharmacodynamics* are those effects which occur once a drug arrives in the vicinity of a receptor.

An analysis of drug binding to receptors involves the relationship of the concentrations of drug, receptor, and drug–receptor complexes with the effect. This is best illustrated using the *law of mass action*. If one assumes (a) that an agonist (*a compound which activates a receptor*) interacts reversibly with its receptor, (b) that the resultant effect is proportional to the number of receptors occupied, and (c) that the maximum effect occurs when all receptors are occupied, then Equation 6.1 holds:

Equation 6.1

$$\text{Ligand (L)} + \text{Receptor (R)} \underset{k_2}{\overset{k_1}{\rightleftharpoons}} \underset{\text{(LR)}}{\text{Ligand–Receptor Complex}}$$

At equilibrium, ligand–receptor complexes form (k_1 = association rate constant) at the same rate as they dissociate (k_2 = dissociation rate constant). Equation 6.1 can be rearranged to define the equilibrium dissociation constant K_d:

Equation 6.2

$$\frac{[L][R]}{[LR]} = \frac{k_2}{k_1} = K_d$$

The K_d is the concentration of ligand which occupies half of the receptors at equilibrium. A small K_d means that the receptor has a high affinity for the ligand ($k_1 >> k_2$, i.e. fewer drug molecules are required to occupy 50% of the receptors). A large K_d means that the receptor has a low affinity for the ligand. The law of mass action also predicts the fractional receptor occupancy at equilibrium as a function of ligand concentration:

Equation 6.3

$$\text{Fractional occupancy (\% [LR])} = \frac{[L]}{[L] + K_d}$$

When $[L]=K_d$, the fractional occupancy = 0.5.

Saturation binding experiments are used to determine total receptor number and affinity for a specific ligand. This is performed by keeping the receptor concentration constant and measuring specific binding of various concentrations of radioligand at equilibrium. A plot of fractional occupancy (%[LR]), or the moles of ligand bound per mole of receptor, versus [L] produces a rectangular hyperbole (adsorption isotherm) that is usually transformed into a logarithmic scale (Fig. 6.2a). Notice that the log scale produces a symmetrical sigmoid curve (Fig. 6.2b); log [L] at half saturation will give log K_d. Specific binding at equilibrium is equal to the fractional occupancy times the total receptor number (B_{max}):

Equation 6.4

$$\text{Specific binding} = \text{fractional occupancy} \bullet B_{max} = \frac{B_{max} \bullet [L]}{K_d + [L]}$$

The B_{max} and K_d can be calculated directly from the saturation binding curve of Fig. 6.2 by fitting the data to Equation 6.4 using nonlinear regression analysis. Historically, before nonlinear regression analysis, data from saturation binding experiments were transformed into a linear graph to aid analysis. One way to linearize data is the Scatchard (or Rosenthal) plot, which is widely used in studying receptor–ligand interactions (Fig. 6.2c). In this plot, the x-axis is specific binding [LR] and the y-axis is the ratio of specific binding to concentration of free ligand [L]; B_{max} is the x-intercept and the K_d is the negative reciprocal of the slope. Although Scatchard plots are useful for visualizing data, they have inherent inaccuracies since linear transformations can distort data.

Competition binding experiments measure binding of a single concentration of radiolabeled ligand (usually $[L] = K_d$) in the presence of increasing concentrations of unlabeled ligand. These experiments are useful in determining whether a drug binds to a specific receptor and with what affinity, and in determining receptor number and affinity (particularly when two or more receptor subtypes are present).

Molecular characterization of receptor protein is difficult since membrane receptors (the majority of clinically important receptors) are present in very small concentrations compared with other membrane proteins. Strategies for studying receptors often require purified receptor protein. Solubilization with detergents is required to release receptor protein from the lipid membrane environment, following which proteins carrying the binding sites can be isolated and purified, and the overall receptor structure determined. Purified receptor protein can then be reconstituted into artificial lipid membranes in order to study receptor function. Since the total amount of receptors present in tissues is extremely low, the development of purification processes with sufficient specificity is essential. Purification usually relies on the use of affinity chromatographic techniques in which solubilized receptors are exposed to a solid resin matrix (column) containing drug that binds the receptor of interest. However purification of receptors was a tedious process until the advent of molecular biology techniques. Molecular cloning of the cDNAs encoding distinct receptors

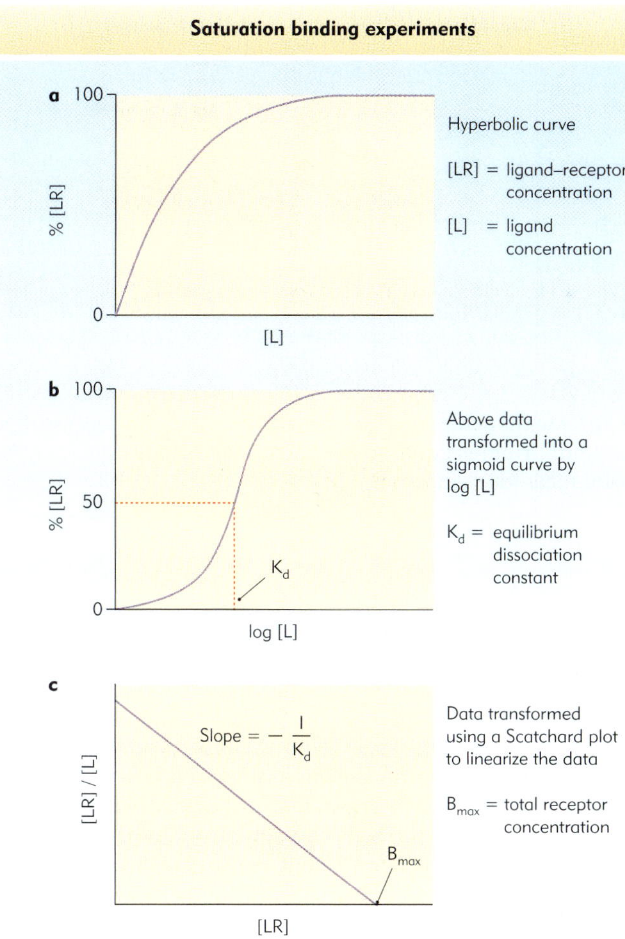

Figure 6.2. Saturation binding experiments. (a) Hyperbolic curve. (b) Above data transformed into a sigmoid curve by log [L]. K_d = equilibrium dissociation constant. (c) Data transformed using a Scatchard plot to linearize the data. The concentration of bound ligand/concentration of free ligand (can be assumed to be equal to [L] if [L] >>[receptor]) is plotted against the concentration of bound ligand. The example shown is for a simple case of one binding site, which yields a linear plot. The x-intercept is the maximum concentration of bound ligand, which is assumed to be the same as the total concentration of the receptor.

has revolutionized receptor biochemistry. cDNA cloning is the process by which the messenger RNA (mRNA) encoding the receptor of interest, in the form of the more stable and manipulable complementary DNA (cDNA), is isolated. The cDNA is placed into bacteria capable of making many copies of the desired DNA fragment, and then extracted from bacteria by cell lysis. DNA encoding a distinct receptor can then be expressed in cells not normally containing the receptor, and the expressed protein tested using classic ligand binding techniques. Receptor 'over expression' (expression at much higher concentrations than normally present in native tissues) in these cells facilitates receptor purification for biochemical studies. An explosion in identification and characterization of receptors and receptor subtypes has occurred using molecular biology techniques, revolutionizing the field of molecular pharmacology (Chapter 4).

RECEPTOR THEORIES

Numerous mathematical, thermodynamic, and biochemical models have been formulated to describe the interactions of receptors and their ligands. However, four main theories have been used over the years to describe drug–receptor interactions.

The preeminent receptor theory is *occupation theory*, which holds that transmembrane receptor activation induced by ligand binding is required for a signal to be transduced to the intracellular space. The essential features of this theory are that drug-mediated responses are dependent on four factors: [R], receptor density; *f*, the efficiency of the process converting receptor stimulus to cellular response; K_d, the equilibrium dissociation constant; and ϵ, the intrinsic efficacy of the drug acting on the receptor. These last two parameters are specific for each drug–receptor interaction, and are generally independent of species, cell type, or tissue response. Therefore these measured parameters form the basis of receptor pharmacology. The theory can be summarized in Equation 6.5. A number of assumptions are used to construct this model. Of particular relevance is the assumption that the concentration of drug in the receptor compartment or biophase (region immediately surrounding the receptor) rises instantaneously to the equilibrium concentration. However many drug–receptor interactions do not adhere to this ideal situation due to pharmacokinetic considerations; as a result, quantitation of these interactions is often hampered.

Equation 6.5

$$\text{Response} = f\left[\frac{\epsilon \bullet [R]}{1 + K_d/[L]}\right]$$

A second drug–receptor interaction model that has both theoretical and practical advantages over the classic occupation theory is the *operational model.* This model originates with the experimental observation that most drug concentration-response curves describe a rectangular hyperbole (Fig. 6.2a). Thus the model is experimentally accessible and can be tested by producing a saturation curve (described previously). This is a simpler model than the occupation model in that drug–receptor interactions can be described in terms of three parameters: K_d, [R], and K_e, the concentration of ligand–receptor complex ([LR]) that elicits half-maximal cellular response.

An alternative model, based on the kinetics of onset and offset of drug binding at a receptor, is referred to as the *rate theory*. This receptor theory specifically addresses the experimental observation that antagonists act more slowly than agonists and that the rate of offset of an antagonist is often inversely proportional to its potency. The underlying premise is that it is the rate of drug–receptor interaction that produces a response, not the occupation of receptor by drug.

A combination of elements from both the rate theory and occupation theory models is accommodated by the fourth model, the *receptor-inactivation model*. This theory of receptor–drug interaction proposes that ligands bind to a receptor with an onset rate k_1 and an offset rate k_2 to form a ligand–receptor complex; formation of the ligand–receptor complex transforms the receptor into an inactive state (incapable of further activation or binding), governed by the rate constant k_3. Receptor inactivation predicts a transient peak receptor response followed by a reduced steady state (fade). This model is difficult to test experimentally on the basis of fade.

In the quest to simplify receptor–ligand binding concepts, a *two-state model* has recently been proposed to explain results from transgenic animals where receptors have been massively over-expressed. This theory suggests that a dynamic equilibrium exists between inactive receptor (R) and activated receptor (R*).

Equation 6.6

$$\mathbf{R} \rightleftharpoons \mathbf{R}^*$$

The ratio of R/R* depends on the tissue studied, and possibly on the receptor itself. In native tissues, although R* is present, it is in such low concentration in the unstimulated state that baseline effects are not seen (equilibrium is toward the left, i.e. toward R). However, in transgenic animals where receptors are over-expressed 1000-fold, effects of R* are seen as increased basal activity of receptor function in the absence of agonist. In this theory, agonists bind selectively to R* and stabilize the activated receptor, while antagonists bind equally to R and R*, and inverse agonists bind selectively to R to stabilize the inactive form of the receptor (Fig. 6.3, Equation 6.7).

Equation 6.7

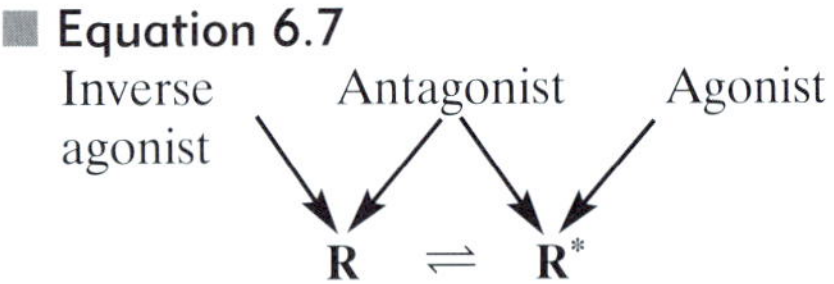

Inherent in this theory is the concept of protein *allosterism* (literally, other site), a property that describes proteins as malleable structures with a range of three-dimensional conformations that may accommodate cooperative interactions between ligands binding at multiple sites. This is well illustrated in the ability of hemoglobin to undergo conformational changes after binding of an oxygen molecule; allosteric effects facilitate cooperative binding of subsequent oxygen molecules. This interaction (e.g. oxygen binding) is mathematically described by a sigmoidal relationship rather than a hyperbolic curve. Recent pharmacologic evidence suggests that instead of two forms of the receptor (R and R*), several gradations may exist between R and R* (Equation 6.8). Although this equation is more physiologically correct, the two-state theory provides an understandable explanation for most receptor–drug interactions observed in the clinical setting.

Equation 6.8

$$\mathbf{R} \rightleftharpoons R^A \rightleftharpoons R^B \rightleftharpoons R^C \rightleftharpoons \mathbf{R}^*$$

CONCENTRATION–RESPONSE RELATIONSHIPS

The binding of ligand to receptor leads to enhancement, inhibition, or blockade of molecular signaling 'downstream' of the receptor. The molecular signal is amplified through a series of biochemical and physical interactions to produce an observable pharmacological response (e.g. epinephrine administration increases heart rate). However, receptor theories thus far presented do not address the amount of drug required to obtain a specific magnitude and duration of clinical response. To answer these questions, concepts of agonist potency and efficacy must be introduced.

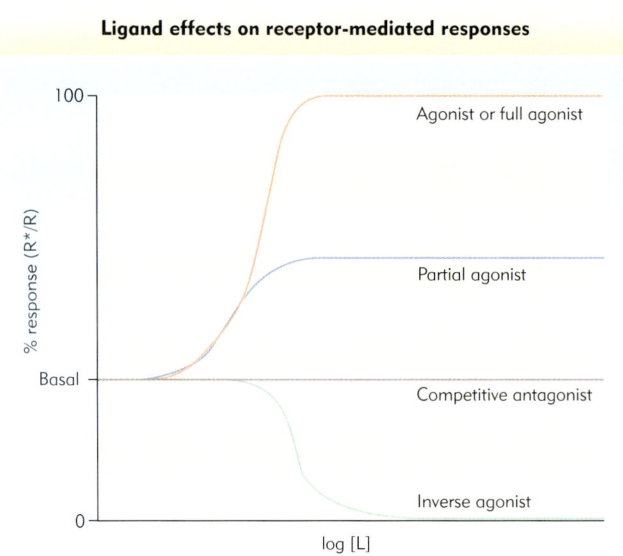

Figure 6.3. Ligand effects on receptor-mediated responses.

Agonists

An *agonist* is defined as a ligand which activates a receptor upon binding. This term is generally applied to a *full agonist*, that is an agonist which causes maximal activation of a receptor (Fig. 6.3). Using the R, R* nomenclature introduced earlier, a full agonist sufficiently stabilizes the active conformation (R*), so that at a saturating concentration it will drive the equilibrium completely to the active state (R*) (Equation 6.6). *Potency* is a term used to differentiate agonists which activate the same receptor but require different concentrations of each drug to achieve the same maximal biological effect (Fig. 6.4). Note, as illustrated in Fig. 6.4, the most potent drug (Drug 1) has the smallest K_d, whereas the least potent drug (Drug 4) has the largest K_d. The term *affinity* is often used instead of *potency*, and refers to the reciprocal of the K_d. *Partial agonists* are defined as drugs that produce submaximal tissue responses (Fig. 6.3); these drugs are able to block the effect of full agonists, sometimes mistakenly giving the appearance of an antagonist (Fig. 6.5). Hence, historically some partial agonists have been described as mixed agonist–antagonist drugs; however, this term is rarely used now.

Efficacy

It is necessary to differentiate the ability of a drug to bind to a receptor, *affinity*, from its ability to produce a change in the receptor resulting in stimulation, *efficacy*. Efficacy refers to the maximum magnitude of effect that can be achieved with a drug (Fig. 6.6), e.g. a partial agonist has lower efficacy than a full agonist. Drugs can alter receptor proteins by either *conformational induction* (whereby energy barriers between possible protein conformations of minimal free energy can be overcome by agonist binding) or *conformational selection* (selective binding of an agonist to one or more coexisting conformations of the receptor in equilibrium, inducing an equilibrium shift to the activated form). Thus, efficacy of a drug may be due to the extent to which an agent produces conformational induction or selection. The term *intrinsic activity* describes the relative maximum effects for a series of compounds, but is often used interchangeably with efficacy.

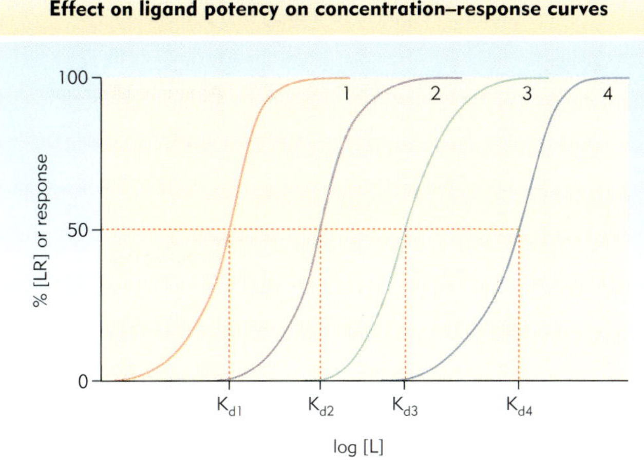

Figure 6.4. Effect of ligand potency on concentration–response curves. All sigmoid curves – parallel, all reacting 100% [LR]. Drug 1 – most potent, with smallest K_d (K_{d1}). Drug 4 – least potent, with largest K_d (K_{d4}). All drugs have same maximal response and differ only in *potency.*

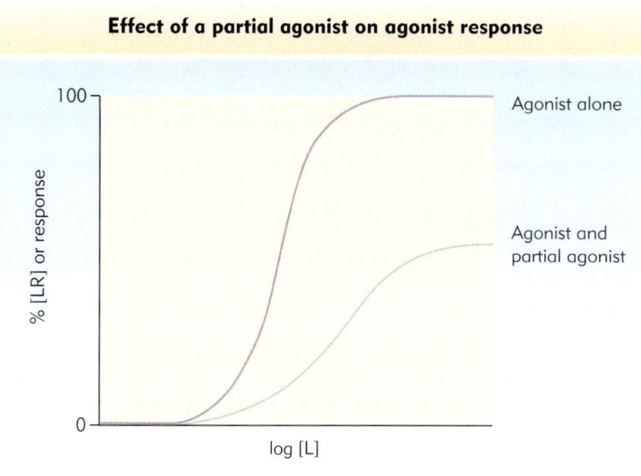

Figure 6.5. Effect of a partial agonist on agonist response. Agonist alone produces 100% response (sigmoid curve). Addition of partial agonist reduces maximal response of agonist.

Spare receptor concept

The relationship between receptor stimulus (percentage receptor occupation) and tissue response is usually nonlinear. This hyperbolic relationship (Fig. 6.7) illustrates the general phenomenon that maximal (or near maximal) responses can often be produced by stimulation of less than all of the receptors present in a given tissue. Further receptor occupancy or stimulation produces no further biological effect. This phenomenon has been given the name *spare receptor concept, receptor reserve, or spare capacity*. An example is provided by the pharmacologic effect of neuromuscular blocking drugs. Receptor occupancy of 70% by these cholinergic receptor antagonists produces no reduction in adductor pollicis muscle twitch in response to ulnar nerve stimulation; 80–90% of receptors need to be occupied before twitch reduction is demonstrated. Thus, activation of only 30% of the receptors is capable of eliciting a full response (Chapter 32).

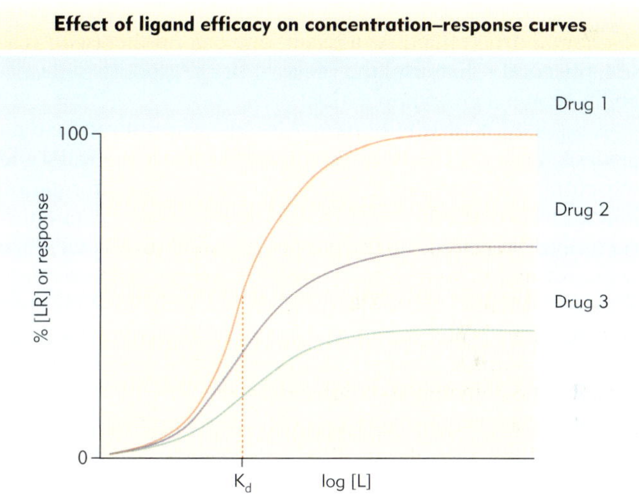

Figure 6.6. Effect of ligand efficacy on concentration–response curves. Series of agonists with constant potency (i.e. curves *not* shifted to left or right), but differing efficacies. Drug 1 is most efficacious, Drug 3 least efficacious.

MEASUREMENT OF BIOLOGICAL RESPONSES

Pharmacological responses can be defined as *graded* or *quantal*. The effect of epinephrine on heart rate is an example of a graded response, characterized by increasing magnitude of drug response with greater concentration of drug at the receptor site. Therefore, graded responses are described by the *magnitude* of the effect (see Fig. 6.4). Although most drugs produce a graded pharmacological response, for some drugs the observable response appears to be an 'all-or-none' event; this action is described as a *quantal* response. Of note, although an overt response may be quantal, underlying molecular mechanisms may still depend on the interaction of the drug with a specific number of receptors in a graded fashion (e.g. an all-or-none quantal response occurs once 50% of receptors are occupied). Since quantal responses are subject to inter-individual variability, whereby different concentrations of drug are required to trigger a biological response, the *frequency* of response in a population becomes the important variable in describing quantal effects. In clinical pharmacodynamic studies, graded responses can be examined in terms of quantal effect, being defined *a priori* in terms of what magnitude of effect would be clinically significant [e.g. anesthetic agents generally produce a graded response when administered, however minimal alveolar concentration (MAC) for inhalational anesthetics is decided using an *a priori* definition of surgical anesthesia, thereby converting a graded response to a quantal response; see Chapters 22 and 24].

Quantal responses require population statistics to describe the biological effect. Results can be plotted by comparing the number of subjects that respond at varying concentrations of drug. This produces a distribution curve with most of the subjects clustered around the central tendency (mean or median, Fig. 6.8a). The distribution is determined (Gaussian or non-Gaussian), which facilitates description of a population response

Relationship between receptor occupancy and biological response

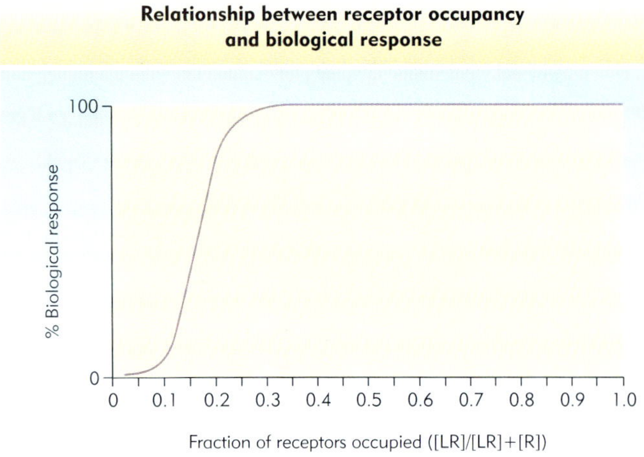

Figure 6.7. Relationship between receptor occupancy and biological response. Maximal (100%) or near maximal response can be achieved with only a small fraction of receptors occupied.

to quantal drug effect. As a result, one can predict (with reasonably good reliability) the range of drug response and variability within a given population.

A population distribution curve is not easily utilized for data analysis, since it is more complex to define mathematically and therefore more complex to interpret; however, the information may be transformed into a function that facilitates data interpretation. The effect can be plotted as cumulative percentage response against dose, transforming Gaussian distribution into a sigmoid curve (Fig. 6.8b). Notice this is similar to the transformation described from Fig. 6.2a to Fig. 6.2b, allowing a linearized portion of data to be represented approximately between the 20th and 80th percentiles.

Some drugs produce quantal population responses that have skewed distributions, that are fitted better using a logarithmic scale for the dose. An example is the effect of a chronotropic agent whereby heart rate can be increased over a much larger range than decreased without lethal consequences. The decision of which distribution function to use, and whether to transform data, must be assessed empirically for each drug and response. Note that in clinical practice these data are often represented as the *effective dose* (ED) at which 50% (ED_{50}) or 95% (ED_{95}) of the subjects respond (Fig. 6.8b). ED_{95} is often used to determine dose of induction agent or muscle relaxant in anesthetic practice. In animal studies a value for *lethal dose* (LD_{50}) may also be obtained; this is the dose resulting in 50% animal mortality. The ratio of LD_{50} to ED_{50} describes the *therapeutic ratio*, which estimates the relative safety of a drug dose that produces a clinical response.

Tolerance

Some individuals require unusually large concentrations of drug to achieve biological effect. This response is termed *hyporeactivity*, although when resulting from chronic exposure to a drug (e.g. alcohol) it is more correctly termed *tolerance*, *desensitization* or *tachyphylaxis*. Tolerance may develop secondary to enzyme induction (e.g. alcohol) or exaggerated/repeated physiologic responses (depletion of presynaptic neurotransmitters by excessive stimulated release). However, cellular tolerance usually involves protein conformational changes resulting from

Quantal response to a drug in a population

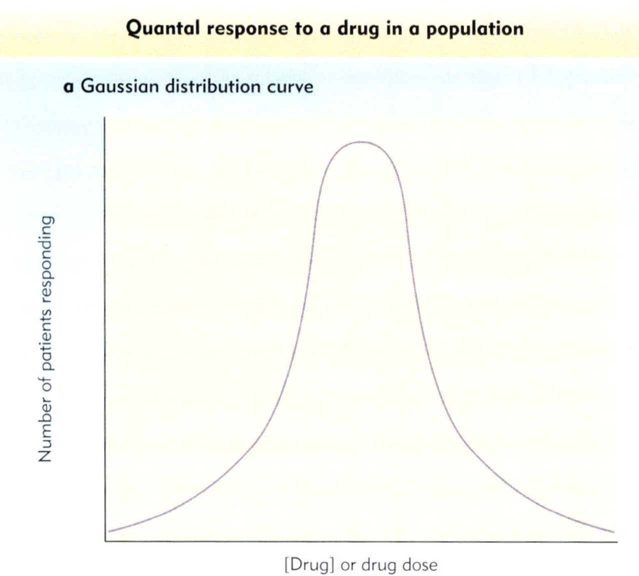

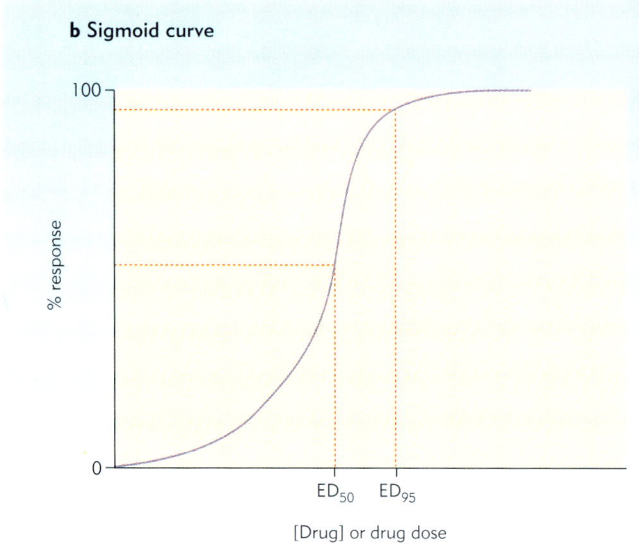

Figure 6.8. Quantal response to a drug in a population. (a) A Gaussian distribution curve, where most subjects are clustered around the mean, describes a quantal dose–response relationship. (b) Transforming the data in (a) by changing the y-axis to *cumulative* % responders produces a sigmoid curve. The effective dose in 50% (ED_{50}) and 95% (ED_{95}) of the population can then be derived.

phosphorylation of the receptor, and/or changes in gene expression, effectively uncoupling the receptor from downstream signal transduction pathways.

Antagonists/inverse agonists

Antagonism is the process by which an agonist-induced response is prevented or attenuated, resulting in the term *antagonists* to describe drugs that produce such effects (see Fig. 6.3). Antagonists can be subdivided by the kinetics and nature of their interactions with receptors. An antagonist that can dissociate (or be displaced) from a receptor produces *reversible antagonism*. An antagonist which forms a chemical bond with a receptor (e.g. alkylating agent) produces *irreversible antagonism*. Of note, 'irreversible' antagonism produced by drugs that dissociate extremely slowly from receptors is better classified as *pseudo-irreversible antagonism*. Some reversible antagonists may bind to a site on the receptor distinct from the agonist recognition site, but through allosteric or other mechanisms, prevent agonist activation of the receptor; this is termed *non-competitive* or *allotopic antagonism*. Alternatively, a reversible antagonist may also bind to the agonist recognition site, thereby competing for binding with the agonist, a process termed *competitive antagonism*.

Inverse agonists preferentially bind to the inactive receptor (R), and stabilize this conformation (see Equation 6.6). Hence inverse agonists actually produce effects opposite to that of agonists (see Fig. 6.3). Recently it has been demonstrated that some 'β-blockers' previously classified as β-adrenergic receptor *antagonists* are actually *inverse agonists,* e.g. timolol, alprenolol, nadolol, and possibly propranolol and metropolol. Inverse agonists have theoretical advantages over antagonists in disease processes where basal activity of a receptor is increased as a result of a conformational change to R* leading to increased signal transduction, since these agents may reverse an underlying mechanism in the disease process.

INTERACTIONS OF AGONISTS WITH ANTAGONISTS

Interactions between agonists and antagonists can be used to describe specific antagonist / receptor interactions. If inhibition by an antagonist can be overcome by increasing concentrations of agonist, ultimately achieving the same maximal agonist effect, the antagonist is by definition competitive. Figure 6.9a illustrates competitive antagonism, in which the log concentration–effect curve for an agonist is shifted to the right by a competitive antagonist, while retaining maximal effect. In contrast, a non-competitive antagonist prevents the agonist, at any concentration, from producing a maximal effect on a given receptor. This results in depression of maximal effect of agonist in the log concentration–effect curve (whether or not it is accompanied by a shift to the right; Fig. 6.9b).

Interactions between agonist and antagonist

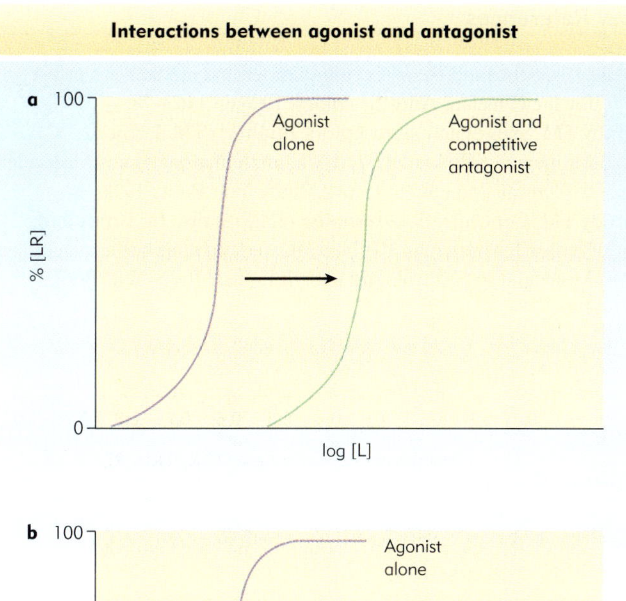

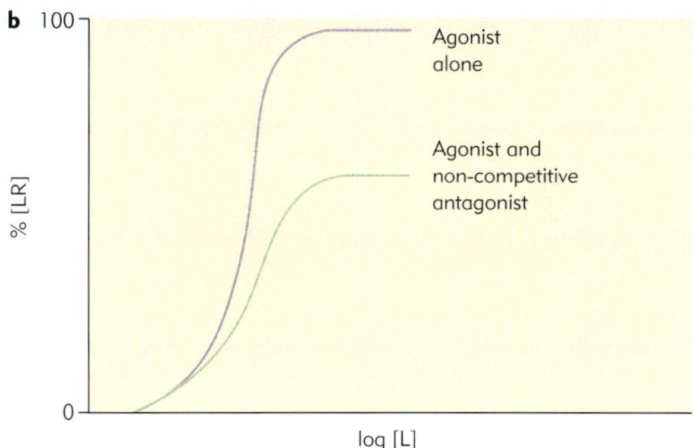

Figure 6.9. Interactions between agonist and antagonist. (a) Sigmoid curve of agonist shifted to right by addition of *competitive antagonist*. Note maximal biological effect remains unchanged, but requires increased agonist concentrations to achieve same maximal effect. (b) Maximal response of agonist is reduced by addition of *non-competitive antagonist* [unlike effect of addition of *competitive antagonist* in (a)].

Key References

Bello EA, Schwinn DA. Molecular biology and medicine: a primer for the clinician. Anesthesiology. 1996;85:1462–78.

Brody TM. Sites of action: receptors. In: Brody TM, Larner J, Minneman KP, Neu HC, (eds). Human Pharmacology: Molecular to Clinical, 2nd edn. St.Louis: Mosby Year Book; 1994.

Brody TM. Concentration–response relationships. In: Brody TM, Larner J, Minneman KP, Neu HC, (eds). Human Pharmacology: Molecular to Clinical, 2nd edn. St.Louis: Mosby Year Book; 1994:25–32.

Kenakin, TP. Pharmacologic Analysis of Drug-Receptor Interaction. New York: Raven Press; 1994.

Ross EM. Pharmacodynamics. In: Hardman JG, Limbird LE, Molinoff PB, Ruddon RW, Gilman AG, (eds). The Pharmacological Basis of Therapeutics, 9th edn. New York: McGraw-Hill; 1996:24–41.

Further Reading

Hulme EC. Receptor-Effector Coupling, 1st edn. Oxford: Oxford University Press; 1990.

Limbird LE. Cell Surface Receptors: A Short Course on Theory and Methods, 2nd edn. Boston: Kluwer Academic Publishers; 1996.

Chapter 7 Principles of pharmacokinetics

Christopher J Hull

Topics covered in this chapter

Drug uptake
Drug distribution
Drug elimination
Factors affecting drug disposition
Plasma concentration decay after single bolus dosing
Simple models of drug disposition
Population modelling

Anesthesia involves delivery of appropriate quantities of drugs to their sites of action to achieve the desired pharmacologic effects, followed by the removal of those drugs from their sites of action in a selective and controlled manner. In order to achieve these objectives, the pharmocokinetic characteristics of those drugs must be understood. Pharmacokinetics describes the uptake of drugs into the body, their distribution within it, and their elimination from the body (Fig 7.1). The sister discipline of pharmacodynamics considers the relation between drug concentration at the site of action and the time course and intensity of pharmacologic action (see Chapter 6).

DRUG UPTAKE

Oral administration

Drug administration by the oral route allows the pharmacist considerable control over the rate at which the drug becomes available for absorption, which makes it preferred under some circumstances. Figure 7.2 illustrates some of the processes involved.

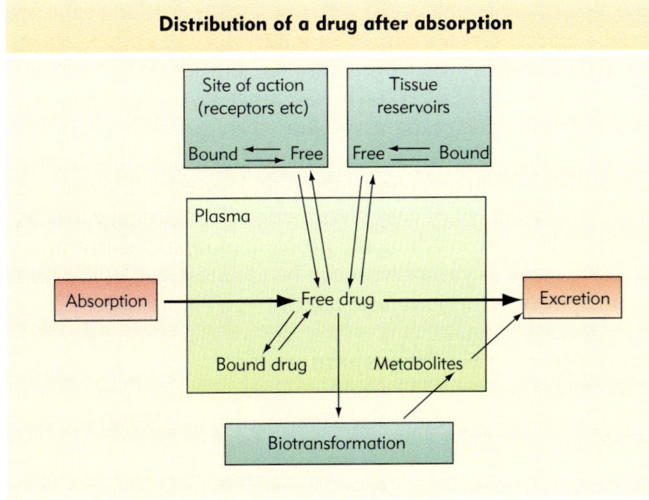

Figure 7.1 Distribution of a drug after absorption. (Adapted, with permission, from Hull, 1991)

Solution and dissolution

Before a drug can be absorbed, it must enter solution. Tablets may be formulated to disintegrate or even effervesce on contact with water, thus facilitating dissolution. Close compaction with binding agents results in much slower disintegration and, therefore, slower absorption. Capsules may have a variety of characteristics. In the simplest form, the envelope is made of gelatin, which prevents unpleasant taste but dissolves rapidly. Enteric-coated capsules resist gastric acid and release drug into the alkaline milieu of the upper jejunum, either to protect the stomach from irritants or to protect drugs such as penicillin from destruction by a strongly acid environment. Sustained-release formulations may be nonhomogeneous, with some elements disintegrating rapidly and others more slowly.

Diffusion

To cross cellular barriers such as the gastrointestinal mucosa, drugs must cross lipid membranes. Drugs do this mainly by passive diffusional transfer (see Fig. 7.2). The main factor that determines the rate of passive diffusional transfer across membranes is lipid solubility. Molecular weight is a less important factor. Many drugs are weak acids or weak bases, and their state of ionization varies with pH according to the Henderson–Hasselbalch equation. With weak acids or bases, only the uncharged species (the protonated form for a weak acid; the unprotonated form for a weak base) can diffuse across lipid membranes; this gives rise to pH partition. This means that weak acids tend to accumulate in zones of relatively high pH, whereas weak bases do the reverse.

The drug must dissolve in water to become diffusible. After this, absorption is enhanced by lipid solubility. Therefore, methadone is absorbed more rapidly than morphine. Many drugs, such as meperidine (pethidine), are almost entirely ionized at gastric pH; these are soluble but unavailable. Only on entering the more alkaline milieu of the small bowel does a significant fraction become free base and, therefore, absorbable. The opposite may also apply, as in the case of aspirin, which is poorly ionized in the acid medium of the stomach and undergoes rapid absorption after oral dosing. Consequently, the behavior of individual drugs depends upon whether they are acids or bases, and upon their pK_a values. In the case of drugs absorbed from the small bowel, the process may be both complex and unpredictable because of variation in the rate of gastric emptying caused by food, drugs, or disease. Food par-

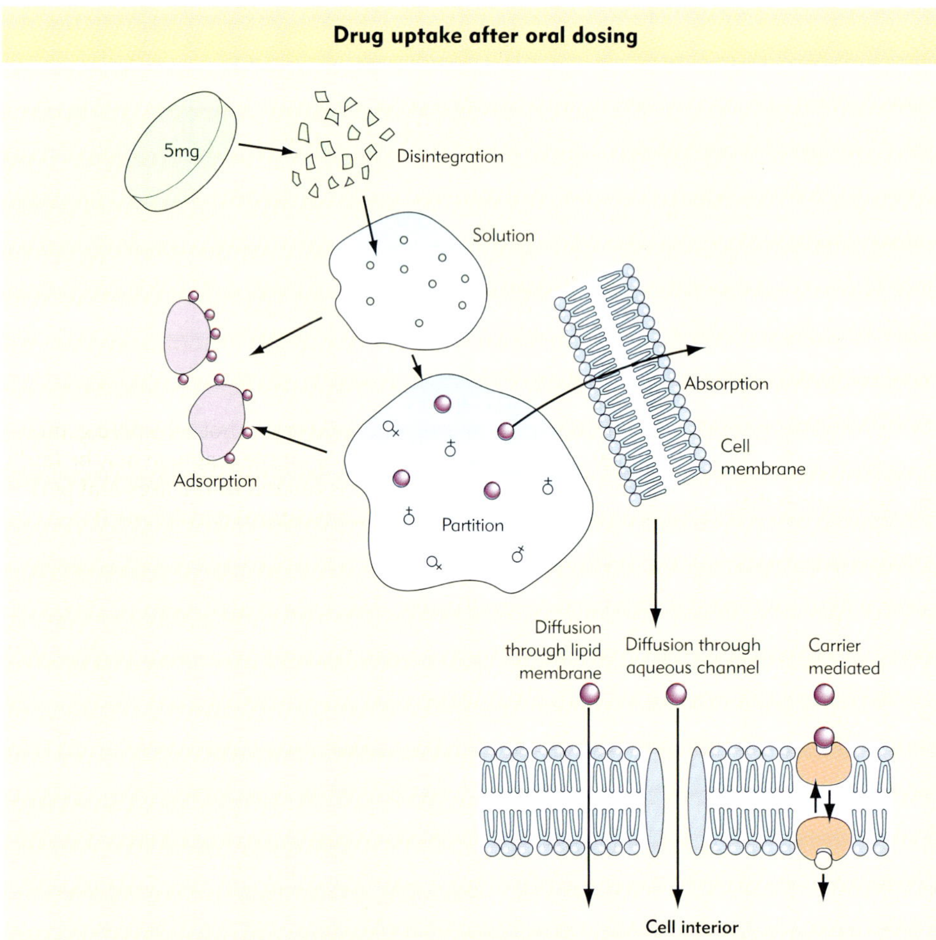

Figure 7.2 Drug uptake after oral administration. (Adapted, with permission, from Hull, 1991)

ticles may also adsorb the drug, thus reducing the dose available for absorption. Other drugs may influence uptake in a variety of ways. They may modify intragastric pH (e.g. histamine H_2 antagonists), promote or delay gastric emptying (e.g. morphine, metoclopramide, and cisapride), or interact in the gastrointestinal tract itself (e.g. antacids may form insoluble complexes with drugs such as digoxin, thereby making them 'unavailable').

Bioavailability

Many drugs, when administered orally, achieve only partial uptake into the bloodstream. *Bioavailability* may be defined as the ratio of effective dose to the administered dose. This permits calculation of an equivalent oral dose from a known systemic dose, and vice versa. Bioavailability is determined by giving the same dose both orally and intravenously (on different occasions), followed by measurement of plasma concentrations throughout the elimination phase (Fig. 7.3). Following estimation of the area under each concentration/time curve (AUC_o and AUC_{iv}, respectively), bioavailability can be calculated as AUC_o/AUC_{iv}.

Sublingual and transmucosal administration

First-pass effects (see below) can be avoided if the drug is absorbed into a tissue that does not drain into the portal circulation, as when an agent is rapidly absorbed from a sublingual tablet or from the nasal, oral, or rectal mucosa.

The *sublingual* route is limited to potent, rapidly absorbed drugs [e.g. nitroglycerin (glyceryl trinitrate), isosorbide dinitrate, and buprenorphine]. Drugs with high lipid solubility have the greatest permeability, but it is also important that the agent is sufficiently water soluble to reach a high concentration in saliva. Drugs with high lipid solubility (e.g. buprenorphine) may be stored at the site of absorption, thus delaying (and prolonging) systemic uptake. An oral transmucosal formulation of fentanyl has been used with some success in children.

Rectal administration is popular in some countries but has the disadvantage that evacuation may precede absorption, or conversely local inflammatory disease may greatly accelerate absorption. The rectal route has been made more reliable with the introduction of hydrogel preparations. A hydrogel is a synthetic material consisting of cross-linked ethylene oxide chains that form a matrix which expands greatly when hydrated. Hydration of the hydrogel allows the enclosed drug to diffuse into the surrounding medium at a controlled rate. Hydrogel suppositories have the advantage of easy placement and retention, with controlled release overcoming the problem of rapid absorption.

Drugs such as vasopressin can be administered in the form of fine powders for *intranasal* use.

Administration via the respiratory tract

The respiratory tract is a traditional route for the administration of anesthetic agents. The kinetics of *inhaled gases* are considered in Chapter 8.

Aerosols

Many drugs are absorbed rapidly from both alveoli and the bronchial mucosa. If the agent is water soluble, a solution can be

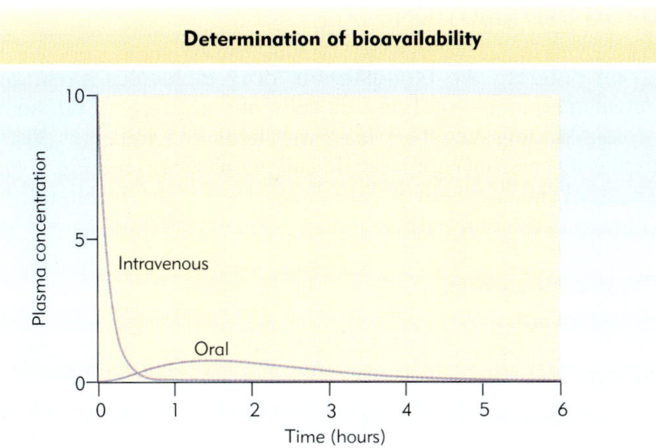

Figure 7.3 Determonation of bioavailability. Areas under the plasma concentration/time curves after intravenous and oral dosing can be compared to determine bioavailability.

finely divided as an aqueous *aerosol*. Particle size is crucial. If greater than 10μm in diameter, particles are trapped in the upper respiratory tract and uptake is minimal. Those in the 2–10μm range are trapped by the small bronchi and bronchioles and are, therefore, ideal for a bronchodilator. Very small particles (such as the <1μm nicotine-carrying droplets in tobacco smoke) pass directly to the alveoli, and a large proportion of any drug delivered in this way is absorbed into the pulmonary capillary blood. Consequently, for a drug such as nitroglycerin, aerosol administration is simply a noninvasive means of giving a small intravenous dose, and very small droplet sizes are used for maximum uptake.

Inhaled solids

If prepared as a finely divided powder, a drug may be inhaled in the same manner as an aerosol. *Inhaled solids* have several possible advantages:

- it is not necessary to formulate the drug as a solution, so particle size can be controlled precisely and the difficulties of formulating some lipid-soluble drugs as aqueous solutions are avoided; and
- weak acids and bases, which are partially ionized in aqueous solution, can be delivered as free acid or free base, which is rapidly absorbed.

The main limitation is that a dry powder causes bronchial irritation; as a result, the method is limited to potent drugs given in very small doses [cromolyn sodium (sodium cromoglycate) is a well-known example].

Endobronchial administration

For lipid-soluble drugs, endobronchial administration is effective. When local anesthetic agents such as tetracaine (amethocaine) are applied to the trachea and bronchi for endoscopic procedures, an appreciable fraction of the dose will be absorbed rapidly. In the absence of venous access, some drugs of small molecular size can be administered simply by injecting them down an endotracheal tube; succinylcholine (suxamethonium) and atropine are good examples. However, bioavailability may be low.

Transdermal administration

If a drug is sufficiently potent, therapeutic quantities may be absorbed directly through the skin. For example, tetracaine is a very potent and lipid-soluble agent and a 4% preparation in carbomer is rapidly acting and highly effective. Less potent and less lipophilic drugs such as lidocaine (lignocaine) present greater difficulties. Although a 5% solution is effective when applied to mucous membranes, it does not penetrate the intact skin because only the small unionized fraction is diffusible. However, a eutectic mixture of lidocaine and prilocaine forms an oil at room temperature, which can be emulsified to a cream without adding any other oils (Brodin et al., 1984) (EMLA™). An 80% free base concentration in the lipid phase ensures rapid transdermal diffusion (Evers et al., 1985). Transdermal uptake results in a shallow zone of local anesthesia involving the dermis and subcutaneous tissues only, with limited systemic uptake.

In the case of a drug whose dosage is not critical (e.g. nitroglycerin), systemic uptake from a simple ointment may be fairly constant. The rate of uptake is related to the area and perfusion of the skin surface and, therefore, may be regulated (to some extent) by choice of site and the quantity applied. In more critical applications, a drug depot may be separated from the skin by a diffusion-limiting membrane and secured by means of an adhesive 'patch'. So long as the depot drug mass is large compared with the delivered dose, the diffusion-limiting membrane will release drug at an almost constant rate for extended periods. Transdermal patches containing scopolamine (hyoscine) are effective in the treatment of motion sickness, and nitroglycerin patches are available for the prophylaxis of angina pectoris. The administration of potent opioids is an obvious application for this technique, and a patch device for delivering fentanyl has been developed. The bioavailability of fentanyl delivered in this way appears to be high.

Intramuscular and subcutaneous administration

Administration by injection can reduce the variation in uptake inherent to oral dosing. The rate of uptake depends upon a number of factors.

Bioavailability

This is often 100% but should not be assumed to be so; some drugs may bind so avidly to tissue constituents as to be sequestered.

Local tissue solubility and binding

High solubility or binding at the injection site may greatly diminish immediate availability (especially when lipid-soluble drugs are injected into subcutaneous fat). Since the processes are reversible, this should not be seen as diminished bioavailability but as partitioning, which diminishes the diffusible concentration.

Water solubility

The drug cannot diffuse to adjacent capillaries except in aqueous solution. As the pH of the drug depot shifts from that of the preparation to that of the tissue, a reduction in ionized fraction may result in lowered water solubility and some drug may come out of solution as crystals. In some depot preparations, the injected drug is dissolved in oil; here, partitioning between oil and water phases results in very slow tissue uptake of the drug.

Permeability

Ability to diffuse through tissues is enhanced by a low molecular weight and high lipid solubility. Rapid uptake is favored by low ionization, *so long as the drug remains in aqueous solution.*

Perfusion

This is responsible for much of the observed variation in uptake rate. Blood flow in different muscle sites may vary considerably, especially when the subject is physically active. Perfusion of subcutaneous sites may be very poor, resulting in slow uptake. Accidental subcutaneous injection is a frequent cause of apparently ineffective intramuscular injections.

Spinal and epidural administration

Both local anesthetic agents and opioids can be administered intrathecally and extradurally (Chapter 28). The term *uptake* is difficult to define in this context, because two quite separate processes are at work. While the drug undergoes systemic uptake in the conventional sense, it also diffuses directly to neural tissues where (presumably) the pharmacologic action occurs. Thus, the pharmacologic site of action is reached without the drug first entering the systemic circulation.

Following intrathecal injection, these two uptake mechanisms occur simultaneously (with heavy emphasis on neural uptake) while the drug disperses through the subarachnoid space under the influence of the specific gravity of the administered solution, the patient position, and mass movements of the cerebrospinal fluid (CSF). Nevertheless, 100% of an injected dose of lidocaine does, eventually, reach the systemic circulation, but the peak blood level occurs after a considerable and variable delay. Neural uptake of such drugs depends largely upon lipid solubility. Lipid-soluble agents such as etidocaine achieve greater penetration than less lipophilic drugs, such as procaine, chloroprocaine, and mepivacaine. Direct diffusion reaches only superficial layers of the cord; penetration of deeper structures depends upon diffusion from CSF in perineural clefts surrounding nerve cell bodies in the substance of the cord.

Disposition after extradural administration is more complex, since the drug disperses into the interstices of the extradural tissues, while at the same time undergoing systemic uptake (much more rapidly than from the CSF) and diffusion both through the dura and into the nerves traversing the epidural space. While neural and systemic uptake are favored by high lipid solubility, the dura acts as a simple diffusion barrier where molecular shape and weight are the determining factors: small, compact molecules diffuse faster than large ones. Drugs may also reach the CSF by diffusion through the arachnoid villi in the dural root sleeves and by uptake into spinal segmental blood vessels. Diffusion into the CSF is often rapid, and peak bupivacaine concentrations have been observed within 10–20 minutes of injection. Uptake of lipophilic drugs (such as fentanyl) into epidural fat may be extensive, thus reducing diffusion into both CSF and the systemic circulation. Sequestration in epidural fat may be very prolonged. Such buffering in the extradural space may explain (at least in part) the long duration of action of opioids such as fentanyl when administered by this route.

Modification of local capillary blood flow, either by direct effects of the drug itself or by the action of some added vasopressor, may greatly modify the balance between systemic and neural uptake. Thus plasma concentrations following intrathecal or epidural lidocaine or diacetylmorphine (diamorphine; heroin) are reduced when epinephrine (adrenaline) is added to the solution. By this means it is possible to limit systemic side effects and prolong the pharmacologic effects of drugs administered by the extradural route.

DRUG DISTRIBUTION

Upon entering the bloodstream, drug molecules partition between aqueous solution, red cells, and a variety of possible protein-binding sites. They leave the circulation and enter other tissues by crossing capillary and cell membranes (see Fig. 7.1). These events are heavily influenced by the physicochemical characteristics of the drug.

Physical properties

Molecular size

Small, uncharged molecules (mw < 100) penetrate the phospholipid–protein bilayers of cell membranes without difficulty, regardless of other characteristics. Larger lipid-soluble molecules can also pass freely, but those with molecular weights above 600 diffuse more slowly. However, charged hydrophilic molecules (see below) can cross such membranes only by passage through specialized channels, fenestrations in capillary membranes or pores between endothelial cells.

Capillaries vary widely in their permeability to drugs. For instance, the renal glomerular capillary is permeable to all non-protein-bound drugs in plasma. Muscle capillaries have intercellular pores through which bulky and highly polar drugs such as neuromuscular blocking agents can pass. In contrast, vascular endothelial cells in the brain are fused together to form *tight junctions*. Consequently, only drugs that are very small or lipid soluble diffuse freely into the brain. The feto–placental membrane has similar but somewhat less efficient characteristics.

Polarity and ionization

Many molecules carry electrostatic charges that prevent passage across lipid membranes. This may be because of ionization, or nonuniform electron distributions, which cause the molecule to behave as a dipole (Chapter 1). Such polarity is a feature of small molecules containing hydroxyl, amino, or carboxyl groups. Some drugs, such as quaternary ammonium compounds, are fully ionized and, therefore, cross capillary membranes relatively slowly and cannot cross brain capillaries or cellular membranes at all. Many organic compounds, such as the volatile anesthetic agents, are small, un-ionized, and highly diffusible molecules.

Weak acids and bases in aqueous solution dissociate into ionized and un-ionized forms, with the relative proportions depending upon the pH and the pK_a of the drug (Fig. 7.4). With increasing pH, acids become increasingly ionized, whereas bases become increasingly un-ionized. Strong bases have high pK_a values; strong acids have low values. Both are highly ionized at pH 7.4. Weak acids and bases with pK_a values in the range 6.5–8.5 are partially ionized at pH 7.4 (e.g. thiopental is 40% ionized) and may show marked changes in ionization following small variations in pH. Since un-ionized molecules cross lipid membranes far more readily than ionized molecules, partitioning between the two species is of great importance.

Lipid solubility

The diffusibility of any drug across a lipid membrane is closely related to its lipid solubility. Thus the free acidic (un-ionized) form of thiopental (thiopentone), with high lipid solubility, is much more diffusible than that of phenobarbital (phenobarbitone). Similarly, fentanyl base is much more diffusible than morphine base. The rapid onset of action of both thiopental and fentanyl are closely related to the lipid solubility of the un-ionized form, which permits rapid diffusion into the brain.

Values of pK_a and un-ionized proportions at pH 7.4					
Bases	pK_a	Un-ionized (%)	Acids	pK_a	Un-ionized (%)
Pancuronium	–	0	Furosemide (frusemide)	3.9	0.03
Atropine	9.7	0.5	Warfarin	5.0	0.4
Propranolol	9.4	1.0	Chlorothiazide	6.8	20.1
Fentanyl	8.4	9.1	Phenobarbital (phenobarbitone)	7.4	50
Bupivacaine	8.1	16.6	Thiopental (thiopentone)	7.6	61.3
Morphine	7.9	24.0	Phenytoin	8.3	88.8
Ketamine	7.5	44.3	Isoproterenol (isoprenaline)	10.1	99.8
Alfentanil	6.5	89.0	Propofol	11.0	99.97
Diazepam	3.3	99.99			

Figure 7.4 Values of pK_a and ionization at pH 7.4 of some commonly used drugs.

Plasma protein binding

Many drugs bind reversibly to plasma proteins (Fig. 7.5). Generally, acidic drugs (such as salicylates and barbiturates) bind to albumin, but basic drugs (such as fentanyl, propranolol, and diazepam) also bind extensively to globulins, lipoproteins, and glycoproteins. A number of drugs (such as alfentanil, bupivacaine, and propranolol) bind to acute-phase proteins such as α_1-acid glycoprotein (AGP). Because of wide variation in plasma AGP concentrations owing to age and disease, this is a major source of pharmacokinetic variation. Many drugs reversibly bind to both plasma and tissue proteins.

Only free, unbound drug can diffuse across lipoprotein membranes. As free drug diffuses out of the plasma, drug–protein complexes dissociate to restore the binding equilibrium. Therefore, all the drug in plasma, both free and bound, is available for diffusion. However, the equilibrium across a membrane is of free, diffusible drug, so that protein binding may have a major influence on drug distribution to individual tissues. The free, unbound concentration of a highly protein-bound drug (such as midazolam) is a tiny fraction of the plasma concentration and, therefore, it is very sensitive to variations in the binding ratio. In situations such as renal failure, reduced protein binding almost doubles the free fraction of midazolam. In contrast, poorly protein-bound drugs (such as ketamine and muscle relaxants) are relatively insensitive to changes in protein binding.

Tissue binding and sequestration

Most drugs that bind to plasma proteins also find binding sites in the tissues themselves. Were this not the case, the disposition of drugs with high plasma protein binding – such as diazepam – would be almost entirely restricted to the circulation. Binding to lung tissue provides important examples (see below). Tissue binding is responsible for much of the interindividual variation in distribution volume.

Most drugs bind reversibly to tissue components; as a result, when the unbound concentration declines the bound fraction rapidly dissociates to maintain a dynamic equilibrium. However, some drugs bind with such high affinity that they remain *sequestered* in the tissue concerned for an extended period. The best known example is the antimalarial quinacrine, which binds to nuclear proteins of liver cells to form a long-lasting drug depot. Heavy metals and tetracyclines are sequestrated in bone, and *d*-tubocurarine binds avidly to chondroitin and other mucopolysaccharides.

Percentage binding to plasma proteins			
Drug	Binding (%)	Drug	Binding (%)
Warfarin	99	Thiopental (thiopentone)	80
Diazepam	98	Etomidate	75
Propofol	98	Lidocaine (lignocaine)	65
Bupivacaine	95	Atracurium	51
Furosemide (frusemide)	95	*d*-Tubocurarine	45
Sufentanil	92.5	Morphine	40
Alfentanil	91	Vecuronium	30
Propranolol	90	Ketamine	12
Fentanyl	82	Caffeine	<5

Figure 7.5 Binding to plasma proteins of some commonly used drugs.

First-pass effects

Many drugs undergo quite different patterns of disposition depending on the route of administration. For instance, when a drug is administered by rapid intravenous injection, the administered dose arrives at the pulmonary artery in very high concentration and then must pass through the pulmonary capillary bed before reaching the systemic circulation. While highly ionized drugs (such as muscle relaxants) remain in the bloodstream, un-ionized molecules are likely to diffuse into the lung tissue. In particular, basic drugs bind reversibly to pulmonary tissue proteins, leading to high pulmonary uptake during the first circulatory pass. In this way, more than 80% of a rapidly injected dose of fentanyl may undergo first-pass pulmonary uptake. The lung, therefore, may have a major influence on early drug distribution. It must be emphasized, however, that much of the drug taken up by lung tissue returns to the circulation very rapidly as plasma concentrations decline behind the initial front; this has the effect of flattening and spreading the drug pulse. The overall effect is both to delay and to attenuate the peak initial concentration reaching the brain. Other basic drugs such as lidocaine, bupivacaine, and propranolol also bind avidly to lung proteins, and it has been found that pulmonary uptake of fentanyl is reduced from 80 to 20% by pretreatment with propranolol.

Apparent volume of distribution

When a dose of a drug is injected intravenously, it first mixes with the plasma and some may diffuse into erythrocytes. If no other processes were involved, this might be completed within two or three circulation times. However, most drugs also diffuse into the extracellular space and some penetrate cells. Therefore the *physical volume of distribution* may range between the volume of the plasma alone (60mL/kg) and that of total body water (600mL/kg). However, in most cases, drug distribution is infinitely more complex because of factors such as ionization and reversible binding in both plasma and tissues. For these reasons, the physical volume of distribution may be a very poor predictor of drug concentrations following administration.

A drug can be considered to occupy a certain space that does not necessarily equate with that of the physical volume of distribution. This may be defined as that well-stirred, homogeneous *apparent* space consisting entirely of plasma (or blood) in which the dose of drug *would* have been dispersed in order to explain the observed degree of dilution. That space is known as the *apparent volume of distribution* (V_d = dose/concentration).

For example, 100mg of a drug is dispersed widely throughout a 70kg body and at steady state is found in plasma at a concentration of 1μg/ml. The total physical volume into which the drug could have dispersed could not have exceeded 42L, and this, therefore, would have overpredicted the final concentration as 2.38μg/mL. The apparent volume of distribution is much greater and is calculated as dose/concentration: 0.1/0.001 = 100L. The apparent volume is not constrained by the physical volume, and extensive tissue binding may result in very large values (Fig. 7.6). Similar effects are seen with drugs such as halothane that do not undergo extensive binding but have widely differing solubilities in body tissues.

In pharmacokinetic terms, the apparent volume of distribution is useful because it provides the essential link between dose, volume and concentration. If a certain plasma concentration C is required, the required dose X_d can be calculated easily as $X_d = CV$. Unfortunately, that attractively simple relation is obscured by the fact that drug elimination commences immediately. Thus, by the time a dose of drug has distributed to body tissues, a significant portion is likely to have been eliminated. So, while apparent volume of distribution is a valid, indeed essential, concept, it must be considered in the context of simultaneous elimination.

Apparent volumes of distribution (V_d)

Drug	V_d (L)	Drug	V_d (L)
Halothane	2530	Thiopental (thiopentone)	120
Imipramine	2100	Lidocaine (lignocaine)	110
Chlorpromazine	1400	Midazolam	95
Propofol	1000	Alfentanil	27
Digoxin	750	Vecuronium	12
Fentanyl	330	Remifentanil	20
Propranolol	180	Warfarin	8

Figure 7.6 Apparent volumes of distribution of some commonly used drugs (typical values).

DRUG ELIMINATION

Some drugs (e.g. gallamine, atenolol, sotolol, volatile anesthetic agents) are eliminated unchanged by the kidney or lung, while others (e.g. cisatracurium) undergo spontaneous chemical decomposition within the body. Many drugs are eliminated from the body by means of enzyme-mediated reactions, either in organs such as the liver (e.g. lidocaine, propranolol, propofol) or in the plasma itself (e.g. succinylcholine, diamorphine, mivacurium, esmolol, remifentanil). Many drugs rely on multiple pathways; thus pancuronium is both metabolized in the liver and excreted by the kidney.

Enzyme-catalyzed reactions

Many drugs are subjected to enzymatic processes, by which they may be broken down or transformed into water soluble metabolites. The velocity (v) of enzyme-catalyzed reactions depends on the quantities of enzyme and substrate present, and also upon the efficiency of the enzyme (Chapter 1). The Michaelis constant (K_m) is numerically equal to the substrate concentration (S) at which the reaction proceeds at half the maximum velocity (V_{max}). If C is the substrate concentration:

Equation 7.1

$$\frac{V}{V_{max}} = \frac{C}{C+K_m}$$

When viewed in graphic form, Equation 7.1 represents a hyperbolic function (Fig. 7.3). If the substrate concentration is very low (where $C \ll K_m$), the denominator simplifies to K_m:

Equation 7.2

$$\frac{V}{V_{max}} = \frac{C}{K_m}$$

Since K_m and V_{max} are constants, the reaction velocity (and therefore the rate of metabolism) is proportional to the substrate concentration. At high concentrations (where $C \gg K_m$), the denominator simplifies to C and the equation becomes:

Equation 7.3

$$\frac{V}{V_{max}} = C$$

Under these conditions the rate of reaction remains constant, irrespective of any further rises in drug concentration. Thus in the case of a drug (such as thiopental) whose K_m greatly exceeds the plasma concentrations expected after clinical doses, the rate of metabolism is usually proportional to the plasma concentration. At high concentrations, however, nonlinearity or even saturation may occur.

Extraction ratio and clearance

As blood passes through an organ of elimination such as the liver or kidney, a relatively constant fraction of the drug is extracted for metabolism or excretion. Extraction ratio (ER) is the ratio of extracted drug to that entering the organ and has values in the range 0–1. For the liver, no distinction is made between portal and arterial perfusion.

Drug clearance describes the efficiency of drug elimination. Conventionally, it is defined as the volume of plasma (or blood) which is cleared of drug per unit time. This is a useful approach when considering drug clearance by an organ, but in whole body terms is less useful. Whole body clearance is more usefully

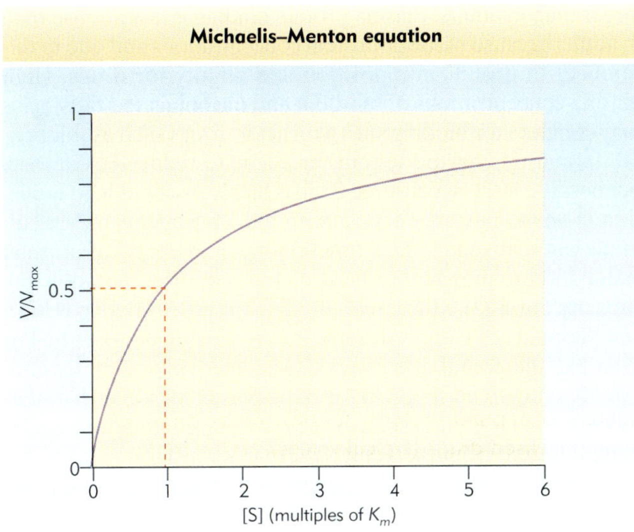

Figure 7.7 The Michaelis–Menten equation. This is a graphical representation of Equation 7.1.

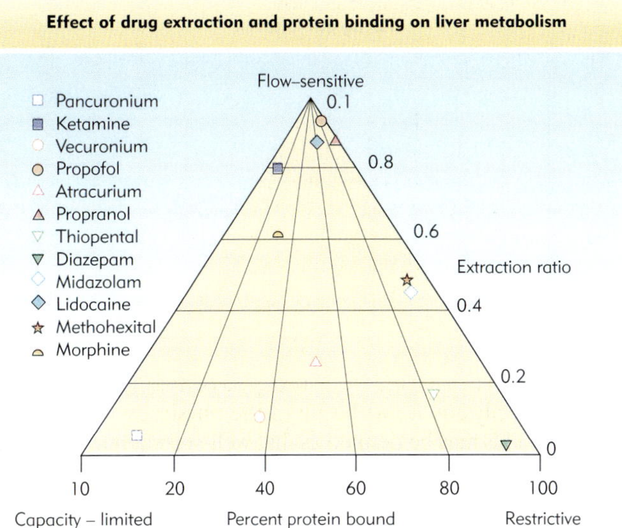

Figure 7.8 The effect of drug extraction and protein binding on hepatic drug metabolism. Drugs with high extraction are sensitive to changes in hepatic blood flow (perfusion limitation). Drugs with low extraction but high protein binding are sensitive to changes in binding (restrictive clearance). Drugs with low extraction and low binding are sensitive to changes in enzyme capacity. (Adapted from Blaschke, 1997).

defined as the rate of drug elimination per unit of drug concentration in plasma. Thus, if drug elimination is expressed as g/h, and concentration as g/L, clearance will be elimination/concentration [i.e. (g/h)/(g/l)] and will have units of L/h.

Some thought will reveal that the two definitions are simply two ways of expressing the same quantity. This concept will be developed further in later sections.

The influence of protein binding on hepatic drug metabolism

The rate of an enzyme-mediated metabolic pathway in the liver depends upon the free drug concentration in the liver cell and, therefore, on the free drug concentration in the hepatic sinusoid (C_f), and on the K_m. If $C_f \gg K_m$ the drug may be consumed so rapidly that the free concentration in blood declines almost to zero. As it does so, the protein binding equilibrium shifts and bound drug dissociates. Consequently, blood in the sinusoid may be stripped of both free and bound drug fractions. Under such high-extraction conditions, the rate of metabolism depends on the supply of drug (i.e. hepatic perfusion). Therefore, highly extracted drugs (e.g. lidocaine and propranolol) are metabolized by high-capacity enzyme systems that consume drug efficiently even when blood concentrations are very low. In the case of a drug with an unbound concentration of the same order of magnitude as (or less than) K_m, the rate of drug consumption may be insufficient to reduce the unbound concentration in the sinusoid. Then, the rate of metabolism is proportional to C_f. Furthermore, because C_f remains unchanged, the protein binding equilibrium also remains unchanged so that bound drug remains bound. If the drug is highly protein bound, the unbound fraction is very low, as is the rate of metabolism. This is known as *restrictive elimination*. The influence of protein binding and drug extraction on hepatic metabolism may conveniently be expressed in graphic form (Fig. 7.8).

Renal drug elimination

In the kidney, glomerular filtration provides a different situation. Since the filtrate comprises all the elements of plasma, bar proteins and protein-bound drugs, its removal does not alter the unbound drug concentration. Therefore, the protein-binding equilibrium remains undisturbed and drug is not removed from plasma proteins. In the case of drugs that are metabolized by the renal parenchyma (e.g. morphine), the role of protein binding is similar to that in the liver.

Presystemic, or first-pass hepatic metabolism

Many drugs that are administered by the oral route reach the systemic circulation via the hepatic portal venous system and, therefore, must pass through the liver. Consequently, some fraction of the dose may be metabolized before reaching the systemic circulation. This is known as *presystemic* or *first-pass* hepatic metabolism. If a large fraction is eliminated in this way, the effective dose may be greatly reduced. As a result, drugs such as propranolol must be given in much larger doses when administered orally.

Presystemic metabolism may also take place in the gut wall. For instance, isoproterenol (isoprenaline) is subjected to extensive sulfate conjugation in the intestinal mucosa and very little reaches the systemic circulation in active form. Chlorpromazine, levodopa, and methyldopa are all affected similarly. Morphine, too, is conjugated, but with glucuronic acid. Nitroglycerin is extensively hydrolyzed in the gut wall and so is almost ineffective if swallowed; hence the conventional sublingual route.

Cumulation

If a drug is administered repeatedly, or by continuous infusion, the mean rate of administration is likely to be greater than the initial rate of elimination. Consequently, the mass of drug in the body must increase until, at equilibrium, the plasma concentration reaches a level at which the rate of elimination equals the mean rate of administration (Fig. 7.9). That increase is called *cumulation* and is a feature of repeated administration

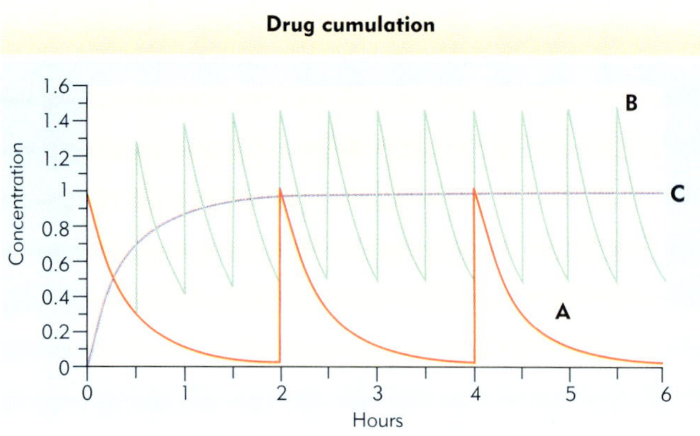

Figure 7.9 Drug cumulation. Line A represents plasma concentrations of a drug ($t_{1/2\beta}$ 30 minutes) administered as intravenous bolus doses at 2 hour intervals. As each dose is administered, the plasma concentration following the previous dose has decayed almost to zero, so that successive doses result in almost identical plasma concentration profiles. Line B shows the result of administering the same dose at 30 minute intervals. Now, cumulation occurs. The plasma concentration at which each dose is given increases, reaching a steady state after some four half-times. Line C shows the result of a continuous infusion. Here, there are no pulses due to bolus dosing, and a steady state is achieved after some four half-times. Concentration decay after prolonged dosing may be context sensitive (see Fig. 7.14).

or infusion of almost every drug used in anesthetic practice. It is particularly likely to occur when the dosing interval is equal to or less than the elimination half-time.

FACTORS AFFECTING DRUG DISPOSITION

Age, sex, and body weight

The disposition of any drug will vary greatly in a normal population. This variation results in part from differences in body size. However, there are strong correlations between body weight and both age and sex; as a result, identifying the actual sources of variation can be a daunting task. In a large study of adult patients taking a small standard dose of propranolol, sex was found to be the most important pharmacokinetic determinant, with age, smoking habit, and racial type also significant. After taking those factors into account, body weight had no significant influence. There are numerous other examples of sex differences, presumably caused by relative differences in the masses of tissues such as muscle and fat. Women also have less efficient clearance of drugs such as temazepam and lidocaine. The reasons are not clear but may result from sex differences in hepatic enzymes such as the cytochrome P450 mixed oxidase system.

In children, body size clearly is a more important factor than in adults. For instance, the distribution volumes of *d*-tubocurarine, thiopental, and alfentanil vary directly with body weight, even in quite young infants. However, body weight has less influence on clearance, which, therefore, should be scaled down with some caution.

Drug disposition in neonates often is quite different from that in older infants. This is not surprising since they have a greater water content and many organs (brain, liver, etc.) are relatively larger than in adults. Plasma protein binding is less intense than in adults because of lower protein concentrations and due to differences in protein composition and affinity for drugs. High plasma concentrations of bilirubin and unconjugated fatty acids may compete for binding sites with acidic drugs such as thiopental. Immature enzyme systems may lead to reduced clearance, but because fetal cytochrome P450 is highly susceptible to induction *in utero*, maternal exposure to inducing agents may result in neonatal mixed oxidase function much in excess of normal. Indeed, there may be dramatic changes in drug-metabolizing capacity during the first week of life. All these influences have complex and often unpredictable effects on drug disposition. For example, thiopental distributes to a smaller volume of distribution than expected on the basis of body weight, while that of *d*-tubocurarine is greater than expected. Drug elimination may be quite different from the adult pattern (Fig. 7.9).

With aging, there is reduction in both muscle and bone mass, and fat occupies a greater relative part of the body mass (Chapter 66). Consequently water-soluble drugs such as muscle relaxants tend to have *decreased* apparent volumes of distribution in elderly patients. In contrast, lipid-soluble drugs (e.g. lidocaine, diazepam, or meperidine) have been shown to have *increased* distribution volumes in the elderly. Since hepatic blood flow progressively decreases in elderly subjects, highly extracted drugs such as lidocaine and propranolol may exhibit reduced clearance. This effect is compounded by the inevitable decrease in presystemic metabolism, leading to greater bioavailability and even greater plasma concentrations. Less efficiently cleared drugs such as diazepam are influenced by the general reduction in hepatic biomass in elderly subjects, but the effect may be offset by reduced plasma protein binding leading to greater unbound plasma concentrations. Since aging is associated with a progressive reduction in renal function (30–50% reduction in creatinine clearance by 65 years of age), drugs dependent on renal excretion are less efficiently cleared in elderly patients. Elderly patients also are subject to a variety of age-related secondary factors. While more prone to debilitating diseases and exposed to a wider range of drugs, they smoke and drink less than young adults.

Pharmacogenetics

The pharmacokinetic profiles of some drugs are heavily influenced by genetic factors. Inherited variation in the characteristics of an enzyme system is called *genetic polymorphism*. The example best known to anesthetists is the genetic variation in cholinesterase characteristics, which has major effects on the rate of hydrolysis of drugs such as succinylcholine and mivacurium (Chapter 32). Drugs that are acetylated in the liver (e.g. hydralazine, procainamide, isoniazid, nitrazepam, phenelzine) show distinct differences in clearance, depending on the acetylator type of the individual. The proportions of 'fast' and 'slow' acetylators vary widely between ethnic groups. The cytochrome P450 enzyme system also is subject to genetic polymorphism, influencing the metabolism of drugs such as phenacetin, metoprolol, and phenytoin.

Pregnancy

Even in early pregnancy, a number of physiologic functions undergo changes that alter drug disposition significantly (Chapter 65). For instance, gastrin uptake of paracetamol is delayed in women who are as little as 12 weeks pregnant. Renal blood flow and glomerular filtration rate are increased from early pregnancy; as a result, the clearances of drugs such as

Elimination half-times of some common drugs		
	Half-time (hours)	
	Neonates	Adults
Bupivacaine	25	1.3
Lidocaine (lignocaine)	3	1–2
Diazepam	25–100	15–25
Meperidine	22	3–4
Morphine	7	2–3
Sufentanil	5–19	3–4
Fentanyl	1–7	3–6
d-Tubocurarine	5.6	2.7

Figure 7.10 Elimination half-times of some common drugs in neonates and adults.

muscle relaxants and antibiotics are increased. Plasma volume increases by some 50%, total body water by up to 8L, and body fat by 3–4kg in the third trimester, leading to large increases in the apparent volumes of distribution of many drugs. These effects are accentuated by reductions in serum albumin and (usually) AGP. These changes are particularly significant in the case of highly bound, poorly extracted drugs such as diazepam and midazolam.

Disease

Many disease conditions are associated with abnormal pharmacokinetics. Changes in drug distribution may often result from loss of body muscle and fat or altered protein binding. Both renal and hepatic disease are associated with disturbed protein binding, and a variety of inflammatory and malignant conditions are associated with increased plasma concentrations of AGP.

Hepatic drug elimination may be compromised in many ways; these include loss of hepatic biomass, reduced hepatic blood flow, altered protein binding, and loss of specific enzyme systems both in the liver and in the blood. The effects are highly variable, depending on the nature and severity of the disease process and the drug concerned.

Renal elimination may be compromised by reduced glomerular filtration and complicated by abnormal protein binding. The kidney has a particularly important role in eliminating the water-soluble metabolites of nonpolar drugs, which do not themselves appear in the urine. For example, renal failure has little effect on the excretion of unchanged morphine but severely restricts the elimination of morphine 6-glucuronide, an active metabolite. Some drugs (such as morphine) are *metabolized* in the kidney, and this may continue despite renal failure so long as organ perfusion is maintained.

Cardiac failure and other low-output states are associated with greatly delayed uptake of drugs administered by any route other than intravenous injection. Even in the latter, slow venous transit may delay the onset of such drugs as thiopental and propofol. Poor tissue perfusion may severely restrict the distribution of drugs; as a result, those organs in which perfusion is maintained (such as the brain) may be exposed to very high drug concentrations. The altered pharmacology of thiopental in a patient who has hemorrhagic shock is an apt example. Both renal and hepatic blood flow tend to decline in proportion to changes in cardiac output; thus the half-time of lidocaine, which is susceptible both to changes in hepatic perfusion and to restricted distribution, may be two to three times greater in patients who have cardiac failure.

Alcohol and tobacco

Several studies have demonstrated pharmacokinetic differences between those who smoke and those who do not. For instance, smokers taking a small standard dose of propranolol have lower plasma concentrations than nonsmokers because of cytochrome P450 induction.

Alcohol has a similar effect on the cytochrome P450 system and regular drinkers may have greater than normal clearance of many drugs. It should be noted, however, that alcohol competes with other drugs for enzyme sites, so the inebriated drinker may have reduced rather than increased metabolic clearance of some drugs. This principally affects poorly extracted drugs such as tolbutamide, phenytoin, and warfarin. As alcoholism progresses towards liver failure, the pattern changes to that of diminished hepatic function, involving loss of biomass, reduced perfusion, altered protein binding, and loss of both muscle and fat. In patients who have alcoholic cirrhosis, the elimination half-time of diazepam may be twice that in normal individuals.

Pharmacokinetic drug interactions

Many drugs influence the uptake of others. For instance, antacids inhibit the absorption of tetracyclines. Drugs such as metoclopramide and cisapride influence uptake of orally administered opioids by modifying the rate of gastric emptying. The uptake of local anesthetics is reduced by the coadministration of vasoconstrictors such as epinephrine, norepinephrine (noradrenaline), and octapressin.

Any drug that binds to plasma proteins is likely to inhibit the binding of other drugs with affinity for the same site(s): thus warfarin competes with salicylates, tolbutamide and sulfonamides for albumin sites.

Drugs that reduce cardiac output are likely to influence the disposition of other drugs, or even their own. Halothane, propranolol, and propofol are good examples. The effects range from altered distribution to reduced clearance owing to the effect on hepatic blood flow.

Many drugs compete for elimination pathways; thus the hydrolysis of succinylcholine is influenced by the coadministration of procaine, cocaine, chloroprocaine, tetracaine, propanidid, diacetylmorphine, or mivacurium.

Some drugs influence the metabolism of others by inducing or inhibiting the cytochrome P450 mixed oxidase enzyme system. Inducing agents include many common drugs as well as chemicals such as benzene; insecticides such as Aldrin, Dieldrin, Lindane, Perthane, and DDT; and fungicides such as hexachlorobenzene. Cimetidine is an example of a P450 inhibitor.

Drugs may also inhibit other metabolic enzymes. Monoamine oxidase inhibitors interfere with the metabolism of amphetamines, ephedrine, methoxamine, cocaine, fenfluramine, atropine, phenytoin, levodopa, phenothiazines, opioids, thiazide diuretics, benzodiazepines and tricyclic antidepressants.

Many other examples of pharmacokinetic interactions are found in the comprehensive review by Runciman (1987).

PLASMA CONCENTRATION DECAY AFTER SINGLE BOLUS DOSING

In many cases, the rate of drug metabolism or excretion is proportional to the plasma concentration. Any variable whose rate of change is proportional to its own magnitude will change exponentially and is said to be a first-order process. The declining plasma concentrations of many drugs can be fitted by mathematical functions comprising one or more exponential terms. In the simplest possible case, the function may be of the form:

Equation 7.4

$$\frac{C}{C_0} = e^{-kt}$$

where C_o and C represent the concentration at times zero and t, respectively, k is a rate constant, and e the base of the natural logarithm (2.7183...). A basic property of exponential decay is that the variable (i.e. concentration) declines by a constant proportion per unit time (Fig. 7.11).

An exponentially declining plasma concentration can be characterized by its rate constant. Rate constant k expresses the gradient at any time (i.e. rate of concentration decline) as a fraction of the concentration at that time and has the dimension reciprocal time (i.e. h^{-1}). It can also be expressed in the time domain as the time constant, calculated as $1/k$, which states the time taken for the variable to decline to 36.8% (or, more precisely, 1/e) of its original value (see Fig. 7.10).

While the time constant describes the process in convenient units, the fraction 1/e is not easy to grasp. The use of half-time ($t_{1/2}$) overcomes the difficulty. This is the time taken for C to decline from any initial concentration C_0 to half that value. Thus at 1 half-time $C/C_0 = 0.5$. Now Equation 7.4 is easily solved to determine t, which is the only unknown. Taking natural logarithms (symbol ln) on both sides, $\ln 0.5 = -kt$. then: $t = 0.693/k$.

An exponential decay always declines by 50% in one half-time and then continues to do so in successive half-times to infinity.

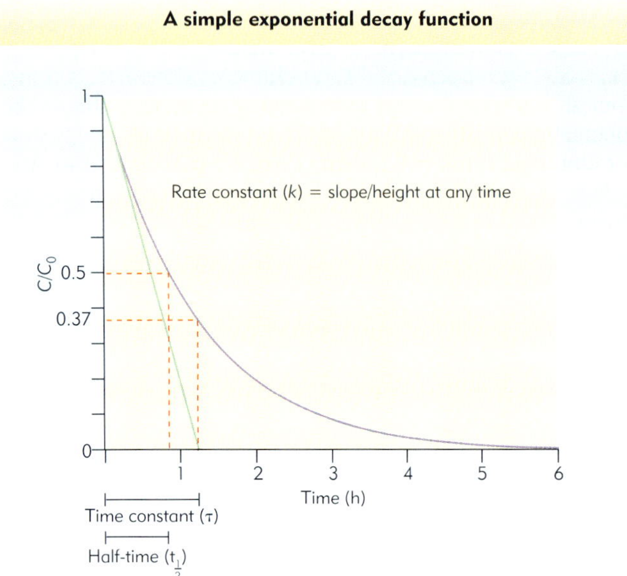

Figure 7.11 A simple exponential decay function.

In many cases, plasma concentrations decay in a more complex manner. For instance, it is often found that the initial decay is faster and the final decay slower than accounted for by a simple exponential decay. In such cases, a better fit may be obtained by a function comprising the sum of two or more exponential terms. Figure 7.12a shows such a decay, where an exponential function fitted to the later plasma concentrations clearly does not satisfy the early data points. Figure 7.12b shows a bi-exponential function of the form:

Equation 7.5

$$C_0 = Ae^{-\alpha t} + Be^{-\beta t}$$

fitted to the same data.

Single and bi-exponential curves may, when plotted on linear coordinates, appear somewhat similar. However, since taking natural logarithms transforms $C/C_0 = e^{-kt}$ to $\ln(C/C_0) = -kt$, a plot of lnC against time yields a straight line (Fig. 7.13a).

Bi-exponential functions cannot be transformed to linear equations, so that plots of log-concentration against time are

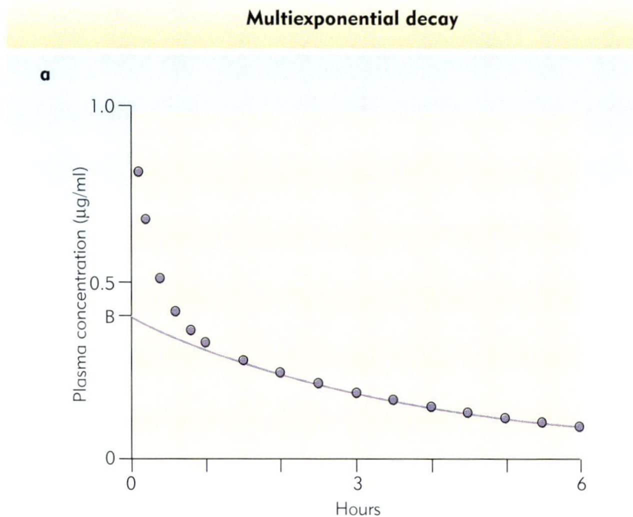

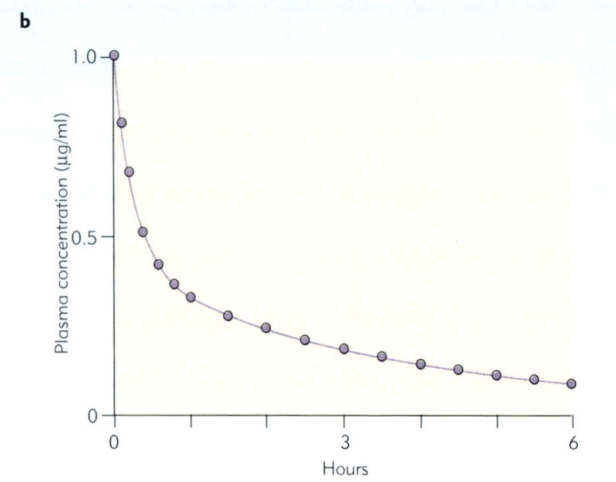

Figure 7.12 Multiexponential decay. (a) An exponential decay function fitted to the last eight data points will not satisfy the early data. Whereas (b) a function comprising two exponential terms fits all the data points.

not straight lines (Fig. 7.13b). It should, however, be noted that because $A.e^{-\alpha t}$ quickly diminishes to a negligible value, a bi-exponential function then simplifies to $B.e^{-\beta t}$. Therefore, the terminal phase of such a plot approximates very closely to a straight line.

In some cases, even more complex functions, comprising three or more terms, may be required.

Each of the terms in Equation 7.5 is an exponential decay, characterized by its individual rate constant (α, β). Each, therefore may be expressed as a half-time ($t_{1/2\alpha}$, $t_{1/2\beta}$). Although Equation 7.5 is the sum of the two terms, the first term quickly decays to negligible values. As a result, during the elimination phase the equation simplifies to:

Equation 7.6

$$C = Be^{-\beta t}$$

The half-time $t_{1/2\beta}$ is often described as the elimination, or terminal, half-life and gives a useful indication of the time taken to eliminate drug from the body. The term $t_{1/2\alpha}$ is not so useful because the contribution of $Ae^{-\alpha t}$ to the decay curve depends on the dosing history (see below on context-sensitive half-time).

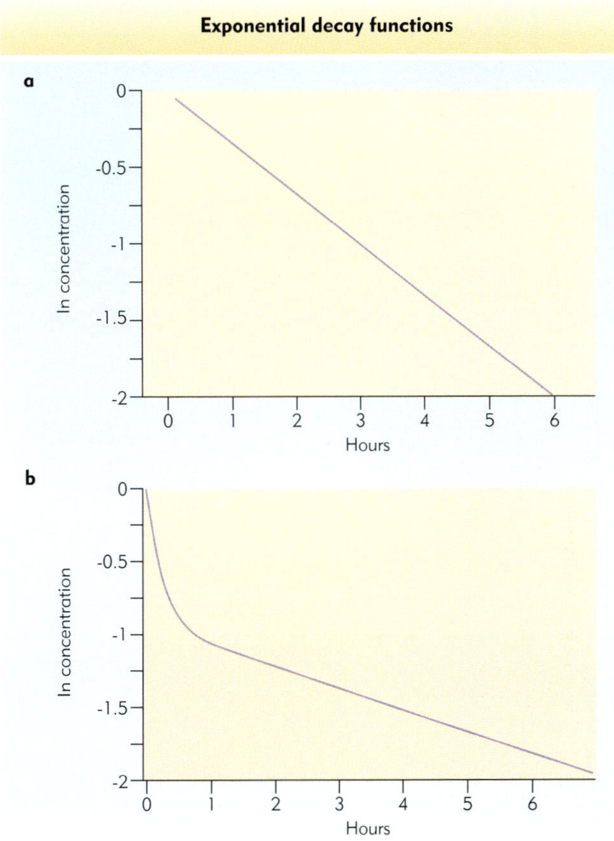

Figure 7.13 Exponential decay functions. (a) shows an exponential decay function (data of Fig. 7.11) re-plotted in semi-logarithmic form, with the x axis representing natural logarithms of drug concentration. (b) shows a bi-exponential decay function (see Equation 7.5) plotted in the same way.

SIMPLE MODELS OF DRUG DISPOSITION

Since our objectives are to predict the time course of drug concentrations after stated dosing regimens, and to determine the optimum dosing regimens for stated outcomes, it is essential to have mathematical models which can be solved to yield such information.

Physiologic models

So-called 'physiologic' models of drug disposition attempt to simulate mathematically the actual movement of drug in the circulation and a number of organ groups. The complexity of such a model is limited only by the physiologic detail available and the availability of reliable data on drug affinity for a wide range of tissues.

Physiologic models consist of a circulation and one or more compartments, each of which is considered to be homogeneous. Drug equilibrates between blood and each compartment according to a rate constant and a partition coefficient. Elimination from such a model illustrates some important principles.

Figure 7.14 shows a circulatory pool that perfuses an organ of elimination such as the liver. 'Plasma' containing drug at concentration C_a is passed at rate Q through the organ. The effluent plasma concentration is C_v. The amount of drug removed from each milliliter of plasma is $C_a - C_v$, and so the overall rate of drug elimination must be $Q(C_a - C_v)$. The extraction ratio (ER) can be calculated as the fraction of drug extracted from each milliliter of plasma as it passes though the organ:

Equation 7.7

$$\mathrm{ER} = \frac{C_a - C_v}{C_a}$$

While extraction ratio is a most informative measure, it ignores perfusion and, therefore, is not an index of elimination performance by the organ as a whole. This is provided by clearance (Cl), which is the product of extraction ratio and organ perfusion:

Equation 7.8

$$\mathrm{Cl} = \mathrm{ER}.Q$$

If ER = 1, clearance must equal perfusion Q and, therefore, represents that volume of plasma entirely cleared of drug per unit time. Since the dimension of Q is volume/time and ER is dimensionless, it follows that the dimension of clearance also must be volume/time. If ER = 0.5, then Q/2L *appear* to be cleared of drug per unit time. If ER = 0.1, then Q/10L are cleared, and so on.

Now consider Equation 7.8 in an expanded form, expressing ER in terms of afferent and efferent concentrations:

Equation 7.9

$$\mathrm{Cl} = Q\frac{(C_a - C_v)}{C_a}$$

Since $Q(C_a - C_v)$ expresses the rate of drug elimination, Equation 7.9 can be restated as:

Equation 7.10

$$\text{Clearance} = \frac{\text{Rate of elimination at time } t}{\text{Concentration at time } t}$$

This is a much more satisfactory expression of elimination efficiency because it expresses the rate of elimination in terms of

Circulation model with one organ of elimination

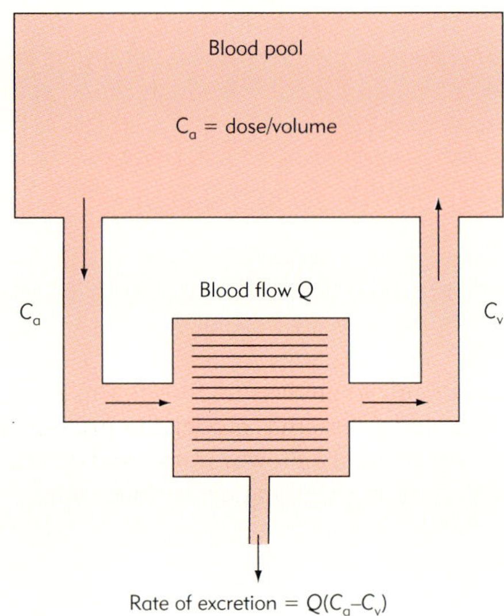

Figure 7.14 A circulation model with one organ of elimination.

prevailing drug concentration; the greater the rate of elimination for a given concentration, the more efficient the process.

Compartmental models

An even simpler approach is to consider the body as one or more homogeneous compartments in which blood:tissue partition coefficients are assumed to be 1. Consider a one-compartment model of this type. The route of elimination is directly from the compartment and is available to all drug in the body at all times (Fig. 7.15a).

The apparent volume of distribution (V_d) is expressed simply in terms of dose (X_d) and initial concentration (after dosing) C_0:

Equation 7.11

$$V_d = \frac{X_d}{C_0}$$

At any time, the rate of elimination may be expressed as the rate of decline in plasma concentration (ΔC) times the volume of distribution (V_d). Clearance is the rate of elimination per unit concentration:

Equation 7.12

$$\text{Cl} = \frac{\Delta C V_d}{C}$$

Note, however, that a rate constant is the rate of change of a variable per unit of magnitude (i.e. $k = \Delta Y/Y$). So:

Equation 7.13

$$\text{Cl} = kV_d$$

After a single dose, drug concentration will decline exponentially according to Equation 7.4 and this can be developed to solve for any combination of dose and/or infusion, and for any specified initial condition before dosing. Now,

Equation 7.14

$$X = \left[X_d + X_\Phi - \frac{k'}{k}\right]e^{-kt} + \frac{k'}{k}$$

where X is the mass of drug in the body at any time t, X_Φ is the mass of drug in the body before dosing, and k' is the rate of an infused drug input. Drug concentration at any time is simply X/V.

One- and two-compartment models

a

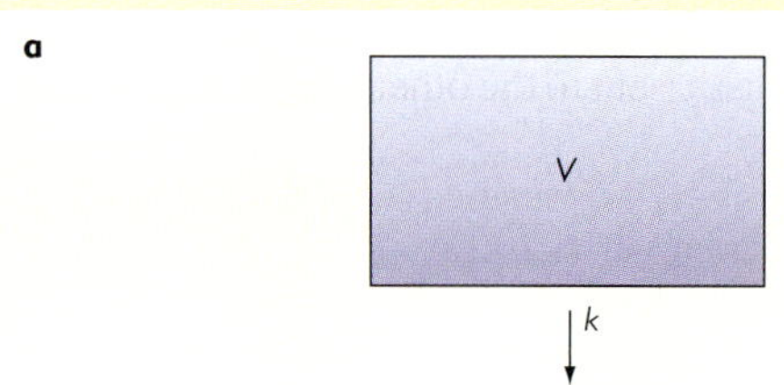

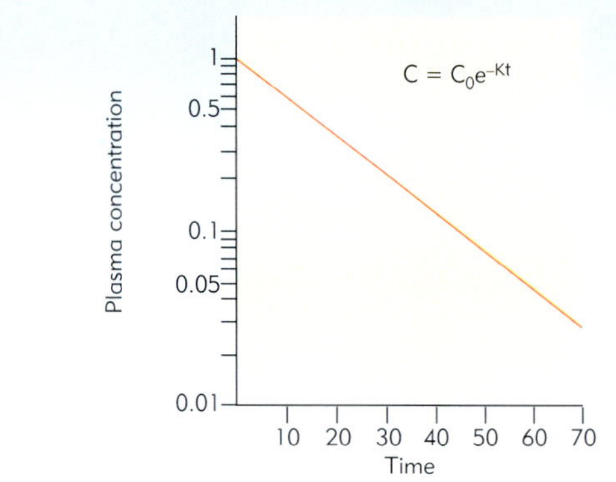

b

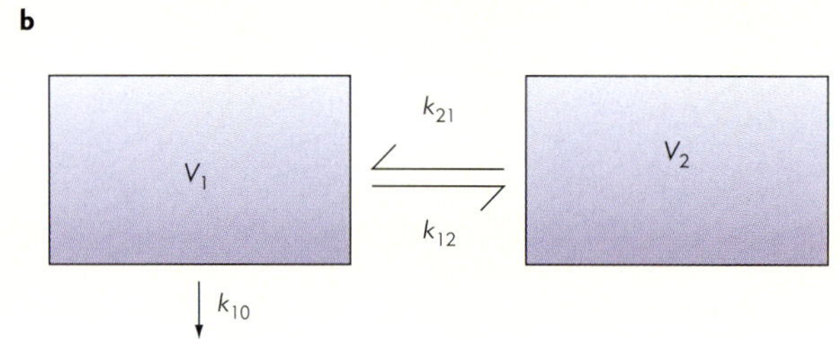

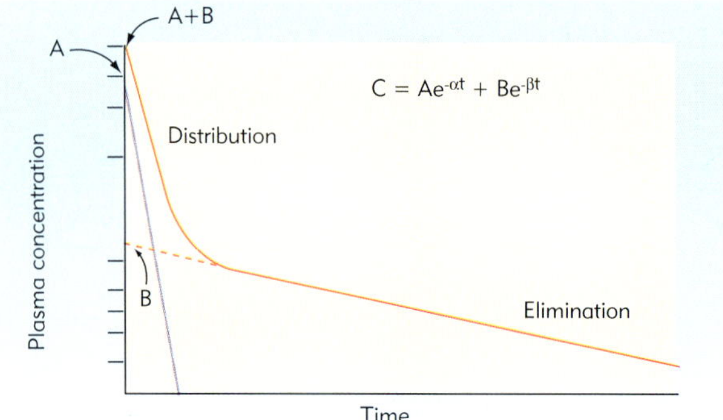

Figure 7.15 One- and two-compartment models. See the text for details.

If the plasma concentrations following a single dose are best fitted by a function comprising two exponential terms (see Fig. 7.13b) and having the form described by Equation 7.5, the corresponding model must have two compartments (Fig 7.15b). It is conventional to specify that dosing and elimination are restricted to the central compartment (V_1).

The model now has three rate constants and two volumes, which can be calculated from A, B, α, and β using standard equations. These also may be expressed as clearances. Whole body clearance is as in the one-compartment model:

Equation 7.15

$$Cl = k_{10}V_1$$

Intercompartmental clearance, which expresses the efficiency of transfer from one compartment to the other, may be expressed as:

Equation 7.16

$$Cl = k_{12}V_1 = k_{21}V_2$$

This equality is inevitable in any real model. The apparent volume of distribution at steady state (V_{ss}) is simply the sum of V_1 and V_2. This parameter can be estimated directly at an infusional steady state as the ratio of mass of drug in the body to plasma concentration.

As with the one-compartment model, it is possible to solve for any combination of bolus and infusional doses, commencing with any initial conditions. The equations are cumbersome, and the reader is referred to more detailed accounts (Hull, 1991, 1994). Three- and even four-compartment models are possible, but the mathematics become even more unpalatable as model complexity increases.

Context-sensitive half-time

If a drug with two-compartment kinetics, such as alfentanil, is given as a single dose, plasma concentrations decline by 50% within a few minutes. If an infusion of the same drug was administered for many hours so as to reach the same peak plasma concentration and then discontinued, the plasma concentration would decline more slowly than before because of the much larger mass of drug in the deep compartment (Fig. 7.16). This has obvious implications with regard to the rate of recovery.

The time taken for plasma concentration to decline to half the peak concentration depends on the initial mass of drug in the deep compartment(s) and, therefore, is highly sensitive to the preceding dosing pattern. This period has become known as the context-sensitive half-time. Unfortunately, this term may easily be confused with exponential half-time. It is important to note that in an exponential decay, the variable declines to 50% at $t_{1/2}$, and then to 25% at $t_{1/2} \times 2$, whereas the context-sensitive half-time makes no prediction as to the value at $t_{1/2} \times 2$. It is, however, useful in that it indicates the likely increase in recovery time after repeated dosing or infusions. For example, the context-sensitive half-time of alfentanil extends markedly after a long infusion, whereas that of remifentanil, which is destroyed rapidly in the plasma, does not.

Physiologic or compartmental models?

We have seen how drug disposition can be modeled using two quite different approaches. However, so long as our assumptions regarding a well-stirred single compartment remain valid, these models simply are different ways of expressing the same thing.

While the perfusion model certainly has the advantage of being more realistic, it also has more parameters. If it is extended to comprise all major organs, the number of parameters may become very large and some may be very difficult to estimate.

The compartmental model has appealing simplicity, at least at first glance, and requires no more than a set of plasma concentrations after a single dose or short infusion in order to calculate its parameters. However, it has many limitations, which become very obvious when faced with questions such as the influence of changing organ mass, cardiac output or individual organ failure on the pattern of disposition.

POPULATION MODELLING

It is not too difficult to analyse a set of plasma concentration data to yield a compartmental model comprising one, two or even three compartments. However, the real difficulties begin when deciding what may legitimately be done with such a model. In truth it does little more than indicate what might be expected to happen if the same dosing regimen were administered to the same subject again. If applied to other individuals it could (and probably would) be wildly inaccurate because of large differences in pharmacokinetic profiles. To be of predictive value in other individuals it is essential that all sources of pharmacokinetic variation are accounted for.

We could take a set of models derived for a group of broadly similar individuals, and then average each of the parameters to yield a 'mean model'. Such a model would represent patients of that age, sex, weight, smoking habits, etc. Unfortunately, this approach has limitations.

First, the confidence with which the individual models were derived from sets of concentration data will have varied considerably, but all the results are averaged with equal weighting to yield an aggregate model. Clearly, one or two ill-defined models could introduce major errors.

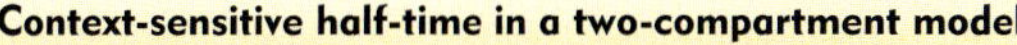

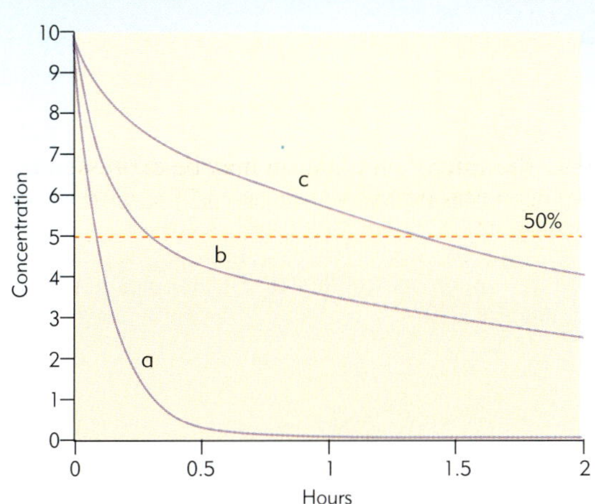

Figure 7.16 Context-sensitive half-time in a two-compartment model following (a) a single dose, (b) a short infusion, and (c) a long infusion. The time taken to reach 50% of the initial concentration varies according to the context (i.e. dosing pattern).

Second, such an aggregate model can only hope to emulate the mean behavior of a group of similar subjects; faced with an individual the predictive power must be poor unless he or she has characteristics very close to the mean in every respect.

Third, it is commonplace for investigators to take the model parameters from each subject, scale the distribution volumes by body weight, and then average them all together to produce what he calls a 'weight-corrected' model. To apply the model to some other individual, the distribution volumes are scaled up according to body weight. If distribution volume is not proportional to body weight (and in the adult population it is most unusual for it to be so), this procedure may, with the intention of being more scientific, have the opposite effect.

A better alternative is to derive a population model for the drug concerned. In its simplest form this is just a better way of determining an aggregate model for a group of subjects; the curve-fitting procedure considers the raw data from all the subjects simultaneously, so that the problem of weighting is eliminated. Notwithstanding the limitations, this can be surprisingly effective.

A more sophisticated approach is to take plasma concentration data from a large number of subjects, noting also those factors which might possibly contribute to variation in model parameters. Then, a non-linear multiple regression is performed on both the concentration data and the putative influencing factors. This not only identifies those characteristics which influence model parameters but also determines the weighting factors. This is especially important with regard to body weight, which is usually significant but with a weighting factor much less than 1. The problem with this method is that many data sets are required from a wide range of subjects. The computer program NONMEM has become the standard method of performing such analyses.

Models of this type will increasingly become feasible as pharmacokinetic databases become larger and wider-ranging.

Key References

Axelsson K, Widman B. Blood concentration of lidocaine after spinal anaesthesia using lidocaine with adrenaline. Acta Anaesth Scand. 1981;25:240–5.

Blaschke TF. Protein binding and kinetics of drugs in liver diseases. Clin Pharmacokinet. 1997;2:32–44.

Brodin A, Nyqvist–Mayer A, Wadsten I, et al. Phase diagram and aqueous solubility of the lignocaine-prilocaine binary system. J Pharmaceutical Sci. 1984;73:4.

Burm AGL, van Cleef JW, Gladines MPRR, et al. Epidural anesthesia with lidocaine and bupivacaine: effects of epinephrine on the plasma concentration profiles. Anesth Analg. 1986;65:1281–4.

Burm AGL, van Cleef JW, Vermeulen NPE, et al. Pharmacokinetics of lidocaine and bupivacaine following subarachnoid administration in surgical patients: simultaneous investigation of absorption and disposition kinetics using stable isotopes. Anesthesiology. 1988;69:584–92.

Cousins MJ, Bridenbaugh PO, (eds). Neural blockade in clinical anaesthesia and management of pain. 2nd edn. Philadelphia: JB Lippincott Co. 1988;57.

Evers H, Von Dardel O, Juhlin L, et al. Dermal effects of compositions based on the eutectic mixture of lignocaine and prilocaine (EMLA). Studies in volunteers. Br J Anaesth. 1985;57:997–1005.

Hughes MA, Glass PS, Jacobs JR. Context-sensitive half-time in multicompartment pharmacokinetic models for intravenous anesthetic drugs. Anesthesiology. 1992;76:334–41.

Jamous MA, Hand CW, Moore RA, et al. Epinephrine reduces systemic absorption of extradural diacetylmorphine. Anesth & Analg. 1986;65:1290–4.

Kremer JMH, Wilting J, Janssen LHM. Drug binding to human alpha-1-acid glycoprotein in health and disease. Pharmacol Rev. 1988;40:1–47.

McCafferty DF, Woolfson AD, Boston V. *In vivo* assessment of percutaneous local anaesthetic preparations. Br J Anaesth. 1989;62:17–21.

Moore RA, Bullingham RSJ, McQuay HJ, et al. Dural permeability to narcotics: *In vitro* determination and application to extradural administration. Br J Anaesth. 1982;54:1117–28.

Roerig DL, Kotrly KJ, Ahlf SB, Dawson CA, Kampine JP. Effect of propranolol on the first pass uptake of fentanyl in the human and rat lung. Anesthesiology. 1989;71:62–8.

Sear JW. Metabolism and elimination of drugs: influence of disease states. In: Prys-Roberts C, Brown BR Jr, (eds). International practice of anaesthesia. Oxford: Butterworth Heinemann; 1996:1/14/3.

Sheiner LB. The population approach to pharmacokinetic data analysis: rationale and standard data analysis methods. Drug Metabolism Rev. 1984;15:153–71.

Vinik HR, Reves JG, Greenblatt DJ, et al. The pharmacokinetics of midazolam in chronic renal failure patients. Anesthesiology. 1983;59:390–4.

Walle T, Byington RP, Furberg CD, et al. Biologic determinants of propranolol disposition: results from 1308 patients in the beta-blocker heart attack trial. Clin Pharmacol Ther. 1985;38:509–18.

Wilkinson GR, Lund PC. Bupivacaine levels in plasma and cerebrospinal fluid following peridural administration. Anesthesiology. 1970;33:482–6.

Further Reading

Hull CJ. Pharmacokinetics for anaesthesia. Oxford: Butterworth Heinemann; 1991.

Hull CJ. Compartmental models. Anaesth Pharmacol Rev. 1994;2:188–203.

Runciman WB, Mather LE. Effects of anaesthesia on drug disposition. In: Feldman SA, Scurr CF, Paton W, eds. Drugs in anaesthesia: mechanisms of action. London: Arnold; 1987:87–122.

Whiting B, Kelman AW, Grevel J. Population kinetics. Theory and clinical application. Clin Pharmacokinetics. 1986;11:387–401.

Chapter 8 Pharmacokinetics of inhalation anesthetics

Jerrold Lerman

Topics covered in this chapter

DRUG DELIVERY SYSTEMS

Circuits

The anesthetic circuit serves several purposes, including the delivery of anesthetic, oxygen, heat, and humidity to the patient, and the removal of anesthetics and carbon dioxide from the patient. The circuit also facilitates ventilation, either spontaneous or mechanical. The classification of anesthetic circuits can be confusing, but a simple approach classifies circuits as:

- circuits that include a carbon dioxide absorber (e.g. circle systems);
- rebreathing circuits where inspired and exhaled gases can mix (e.g. Ayre's T-piece or the Bain circuit).
- nonrebreathing circuits in which a one-way valve separates the inspired and exhaled gases (e.g. the resuscitation self-inflating bag);

Circle systems are made up of a fresh gas hose from the anesthetic machine, a canister (which contains a carbon dioxide absorbent such as soda lime or barium hydroxide lime), a reservoir bag for spontaneous or manual ventilation, two unidirectional valves (one on each of the inspiratory and expiratory limbs of the circuit), inspiratory and expiratory hoses, and a Y-piece to connect the hoses to the mask or tracheal tube. They may be used with either spontaneous or controlled ventilation, at any fresh gas flow (the lowest flow being 4mL/min per kg body weight oxygen flow), for prolonged periods, and with patients of any age. The absorbent removes carbon dioxide from the exhaled gas in an exothermic reaction that produces an alkaline medium, heat, and water (Fig. 8.1). When the absorbent is expended, an indicator changes color. After leaving the canister, the exhaled gas mixes with fresh gas in the inspiratory limb of the circuit. These circuits are efficient, inexpensive, and environmentally friendly. However, they suffer from several disadvantages including a slow wash-in and wash-out of anesthetic (see below), bulky and heavy tubing, and, if high-compliance hoses are used with positive pressure ventilation, wasted ventilation. Furthermore, unidirectional valves can fail and cause unanticipated rebreathing of exhaled gases or the inability to ventilate with positive pressure. Finally, concerns exist regarding the degradation of inhaled anesthetics in the presence of absorbents.

Reactions involved in the chemical absorption of carbon dioxide

Reaction of carbon dioxide with barium hydroxide lime

$Ba(OH)_2 + 8H_2O + CO_2 \rightleftharpoons BaCO_3 + 9H_2O + \text{heat}$

$9(H_2O) + 9CO_2 \rightleftharpoons 9H_2CO_3$

Then by direct reactions and by KOH and NaOH

$9H_2CO_3 + 9Ba(OH)_2 \rightleftharpoons 9BaCO_3 + 18H_2O + \text{heat}$

Reaction of carbon dioxide with soda lime

$CO_2 + H_2O \rightleftharpoons H_2CO_3$

$H_2CO_3 + 2NaOH(KOH) \rightleftharpoons Na_2CO_3(K_2CO_3) + 2H_2O + \text{heat}$

$Na_2CO_3(K_2CO_3) + Ca(OH)_2 \rightleftharpoons CaCO_3 + 2NaOH(KOH)$

Figure 8.1 Reactions involved in the chemical absorption of carbon dioxide. The reaction with barium hydroxide lime involves a direct reaction of barium hydroxide and carbon dioxide and liberates more water than the reaction with soda lime.

Inhaled anesthetics that degrade in the presence of absorbents include halothane, isoflurane, enflurane, and sevoflurane. At high temperatures, halothane is degraded to 2-bromochloroethylene, although the concentration of this degradation product is less than 3% of its lethal concentration. Isoflurane, enflurane, and desflurane are absorbed and degraded to small extents in the presence of soda lime. Sevoflurane also undergoes alkaline hydrolysis to produce five compounds, of which compound A, a halogenated alkene, is the most abundant (Fig. 8.2). Several factors increase the rate of degradation of sevoflurane and thus increase the production of compound A in the presence of carbon dioxide absorbents. These include high concentrations of sevoflurane, very low fresh gas flows (i.e. closed circuits), high absorber temperature, prolonged exposure, and dry absorbent. The degradation is greater with barium hydroxide lime than with soda lime and in adults compared with infants. Concern regarding the generation of compound A stems from the fact that it causes histologic and biochemical changes in rat kidney, although similar changes have not been demonstrated in primates or humans. A minimum fresh gas flow of 2L/min is recommended with sevoflurane in the presence of a carbon dioxide absorbent.

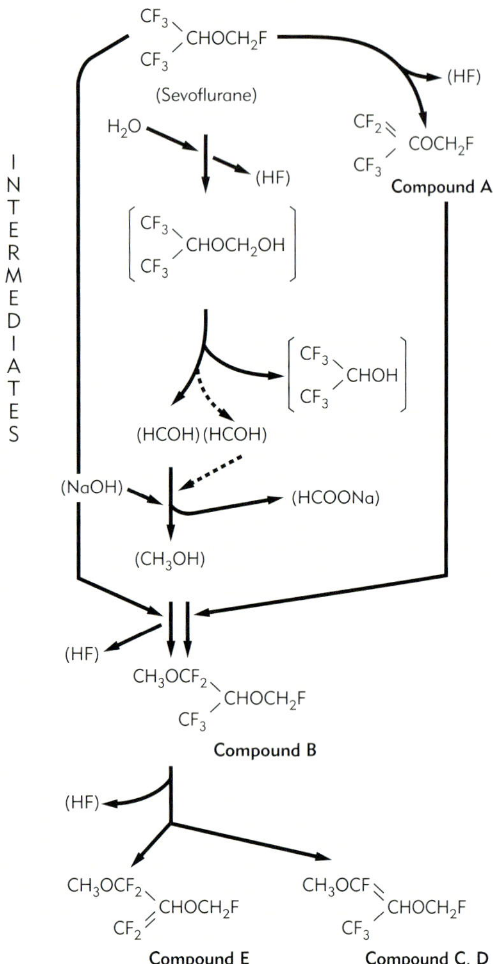

Figure 8.2 Possible mechanism for the decomposition of sevoflurane by soda lime.

Carbon monoxide is another product of the degradation of inhaled anesthetics in the presence of carbon dioxide absorbents. Carbon monoxide can be formed after volatile anesthetics interact with very dry absorbent. The amount formed depends in part on the anesthetic (desflurane > enflurane > isoflurane >>> halothane = sevoflurane). Factors that increase degradation include low moisture content, high temperature, and the use of barium hydroxide lime rather than soda lime. To avoid drying out the absorbent, it is essential that the fresh gas flow is disconnected from the anesthetic machine when the machine is not in service, that the anesthetic machine is turned off before long periods of disuse, and that, if the circle circuit is left intact, the reservoir bag also remains in place.

Rebreathing circuits have been further classified by Mapleson according to their design and function during spontaneous respiration (designated A–F). The most common rebreathing systems in use belong to the Mapleson E or F category. Examples are the Jackson–Rees modification of the Ayre's T-piece and the Bain circuit, which is a valved coaxial version. Rebreathing is always possible with these circuits depending on the minute ventilation and fresh gas flow. These circuits deliver rapid wash-in and wash-out of anesthetic (see below). In the past, large fresh gas flows were used to prevent rebreathing carbon dioxide. With the widespread availability of capnography, much lower fresh gas flows may be used to maintain end-tidal carbon dioxide tensions within normal limits. Accurate end-tidal carbon dioxide tension assessment is possible even in small infants with the use of a catheter inserted into the lumen of the tracheal tube. Disadvantages of rebreathing circuits include the apparent high cost (because of the large fresh gas flows used in the past), environmental concerns (because of the wasted large fresh gas flow, including nitrous oxide), minimal heat conservation, and negligible humidity.

Vaporizers

Vaporizers are devices that deliver the desired concentration of anesthetic vapor. They are situated on the anesthetic machine, upstream from the fresh gas outlet. Functionally, vaporizers fulfill two roles: they act as both reservoirs and controllers. As reservoirs, vaporizers store a volume of liquid anesthetic. As controllers, they add a calibrated volume of anesthetic vapor to the fresh gas to yield the desired inspired concentration of anesthetic. Most modern vaporizers are temperature-compensated, concentration-calibrated variable bypass devices designed for use with a specific anesthetic (Fig. 8.3). The desflurane vaporizer is not a variable bypass vaporizer and depends on electricity to maintain high temperature and pressure within the vaporizer, as described below.

Delivery of a known concentration of anesthetic vapor is achieved using a variable bypass system. Fresh gas is split into two streams: a smaller stream that passes through the vaporizer and a larger stream that bypasses the vaporizer. The concentration-calibrated controller directs a fraction of fresh gas into the vaporizer where it becomes saturated with anesthetic vapor. Upon exiting the vaporizer, this smaller stream mixes with the larger bypass stream to yield the inspired concentration set on the controlling dial. The low boiling point of desflurane precludes delivery by a variable bypass system. Instead, desflurane is delivered via an electrically heated (39°C) and pressurized (1500mmHg) vaporizer that injects a known volume of desflurane vapor into the fresh gas flow to yield the dialed inspired concentration.

Several techniques are used to control vaporizer output during changes in vaporizer temperature, including expandable bellows and bimetallic strips (composed of nickel and brass). As vaporizer temperature increases, the bellows expand or the strip bends to increase bypass flow. This increase in bypass flow compensates for the increase in anesthetic concentration in the effluent that results from the increase in temperature. Because the relationship between temperature and vapor pressure of volatile anesthetics is nonlinear, vaporizers are calibrated within a narrow operating temperature range.

Each vaporizer is calibrated for use with one inhaled anesthetic. Anesthetic-specific filling keys can be used to ensure that the vaporizer is filled with the intended anesthetic. If a vaporizer is filled with an anesthetic for which it was not intended, output may be greater, less, or no different than the 'dialed' concentration, depending on the characteristics of both the vaporizer and the anesthetic. The volume of liquid anesthetic vaporized per hour may be estimated by the simple expression: 3 × dialed% × fresh gas flow (L/min) (where 3 is a factor that corrects for time and volume units). Thus, 1% halothane at a gas flow of 6L/min vaporizes 18mL of liquid halothane per hour.

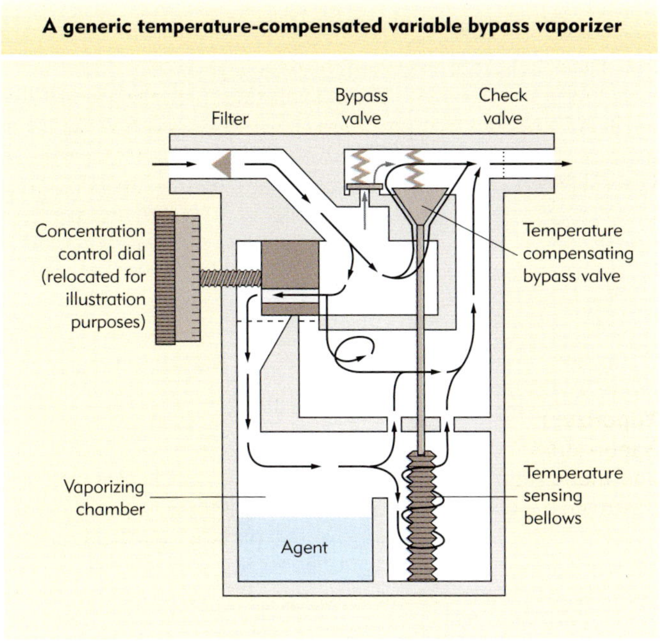

A generic temperature-compensated variable bypass vaporizer

Figure 8.3 A generic temperature-compensated variable bypass vaporizer. Temperature compensation is achieved by a gas-filled temperature-sensing bellows that controls a temperature-compensating bypass valve. Other vaporizers use a bimetallic strip incorporated into a flap valve in the bypass gas flow. (With permission from Eisenkraft, 1993.)

Modern vaporizers are well-engineered devices capable of delivering the dialed inspired concentration from 0.2 to 15L/min for most anesthetics and concentrations. However, the dial indicator may overestimate the delivered concentration at higher dial settings when fresh gas flow exceeds 5L/min. Vaporizer performance can be affected by factors other than fresh gas flow rate, including carrier gas composition (nitrous oxide dissolves in the liquid anesthetic and decreases vaporizer output during the early period of administration), atmospheric pressure (at high altitude, vaporizer output increases substantially in terms of volume percentage but increases much less in terms of potency), filling the vaporizer with an anesthetic for which it is not calibrated, and back pressure in the fresh gas circuit (although most vaporizers and anesthetic machines have back-pressure compensation valves). The maximum inspired concentration that a vaporizer can deliver is determined by a number of characteristics of the anesthetic including the concentration at which it is flammable, its potency, its wash-in profile, and its lethal concentration.

PHARMACOLOGY

This subject is covered in detail in Chapter 24. The potent inhalational (volatile) anesthetics are polyhalogenated alkanes (halothane) or ether derivatives [methylethyl ethers (methoxyflurane, enflurane, isoflurane, desflurane) or methylisopropyl ethers (sevoflurane)]. They share physicochemical properties including reduced flammability, boiling point at approximately 50°C [with the exception of methoxyflurane (104°C) and desflurane (23°C)] and stability in the liquid and vapor phases (Fig. 8.4).

The potency of inhalational anesthetics is measured by the minimum alveolar concentration (MAC), which is that concentration that prevents movement in response to a standardized skin incision in 50% of subjects (Chapter 24). The MAC values for volatile anesthetics in neonates and adults are shown in Figure 8.4. Minimum alveolar concentration decreases with increasing age; it is maximal in infancy and decreases thereafter and with decreasing gestational age to 24 weeks (Fig. 8.5). For sevoflurane, MAC appears to vary less with age; the MAC in neonates and infants (1–6 months of age) is 3.2% and that in older infants and children up to 12 years of age is 2.5%. Minimum alveolar concentration varies

Properties of inhalation anesthetics

Physical properties	Halothane	Enflurane	Isoflurane	Sevoflurane	Desflurane
Chemical structure	F Br F-C-C-H F Cl	F F Cl H-C-O-C-C-H F F F	F Cl F H-C-O-C-C-F F H F	H CF_3 F-C-O-C-H H CF_3	F F F H-C-O-C-C-F F H F
Molecular weight	197.4	184.5	184.5	200.1	168
Boiling point (°C)	50.2	56.5	48.5	58.6	23.5
Vapor pressure (mmHg)	244	172	240	185	664
Percent metabolized (*in vivo*)	15–20	2.4	0.2	5.0	0.02
Solubility					
Blood:gas ratio in adults	2.4	1.9	1.4	0.66	0.42
Blood:gas ratio in neonates	2.1	1.8	1.19	0.66	–
Fat:blood ratio in adults	51	–	45	48	27
Minimum alveolar concentration (MAC)					
MAC in adults	0.75	1.7	1.2	2.05	7.0
MAC in neonates	0.87	–	1.6	3.2	9.2

Figure 8.4 Properties of the inhalation anesthetics. The data regarding the percentages of compounds metabolized *in vivo* are from studies in both humans and animals.

with a number of factors in addition to age, including coadministration of other agents (e.g. nitrous oxide, opioids, α_2-agonists, etc.), temperature, and pregnancy.

PHARMACOKINETICS

General principles

The increase in the ratio of inhaled anesthetic fraction or partial pressure in the alveoli (FA) to that in inspired (FI) fresh gas with time is known as wash-in. The relationship between FA/FI and time during this wash-in period is described by the differential equation:

Equation 8.1

$$\frac{dFA}{dFI} = -t/\tau$$

where t is time and τ is the time constant. The units of τ are time and thus the ratio dFA/dFI is dimensionless. The time constant for wash-in of inhaled anesthetics is defined as the ratio of the capacity of the reservoir (V) into which the anesthetic is delivered to the flow rate of anesthetic (Q) into the reservoir:

Equation 8.2

$$\tau = \frac{V}{Q}$$

To solve Equation 8.1, the ratio FA/FI, must be defined at the extremes of time: at $t = 0$, when FA/FI is zero, and at $t = \infty$, when FA/FI approaches 1.0. Equation 8.1 is then integrated to yield:

Equation 8.3

$$\frac{FA}{FI} = 1 - e^{-t/\tau}$$

Using Equations 8.2 and 8.3, we can estimate the time to equilibration of FA and FI in the lungs, assuming uptake of anesthetic from the lungs is negligible. For adults, the functional residual capacity (FRC) is 2L and alveolar ventilation is 4L/min. Hence, τ is 2/4 or 0.5 minutes. When t equals 1τ, FA/FI $= 1 - e^{-1}$ or 0.63. Thus, the alveolar fraction is 63% of the inspired fraction. The values for FA/FI for larger multiples of 2, 3, and $4t$ are 84, 92, and 96%, respectively. Based on these values, it takes four half-lives or approximately 2 minutes to reach 96% equilibration of FA with FI in the adult.

Determinants of wash-in

The rate of increase in FA/FI (wash-in) depends on a balance of the rate of anesthetic delivery to and removal (or uptake) from the lungs. If delivery to the lungs is unopposed (negligible uptake), then the increase in FA/FI progresses unopposed and rapidly towards equilibration (i.e. unity) as for the wash-in of nitrous oxide and desflurane (and of other inhalation anesthetics in the first 2 minutes of wash-in). This interval represents unopposed wash-in of anesthetic into the lungs and has implications for the maximum deliverable inspired concentration by a vaporizer (see below). However, if delivery to the lungs is opposed by rapid removal (as in the case of a more soluble anesthetic such as halothane), then FA/FI increases more slowly (Fig. 8.6a). The wash-in of inhalational anesthetics depends upon six factors. The first three factors determine the rate of anesthetic delivery to the lungs: ventilation, FRC, and inspired concentration. The second three determine its rate of removal from the lungs: solubility, cardiac output, and alveolar-to-venous partial pressure gradient.

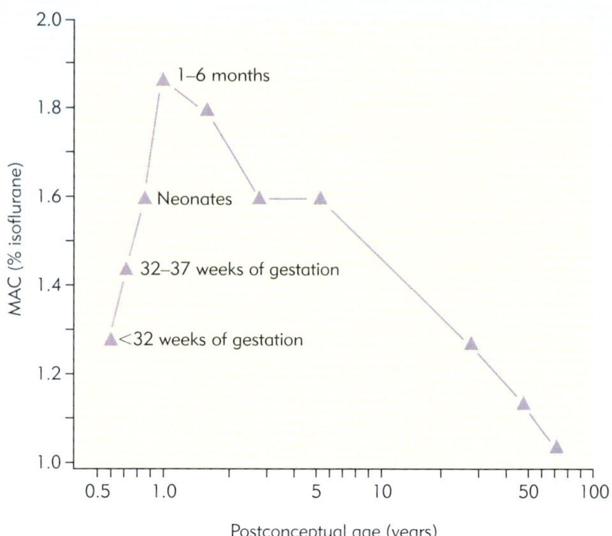

Figure 8.5 Relationship between age and the minimum alveolar concentration (MAC) for isoflurane. MAC increases throughout gestation, reaching a maximum in infants 1–6 months of age. Thereafter, MAC decreases with increasing age.

Ventilation

The fraction of the minute ventilation that determines anesthetic delivery to the lungs is that fraction involved in gas exchange, that is, alveolar ventilation (Chapter 44). Throughout this chapter, ventilation refers exclusively to alveolar ventilation, which directly affects the wash-in of inhalation anesthetics in the lungs. That is, changes in alveolar ventilation result in parallel changes in the rate of increase in FA/FI (Fig. 8.6b).

Functional residual capacity

The value of τ depends on the ratio of the volume of the reservoir into which the gas flows, the FRC (V), to the alveolar ventilation (Q), as in Equation 8.2. Changes in FRC lead to parallel changes in τ during wash-in, provided alveolar ventilation remains constant. In clinical situations such as obesity and restrictive lung defects in which FRC is reduced, wash-in is more rapid.

Inspired concentration

The inspired concentration of an inhalational anesthetic is the driving force of anesthetic into the lungs, blood, and tissues. The greater the inspired concentration, the greater the driving force and the more rapid the increase in the ratio FA/FI. This factor significantly affects only nitrous oxide because it is given in concentrations greater than 50%.

Uptake of anesthetic from the lungs

Uptake of anesthetic from the lungs is the product of three factors: cardiac output, solubility or the blood/gas partition coefficient (λ), and the alveolar-to-venous partial pressure gradient. If any of these factors decrease, uptake decreases in parallel. As

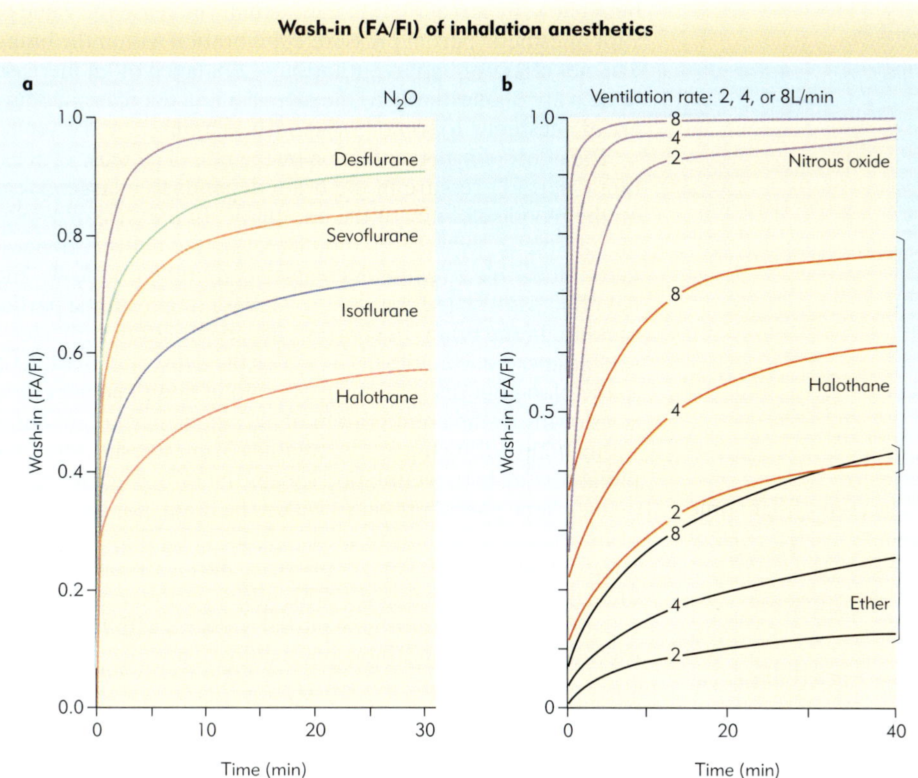

Figure 8.6 Wash-in (FA/FI) of inhalation anesthetics. (a) The wash-in of anesthetics increases as their solubility in blood decreases. (b) Increasing alveolar ventilation at a fixed cardiac output increases wash-in. The effect of ventilation on wash-in increases with increasing anesthetic solubility in blood.

a consequence, the partial pressure of anesthetic remaining in the lungs increases more rapidly until it equilibrates with the inspired partial pressure.

Solubility

Inhalational anesthetics partition from the gas phase into two physiologic compartments: an aqueous phase and a protein/lipid phase. This is analogous to the distribution of oxygen and carbon dioxide in blood between the aqueous phase and hemoglobin. The fraction of anesthetic that is dissolved in the aqueous phase determines the *partial pressure* of the anesthetic (Fig. 8.4). The remainder of anesthetic is bound to proteins and lipids in liquids and tissues. The solubility of inhalational anesthetics is defined as the ratio of the concentrations of anesthetic in two phases when the partial pressure of the anesthetic in the two phases has equilibrated.

The rate of increase of wash-in is inversely related to anesthetic solubility in blood; anesthetics that are less soluble wash-in more rapidly than those that are more soluble. This occurs because the diminished uptake of less-soluble anesthetics from the lungs results in the accumulation of more anesthetic within the lungs and its partial pressure increases more rapidly than for the more soluble anesthetics (Fig. 8.6). Thus, the alveolar partial pressure of less-soluble anesthetics equilibrates more rapidly with inspired partial pressure than does the alveolar pressure of the more-soluble anesthetics. The same holds true for the tissue partial pressure of anesthetics.

Cardiac output

Uptake of inhalational anesthetic from the lung involves movement of anesthetic across the alveolar capillary membrane and removal of anesthetic by blood traversing the pulmonary capillaries. The alveolar–capillary membrane offers negligible resistance to anesthetic movement. Removal of anesthetic from the lungs depends on two remaining factors: pulmonary blood flow (or cardiac output) and the alveolar-to-venous partial pressure gradient. The greater the pulmonary blood flow, the greater the uptake of anesthetic by blood, which in turn increases the quantity of anesthetic delivered to tissues. However, the greater uptake of anesthetic from the lungs actually slows the rise of wash-in. Because the difference in anesthetic partial pressures (not concentrations) between the lungs or blood and tissues is the driving force along which anesthetics move from lung into blood and from blood into tissues, the slower rate of increase of alveolar partial pressure slows the accumulation of anesthetic in fluids and tissues. Thus, an increase in cardiac output actually slows the rate of increase of both wash-in and the partial pressure of anesthetic in tissues (Fig. 8.7). Conversely, as cardiac output decreases, so too does the uptake of anesthetic from the lungs. This speeds the equilibration of FA and FI. When the blood flow to brain and heart is preserved in states with low cardiac output, the rapid increase in alveolar and blood anesthetic partial pressures rapidly depresses vital organ function.

Alveolar-to-venous partial pressure gradient

The alveolar-to-venous partial pressure gradient is the force that drives inhalational anesthetics from the alveolus to the venous blood. As the anesthetic partial pressure in tissues approaches that in blood, so too does the partial pressure of anesthetic in the venous blood returning to the lungs approach alveolar values. The net effect is a decrease in the alveolar-to-venous anesthetic partial pressure gradient and, therefore, a decrease in the uptake of anesthetic from the lungs. As this gradient approaches zero (i.e. the partial pressures of anesthetic in tissues, blood, and lungs equilibrate), uptake of anesthetic also approaches zero. This occurs earlier for less-soluble anesthetics.

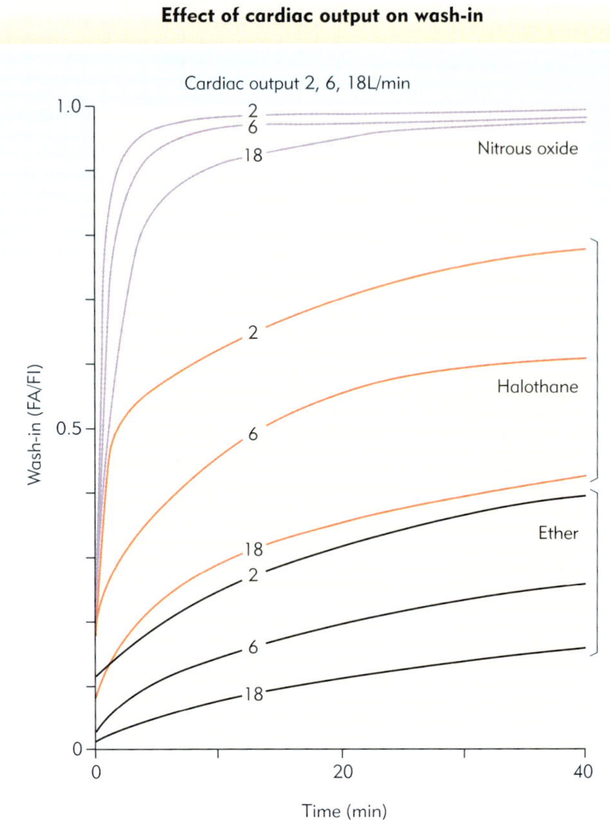

Figure 8.7 Effect of cardiac output on wash in. Increasing cardiac output at a fixed alveolar ventilation decreases wash-in. The effect of cardiac output increases with increasing anesthetic solubility in blood.

SPECIFIC CONDITIONS

Ventilation

Changes in ventilation

Changes in ventilation affect the rate of increase of wash-in of more soluble inhalational anesthetics to a greater extent (Fig. 8.6b). The rate of increase of wash-in of less-soluble anesthetics is rapid because there is little uptake of anesthetic from the lungs, and FA/FI equilibrates rapidly. In contrast, the rate of increase of wash-in for more-soluble anesthetics is slow. This slow wash-in may be attributed to the rapid removal of anesthetics from the alveoli because of their high solubilities in blood and tissues. If the delivery of the soluble anesthetic was increased, the balance of the delivery to and uptake from alveoli would favor an increased delivery and, therefore, an increase in the rate of wash-in of anesthetic.

Hyperventilation

On the basis of the above discussion, increases in ventilation (or hyperventilation) should speed the rate of alveolar-to-blood-to-tissue anesthetic movement and, thus, reduce the time for equilibration of anesthetic pressures within tissues. However, increases in alveolar ventilation may also affect tissue blood flow. For example, hyperventilation decreases arterial carbon dioxide tension, which in turn decreases cerebral blood flow. Because the delivery of anesthetic to the brain depends on its blood flow, hyperventilation may actually increase the value of τ for anesthetic partial pressure equilibration within the brain. The net effect of hyperventilation is a balance of an increase in delivery of anesthetic to the alveoli and a decrease in delivery of anesthetic to some tissues such as brain.

The effect of hyperventilation on the rate of increase of anesthetic partial pressure in the brain depends to a large extent on the blood solubility of the anesthetic. In the case of a soluble anesthetic, hyperventilation increases the delivery of anesthetic to the blood while decreasing cerebral blood flow. The net effect is to speed the rate of increase of anesthetic partial pressure in the brain. In contrast, hyperventilation with a less-soluble anesthetic minimally increases the delivery of anesthetic to the blood but decreases cerebral blood flow. The net effect is a slowing of the equilibration of anesthetic partial pressures within brain during the first 15 minutes of anesthesia. After this initial period, hyperventilation speeds the rate of equilibration of anesthetic partial pressures within the brain. For anesthetics of intermediate solubility such as halothane, these opposing effects of hyperventilation are offsetting during the initial period of anesthesia (Fig. 8.8). After this initial period, however, the rate of increase of anesthetic partial pressure within the brain exceeds that during normocapnic ventilation.

Modes of ventilation

Two feedback mechanisms exist in response to inhalational anesthesia: respiratory and cardiovascular. The respiratory feedback mechanism is a negative feedback loop in which *spontaneous ventilation* decreases as the depth of anesthesia increases, owing to respiratory depression. This limits the depth of anesthesia by attenuating the delivery of anesthetic to the lungs. Although the delivery of anesthetic to the lungs subsides, anesthetic present in tissues redistributes from organs in which it is present at a high partial pressure (such as the brain) to others in which it is present at a low partial pressure (such as muscle). When the partial pressure of anesthetic in the brain has decreased to a threshold level, respiration increases. This feedback loop is a protective mechanism that prevents anesthetic overdose by limiting delivery of anesthetic to vital organs.

The second feedback mechanism is a positive feedback loop in which cardiac output decreases as the depth of anesthesia increases. As cardiac output decreases, the uptake of anesthetic from the lungs decreases and, thus, the rate of increase of alveolar-to-inspired anesthetic partial pressure increases further. This increase in alveolar partial pressure is reflected in an increase in the partial pressure of anesthetic in blood and a greater driving force for anesthetic delivery to tissues. The increase in anesthetic partial pressure in tissues further depresses organ function such as cardiac output, with a further increase in anesthetic partial pressure in alveoli, blood, and tissues.

The significance of these two feedback loops on the pharmacokinetics of volatile anesthetics has been investigated in adult dogs. Dogs were allowed to breathe spontaneously while anesthetized with halothane in concentrations between 0.3 and 4%. FA/FI increased to approximately 0.65 after 15 minutes, where it remained for up to 50 minutes. All of the dogs survived. In a second experiment, dogs were ventilated mechanically while anesthetized with halothane at similar inspired concentrations. The FA/FI plateaued only in those dogs given an inspired concentration of 1.5% or less. The FA/FI increased relentlessly to approximately 1.0 in those dogs

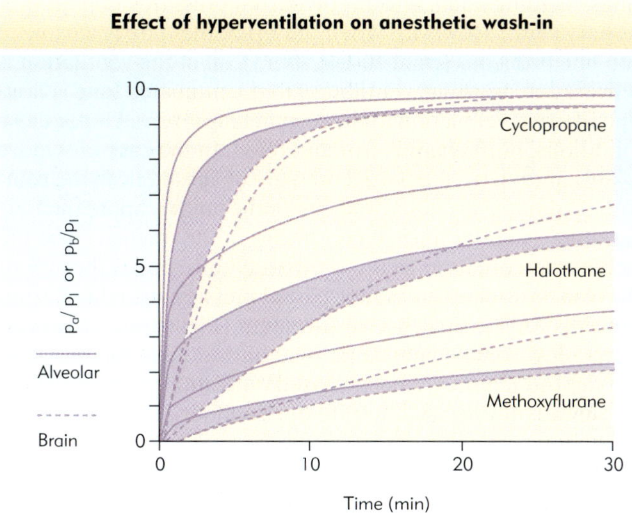

Figure 8.8 The effect of hyperventilation on the wash-in of three inhalational anesthetics of different solubilities: cyclopropane (less soluble), methoxyflurane (very soluble), and halothane (intermediate solubility). Two conditions are delineated: normocapnia (denoted by the curves joined by the purple shading) and hypocapnia induced by hyperventilation (other curves). Compared with the normocapnic state, hyperventilation speeds the rise of alveolar anesthetic partial pressure for all three anesthetics, although the effect is greatest with the most soluble and least with the least soluble anesthetic. In contrast, hyperventilation delays the rise of brain anesthetic partial pressure most with the least soluble and least with the most soluble anesthetic. The effect on halothane is intermediate. Pa, alveolar partial pressure; Pb, brain partial pressure; PI, inspired partial pressure of anesthetic. (Adapted with permission from Munson and Bowers, 1967.)

that were anesthetized with 4 and 6% halothane; within 1 hour most of those dogs experienced circulatory collapse (Fig. 8.9). Thus, spontaneous ventilation remains an effective negative feedback mechanism for preventing an overdose of a volatile anesthetic. In contrast, *controlled ventilation* exposes patients to a positive feedback mechanism that may result in a relentless downward spiral of circulatory depression unless anesthetic partial pressure is reduced.

The concentration effect

The concentration effect results from two factors: a concentrating effect and an augmentation in effective ventilation. When an inhalational anesthetic is administered in a small concentration (1%), uptake of half of this anesthetic results in a concentration of approximately 0.5%. The net effect of the uptake of this small volume on the alveolar gas volume is small; ventilation is minimally affected. If, however, the anesthetic is administered in an 80% concentration, uptake of half of the anesthetic contracts the residual gas volume. The net concentration is not 50% of the original concentration but rather it is 66%, because of the concentrating effect on the smaller residual gas volume. This effect along with the additional ventilation that follows the contracted alveolar volume leads to a concentration that exceeds 70%. The only anesthetic administered today that is subject to the concentration effect is nitrous oxide.

Second gas effect

When two anesthetics are administered one in a large concentration and another in a small concentration, the concentration effect of the first anesthetic may increase the concentration of the second anesthetic. This effect, which is produced by the same two mechanisms that explain the concentration effect above, has been demonstrated in dogs, but its clinical relevance has been questioned.

Overpressure technique

In order to establish rapidly the desired partial pressure of anesthetic in the alveoli or brain, its inspired partial pressure may be adjusted to a value that is severalfold greater than the desired alveolar partial pressure (known as the overpressure technique). For example, if the target alveolar (or brain) partial pressure of an anesthetic is 1.0%, then the inspired partial pressure of anesthetic could be adjusted to a value of 3%. During the early period of anesthesia, FA/FI increases rapidly, reaching a ratio of 0.3 (Fig. 8.6a) and, thus, achieving the target alveolar or brain partial pressure of 1%.

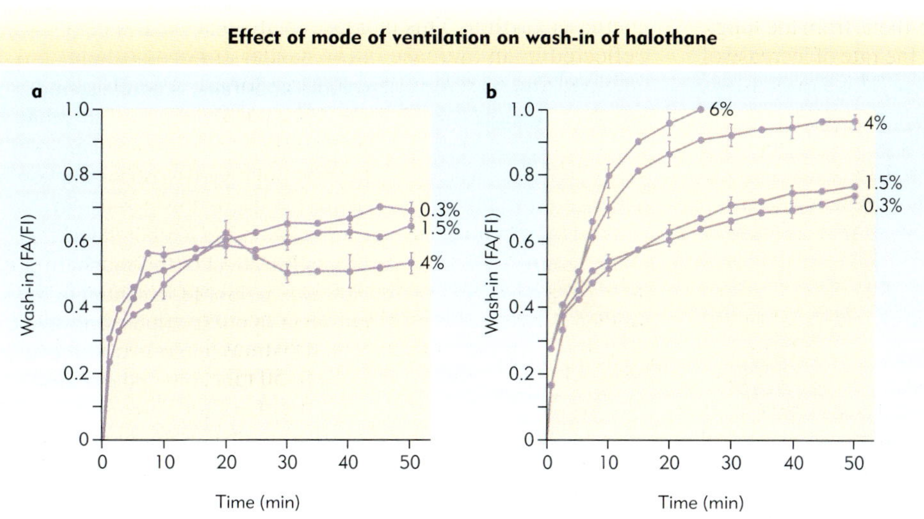

Figure 8.9 Effect of mode of ventilation on wash-in of halothane. Wash-in [the rate of rise of the ratio of alveolar (FA) to inspired (FI) anesthetic partial pressure] is shown for (a) spontaneous and (b) controlled ventilation. The negative feedback effect of spontaneous ventilation limits the rate of rise of FA/FI. All dogs survived. The positive feedback effect of decreased cardiac output during controlled ventilation, resulted in death in those dogs anesthetized with 4 or 6% halothane.

Vital capacity inductions

Although the traditional technique used for induction of anesthesia by inhalation is a stepwise increase in inspired concentration every few breaths, single-breath vital capacity inductions have become popular with the introduction of sevoflurane. The stepwise technique was conceived out of concerns that laryngospasm and breathholding might occur if high concentrations of halothane were administered too rapidly. These concerns have not been supported with recent evidence. To perform a single-breath induction, the anesthetic circuit is first primed with the maximum deliverable concentration of anesthetic and the patient then performs one or more vital capacity inhalations. These inductions are more rapid than graded stepwise inductions.

Cardiac output

Changes in cardiac output affect the rate of increase in alveolar-to-inspired anesthetic partial pressure of soluble anesthetics to a greater extent than less-soluble anesthetics. Soluble anesthetics are removed from the alveoli in greater quantities and, therefore, in the presence of an increased cardiac output, the rate of rise of alveolar-to-inspired partial pressures of soluble anesthetics is slower than that of less-soluble anesthetics. This is reflected in parallel changes in the partial pressure of more soluble anesthetics in tissues, since the anesthetic partial pressure in the blood equilibrates with that in the alveoli.

Shunts

Left-to-right shunts (where blood is recirculated through the lungs) do not usually affect wash-in of inhalational anesthetics provided cardiac output and its distribution remain unchanged. In contrast, right-to-left shunts (where venous blood bypasses the lungs and mixes with arterial blood) exert a significant effect on wash-in of inhalational anesthetics. The magnitude of this effect depends on the solubility of the anesthetic: right-to-left shunts affect less-soluble anesthetics (i.e. nitrous oxide, desflurane, and sevoflurane) to a much greater extent than they affect the more soluble anesthetics (i.e. halothane and methoxyflurane). In the model shown in Figure 8.10, each lung is represented by one alveolus and is perfused by one pulmonary artery. When the tracheal tube is positioned at the mid-trachea level (i.e. no shunt), ventilation is divided equally between both lungs, yielding equal anesthetic partial pressures in both pulmonary veins. However, when the tip of the tube is advanced into one bronchus (right-to-left shunt), all of the ventilation is delivered to one lung; ventilation to the intubated lung is doubled whereas ventilation to the second lung is zero. Under these conditions, normocapnia is maintained. In the case of a more soluble anesthetic, the partial pressure of anesthetic in the combined pulmonary venous drainage of the lungs is approximately the same as under normal conditions in the trachea since the increased ventilation to the intubated lung speeds the rise of alveolar-to-inspired anesthetic partial pressure such that it compensates for the presence of the shunt (Fig 8.10b). However, when a less-soluble anesthetic is administered in the presence of a right-to-left shunt, the increased ventilation to the intubated lung minimally affects the rate of rise of alveolar-to-inspired anesthetic partial pressures in that lung since changes in ventilation do not appreciably affect the wash-in of less-soluble anesthetics (Fig 8.10c). In this case, the anesthetic partial pressure in the combined pulmonary venous drainage lags behind that which would occur in the absence of a right-to-left shunt.

Temperature

The solubility of inhalational anesthetics in blood and tissues is inversely related to temperature: as the temperature decreases, the solubility increases. Solubility increases 4–5% for every 1°C decrease in temperature. Temperature has a predictable effect on the pharmacokinetics of inhalational anesthetics. As temperature decreases and solubility increases, the rate of rise of alveolar-to-inspired anesthetic concentration slows. This effect is most prominent during cardiopulmonary bypass, when temperatures as low as 10–15°C are used.

TISSUE UPTAKE

The uptake of anesthetic by the body is the sum of uptake by all tissues in the body. Initially, the uptake of anesthetic by tissues is great and the partial pressure of anesthetic in the venous blood returning to the lungs is low. As the partial pressure of anesthetic in tissues approaches that within the alveoli, the partial pressure of anesthetic in venous blood also increases. This diminishes the alveolar-to-venous partial pressure gradient, one

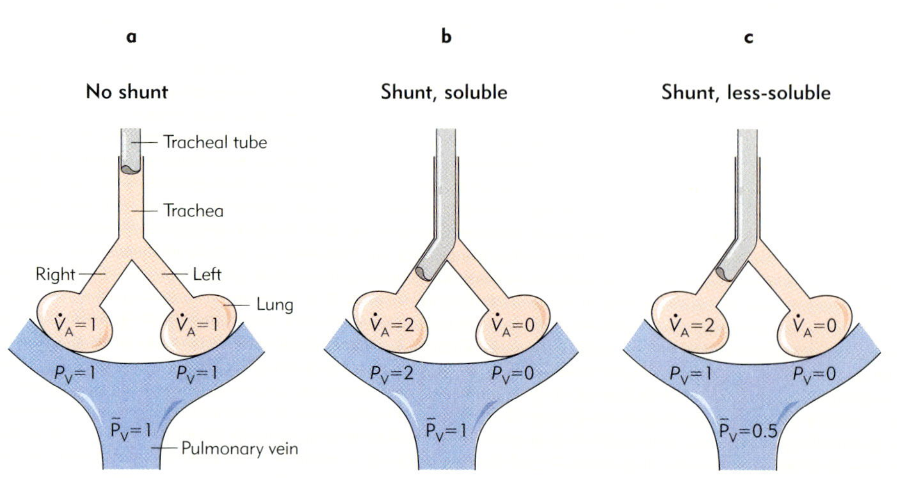

Figure 8.10 The effect of shunts on the rate of increase of pulmonary vein anesthetic pressures varies with the solubility of the anesthetic. If a soluble anesthetic is administered in the presence of a right-to-left shunt (b), normocapnia is maintained and hypoxic pulmonary vasoconstriction is negligible. Here, the increase in ventilation to the intubated lung offsets the effect of the shunt. However, a right-to-left shunt in the presence of a less-soluble anesthetic (c) limits the increase in anesthetic partial pressure in the pulmonary vein (P_V). Since an increase in alveolar ventilation does not affect the wash-in of a less-soluble anesthetic substantially, the shunted blood slows the rate of rise of P_V.

of the determinants of anesthetic uptake from the lungs, and anesthetic uptake diminishes.

Anesthetic uptake can be estimated by grouping tissues according to the time to anesthetic partial pressure equilibration within the tissues; this is related to the relative solubility of the inhalational anesthetics in those tissues and the perfusion to the tissues. Tissues have been divided into four groups: the vessel-rich group (VRG), muscle group (MG), fat group (FG), and vessel-poor group (VPG). The VRG comprises five organs: brain, heart, kidney, splanchnic (liver), and endocrine glands. The VPG includes bone.

The time constant for equilibration of anesthetic partial pressure in a tissue is defined as the ratio of the capacity of the organ and the blood flow to the organ. The capacity of the tissue reservoir for anesthetic is the product of the volume of the tissue and the solubility of the anesthetic in that tissue (tissue:blood partition coefficient). The time constant for organs is thus defined as:

Equation 8.4

$$\tau = \frac{V\lambda_{t/b}}{Q}$$

where $\lambda_{t/b}$ is the tissue:blood partition coefficient, V is tissue volume and Q is tissue blood flow. Since the volume of most tissues and their blood flow is constant, changes in the value of τ of a tissue are determined by its partition coefficient. For example, the time to equilibration of anesthetic partial pressures in tissues such as the brain may be expressed in terms of τ as follows:

Equation 8.5

$$\tau = \frac{\text{Volume of the brain (mL)} \times \text{brain/blood solubility}}{\text{Brain blood flow (mL/min)}}$$

The rate of rise of anesthetic partial pressure in tissues follows a pattern that is determined by the delivery of anesthetic to these tissues. That is, tissues that are perfused with a greater fraction of the cardiac output equilibrate more rapidly: VRG > MG > VPG > FG.

Uptake of anesthetic by the VRG is denoted by the initial flattening of the wash-in curve for inhalational anesthetics. Without uptake by the VRG, wash-in would continue to increase as rapidly as it did during the first minutes of wash-in. The effect of uptake of anesthetic by the VRG is to slow the rate of rise of alveolar-to-inspired partial pressure.

Wash-in of inhalational anesthetics into the VRG is usually complete within the first 15–20 minutes of anesthesia. In adults, these tissues comprise 8% of body weight but receive 75% of cardiac output. Accordingly, τ for the VRG is small and anesthetic partial pressures equilibrate rapidly in these organs. For example, the time to 1τ or 66% equilibration of halothane partial pressure in the VRG is 3 minutes and the time to 96% is 12 minutes. The wide range of values of τ for different tissues is attributable to tissue:blood solubility; the greater the solubility, the greater the value of τ and vice versa.

After equilibration of anesthetic partial pressure in the VRG, wash-in should increase rapidly. However, the rate of increase of wash-in is slower than expected because of the uptake of anesthetic by the MG. Uptake by this group becomes prominent approximately 20 minutes after induction of anesthesia and continues for approximately 200 minutes. The value of τ for anesthetic in the MG is greater than that in the VRG by 10- to 30-fold. This may be attributed to a relatively lower cardiac output per unit muscle mass and a greater solubility of anesthetics in muscle. The time to equilibration of anesthetic partial pressure in muscle is 2–6 hours depending on the anesthetic.

After equilibration of anesthetic partial pressure in the MG, uptake continues by the VPG and FG, as reflected by their large τ values. Fat represents 20% of body weight but receives only 6% of cardiac output in the healthy adult. Although perfusion of fat per unit volume is only 10–20% less than that of muscle, the solubility of anesthetics in fat is 10–30 times greater than that in muscle. On the basis of Equation 8.4, the value of τ for fat is 10–30 times that in muscle, or 1.5–40 hours depending on the anesthetic. With τ values of this duration, uptake of anesthetic by fat usually contributes minimally to the total tissue uptake.

PHARMACOKINETICS IN INFANTS AND CHILDREN

The rate of rise of alveolar-to-inspired partial pressures of inhalational anesthetics is more rapid in neonates and infants than in adults. This observation has been attributed to four differences between infants and adults. The order of these four factors reflects their relative contributions to this effect. The net effect of these differences between neonates and adults is to speed the equilibration of anesthetic partial pressures in alveoli and tissues and thereby speed the rate of rise of wash-in in infants and children compared with adults.

Factor 1: alveolar ventilation to functional residual capacity ratio

The greater the ratio of alveolar ventilation to FRC, the more rapid the wash-in of anesthetic (Fig. 8.6). In neonates, this ratio is approximately 5:1 compared with only 1.5:1 in adults. The greater ratio in neonates is attributable to the threefold greater metabolic rate and concommitant oxygen consumption in neonates compared with adults (Fig. 8.4).

Factor 2: solubility in blood

The solubility of inhalational anesthetics in blood varies with age. The blood solubilities of halothane, isoflurane, enflurane, and methoxyflurane are 18% less in neonates and the elderly than in young adults. These differences may be attributed to differences in blood constituents: blood:gas partition coefficients of isoflurane and enflurane correlate directly with serum albumin and triglyceride concentrations; that of halothane correlates directly with serum cholesterol, albumin, triglyceride, and globulin concentrations; and that of methoxyflurane correlates directly with serum cholesterol, albumin, and globulin concentrations.

Factor 3: solubility in tissues

The solubilities of halothane, isoflurane, enflurane, and methoxyflurane in tissues of the VRG in neonates are approximately 50% of those in adults. The decreased tissue solubilities are attributable to greater water content and decreased protein and lipid concentrations in neonates.

The solubilities of volatile anesthetics in muscle increase with age from neonates to the elderly. The reduced solubility of anesthetics in the muscle of neonates may be attributed to the low protein content of muscle in the first few months of life, whereas the increased solubility in the elderly reflects the increased protein and fat content of muscle in this age group. The reduced solubility in the muscle of neonates speeds equilibration of anesthetic partial pressure in muscle during the interval when uptake by muscle is greatest, that is, between 20 and 200 minutes.

Factor 4: cardiac output

The greater cardiac index in neonates compared with adults speeds equilibration of alveolar and inspired anesthetic partial pressures. This may be explained by the preferential distribution of cardiac output to the VRG in neonates. The VRG receives a greater proportion of the cardiac output in neonates because it comprises 18% of the body weight in neonates compared with only 8% in adults.

ELIMINATION

General principles

The wash-out of inhalational anesthetics follows an exponential decay (the inverse of wash-in) and varies inversely, with the blood:gas solubility; that is, the lower the solubility, the more rapid the wash-out (Fig. 8.4). However, elimination of inhalational anesthetics depends on other factors as well, including duration of anesthetic exposure and metabolism. Recovery from anesthesia parallels the wash-out of inhalational anesthetics.

Wash-out of inhalational anesthetics differs from wash-in in two respects. First, during wash-in, the inspired concentration of anesthetic can be increased to compensate for the rapid uptake of anesthetic from the lungs. However, during wash-out, the minimum partial pressure of the anesthetic cannot be less than zero. Therefore, the inspired concentration of anesthetic cannot increase the rate of wash-out of inhalational anesthetics. Second, during wash-out, anesthetic exits tissues in sequence (VRG, MG, VPG and FG) but may also redistribute from any one of these tissues into another tissue group. This may be particularly relevant for the more-soluble anesthetics.

The effect of the duration of anesthesia on the rate of wash-out depends in part on the solubility of the anesthetic. For anesthetics with low solubilities, wash-out is rapid and the duration of anesthesia has an attenuated effect. For anesthetics that are very soluble, the rate of wash-out varies inversely with the duration of anesthesia.

Percutaneous loss of inhalational anesthetics is small compared to expired and metabolic losses. These losses depend on the blood solubility of the anesthetic. Quantitatively, percutaneous losses of inhalational anesthetics do not affect their pharmacokinetics.

Metabolism

Metabolism of inhalational anesthetics depends primarily on cytochrome P450 enzyme systems located in the endoplasmic reticulum of hepatocytes (Chapter 7). The two major pathways for metabolism are the oxidative and reductive pathways. Of the oxidative pathways, dehalogenation and *O*-dealkylation have been implicated. Dehalogenation is the result of hydroxylation of the halogenated carbon, which decomposes to a carboxylic acid and inorganic halogens. The presence of two halogens on the terminal carbon provides optimal conditions for dehalogenation, whereas the presence of three halogens dramatically reduces the probability of dehalogenation. *O*-Dealkylation is the result of hydroxylation of an alkyl group adjacent to the oxygen of the ether bond. The intermediate compound rapidly decomposes to an alcohol and an aldehyde. The aldehyde may be oxidized by aldehyde oxidase to carboxylic acid or reduced by alcohol dehydrogenase to an alcohol. The reductive pathway has only been demonstrated for halothane.

The extent of *in vivo* metabolism of inhalational anesthetics ranges from 50% for methoxyflurane to 0.02% for desflurane (Fig. 8.4). With the exception of halothane and methoxyflurane, metabolism of inhalational anesthetics accounts for the elimination of 5% or less of the anesthetic administered; consequently the contribution of metabolism to their pharmacokinetics is small.

Methoxyflurane

Methoxyflurane is an ether anesthetic that is oxygenated either at the methyl carbon or at the dichloroethyl carbon, with the release of large quantities of inorganic fluoride, dichloroacetic acid, and, possibly, methoxydifluoroacetic acid. Defluorination of methoxyflurane occurs in the presence of cytochrome P450, glutathione *S*-transferase, and may also occur by a nonenzymatic pathway that requires vitamin B_{12} and glutathione. Plasma inorganic fluoride concentrations in excess of 95μg/dL (50μmol/L) have been associated with high-output renal insufficiency. Metabolism of methoxyflurane is increased after pretreatment with phenobarbital (phenobarbitone), diphenylhydantoin (phenytoin), ethanol, diazepam, and isoniazid.

Halothane

Halothane is extensively metabolized oxidatively and reductively via the cytochrome P450 system. The products of the oxidative pathway are inorganic bromide, chloride, and trifluoroacetic acid; the products of the reductive pathway are inorganic bromine and fluoride. An alternate reductive pathway requires an electron donor (usually cytochrome P450 enzyme system) and an anaerobic milieu. This pathway results in several volatile halogenated compounds (1,1-difluoro-2-chloroethylene, 1,1,1-trifluoro-2-chloroethane, and 1,1-difluoro-2-bromo-2-chloroethylene). Inorganic fluoride is also released with the first metabolite. Peak plasma inorganic fluoride concentrations are low [<28.5μg/dL (<15μmol/L)] even after 19.5MAC.h halothane in adults. Metabolism of halothane is increased after administration of phenobarbital or isoniazid and after prolonged exposure to subanesthetic concentrations of halothane.

Sevoflurane

Sevoflurane is metabolized by cytochrome P450 2E1 via oxidation of the α-carbon. The profile of plasma inorganic fluoride production after sevoflurane anesthesia in adults without hepatic enzyme induction is similar to that of enflurane. Maximum fluoride concentrations reach 47.5–66.5μg/dL (25–35μmol/L) within 1 or 2 hours of discontinuation of the anesthetic but decrease to less than 9.5μg/dL (5μmol/L) within several hours. The rapid decrease in serum inorganic fluoride after discontinuation of the anesthetic is attributed to the rapid wash-out and minimal metabolism of sevoflurane. Plasma inorganic fluoride concentrations are approximately 20% greater after prolonged exposure (13.4 ± 0.9 hours) to sevoflurane and in mildly obese patients compared with concentrations after brief exposures in nonobese adults. Recent data indicate that metabolism of inhalational anesthetics within the kidney may explain why some anesthetics that release inorganic fluoride cause high output renal insufficiency (i.e. methoxyflurane) and others (sevoflurane) do not. The reduced affinity of renal cytochrome P450 2E1 for sevoflurane compared with that for methoxyflurane results in a subtoxic intrarenal concentration of inorganic fluoride and, therefore, less damage to renal tubular cells. Defluorination of sevoflurane is increased after pretreatment with phenobarbital, diphenylhydantoin, ethanol, and isoniazid.

Enflurane

Enflurane is metabolized to only a small extent *in vivo*. It is metabolized via oxidative dehalogenation at the chlorofluoromethyl carbon by cytochrome P450 2E1. The resultant inorganic fluoride yields serum concentrations that are considered subtoxic.

Isoflurane

Isoflurane is metabolized to a small extent. Metabolism occurs via oxidation of the α-carbon, yielding trifluoroacetic acid, inorganic fluoride, and several intermediate compounds. The maximum serum concentration of inorganic fluoride after isoflurane is less than 9.5μg/dL (5μmol/L), although plasma fluoride concentrations in excess of 95μg/dL (50μmol/L) have been reported after prolonged administration (19.2MAC.h). Enzyme induction increases metabolism of isoflurane, although metabolism does not contribute significantly to its elimination.

Desflurane

Of the inhalational anesthetics, desflurane is the least metabolized *in vivo*. The reduced metabolism is attributed to the substitution of fluoride for chlorine on the α-carbon, thereby decreasing the affinity of this substrate for cytochrome P450 enzymes. Inorganic fluoride levels after desflurane anesthesia are less than 5.7μg/dL (3μmol/L) even after prolonged exposure.

Infants and children

Age significantly affects the rate of metabolism of inhalational anesthetics. Metabolism of inhalational anesthetics in neonates and infants is less than in adults. This has been attributed to reduced activity of hepatic microsomal enzymes, reduced fat stores, and more rapid exhalation of the anesthetics. After 131MAC.h isoflurane, plasma inorganic fluoride levels are not elevated.

PHARMACOKINETICS AND CIRCUITS

Wash-in

The rate of wash-in of anesthetic into the anesthetic circuit is determined by fresh gas flow and the volume within the anesthetic circuit. In the case of the Mapleson D and F (i.e. the Bain and Ayre T-piece) circuits, wash-in is fast even under low fresh gas flow conditions (0.5–2.0L/min) because the volume of these circuits is small. In circle circuits, the volume of the circuit is large. These circuits consist of a large reservoir bag (2L), carbon dioxide canister, and large bore corrugated tubing with gas volumes approaching 7–10L. Under low flow (0.5L/min) conditions, the gas volume of the circuit is 14-fold greater than the fresh gas flow. This results in a time to 96% equilibration of anesthetic concentration of 56 minutes, which illustrates the difficulty in effecting rapid changes in anesthetic partial pressures with a low fresh gas flow in this type of circuit. Increasing the fresh gas flow to 3.5L/min decreases the time to 96% equilibration by fivefold, to 8 minutes. With these circuits, large fresh gas flows are required for a rapid increase or decrease in anesthetic partial pressure.

Anesthetic loss to circuitry and carbon dioxide absorbers

Inhalational anesthetics may be removed from the fresh gas flow at several sites in the delivery circuit, including the gas tubing, the carbon dioxide absorber, and the bag. All inhalational anesthetics are soluble in the plastic and rubber components of the circuit. This poses a serious problem for the soluble anesthetics methoxyflurane and halothane, which are both soluble in polyethylene, rubber, and polyvinyl chloride endotracheal tubes. This is not an issue for other less-soluble anesthetics.

Closed circuit or low flow anesthesia

Closed circuit anesthesia is based on the principle that anesthetic requirements can be predicted by the wash-in of inhalational anesthetics and that, based on the uptake, no more and no less anesthetic need be administered. This technique requires a measure of the oxygen partial pressure within the circuit, particularly in the presence of nitrous oxide, and a measure of the partial pressure of anesthetic being delivered. Today, both of these monitors are available and should not prevent the safe use of this technique.

Empiric formulae were developed to predict the anesthetic requirements of patients during closed circuit anaesthesia. The uptake of anesthetic during the first minute of anesthesia can be predicted from the modified uptake equation:

Equation 8.6

$$U_1 = \frac{\lambda QA}{\mathrm{BP}}$$

where U_1 is the uptake in the first minute, λ is the blood:gas solubility of the anesthetic, Q is the cardiac output, and A is the alveolar partial pressure corrected for barometric pressure (BP). The A/BP is abbreviated from $(A - v)$/BP, where v is the anesthetic partial pressure in the venous blood, which is zero at the commencement of anesthesia. The uptake at any time U_t may be expressed as:

Equation 8.7

$$U_t = U_1 t^{-1/2}$$

Although these formulae provide an estimate for the amount of liquid anesthetic required each minute in the circuit, interindividual variability in the dose required is substantial. Factors that contribute to this variability include body mass and surface area, anesthetic requirements, and pathophysiologic conditions.

Key References

Eger EI II. Anesthetic uptake and action. Baltimore, MD: Williams & Wilkins; 1974.

Eisenkraft JB. Anesthesia vaporizers. In: Ehrenwerth J, Eisenkraft JB, eds. Anesthesia equipment: principles and applications. St Louis, MO: Mosby; 1993:57–88.

Ledez KM, Lerman J. The minimum alveolar concentration (MAC) of isoflurane in preterm neonates. Anesthesiology. 1987;67:301–7.

Munson ES, Bowers DL. The effects of hyperventilation on the rate of cerebral anesthetic equilibration. Anesthesiology. 1967;28:377–81.

Smith TC. Anesthesia breathing systems. In: Ehrenwerth J, Eisenkraft JB, eds. Anesthesia equipment: principles and applications. St Louis, MO: Mosby; 1993:89–113.

Yasuda N, Lockhart SH, Eger EI II, et al. Comparison of kinetics of sevoflurane and isoflurane in humans. Anesth Analg. 1991;72:316–24.

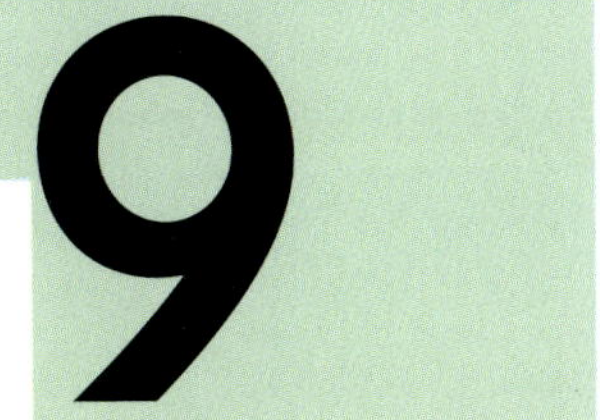

Chapter 9 Anesthetic drug interactions

H Ronald Vinik

Topics covered in this chapter

The state of general anesthesia can be achieved with a single drug, which is usually a potent inhalational agent. However, general anesthesia has several components, including analgesia, amnesia, unconsciousness, and suppression of somatic motor, cardiovascular, and hormonal responses to surgery (Chapter 22). The actions of intravenous agents are more easily recognized because they often have a predominant, if not a specific, action influencing particular receptors. For example, opioids have a dominant analgesic effect, as well as a sedative hypnotic component at higher doses. This 'pure' opioid action is not complete general anesthesia and patients can be pain free, immobile, and yet still aware. However, the addition of a subhypnotic dose of a benzodiazepine with the opioid combines to produce a state of general anesthesia.

A spectrum of pharmacologic actions via different drugs can be used to create the state of general anesthesia by targeting the components of anesthesia including hypnosis, analgesia, amnesia, and suppression of reflexes. The spectrum of effects that constitutes the state of general anesthesia should not be considered to result from a single anesthetic action even if produced by one drug, that is, an inhalational agent. These effects are produced by separate pharmacologic actions that are not easily recognized because of insufficient specificity of the actions of inhalational agents (Chapter 24). Intravenous agents, by comparison, have more specific actions that can be more easily identified.

SPECIFICITY OF ACTION

Classic theories of inhalational anesthesia are based on unitary mechanisms of anesthetic action where one anesthetic may be freely replaced by another. This predicts that combinations of anesthetic agents should have an additive effect. This has been confirmed for several inhalational agents. Because intravenous agents have different and apparently more specific mechanisms of action, one can expect drug interactions to be additive, synergistic, or even antagonistic.

Several groups of intravenous drugs can provide anesthesia similar to that of inhalational agents by acting on specific receptors. Receptor-mediated action is defined by a specific response that is dose dependent and may be reversed with a specific antagonist. Intravenous anesthetic agents, including barbiturates, benzodiazepines, etomidate, ketamine, propofol, and steroid anesthetics have well-defined receptor-mediated actions, although specific antagonists are available only for benzodiazepines (Chapter 23).

DRUG INTERACTIONS

Intravenous anesthetics are commonly combined in anesthesiology to achieve effects that no single agent can achieve alone. To maximize safety and efficacy of combined drug use, however, drug interactions that contribute to the desired effects must be characterized. The commonly described drug interactions in anesthesia usually relate to the potential for toxicity; however, drug interactions need not be detrimental. Interactions may be beneficial if they are quantitatable, predictable, consistent, and controllable.

Drug interactions can be additive, supra-additive (synergistic), or antagonistic. Additive means that the effect of the combination of the drugs is just a summation of the actions of each drug with no other specific interaction. Synergistic means that the effect of a drug is enhanced by the presence of another drug so that the combined effect of the two drugs is greater than the sum of their individual actions. Antagonistic means that one drug reduces the effectiveness of the other. Drug interactions can occur by a number of distinct mechanisms.

- Physicochemical: drugs may be incompatible when mixed, for example because of large pH differences that cause precipitation [e.g. thiopental (thiopentone) and vecuronium].
- Pharmacokinetic: a drug may change or compete for protein-binding sites and consequently alter the availability of the active unbound form of another drug at the receptor site, or it may alter the distribution, absorption, metabolism, or excretion of another drug.
- Pharmacodynamic: a drug may modulate the receptor sensitivity to another drug at a common receptor site [e.g. the interaction between barbiturates and benzodiazepines at the γ-aminobutyric acid($GABA_A$) receptor]. A drug interaction may also occur at separate receptor sites, mediated by different neurotransmitter pathways (e.g. the potent interaction between benzodiazepines and opioids).

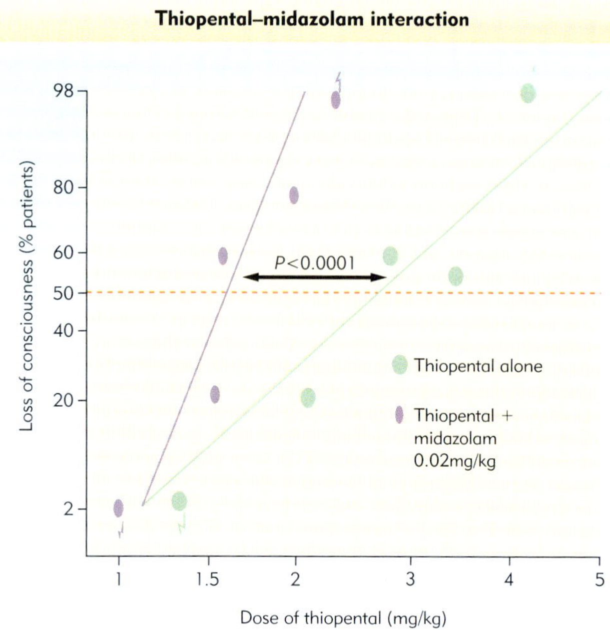

Figure 9.1 Dose–response curve of thiopental–midazolam hypnotic interaction determined by probit analysis. The abolition of the ability to open eyes on command and loss of eyelash reflex, which correlates with loss of consciousness, was used as an end point of anesthesia. A fixed dose of midazolam or saline was injected intravenously first, followed 1 minute later by thiopental. The degree of synergism resulted in a 49% reduction in the ED_{90} of thiopental, from 3.87 to 1.97mg/kg. (With permission from Vinik and Kissin, 1990.)

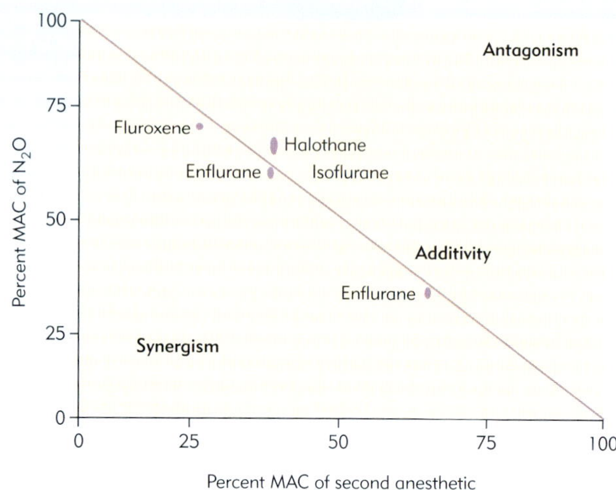

Figure 9.2 Isobologram for the interaction of various inhalational anesthetic agents. The interaction between various volatile anesthetics and nitrous oxide is plotted as percent MAC to reveal additive interactions. (With permission from Quasha, 1980.)

- Physiologic: drugs acting at different receptors do not interact *per se* but may produce the same physiologic effect (e.g. a cholinergic agonist and a β-adrenoceptor antagonist will both produce bradycardia but mediated by different mechanisms).

Pharmacokinetic and pharmacodynamic interactions are most relevant for quantitating anesthetic drug interactions.

QUANTITATION OF DRUG INTERACTIONS

To measure the effect of combining two agents, dose–response curves are determined for the individual agents separately and then for the combination using a probit procedure (Fig. 9.1). If the plotted curve shifts significantly to the left or the slope becomes significantly steeper when a combination is assayed, a synergistic interaction has occurred. Interactions can also be compared by isobolographic analysis, a more precise and commonly used technique of measuring drug interactions. On an isobologram, points on the *x* and *y* axes represent the potency expressed as the 50% effective dose (ED_{50}) for a particular effect of each of two agents alone. A straight line defines the fractional combinations of the two agents that would have the same potency if the interaction between them were additive. Figure 9.2 shows an isobologram for combinations of inhalational agents using minimum alveolar concentration (MAC; that concentration which prevents movement to a painful stimulus in 50% of patients) as an end point. Synergistic interactions fall below and antagonistic interactions fall above the line of additivity. The combinations fall near the additive (diagonal) line, confirming that the effects of combining these drugs are additive. In contrast, an intravenous combination of a benzodiazepine and an opioid is clearly synergistic (Fig. 9.3). These isobolograms were constructed using drug doses required to produce a particular effect, but steady-state plasma concentrations of modeled effect-site concentrations could also be used.

TYPES OF INTERACTIONS

Synergistic interactions

Anesthetic synergism between benzodiazepines and barbiturates has been reported in both animal experiments and surgical patients. Barbiturates allosterically enhance benzodiazepine binding to the benzodiazepine site on the $GABA_A$ receptor (Chapter 23). Therefore, the potentiating effect of thiopental can be explained by an interaction with benzodiazepines at this receptor. The benzodiazepine–barbiturate anesthetic synergism is mutual. In rats, very small doses of midazolam potentiate the hypnotic effect of pentobarbital (pentobarbitone) to the same extent that pentobarbital potentiates the hypnotic effects of midazolam. A study evaluated the hypothesis that a very low subhypnotic dose of midazolam (0.02mg/kg, less than one tenth of the ED_{50} value for midazolam-induced unconsciousness) potentiates thiopental-induced unconsciousness in humans (Fig. 9.1). A 96% increase in hypnotic potency was obtained with the combination of thiopental and midazolam compared with thiopental alone. The addition of midazolam changed the position of the curves so that the ED_{50} was shifted to the left along the dose axis and the slope of the curve became steeper. The effect of midazolam was more

Isobologram for the interaction of midazolam and morphine

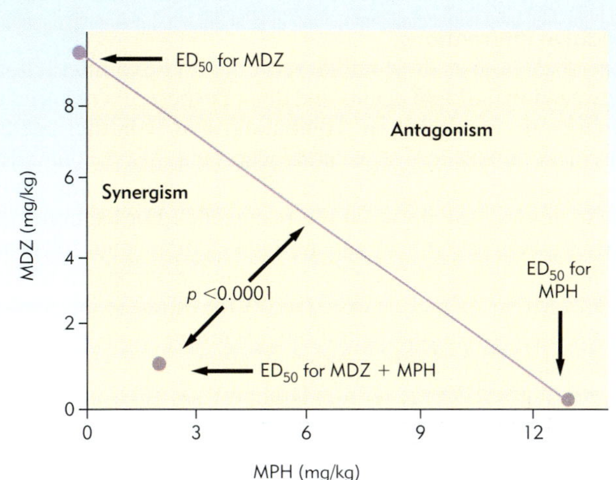

Figure 9.3 Isobologram for the interaction of morphine (MPH) and midazolam (MDZ). Data are for the ED_{50} for loss of righting reflex, which corresponds to loss of consciousness (hypnosis), in rats. (With permission from Kissin, 1990.)

Alfentanil–midazolam hypnotic interaction

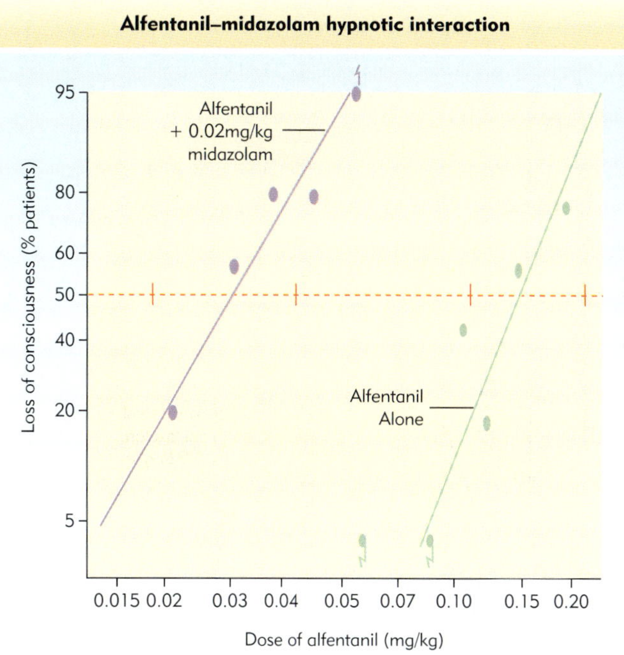

Figure 9.4 Dose–response curve of alfentanil–midazolam hypnotic interaction. The study design was similar to that described in Figure 9.1, using the loss of eyelash reflex (hypnosis) for the response. (With permission from Vinik and Kissin, 1989.)

pronounced at the upper end of the curve. Consequently, the least sensitive patients showed the maximum synergism.

A marked degree of mutual hypnotic synergism has also been demonstrated with opioids and benzodiazepines. Figure 9.4 shows that the ED_{50} for induction of hypnosis with alfentanil is 0.13mg/kg, which can be reduced to 0.027mg/kg by adding a small dose of midazolam (0.02mg/kg) 1 minute before the alfentanil. Figure 9.5 demonstrates that the synergism is mutual and very potent. A subanalgesic dose of alfentanil (3μg/kg) significantly potentiates the hypnotic effect of midazolam. Alfentanil, primarily an analgesic, can have potent hypnotic effects when combined with a benzodiazepine. A dose of 0.02mg/kg alfentanil reduced the ED_{50} of midazolam to 0.07mg/kg, a premedication dose if used alone.

The interaction between alfentanil (0.02mg/kg) and propofol is additive, not synergistic, for hypnosis (Fig. 9.6). The difference between propofol alone and the combination of propofol and alfentanil was not significant at the ED_{50} level. The midazolam–propofol interaction, however, is synergistic (Fig. 9.7) and is similar to the midazolam–thiopental interaction. This probably reflects a similar interaction of thiopental and propofol with barbiturates at the $GABA_A$ receptor. A synergistic interaction between propofol and the benzodiazepine flurazepam has been demonstrated in the facilitation of GABA receptor-mediated Cl^- current using recombinant human $GABA_A$ receptor constructs.

The α_2-adrenoceptor agonist–benzodiazepine combination (dexmedetomidine–midazolam) in a rat model results in profound synergism for hypnotic effect. The data support a pharmacodynamic mechanism of interaction because the blood concentration and the receptor-binding site concentrations of each drug did not change in the combination. Possible mechanisms to explain the synergistic hypnotic interaction between midazolam and dexmedetomidine include facilitation of release or binding of GABA to its receptor; inhibition of adenylyl cyclase, thereby reducing the activity of cyclic adenosine monophospate (cAMP)-dependent protein kinase and altering the conductance properties of the Cl^- channel of the GABA

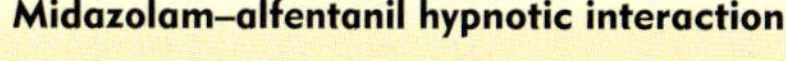
Midazolam–alfentanil hypnotic interaction

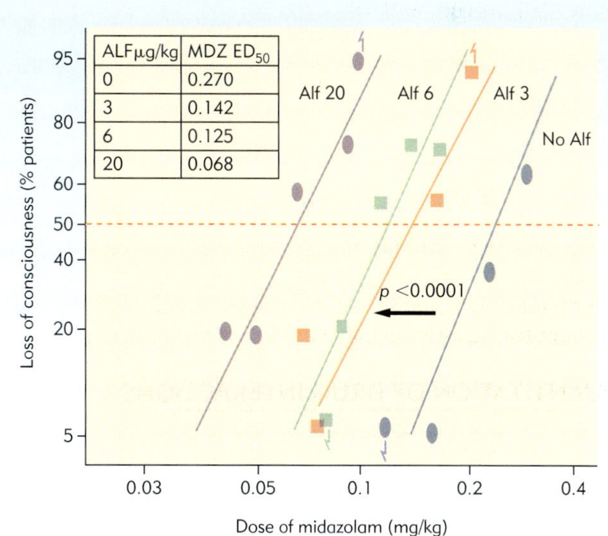

Figure 9.5 Dose–response curve of midazolam (MDZ)–alfentanil (ALF) hypnotic interaction The study design was similar to that described in Figure 9.1, using the loss of eyelash reflex (hypnosis) for the response. The inset shows the ED_{50} of midazolam at each dose of alfentanil (With permission from Kissin and Vinik, 1990.)

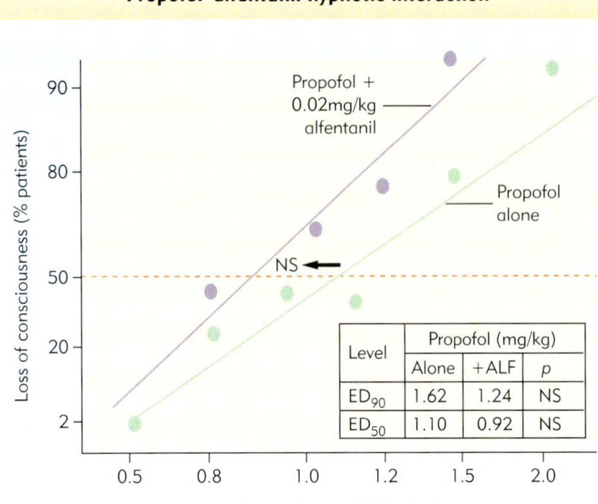

Level	Propofol (mg/kg)		
	Alone	+ALF	*p*
ED_{90}	1.62	1.24	NS
ED_{50}	1.10	0.92	NS

Figure 9.6 Dose–response curve of propofol–alfentanil (ALF) hypnotic interaction. The study design was similar to that described in Figure 9.1, using the loss of eyelash reflex (hypnosis) for the response. The inset shows the ED_{90} and ED_{50} values of propofol with or without alfentanil. (With permission from Vinik, 1991.)

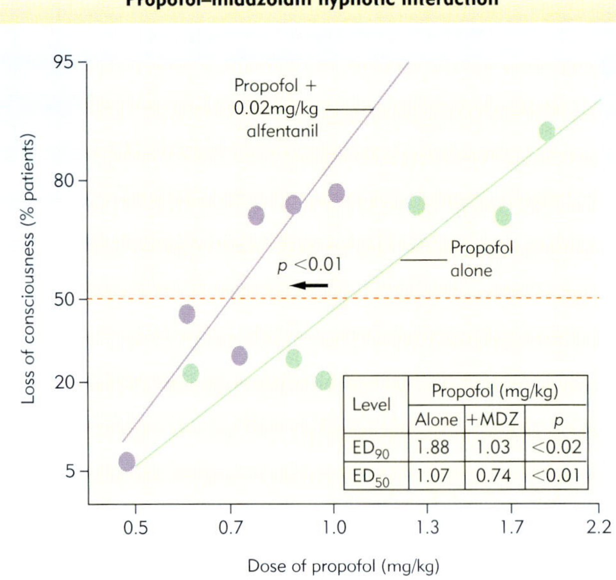

Level	Propofol (mg/kg)		
	Alone	+MDZ	*p*
ED_{90}	1.88	1.03	<0.02
ED_{50}	1.07	0.74	<0.01

Figure 9.7 Dose–response curve of propofol–midazolam (MDZ) hypnotic interaction. The study design was similar to that described in Figure 9.1, using the loss of eyelash reflex (hypnosis) for the response. The inset shows ED_{90} and ED_{50} values of propofol with or without midazolam. (With permission from Vinik, 1991.)

receptor; and/or the convergence of the two receptor–effector systems to enhance membrane hyperpolarization. A reduction in MAC by α_2 agonists also occurs by a pharmacodynamic interaction and is not explained by pharmacokinetic alteration of volatile agents by dexmedetomidine.

Additive interactions

Anesthesiologists are familiar with the additive interactions between inhalational agents and do not expect an enhanced or synergistic result when combining two volatile agents. Interactions between intravenous agents may also be only additive. Additive interaction implies that there is no pharmacodynamic interaction between the two agents. For example, the interactions ketamine–thiopental and ketamine–midazolam are additive for hypnotic as well as for antinociceptive effects. This lack of synergism may be explained by the different mechanism of action of ketamine: it inhibits excitatory transmission by decreasing depolarization through blockade of *N*-methyl-D-aspartate (NMDA) receptors (Chapter 23). This mechanism differs from the allosteric potentiation of the $GABA_A$ receptor by barbiturates and benzodiazepines.

Antagonist interactions

Although diazepam–opioid combinations are synergistic for hypnosis, the interactions between morphine and fentanyl with diazepam in producing antinociception demonstrate relative antagonism in rats. The antagonism observed is relative in that there was no increased need for one drug when the other was added. This might more accurately be referred to as infra-additive rather than antagonistic. A mechanism for diminishing an effect of another drug by adding a second drug can be seen with morphine antinociception. Morphine has a dual antinociceptive action comprising both spinal and supraspinal actions (Chapters 21 and 26). A second agent can diminish the supraspinal component by inhibiting the activation of descending pain-inhibition pathways. The interaction of morphine and halothane or morphine and thiopental to suppress the heart rate increase to noxious stimuli is probably an example of this type of antagonism.

MECHANISMS OF INTERACTIONS

Pharmacokinetic interactions

Pharmacokinetic drug interactions occur when one drug alters the availability of another drug at its site of action. An example is the effect of myocardial depressants on cardiac output (e.g. a bolus dose of thiopental). The hemodynamic depression slows redistribution and consequently increases the plasma-to-effect site ratio of concurrently administered drugs. For example, two equal doses of thiopental administered intravenously 80 seconds apart produce a much higher plasma concentration after the second dose (Fig. 9.8).

Protein binding affects the amount of free active drug available at the effect site. When a highly protein bound drug is rapidly administered intravenously, the binding capacity of plasma proteins may be temporarily exceeded, resulting in a relatively high concentration of unbound active drug that will produce a more intense reaction at the receptor site. Consequently, competitive displacement by one drug of another from plasma protein-binding sites will magnify the effect of the other drug, which is freed to react at the effector site.

The α_2-adrenergic agonists such as clonidine and dexmedetomidine can be used to reduce the dose requirement of intravenous and volatile anesthetics. Dexmedetomidine reduces the MAC of volatile agents by a pharmacodynamic interaction. The mechanism of interaction between dexmedetomidine and

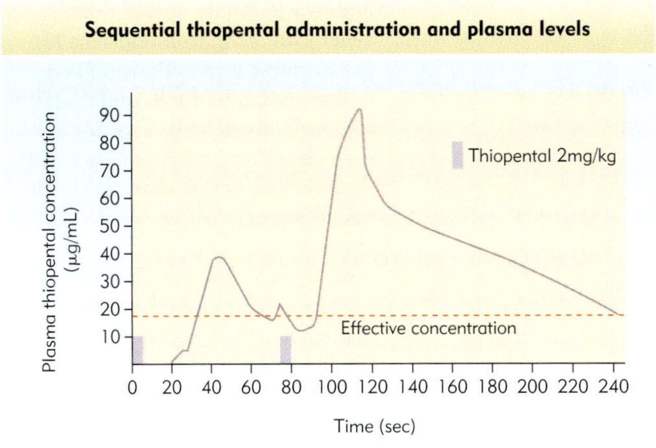

Sequential thiopental administration and plasma levels

Figure 9.8 Effect of sequential thiopental administration on its plasma concentration. Two equal doses were given 80 seconds apart. The first dose produced a peak plasma concentration of 40μg/mL, followed by a rapid fall resulting from redistribution. The second dose produced a much higher peak concentration with a slower decline as a result of the prolonged redistribution caused by the reduced cardiac output and possibly saturation of binding sites produced by the first doses. (With permission modified from Crankshaw, 1987.)

thiopental appears to be related to altered pharmacokinetic distribution. A combination of thiopental and dexmedetomidine results in a 30% decrease in the dose of thiopental necessary for equal suppression of the electroencephalogram (EEG). The calculated plasma concentration at the effect site was the same in both groups, indicating that the interaction was not pharmacodynamic (i.e. dexmedetomidine did not change the CNS sensitivity to thiopental). Rather, the effect was pharmacokinetic in that blood pressure, heart rate, and cardiac output are decreased by α_2 agonists, which then alter the volume of distribution (V_d) and intercompartmental shifts of thiopental. Similar effects are seen with concurrent β blocker administration.

Important pharmacokinetic interactions may occur at the level of drug metabolism (Chapter 7). One drug may induce the metabolism of another drug (e.g. the induction of hepatic microsomal P450 enzymes by barbiturates). Enzyme induction takes days to develop and is not usually of concern with acute drug interactions but may be relevant in patients on chronic medication [e.g. the increased requirement for vecuronium in patients taking diphenylhydantoin (phenytoin)]. Alternatively, enzyme inhibition by one drug may inhibit the metabolism of another drug and potentiate its effect [e.g. the inhibition of midazolam, diazepam, fentanyl, and meperidine (pethidine) metabolism by inhibition of the cytochrome P450 isozyme CYP3A by nelfinavir and other human immunodeficiency virus (HIV) protease inhibitors].

ANALYSIS OF ANESTHETIC DRUG INTERACTIONS

Since drug concentrations at the site of action in the CNS cannot be measured directly, they must be estimated. These estimates are based on steady-state concentrations that are achieved over time, which allows for equilibration between plasma and the site of effect. Equilibration can be facilitated by using computer-assisted pharmacokinetic model-driven infusions for rapid equilibration of the plasma and the effect-site concentrations of drug.

Evidence for drug interactions can be obtained by dose–response analysis (see above) or by analysis of estimated brain concentration of drugs (using steady-state blood concentrations). If both analyses show the same degree of synergism, the interaction is mediated by pharmacodynamic mechanisms. If the synergism is manifested only by the dose-related analysis, then the mechanism is pharmacokinetic. For example, the hypnotic synergism between morphine and diazepam was evident both when the effective concentrations were expressed as fractions of the brain concentration and in the dose-related analysis, indicating that the diazepam–morphine interaction is pharmacodynamic in nature. Further evidence for the pharmacodynamic nature of the interaction was obtained by analyzing the interaction for different components of anesthesia. In a rat study assessing the interaction for a combination of morphine and thiopental, a synergistic interaction was observed for the righting reflex (hypnotic effect), while an antagonistic interaction was observed for the ability of the combination to block the motor response to a noxious stimulus. This difference is obviously not related to a pharmacokinetic mechanism.

When combinations of intravenous anesthetic agents are given, the degree of sedation/hypnosis cannot be predicted from the doses of the individual drugs unless the effect of a possible interaction is known and measured. There is some disagreement in the reports of the mechanism of interaction between propofol and opioids. Administration of propofol–alfentanil in bolus doses for induction of anesthesia indicates additivity or borderline synergism. Propofol–fentanyl combinations were only additive. However, when using steady-state plasma concentrations, reports indicate that propofol blood concentrations required for loss of consciousness are markedly reduced by alfentanil. A similar effect was described for fentanyl. When different methods of analysis are used, results can be difficult to compare; however, the pharmacodynamic propofol–opioid interaction when determined using blood concentration analysis is clearly more synergistic than that determined using dose-related analysis. Possible explanations for this discrepancy may be pharmacokinetic effects of drugs given in bolus doses on cardiac output, altered volume of distribution, or overwhelming of the protein-binding capacity of highly bound drugs. These effects will enhance the effect of the concomitantly administered drug through a pharmacokinetic interaction rather than a pharmacodynamic interaction.

ADVANTAGES OF SYNERGISTIC DRUG INTERACTIONS

Drug interactions significantly enhance the hypnotic effects of certain combinations of anesthetics when given concurrently for peak effect. The nature and degree of side effects provoked by the interactions between intravenous anesthetics determine whether hypnotic synergism is of any clinical value. It may be possible to use smaller, less toxic doses if the synergism has a greater effect on hypnosis than on undesired end points such as cardiovascular depression. The combination of propofol and ketamine has been used for total intravenous anesthesia. There is an additive interaction between propofol and ketamine when used for induction of anesthesia for either an hypnotic or an anesthetic effect. The clinical effect of this additive interaction was complimentary for hemodyamic effects. The usual increase

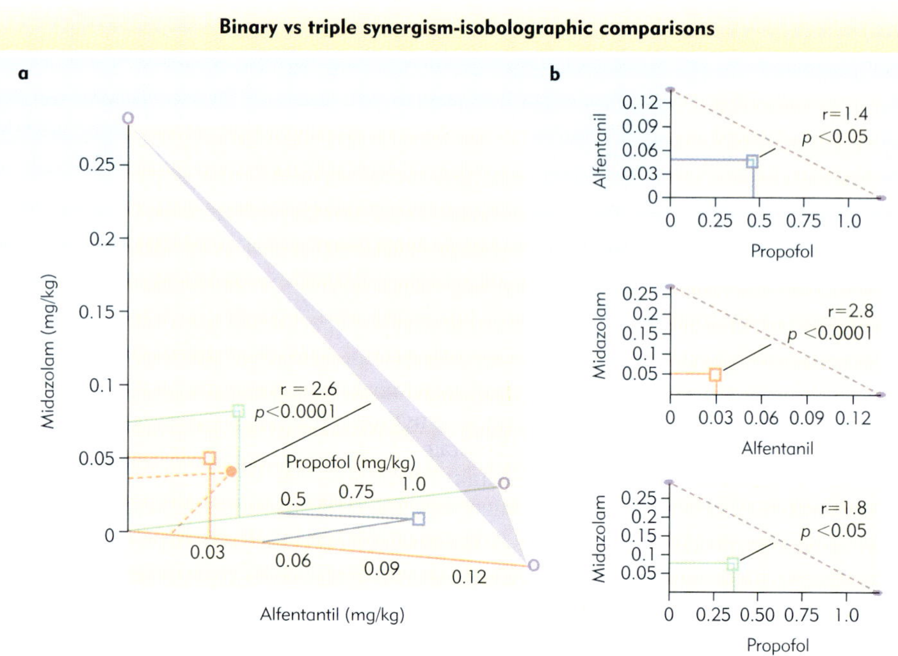

Figure 9.9 Binary versus triple synergism: ED_{50} isobolograms for the hypnotic interactions among midazolam, alfentanil, and propofol. (a) Triple interactions. The dotted area shows an additive plane passing through three single-drug ED_{50} points (small open circles, o); the closed circle (•) is an ED_{50} point for the triple combination, and the open squares are ED_{50} points for the binary combinations. The ratio (R) of the single-drug dose (ED_{50} = 1) to combined fractional dose (in fractions of single-drug ED_{50} values), reflects the degree of synergism. The *p* value is signficance of the difference from the additive effect. (b) Binary interactions: the dotted lines are lines of additivity. (With permission from Vinik et al., 1994.)

in heart rate and blood pressure induced by sympathetic stimulation with ketamine was opposed by the effect of propofol, which decreases hemodynamic response by decreasing systemic vascular resistance and myocardial contractility, with resulting improved cardiovascular stability.

The view that a combination of intravenous anesthetics should be regarded as a 'new' drug with individual properties rather than merely reflecting the known properties of the individual agents deserves serious consideration. Synergistic drugs will significantly reduce the component doses required for a hypnotic effect. In the thiopental–midazolam combination, patients who were least sensitive to thiopental showed the greatest degree of synergism, so that those who originally required 5mg/kg thiopental needed only 2mg/kg when 0.02mg/kg midazolam was given concurrently. This has the effect of reducing interpatient variability and makes the patient hypnotic response more predictable and consistent.

Benzodiazepine–opioid hypnotic interactions are markedly synergistic. Figure 9.9 indicates that the midazolam–alfentanil combination reduces each component by 74% for the hypnotic end point of loss of consciousness. The addition of propofol, however, did not significantly increase the degree of synergism. The propofol–midazolam–alfentanil interaction provides profound synergism, but this is not significantly different from that of the midazolam–alfentanil combination. However, the combination of midazolam, alfentanil, and propofol when given in reduced doses rapidly has clinical applications because of the following pharmacologic effects: the dose of propofol is markedly reduced; the onset of action is accelerated compared with that seen with the individual drugs (induction is consistently achieved in 45 seconds or less with individually subhypnotic doses); hemodynamic response to intubation is markedly blunted even when intubation is 60 seconds after induction; and intraocular pressure is controlled to below baseline after succinylcholine administration.

ADVERSE DRUG INTERACTIONS

Numerous adverse drug interactions have been documented that are pertinent to the anesthesiologist. Many of these are pharmacokinetic interactions leading to reduced metabolism and enhanced effects (Chapter 7). These range from the adverse reactions of combining monoamine oxidase (MAO) inhibitors with the analgesic meperidine to the enhancement of action of the anticoagulant warfarin by the concurrent use of drugs such as sulfonamides, salicylates, metranidazole, and the histamine H_2 blocker cimetidine. The explosion in development of new drugs requires constant attention to identify potentially toxic drug interactions. An interesting example is the interaction between benzodiazepines and indinavir, a new HIV protease inhibitor. They both undergo oxidative metabolism by cytochrome P450 CYP3A4; as a result, the sedative and respiratory depressive effects of the benzodiazepines can be intensified and prolonged.

This chapter has focused on the synergy between concurrently used intravenous anesthetic agents that can be used to achieve desired end points. However, synergism can also be detrimental. An example is the potentiation of respiratory depression by relatively modest doses of a benzodiazepine or volatile anesthetic with an opioid. Marked hypoxemia can occur with a combination of midazolam and fentanyl in contrast to the unremarkable effects when these drugs are used separately. The consequences of drug interactions range from serious toxicity (including fatalities, which have been reported with the combination of MAO inhibitors and meperidine) to the relatively insignificant prolongation of mild sedation. The aware clinician can often use a particular interaction therapeutically to reduce the amount of drug required for a desired effect and to avoid potential undesired interactions.

ANALGESIC DRUG INTERACTIONS

Combinations of opioids and nonsteroidal anti-inflammatory drugs (NSAIDs) are commonly used to control pain in the perioperative period (Chapter 27). An opioid-sparing effect by the concurrent use of NSAIDs occurs following gynecologic and abdominal surgery, which suggests that NSAIDs have an antinociceptive action in visceral pain. A visceral antinociceptive synergistic interaction between ketorolac and morphine has been demonstrated in rats. Ketorolac potentiates morphine antinociception despite a lack of discernible antinociception when used alone.

Previously, the primary mechanism of antinociception of NSAIDs was believed to be a peripheral anti-inflammatory effect; however, a central action also exists. Intrathecal ketorolac potentiates the antinociception produced by intrathecal morphine in rats. Nonsteroidal anti-infammatory drugs (NSAIDs) may modulate opioid receptor function through prostaglandin synthesis or neuropeptides. The antinociceptive response of a combination of morphine and ketorolac was completely reversed by the administration of naloxone, indicating the primary role of opioid receptor action. These results have clinical implications because the dose-dependent side effects of both drugs can be minimized by the reduced component doses.

CONCLUSIONS

A clear understanding of pharmacodynamic principles in drug interactions enables the clinician to maximize efficacy and minimize toxicity of drug combination therapy. The underlying rationale for using drugs with different mechanisms of action include promotion of synergistic beneficial pharmacologic effects, avoidance of additive side effects by dose reductions, and possibly decreasing tolerance (e.g. in infusions for sedation in intensive-care units).

Well-designed studies to elucidate the mechanisms of drug interactions should be encouraged because anesthesiologists have been slow to explain and exploit synergistic drug interactions. Oncologists have used synergistic combinations of chemotherapeutic agents with great success and combinations of antibiotics have major therapeutic advantages in cases of resistant infections. The application of rigorously defined pharmacologic and pharmacokinetic principles should enhance patient care by reducing anesthetic toxicity, increasing dosing predictability, and reducing costs.

Key References

Berenbaum MC. What is synergy? Pharmacol Rev. 1989;41:93–141.
Crankshaw DD. Hypnotics in infusion anesthesia with particular relevance to thiopentone. Anesth Intens Care. 1987;15:90–6.
Kissin I. General anesthetic action: an obsolete notion? Anesth Analg. 1993;76:215–18.
McKay AC. Synergism among i.v. anaesthetics. Br J Anaesth. 1991;67:1–3.
Vinik HR, Bradley EL Jr, Kissin I. Triple anesthetic combination: propofol–midazolam–alfentanil. Anesth Analg. 1994;78:354–8.

Further Reading

Buhrer M, Mappes A, Lauber R, Stanski D, Maitre P. Dexmedetomidine decreases thiopental dose requirement and alters distribution pharmacokinetics. Anesthesiology. 1994;80:1216–27.
Finney DJ. Probit analysis, 3rd edn. London: Cambridge University Press; 1971.
Gillies GWA, Kenny GNC, Bullingham RES, McArdle CS. The morphine sparing effect of ketorolac tromethamine. Anaesthesia. 1987;42:727–31.
Hui TW. Additive interactions between propfol and ketamine when used for anesthesia induction in female patients. Anesthesiology. 1995;82:641–8.
Kissin I, Brown PT, Bradley EL Jr. Morphine and fentanyl anesthetic interacts with diazepam: relative antagonism in rats. Anesth Analg. 1990;71:236–41.
Kissin I, Vinik HR. Midazolam potentiates thiopental sodium anesthetic induction in patients. J Clin Anesth. 1991;3:367–70.
Leeb-Lundberg F, Snowman A, Olsen RW. Barbiturate receptors are coupled to benzodiazepine receptors. Proc Natl Acad Sci USA. 1980;77:7468–74.
Malmberg AB, Yaksh TL. Pharmacology of the spinal action of ketorolac, morphine, ST-91, U50488H, and L-PIA on the formalin test and an isobolographic analysis of the NSAID interaction. Anesthesiology. 1993;79:270–81.
Maves T, Pechman P, Meller S, Gebhart GF. Ketorolac potentiates morphine antinociception during visceral nociception in the rat. Anesthesiology. 1994;80:1094–101.
Reynolds JN, Maitra R. Propofol and flurazepam act synergistically to potentiate $GABA_A$ receptor activation in human recombinant receptors. Eur J Pharmacol. 1996;314:151–6.
Salonen M, Reid K, Maze M. Synergistic interaction between $\alpha 2$ adrenergic agonists and benzodiazepines in rats. Anesthesiology. 1992;76:1004–11.
Vangen O, Doessland S, Lindback E. Comparative study of ketorolac and paracetamol/codeine in alleviating pain following gynaecological surgery. J Int Med Res. 1988;16:443–51.

Chapter 10 Basic physical principles

Paul CW Beatty

Topics covered in this chapter

What is physics?
Mass, force, work, and energy
Pressure and density
States of matter and latent heat
Gas laws
Avogadro's hypothesis
Calorimetry and heat transfer
Solubility and diffusion

WHAT IS PHYSICS?

Physics is natural sciences' attempt to describe the fundamental laws of the world around us. That may seem a rather grandiose way of starting a chapter in a book devoted to explaining the application of the basic sciences in anesthesia, but it is the very nature of physics that often most foxes medical scientists. Physics asks and answers simple fundamental questions. It follows the implications of those questions to their logical and sometimes extraordinarily strange conclusions. The key to understanding it is to do the same. When in doubt ask simple questions! It describes in detail what it finds using the clarity and economy of mathematics. As a result, descriptions in the physical sciences require precision. The starting point for many physical descriptions is a few basic concepts inspired by experimental observation. These concepts lead to basic definitions of quantities defined by number and unit. In the end, however, physics resolves into a single theme. It is the description of the natural laws that govern energy transfer. All the topics to be covered in this chapter are concerned with energy in one form or another.

MASS, FORCE, WORK, AND ENERGY

The first major problem that was addressed by physics was how and why things move. Intuitively we know that heavy objects require more effort to pick up from ground level. People also noted that when dropped from a height, objects moved faster and faster until they hit the ground. Initially, it was thought that the heavier the object the faster it would fall, but Galileo proved that this rate of increase in speed (acceleration) was independent of the weight of the object. Therefore, the next question was, what makes objects fall? When objects fall or move in any way what controls how they move? Does the motion of things on earth say anything about how the planets move in the heavens? One other observation was important. Intuitively, people realized that the same volumes of different materials had different weights. However, Archimedes showed that the weight of an object immersed in water was reduced by the equivalent of the weight of water it displaced. Is there some property of materials that makes the weight of the water and the reduction in weight of the object equivalent?

It was Newton, through his Laws of Motion and Theory of Gravity, who answered all these questions and by doing so founded physics as we think of it. The definitions and principles he used are shown in Figure 10.1.

The ultimate concept derived from Newton's laws is that of energy. Energy can be defined as the capacity to perform work. However, since work is about moving forces and forces are about creating motion, energy can be thought of as the property of an object to create motion. In the case of gravity, when an object is dropped from a high tower it has a far higher velocity at impact than if dropped only a few meters. Thus, it can create more change in motion in other bodies at impact. The faster it moves, the more capacity for creating motion it has. This energy that the object has by virtue of its motion is *kinetic energy*.

The capacity to do work was in the object before it fell. The higher the tower from which the object falls, the further is the separation of the object from the ground, and the more work is done against gravity. Thus, there is an energy that an object has by virtue of its position in a region over which a natural force acts. This is *potential energy*. Potential energy can be converted into kinetic energy and vice versa. In a closed system, one in which energy does not flow out or in, energy is always conserved. The nature of the energy in a system leads to energy being referred to in different ways in different circumstances. For instance, the energy associated with motion may be called mechanical energy, or that with chemical reactions, chemical energy, and so on, but all energy ultimately is the same and in the SI system has the unit joule (J).

PRESSURE AND DENSITY

As physical quantities, pressure and density are also related to gravity and Newton's laws. Torricelli, an Italian scientist, performed the classic experiment that revealed this in 1643 and invented the barometer at the same time (Fig. 10.2). He filled a closed glass tube with mercury and placed the open end of the tube in an open dish of mercury. With the tube inclined from the vertical he noted that the mercury filled the tube. However, as the tube was raised to the vertical, when the length of the mercury column above the surface of the mercury in the dish reached a specific length (0.76m) a space formed at the top of the tube (known as Torricelli's vacuum). His explanation was that atmospheric

Definitions and principles of physics

Newton's Laws of Motion:

I An object remains at rest or continues in motion in a straight line unless acted on by an external force

II The rate of change of momentum of an object is proportional to the applied force

III To the action of every force, there is an equal and opposite opposing force generated

Force – That which causes or changes motion (SI unit: newton, N = kg m/s^2)

Mass – A measure of the amount of matter in a body (SI unit: kilogram, kg)

Velocity – The rate of change of position of an object (speed of motion) in a given direction (SI unit: meter per second, m/s)

Force of gravity – The force that causes objects to fall toward a body and controls the motions of the planets; it is proportional to the product of the masses of the two objects involved and inversely proportional to their distance apart

Momentum – The mass of an object in motion multiplied by its velocity (SI unit: kilogram meter per second, kg m/s)

Acceleration – The rate of change of the velocity of an object in motion. Thus, Newton's second law of motion means that force equals mass multiplied by acceleration

Work – Work is done when the point of application of a force moves; the work done equals the force multiplied by the distance moved by the force's point of application (SI unit: joule, J); the concept of work is fairly intuitive, as is the concept of power

Power – The rate of doing work or the work done per unit time; power equals the work done divided by the time taken to do it (SI unit: watt, W)

Kinetic energy – The energy an object has by virtue of its motion (SI unit: joule, J)

Potential energy – The energy an object has by virtue of its position or state (SI unit: joule, J)

Law of Conservation of Energy – In a closed system for which no energy leaves or enters, the amount of energy in the system is constant

Law of Conservation of Momentum – When two or more objects act upon one another their total momentum does not change unless external force is applied; this is derived from Newton's Third Law of Motion

Pressure – Force per unit area of application (SI unit: pascal, Pa = N/m^2)

Density – The mass per unit volume of a substance (SI unit: kilogram per cubic meter, kg/m^3)

Absolute pressure measurement – A pressure measurement made with reference to vacuum

Relative or gauge pressure – A pressure measurement made with reference to atmospheric pressure

Latent heat – The latent heat of X (e.g. vaporization) is the energy required to convert 1kg of a substance from one phase to another without change in temperature at a given pressure (SI unit: joules per kilogram, J/kg).

Fick's Law – The rate of diffusion is proportional to the gradient of concentration

Graham's Law – The rate of diffusion through a permeable material is inversely proportional to the square root of the molecular weight of the diffusing molecules

Henry's Law – Given an inert gas in contact with a liquid, the mass of gas that dissolves in the liquid is directly proportional to the partial pressure of the gas above the liquid

Figure 10.1 Definitions and principles of physics.

pressure kept the column of mercury in the tube. He also noted that the upper level of the mercury varied from day to day.

Consider the basic mechanical unit of the mercury, an atom, to be a solid ball. The atoms of the mercury in a barometer do not move perceptibly. Therefore, by Newton's Third Law of Motion, they must experience no net force. Consider the forces that act on a mercury atom about half way up and near to the center of the tube of the barometer. The forces the atom experiences in a horizontal plane from neighboring atoms must be equal, otherwise it would move. Similarly, all the oblique forces it receives from the layers above and below must balance and be equal. The force it experiences from the layer of atoms vertically above it is slightly less than the force it bears down with upon the layer of atoms below, but is still balanced. The difference is the force caused by gravity on its own mass. The force that bears down is the force caused by the weight of all the atoms above this atom. The net force upward, which supports the column of mercury above the layer in which our atom lies, is the sum of all the infinitesimal forces experienced by all the atoms in the layer which, except at the contact point between the mercury and the tube, must be equal. The size of the atoms and the cross-sectional area of the tube limit the number of atoms that can be packed into one horizontal layer. Thus, the net force upward is proportional to the cross-sectional area of the tube, or (in other words) the force per unit area across the layer is constant. This gives the basic definition of pressure (see Fig. 10.1).

Torricelli's mercury barometer experiment

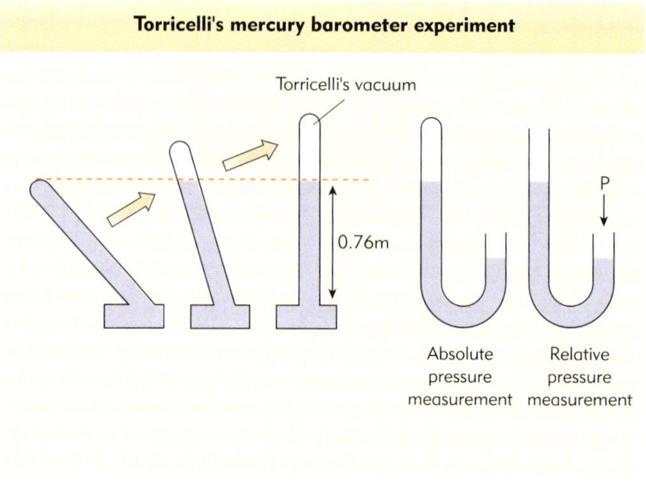

Figure 10.2 Torricelli's mercury barometer experiment.

The actual value of the pressure is determined by the weight of the column of mercury above the point of measurement. In the barometer, all the infinitesimal forces are resolved and it is the atmospheric pressure at the surface of the mercury in the dish that supports the column of mercury and balances the pressure at the bottom of the barometer tube. The weight of the mercury column is given by the number of atoms in the column, which is determined by the mass of the individual atoms and the number that can be packed into the volume of the column. This is the density (ρ) of the substance.

The pressure P is given by Equation 10.1, in which h is the column height, a the cross-sectional area, and ρ the density of mercury.

Equation 10.1

$$P = \frac{(hag\rho)}{a} = hg\rho$$

Equation 10.1 means that, since density and acceleration caused by gravity (g) are constant in the barometer, atmospheric pressure can be measured by reference only to the height of the mercury column above the surface of the mercury in the dish. Hence units of pressure measurement such as mmHg are used.

Since Torricelli's barometer has essentially a vacuum at one end of its column of mercury, it measures pressure with reference to this vacuum, a true zero pressure, to give an absolute pressure measurement. Torricelli's vacuum is not actually a vacuum since it contains a saturated vapor of mercury, which exerts a saturated vapor pressure.

Absolute pressure measurements are most often found in hyperbaric medicine or in the measurement of vacuum itself. If a barometer's mercury column and dish is replaced by an open-ended 'U'-tube, one end of which is connected to a pressure source to be measured, then the pressure measurement made is relative to atmospheric pressure (fig. 10.2).

STATES OF MATTER AND LATENT HEAT

Three states of matter are of interest to anesthetists – solid, liquid, and gas. These are three stable states in which molecules exhibit distinctly different bulk physical characteristics. The difference between the states is the degree of intermolecular bonding that exists. In gases the molecules move around freely and are very unstructured, and virtually no intermolecular forces exist. In liquids molecules still move easily, but they display some evidence of wanting to cohere, like forming droplets under surface tension; slight but significant intermolecular forces exist. Solids are hard and resist deformation. The molecules within them can form regular, ordered patterns called crystal structures; the intermolecular forces are strong.

In all three states, thermal energy is held in the molecules as the kinetic energy associated with the velocity of their random motions. In the gas phase these motions involve collisions, both with the sides of the vessel containing the gas and with other molecules. The more heat there is in the gas, the higher the molecular velocities. In the liquid or solid phases kinetic energy is associated with molecular vibration or limited molecular motion. The more heat, the greater the amplitude of the vibrations and the more kinetic energy present in that form of motion. The amount of thermal energy present is expressed as temperature.

To change from one state of matter to another, for example from liquid to gas, the kinetic energy of the vibrations must be increased until the intermolecular forces can no any longer hold the molecules together as liquid and they break free. This can be achieved by heating the liquid. As the liquid heats up, the vibrations increase until the point is reached at which the kinetic energy in the vibrations is equal to the kinetic energy the molecules would have in the gaseous state at the same temperature. However, gas does not form. The intermolecular forces still exist, so a residual potential energy must be supplied to the molecules for the gas to form. This energy is *latent heat*. It does not result in extra vibrations in the molecules and therefore is supplied at the volatilization temperature or boiling point. The difference between these two is simply the conditions. In boiling, heating is vigorous enough to cause the conditions to be met for gas formation throughout the liquid volume all at once. Thus bubbles of gas form spontaneously in the bulk of the liquid.

The same principles apply to cooling a liquid or gas. If the vibrations are reduced sufficiently, intermolecular forces can establish themselves. So a practical way of solidifying a liquid is to remove thermal energy (heat) by cooling the liquid. If the temperature change in the liquid is plotted against time, as this process proceeds a point occurs at which the temperature of liquid ceases to fall but the liquid begins to solidify. At this point

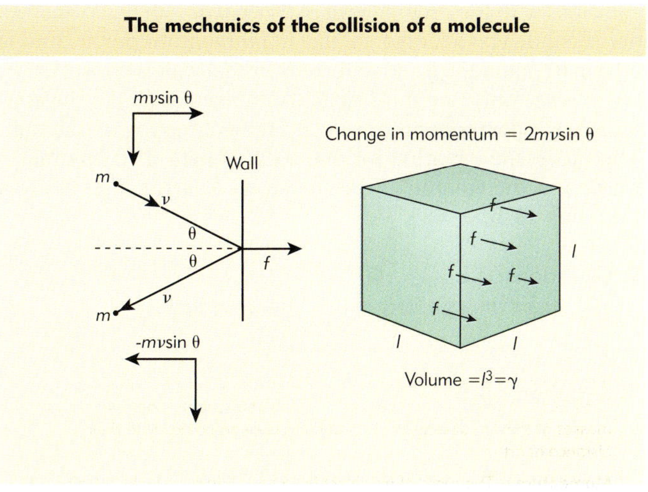

Figure 10.3 The mechanics of the collision of a molecule of an ideal gas with the wall of the container holding the ideal gas.

the molecular vibrations have been reduced to a level such that the only energy that must be removed for solidification is the latent heat. As cooling proceeds this occurs and solidification takes place at the same temperature, the freezing point. In the opposite direction, it is the melting point.

GAS LAWS

In explaining latent heat, the concept of molecular kinetic energy in gases was introduced. It is the basis of the kinetic theory of a gas, which considers the molecules in a gas as a collection of elastic balls in free, random motion inside a container. They obey Newton's laws of motion and therefore travel in straight lines unless they hit each other or the vessel walls. No energy is lost in any collision, that is the collisions are perfectly elastic. No intermolecular forces are present, and gravity does not affect the system. These assumptions do not hold for real gases, but they hold well enough to be useful.

Kinetic theory links Newton's laws of motion and the gas laws through a molecular description of the source of pressure in gases. When a molecule strikes the wall of the vessel that contains the gas, it bounces off the wall. Figure 10.3 shows what happens to a molecule (mass m) as it strikes the wall at an angle θ. It is reflected off the wall at the same angle and, since no energy is lost in the collision, it leaves at the same velocity (v) as it had on striking the wall. If we resolve its momentum into a part perpendicular to the wall and a part parallel to the wall before and after the collision, then since the direction of flight has changed, the change in momentum in the direction of the wall is $2mv\sin\theta$. Since momentum is conserved, Newton's laws show that the result of the collision is the creation of a tiny instantaneous force (f) that acts on the wall of the container. In a real gas container billions of such collisions occur each second. The average force they exert in 1 second over a unit area of one wall of the vessel volume (V) is the average force per unit area, or pressure (P).

To quantify P, we need to know how many collisions occur per second. In a cubic container of side length l, a molecule that collides perpendicularly with one wall will, after recoil, travel back to the opposite wall and there be reflected back before striking the first wall again. Therefore, the average time between collisions with the original wall is $2l/v\sin\theta$ or $v\sin\theta/2l$ collisions per second. The average change in momentum per second is $m(v\sin\theta)^2/l$ and the average force over that wall is $m(v\sin\theta)^2/l^3$. On average only one third of all the molecules (N) in the container have components of velocity in the direction of one wall. Therefore, the equation for one wall (Equation 10.2) applies, where V is the volume of the container. Rearrangement gives Equation 10.3.

Equation 10.2

$$P = \frac{[0.33Nm(v\sin\theta)^2]}{l^3} = \frac{[0.33Nm(v\sin\theta)^2]}{V}$$

Equation 10.3

$$PV = 0.33Nm(v\sin\theta)^2$$

The motion of the molecules in the gas is clearly governed by statistical considerations. Thus, to derive bulk properties such the gas laws from kinetic theory, average measures applicable to the whole gas need to be used in the model. For instance, what should the value of the average molecular velocity be? The answer is the root mean square velocity, c, which replaces $v\sin\theta$ in Equations 10.2 & 10.3. The kinetic energy for the whole of the gas, E, in the container is $0.5Nmc^2$, where N is the total number of molecules of mass m, which gives Equation 10.4, in which R is a constant (*the gas constant*) and T is a variable proportional to the average kinetic energy of the molecules, known as temperature.

Equation 10.4

$$PV = 0.33Nmc^2 = 0.67E = RT$$

Equation 10.4 is the ideal gas equation, which summarizes all the gas laws determined empirically.

Given this development of the concept of temperature, when T=0, no molecular motion occurs. This is the definition employed in the SI system, in which temperature is measured in degrees Kelvin (°K). The freezing point of water is 0°C or 273.16°K.

Boyle's Law states that at a constant temperature, pressure varies inversely with volume. If temperature T is held constant, it follows from the ideal gas law that the pressure P is inversely proportional to volume V (Equation 10.5).

Equation 10.5

$$P \propto \frac{1}{V}$$

As the volume of the container is reduced the molecules have less distance to travel between collisions with the walls and thus the rate of collisions rises and therefore so does pressure.

Charles' Law, or Gay Lussac's Law, states that at a constant pressure the volume of a given mass of gas varies directly with the absolute temperature. In contrast, at constant volume V, the pressure P is directly proportional to absolute temperature T (Equation 10.6).

Equation 10.6

$$P \propto T$$

As temperature rises the amount of kinetic energy of the gas increases and the average velocity of the molecules increases, so the change in momentum for each collision increases and the pressure rises.

AVOGADRO'S HYPOTHESIS

Avogadro's Hypothesis states that equal volumes of gas at the same temperature and pressure contain the same numbers of molecules. Avogadro's Hypothesis is implicit in the kinetic theory description of the gas laws. Since temperature is the measure of internal energy, if temperature, volume, and pressure are constant then the number of molecules in the given volume must be the same, irrespective of the mass of the molecules.

In SI units, 1 mole (mol) of a substance is the quantity that has a mass equal to its molecular mass. Molecular mass is the ratio of the mass of a substance's molecule to one-twelfth the mass of an atom of carbon 12 (^{12}C).

The number of molecules in a mole of anything is thus the molecular mass of the substance divided by the mass of one molecule of the substance, which is the molecular mass multiplied by one-twelfth the mass of a carbon-12 atom. That is always a constant and the number is Avogadro's number, 6.02×10^{23}. Thus 1mol contains Avogadro's number of molecules. At standard temperature and pressure (s.t.p. i.e. 0°C and 760mmHg) one mole of gas occupies 22.4L.

If the total mass of the gas is M (= Nm) and the atomic mass of the gas is M_a, then the number of moles of the gas is M/M_a. As 1mol of gas contains Avogadro's number of molecules, N_a, Equation 10.7 is another form of the ideal gas equation.

Equation 10.7

$$PV = \left(\frac{M}{M_a}\right)N_a kT$$

If we define a new constant R [J/(°Kmol)] as the gas constant ($N_a k$), then the most familiar form of the ideal gas equation is given (Equation 10.8).

Equation 10.8

$$PV = \left(\frac{M}{M_a}\right)RT = \text{n}RT$$

Dalton's Law of partial pressures states that in a mixture of gases the pressure exerted by one gas is the same is it would exert if it occupied the container alone. From kinetic theory, in a mixture of two gases the collisions of the molecules of each gas with the container can be considered separately. So the pressure that results from one gas can be derived from the ideal gas equation and added to the pressure from the other to give the total pressure (Equation 10.9).

Equation 10.9

$$P_t = P_a + P_b = \left(\frac{RT}{V}\right)\left[\left(\frac{M}{M_a}\right) + \left(\frac{M}{M_b}\right)\right]$$

CALORIMETRY AND HEAT TRANSFER

Calorimetry is the measurement of the amount of heat evolved, absorbed, or transferred. The techniques used for calorimetry vary with the mechanisms of heat transfer. To understand these mechanisms it is best to start with the kinetic theory and gases.

Kinetic theory assumes that the total kinetic energy in a gas is simply the sum of all the molecular kinetic energies. Thus, the higher the temperature, the higher the average velocity of the molecules. Since the number of collisions that a molecule can have increases with its velocity, the higher the temperature of a gas, the higher the number of collisions averaged over time. This energy is transferred in collisions between the molecules and the walls of the vessel. Momentum and energy are conserved in these collisions, but molecules can still change their velocities. In collisions of molecules of the same gas in which one molecule is of higher velocity than the other, on average the velocity of the faster molecule is reduced by the collision and the velocity of the slower molecule is increased. Thus, if a body of gas of a higher temperature mixes with a gas of a lower temperature the collisions tend to heat the cooler gas and cool the hotter gas. In this way, the transfer of molecular kinetic energy from molecule to molecule can pass heat.

In gases it is the collisions between free mobile molecules that transfer the energy, but in liquids and solids the molecules are constrained by intermolecular forces. However, they can still possess kinetic energy, either as a more limited motion similar to that of gas molecules or as vibrational kinetic energy while still held in place in a solid crystal lattice. This kinetic energy can be coupled from molecule to molecule by intermolecular forces. Coupling of kinetic energy by molecular coupling is the first mode of heat transfer – *conduction*.

The speed at which heat spreads is indicated by the thermal conductivity of the substance. In gases thermal conductivity is closely allied to the process of diffusion (described later). Conduction in solids is much more complex than this simple treatment allows, but can be described by quantum mechanics.

The calorimetry of conduction is concerned with bringing objects of different temperatures together and measuring their common temperature after heat transfer has ceased. This raises the concept of objects having a capacity to hold heat.

Thermal or heat capacity

The thermal capacity of a body is the quantity of heat required to raise its temperature by 1°K (SI unit is the joule, J). The thermal capacity divided by the mass of the object is the specific thermal capacity. The thermal capacity of 1mol of a substance is the molar thermal capacity.

For the most part, calorimetry is carried out to determine an unknown quantity of heat or the details of heat flow in a specific physical or chemical process. Thus, calorimetry can be used only to measure heat flow within a closed system (i.e. heat does not flow to the outside world). If heat flow cannot be prevented by insulation or placing the calorimeter in a vacuum, corrections for heat flow into or out of the calorimeter have to be made.

If we take two metal objects of thermal capacities C_1 and C_2, heat them to two different temperatures T_1 and T_2, and place them in contact in a well-insulated calorimeter, heat flows between them by conduction and eventually they come to a single temperature T_A. Since no heat is lost (assuming a perfect calorimeter), the heat balance in the system can be represented by Equation 10.10.

Equation 10.10

$$T_1C_1 + T_2C_2 = T_A(C_1 + C_2)$$

Convection is also explained in terms of kinetic theory and the gas laws, but a twist is that in practice it can only occur naturally in bodies of fluids under gravity. In a container of gas under gravity at constant pressure, if part of the gas is heated locally it effectively occupies more volume and is less dense. It thus tends to rise as a body and mix with the cooler gas around it. If it rises and is cooled by coming into a colder part of the container, it then sinks and a circulating current is formed that mechanically mixes the gases and thus transfers heat more rapidly. In calorimetry, convection effects aid heat transfer if fluids are involved. Stirring or otherwise mixing the fluids is even more effective and quicker, which can be thought of as forced convection.

While convection is a bulk effect and conduction is governed by molecular considerations, *radiation*, the final physical heat-transfer process, is exhibited on a submolecular basis. Some of the kinetic energy in a heated molecule is stored as vibrations of the molecular structure itself and of the electrons that surround it. Thus, some of the kinetic energy results in motions of charged particles and this movement creates electromagnetic fields that can radiate electromagnetic waves in the infrared range. (Electromagnetic radiation is considered in Chapter 11.) If this infrared radiation intercepts another molecule it can interact with that molecule and increase that molecule's internal kinetic energy and hence temperature. This heat transfer mechanism is the only one that can take place in a vacuum. Since infrared radiation has a relatively short wavelength, like visible light it effectively travels in straight lines. Radiative heat transfer is thus a line-of-sight phenomenon. Again, a detailed description of radiation requires some appreciation of quantum mechanics and is very complex.

Conduction, convection, and radiation are the three physical methods of heat transfer from one body to another. However, heat is only a specific form of energy. If heat locked up as potential energy in any way is transferred to another place and released as heat again, then heat transfer has, in a very general sense, taken place. In the body, heat generation is biochemical from the chemical potential energy in food and oxygen in respiration. The heat generated is transferred from the body by conduction to the air, convection of air at the skin, losses from chemical binding of energy in exhaled carbon dioxide, and losses from latent heat changes in sweating or humidification of ventilatory gases in the upper respiratory tract (Chapter 64).

Calorimetry of heat transfer of the body as a whole aims to account for all the sources of energy transfer and measure them. This is carried out in a whole body calorimeter for metabolic studies.

SOLUBILITY AND DIFFUSION

The process of diffusion can be explained very simply from kinetic theory. If two different gases (or any fluids in any sense) are separated by a physical barrier and that barrier is removed, the kinetic motion of the molecules of the gases mixes them and equalizes their energy until both are perfectly mixed. At this point they are constrained only by the walls of the vessel that contains them.

Of more interest in medicine is how fast this mixing proceeds, which can be expressed in terms of the number of molecules transported through a given area in a given time. This rate of mass transport through another gas or liquid per area per second (M) is proportional to the density gradient ($\partial P/\partial z$). This is Fick's Law (Equation 10.11), in which D is the diffusion coefficient and is proportional to how far molecules travel before collisions. It is thus inversely proportional to gas density and proportional to mean molecular velocity (and hence absolute temperature). Mass transport is one of the fundamental physical principles that underlie gas exchange during respiration throughout the body.

Equation 10.11

$$M = D\left(\frac{\partial P}{\partial z}\right)$$

If a membrane permeable to the gas is placed in the way of diffusing molecules, molecular motion is limited by the channels or pores through which the gas can diffuse. In this situation the rate of diffusion becomes dependent on the molecular weight of the gas (Graham's Law).

The other limiting factor to gas transport is the solubility of the gases in blood. Henry's Law governs this when gases are not bonded chemically in the liquid, such as oxygen in hemoglobin. Even in this case, the gas bound by hemoglobin in red cell bodies is exchanged first with plasma and then the cells of tissue or the alveoli, so Henry's Law still plays a part in diffusion limitations to the exchange of oxygen.

The kinetic theory explanation of Henry's Law is the mirror image of the kinetic theory explanation of how saturated vapors are formed. The gas molecules in the liquid have kinetic motion and some have enough velocity to leave the surface of the liquid. When in the gas phase above the liquid, molecules collide with the gases present and some fall back into the liquid. Eventually the rate of loss of molecules from the gas phase equals the rate of emergence of molecules from the liquid, which is a dynamic equilibrium. The partial pressure exerted by the gas at this point is the saturated vapor pressure of the gas.

Henry's Law describes the same equilibrium from the point of view of dissolving the gas. At the equilibrium point the liquid has become saturated with all the gas it can hold. The concept of partial pressure can be applied to its state in the liquid – hence the idea of partial pressures or tensions to measure saturated and other concentrations of gas in a liquid. The pressures involved are temperature dependent, with the amount of gas dissolved decreasing with increased temperature.

Henry's Law is couched in terms of the mass of gas or the partial pressure, but it is possible to express the amount of gas dissolved in terms of the volume of gas in the liquid phase to the gas present in the same volume of the gas phase. This gives a ratio called the partition coefficient or Ostwald solubility coefficient (λ).

The partition coefficient has the advantage that it allows gas exchange to be expressed in terms of volumes directly related to other physiologic volumes, such as tidal volume. It is of particular use in compartmentalized models of gas exchange. Since gases dissolve inertly in many tissues (as if these tissues were liquids), a partition coefficient for a complex tissue can be estimated from the weighted sum of the partition coefficients of the tissues' basic chemical constituents. Thus, the partition coefficient of blood can be estimated by combining the coefficient for olive oil to represent lipids, saline to represent plasma.

Further Reading

Bragg M. On giant's shoulders. London: Hodder & Stoughton; 1998

Davis PD, Parbrook GD, Kenny GNC: Basic physics and measurement in anaesthesia, 4th edn. Oxford: Butterworth–Heinemann; 1995.

Macintosh R, Mushin W, Epstein HG. Physics for the anesthetist, 3rd edn. Oxford: Blackwell; 1963.

Ohanian HC. Principles of physics. New York: WW Norton; 1994

Chapter 11 Electromagnetism, light, and radiation

Paul CW Beatty

Topics covered in this chapter

Electricity
Charge, potential, and electromotive force
Resistance, Ohm's law, inductance, and impedance
Amplifiers
Electrical hazards and safety measures
Electromagnetic radiation and light
Radioactivity and radiation

ELECTRICITY

Electricity is a general term for phenomena associated with charged particles (usually electrons or protons) at rest or in motion. (The word electron derives from the Greek *elektron* meaning amber.) Electromagnetic theory is the physics of charged particles in electromagnetic fields. It extends beyond simple electrical phenomena and circuit theory to radio transmission, light waves, X-rays, nuclear magnetic resonance (NMR), and other forms of electromagnetic radiation.

CHARGE, POTENTIAL, AND ELECTROMOTIVE FORCE

Charge is the total quantity of electricity in an object, and can be thought of as the number of charged particles in a body (SI unit is the coulomb, C). Charges can have signs, that is positive or negative. An attractive force exists between opposite charges and a repulsive force between charges of similar sign. As with gravity, work is carried out when charges are moved against electrostatic forces and bodies having charge can have potential energy because of the electrostatic field.

The electrostatic measure of potential energy is the electric *potential*. It can be positive or negative depending on the sign of the charge on the body. The earth is assigned a potential of zero, so that the difference in electric potential between two different bodies is simply the sum of the electric potential of the two bodies above the earth, the potential difference (Fig. 11.1).

When a conductor connects two points of different potential difference, a current flows between them. For this to occur a source of energy is required to make the electrons flow in the conductor; this is called the electromotive force (EMF) and has the same SI unit as potential (V).

The difference between potential difference and EMF can be very important in physiologic measurements and hence in anesthesia. Electrical energy is dissipated in an electrical circuit by the resistance and impedance of that circuit only when current flows. Bioelectric phenomena, such as those measured using the electrocardiogram (ECG), electroencephalogram, etc., are generated deep in the body. Inevitably, resistances between the source of these bioelectric potentials and the skin makes it harder to measure the signals. Accurate measurement of these requires as little energy dissipation as possible. Thus, we would like to make measurements potentiometrically (when no current flows).

Definitions in electromagnetism

Potential difference – The work performed when one positive electric charge is moved from one point to another (SI unit: volt, V)

Electromotive force – The rate at which energy is drawn from a source and dissipated in an electrical circuit when unit current flows (SI unit: volt, V)

Volt – The potential difference between two points on a conducting wire carrying 1A of current between which 1W of power is dissipated

Current – Overall movement of electrons through a conductor, or charge flow per unit time

Ampere – The current that produces a force of 2×10^{-7}/N.m^{-1} when flowing in two straight infinitely long parallel conductors 1m apart in a vacuum

Farad – The capacitance of a capacitor across which exists a potential difference of 1V when storing 1 coulomb of charge

Power – The power dissipated in a resistance is equal to the product of the potential difference across the resistor and the current flowing through the resistor (SI unit: watt, W)

Inductance – That property of an electrical circuit as a result of which an EMF is generated by a change in current flowing in the circuit (self inductance) or by a change in current in a neighbouring circuit that is magnetically linked to the first circuit (mutual induction)

Henry – The SI unit of an inductance in a closed electrical circuit, such that a change in current of 1A produces a change in EMF of 1V

Becquerel – A radioactive source with a disintegration rate of one disintegration per second is said to have an activity of 1 Bq (1 Curie, Ci = 3.7×10^{10} Bq)

Gray – When a source of radiation transfers 1 J.kg^{-1} of energy to a body then the absorbed dose is 1 Gray (Gy)

Figure 11.1 Definitions in electromagnetism.

Charge may be transferred from object to object by electrostatic contact without a conductor, but it is most commonly transferred using conduction through metals, which allow electrons to flow from one body to another. When charge moves or flows it is a current, or charge transferred per unit time. When current flows in a wire a magnetic field is created around the wire and deflects a compass needle in a direction depending on the direction of flow of the current. Attractive or repulsive magnetic forces can be established between parallel wires with currents flowing in the appropriate direction, an effect that is used to define the unit of current (ampere).

Returning to electrostatics, the property that relates electric potential to the amount of charge that an object holds is its capacitance, C, given by Equation 11.1.

Equation 11.1

$$C = \frac{Q}{V}$$

It is this property of a system of electrical conductors and insulators that allows the system to store electrical charge. Capacitance varies with object shape, since the field intensity around an object and hence the work required to place charge on the object against the field varies with its shape. Figure 11.2 shows a parallel plate capacitor with one plate connected to earth and a positive charge placed on the other plate. This induces negative charges to flow from earth to balance this charge. The force that exists between the plates as a result follows the general form of all electrostatic forces, Equation 11.2, in which E is the field strength or force on a unit charge a distance r from a charge Q; ϵ is the *permitivity* of the space between the charges.

Equation 11.2

$$E = \frac{Q}{(4\pi r^2 \epsilon)}$$

The permitivity of vacuum, or free space, ϵ_0, is a constant, but other insulators can increase the permitivity if placed between the charges. Thus, placing an insulator between the plates of a parallel plate capacitor decreases the force between the plates, decreases the work required to move charge onto the plates, decreases the potential difference induced across the capacitor, and therefore increases capacitance.

The capacitance of a parallel plate capacitor of which A is the plate area, ϵ the permitivity of the dielectric in the space between the plates, and d the separation of the plates, is given by Equation 11.3.

Equation 11.3

$$C = \frac{A\epsilon}{d}$$

To increase capacitance, either area or permitivity can be increased or plate separation reduced.

The energy stored in the electric field of a capacitor can be released through a resistor to earth. If this is carried out using a switch, the voltage (V_t) from the capacitor falls exponentially with time to zero from a maximum (V_0) before the switch is thrown (Equation 11.4, in which RC is the time constant of the circuit).

Equation 11.4

$$V_t = e^{-t/RC}$$

RESISTANCE, OHM'S LAW, INDUCTANCE, AND IMPEDANCE

How dissipation of energy supplied by a source of EMF occurs depends on whether current flows steadily through conductors in one direction all the time (direct current, DC) or whether it oscillates in direction (alternating current, AC).

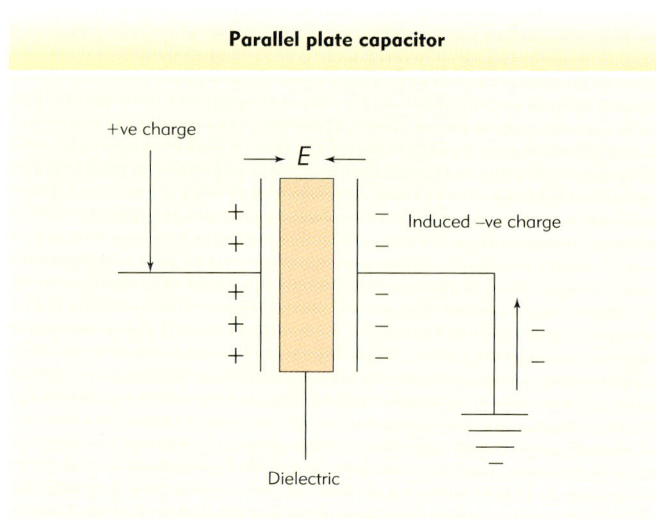

Figure 11.2 The parallel plate capacitor.

Resistance is the simplest process of dissipation. All conductors exhibit resistance, except superconductors below specific, extremely low temperatures. Resistance can be thought of simplistically as the result of collisions between the moving electrons that carry the current in a conductor and the molecules or atoms of the main crystal lattice that make up the conductor. The collisions result in transfer of energy that eventually is dissipated as heat within the conductor.

Resistance (SI unit is the ohm, Ω) for a conductor relates current (I) to potential difference (V) across the conductor (Equation 11.5).

Equation 11.5

$$R = \frac{V}{I}$$

This is Ohm's Law, given in a more familiar form in Equation 11.6.

Equation 11.6

$$V = IR$$

Resistance depends on the shape of the conductor, since current flow is not uniformly distributed even in a uniform conductor. Resistance is proportional to conductor length and inversely proportional to conductor cross-sectional area. Stretching a conductor increases its length, and the resultant increase in resistance is the basis of strain gauges.

Temperature increases can cause conductors to expand, which leads to an increase in resistance by this mechanical effect as well as affecting electron flow. Resistors used in electronic circuitry are made from metal alloys or films or carbon compounds designed to reduce the effects of changes in ambient temperature.

Different materials have different specific resistances or resistivities. Resistivity (ρ) is the resistance of a unit cube of the conductor at 0°C (SI unit is ohm meters, Ωm), and generally is given by Equation 11.7.

Equation 11.7

$$\rho = \frac{RA}{l}$$

For resistances in series (Fig. 11.3a), the total potential difference across the resistors is the sum of the potential differences across the individual resistors (Equation 11.8). For resistances in parallel (Fig. 11.3b), Equation 11.9 applies.

Equation 11.8

$$V = V_1 + V_2 + V_3 = IR_1 + IR_2 + IR_3$$

Equation 11.9

$$I = I_1 + I_2 + I_3 = \left(\frac{V}{R_1}\right) + \left(\frac{V}{R_2}\right) + \left(\frac{V}{R_3}\right)$$

The way in which resistances dissipate electrical energy is independent whether the current flow is AC or DC, but this is not true of inductances or capacitances.

In the same way that moving charge into an electrostatic field against electrostatic forces requires work, so moving magnetic poles into a magnetic field requires work. There are no single magnetic poles so, unlike the electrostatic example, moving magnetic poles is more like forcing together two magnetic fields than placing single charges on bodies in the field. Faraday found that if a wire was placed in a permanent magnetic field between the poles of a 'U'-shaped magnet and a current was made to pass along the wire, the wire would kick out of the field. The magnetic field created by the current around the wire opposes the magnetic field of the permanent magnet, which produces a force and hence motion. The direction of motion is given by Fleming's Left Hand Rule (Fig. 11.4).

If a conductor is moved through a magnetic field a current is induced in the conductor (the dynamo effect). If the conductor is placed in a magnetic field that can vary in intensity with time, which is equivalent to moving it in and out of a fixed field, both a time-varying current and an associated magnetic field are induced in the conductor. Time varying (i.e. AC) currents can induce currents in other conductors placed within the influence of the magnetic fields created by those currents (*electromagnetic induction*). If two coils or conductors are used energy is transferred by induction from one coil to the other. This is the principle of the transformer (Fig. 11.5) in which two coils are wound on either side of a circular metal ring composed of a magnetic material such as iron. This core channels the magnetic field produced by the coil that is excited with the AC and transfers it efficiently to the other coil, in which is induced another AC (*mutual induction*).

The coil that is excited in a transformer is termed the *primary*, and the one in which the current is induced is termed the *secondary*. The number of turns in the primary (N_P) and the secondary (N_S) can be different. If this is the case, ignoring losses in the transformer, the EMF (V_S) that the secondary coil can provide is related to the EMF (V_P) used to excite the primary (Equation 11.10)

Equation 11.10

$$\frac{V_S}{V_P} = \frac{N_S}{N_P}$$

A conductor has *self-inductance* as well. In a coil, this exists because one turn of the coil sits in the magnetic field of the next turn, and so on. When an AC is applied the changing magnetic fields in one turn produce opposing currents in the neighboring turns, and thus energy is dissipated.

So far we have not discussed the nature of the AC. Any time-varying current causes inductive effects. However, the term AC is conventionally applied to sinusoidal current flows. A sinusoidal wave form is defined by its amplitude and frequency (*f*). Given a regular waveform such as a sinusoid, is there an AC equivalent for inductors for resistance. The faster the magnetic fields in the inductor reverse, the more energy is dissipated, so any equivalent term must be frequency dependent. The overall

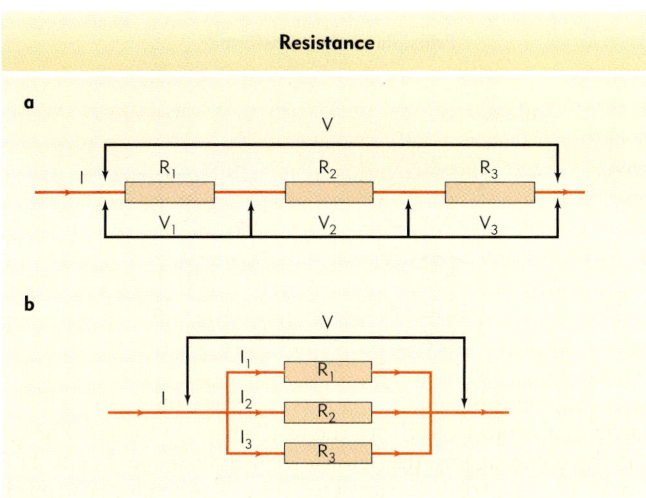

Figure 11.3 Resistance. (a) Resistors in series. (b) Resistors in parallel.

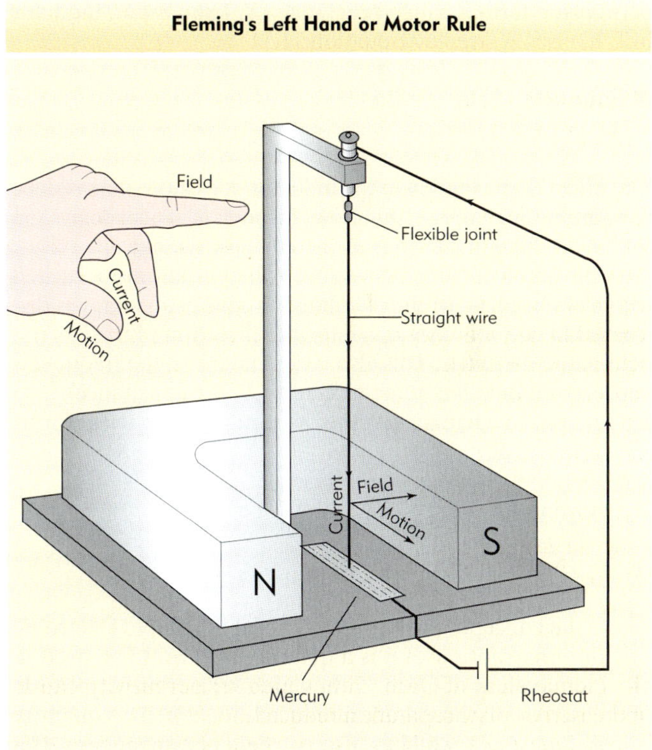

Figure 11.4 Fleming's Left Hand or Motor Rule. The first finger, thumb, and second finger of the left hand are held at right angles to each other; if the direction of the first finger is taken to indicate the direction of a fixed magnetic field and the second finger the direction of current flow in a conductor placed in that field, then the direction of the thumb indicates the direction of force experienced by the conductor in the field.

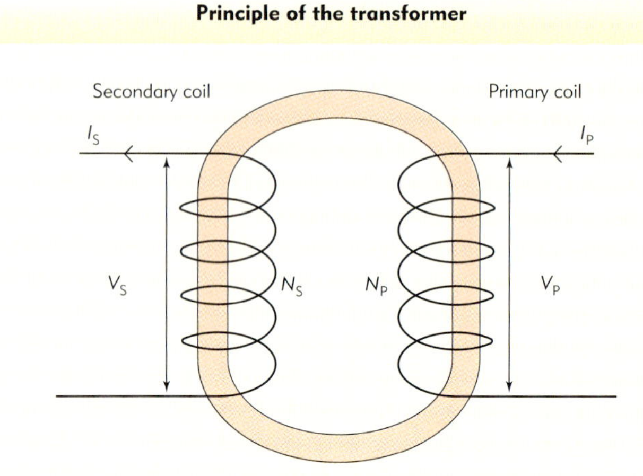

Figure 11.5 The principle of the transformer.

dissipation term is called reactance (X_L) and for an inductor of L henries is given by Equation 11.11.

Equation 11.11

$$X_L = 2\pi fL$$

The effect of dissipation in the inductor does more than reduce the amplitude of the AC that flows through it. It also delays the sinusoidal current, which is termed a phase change.

A similar line of argument applies when a capacitor is excited with a sinusoidal current or voltage. In this case energy is dissipated in continuously reversing the direction of the electric field in the dielectric. This also is dependent on the frequency, and capacitance has reactance too (X_L). Capacitances also induce phase changes in the AC and voltage waveforms (Equation 11.12).

Equation 11.12

$$X_C = \frac{1}{2\pi f}$$

While the concept of reactance is useful for simple electronic calculations, more useful is a quantity that could be used in an AC equivalent of Ohm's law, which relates the amplitude of the current to the voltage across an inductor. This quantity is impedance (Z), which is also is frequency dependent. If a resistor, capacitor, and an inductor are connected in series the impedance of the three together to AC is given by Equation 11.13.

Equation 11.13

$$Z = \{R^2 + [2\pi fL - 1/(2\pi C)]^2\}^{0.5}$$

AMPLIFIERS

The main way that signals and physiologic measurements are processed in medicine is as electrical signals. Even for original signals that are not electrical, transducers or sensors of one form or another are employed to convert them into electrical signals (Chapters 12–14). In any instrument the amplifier is the vital circuit component.

The performance of an amplifier is defined by its gain (A), which is the ratio of the output signal amplitude (v_o) to the input signal amplitude (v_i) (Equation 11.14). A negative gain indicates that the signal is inverted.

Equation 11.14

$$A = \frac{v_o}{v_i}$$

Bandwidth is the range of frequencies of signal over which the amplifier amplifies without distortion in frequency (amplifying one frequency more than another) or introducing phase shifts in the signal or components of the signal.

If small signals are to be amplified, the higher the input impedance (Z_i), the more sensitive the amplifier can be. However, input impedance should be resistive so as not to introduce phase shifts, etc.

Output impedance (Z_o) should be low so that the amplifier can provide adequate EMF to drive any form of load or other type of electronic circuit. An amplifier should not produce offset voltages at its own inputs.

The amplifiers used in medical instrumentation are almost entirely operational amplifiers. These are integrated circuits in which the transistors, resistors, and all other components required to construct the amplifier have been manufactured on a single piece of silicon (chip).

An operational amplifier (op-amp) has three terminals – inverting input, noninverting input, and output. Voltage signals applied to the inverting input (v_1) with the noninverting terminal (v_2) connected to earth (ground) are amplified and appear at the output inverted, and vice-versa for the noninverting input. If signals are applied simultaneously to both, the difference between the signals is amplified and appears at the output. In the latter configuration the amplifier is acting as a differential amplifier.

Operational amplifiers have the following ideal characteristics:

- linear in response both in gain (infinite gain) and phase;
- accurately amplify signals with a very wide range of frequency components (infinite bandwidth);
- stable with temperature;
- very low offset voltages (when $v_1 = v_2$, $v_o = 0$);
- very high (infinite) common mode rejection ratio (CMRR);
- very high (infinite) input impedance; and
- very low (zero) output impedance.

An amplifier with an infinite gain is not very useful. The slightest signal would send it off to infinite gain, which in practice means that the output would immediately saturate at the value of the supply voltage to the device. In practice the gain and performance of the op-amp is controlled by negative feedback to produce a usable amplifier of known performance that still preserves many of the ideal op-amp characteristics. Negative feedback is applied to the op-amp using two or three external resistors connected to the op-amp terminals.

High CMRR is of particular importance in anesthesia and medical instrumentation. Much of the interference suffered in operating rooms is associated with mains electricity supply and currents flowing in the power supplies of equipment connected to it. The magnetic fields created by these currents induce currents at the mains supply frequency in any conductor within range. These currents are very small but are of the same order as some of the bioelectric potentials, such as the ECG. Since these interfering currents are likely to be of the same size in all leads of an ECG or other measuring leads, they should appear as common mode signals at the inputs of any preamplifier used. High CMRR should therefore eliminate these interfering signals.

However, even with precision components, no pairs of resistors can be matched exactly, and if the match is not achieved, CMRR is reduced.

ELECTRICAL HAZARDS AND SAFETY MEASURES

Electricity has three damaging effects on the body and living tissue:

- electrolysis that causes local chemical breakdown of tissue;
- heating that causes burns; and
- stimulation of excitable cells (i.e. shock).

Electrolysis

The least well-described hazard is electrolysis. It is a purely local effect and is not life threatening. It can occur wherever a low DC of a few milliamps is applied to the skin for a sufficient time. The skin breakdown that occurs has many of the characteristics of a chemical burn. The effect is proportional to current density, but occurs readily at a few volts. Battery-powered equipment is capable of producing this effect.

Burns

In anesthesia burn injuries to patients are most likely to occur because of faulty or badly applied electrocautery (diathermy) equipment. Surgical electrocautery equipment uses a high frequency current at about 1MHz to disrupt or destroy tissue. At these frequencies no neuromuscular effects are produced. Monopolar electrocautery uses a small cutting and/or coagulating electrode in which the current density is high. The cutting effect is proportional to current density, since it is simply the result of dissipating electrical energy in a small volume of tissue. To reduce the current density at exit of the current from the body, a large-area electrode is used, usually strapped tightly to the thigh. If this electrode is badly fitted or damaged, local hot spots may develop on the plate or the current may find a lower impedance return path through ECG electrodes or chance contact between the patient's skin and objects connected to earth (like the operating table or anesthetic equipment). If these contact areas are small enough and the exit current density high enough a burn occurs at these sites. Staff can also receive small shocks in these circumstances if they complete the earth return circuit by having contact with the patient. The shock arises because the patient's potential may rise above that of earth until contact is made as the return current tries to find a suitable return path. Bipolar cautery uses two electrodes of similar small size in the form of tweezers. The burning effect takes place between the electrodes and no large earth return electrode is required.

The other indirect burn risk associated with electrical equipment is explosion. When inflammable anesthetic agents were commonly used this was a major hazard. Static electrical discharges and electrical equipment that could cause sparking were potential sources of ignition. Anesthesia is still carried out using gases that readily support combustion (oxygen and nitrous oxide) and there are plenty of paper or cloth drapes and alcohol based skin preparations to burn. Electrical equipment is still a source of ignition for these fuels. The possibility also exists for ignition from hot components inside anesthetic equipment or monitoring equipment.

Electrical shock	
Current	**Effect**
Macro shock:	
1mA	Threshold of perception
5mA	Accepted maximum harmless current
10–20mA	'Let-go' current. Threshold of tetanic contraction of skeletal muscle. The point at which the individual can just let go of a current carrying conductor
50mA	Pain, fainting, mechanical injury
100–300mA	Ventricular fibrillation Respiration center remains intact
6000mA	Sustained ventricular contraction Defibrillation effect Burns if the current is high enough
Micro-shock:	
10μA	Recommended safe current limit for directly applied cardiac equipment
50μA	Maximum fault condition current for cardiac equipment
100μA	Ventricular fibrillation

Figure 11.6 Electrical shock.

Shock

The source of electrical hazard that is most important to anesthetists is shock. The severity of shock is determined by the current involved and the frequency. The maximum neuromuscular effects of electrical currents occur in the frequency range in which cells produce action potentials. This tends to be about 50–60Hz, the frequency of AC mains supplies.

In terms of life-threatening shock, the heart is the susceptible organ. A sufficient current flow through the heart produces ventricular fibrillation. In *macroshock* an externally applied current produces a sufficient current flow in the thorax to induce fibrillation. However, the other main determinants of shock severity are whether the skin is broken at the point of application of the current and whether the heart is exposed to direct application of the current (*microshock*). The skin provides a relatively high impedance, which underlying tissues do not. The removal of this protection reduces the fibrillation threshold by 10,000 (Fig. 11.6).

Limitation of current flow from equipment to patients and staff, under normal operating and fault conditions, is the primary method of preventing shock hazard. To do this both the design of the instrument and the design of the mains supply to that instrument are important (Fig. 11.7).

ELECTROMAGNETIC RADIATION AND LIGHT

Electromagnetic radiation is the collective term for all the electromagnetic fields that propagate across space. The nature of the field follows from considering electrostatic and electromagnetic induction. If an oscillating EMF is applied to a conductor, then associated with the induced current flow is a local electric and magnetic field, both of which vary in time. The laws of induction dealt with above are concerned with those fields

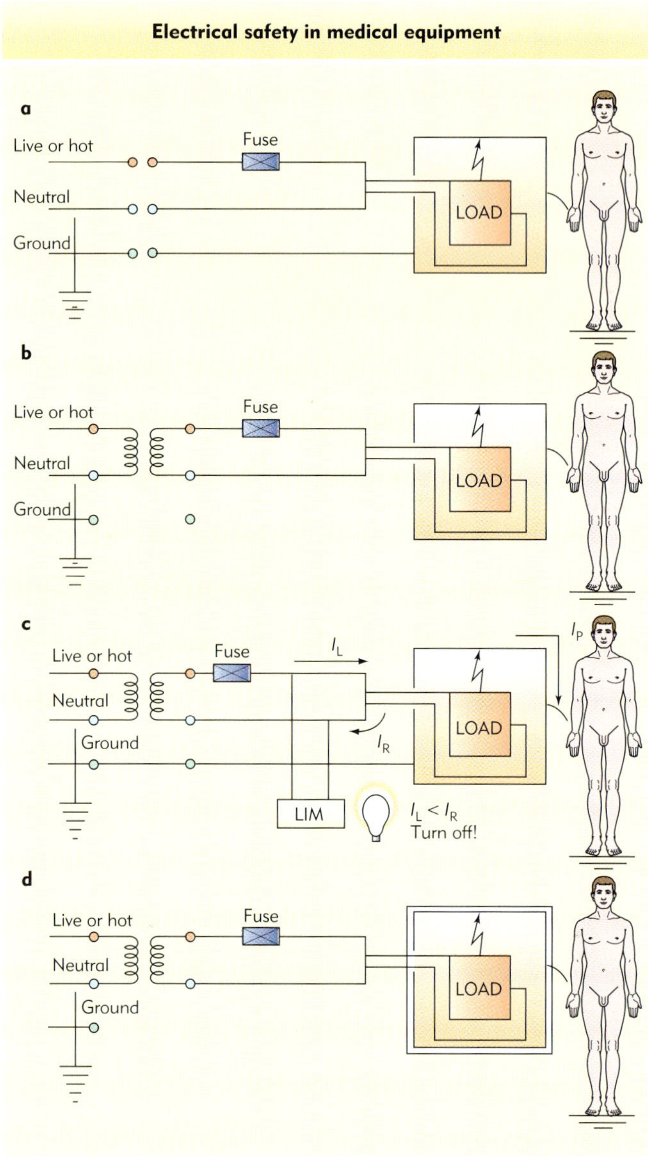

Figure 11.7 Strategies for electrical safety used in medical equipment. (a) Using a simple earth, the earthed case of the instrument conducts the current from the internal instrument fault that shorted the load to the case away from the patient or operator to earth by providing the lowest impedance conduction path. (b) With an isolation transformer (earth-free system), the transformer eliminates the connection between the earth at the supply and the neutral as far as the instrument is concerned. Under a fault, the patient simply grounds the neutral side of the transformer, but no current flows through the patient. Isolation transformers can be incorporated into the instruments instead of the supply. (c) With an isolation transformer and a line isolation monitor (LIM; residual current detector), the isolation transformer is provided in the supply but an earth connection is maintained. In the event of a fault the LIM detects the difference in current (I_L) between the live (hot) wire and the neutral wire (I_R) created by the current flowing through the patient (I_P). It then cuts the power quickly enough to prevent shock. (d) In double insulation (earth-free system), physically isolating the load twice over from the case makes the instrument safe with the fault.

local or near to the conductor. Also a field is created at a distance or far from the conductor. This field is a combined electric–magnetic field that propagates away from the conductor at the speed of light. Like the near field it is capable of inducing currents and EMF in other conductors.

Electromagnetic radiation is a continuous spectrum of waves of different frequencies. These are divided up into sections largely related to their interactions with matter, the characteristics of which change with frequency (or wavelength). The common divisions of this spectrum are shown in Figure 11.8.

Energy is transmitted in electromagnetic radiation governed by laws given in Equations 11.15 & 11.16, in which λ is the radiation wavelength, f is frequency, c is the speed of light, E is energy, and h is Plank's constant.

Equation 11.15

$$\lambda f = c$$

Equation 11.16

$$E = hf$$

This description of electromagnetic radiation views the field as a wave motion. However, when electromagnetic radiation interacts with matter it exhibits particle-like properties as well as wave-like properties. Some effects are best described in terms of wave motion and some by a particle model. The name given to the electromagnetic radiation particle is the *photon*.

Bohr developed a description of the interaction of photons with matter. The idea that electromagnetic radiation carries energy in specific packets or quanta is summarized by Plank's equations above. Einstein explained the photoelectric effect using this idea. He explained why the electrons emitted from metal surfaces when illuminated with light were of a specific energy when the energy from the light reached a specific threshold. Finally, Bohr knew that observation of the details of the spectra of light emitted by elements showed discrete lines of light of specific frequencies.

Bohr combined these facts with Rutherford's view of the structure of the atom (as a small positively charged nucleus with electrons in orbits around this nucleus) and suggested that the electrons of the atom orbited the nucleus only at specific distances. This meant that the kinetic energy of the electrons in orbit could not take up *any* value but only *permitted* values. Thus, for an electron to be raised to a new orbit of higher energy, the energy supplied has to reach the threshold between the two orbits. If the energy is below this threshold the electron stays in the same orbit. This explains the photoelectric effect. If a high-energy electron decays to a lower energy orbit, a photon of the energy difference is emitted, since energy has to be conserved. This explains the discrete nature of the spectral lines.

Bohr's simple atomic model was soon modified by quantum mechanical explanations. However, the basic quantum mechanical nature of photon absorption or emission by electrons in atomic or molecular structures remains a key idea of present day physics. To atomic properties can be added molecular properties, since we now know that the electrons of constituent atoms in molecules can be shared so they have quantum levels that are a property of molecular structure (Chapter 1).

Absorbance and Beer's Law

Consider a beam of monochromatic light (light of single wavelength and therefore photon energy) incident on a sample of

Electromagnetic radiation		
Wavelength (m)	Type	Frequency (Hz)
10^{-13}		10^{19}
10^{-12}	γ rays	
10^{-11}		
10^{-10}		10^{16}
10^{-9}	X rays	
10^{-8}	Ultraviolet light (violet)	
10^{-7}		
10^{-6}	Visible light (white)	10^{12}
10^{-5}		
10^{-4}	Infrared light (red)	10^{9}
10^{-3}		
10^{-2}	Microwaves	
10^{-1}		
1	Radio waves UHF	
10	VHF	
10^{2}		
10^{3}		
10^{4}		

Figure 11.8 Electromagnetic radiation.

substance known to absorb light of this wavelength, termed a *chromophore*, mixed in a nonabsorbing matrix. The amount of absorption of the incident light is the number of photons absorbed, which depends on the probability of a photon interacting with an electron of the correct quantum state. Thus the amount of absorption is proportional to the thickness of the sample, the concentration of the chromophore, and the efficiency of the chromophore at absorbing the light. In such situations slices through the sample of equal width absorb the same proportion of light, which means that the intensity of light falls exponentially with path length through the sample. This is given by Equation 11.17, in which I is the emergent light intensity, I_0 is the incident light intensity, k is a constant, and l is the path length. Taking logarithms of Equation 11.17 and rearranging gives Equation 11.18.

Equation 11.17

$$I = I_0 e^{-kl}$$

Equation 11.18

$$\log_{10} \frac{(I_0)}{I} = \frac{kl}{2.303}$$

The term $\log_{10} (I_0/I)$ is called variously the absorbance, the extinction coefficient, or the optical density. The expression states that absorbance is proportional to absorbing layer thickness, which is Lambert's Law. Chromophore concentration is implicitly present as part of the constant k. Rewriting Equations 11.17 & 11.18 to show it explicitly gives Equations 11.19 & 11.20, in which ϵ is the absorption coefficient, c is concentration, and A is absorbance; the latter is Beer's Law.

Equation 11.19

$$I = I_0 e^{-k'l}$$

Equation 11.20

$$\log_{10} \frac{(I_0)}{I} = A = \epsilon cl$$

Fluorescence

The energy absorbed by the electrons of the chromophore may remain in the chromophore as an excited state. However, one of the following is more likely to result:

- a chain of internal excitations and electron transitions that results in dissipation of the energy as heat to neighboring molecules;
- the excited state may be so energetic that chemical breakdown occurs; or
- after one or two internal transitions the energy is radiated from the molecule as light of a different wavelength or group of wavelengths (*fluorescence*).

If this emitted light is not absorbed by the chromophore its intensity and other properties are measurable. The fluorescent light is emitted in all directions at a lower wavelength than that of the original light. Fluorescence is very useful as it is specific to the chemistry of the chromophore and may accompany chemical changes. As an alternative measurement to absorbance it has the advantage of greater sensitivity. This arises because, although the light has lost its directionality and is of a lower intensity, it is measured with reference to a true zero light condition.

Lasers

The action of a laser (light amplification by stimulated emission of radiation) in many ways is similar to the process of fluorescence. The energy state from which the fluorescent light is emitted is very often a *metastable* electron state. Electrons are temporarily held in this orbit until some process triggers their decay back to an unexcited energy state and a photon associated with the transition is emitted. In the case of fluorescence the delay is small and the metastable state very 'unstable'. However, in laser action the metastable state is relatively 'stable' and the trigger to decay the electron is very specific – emission of a photon from the metastable state itself.

The original type of laser shown in Figure 11.9 is made from a crystal of ruby. A mirror is placed at one end of the ruby crystal and a half-silvered mirror at the other, all surrounded by a helical flash tube. This tube emits a broad spectrum of visible light, which enters from the sides of the crystal and is reflected up and down the crystal many times by the mirrors. The photons in the blue and green parts of the flash tube spectrum raise unexcited electrons into two ranges of closely packed excited states, called *bands*. However, the electrons rapidly decay from these states to a single metastable state of lower energy. Electrons accumulate in this metastable state as the pumping action continues until so many electrons are in it that the normal population of electrons between this state and the normal unexcited state becomes inverted. At this point a single decay is enough to start an avalanche of electron decays, since the emission of one photon *stimulates* another electron emission and so on. What is very particular about the light emitted, however, is that it is not emitted in a random fashion. The stimulation process leads to photons that are in-phase, or coherent. The avalanche emission therefore behaves as one wave motion, emerging from the half-silvered end of the crystal as a highly focused, single wavelength and highly energetic beam.

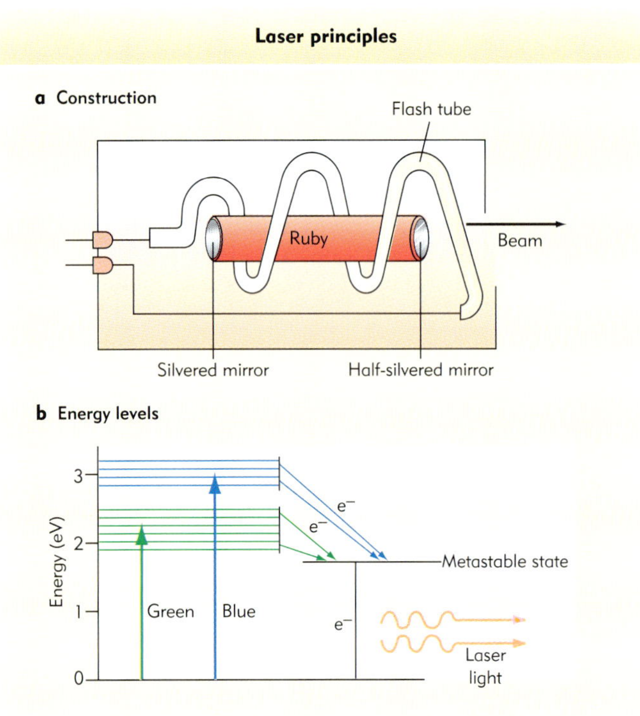

Figure 11.9 The construction of an early ruby laser and the energy levels associated with its action.

Laser action has been demonstrated in a wide variety of substances and at a wide range of wavelengths, including microwaves (masers). Gas lasers, such as the helium–neon laser (which gives red light for plastic surgery), use an electric discharge to pump the electrons in the gas mixture. Considerable power is possible. Laser light interacts with tissue in four ways – thermal heating, photochemically, thermoacoustically, and to produce photoablation. Medical lasers are often very powerful and can be used to cut, weld, or ablate tissues. Medical laser light is often of sufficient intensity to be an ignition risk.

Nuclear magnetic resonance

In the nucleus of an atom each positively charged proton can have a 'spin', a property that can be thought of as if the proton spins on its axis. Associated with this spin is a magnetic field. In the nucleus, protons usually align themselves in pairs of opposite spin to neutralize the overall magnetic field, but in atoms with an odd number of protons this is not possible. This occurs in ^{1}H, ^{3}C, ^{14}N, ^{17}O, ^{23}Na, and ^{31}P, all of which are biochemically important elements common in the body.

Under normal circumstances the orientations of the nuclear fields for individual atoms are random, but when an external magnetic field is applied these orientations align with the field such that the North (N) pole of the particle lines with the South (S) pole of the field. Aligning N–N is also possible, but this state has a higher quantum energy than the N–S orientation and is therefore somewhat like the excited state of an electron in an atom. Nuclei in the magnetic field are not stationary but *precess*, that is wobble rather like a top or a gyroscope. The frequency at which they precess is fixed by the magnetic field strength. If the nuclei are irradiated with an electromagnetic field at this frequency in the N–S state, they resonate with that field, absorb energy, and can flip to the N–N state. If the electromagnetic radiation is removed, the nuclei decay back to the N–S state in a time that depends on their binding with the atoms around them (effectively the chemistry of the molecules around them). The time constants for these relaxations are quite long (from milliseconds to seconds). The associated electromagnetic radiation can be detected and if pulses of electromagnetic radiation are used to excite the nuclei, the resultant spin echoes can be gated in time. Since the excitation frequency is atom specific and the echoes have time constants characterized by their interactions, NMR is a very specific analysis tool. It enables the study of one atom type within a sample and it can be carried out *in vivo* as well as *in vitro*.

The principle of NMR applies to any spinning, charged atomic particle including electrons, in which case the equivalent effect is electron spin resonance (ESR). The NMR equipment used to create images of body sections (similar to computed tomography images) can also be used to examine ESR effects and is thus given the general name of magnetic resonance imaging (MRI). To reconstruct an image from all the possible echoes in a volume slice of tissue requires sophisticated pulse and gating sequences.

Fiberoptics

In many medical measurement applications it is useful to transmit into or gather light from the body over relatively long path lengths and through small openings or orifices without undue losses. Fiberoptics is a convenient way of achieving this. Fiberoptic cables rely on the principle of total internal reflection of visible light.

A fiberoptic cable is made up of 400–500 individual fibers. The fibers can be made of plastic or glass and each has a coating that increases the internal reflection of the fiber. When light is injected into the end it is trapped by the multiple internal reflections and transmitted from one end to the other. The fibers themselves are flexible and thus the whole cable can be bent and shaped as needed. Glass fibers have transmission efficiencies of 60% over 50cm for wavelengths of 400–1200nm. Plastic fibers have 70% transmission efficiencies for the same distance, but at a more limited range of wavelengths (500–850nm).

Fiberoptic cables come in two forms. In *noncoherent* cables (called *light guides*) the fiber diameter is 13–100nm and no correlation exists between a fiber's spatial position at the entrance to the cable and where it emerges. These are used for transmission of light into the body only. In *coherent* fiber bundles or cables the fibers occupy the same spatial position at entrance and exit, so image can be transmitted faithfully through the bundle. These cables are used for endoscopy.

Fiberoptic cables are relatively more energy efficient at transmitting pulses of information than the equivalent wire conductor, although efficiency is lost in having to create the light pulses initially and to convert the light pulses back into electricity at the end of the cable. Fiberoptic cables have the added advantage that the pulses transmitted down the fiber are less distorted by the transmission, which means that the fiber has a greater bandwidth and can transmit more pulses per second than a wire. Fiberoptics is becoming the standard method of transmitting digital information over long distances. In medicine this technology is very attractive as a way of transmitting information from inside the body. Information in the form of light pulses in the fiber is immune from electrical interference and the fibers themselves provide electrical isolation from the patient.

RADIOACTIVITY AND RADIATION

Elements are characterized by the number of protons and neutrons in their nuclei. The number of protons is the atomic number, Z, of the element. The atomic number equals the number of electrons in orbit around the nuclei. The number of electrons determines the chemistry of the element. Developing the Bohr model of the atom a little further, more than one electron can exist in each of the orbitals with the same quantum energy. It is found that the greatest chemical stability exists when the outer orbital or *shell* of an atom has an even number of electrons. The shells are given letters to distinguish them and the maximum number of electrons allowed in each shell rises with the number of shells. The innermost shell, the K-shell has a maximum of two electrons, the L-shell a maximum of eight, the M-shell a maximum of 18, and so on. It is the configuration of the electrons in the outer shell of the element that determines its position in the *periodic table*. Hydrogen, lithium, sodium, rubidium, and francium all have outer shells with one electron. Their ability to lose this electron to form positive ions therefore tends to dominate their chemistry and makes their chemistry similar in many respects.

The number of neutrons in the nucleus of the element does not affect the chemistry of the element, but does affect its mass number, A, which is the total number of neutrons and protons in the nucleus. Elements with the same Z but different A values are isotopes of the same element. To distinguish different isotopes in chemical equations, the A value (mass number) is added as a superscript before the chemical symbol and the Z value (atomic number) as a subscript. Thus the three isotopes of hydrogen are given the nomenclature ${}^{1}_{1}H$ (hydrogen), ${}^{2}_{1}H$ (deuterium), and ${}^{3}_{1}H$ (tritium).

The nucleus is held together by strong and weak nuclear forces that are very short range. As with electrons in the shells, protons and neutrons in the nucleus can exist in excited or other states that are described by quantum mechanics. Thus decay of the nucleus is possible just as ionization of an atom is possible. Spontaneous nuclear breakdown leads to radioactivity.

Most naturally occurring isotopes exist as mixtures of *stable isotopes* that do not exhibit radioactivity. However, some *unstable isotopes* (*radioactive isotopes*) do exist naturally, and others can be created by bombarding stable isotopes with charged subatomic particles.

Types of radioactivity

Disintegration of the nucleus may be accompanied by emission of particles and/or energy. The three types of radiation associated with nuclear decay are α-radiation, β-radiation, and γ-radiation.

α-Radiation

α-Radiation consists of heavy, positively charged particles with a mass number 2 and an atomic number 4 (i.e. helium nuclei ${}^{4}_{2}He$). A typical transition that emits α-particles is the breakdown of radium (Ra) into radon (Rn) (Equation 11.21).

Equation 11.21

$${}^{226}_{88}Ra \rightarrow {}^{222}_{86}Rn$$

Since α-particles are heavy they do not have high velocity. They are easily absorbed by passage through a few millimeters of air, tissue, or other material. However, they carry quite a lot of kinetic energy because of their mass and deposit this effectively in biologic tissues, which results in considerable cellular damage. An α-particle is quite capable of entirely smashing the nucleus of a cell!

β-Radiation

β-Radiation consists of electrons or positrons, but the majority of isotopes decay by β-particle emission. Isotopes with an excess of neutrons usually decay by this pathway. Loss of a negative charge from the nucleus effectively converts a neutron into a proton, and so the atomic number of the element increases. A typical decay of this type that emits β-particles is the decay of phosphorus-32 into sulfur-32 (Equation 11.22).

Equation 11.22

$${}^{32}_{15}P \rightarrow {}^{32}_{16}S + {}^{0}_{-1}\beta$$

Neutron-deficient nuclei can emit a positron (a positively charged electron, the antiparticle of the electron) which reduces atomic number by 1, as with the decay of iron-18 (Equation 11.23).

Equation 11.23

$${}^{18}_{9}Fe \rightarrow {}^{18}_{8}O + {}^{0}_{1}\beta$$

Since β-particles have low mass they have high velocities and are harder to absorb than α-particles. However, their range in tissue is only a few millimeters. Thus, if a β-active isotope is injected into the body, external detection is not possible. Such isotopes are used for tracer studies in which the radioactivity is measured in samples removed from the body, for example the use of tritiated water (${}^{3}H_2O$) as a tracer for the measurement of lung water.

Positron decay isotopes are the basis of a relatively new form of functional imaging of tissue – positron emission tomography (PET). In PET, biochemically active isotopes are prepared that decay by positron emission (e.g. glucose). The isotope is injected and taken up by the targeted tissues. Positrons emitted from the isotope are slowed by their interactions with tissue. When a positron encounters an electron, its antiparticle, they annihilate each other and the energy is released as photons, in this case two γ-rays. Since at annihilation neither the electron nor the positron has much momentum, the γ-rays are emitted at 180° from each other. Thus they arrive at two γ-ray detectors on opposite sides of the body at the same time, which can be used to determine where they came from.

Since β-particles have low mass they deposit little energy in tissue, and until relatively recently were considered the least dangerous form of radiation. However, it is now recognized that while they do not cause widespread cellular damage, they can break DNA strands in the nuclei of cells and may thus be more dangerous mutagens if ingested than had previously been thought.

γ-Radiation

γ-Radiation (γ-rays) consists of photons and thus is part of the electromagnetic spectrum. It is given off by radioactive decay as a way of removing excess energy or as the result of a secondary annihilation (as with the electron–positron example given above). In common with all electromagnetic radiation, γ-rays are very difficult to stop and penetrate many centimeters of tissue (if they do not pass straight through the body). They are highly energetic.

Units of measurement

The amount of radioactivity of a source or its activity is measured in terms of the number of disintegrations per unit time (SI unit is the becquerel, Bq). Of great clinical importance is the absorbed dose of radioactivity, which is measured by the energy transferred to a substance by the radiation (SI unit is the gray, Gy). The absorbed dose needs to be adjusted for the biologic effectiveness of the radiation, which depends on radiation type and target organ. The effective dose is the absorbed dose weighted by terms for radiation type and organ sensitivity (SI unit is sievert, Sv).

Mathematics of radioactivity

Radioactivity is a probabilistic effect. When an individual atom will decay is not known, but in a given time the number of atoms that decay is a fixed proportion of the number of atoms capable of decaying; this is defined by an exponential decay curve that has the mathematical form of Equation 11.24, in which N is the number of atoms left that can disintegrate, N_0 is the number at the start, k is a constant, and t is time.

Equation 11.24

$$N = N_0 e^{-kt}$$

The rate at which an exponential curve falls can be defined using two indices: the time constant (k), and the half-life ($t_{1/2}$). Half-life is the time required for the initial number of atoms to drop to 50% of its initial value (Equation 11.25).

Equation 11.25

$$t_{1/2} = \frac{(\log 0.5)}{-k} = \frac{0.698}{k}$$

Further Reading

Ohanian HC. Principles of physics. New York: WW Norton & Company; 1994.

Webster J. Medical instrumentation, 3rd edn. New York: John Wiley & Sons; 1998.

Chapter 12 Electrocardiography

Martin J London

Topics covered in this chapter

Technical aspects of the electrocardiograph
Digital signal processing and computed electrocardiography
Lead systems
Detection of myocardial ischemia

Although cardiologists are recognized as the ultimate authorities in electrocardiography (ECG), all clinicians involved in perioperative and critical care may obtain valuable information from it either in the form of a standard 12-lead tracing or as a continuous monitor (Fig. 12.1). With recent advances in ECG and computer technology, the distinction between 'diagnostic' and bedside 'monitoring' units has blurred. Newer bedside units can record diagnostic quality 12-lead tracings and automatically transfer them over a hospital network to a central storage and retrieval work station.

The diagnostic and monitoring capabilities of ECG continue to develop and expand (Fig. 12.2). The routine use of digital signal processing (DSP) facilitates continuous ECG monitoring inexpensively with minimal invasiveness or discomfort to the patient. However, there are limitations defined by the relationship between sensitivity and specificity (usually inversely related) for detecting certain disease processes, particularly coronary artery disease and its consequences. Electrocardiagraphy may suffer from an unacceptably high false-positive (low specificity) or false-negative (low sensitivity) rate, thus necessitating other diagnostic modalities.

The practicing anesthesiologist relies heavily on ECG to make critical decisions in the perioperative period in patients undergoing cardiac and noncardiac (particularly vascular) surgery. This chapter reviews the theory behind, and operating characteristics of, selected ECG hardware used in the perioperative period. In the near future, newer monitoring systems specifically designed for cardiovascular suites and intensive-care units (ICUs) will likely utilize multiple-lead data processing, sophisticated trending and alarm capabilities, and, ultimately, artificial intelligence techniques to assist in detecting ischemia, arrhythmias, and other cardiovascular information.

Clinical information available from electrocardiography

Anatomy/morphology
- Infarction
- Ischemia
- Hypertrophy

Physiology
- Automaticity
- Arrhythmogenicity
- Conduction
- Ischemia
- Autonomic tone
- Electrolyte abnormalities
- Drug toxicity/effect
- Ejection fraction (?)

Figure 12.1 Clinical information available from electrocardiography. (With permission from London and Kaplan, 1999.)

Electrocardiographic data for clinical use

P wave
- Polarity
- Duration
- Mean amplitude
- Area
- Frequency content

P–R segment
- A–H interval
- H–V interval

QRS complex
- Polarity
- Duration
- Area
- Mean amplitude
- Frequency content
- Late potential-power spectrum

ST–T wave
- Slope of ascending/descending limbs
- Area
- Ratio of area to peak, duration to peak

Power spectrum of variation

Arrhythmias
- Morphology
- Coupling interval

Figure 12.2 Data extraction from the electrocardiography to support current and future clinical uses. Data derived with and without ancillary corrective modalities. (With permission from London and Kaplan, 1999.)

TECHNICAL ASPECTS OF THE ELECTROCARDIOGRAPH

Power spectrum

The ECG signal can be considered in terms of its amplitude (or voltage) and frequency components (generally termed 'phase'). Voltage considerations differ depending on the source of the ECG. Surface recording involves amplification of considerably smaller voltages (in the order of 1mV) than recording sites closer to the heart (i.e. endocardial, esophageal, and, recently, tracheal leads). Figure 12.3 presents the power spectrum of the ECG frequency components based on Fourier transformation, in which a periodic waveform is analyzed mathematically by decomposition to its harmonic components (sine waves of varying amplitude and frequency). Also represented are the spectra of some of the major sources of artifact, which must be eliminated during processing and amplification of the QRS complex. The frequency of each of these components can be equated to the slope of the component signal. The R wave with its steep slope is considered a high-frequency component, whereas P and T waves have lesser slopes and, therefore, are lower in frequency. The ST segment has the lowest slope or frequency, not much different from the 'underlying' electrical (i.e. isoelectric) baseline of the ECG.

Before the introduction of DSP, accurate display of the ST segment presented significant technical problems, particularly in operating room or ICU environments (see below). Although the overall frequency spectrum of the QRS complex in Figure 12.3 does not appear to exceed 40Hz, many components of the QRS complex, particularly the R wave, exceed 100Hz. Very-high-frequency signals of clinical significance are pacemaker spikes. Their short duration and high amplitude present a technical challenge because they must be properly recognized and rejected to allow accurate determination of the heart rate (HR). The range of frequencies of greatest importance for optimal processing in ECG monitors is presented in Figure 12.4.

Artifacts

Motion artifact and 'baseline wander' result from several causes. Intrinsic or physiologic artifacts include the electrical potentials generated by the skin. Skin impedance varies at different skin sites, at different times of the day as well as seasonally, and may be 50% higher in females. With application of a silver–silver chloride electrode, impedance decays with a time constant of 6.9 minutes as the conductive gel penetrates the skin. Deformation of the stratum granulosum generates significant electrical potentials of several millivolts as cells slide over each other or are stretched. Skin potentials up to 64mV are measurable between any two electrodes on the skin surface, varying with the type of electrolyte used. An additional factor is the direct current (DC) potential stored by the electrode itself, termed *offset potential,* which varies with the type of electrode used. A striking example of an offset potential is the transient obliteration of the ECG that occurs immediately following electrical defibrillation. Poor electrode contact enhances pickup of power-line interefence.

Another major physiologic artifact is electromyographic (EMG) noise produced by motor activity, either conscious (i.e. during treadmill testing or ambulatory ST segment monitoring) or unconscious (i.e. shivering or Parkinsonian tremor). Electromyographic noise is similar in amplitude to the ECG but is of higher frequency. Since it is a totally random signal, in contrast to the regular repetitive ECG signal, it is generally amenable to significant reduction using DSP techniques (see below).

Power spectrum of the electrocardiograph signal

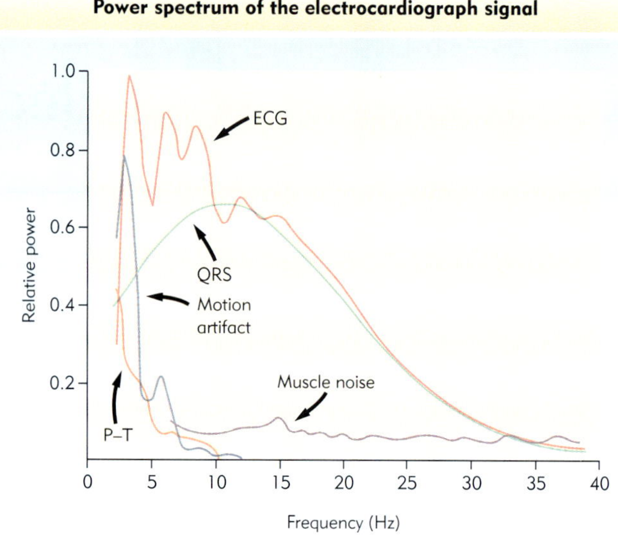

Figure 12.3 Power spectrum of the electrocardiography signal including its subcomponents and common artifacts (i.e. motion and muscle noise). The power of the P and T waves are low frequency, while the QRS complex is concentrated in the midfrequency range. (Reproduced from Thakor NV: From Holter monitors to automatic defibrillators: Developments in ambulatory arrhythmia monitoring. IEEE Trans Biomed Eng. 31:770, 1984, with permission © 1984, IEEE.)

Range of signal frequencies included in different phases of processing in an ECG monitor

Processing	Frequency range (Hz)
Display	0.5 (0.05)–40
QRS detection	5–30
Arrhythmia detection	0.05–60
ST segment monitoring	0.05–60
Pacemaker detection	1500–5000

Figure 12.4 Range of signal frequencies included in different phases of processing in an electrocardiographic monitor. (With permission from London and Kaplan, 1999.)

There are also nonphysiologic or extrinsic causes of artifact. An important one is termed 'common-mode rejection'. The ECG signal is the difference in potential between two electrodes and is, therefore, a differential signal. Furthermore, the body is not at absolute ground potential, which is why the right leg lead is used as a reference electrode. This higher potential (over that of an absolute ground) is termed *common-mode potential* because it is common to both of the electrode inputs to the differential amplifier used to amplify the ECG signal. Common-mode potential must be rejected or it may alter the ECG signal. The ability of a differential amplifier to reject these potentials (relative to the differential inputs) is determined by the common-mode rejection ratio (CMRR) and is of great importance in significantly attenuating a variety of environmental factors. In modern amplifiers, the CMRR should be at least 10^5; in newer diagnostic digital ECG units, it is at least 10^6.

Power line interference (e.g. 60Hz in the USA, 50Hz in the UK) is a common environmental problem. Power lines and other electrical devices radiate energy, which may enter the monitor via poor electrode contact or cracked or poorly shielded lead cables. It may also be electromagnetically induced as these signals radiate through the loop formed by the body, the lead cables, and the monitor. This type of interference may be reduced by twisting the lead cables together, although this suggestion is impractical for intraoperative monitoring. At the very least, the distance between lead cables should be minimized. In newer diagnostic ECG machines, analog-to-digital (A/D) signal conversion occurs in an acquisition module close to the patient, which effectively reduces the length of the lead cables and, thus, the amount of induction possible. A line frequency 'notch' filter is also often used to remove interference.

Electrocautery (electrosurgery) units generate radiofrequency currents at very high frequencies (800–2000kHz) and high voltages (1kV, which is one million times greater than the ECG signal). Older units used a modulation frequency of 60Hz, which spreads electrical noise into the frequency range of the ECG signal. However, newer units have increased the modulation frequency to 20kHz, minimizing spread into the QRS frequency range. In order to minimize electrocautery artifact, the right leg reference electrode should be placed as close as possible to the grounding pad. In addition, the ECG monitor should be plugged into a different power outlet to the electrosurgical unit.

Monitoring electrodes should be placed directly over bony prominences of the torso (i.e. clavicular heads and iliac prominences) to minimize excursion of the electrode during respiration, which can cause baseline wander. To avoid loss and alteration of the signal, electrode impedance must be optimized. By removing a portion of the stratum corneum (gentle abrasion with a dry gauze pad works well, resulting in a minor amount of surface erythema), skin impedance can be reduced by a factor of 10 to 100. Optimal impedance is 5000Ω or less.

Clinical devices with which the patient is in physical contact, particularly via plastic tubing, may at times cause significant ECG artifact. Although the exact mechanism is uncertain, two likely explanations are either a piezoelectric effect owing to mechanical deformation of the plastic, or buildup of static electricity between two dissimilar materials, especially those in motion. This has been noted with the use of cardiopulmonary bypass and can mimic atrial arrhythmias. Other clinical devices associated with ECG interference, albeit rarely, include infusion pumps and blood warmers. Isolated power supply line isolation monitors (LIMs) have also been associated with 60Hz interference. This can be diagnosed by removing the LIM fuses to see if the artifact disappears.

Frequency response: monitoring and diagnostic modes

Given the importance of the ECG in diagnosing myocardial ischemia, it is important to realize that significant ST segment depression or elevation can occur as a result of improper signal filtering. This artifact was a significant problem before the introduction of DSP. As noted above, ECG signals must be amplified and filtered before display. To reproduce component frequencies accurately, each must be amplified equally (i.e. the monitor must have a flat amplitude response over the wide range of frequencies present). Similarly, because the slight delay in a signal as it passes through a filter or amplifier may vary in duration with different frequencies, all frequencies must be delayed equally (i.e. have a linear phase response). If the response is nonlinear, various components may appear temporally distorted (termed *phase shift*).

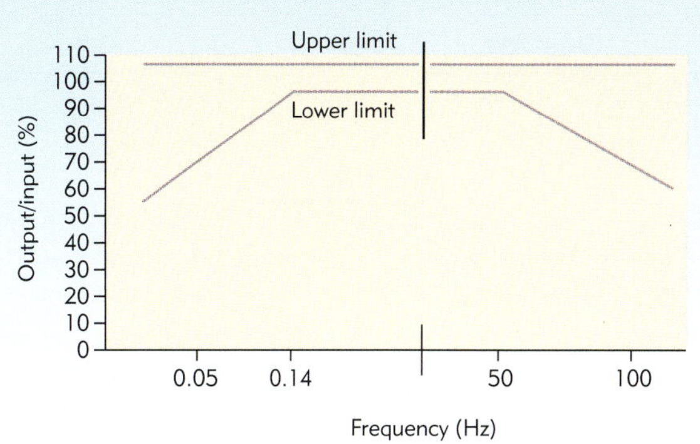

Figure 12.5 Frequency response for direct-writing electrocardiography, recommended by the American Heart Association. The bandwidth is demarcated by the upper and lower corner frequencies (in this example 0.05 and 100Hz); which are located –3dB (approximately a 30% decrease in voltage) relative to the amplification at a frequency near the middle of the bandwidth (heavy vertical bar). (Reproduced from Pipberger HV, Arzbaecher RC, Berson AS, et al. Recommendations for the standardization of leads and of specifications for instruments in electocardiography and vectorcardiography. Report of the Committee on Electrocardiography, American Heart Association. Circulation. 1975;52:11, with permission; copyright American Heart Association.)

Nonlinear frequency response in the low-frequency range (0.5Hz) can cause artifactual ST depression, whereas phase delay in this range may cause ST segment elevation. Although a completely linear response is desirable, with analog filters it is not generally possible and a bandwidth of 0.05–100Hz (at 3dB) is recommended (Fig. 12.5). The response at 0.05Hz should not be reduced by more than 30% (at 3dB) from the response at 0.14Hz. Phase response is not well described but is generally considered adequate when amplitude response criteria are met. Since a greater amount of baseline noise is present when a 0.05Hz cutoff is used, the 0.5Hz cutoff is often used to display a more stable signal. This is commonly referred to as 'monitoring mode', while use of a 0.05Hz low-frequency cutoff is known as 'diagnostic mode'. The difference in ST segment morphology at different low-frequency cutoffs is illustrated in Figure 12.6. Most new monitors use signal-averaging techniques that are very effective in eliminating most artifact even in the diagnostic mode.

High-frequency response is of less importance since the ST segment and T wave reside in the low-frequency spectrum. However, at the commonly used high-frequency cutoff of 40Hz, the amplitude of the R and S waves may diminish significantly, making it difficult to diagnose ventricular hypertrophy.

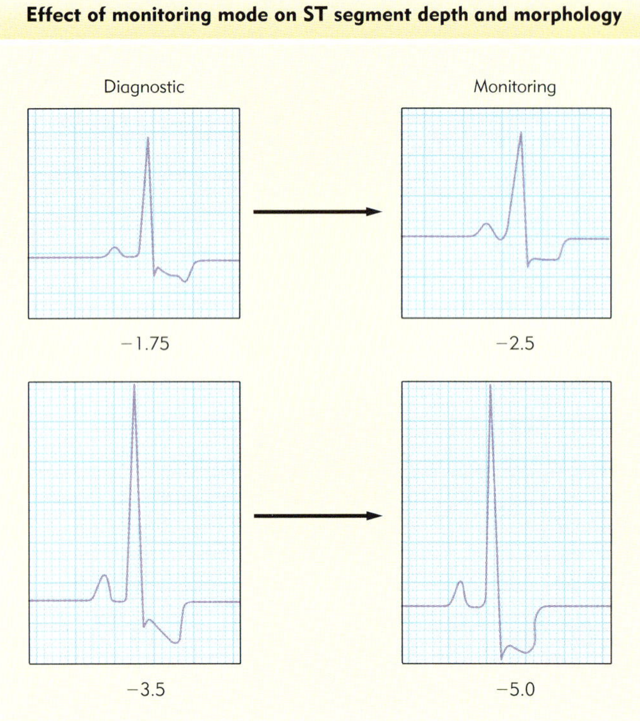

Figure 12.6 The effects of the monitoring mode on ST segment depth and morphology using a digital electrocardiography simulator. A SpaceLabs PC2 monitor (Redmond, WA) was switched from monitoring (0.5–40Hz) to diagnostic mode (0.05–70Hz). Note the increase in the depth of ST segment depression and the alteration of slope in both leads. (With permission from London, 1993.)

DIGITAL SIGNAL PROCESSING AND COMPUTED ELECTROCARDIOGRAPHY

The foundation of DSP is the A/D converter, which samples the incoming continuous analog signal (characterized by variable amplitude or voltage over time) at a very rapid rate and converts the sampled voltage into binary numbers, each of which has a precise time index or sequence. The 'bit size' of the A/D converter controls the number of measurements possible within a given voltage range according to the formula 2^n–1 (i.e. an 8-bit converter divides the input range into 255 intervals). The larger the bit size, the greater the resolution of the signal. However, greater bit size and higher sampling rates require more powerful microprocessors and more computer memory. Most commercially available units use minimum sampling rates of 256Hz (resulting in 4ms increments) with at least 12-bit resolution. Use of lower sampling rates may result in a slight difference in the time at which digitization of each QRS complex begins (phase shift), which can distort the signal as noted above. Newer diagnostic ECG units are capable of sampling at 1000Hz (termed *high-resolution* or *high-res* ECG).

Following A/D conversion, the resultant data bits are inspected by a microprocessor using a mathematical construct to determine where reference points ('fiducial points') are located. A common method locates the point of most rapid change in amplitude (located on the downslope of the R wave). This process characterizes the baseline QRS complex (QRS recognition) and provides a template on which subsequent beats are overlaid (beat alignment) and averaged (signal averaging). This allows visual display of the QRS complex and quantitation of its components, as well as elimination of random electrical noise and wide complex beats that fail to meet criteria established by the fiducial points.

Signal averaging is a critical component of this process. Using this technique, noise is reduced proportionally by the square root of the number of beats averaged. Thus, a tenfold reduction in noise is accomplished by averaging only 100 beats. Because of the proprietary nature of this technology (the specific algorithms used are patented), the method used may vary by manufacturer. Consequently, the processed QRS complexes may vary in the 'quality' of representation (i.e. if noise or aberrant beats are averaged into the complex, it will vary from the raw analog complex).

The averaging process involves comparison of the voltages at a particular time point between the incoming complex and the template. Although the easiest method is to use the mean difference between voltages to update the template, the most accurate method is to use the median (because it is less affected by outliers, such as aberrant beats or other signals that have escaped QRS matching). The disadvantage is that median averaging is computationally more complex (i.e. memory intensive) and may have slightly higher baseline noise content. Because median averaging is impractical for continuous data acquisition, another technique that minimizes the influence of outliers is used, termed incremental averaging. When the incoming value is above the value of the template (by any amount), a small, fixed voltage increment is added to the template (generally 10mV/beat); when it is below the previous beat, the same value is subtracted.

Most monitors display a visual trend line from which deviations in the position of the ST segment can be rapidly observed to aid on-line detection of ischemia. For example, a trend line can be generated by summing the absolute values of the ST segment location in three leads (I, II, and a V lead, which represent a quasi-orthogonal lead set). In addition, nearly all monitors display on-screen numerical values for the position of the ST segment used for ischemia detection (generally 60–80ms following the J point), although the specific point used can usually be adjusted by the clinician.

LEAD SYSTEMS

Placement of ECG electrodes is a critical determinant of the morphology of the ECG signal. Lead systems have been developed based on theoretic considerations (i.e. the orthogonal arrangement of the Frank XYZ leads) and/or references to anatomic landmarks that facilitate consistency between individuals (i.e. the standard 12-lead system). Figure 12.7 describes basic mathematical relations between the components of the 12-lead system and the Frank–Lewis orthogonal lead system.

Einthoven (1845) established ECG using three extremities as references: the left arm (LA), right arm (RA), and left leg (LL). He recorded the difference in potential between the LA and RA (lead I), LL and RA (lead II), and LL and LA (lead III). Since the signals recorded were differences between two electrodes, these leads were termed bipolar. The RL served only as a reference electrode. Since Kirchoff's loop equation states that the sum of the three voltage differential pairs must equal zero, it is easily derived that the sum of leads I and III must equal lead II, which is, therefore, redundant. The positive or negative polarity of each of the limbs was chosen by Einthoven to result in positive deflections of most of the waveforms and has no innate physiologic significance. He postulated that the three limbs defined an imaginary

Definition of electrocardiography leads

Lead type	Electrodes used	Definition
Bipolar or limb leads (Einthoven)	LA, RA, LL, RL	I = LA − RA II = LL − RA III = LL − LA
Augmented (Goldberger)	LA, RA, LL, RL	aV_R = RA − 0.5 (LA + LL) aV_L = LA − 0.5 (LL + RA) aV_F = LL − 0.5 (LA + RA)
Unipolar chest leads (Wilson)	V_1–V_6	$V_1 = v_1$ − (LA + RA + LL)/3 $V_2 = v_2$ − (LA + RA + LL)/3 $V_3 = v_3$ − (LA + RA + LL)/3 $V_4 = v_4$ − (LA + RA + LL)/3 $V_5 = v_5$ − (LA + RA + LL)/3 $V_6 = v_6$ − (LA + RA + LL)/3
Orthogonal vector leads (Frank)	I, E, C, A, M, H, F	X = 0.610A + 0.171C − 0.781I Y = 0.655F + 0.345M − 1.000H Z = 0.133A + 0.736M − 0.264I − 0.374E − 0.231C

v, precordial voltage (before input to central terminal of Wilson).

Figure 12.7 Definitions of electrocardiography leads. (With permission from London and Kaplan, 1999.)

Locations of precordial leads

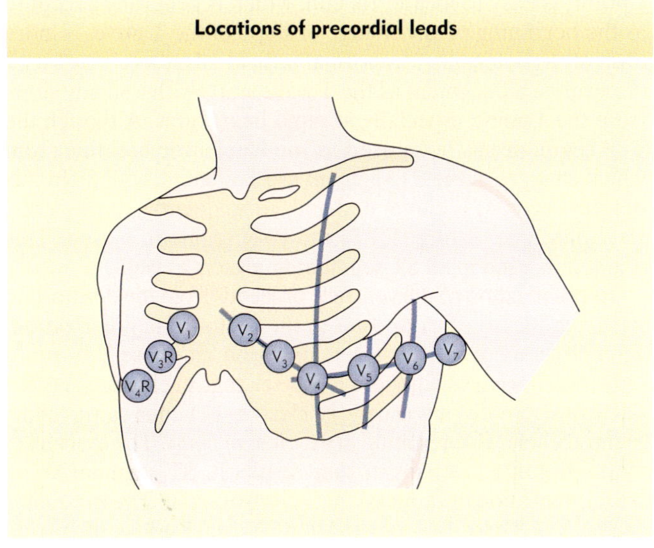

Figure 12.8 The locations of the precordial leads. Heavy vertical lines represent the midclavicular, anterior axillary, and midaxillary lines, respectively (from left to right). V_1 and V_2 are referenced to the fourth intercostal space and V_4 to the fifth space. V_3 lies on a line between V_2 and V_4. V_5 and V_6 lie on a horizontal line from V_4. Additional precordial leads can be obtained on the right side (V_3R, V_4R), as well as extending further left from V_6 (V_7). (With permission from Friedman, 1985.)

equilateral triangle with the heart at its center. Given the influence of Einthoven's vector analyses of frontal plane forces, it was only a matter of time before others incorporated the other two orthogonal planes (transverse and sagittal).

Wilson refined and clinically introduced the unipolar precordial leads. He postulated a mechanism whereby the electrical potential could be measured at the site of the exploring precordial electrode (the positive electrode). A negative pole with zero potential was formed by joining the three limb electrodes in a resistive network in which equally weighted signals cancel each other out. He termed this the 'central terminal' and, in a fashion similar to Einthoven's vector concepts, postulated it was located at the electrical center of the heart, representing the mean electrical potential of the body throughout the cardiac cycle. He described three additional limb leads (V_L, V_R, and V_F). These leads measured new vectors of activation and, thus, established the hexaxial reference system for determination of electrical axis. He subsequently introduced the six unipolar precordial V leads in 1935 (Fig. 12.8). Clinical application of the unipolar limb leads was limited because of their smaller amplitude in relation to the bipolar limb leads from which they were derived. Goldberger (1942) augmented their amplitude (by a factor of 1.5) by severing the connection between the central terminal and the lead extremity (which he termed 'augmented limb leads'). These three lead groups, the bipolar limb leads, the unipolar precordial leads, and the augmented unipolar limb leads, form the conventional 12-lead ECG system.

Mann (1920) introduced the concept of vectorcardiography (VCG), which measures the time course of the mean instantaneous spatial cardiac vectors. This was represented by a loop in the frontal plane, although it was not until the invention of the cathode ray oscilloscope that it could be directly recorded. However, use of the frontal plane bipolar leads had limitations. Lead I, although oriented horizontally (the *x* direction), is only an approximation since current flow in the lead field is not uniform or solely in the *x* direction (based on the dipole theory). Therefore, a number of alternative lead systems allowing more accurate depiction of the vector loop in the three orthogonal axes (transverse *x*, vertical *y*, and sagittal *z* leads) were investigated. The most widely accepted is that of Frank, which uses seven exploring electrodes interconnected by a resistor network to derive approximately uniform vector fields of equal magnitude in the *x*, *y*, and *z* axes. It is properly termed a 'corrected orthogonal lead system', given that it takes into account assumptions that the body volume conductor is nonuniform, the heart is eccentric as a source, there are a number of dipoles, and there is variation in the vectorial expression of the magnitude of an electrical signal. The Frank lead system allowed standardized recording of the VCG, although it has never been widely accepted clinically because of its complexity. Nonetheless, the VCG may be superior to the 12-lead ECG in diagnosing myocardial infarction. Also the VCG may have advantages in detecting right ventricular hypertrophy and atrial enlargement. With renewed clinical interest in continuous computed VCG and ventricular potential analysis, both of which require Frank lead placement, this lead system may be used clinically in the near future.

DETECTION OF MYOCARDIAL ISCHEMIA

Pathophysiology of ST segment responses

The ST segment is the most important portion of the QRS complex for evaluating ischemia. The origin of this segment, at the

J point, is easy to locate. Its end, which is generally accepted as the beginning of any change of slope of the T wave, is more difficult to determine. In normal individuals, there may be no discernible ST segment as the T wave starts with a steady slope from the J point, especially at rapid heart rates. Although the T–P segment has been used as the isoelectric baseline from which changes in the ST segment are evaluated, with tachycardia this segment is eliminated and, consequently, during exercise tolerance testing (ETT) the P–R segment is used. This segment is used in all ST segment analyzers as well.

Repolarization of the ventricle proceeds from the epicardium to the endocardium, opposite to the vector of depolarization. The ST segment reflects the midportion, or phase 2, of repolarization during which there is little change in electrical potential. Consequently, it is usually isoelectric. Ischemia causes a loss of intracellular K^+, resulting in a *current of injury.* The exact electrophysiologic mechanism that results in ST segment shifts (either elevation or depression) is controversial. The two major theories are based on postulation of either a loss of resting potential as current flows from the uninjured to the injured area (*diastolic current*) or a true change in phase 2 potential as current flows from the injured to the uninjured area (*systolic current*). With subendocardial injury, the ST segment is depressed in the surface leads. With epicardial or transmural injury, the ST segment is elevated. When a lead is placed directly on the endocardium, opposite patterns are recorded.

ST segment depression as a marker of ischemia

With ischemia or infarction, later portions of the ST segment (i.e. delayed repolarization) are affected, causing downsloping or horizontal depression. Varying local effects and differences in vectors during repolarization result in different ST morphology recorded by different leads. It is generally accepted that ST changes in multiple leads are associated with more severe ischemia. The generally accepted criterion for ischemia, derived from exercise testing, is 0.1mV (1mm) depression measured at 80ms after the J point. The slope of the segment must be horizontal or downsloping such that this degree of depression is maintained for at least 80ms. Downsloping depression is associated with more diseased vessels and a worse prognosis than horizontal depression. It is generally accepted that slowly upsloping depression with a slope of 1mV/s or less represents ischemia. Although 80ms after the J point is the point most commonly used, 60 or 40ms is also used.

Despite the clinical focus on the ST segment for monitoring, the earliest ECG change at the onset of transmural ischemia (e.g. ligation of a coronary artery in an animal or in the hyperacute phase of myocardial infarction) is the almost immediate onset of a tall, peaked T wave, a so-called primary change. This phase is usually very transient and is often missed. A significant increase in R wave amplitude may also occur at this time.

Detection of perioperative myocardial ischemia, indicated by significant ST segment responses, has been facilitated by technical advances in operating room and ambulatory monitoring techniques, which allow capture and analysis of ECG data over several days or weeks. Studies have demonstrated significant associations of perioperative ischemia with adverse cardiac outcomes in adults undergoing a variety of cardiac and noncardiac surgical procedures, particularly major vascular surgery. However, ease of use of new ST segment trending has resulted in its nearly routine use in many low-risk surgical patients, leading to a number of false-positive responses. Based on recent data showing a very low incidence of positive responses (all of which appeared to be false positive in a large cohort of patients with only one risk factor for coronary artery disease), minor ST segment changes must be interpreted with appropriate caution to avoid costly diagnostic tests being performed based on perioperative ECG responses.

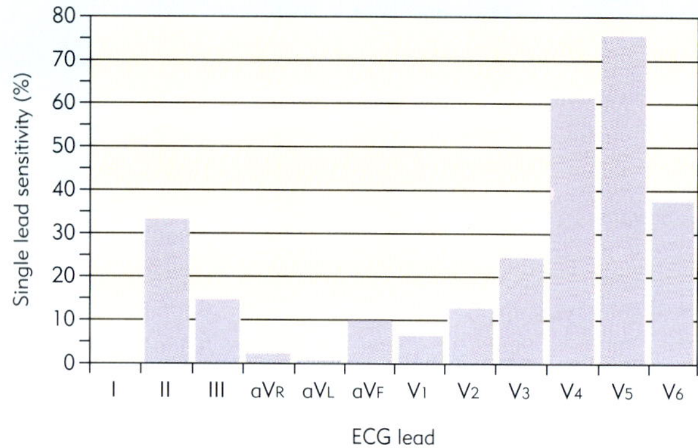

Figure 12.9 Single-lead sensitivity for the intraoperative detection of ischemia. This was based on 51 episodes detected in 25 patients undergoing noncardiac surgery. Sensitivity was calculated by dividing the number of episodes detected in that lead by the total number of episodes. Sensitivity was greatest in lead V_5; the lateral leads (I, aV_L) were insensitive. (With permission from London et al., 1988.)

Lead systems

Although the factors responsible for precipitating ischemia during ETT and surgical settings differ (i.e. increased cardiac output and heart rate during ETT versus various adverse combinations of heart rate/bloodpressure/cardiac output or hemodynamically 'silent' myocardial ischemia during surgery), the leads found to be most sensitive during ETT are clearly useful in the operating room.

Lead V_5 was found to detect about 90% of positive responses in the earliest studies. Use of all 12 leads with the limb electrodes moved to the shoulders and iliac crests to allow a stable signal permitted better evaluation of lead sensitivity and specificity. Using this array (which is now clinically routine), the lateral precordial leads were most sensitive (54–82%), followed by the inferior leads (32–44%). Lead I is generally insensitive (10%). Most false-positive responses occur in the inferior leads.

The recommended leads for intraoperative monitoring, based on several clinical studies, do not to differ from those used during ETT. In the largest clinical study using continuous, computed 12-lead ECG analysis, nearly 90% of responses involved ST segment depression alone and approximately 70% were noted in multiple leads (Fig. 12.9). The use of both leads V_4 and V_5 had a sensitivity of 90%, whereas the standard clinical combination, II and V_5, was 80% sensitive.

Electrocardiography noise reduction can be aided (but not eliminated) by proper skin preparation before placement of electrodes. Digital sound processing can markedly improve signal quality in certain situations. For example, preinduction or early postoperative shivering can obscure the QRS complex. With the marked increase in whole body and myocardial oxygen consumption that results, the risk for myocardial ischemia increases.

Reduction of muscle artifact by digital signal processing

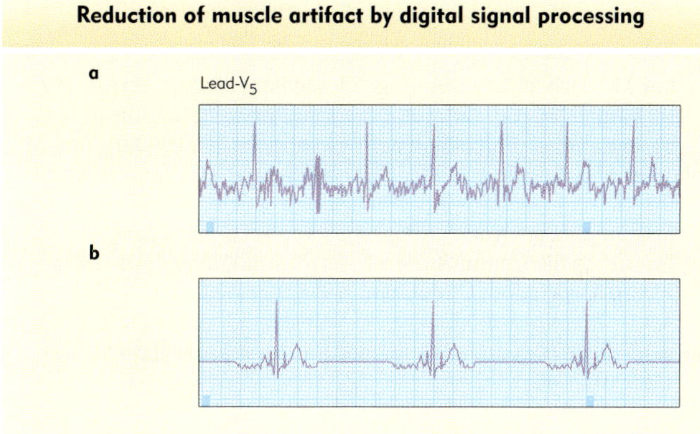

Figure 12.10 Reduction of muscle artifact (simulated) by digital signal processing using signal averaging. This was achieved using a PC2 Bedside Monitor (SpaceLabs, Inc., Redmond, WA). (a) The initial learned complex ('dominant') on the left is followed by real-time complexes. (b) Median complexes smoothed by signal processing. The degree of noise reduction is proportional to the square root of the number of beats averaged.

ST segment trending

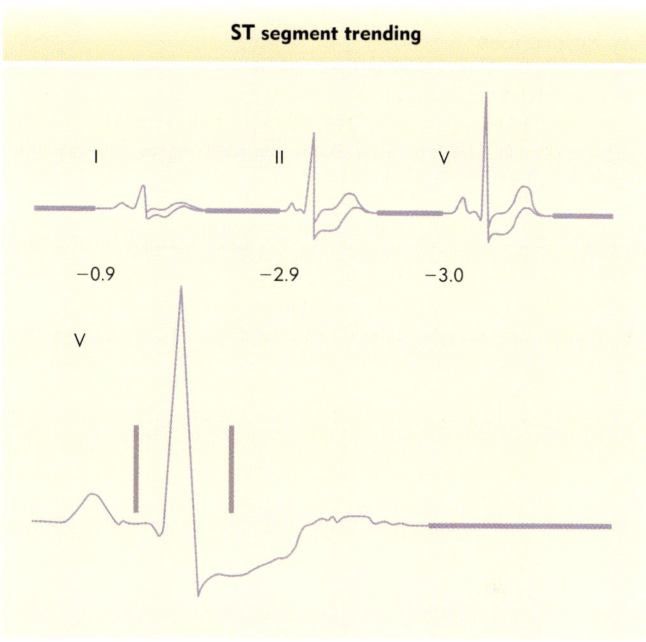

Figure 12.11 ST segment trending. The graphic output of the 'ST adjustment' window from a Marquette Electronics (Milwaukee, WI) ST segment analyzer (Series 7010 monitor) is displayed. This software allows trending and display of three leads (I, II, and any one V lead). In this window, the initial complex ('learned' when the program was activated) is displayed along with the current complex. Two complexes are superimposed with different intensities to facilitate comparison. ST analysis is performed automatically at 80ms after the J point, although this point can be manually adjusted by the user. The left vertical line indicates the reference potential and the right vertical line indicates the point for ST analysis

Digital sound processing can detect ischemic episodes under these conditions better than conventional monitoring (Fig. 12.10).

Most episodes of perioperative ischemia go undetected by the clinician. It is impossible to monitor the ST segment continuously without some type of automated system. The ability of monitors with trending capabilities to display trend lines and present abnormal complexes concurrently with the baseline complex enhances the ability to detect episodes of ischemia on-line (Fig. 12.11).

Since the late 1980s, ST trending capability has been incorporated directly, or as a low-cost option, into most operating room monitors. However, there are few data available on the validation of the accuracy of these devices and there are no specific standards for their performance.

Accuracy has been verified over a wide range of ST segment depression or elevation; however, errors were noted that arose either from improper filtering by the software's algorithm of ectopic, paced, or wide complex beats or from occasional 'idiosyncratic' errors in normal complexes. Changes should be verified based on an actual printout of the ECG on a recorder using the 'diagnostic' filtering mode.

Currently, most monitors have the capability to analyze at least three leads and some can analyze all leads inputting to the monitor (including 12 leads via appropriate cables). All monitors allow the user to reposition the analysis points, presumably to account for abnormal complexes (Fig. 12.11). When the ST analysis feature is activated, the monitor frequency response is automatically placed in the diagnostic mode (0.05Hz). Configurable ST segment alarms are available on most units, although again the utility and operating characteristics of these functions have not been validated.

The greatest problem with these devices and their alarms may not be a lack of validation data but rather their improper use (lack of skin preparation, improper lead placement).

Key References

Friedman HH. Diagnostic electrocardiography and vectorcardiography. New York: McGraw-Hill; 1985:41.

Garfein OB. The promise of electrocardiography in the 21st century. Ann N Y Acad Sci. 1990;601:370.

London MJ, Hollenberg M, Wong MG, et al. Intraoperative myocardial ischemia: localization by continuous 12 lead electrocardiography. Anesthesiology. 1988;69:232–41.

London MJ, Kaplan JA. Advances in electrocardiographic monitoring. In: Kaplan JA, ed. Cardiac anesthesia. 4th edn. Philadelphia, PA: Saunders; 1999:359–400.

London MJ. Ischemia monitoring: ST segment analysis versus TEE. In: Kaplan JA, ed. Cardiothoracic and vascular anesthesia update, Vol. 3. Philadelphia, PA: Saunders; 1993:1–20.

Pipberger HV, Arzbaecher RC, Berson AS, et al. Recommendations for the standardization of leads and of specifications for instruments in electocardiography and vectorcardiography. Report of the Committee on Electrocardiography, American Heart Association. Circulation. 1975;52:11–31.

Plonsey R. Electrocardiography. In: Webster JG, ed. Encyclopedia of medical devices and instrumentation. New York: John Wiley; 1988:1017–40.

Further Reading

Bailey JJ, Berson AS, Garson A Jr, et al. Recommendations for standardization and specifications in automated electrocardiography: bandwidth and digital signal processing. A report for health professionals by an ad hoc writing group of the Committee on Electrocardiography and Cardiac Electrophysiology of the Council on Clinical Cardiology, Am Heart Assoc. Circulation. 1990; 81:730–9.

Barr, RC. Genesis of the electrocardiogram. In: Macfarlane PW, Veitch Lawrie TD, eds. Comprehensive electrocardiology. theory and practice in health and disease, Vol. 1. New York: Permagon Press; 1989:129-49.

Laks MM, Arzbaecher R, Bailey JJ, Geselowitz DB, Berson AS. Recommendations for safe current limits for electrocardiographs. A statement for healthcare professionals from the Committee on Electrocardiography, American Heart Association. Circulation. 1996;93:837–9.

London MJ, Ahlstrom LD. Validation testing of the spacelabs PC2 ST-segment analyzer. J Cardiothorac Vasc Anesth. 1995;9:684–93.

Macfarlane PW. Lead systems. In: Macfarlane PW, Veitch Lawrie TD, eds. Comprehensive electrocardiology. theory and practice in health and disease, Vol. 1. New York: Permagon Press;1989:316–50.

Mirvis DM, Berson AS, Goldberger AL, et al. Instrumentation and practice standards for electrocardiographic monitoring in special care units. A report for health professionals by a Task Force of the Council on Clinical Cardiology, American Heart Association. Circulation. 1989;79:464–71.

Mirvis DM. The QRS complex: ventricular activation. In: Electrocardiography: a physiologic approach. St Louis, MO: Mosby;1993:138–49.

Schlant RC, Adolph RJ, DiMarco JP, et al. Guidelines for electrocardiography. A report of the American College of Cardiology/American Heart Association Task Force on Assessment of Diagnostic and Therapeutic Cardiovascular Procedures (Committee on Electrocardiography). Circulation. 1992; 85:1221–8.

Thakor NV. Electrocardiographic monitors. In: Webster JG, ed. Encyclopedia of medical devices and instrumentation. New York: John Wiley;1988:1002–17.

Thakor NV. From Holter monitors to automatic defibrillators: developments in ambulatory arrhythmia monitoring. IEEE Trans Biomed Eng. 1984;31:770.

Chapter 13 EEG, EMG and evoked potentials

Tod B Sloan

Topics covered in this chapter

Electroencephalography
Evoked potentials
Electromyography
Sleep and anesthesia

The nervous system functions by electrical activity. This allows diagnostic and monitoring approaches to assess its structural and functional integrity. Although not a replacement for the neurologic examination, the results of electrophysiologic studies can enhance diagnosis of neurologic dysfunction. In states of altered consciousness or during anesthesia, electrophysiological monitoring can greatly improve the understanding of neurologic functioning and integrity. Electroencephalography (EEG), evoked potential (EP) measurement, and electromyography (EMG), have many aspects in common and will be discussed in this chapter in the context of their intraoperative applications.

ELECTROENCEPHALOGRAPHY

Electroencephalography is based on the spontaneous electrical activity of the cerebral cortex. It represents the summated voltage changes resulting from activity in excitatory and inhibitory synapses in the pyramidal layers II, III, and V of the outer cortex. The activity recorded at an individual scalp electrode represents the synaptic activity within 2–2.5cm from the recording electrode. This local activity may be from intrinsic activity of the local cortex or it may be the result of the influence of other neural regions (most notably the pacemaker-like influence of deeper structures on the background rhythm).

The EEG is recorded by amplifying the electrical activity in a pair of scalp electrodes (referred to as a 'montage'). The signals from these brain regions are amplified through a differential amplifier, and noise is removed by common mode rejection. In essence, the activity from one electrode is subtracted from the other, eliminating any activity that is present in both electrodes. Filtering out low- and high-frequency activity that is not within the EEG range (0.5–30Hz) allows further signal improvement. The resulting signal (referred to as time domain) is then displayed visually on a screen or on paper as a plot of amplitude versus time (Fig. 13.1).

Traditional methods of EEG analysis involve visual inspection of the tracings. Frequency content, amplitude, patterns of activity, and relationship of activity between channels are a few of the factors analyzed. Several rhythms or patterns of activity have been identified in awake patients. These are of limited importance during anesthesia except for the changes related to anesthesia or physiology (especially ischemia), discussed below, and spike activity associated with seizures. The ability to detect seizure spike activity is unique to monitoring with the EEG and forms the basis of intraoperative monitoring during seizure focus resection.

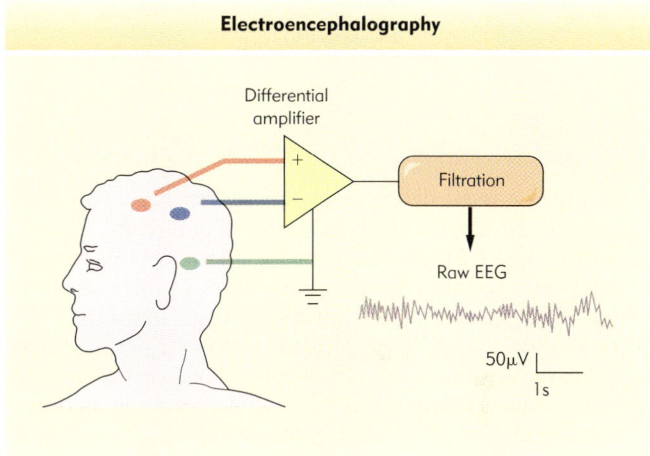

Figure 13.1 Diagram of EEG recording system. The EEG is amplified from two scalp electrodes by a differential amplifier. The activity is filtered to remove unwanted signals such as 60Hz line frequency and displayed as a plot of amplitude versus time.

For intraoperative monitoring, three aspects of the EEG are primarily considered: frequency, amplitude (in microvolts), and symmetry. Quantitative methods of EEG analysis have also been developed. These focus most commonly on frequency, amplitude, and more complex mathematical analysis.

Frequency content of the EEG is usually described by four frequency bands. β frequencies (13–30Hz) are fast frequencies typical of a normal subject who is awake and alert. The α frequencies (8–12Hz) are typical of a patient who is relaxed and has his or her eyes closed. Here the EEG shows an underlying rhythm as if a pacemaker in the thalamus is driving the cortex. Slower EEG frequencies in the θ (4–7Hz) or δ range (0–3Hz) are seen during sleep but are usually considered abnormal when awake. In the anesthetized subject, they may result from drug effects (such as with opioids or deep anesthesia) or may be an indication of impending injury (such as ischemia).

Symmetry of activity is an extremely important component of EEG analysis. In general, activity is usually symmetric about the midsagittal line. Any focal increase in activity (such as with

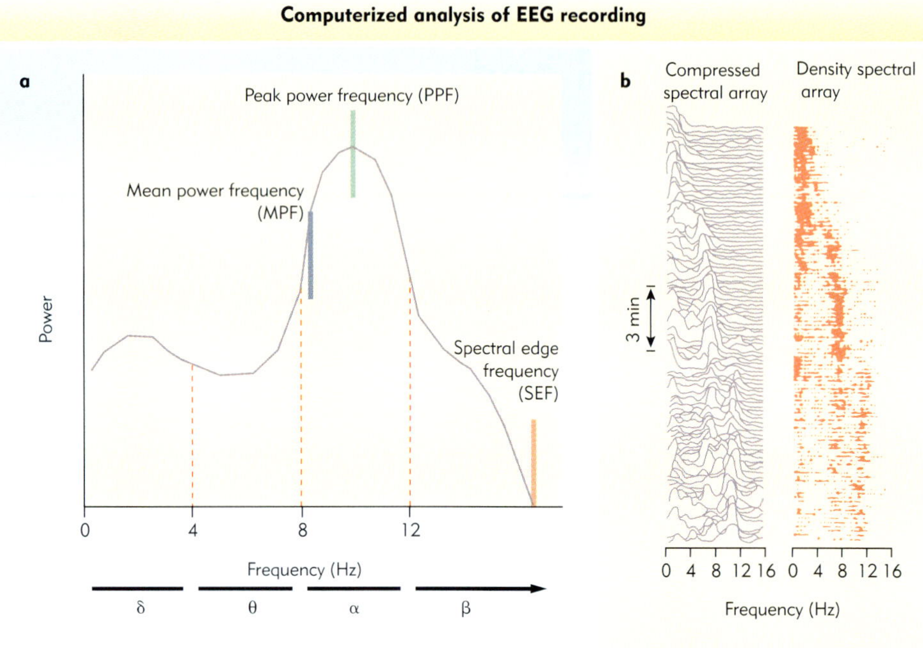

Figure 13.2 Computerized analysis of EEG recording. (a) Frequency amplitude plot after Fourier series analysis. The spectral edge frequency (SEF) is the frequency where 95–99% of the power is contained in lower frequencies. (b) Compressed and density spectral arrays of EEG signals subjected to Fourier series analysis are given for a patient during deepening halothane anesthesia (earlier times in front). Note the progressive loss of high frequency activity. (With permission from Levy et al., 1980.)

a seizure) or focal decrease in activity (such as with local ischemia or stroke) is usually indicative of pathology.

A diagnostic EEG is usually conducted with a large number of electrodes so that recording pairs allow evaluation of the entire cerebral cortex. For intraoperative monitoring, the recording pairs may be limited to the specific regions of interest, as in intracranial aneurysm clipping. For vascular surgery, symmetrically spaced leads allow differentiation between ischemia and deep anesthesia by the evaluation of symmetry. Hence, carotid endarterectomy monitoring might utilize symmetrically placed electrode pairs over the distributions of the right and left anterior, middle, and posterior cerebral arteries.

As with many monitoring techniques, computer processing of the EEG can allow enhancement of the specific variables of interest, although the processed EEG is only as good as the raw data. Early processing methods used simple techniques to determine average amplitude and frequency. Perhaps the most successful was the cerebral function monitor, which determined the amplitude between 2 and 15Hz with emphasis around 10Hz from a single electrode pair and allowed ready recognition of low-frequency activity.

The most commonly employed technique of computed EEG analysis in current use is based on the mathematical technique of Fourier series analysis. This technique takes a complex wave and determines the amplitudes of a series of sine waves that can mathematically reconstruct the wave. A smoothed x–y plot results (Fig. 13.2) that shows the relative amplitude (or power) of each of the component frequencies. These plots give an excellent perspective of both the amplitude and frequency content of the EEG. Spectral edge frequency (SEF) is frequently derived from these data; this is the frequency below which the majority (i.e. 95–99%) of the activity is located. The compressed spectral array (CSA) is a useful variation of this plot in which the effect of time is shown by stacking those x–y plots in a third dimension (time). The density spectral array (DSA) can reveal some data hidden in the CSA by showing increased amplitude as dark regions (see Fig. 13.2)

Several other displays and mathematical signal-processing techniques have been used and have a variety of advantages and disadvantages. In bispectral analysis, the relationship of different frequencies is analyzed. This technique not only analyzes the frequency content but also evaluates the interaction (phase relationships) of waves that produce additional waves to quantitate the degree of phase coupling. Using this technique, a proprietary mathematical index called the bispectral index (BIS) has been formulated that holds promise for quantitating sedation and depth of anesthesia independent of drug type. The BIS is measured using EEG electrodes over the frontal cortex, an area that has been implicated with explicit auditory memory. Other potential monitors of anesthetic depth include midlatency auditory EP (AEP), semilinear canonized analysis, aperiodic analysis or delta power of the EEG, and 40Hz steady-state EPs.

Anesthetic drugs tend to produce either excitation or depression of the EEG (Fig. 13.3). Most agents produce an initial excitatory stage of the EEG characterized by desynchronization (perhaps through loss of inhibitory synaptic function). Amplitude increases as the EEG becomes synchronized, with a predominance of activity in the α range. Increasing doses cause progressive slowing until the EEG achieves burst suppression (activity with interspersed periods of silence) and finally electrical silence. The potent inhalational agents show these typical effects, although they are not equivalent in the degree of their effects. Isoflurane can produce a flat (isoelectric) EEG at clinically usable concentrations, whereas halothane must be increased to toxic levels (of the order of 10% by volume) to produce a flat EEG.

Some anesthetic agents produce further activation rather than depression of the EEG after the initial excitatory effect, such as spike and seizure activity, but eventually produce EEG depression at higher doses. For example, enflurane at higher doses produces spike activity (especially with hyperventilation). Nitrous oxide also increases activity by producing a high-frequency (34Hz) activity in the frontal area but does not usually produce spike activity. Nitrous oxide can also reduce

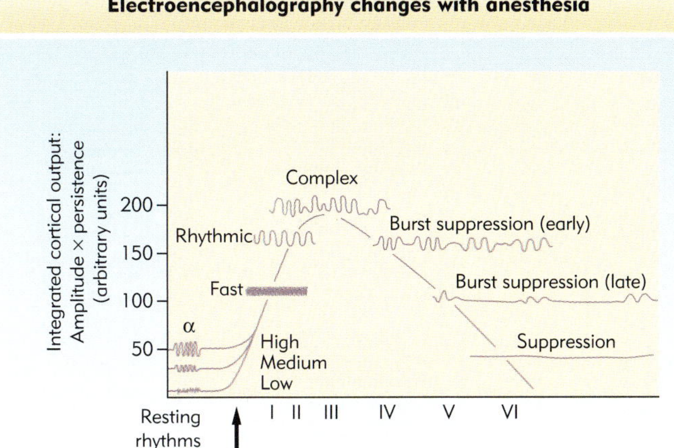

Figure 13.3 Typical changes in the EEG with anesthesia. With increasing depth of anesthesia with an inhalation anesthetic, initial organization into fast frequencies occurs with the formation of rhythmic waves in the α range. Increasing depth of anesthesia causes reduction in frequency and amplitude until burst suppression and a flat EEG are produced. (With permission from Martin, 1959.)

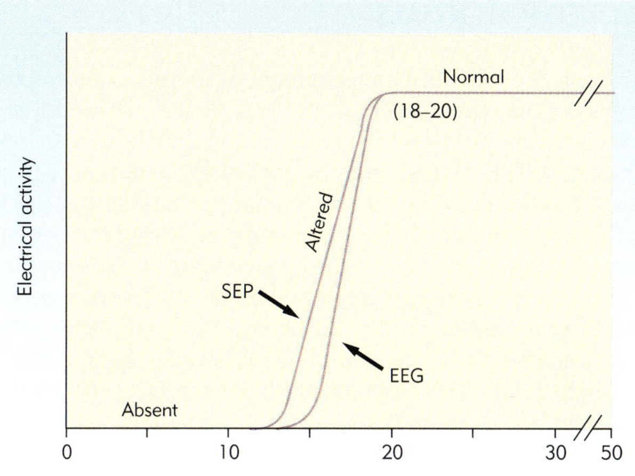

Figure 13.4 Relationship between regional cerebral blood flow, SEPs, and EEG measurements. As regional cerebral blood flow is reduced below 18–20mL/min per 100g tissue, the EEG and SEPs become abnormal. The EEG becomes silent below 12–15mL/min per 100g; SEPs are lost at slightly lower values because subcortical components of the SEP are more tolerant of ischemia. (With permission from Sloan, 1985.)

the degree of slowing produced by the concomitant administration of a volatile anesthetic agent.

Most intravenous sedative agents also follow this pattern of excitation followed by depression, including the barbiturates, benzodiazepines, propofol, and etomidate. Barbiturates produce a flat EEG at higher doses and have been used to produce a pharmacologic coma since the decrease in synaptic metabolic rate improves the balance of nutrient and oxygen supply and demand in head injury and cerebral ischema. Low doses of methohexital (methohexitone) (0.5mg/kg) and etomidate (0.1mg/kg) can enhance epileptic activity and propofol can enhance interictal activity in some seizure patients, but electrical silence follows at high doses. The benzodiazepines produce spike-like activity at low doses in some patients but are frequently used as anticonvulsants.

The opioids do not appear to produce an initial excitement phase but produce a steady decline in EEG frequency, with maintenance of amplitude in the δ range and without producing burst suppression or electrical silence. The effects of ketamine also differ from those of inhalational agents. Ketamine produces high-amplitude θ activity with an accompanying increase in β activity. It has been reported to provoke seizure activity in individuals who have epilepsy but not in normal individuals. Muscle relaxants generally have little effect on the EEG, although succinylcholine (suxamethonium) has an activating effect on the central nervous system during muscle facilitation. Laudanosine, an atracurium metabolite, is a convulsant, but this is not clinically significant with usual doses.

In addition to anesthesia, the EEG is affected by many physiologic variables. Frequency slowing is usually associated with depressed neuronal function. For example, hypoxia, hypotension, hypocarbia, hypoglycemia, and ischemia cause slowing and flattening of the EEG. Hypercarbia [arterial carbon dioxide tension ($PaCO_2$) over 90mmHg] causes high frequency EEG activity; higher levels are associated with findings similar to those of hypocarbia, and very high levels produce a flat EEG. Hypothermia produces slowing below 35°C, with electrical silence at 7–20°C. Hypothermia is associated with reductions in metabolic rate (both basal and activity dependent) and is protective against cerebral ischemia. The EEG also varies with age, with an adult pattern appearing by 10–15 years of age. Since the effects of many pharmacologic and physiologic factors on the EEG are a reduction in frequency and decreased amplitude, the EEG cannot be used as an isolated monitor but must be interpreted in the context of other information, including anesthetic and physiologic variables.

The EEG can be used for intraoperative monitoring during several procedures. Perhaps the most common use of the EEG is in the detection of ischemia (Fig. 13.4). The response to ischemia is rapid; a flat EEG occurs within 20 seconds following complete ischemia. With partial ischemia, the EEG slows at blood flows below 18–20mL/min per 100g tissue and becomes flat at 12–15mL/min per 100g. Since cell death does not occur until lower levels of blood flow are reached (below 10mL/min per 100g), the EEG can be used to signal ischemia. The time to infarction is related to the rate of residual blood flow: the more residual flow that is present, the longer the time to infarction. As much as 10–15 minutes may elapse before infarction after graded ischemia produces EEG changes. Hence the EEG may serve to warn of impending stroke and allow attempts to correct the blood flow prior to irreversible injury.

This warning function has made EEG monitoring a component of carotid endarterectomy and intracranial vascular surgery in many centers. Several studies have shown that EEG monitoring can be used to identify patients who may benefit from shunting during carotoid endarterectomy and who cannot tolerate temporary clipping of intracranial aneurysms, although the effects are controversial. Similarly, EEG has been used to monitor patients undergoing cardiopulmonary bypass to determine whether adequate blood flow is present, although concomitant hypothermia may reduce the effectiveness of EEG monitoring.

EVOKED POTENTIALS

Whereas the EEG is a measurement of spontaneous electrical activity of the brain (cerebral cortex), EPs are measurements of the electrical potentials produced in response to a stimulus ('evoked'). These stimuli may be physiologic in nature (e.g. light flashes to the eyes) or they may be nonphysiologic (e.g. electrical pulses to peripheral nerves). Since stimulation focuses testing on a specific neural tract, assessment is also specific.

Evoked potentials are measured using differential amplifiers and filtering, similar to the EEG. Since the amplitude of EPs is very small (<10μV), a technique known as signal averaging is used to resolve EPs from the much greater EEG (10–1000μV) and electrocardiogram (ECG) activity. Signal averaging involves repeatedly stimulating the nervous system and measuring the response during the period of stimulated neural activity. The recorded activity is digitized and averaged at each poststimulus time point. After averaging 10^2–10^3 windows (the signal/noise ratio increases by the square root of the number of windows averaged), the evoked response becomes apparent since the desired signal is related to the stimulation but the other activity is not and averages out (Fig. 13.5a).

A typical evoked response output is a plot of voltage versus time (Fig. 13.5b). The electrical response at an active electrode (placed near the neural structure producing the desired electrical activity) is compared with that at a reference electrode. An artifact of stimulation occurs at time zero (coincident with the stimulation), followed by a subsequent series of peaks (both positive and negative) and valleys at later times. The peaks (and valleys) are thought to arise from specific neural generators and, therefore, can be used to follow the response at various points along the stimulated tract. The information recorded is usually the amplitude (peak to adjacent trough), the time from the stimulation to the peak (latency), and, occasionally, the time between peaks (interwave latency or conduction time).

Visual evoked responses

Visual EPs (VEPs) are produced by light stimulation of the eyes. For diagnostic purposes, stimulation using a checkerboard on which squares alternate between white and black is used; for intraoperative monitoring, light flash stimulation through closed eyes is used. Traditional VEPs are recorded by electrodes over the occiput and are generated by the visual cortex. The retinal response to visual stimulation (electroretinogram; ERG) can also be recorded by electrodes placed near the eye. By manipulating the color and intensity of the stimulus, the responses of the rods and cones can be separated.

Monitoring of VEPs helps to confirm the structural integrity of the optic tracts, but results may not correlate well with postoperative vision. Furthermore, as a cortically generated response, anesthesia will depress the response in a similar manner to the effect on the EEG. Hence depressant agents (such as inhalational agents) may need to be restricted during monitoring.

Auditory brainstem responses

The auditory brainstem response (ABR) or the brainstem auditory evoked response (BAER) is produced when sound activates the cochlea following transmission through the external and middle ear. Vibrations activate the hair cells in the cochlea, which initiates nerve impulses that travel to the brainstem via cranial nerve VIII. The nerve impulse travels via the brainstem acoustic relay nuclei and lemniscal pathways to activate the cortical auditory cortex. The neural pathway of the ABR appears to follow the normal hearing pathway. In the first 10ms after stimulation, three major peaks are usually seen: wave I is generated by the extracranial portion of cranial nerve VIII; wave III

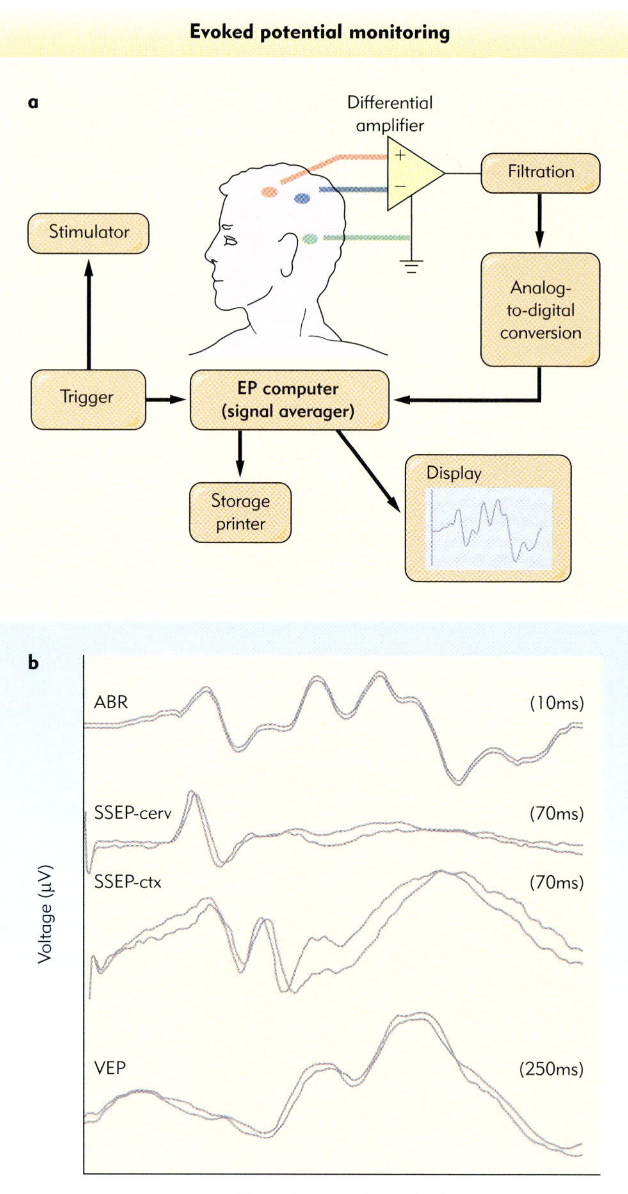

Figure 13.5 Evoked potential (EP) monitoring. (a) EP recording requires a digital computer to conduct signal averaging. A trigger repeatedly causes a stimulus; recording of the voltage change for a set period after each stimulus allows formation of the EP to be demonstrated. (b) Typical sensory evoked responses include the auditory brain stem response (ABR), somatosensory evoked response to median nerve stimulation recorded at cervical (SSEP-cerv) and cortical (SSEP-ctx) locations, and the visual evoked potential (VEP). The time scale is shown at the right for each tracing.

is generated by the auditory pathway nuclei in the pons; and wave V is generated by the high pons or midbrain (lateral lemniscus and inferior colliculus). Occasionally a wave II is seen, and wave IV may be resolvable from V (IV and V often blend together). Responses to auditory stimulation can also be recorded over the auditory cortex (cortical AEP) or cortical association areas (response about 300ms after auditory stimulation; P300). These responses appear to be related to the auditory sensory cortex and cerebral cognitive function areas, respectively.

Testing of ABR is frequently conducted using stimulation with 'clicks' delivered by headphones. Other types of sound have also been used for stimulation, including tone 'pips', which have a more defined frequency content. Usually one ear is stimulated at a time to focus on that neural pathway, with 'white noise' delivered to the other ear to mask stimulatory conditions.

Monitoring of ABR can be used to find the anatomic location of a neural insult and to assist the surgeon during an operation. Procedures in which ABR has been used include surgery on or near the auditory pathways or brainstem (e.g. acoustic neuroma, cerebellopontive angle tumors, posterior fossa procedures). Examination of effects on waves I, III, and V may allow identification of brainstem injury and determine the general anatomic location based on the specific waves that are altered. Recordings can also be taken from the cochlea and intracranial portion of cranial nerve VIII.

In general, anesthetic effects on the ABR are not dramatic. Latency increases may be seen as the concentration of potent inhalational agents increases. Nitrous oxide is generally benign unless it causes changes in middle ear pressure. Some changes can be seen with shifts in body temperature and if cold irrigation fluids are applied into the surgical field.

Somatosensory evoked responses

In the assessment of somatosensory evoked responses, a peripheral nerve is stimulated (similar to neuromuscular blockade monitoring) and the neural response is measured. Large mixed motor and sensory nerves (e.g. posterior tibial, common peroneal, ulnar, and median) are usually stimulated, which results in mixed motor and sensory responses. The length of the neural tract involved makes the somatosensory EP (SSEP) potentially one of the most generally applicable monitors because of the many neural structures that can be assessed (peripheral nerve, plexi, spinal cord, brainstem, sensory cortex). It is thought that the incoming volley of neural activity from the upper extremity represents activity primarily in the ipsilateral dorsal column pathway of proprioception and vibration. Stimulation of the peripheral nerve initiates an impulse that ascends the ipsilateral dorsal column, synapses near the nucleatus cuneatus, decussates near the cervicomedullary junction, ascends via the contralateral medial lemniscus, synapses in the ventroposterolateral nucleus of the thalamus, and finally projects to the contralateral parietal sensory cortex (Fig. 13.6). Recordings following stimulation of the lower extremity include additional components in the spinocerebellar pathways; these more anterior pathways may underlie the alterations in the SSEP observed in anterior cord ischemia, which correlate with motor function.

Several variations in SSEP monitoring have been developed to overcome some of its limitations. One problem is that the SSEP enters the spinal cord through several roots. Dermatomal EPs (DEPs), produced by stimulation of specified cutaneous dermatomal regions, have been used to evaluate the function of individual nerve roots. Anesthetic effects and poor amplitudes in regions with small cerebral representation (e.g. thoracic) limit this technique to some extent. A second problem is that occasionally peripheral nerve stimulation is not sufficient to produce a usable SSEP. One approach to this problem has been to stimulate both extremities simultaneously to increase amplitude. Another approach has been to stimulate the cauda equina via percutaneously placed electrodes. This approach also allows stimulation at spinal levels where no major peripheral nerve is available for stimulation and produces amplitudes at least twice those of traditional SSEP; however, it may fail to detect unilateral injury. A third problem is that anesthesia can decrease the cortical amplitude. Cortical evoked responses are affected by anesthesia in a fashion similar to the effects on the EEG. Inhalational anesthetic agents (including nitrous oxide) significantly reduce amplitudes and must be used in low concentrations [0.3–0.5 minimum alveolar concentration (MAC)] if at all. Anesthesia based on opioids, ketamine, and/or propofol depresses cortical amplitude to a lesser extent. Etomidate and ketamine appear to increase some cortical amplitudes and have been used to facilitate monitoring in very challenging situations. The effect of anesthetic drugs on sensory responses is most pronounced at the cortical level, with decreasing effects on subcortical responses (e.g. ABR).

Recording locations near the spinal cord have been used since they are less affected by anesthesia. Placement of electrodes in the spinal bony elements, intraspinous ligament, or subdural or epidural space and placement percutaneously or directly by the surgeon are being used. Electrodes can also be used for stimulation, with recording of cortical responses, for peripheral neural or compound muscle acyion potential (CMAP) responses, or for recording following transcranial motor cortex stimulation. Perispinal stimulation has been used in an attempt to monitor motor tracts. However, like epidural recording, both motor and sensory tracts are stimulated. Despite its limitations, the SSEP and its variations have been used in a wide variety of procedures (Fig. 13.7), notably those in which the spinal cord or cerebral cortex is at risk.

Motor evoked responses

Monitoring of a purely motor tract signal [motor evoked potential (MEP)] currently requires stimulation of the motor cortex by electrical impulses applied to the brain or scalp [transcranial electrical motor EP (tcEMEP)] or by magnetic stimulation [transcutaneous magnetic motor EP (tcMMEP)]. The evoked response travels down the lateral corticospinal and ventral corticospinal tracts and is recorded as a peripheral motor nerve response or as CMAP. Contributions of sensory pathways are blocked by synaptic interruptions in the thalamus and brainstem, which prevent transmission down sensory pathways. The major clinical difference between the two cortical stimulation techniques is that the electrical technique is moderately painful, because cutaneous pain receptors are stimulated, whereas the magnetic technique is painless (as long as direct stimulation of the scalp muscles is avoided). These techniques also differ electrophysiologically as tcEMEP activates the corticospinal neurons directly with additional cortical activation from internuncial activity. In contrast, tcMMEP activates internuncial synapses only, except at high magnetic intensities.

Responses to transcranial stimulation recorded in the epidural space are preferred by some, because anesthetic effects at the anterior horn cell or neuromuscular junction may reduce or eliminate peripheral responses. The disadvantage of

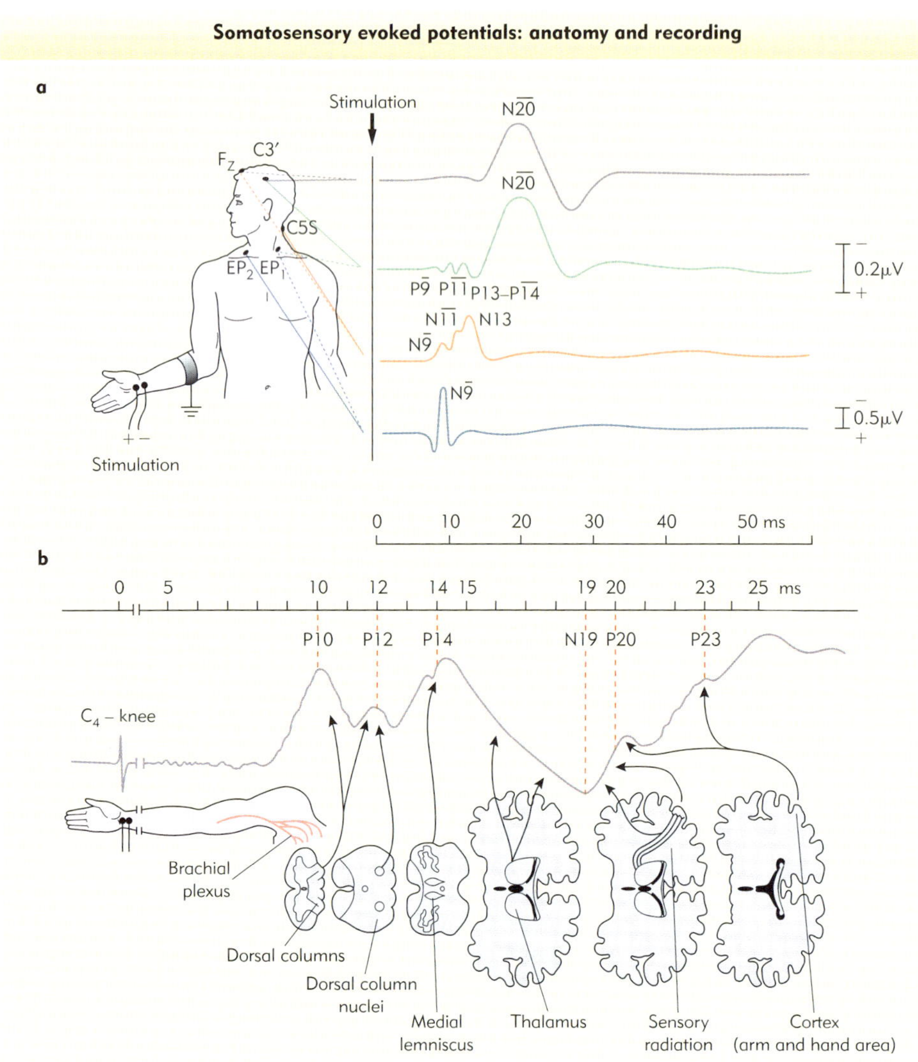

Figure 13.6 Somatosensory evoked potentials: anatomy and recording. (a) Example of evoked potential tracings from various locations for the median nerve SSEP (top). Recordings from Erb's point (EP) over the brachial plexus, cervial spine (C5S), and sensory cortex (C3′, top two tracings) are shown. (With permission from Spehlmann, 1985.) (b) Corresponding anatomy of the nerve and potential peaks. (With permission from Weiderholt et al.,1982.)

epidural recordings is that they probably represent activation of bilateral pathways; as a result, differentiation of a unilateral injury is difficult. In contrast, muscle recordings can differentiate unilateral changes as well as assess potential injury at several nerve root levels simultaneously. A variety of motor nerves and muscle groups can be monitored by varying the stimulator location on the scalp.

Recording methodology is similar for MEP and SSEP, except that CMAP responses are much larger, requiring fewer signal averages to resolve the signal. Onset latency is measured as the time from stimulation to the beginning of the multipeak response. Amplitude is measured as the peak-to-peak voltage of the response. As with the SSEP, the latency or onset is a measure of average conduction velocity. In addition to latency and amplitude, some researchers refer to threshold. The threshold is the lowest amount of magnetic or electrical stimulation that will still elicit a MEP response.

The use of MEP for spinal cord monitoring has increased because of its utility in the detection of vascular insults. Whereas mechanical stress on the spinal cord may affect both sensory and motor pathways, vascular insults may produce localized injury affecting only motor or sensory tracts. Since motor pathways are supplied by anterior spinal arteries from the aorta via penetrating vessels (notably the artery of Adamkiewicz and radicular arteries), the major concern is a loss of motor function without reflection in the SSEP. This problem is most important in the thoracic spinal cord, which is particularly vulnerable to ischemia because it is not well supplied by collateral vessels and may have only one anterior feeding artery between T4 and L4. Despite the potentials for SSEP to miss anterior spinal cord ischemia, studies suggest that it is not completely insensitive. Motor evoked potential have been used for many of the same procedures (notably spinal surgery) where the SSEP is used.

The major drawback of the transcranial techniques has been the effects of anesthesia. Since inhalational agents (including nitrous oxide) may obliterate responses at low concentrations through their effects on the cerebral cortex and anterior horn cells, anesthetic techniques based on opioids, ketamine, or etomidate are useful. If muscle responses are to be recorded, neuromuscular blocking agents must be carefully controlled or avoided (see below). For epidural or peripheral nerve responses, neuromuscular blocking drugs may be advantageous in minimizing patient movement during testing and reducing

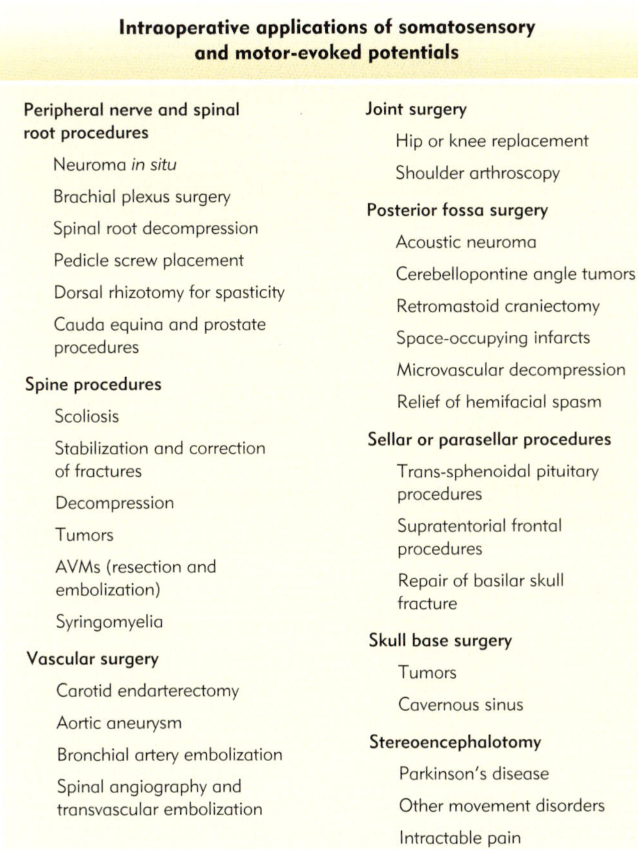

Intraoperative applications of somatosensory and motor-evoked potentials

Peripheral nerve and spinal root procedures
- Neuroma *in situ*
- Brachial plexus surgery
- Spinal root decompression
- Pedicle screw placement
- Dorsal rhizotomy for spasticity
- Cauda equina and prostate procedures

Spine procedures
- Scoliosis
- Stabilization and correction of fractures
- Decompression
- Tumors
- AVMs (resection and embolization)
- Syringomyelia

Vascular surgery
- Carotid endarterectomy
- Aortic aneurysm
- Bronchial artery embolization
- Spinal angiography and transvascular embolization

Joint surgery
- Hip or knee replacement
- Shoulder arthroscopy

Posterior fossa surgery
- Acoustic neuroma
- Cerebellopontine angle tumors
- Retromastoid craniectomy
- Space-occupying infarcts
- Microvascular decompression
- Relief of hemifacial spasm

Sellar or parasellar procedures
- Trans-sphenoidal pituitary procedures
- Supratentorial frontal procedures
- Repair of basilar skull fracture

Skull base surgery
- Tumors
- Cavernous sinus

Stereoencephalotomy
- Parkinson's disease
- Other movement disorders
- Intractable pain

Figure 13.7 Intraoperative applications of somatosensory and motor evoked potentials.(AVM, arteriovenous malformation.)

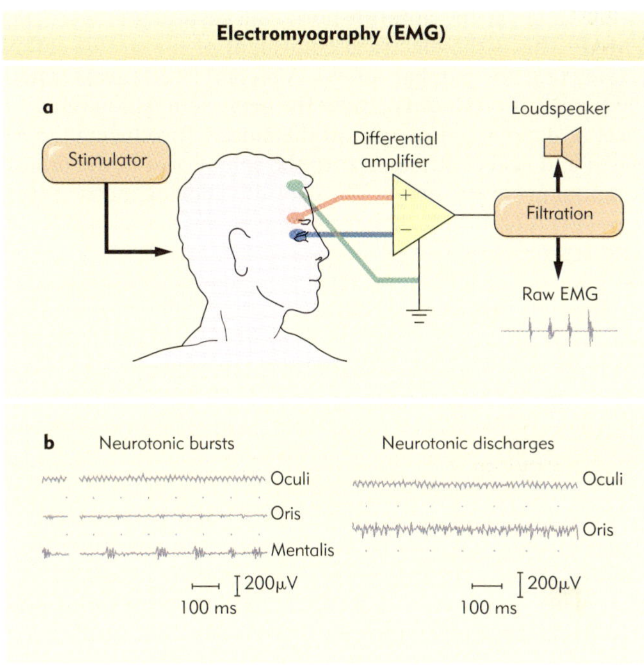

Figure 13.8 Electromyography (EMG). (a) The recording system for orbicularis oculi. (b) Spontaneous EMG activity observed in the operating room is usually one of two types. Neurotonic bursts of activity usually represent mechanical irritation of the nerve (left). Sustained discharge (right) may indicate impending injury as nerve irritation leads to continuous depolarization. (With permission from Cheek, 1993.)

interference in the recording electrodes from nearby muscle activity. The effects of anesthetic depression are partially overcome by newer multipulse techniques in which magnetic or electrical impulses are delivered to the scalp at 200–500Hz. Trains of three to five pulses allow detection of CMAP responses at concentrations of inhalational agents that obliterate responses to single pulses.

ELECTROMYOGRAPHY

Electromyography is the recording of muscle electrical activity by placement of needles within the muscle. This procedure can detect muscle disorders as well as disorders of the nerves that supply the muscle. It is recognized as an invaluable aid to the neurologic diagnosis of diseases affecting the motor unit. Studies frequently allow localization of a lesion to the muscle, neuromuscular junction, or motor nerves.

The traditional needle electrode examination is conducted by placing a recording electrode within a muscle and examining the electrical activity it produces using equipment similar to that used in EEG (Fig. 13.8). The activity is displayed on an oscilloscope and played through a loudspeaker, as characteristic sounds assist in diagnosis. Normally, a resting muscle is electrically silent after mild reactivity to the needle insertion. Neuromuscular abnormalities can increase this insertional reactivity and may help to identify hereditary myopathies and axonal loss in the peripheral nerve supplying the muscle. Reduced insertional activity can be seen with muscle diseases associated with fibrosis or fatty replacement of muscle and in metabolic diseases that reduce electrical excitability of the muscle.

In a resting muscle, spontaneous activity is not normally seen when the needle electrode is immobile. Irregular spike activity, known as spontaneous fibrillation potentials, are thought to result from recently denervated muscle. Other types of activity are seen with other neuromuscular diseases, including fasciculation potentials (in neuropathies and motor neuron disorders), myokymic discharges (in chronic compressive neuropathies and radiation damage to muscles), and complex repetitive discharges (in chronic neuropathic or myopathic processes).

For nerve conduction velocity measurement, an electrical stimulation of a motor nerve elicits a muscle contraction measured electrically as a CMAP. By measuring the time from stimulation and the distance from the stimulation site to the muscle, the speed of conduction through the nerve can be determined. By moving the stimulation point along the nerve, the location of a conduction block can be determined. As an example, this technique is used to identify conduction block in the median nerve in carpel tunnel syndrome. A similar method can be used with the SSEP to determine conduction velocities in peripheral nerves, the spinal cord, or central areas (brainstem to sensory cortex: central conduction time).

The CMAP recorded in nerve conduction studies is termed the M response. A later response, termed the H response, can also be recorded at low stimulation intensities. This response is caused by stimulation of sensory fibers in the nerve. These travel centrally to the spinal cord, where a reflex arc activates the motor fibers at the anterior horn cell, resulting in a second CMAP. This is the electrical equivalent of the stretch reflex activity (e.g. the patellar reflex). A second later wave, termed the F wave, is produced because the nerve stimulation causes a wave of depolarization toward the muscle (producing the M wave) and also centrally toward the spinal cord in the motor components of the nerve. The centrally moving motor nerve depolarization is reflected at the spinal cord and results in an outgoing response that produces a second muscle contraction, the F wave, which has limited value in neurologic diagnosis.

Although diagnostic EMG studies have been done during anesthesia, an anesthesiologist is more likely to encounter EMG as a monitor to assess the integrity of the nerve supplying a monitored muscle. Current methods for EMG in the operating room involve recording electrodes in the muscle of interest, with visible and audible presentation of the electrical activity (see Fig. 13.8). These techniques are superior to the older methods of visible or mechanical detection of muscle activity.

This monitoring system usually focuses on two basic types of spontaneous activity (see Fig. 13.8). First are phasic 'bursts' of activity. These neurotonic discharges are brief (<1s), relatively synchronous motor unit discharges that result from single discharges of multiple axons. The discharge is usually caused by mechanical stimulation of the nerve (nearby dissection, ultrasonic aspiration or drilling, retraction) but can also be caused by thermal (irrigation, lasers, drilling, electrocautery) and chemical or metabolic insults. These short bursts of activity are not usually associated with injurious stimuli but often indicate that the nerve remains intact and is in the vicinity of the operative field.

More injurious stimuli can cause longer tonic or 'train' activity, which is an episode of continuous, synchronous motor unit discharges. These have audible sounds with a more musical quality and have been likened to the sound of an outboard motor boat engine, swarming bees, popping corn, or an aircraft engine. These trains are often associated with nerve compression, traction, or ischemia and are usually an indication of enduring nerve injury. The proposed mechanism of the repetitive discharge is a depolarization of the resting membrane potential to near or above the firing threshold.

Electromyography could be used to monitor any nerve with a motor component. The most common application is for facial nerve monitoring during posterior fossa neurosurgery, where tumors commonly grow to involve the facial nerve, although EMG can be used for other cranial nerves with motor components (Fig. 13.9). The frequent involvement of the facial nerve with tumors in the cerebellopontine angle and acoustic neuroma (or vestibular schwannoma) has led to the application of facial nerve monitoring during resection of these tumors in an attempt to salvage function. Monitoring can warn that the nerve is in the immediate operative field and at risk of injury. Using a hand-held stimulator, the surgeon can stimulate the nerve at 1–5Hz. Repetitive bursts in synchrony with the stimulation verify nerve integrity or confirm that structures for removal are not the nerve. If an injury pattern evolves, stimulation can be used to determine which segment of the nerve is injured.

Monitoring of facial nerve function for resection of acoustic neuroma is accomplished by placing closely spaced bipolar recording electrodes in the orbicularis oris and orbicularis oculi. The value of identifying nerve integrity is that over 60% of patients who have intact nerves will regain at least partial function within a few months of the operation, whereas loss of response is associated with a poor outcome. The excellent outcome data obtained when facial nerve monitoring is used during acoustic neuroma has prompted a National Institute of Health (NIH) consensus panel to identify facial nerve monitoring as a routine part of acoustic neuroma surgery.

Recording Locations for Cranial Nerve EMG Monitoring		
c.n.III	Oculomotor	Inferior rectus
IV	Trochlear	Superior oblique
V	Trigeminal	Masseter, temporalis
VI	Abducens	Lateral rectus
VII	Facial	Orbicularis oculi, orbicularis oris
IX	Glossopharyngeal	Posterior soft palate (stylopharyngeus)
X	Vagus	Vocal folds, special endotracheal tubes, cricothyroid muscle
XI	Spinal Accessory	Sternocleidomastoid, trapezius

Figure 13.9 Recording locations for cranial nerve monitoring by electromyography.

Electromyography has also been used during spine surgery. For example, during surgery on the cauda equina, the anal sphincter and various leg muscles can be monitored. It has also been used during selective dorsal rhizotomy, performed to relieve leg spasticity and thereby improve gait in cerebral palsy.

In general, major anesthetic effects on EMG recordings are limited to the use of muscle relaxants. Since most EMG monitoring is for detection of nerve integrity, complete neuromuscular blockade eliminates any response and renders the technique useless. As with MEP recording, EMG responses from intentional electrical stimulation can be monitored during partial neuromuscular blockade. However, concern has been raised about partial blockade masking transient responses from mechanical nerve stimulation, and it may be prudent to avoid paralysis during EMG monitoring if these responses are desired.

Because of its ability to evaluate both structural and functional integrity of the nervous system, electrophysiologic monitoring has become a valuable monitoring tool during surgery in which neural structures are at risk of operative injury. In some cases, monitoring is indispensable (e.g. seizure focus ablation); in others it is a standard of care (e.g. facial nerve monitoring in acoustic neuroma and spinal monitoring during scoliosis correction), and in many others it is a valuable adjunct.

SLEEP AND ANESTHESIA

The natural state of sleep and the induced state of anesthesia both involve alterations in the state of consciousness. Consciousness can be defined as awareness of attention to one's surroundings (concrete) and an ability to reflect on the sensory representation of one's surroundings (abstract). The conscious state depends on interactions between the brainstem reticular formation and the thalamocortical networks. Since consciousness is determined by neuronal networks, it can be pharmacologically manipulated.

Sleep is an essential, readily reversible physiologic state characterized by unconsciousness, reduced muscle tone, analgesia,

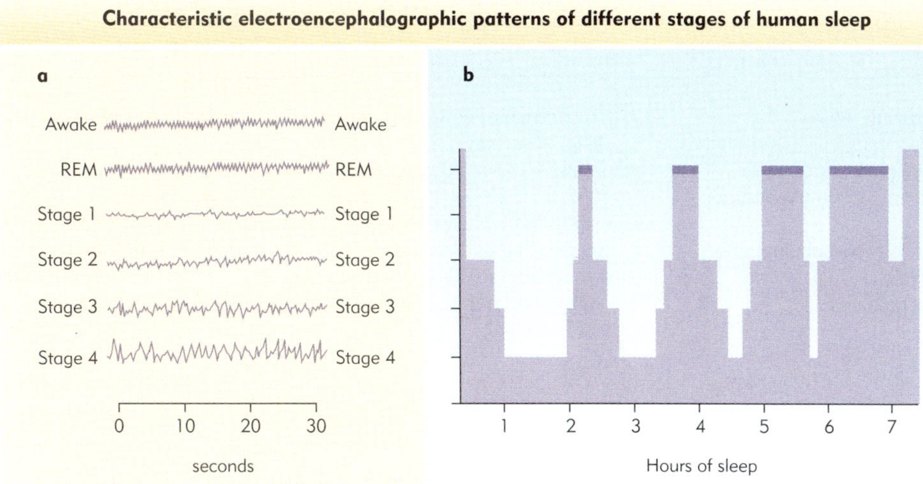

Figure 13.10 Characteristic electroencephalographic patterns of different stages of human sleep. (a) EEG recording during a typical night for a young adult for the waking state and during progressively deeper levels of non-REM sleep. (b) The dark bars represent periods of REM sleep. (Modified with permission from Domino EF., 1994.)

amnesia, respiratory and autonomic disturbances, and dreaming. Sleep has a circadian rhythm (occurs every 24 hours) as well as a more rapid oscillation, which is normally entrained by the light–dark cycle together with many other biologic rhythms. The circadian cycle is directed by the suprachiasmatic nucleus in the hypothalamus (not sensitive to anesthetics), which is linked to a sleep cycle clock in the pontine tegmentum (highly sensitive to anesthetic suppression). The duration of sleep varies widely between individuals (from 5 to 10 hours; average 7.5) and with age, disease states, and drugs. Human sleep is divided into five stages characterized by different motor, autonomic, and polygraphic (EEG, EMG, eye movement) activity (Fig. 13.10). The major distinction is between rapid eye movement (REM) and non-REM (stage I–IV) sleep. The initial stage of sleep is non-REM sleep, during which the EEG progressively becomes more synchronized and slows, the person becomes more difficult to arouse (most difficult during stage IV), pupils constrict, and muscle tone, blood pressure, and heart rate decrease. Rapid eye movement sleep occurs about every 90 minutes, lasting longer later in the sleep period, and is interspersed between periods of non-REM sleep to give a total of 6–8 hours of total sleep. During REM sleep, the EEG is desynchronized in a similar manner to that observed during arousal; there is tonic inhibition of muscle tone interrupted by phasic motor events (e.g. REM), autonomic instability (e.g. irregular respiration, hypotension, and hypertension), and dreaming. The proportion of time spent in REM sleep and in stage III and IV of non-REM sleep decreases with age.

With the onset of sleep, reciprocal thalamocortical connections no longer convey incoming sensory information to the cortex (i.e. there is a functional decortication). This involves diminished firing of brainstem cholinergic, noradrenergic, and serotonergic neurons, which leads to disinhibition of inhibitory GABAergic reticular neurons and causes hyperpolarization of thalamic relay cells. Rapid eye movement is characterized by complete inhibition of noradrenergic locus coeruleus and serotonergic dorsal raphe neurons and by a simultaneous increase in the activity of pontine cholinergic neurons. Therefore, highly localized injections of muscarinic cholinergic agents into the pontine REM sleep-generator network induces REM sleep. Dominance of the aminergic pathways is associated with wakefulness, awareness, and sensitivity to pain, while dominance of the cholinergic system is characterized by dreaming, analgesia, amnesia, and atonia. This physiologic mechanism for the induction of analgesia, amnesia, and atonia may be instructive for future research in anesthetic mechanisms.

Natural sleep and anesthesia share many similarities, but they are clearly distinct. Both are characterized by unconsciousness, impaired thermoregulation, analgesia, amnesia, and atonia (in REM sleep). The EEG in sleep is characterized by predictable rhythmic variations generated endogenously. The effects of anesthetics on the EEG are agent specific (Chapter 23) and dose dependent, but can resemble patterns observed in certain stages of sleep (e.g. the spindles observed with barbiturates). Natural sleep is characterized by autonomic variability, while most anesthetics produce autonomic stability even in the face of painful stimuli. Finally, natural sleep is characterized by easy arousability and spontaneous movements, in contrast to the effects seen in anesthesia.

Key References

Cheek JC. Posterior fossa intraoperative monitoring. J Clin Neurophysiol. 1993;10:412.

Levy WJ, Shapiro HM, Maruchak G, Meathe E, et al. Automated EEG processing for intraoperative monitoring: a comparison of techniques. Anesthesiology. 1980;53:229.

Martin JT, Faulconer A Jr, Bickford RG, et al. Electroencephalography in anesthesiology. Anesthesiology. 1959;20:360.

Rampil IJ. A primer for EEG signal processing in anesthesia. Anesthesiology. 1998;89:980–1002

Sloan T. Refresher courses: Lecture 211. American Society of Anesthesiology; October 1985.

Spehlmann R. Evoked potential primer. Boston, MA: Butterworth; 1985.

Weiderholt WC, Mayer-Harding E, Budnick B, McKeown KL. Stimulating and recording methods used in obtaining short-latency somatosensory evoked potentials (SEPs) in patients with central and peripheral neurologic disorders. Ann NY Acad Sci. 1982;388:349.

Further Reading

Adams DC, Heyer EJ, Emerson RG, et al. The reliability of quantitative electroencephalography as an indicator of cerebral ischemia. Anesth Analg. 1995:57–76.

Chiappa KH. Evoked potentials in clinical medicine. New York: Raven Press; 1990.

Domino EF. Drugs for sleep disorders. In: Brody TM, Larner J, Minneman K, Neu HC (eds). Human Pharmacology: Molecular to Clinical, 2nd edn. St. Louis MO: Mosby; 1994:449–55

Kartush J, Bouchard K (eds). Neuromonitoring in otology and head and neck surgery. New York: Raven Press; 1992.

Moller AR. Evoked potentials in intraoperative monitoring. Baltimore, MD: Williams & Wilkins; 1988.

Neidermeyer E, Lopes de Silva F (eds). Electroencephalography: basic principles, clinical applications and related fields, 3rd edn. Baltimore, MD: Williams and Wilkins; 1993.

Nuwer MR. Evoked potential monitoring in the operating room. New York: Raven Press; 1986.

Rampil IJ. Electroencephalogram. In: Albin MA, ed. Textbook of neuroanesthesia with neurosurgical perspectives, Ch. 6. New York: McGraw Hill; 1997:193–219.

Schramm J, Zentner J, Pechstein U. Intraoperative SEP monitoring in aneurysm surgery. Neurol Res. 1994;16:20–2.

Sloan T. Evoked potentials. In: Albin MA, ed. Textbook of neuroanesthesia with neurosurgical perspectives, Ch. 7. New York: McGraw Hill; 1997:221–76.

Yingling CD. Intraoperative monitoring of cranial nerves in skull base surgery. In: Jackler RK, Brackmann DE, eds. Neurotology. St Louis, MO: Mosby; 1994:967–1002.

Chapter 14 Hemodynamic monitoring

Richard Teplick

Topics covered in this chapter

Patient monitoring systems
Signal reproduction
Pressure monitoring
Interpreting pressures
Measurement of cardiac output

Many therapeutic decisions regarding patient management are based on information gathered from monitors, especially invasive pressure monitors and the electrocardiogram (ECG). However, without fully understanding the principles and limitations of these devices, such data can be inaccurate, imprecise, and misleading. This chapter provides the background for understanding how such devices obtain and process data.

PATIENT MONITORING SYSTEMS

Early bedside patient monitors could usually display one ECG channel and several invasively measured pressures. The ECG was displayed after being processed by filters with different user-selectable bandwidths, and several adjustments were often required to sense the heart rate and calibrate the displayed ECG. Pressures were obtained by amplifying the electrical signal from the transducer, which converts pressures into electrical signals. These signals were displayed on the monitor screen and used to deflect a voltmeter. Pressures could be read from the voltmeter, which was calibrated in pressures rather than volts and swung between systolic and diastolic pressure with each beat, or directly from the display screen. In the latter, horizontal markings had to be placed on the screen corresponding to the pressures in the range of interest, for example 25, 50, and 75mmHg and so on for systemic pressure. The pressure calibration procedure was complex. The pressure amplifiers first had to be adjusted to give the proper deflections on the meter and then the display amplifiers had to be adjusted to yield the proper deflections on the screen.

Since the 1960s, monitors have become much more complex electronically and much simpler to use. They also can monitor many more variables, such as oxygen saturation, temperature, cardiac output, and noninvasive blood pressure. The most important change has been the incorporation of digital computer technology to produce the so-called ‘smart’ monitors. In current-generation monitors, all input signals such as ECG and pressure signals are converted into digital data by rapid sampling. The resultant digitized data are then stored and analyzed by a microprocessor. The incorporation of microprocessors permits selection of an enormous number of display options, plus generation of many derived variables.

There are four characteristics shared by the current generation of monitors. First, they usually process the electrical signal coming from transducers in ways not clearly specified by the manufacturer. Second, the screens are not as tall as they were on many older monitors; as a result, accurate screen calibration is difficult or impossible. This shortcoming is especially evident if several waveforms are displayed simultaneously. Third, the monitors emphasize numeric displays, which are derived by processing the data in a variety of ways usually not clearly defined or characterized. Fourth, relatively simple knobs and buttons have given way to complex software requiring use of ‘soft keys’ or a ‘touchscreen’ to traverse menus.

The impressive display and computational capabilities can mask major limitations in the ability of a monitor to perform some fundamental tasks. For example, as discussed below, there may be considerable error in the numeric values displayed for central pressures. To understand the use and limitations of bedside monitors and the technologic evolution just described, an understanding of the basic principles governing transducers and monitors is necessary. However, the critical question that defines the requisite specifications for monitors is what is the purpose of measuring the different variables.

SIGNAL REPRODUCTION

To assess the fidelity of monitoring devices such as ECG recorders or invasive pressure displays, a method is needed to compare quantitatively the actual electrical signal or intravascular pressures with those displayed on the monitor. However, quantitatively describing the shape of, for example, an arterial pressure waveform is difficult if not impossible. Instead, repetitive patterns such as pressure waveforms can be described completely as the sum of a sequence of sine waves. This type of analysis is often called a Fourier decomposition and the resulting sequence of sine waves is a Fourier series. The general form of a Fourier series representing a waveform $f(t)$ is given by:

Equation 14.1

$$f(t) = \frac{A_0}{2} + \sum_{k=1}^{\infty} A_k \sin\left(\frac{k\pi t}{2} + \alpha_k\right)$$

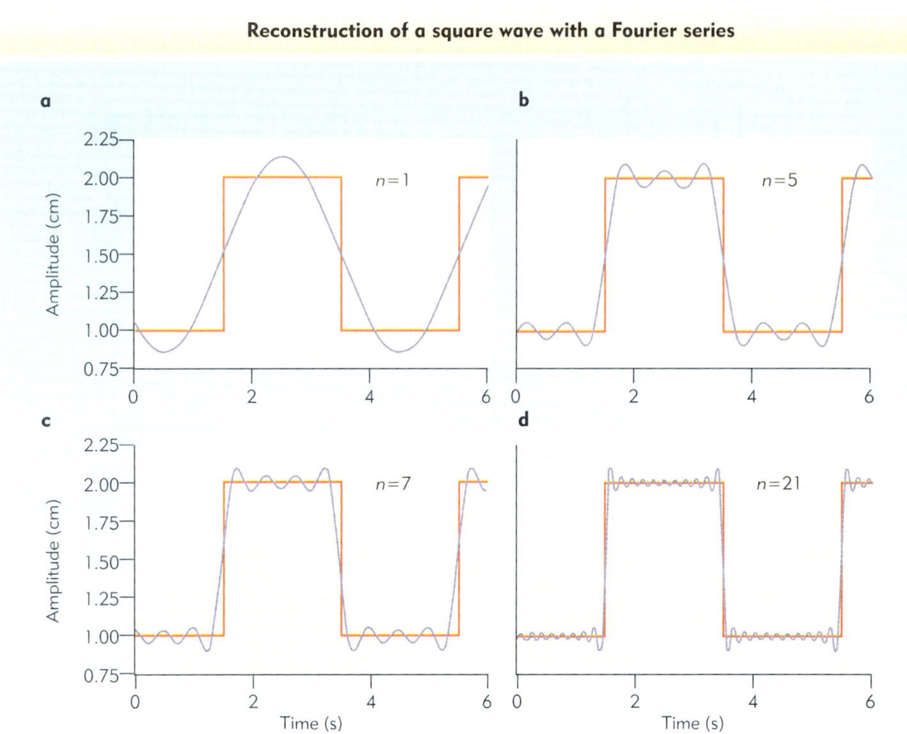

Figure 14.1 Reconstruction of a square wave with a Fourier series. The square wave repeats itself every 4 seconds and has an average amplitude of 1.5cm. The number of harmonics in the Fourier approximation is given by *n*. (a) A single sine wave that also repeats itself every 4 seconds has a frequency of 0.25Hz. This corresponds to the fundamental frequency. Notice that the maximum amplitude of this sine wave is approximately 0.64 so it oscillates between 0.86 and 2.14, providing a relatively poor description of the square wave. (b, c and d) However, this approximation improves as more harmonics (n = 5, 7, and 21) are added. Nonetheless, even with 21 harmonics, the sharp corners are not perfectly reproduced. Typically, sharp corners require very high harmonics to be reproduced accurately.

where t is time, A_k is the amplitude, and α_k are the phases of the series. The kth term in the summation is termed the kth harmonic. The term $A_0/2$ is the average value of the signal represents (e.g. the mean pressure). The amplitude of the kth term determines the size of the kth sine wave and the phase determines the offset of the sine wave from the usual value of zero at $t = 0$. Usually, a waveform can be described precisely with a finite number of terms in the Fourier series. However, this number depends upon the particular waveform and the intended use of the reconstruction. An example of a Fourier series used to describe a square wave is shown in Figure 14.1. The first four sine waves of the series that describe the square wave are shown in Figure 14.2. In this illustration, the values of α_k are such that all of the sine terms always have the value zero at 1.5, 3.5, and 5.5 seconds. The coefficients, A_k, and phases for the first 21 harmonics are shown in Figure 14.3. Notice that these coefficients are only non zero for odd values of k, except for A_0, which equals the mean value of the square wave. In addition, their values decrease rapidly after the first several harmonics. Consequently, very high harmonics add relatively little to defining the shape of the square wave although very high harmonics are required to define the sharp corners. In fact, for waveforms that have abrupt changes such as a square wave, the ripple at the corners will remain constant regardless of the number of terms used in the series. This is known as the Gibbs phenomenon and is the reason that the amplitudes of the high harmonics decrease relatively slowly.

Because essentially any periodic waveform can be represented as a Fourier series, knowledge of the magnitude and phase of each harmonic is sufficient to describe the shape of the waveform quantitatively. Ideally, to avoid distortion of the desired waveform by the monitoring system, the system should maintain the relationships between the magnitudes and phases of each term of the Fourier series describing the measured waveform. Often all waveform features of interest can be accurately reproduced by a limited number of terms in a Fourier series. In this case, the monitoring system need only maintain the relationships of the phases and magnitudes of those frequencies. The range of frequencies that can be transduced without amplitude distortion is termed the *bandwidth* or *frequency response*. The transducing system is said to have a flat frequency response over that range. However, because monitoring systems do not change the amplification of the Fourier terms abruptly outside of the bandwidth, by convention the bandwidth is defined as the range of frequencies over which the amplification does not vary by more than 3 decibels (dB), which is approximately 50% [the power ratio in decibels is defined as $20 \times \log(\text{amplification})$; as a result, at half power, $-3\text{dB} = 20\log{}^{1}/_{\sqrt{2}}$].

The lowest frequency that needs to be amplified without amplitude distortion is usually dictated by the lowest or fundamental frequency of the signal to be monitored. For example, an ECG monitor may be designed to display heart rates that are always expected to be greater than 30 beats/min. This corresponds to a fundamental frequency of 0.5Hz [Hz or hertz is the number of cycles (in this case beats) per second]. Consequently, ECG systems are often designed to reproduce accurately frequencies above 0.5Hz. Below this frequency, amplification decreases rapidly. However, a consequence of such a rapid change in amplification is that the phase of the terms near 0.5Hz also changes. This will produce phase distortion of the reproduced signal. To surmount this, the low end of the bandwidth of most ECG systems is 0.05Hz. The effects of phase distortion have generally not been quantitatively addressed in ECG or invasive pressure monitoring. However, it is known that phase distortion has little effect on audio signals because the human ear is insensitive to such distortions. In contrast, such distortion can be very important in video or digital signals. To avoid phase delay, the phase must either be constant or a linear function of frequency.

The first seven harmonics of the Fourier series for a square wave

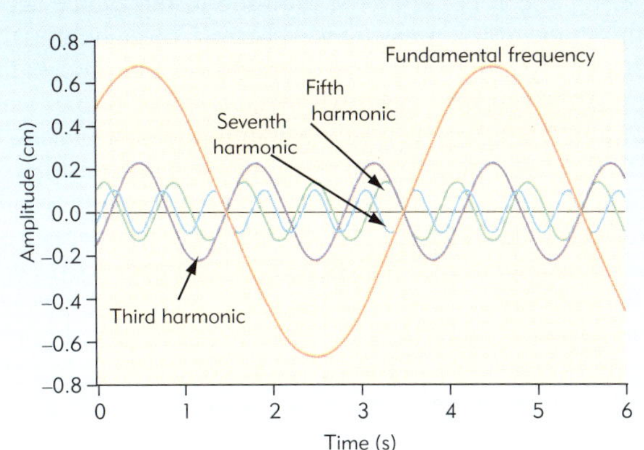

Figure 14.2 The first seven harmonics of the Fourier series for a square wave. The square wave is that shown in Figure 14.1. The mean of 1.5 for the square wave is subtracted from each sine wave so they are shown oscillating around zero. For a square wave all even harmonics are zero. Notice that to reconstruct the square wave, the different harmonics have different heights (amplitudes) and lead or lag each other by differing amounts (phase). Also, the higher harmonics have smaller amplitudes so that eventually addition of higher harmonics would contribute very little to the shape of the square wave

Phases and amplitudes of the first 21 harmonics of square wave in Figure 14.1

Harmonic	Amplitude (cm)	Phase
0	1.5	
1	0.64	0.79
3	0.21	−0.79
5	0.13	0.79
7	0.09	−0.79
9	0.07	0.79
11	0.06	−0.79
13	0.05	0.79
15	0.04	−0.79
17	0.04	0.79
19	0.03	−0.79
21	0.03	0.79

Figure 14.3 Phases and amplitudes of the first 21 harmonics of the square wave shown in Figure 14.1.

PRESSURE MONITORING

Pressure monitoring can be invasive, auscultatory (following auditory changes), or oscillatory (following volume changes).

Invasive pressure monitoring

Transducers

Intravascular transducing systems convert pressure into an electrical signal by exposing one side of a diaphragm within a transducer to the intravascular pressure and the other to atmospheric pressure. This causes the diaphragm to flex and its displacement is converted into an electrical signal, usually by changing the length or property of a material so that its resistance changes. This causes a change in a voltage, termed the excitation voltage, that is applied to an electronic circuit incorporating this variable resistance. The relationship between applied pressure and changes in this measured voltage defines the sensitivity of the transducer. Most new transducers used for hemodynamic monitoring are standardized to produce a change of 50μV/V per 10mmHg (1cmHg) if the excitation voltage is 1V. That is, their sensitivity is 50μV/V per cmHg. Because the diaphragm is stiff (typically, 10cmHg pressure causes a volume displacement of 0.001mm^3), its movement can track even rapidly changing portions of pressure pulses.

The sensitivity of older transducers varied not only between manufacturers but also among transducers produced by the same manufacturer. Consequently, older monitoring equipment had to incorporate circuitry that the user could adjust to compensate for these differences. Fortunately, the sensitivity of most new transducers does not vary significantly from 50μV/V per cmHg. Older transducers also changed their sensitivity with temperature whereas most new transducers have circuitry that compensates for this problem.

Transducer calibration

Invasive transducing systems (i.e. the arterial, central venous, or pulmonary artery cannulae, the associated tubing, the transducer, and the monitor) have to meet three criteria to measure blood pressure accurately: static calibration, linearity, and dynamic calibration.

Static calibration

Primarily because of variations in the sensitivity of transducers, older monitors had to be calibrated to ensure that a given pressure produced the corresponding reading on the monitor. Functionally, almost all pressure monitors have three amplifiers. First, a preamplifier compensates for differences among transducers. The signal from the preamplifier is fed to a second amplifier that is adjusted to produce the proper deflections on a meter, numeric display, or chart recorder. The output of the second amplifier goes to a third amplifier that is adjusted to produce the proper deflections on the screen. Newer monitors usually are designed assuming a transducer sensitivity of 50μV/V per cmHg, stable amplifiers, and a screen amplification that can only be varied in preset increments. Consequently, some or all of their amplifiers cannot be adjusted. However, on occasion transducer sensitivity drifts, the cable develops short circuits, or the amplifiers fail. Consequently, the measured pressures become inaccurate although this might not be apparent to the user. This can be detected easily by performing a static calibration.

For new monitors, there are two steps to this process: zeroing and calibration with a known pressure source. A transducer must be zeroed to ensure that it reads zero pressure in the absence of any applied pressure. To zero a transducer, both sides of the diaphragm are exposed to ambient pressure and the monitor is adjusted to show zero pressure. This usually entails opening the stopcock closest to the transducer to expose the transducer to atmospheric pressure. For older monitors zeroing was accomplished by turning a knob that adjusted part of the electronic bridge used to make the pressure measurement. New monitors do this automatically when requested.

Zeroing the transducer was particularly important in measuring central pressures with transducers that had domes above the diaphragm. The weight of the flush solution in these domes caused a significant offset in central pressures that was corrected by zeroing the transducer. This is less of an issue with current transducers because the fluid-containing portion is very small. Nonetheless, zeroing is also needed to compensate for slight differences in sensitivity resulting from manufacturing factors or temperature.

Once zeroed, the static gain (sensitivity) of the system can be checked by applying a known pressure to the transducer. This can be done by attaching a mercury manometer to the transducer or by filling tubing with saline to a fixed height above the transducer. For example, a column of saline 68cm high corresponds to approximately 50mmHg. If the corresponding pressure is not displayed on the monitor, the cable and then the transducer should be changed in succession. Because the gain of current monitors cannot usually be adjusted by the user, if the problem remains after the above steps, the monitor must be serviced. Because of improved manufacturing, the static gain usually does not have to be checked.

A transducing system must not only read an applied pressure correctly, it must also be linear. This means that if a multiple of the pressure used for static calibration is applied to the transducer, the monitor should read the same multiple of the pressure. Nonlinearity is seldom, if ever, a problem with current equipment.

Signal definition and dynamic performance

A successful static calibration does not guarantee accurate reproduction of pressure waveforms. The transducing system must also be able to reproduce accurately the rapid pressure changes that occur in the systemic and pulmonary circulation. To ensure that these pressures are transduced with high fidelity, dynamic performance must be tested.

The shape of pressure waveforms varies considerably between patients and even within the same patient over time. These shapes often do not conform to the expected or accustomed appearance. For example, waveforms may actually have narrow sharp systolic peaks, although this can also be an artifact. Fortunately, systems can be tested easily to determine whether they are introducing artifacts into displayed waveforms. Testing of this aspect of the system, called the *dynamic response*, is based on the principles of Fourier analysis described above. For example, if the heart rate were 120 beats/min, the fundamental frequency would be 120 beats/min divided by 60 seconds, which is 2 cycles (i.e. 2Hz). The second harmonic would have a frequency of 4Hz, the third 6Hz and so on. The number of harmonics required to describe the pressure waveform depends upon the features of interest. Rapidly changing aspects of a pressure waveform, such as the dicrotic notch, require higher harmonics. If the transducing system distorts the phase or, particularly, the amplitude relationships between the requisite harmonics, the displayed waveform will be distorted. For accurate visualization and determination of systolic and diastolic pressures of most arterial pressure waveforms, only the first six to eight harmonics are required. Higher harmonics usually have amplitudes that are sufficiently small that they may be neglected without distorting the waveform. However, additional harmonics may be required to describe arterial waveforms that have unusual shapes, such as sharp spikes, or other features such as the rate of change of pressure with time, dP/dt, which may require harmonics as high as 90Hz. Therefore, for a heart rate of 120 beats/min, sine waves that have frequencies of at least 2, 4, 6, 8, 10, and 12Hz would be required to reproduce accurately the shape of the pressure waveform. Consequently, the measurement system would have to transduce and process the mean pressure and sine waves with frequencies up to at least 12Hz without changing their relative amplitudes or phases. If this were the case, the pressure waveform would be displayed on the screen without significant shape distortion and would, thus, reflect accurately the actual intra-arterial pressures. However, if the waveform had sharp peaks, higher harmonics would be required.

Although most amplifiers can easily meet these requirements, the transducer and tubing themselves may distort the amplitude and phase relationships of even the low-frequency Fourier series components of a pressure waveform. This occurs because of the relatively high compliance and low resistance of the tubing and the inertia of the flush solution. This distortion may be quantitated by modeling the response of the transducer and tubing to intra-arterial pressure, $P(t)$, by the second-order differential equation

Equation 14.2

$$P(t) = \frac{d^2I(t)}{dt^2} + 2\alpha\omega\frac{dI(t)}{dt} + \omega^2 I(t)$$

where $I(t)$ is the current output from the transducer and α and ω are, respectively, the damping coefficient and resonant frequency of the system. The solution is completely characterized by its ω and and α values. If the value of α is less than 1, a condition termed underdamping, the system will resonate (oscillate) at a frequency close to ω. The actual oscillation frequency, termed the damped natural frequency (DNF), is affected by the α so that

Equation 14.3

$$\text{DNF} = \omega\sqrt{1-\alpha^2}$$

The value of α determines how rapidly the oscillations stop.

If the arterial cannula were abruptly exposed to atmospheric pressure, these oscillations would be visible on the monitor. This is the basis of the 'pop test' described below and is used to determine α and ω. These values can be found by solving Equation 14.2 for this change by setting $P(t)$ to 0 and specifying that the pressure at time zero, $P(0)$, equals the pressure just before the pressure drops to zero and that the first derivative of pressure at time 0 is zero.

Clinical pressure-transducing systems are always underdamped. Because of this tendency to oscillate, the transducing system amplifies or attenuates the magnitudes of the Fourier harmonics of the pressure waveform near the DNF, depending on the value of α. This can cause distortion of the displayed waveform.

The frequency versus amplification plot for a typical transducing system with a value of ω of 20Hz and a value of α of 0.3 is shown in Figure 14.4. Notice that there is little amplification of sine waves below approximately 5Hz. However, there is progressive amplification of the amplitudes of harmonics with frequencies near the DNF. The amplitude is increased by 3dB (an amplification of approximately 1.41) at 12.7Hz. From Equation 14.3, the DNF can be calculated to be 19Hz rather than the value of ω, which is 20Hz. This simulated system also shows a 3dB attenuation for sine waves with frequencies above 29Hz. Assuming a

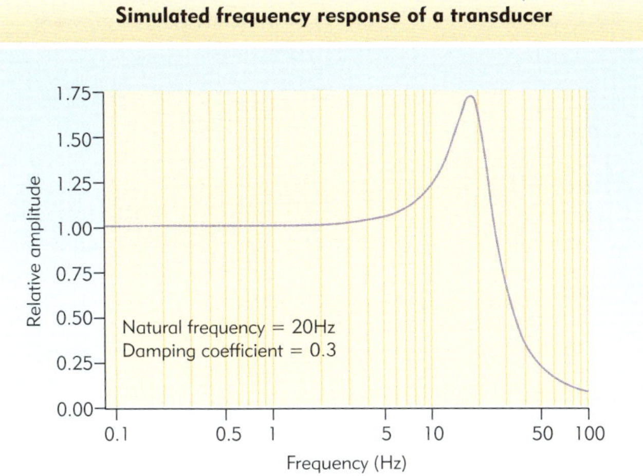

Figure 14.4 Simulated frequency response of a transducer. Simulated response in a transducer with a resonant frequency of 20Hz and a damping coefficient of 0.3. Note that as the frequency approaches 19Hz, the damped natural frequency (DNF), there is progressive amplification. The importance of this amplification, which will distort the resultant pressure waveform, depends on what features are of interest. Amplification exceeds 3dB (an amplification of 1.41), the conventional definition of bandwidth, at approximately 13Hz. Frequencies higher than the DNF are attenuated rapidly so that above approximately 29Hz the amplitudes are less than 1. The width of the resonant peak is determined by the damping coefficient, which does not vary widely among transducers. In this example, if a patient had a heart rate of 120 beats/min, the arterial pressure waveform probably would not be greatly distorted because the amplitude of all Fourier coefficients below the sixth harmonic (12Hz) would undergo less than 3dB amplification. However, certain features such as sharp peaks would not be reproduced because they require higher frequencies to reconstruct. Such distortion could be avoided if the DNF or damping coefficient (see text) were higher.

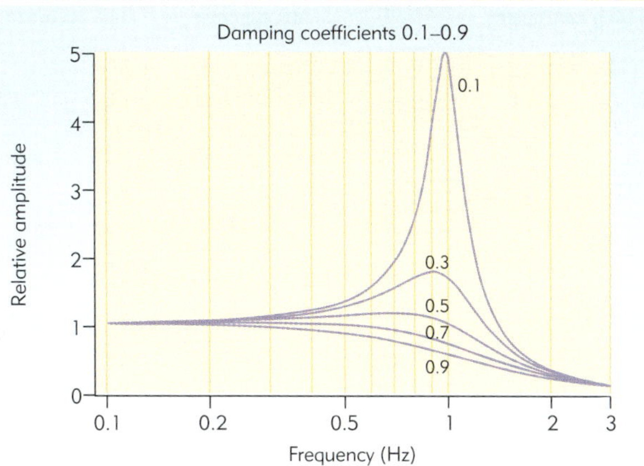

Figure 14.5 Effects of damping coefficient on relative amplification at different frequencies. All of these simulated systems have a resonant frequency of 1.0Hz. However, as the damping coefficient decreases, the damped natural frequency (DNF) also decreases according to Equation 14.3. Frequencies above approximately 0.55Hz are markedly amplified if the damping coefficient is less than 0.3. For damping coefficients between approximately 0.4 and 0.7, amplification never reaches 3dB and the bandwidth is relatively flat. The flattest bandwidth is achieved with a damping coefficient of 0.71. Above a damping coefficient of 0.71, 3dB attenuation occurs at progressively lower frequencies. From this figure, it appears that transducing systems with damping coefficients in the 0.4–0.71 range can accurately reproduce pressure waveforms with frequency components close to the true resonant frequencies of the system.

3dB amplification would be acceptable, the maximum fundamental frequencies that would not distort a pressure waveform using the system in Figure 14.4 would be 2.1 if six harmonics were adequate and 1.6 if eight harmonics were required. The corresponding heart rates would be 127 and 95 beats/min, respectively.

As shown in Figure 14.5, as the damping ratio increases, progressively less amplification occurs near the DNF until, above 0.7071, there is a progressive attenuation with increasing frequency. The relationships between α, the DNF, and the frequencies at which 3dB changes occur are shown in Figure 14.6. This table indicates that a value of α in the range 0.4–0.7 yields the highest frequency response. Unfortunately, α in most transducing systems is seldom greater than 0.25 and often is less than 0.2, for which 3dB amplification occurs at 55% of the DNF. Therefore, for such systems, six to eight times the fundamental frequency should be less than approximately 55% of the DNF. For example, for a heart rate of 60 beats/min, the eighth harmonic is 8Hz so the system should resonate at least at 15Hz. If, however, the heart rate were 120 beats/min, the eighth harmonic would be 16Hz so the system should resonate at least at 29Hz. If the value of α were lower, the value of ω should be higher.

Distortion of the pressure waveform is generally manifest as a spurious increase in systolic pressure if the higher harmonics of the pressure waveform are close to the value for ω. This occurs because high frequencies are needed to reproduce abrupt changes in pressures and these harmonics would be amplified more than lower harmonics (Fig. 14.7). In contrast, if the frequencies of the higher harmonics are sufficiently greater than the DNF they will be attenuated and, therefore, fine definition of the waveform would be lost. Consequently, the systolic pressure would probably be underestimated, the waveform would appear sluggish, and abrupt changes such as the dicrotic notch may disappear.

The dynamic performance of the combined tubing–transducer system can be determined easily by measuring the response to an abrupt change in pressure. This pop test, shown in Figure 14.8, is performed as follows. First, the transducer catheter system is closed to air and to the patient at the patient end by turning the stopcock nearest the arterial cannula to a 45° position. The system is pressurized with the flushing solution (usually to 300mmHg). Finally, the occluded stopcock is rapidly opened to air, and oscillations in the subsequent waveform are observed. The values for DNF and α of the system can be calculated as shown in Figure 14.8.

Gardner studied the dynamic performance characteristics required for accurate measurement of blood pressure and described the pop test in detail. He used an analog computer to simulate transducing systems with different natural frequencies

Effects of damping coefficient on damped natural frequency

Damping coefficient	DNF	3dB increase		3dB decrease
0.1	0.99	0.55	1.29	1.54
0.2	0.98	0.57	1.23	1.51
0.3	0.95	0.64	1.11	1.45
0.4	0.92			1.37
0.5	0.87			1.27
0.6	0.80			1.15
0.7	0.71			1.01
0.8	0.60			0.87
0.9	0.44			0.74
1.0	0.00			0.64

Figure 14.6 Effects of damping coefficient on damped natural frequency. These effects are illustrated together with the frequencies for 3dB changes in amplitude for a transducing system simulated as a second-order system with a resonant frequency of 1.0.

Effect of low resonant frequency on systemic arterial pressure

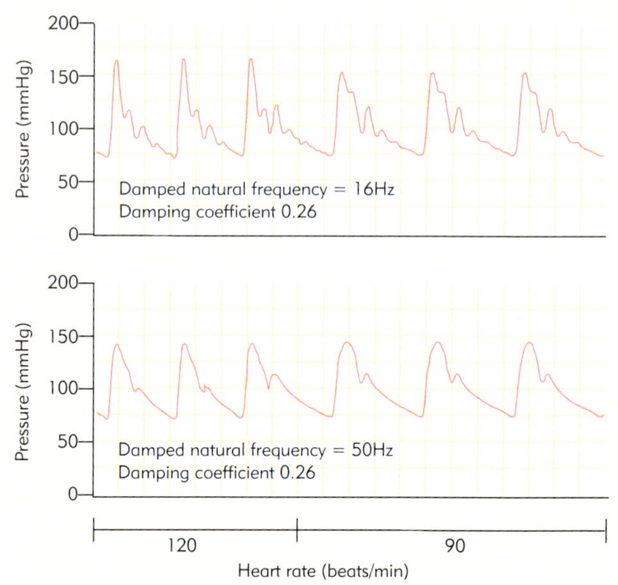

Figure 14.7 Effects of a low resonant frequency of the transducing system on systemic arterial pressure at two different heart rates. Diastolic pressure and mean pressure (not shown) are virtually unaffected by the frequency response of the transducing system. However, the increase in systolic pressure by almost 25mmHg at a heart rate of 120 beats/min (left half of top trace) and 15mmHg at a heart rate of 90 beats/min are artifacts resulting from the low damped natural frequency. This distortion is accompanied by marked oscillations of the waveform (ringing). The improvement in accuracy at a rate of 90 beats/min results from the lower frequency response required at lower heart rates.

and α values. Two patient arterial waveforms were applied to this simulated system. He determined a relationship between the natural frequency and α that appeared to reproduce these two waveforms adequately (Fig. 14.9). Notice that, as expected, as the natural frequency decreases the limits on the acceptable value for α become narrower. Below approximately 13Hz, the waveform was viewed as distorted regardless of the value of α. Because the heart rate was 118, this corresponds to approximately the sixth harmonic. That is, apparently adequate reproduction of the original waveform could be achieved if the first six harmonics could be transduced without amplitude distortion. However, it should be noted that acceptable reproduction in this study was based on appearance rather than any quantitative measure.

The most common cause of low values for ω is air in the tubing, especially near the transducer because it increases the compliance of the system. This effect is magnified when the tubing between the cannula and transducer is long because of the decrease in resistance and increases in compliance and inertia. With the older disposable dome transducers, resonant frequencies above 12–15Hz were generally not achievable, probably because of the compliance of the dome. In contrast, disposable systems may easily resonate above 40Hz if carefully set up because the pressure transducer itself usually has a very broad bandwidth. The limiting factors are the indwelling cannula, the tubing, stopcocks, and air in the system, especially near the transducer. Tubing length, stopcocks, and flush devices are the major factors decreasing the value of ω.

Many newer monitors use filters to try to compensate for the frequency responses of transducing systems. These filters also prevent the spikes often seen on arterial pressure waveforms, erroneously thought to be artifacts. Although such spikes can be artifacts, if the frequency response of the system is adequate, as defined above, the spikes are real. Most of these filters prevent amplification of frequencies much above 12Hz. It is hard to understand how such filters could compensate for all systems, as resonant frequencies may vary widely. However, this issue has not been studied carefully, and the effects of such filters on displayed waveforms have not been well defined. The presence of such filters may prevent the use of a pop test because high-frequency oscillations cannot be visualized. Many new monitors allow the high-frequency cutoff to be set by the user although the default is usually still 12Hz. Manufacturers should be asked about the presence and characteristics of such filters.

Numeric displays

With advances in technology, the original meters used to indicate beat-by-beat pressures were replaced with devices that displayed the desired pressures numerically. Current monitors usually dedicate part of the screen to the numeric display of systolic, diastolic, and mean blood pressures. Because these displayed pressures would be distracting and difficult to read if they were updated with each beat, all monitors display pressures determined by some type of averaging scheme. Older devices used a moving average in which the pressures from each new beat were used to update the average pressures. Specifically,

Equation 14.4

$$Pd_i = Pd_{i-1} + \frac{Pm_i - Pd_{i-1}}{K}$$

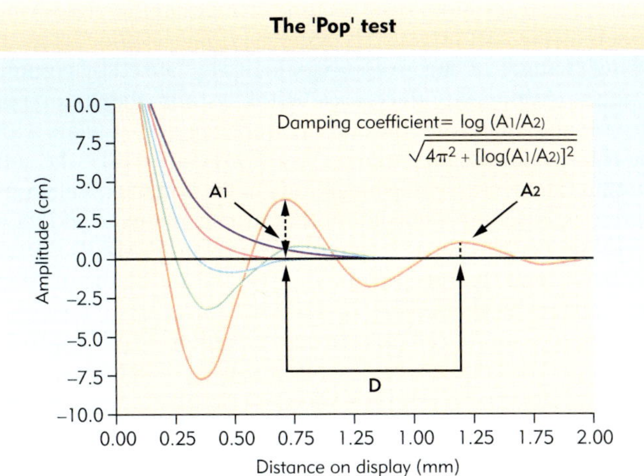

Figure 14.8 A 'pop' test for transducers with the same resonant frequency but different damping coefficients. As the damping coefficient increases towards 1, the oscillations die out more rapidly and the damped natural frequency (DNF) decreases. The pop test can be used to determine the DNF and damping coefficient of a catheter-transducer system. This is illustrated for the pop test yielding the largest oscillations (e.g. the smallest damping coefficient). The system is pressurized as described in the text and is then abruptly opened to air. This process, which is analogous to striking a tuning fork, causes the system to oscillate at its DNF. The DNF can be determined by dividing the rate at which the waveform moves across the screen, the sweep speed, by the distance between the peaks (*D*). In this example *D* is approximately 0.5mm on the display screen, which has the usual sweep speed of 25mm/s. Therefore, the DNF is 25/0.50 = 50Hz. The damping coefficient, which describes how rapidly the oscillations die out, can be calculated from the ratio of the amplitudes of two successive oscillations, A_1 and A_2. In this example, the ratio is approximately 4.25, so the damping coefficient is 0.23. If the sixth or eighth harmonic of the pressure waveform is higher than approximately 18Hz, which is 55% of the DNF, Figures 14.5 & 14.6 indicate that inaccuracies in the pressure waveform will become evident. Consequently, the heart rate should be below 135 or 180 beats/min to keep the eighth or sixth harmonic, respectively, within this range.

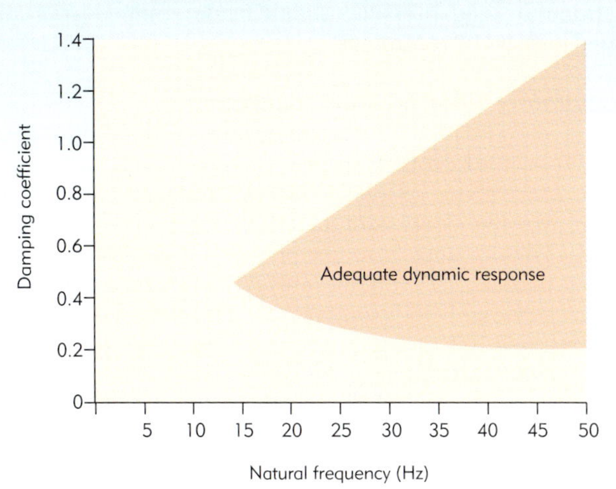

Figure 14.9 Relationship between natural frequency and damping coefficient suggested for accurate transduction of waveforms. A computer was used to simulate transducing systems with different natural frequencies and damping coefficients. The region labeled 'adequate dynamic response' shows the relation between natural frequency and damping coefficient required for accurate visual reproduction. (Adapted from Gardner, 1981.)

where Pm_i and Pd_i are the measured and displayed pressures (systolic, diastolic, or mean) for beat *i*; Pd_{i-1} is the pressure displayed for the previous beat (*i*–1), and *K* is a constant. For larger values of *K*, the displayed pressure is affected less by beat-to-beat changes in Pm_i. Following a sustained abrupt change in pressure, the change in displayed pressure at beat would be

Equation 14.5

$$Pd_i = Pm_n - (Pm_n - Pd_0)\left(\frac{K-1}{K}\right)^i$$

where Pm_n is the new measured pressure and Pd_0 is the original displayed pressure. If *K* were 1, the displayed pressure would be updated to the new pressure with each beat. As *K* increases above 1, the displayed pressure will change more slowly with each beat. For example, using Equation 14.4, if the displayed systolic pressure were 100mmHg and the new beat had a systolic pressure of 120mmHg, for a *K* of 5, the first updated pressure would be 100 + (120 – 100)/5 = 104mmHg. The next pressure would be 104 + (120 – 104)/5 = 107mmHg. After 17 beats, using Equation 14.4, the displayed pressure would be 119.5mmHg. If *K* were only 3, the displayed pressure would be 119.5mmHg after only nine beats. Although it takes longer to display a sustained pressure change with larger values of *K*, the displayed pressure also will not change much with transient pressure changes.

Although usually proprietary, a *K* value of 8 has been recommended for systemic arterial pressures. However, this will generally not correctly display end-expiratory central pressures (see below). To surmount this, an algorithm was developed for which *K* varies according to how much the mean arterial pressure (MAP) of the new beat varies from that of the preceding beat. For bigger differences, larger weighting factors are used so that the displayed pressures are affected to a lesser degree.

Numeric displays have two problems that render them inaccurate and imprecise. First, because of the averaging system, when pressures are changing, the numbers displayed may differ substantially from the actual pressures at the instant of measurement. For example, the pressure displayed just before the onset of respiration may differ markedly from the actual pressure at this time, because the displayed pressure incorporates pressures from a number of preceding beats. The magnitude of this difference depends on the weighting scheme used, the true change in pressure, and the respiratory rate. Second, the actual weights and schemes for changing these numbers for central vascular pressure measurements vary among manufacturers. The information about weighting algorithms is rarely available from the manufacturer, and performance specifications are generally not supplied. For these reasons, if accurate pressures are desired at a particular instant, such as end-expiration or the onset of the QRS complex of the ECG, the numeric pressures should be disregarded. Instead, pressures should be determined from calibrated displays or recordings.

Auscultatory blood pressure monitoring

The standard method for measuring arterial blood pressure is auscultation for Korotkoff sounds. This entails inflating the cuff to a pressure above systolic, slowly deflating the cuff, and listening over the artery with a stethoscope for the Korotkoff sounds. These sounds have five phases: a clear tapping sound (systolic pressure) (I), soft murmurs (II), louder murmurs (III), muffling (IV), and disappearance (V). The genesis of phase I is controversial. It is thought to reflect either turbulent flow or rapid opening and closing of the artery. Phases II and III reflect the gradual increase in flow as the arterial constriction is relieved. Phase V corresponds most closely to invasively measured diastolic pressure. The auscultatory technique has multiple potential sources of error. First, because the sounds depend upon flow, if flow is limited or absent (as might occur with severe vasoconstriction or outflow obstruction), the sounds will be difficult to hear or not heard at all. Second, the pressures obtained depend upon the cuff size, its application, and transmission of the cuff pressures to the underlying artery. In general, cuffs that are too small for the circumference of the arm lead to spuriously increased pressures. Third, if the cuff is deflated rapidly, relative to the heart rate, systolic pressure can be underestimated and diastolic pressure overestimated. For these reasons, this method cannot be considered the 'gold standard' for pressure measurement. In general, auscultated pressures tend to underestimate invasively measured systolic pressures and overestimate diastolic pressures. The importance of this depends upon the purpose of the measurement. Such errors are probably relatively unimportant in monitoring acute changes such as those that might occur during anesthesia or in intensive-care units, where the magnitude rather than the precise value of the change is important. However, these errors can be important for chronic measurements such as the diagnosis of hypertension.

Invasively measured arterial pressure waveforms often have unusual shapes. For example, a radial arterial waveform may show a large spike indicating systolic pressure. However, if auscultation indicates that systolic pressure occurs during the 'shoulder' of such a waveform, the spike might be ignored because it is considered to be 'overshoot'. If the transducing system is calibrated accurately and the dynamic response is sufficiently high, there is no reason not to accept the spike rather than the auscultated pressure as the true systolic pressure. The lower pressure determined by auscultation probably occurs because there is inadequate energy or flow associated with the pressure peak to cause the turbulence or 'flapping' of the vessel wall required to produce the Korotkoff sounds. Consequently, rather than ignoring the spike or calling it overshoot, the spike should be recognized as real if the dynamic characteristics of the transducing system are adequate. Although usually related, directly measured and auscultated pressures can be quite different.

Oscillometrically determined blood pressure

The most common method for determining blood pressure today is probably by automated oscillometry. This technique essentially measures the volume changes in a standard blood pressure cuff resulting from volume changes in the underlying vessels as the cuff pressure is decreased. This is done by measuring changes in cuff pressure, which are caused by volume changes. As pressure decreases below systolic, the volume of the cuff and, therefore, the cuff pressure begin to oscillate with the changes in vascular volume. As the pressure within the cuff continues to decrease, the magnitude of the volume oscillations increases, reaching a maximum that usually plateaus and then decreases back to zero. Mean arterial pressure (MAP) is usually determined as the lowest cuff pressure during the plateau of maximum oscillations.

Although all automated devices calculate MAP approximately as described above, the method used to determine systolic and diastolic pressures varies between companies and even with software revisions within the same company. Criteria used to detect systolic and diastolic pressures often are based on the change in shape of the envelope defining the increase and decrease in the initial and final oscillations. Unfortunately, the specific criteria used are seldom available from the manufacturers. Moreover, they are affected by the methods used to reject artifacts. Consequently, automated devices developed by different companies may yield clinically relevant differences in measured pressures. There have also been many comparisons of auscultated with intra-arterial pressures. Most of these studies show relatively small discrepancies, which, as mentioned, are probably not clinically important in the acute setting. Moreover, although most studies show an oscillometric underestimation of systolic pressure relative to invasively measured arterial pressures, this may be a result of inadequate frequency response of the invasive measurement system. However, this problem may be accentuated and is of greater clinical relevance in the hypotensive or hypertensive patient and for ambulatory monitoring.

INTERPRETING PRESSURES

Systemic pressures

Questions about how or when to measure pressures can usually be easily answered once the purpose of making the measurements is defined clearly. Rather than trying to create hemodynamic profiles, it would seem more constructive to use the data to test hypotheses about the state of the cardiovascular system.

The shape of the arterial pulse is determined by the properties of ventricular contraction and the characteristics of (and changes in) the vascular system as the pressure wave travels down the vascular tree (Fig. 14.10). These changes, caused by reflected waves within the vascular system, generally decrease the width of the pressure waveform and increase systolic pressure as distance from the aortic root increases. However, the magnitude of these changes varies among patients and within a patient when conditions such as temperature or sympathetic tone change. These effects become less marked with age, but in children they have been reported to increase systolic pressure between the aortic root and iliac artery by more than 50%. In contrast to systolic pressure, mean and usually diastolic pressures are slightly lower in peripheral arteries than in the root of the aorta. Changes in the characteristics of either the heart or the vascular system can produce changes in the features of the arterial pulse.

Intravascular systemic arterial pressure tracings may exhibit considerable variation, especially in systolic pressure, during the respiratory cycle. Usually, there is a decrease during spontaneous

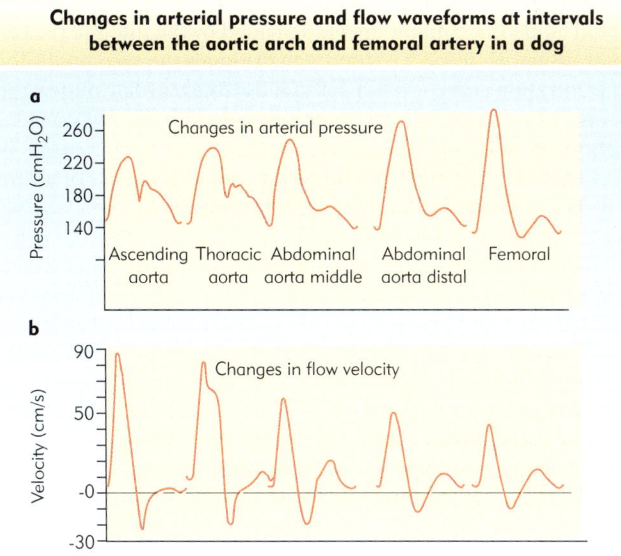

Figure 14.10 Changes in arterial pressure and flow waveforms at intervals between the aortic arch and femoral artery in a dog. (a) Systolic pressure increases with distance from the arch, whereas diastolic pressure remains relatively constant. Also, the shape of the waveform changes, with transformation of the dicrotic notch into a dicrotic wave. (b) Because of the compliance of the vasculature, the relationship between pressure and flow at any instant varies with location, such that flow during diastole becomes more pronounced at more distal locations in the circulation. (With permission from McDonald, 1974.)

breaths. In contrast, during mechanical breaths, systemic arterial pressure usually increases initially, then decreases (the nadir occurs at about the time that airway pressure returns to baseline), and finally gradually rises back to baseline. The length of time required for this last phase varies considerably, ranging from a few beats to 12 beats or more. The exact mechanisms for these variations in pressure are complex and depend on respiratory effects on venous return, pulmonary vascular blood volume, and ventricular loads.

Central pressures

Alterations during respiration

The correct method for measuring central vascular pressures [central venous pressure (CVP), right atrial pressure (RAP), pulmonary artery pressure (PAP), pulmonary capillary wedge pressure (PCWP), and left atrial pressure (LAP)] depends upon the purpose of the measurement. Unlike the respiratory variations in systemic arterial pressures, respiratory changes in central pressures are artifacts. If the purpose is to estimate end-diastolic pressure (EDP), measurements made just before inspiration (i.e. at end-expiration) provide more accurate and precise estimates. However, this cannot be done using the numeric displays because they reflect some form of average over the respiratory cycles and are, therefore, are unlikely to be accurate reflections of EDP. These pressures can, however, be determined accurately from a waveform displayed on a calibrated screen.

Waveform features

The presence of atypical or abnormal configurations in central pressure waveforms can lead to errors in measurement. For example, the typical atrial waveform consists of an A wave, caused by right atrial contraction; a C wave, caused perhaps by bulging and downward movement of the atrioventricular (AV) valves during isovolumic contraction; and a V wave, which occurs during atrial filling. Because the AV valves are closed from approximately the onset of systole until the peak of the V wave, atrial pressures during this time interval cannot reflect ventricular EDP. Also, because end-diastolic volume (EDV) and EDP increase with atrial contraction, the only time that atrial pressures can reflect EDP is after the A wave and before the onset of systole. Therefore, it is logical to measure atrial pressures at approximately the onset of the QRS complex of the ECG. Because A, C, and V waves usually have small amplitudes (of only a few mmHg), their importance in measuring pressures is usually minimal. However, the A and V waves can have large amplitudes that cause error in numeric displays independent of their unreliability in displaying end-expiratory pressures. These errors are apparent and can be readily avoided if the waveform is displayed on a calibrated screen.

Other sources of central pressure measurement error

Occasionally, overinflation of the balloon in a pulmonary artery catheter can yield an erroneous PCWP. This error probably results from transient obstruction of the catheter tip by the balloon or vascular wall, allowing pressure from the pressurized flushing system to build up within the transducer. Because correctly measured PCWP never exceeds diastolic PAP, this problem is readily detected by such a discrepancy. Balloon deflation, flowed by slow reinflation, usually corrects this problem.

The term catheter whip is commonly used to describe pulmonary and systemic arterial waveforms having unusually sharp peaks (spikes) or oscillations (ringing) of uncertain origin. Catheter whip also implies that such features are caused by mechanical motion of the catheter during the cardiac cycle or by a low value of ω for the transducing system. Because a pulmonary artery catheter passes through the right side of the heart into the pulmonary artery inflow tract, the former explanation seems plausible. Moreover, because of the length and relative elasticity of the catheter lumen, it is difficult to obtain a value of ω much above the low teens. This low value could produce the oscillations described as ringing. Ringing that persists throughout the cardiac cycle suggests that a low ω may be the cause. Ringing may pose a substantial problem in measuring diastolic PAP, often used as a surrogate for the wedge pressure, because it makes a displayed waveform difficult to read and may produce very large errors in the numeric displays. One solution is to 'eyeball' the most stable point in the oscillations and use this as the diastolic pressure. It is also possible that filtering or increasing the value of α could minimize this problem. Incorrect values should be suspected if the measured diastolic PAP is lower than the PCWP.

It has been asserted that if the tip of a pulmonary artery catheter lies in zone 1 or 2 of the lungs (described by West et al., Chapter 44), the PCWP may systematically overestimate LAP. Measurement of LAP from the PCWP theoretically depends on a static column of blood between the catheter tip and left atrium. This implies that the venous resistance must be low so that the pressure drop due to continued venous flow is small. It seems improbable that placement of the catheter tip in zones 1 or 2 is a source of error in estimating LAP. First, placement of the catheter tip in a zone 1 region is unlikely because of the low blood flow although changes in ventilation or position may convert other zones to zone 1 areas. Regardless, although blood flow through alveoli may be absent in zone 1, flow to extra-alveolar (corner) vessels should still exist, thus providing the rquisite continuity between the catheter tip and the left atrium. If such continuity were lost, A, C, and V waves should not be observed on the PCWP trace and the PCWP should, by definition, be considerably higher than pulmonary artery diastolic pressure. Therefore, by definition, there must be continuity between the catheter tip and the left atrium, even disregarding the extra alveolar vessels. If inflation of the balloon caused all venous channels in this zone to collapse, vascular continuity to the left atrium would be lost and the PCWP should reflect alveolar pressure rather than LAP. This is unlikely because of the multiple arteriovenous pathways. Nonetheless, the literature is confusing on this issue because studies have implied incorrectly that there is no flow and thus no patent arterial-left atrial channel in these regions. As in a zone 1 region, A, C, and V waves would not be observed if such continuity were lost, but this has not been reported. The discrepancies between PCWP and LAP attributed to the catheter tip lying in zone 2 could be a result of increased venous resistance caused by the partial collapse of the pulmonary veins in these zones. This would result in a relatively large pressure drop between the catheter tip and the left atrium due to continued venous flow after balloon inflation. An additional source of confusion is the use in some studies of values for PCWP and LAP that are averaged over respirations. These considerations suggest that having a catheter tip in zones 1 or 2 is unlikely to be the source of spuriously large PCWP/LAP differences. Nonetheless, the possibility of this occurrence underscores the importance of visually examining the PCWP waveform for A, C, and V waves.

MEASUREMENT OF CARDIAC OUTPUT

Cardiac output is usually measured clinically by indicator dilution. The method involves measurement of pulmonary or systemic arterial changes in the concentration of an indicator (such as color or cold) injected into venous blood. Thermal indicators are the most common indicators used clinically. Thermodilution depends upon measuring changes in blood temperature in the pulmonary artery with a thermistor. Less commonly, indocyanine green, a dye, is used. Its concentration is measured at a site in the arterial circulation. Although other noninvasive techniques based on Doppler flow or changes in impedance are available, the validity of these methods is controversial.

Dilution methods for calculating cardiac output are based on the Stewart–Hamilton equation, which is an expression of conservation of mass. If none of the indicator were lost from the circulation, the amount that would be recovered at the detection site if all blood flow passed by this site would equal the total amount injected (C_i). Consequently,

Equation 14.6

$$C_i = \int_0^{\infty} q(t)c(t)\mathrm{d}t$$

where $q(t)$ and $c(t)$ are the blood flow and concentration as functions of time, t, at the detection site. If $q(t)$ were nearly constant, Equation 14.6 becomes:

Equation 14.7

$$C_i = Q\int_0^{\infty} c(t)\mathrm{d}t$$

where Q is the cardiac output. Therefore, the cardiac output would equal the amount injected divided by the integral of concentration with respect to time, which equals the area under the concentration curve (AUC). Even if the total cardiac output did not pass by the sampling site, the change in indicator concentration would be the same in every arterial branch. Consequently, the AUC would be the same regardless of where it is measured and, therefore, cardiac output can still be estimated using Equation 14.7.

There are three important assumptions made in indicator dilution techniques. First, at some point distal to the injection site of the indicator and proximal to the measurement site, all blood passes through a single channel or at least intermixes. This ensures that the indicator is diluted by the total blood flow. Second, any changes in flow during the measurement period must occur rapidly and the average flow must not change during the measurement period. This assumption may be violated by respiration because it may be slow relative to the measurement period. Finally, the indicator must remain in the vascular space, and large shifts of fluid to or from the vascular space cannot occur during the measurement period. If the third assumption were not true, the concentration of the indicator would change independently of blood flow.

Thermodilution method

Cardiac output

The thermodilution method entails injecting a known amount of cold fluid, usually normal saline or 5% dextrose in water, at a known temperature below blood temperature (most often room temperature but occasionally 0°C) into the right atrium. The resulting change in temperature of pulmonary arterial blood is measured by a thermistor on the tip of a pulmonary artery catheter. These data are used to produce a thermodilution curve of blood temperature versus time. Cardiac output is then calculated from a variant of Equation 14.7:

Equation 14.8

$$Q = \frac{K(T_{\mathrm{bi}} - T_{\mathrm{i}})60V}{\int_0^{\infty} T_{\mathrm{b}}(t)\mathrm{d}t}$$

where T_{bi} and T_i are the initial blood and injectate temperatures, respectively; $T_b(t)$ is the blood temperature as a function of time (t); V is the volume of injectate; and K is a constant, usually 1.08, that depends upon volume, specific gravity, specific heat of the injectate and the blood, and heat loss within the catheter. The terms in the numerator of this equation, which define the amount of cold injected, are incorporated into the calibration number set on the cardiac output computer.

Recirculation is usually not a problem with thermodilution. However, the different temperatures in the superior and inferior vena cavae cause the pulmonary artery temperature to vary with respiration. Consequently, it is difficult to determine when the temperature curve returns to baseline. To surmount this problem, the AUC for the temperature difference curve usually is computed by halting the calculation when the washout curve has decayed to approximately 25–30% of the peak value. Then, assuming an exponential return to baseline, a constant is added to the AUC calculated up to this point.

An exponential decay is based on the following model. Assume that a bolus of indicator, b, is injected into the right ventricle and mixes with the blood instantaneously to yield a concentration C_1 equal to b/EDV. Given an ejection fraction (EF), the first beat will eject an amount of indicator equal to

EDV × EF × C_1. After the ventricle refills to the EDV, the concentration of indicator (C_v) will equal the original amount minus the amount ejected divided by the EDV:

Equation 14.9

$$C_v = \frac{C_1 \times EDV - C_1 \times EDV \times EF}{EDV} = C_1(1-EF)$$

On the next beat, the amount of indicator ejected would equal EDV × EF × C_v (the ventricular concentration given by Equation 14.9). The concentration of indicator after refilling back to the EDV would then be

Equation 14.10

$$\frac{C_1(1-EF) \times EDV - C_1(1-EF) \times EDV \times EF}{EDV} = C_1(1-EF)^2$$

This process would repeat itself with each beat until the concentration remaining in the ventricle was infinitesimal. If *b* were the amount of cold saline injected into the right ventricle, a thermistor in the pulmonary artery would detect a temperature given by Equation 14.9 after the first beat. On the second beat, the temperature change relative to baseline would be given by Equation 14.10. Therefore, after each beat, the temperature would decrease by an amount proportional to 1 – EF; as a result, after *n* beats the ejection temperature would be proportional to $C_1(1-EF)^n$. In fact, this theoretic decrease in temperature by 1 – EF is the basis of the right ventricular ejection fraction thermodilution catheter (see below). If the EF became progressively smaller while the number of beats increased, in the limit of an infinitely small EF and infinitely many beats, the temperature would rise towards baseline exponentially. This formulation does not account for the gradual rather than abrupt drop in temperature following the bolus injection. However, both portions of the curve can be described using a two-compartment kinetic model with pulmonary blood representing the peripheral compartment.

The theoretic problem with thermodilution cardiac-output measurement is that the increase in temperature back towards baseline should not be monoexponential if the stroke volume varies slowly over the measurement period (the second assumption above). This would be expected with, for example, respiration. Moreover, a monoexponential increase in temperature back towards baseline has not been validated *in vivo* in the presence of such variations. In fact, because the changes in stroke volume with respiration occur slowly with respect to the measurement period, thermodilution outputs may vary by as much as 70% when injection is performed at different times during the respiratory cycle. To solve this problem, the injection can be made at the end of expiration. Cardiac-output measurements have been observed to vary from 5.0 to 8.4L/min if injections were made randomly during respiration. If injections were made at end-expiration, the range was reduced to 6.3–7.1L/min. Clinically significant differences between sets of three measurements can only be detected for differences of 12–15%. Nonetheless, if the average output is desired, it may be more appropriate to average multiple injections randomly distributed throughout the respiratory cycle. As is the case for pressure measurements, changes in output (more specifically stroke volume) are more useful than the absolute number. Therefore, when measuring cardiac output, precision is more important than accuracy.

Thermodilution has often been shown to overestimate low cardiac outputs. Although this has usually been ascribed to excessive heat loss relative to the cardiac output, more recent data indicate that it is a result of an increase in cardiac output resulting from the cold bolus. It is also possible that the reduced temperature in the coronary circulation increases cardiac contractility, thereby increasing stroke volume. Errors in thermodilution cardiac outputs may also occur in the presence of tricuspid valve insufficiency. Such errors might occur because of heat loss in the regurgitant volume (in effect less cold is injected) or because the downslope of the curve is not monoexponential, thereby causing errors in the extrapolated portion of the area. With the former source of error, cardiac output should be overestimated while in the latter it would probably be underestimated because of a slower than predicted return to baseline. Interestingly, outputs were overestimated by thermodilution in a dog model, whereas in humans they were underestimated. This difference may have arisen because of different standards of comparison; a pulmonary flowmeter in dogs and indocyanine green or the Fick method in humans.

Ejection fraction

Interestingly, the theoretic increase in blood temperature by an amount proportional to 1 – EF with each beat predicted for bolus thermodilution cardiac output measurement is the basis of the right ventricular ejection fraction (RVEF) measurement by thermodilution. The RVEF catheter originally depended on a thermistor that could respond to temperature changes rapidly enough to detect the predicted plateaus in temperature with each ejection, which should have a constant ratio of 1 – EF. This was done by triggering the temperature measurement with the QRS of the ECG sensed using electrodes within the catheter. Eventually, this gave way to methods using slower thermistors and identifying the points on the exponential portion of the curve from the QRS complex. There are, however, several problems with these techniques. First, there is no 'gold standard' for right ventricular volume. Consequently, validation is very dependent upon the standard of comparison for RVEF. Second, although it has been asserted that the accuracy of thermodilution-measured ejection fraction has been validated, this does not seem to be the case. For example, comparisons with biplane angiography yielded an r^2 value of only 0.69 with a regression slope and intercept of 0.76 and 15.5, respectively, indicating an underestimation of EF that increased as EF decreased. Both better ($r^2 = 0.85$) and worse ($r^2 = 0.45$) relationships have been found with first-pass radionuclide scanning. Tricuspid insufficiency, as expected, also interferes with the measurement of RVEF. However, it is unclear whether this is a result of indicator loss, as described above, or invalidation of the assumptions of the thermodilution method because of the addition of progressively diluted indicator to the right ventricle with each beat from the regurgitant volume. Collectively, these data and theoretic calculations suggest that measurement of RVEF by thermodilution is unlikely to be accurate or precise. However, it might be useful in distinguishing between high and low EF in situations when stroke volume is low and RAP is elevated, which could be secondary to, for instance, high transmural pressures or right ventricular dysfunction. In the former the EF should be high, and in the latter it should be low.

Continuous cardiac output

One of the perceived limitations of thermodilution cardiac-output measurement is that it is not continuously measured. To surmount this, the basic principles have been adapted to provide continuous measurement using heat instead of cold as an indicator. The major obstacles to continuous measurement were the excessive heat required and the thermal noise spectrum from intrinsic blood temperature changes, particularly from respiration, and slow baseline temperature changes. These problems were solved by using pseudorandom binary coded temperature pulses that resembled white noise to form cross-correlations with the resultant temperature measurements. The continuous cardiac-output pulmonary artery catheter uses a 10cm heating coil placed between the right atrium and ventricle to produce these temperature pulses. Each binary code must last longer than the duration of the corresponding bolus thermodilution washout curve. Because of thermal noise, this process must be repeated at least 10 times before a reliable output can be calculated. Consequently, the minimum time to obtain an output is approximately 5 minutes. Numerous clinical studies have compared continuous cardiac-output measurements with both bolus thermodilution and indocyanine green measurements with generally good agreement. The major disadvantage to the continuous system is that it cannot respond rapidly to changes in cardiac output. Response time to display a change of 0.9L/min following a 1L/min abrupt change in output is between 10 and 12.5 minutes. Therefore, it would not be useful in determining the cause of an acute change in hemodynamics as its response is much too slow.

Key References

Ellis DM. Interpretation of beat-to-beat blood pressure values in the presence of ventilatory changes. J Clin Monit. 1985;1:65–70.

Gardner RM. Direct blood pressure measurement – dynamic response requirements. Anesthesiology. 1981;54:227–36.

Klienman B. Understanding natural frequency and damping and how they relate to the measurement of blood pressure. J Clin Monit. 1989;5:137–47.

McDonald DA. Blood Flow in Arteries, 2nd edn. Baltimore, MD: Williams & Wilkins; 1974:356.

Maran AG. Variables in pulmonary capillary wedge pressure: variation with intrarthoracic pressure, graphic and digital recorders. Crit Care Med. 1980;8:102–5.

Ramsey III M. Blood pressure monitoring: automated oscillometric devices. J Clin Monit. 1991;7:56–67.

Yelderman M. Continuous measurement of cardiac output with the use of stochastic system identification techniques. J Clin Monit. 1990;6:322–32.

Further Reading

Bruner JMR, Krenis LJ, Kunsman JM, Sherman AP. Comparison of direct and indirect methods of measuring arterial blood pressure. Med Instrum. 1981;15:11–21.

Haller M, Zöllner C, Briegel J, Forst H. Evaluation of a new continuous thermodilution cardiac output monitor in critically ill patients: a prospective criterion standard study. Crit Care Med. 1995;23:860–6.

Hamilton WF. Measurement of the cardiac output. In: Handbook of physiology: Circulation. Vol. 1, Section 2. Washington, DC: American Physiology Society; 1962:551–84.

Kaufmann MA, Pargger H, Drop LJ. Oscillometric blood pressure measurements by different devices are not interchangeable. Anesth Analg. 1996;82:377–81.

Ladin Z, Trautman E, Teplick R. Contribution of measurement system artifacts to systolic spikes. Med Instrum. 1983;17:110–2.

Posey JA, Geddes LA, Williams H, Moore AG. The meaning of the point of maximum oscillations in cuff pressures in the indirect measurement of blood pressure. Part I. Cardiovasc Res Bull. 1969;8:15–25.

Chapter 15 Monitoring of anesthesia gases, capnography, and pulse oximetry

Emilio B Lobato and Nikolaus Gravenstein

Topics covered in this chapter

Gas analysis
Analyzers
Capnography: carbon dioxide analysis
Pulse oximetry

GAS ANALYSIS

Measurement of gas concentrations is of importance to the anesthesiologist. Analysis of O_2 with an alarm to detect a low fraction of inspired O_2 (F_IO_2) ensures adequate delivery to the patient from the source, while detection of CO_2 verifies ventilation and cardiac output. Monitoring of both O_2 and CO_2 is a standard of care during intraoperative management of intubated patients. While monitoring anesthetic gases is not a universal standard of care, it allows identification of inhalation agents, titration of anesthetic dose, early recognition of overdose, and provides evidence of anesthetic elimination during emergence. Agent monitoring also aids in the understanding of the principles of uptake and distribution. In addition, the sudden appearance of N_2 can provide an early indication of venous air emboli with some systems. Interpretation of gas analysis data is enhanced by an understanding of the principles involved in the devices used.

Data acquisition

Modern gas analyzers function by analyzing gas either at the main breathing circuit (mainstream analyzers) or by extracting a gas sample via a small-bore tube and analyzing it away from the breathing circuit (sidestream analyzer or diverting system). Currently, mainstream analyzers are only used to detect O_2 in the breathing circuit and CO_2 at the airway connection. Their advantages include the lack of any delay in measurements caused by transport time, no need for a gas sampling line, and relatively easy maintenance. Disadvantages include the added weight at the airway, relative fragility, and the inability to identify other gases in the circuit.

Sidestream analyzers can analyze several gases simultaneously, provide minimum weight at the airway, and are durable. Disadvantages include transport delay time and susceptibility to obstruction of the gas sampling line by water and secretions.

Data analysis

Data can be displayed as concentration (% volumes) or partial pressure (mmHg or kPa: 1mmHg = 0.133kPa). If the ambient partial pressure is known, concentration and partial pressures can be derived from measurement of one parameter.

Partial pressure

Systems that utilize infrared light (infrared spectrometry) or laser emission (Raman spectroscopy) measure the number of molecules of gas present in a mixture. Since pressure is dependent on the number of molecules, these systems identify the absolute partial pressure. When the ambient pressure is known, concentration can be derived as:

% volume = partial pressure/ambient pressure (mmHg).

If the ambient pressure differs from the value used for calibration of the instrument, the true concentration will be different from the one displayed. The system must also correct for the presence of water vapor (partial pressure 47mmHg at sea level). The following examples illustrate the importance of proper calibration. If the analyzer at sea level is calibrated to report as a fraction of 760mmHg (dry gas) rather than at 713mmHg (water-saturated alveolar gas), the device will overestimate the actual alveolar gas concentration. If the partial pressure of halothane is 7.6mmHg and is reported as 1% by a system analyzer calibrated at sea level (ambient pressure of 760mmHg), it will still be displayed by this analyzer as 1% in Denver (atmospheric pressure 580mmHg) although the true concentration will be much higher, namely 1.75% (7.6mmHg = 1.75% of 580mmHg).

Concentration

Systems that report values as concentration (%) identify components of a gas mixture and determine the percentage contributed by each gas to the total mixture. These systems do not measure partial pressure; using a value for ambient pressure allows calculation of the corresponding partial pressure. Unidentified gases are not recognized and, therefore, their presence will artificially elevate the concentration of the remaining components in the mixture. For example, in a patient receiving 1% isoflurane in 100% O_2, the addition of 50% helium, which is not recognized by the system, will artificially elevate the reported concentration of isoflurane to 2% since the values are read in half the volume of gas. In contrast, a Raman spectroscopy analyzer will provide accurate values by reading the partial pressure of each anesthetic gas.

ANALYZERS

There are a number of different techniques available for measuring gases; each method measures a particular range of gases.

Infrared analyzers

Infrared analyzers detect the absorption of energy from infrared light passing through a mixture of gases. Only compounds with significant dipoles such as CO_2, nitrous oxide (N_2O), water, and volatile agents are measured; nonpolar compounds such as O_2 and N_2 are not detected. These analyzers measure partial pressure since the absorption of infrared light depends on the number of molecules. The potential overlap between gases with very similar infrared absorption characteristics (e.g. CO_2 4.3μm, N_2O 4.4μm, and most volatile agents) has required analyzers with better resolution of absorption peaks to allow separation of various compounds (Fig. 15.1).

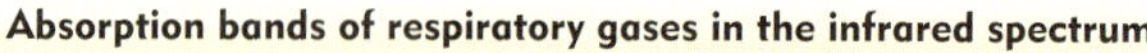

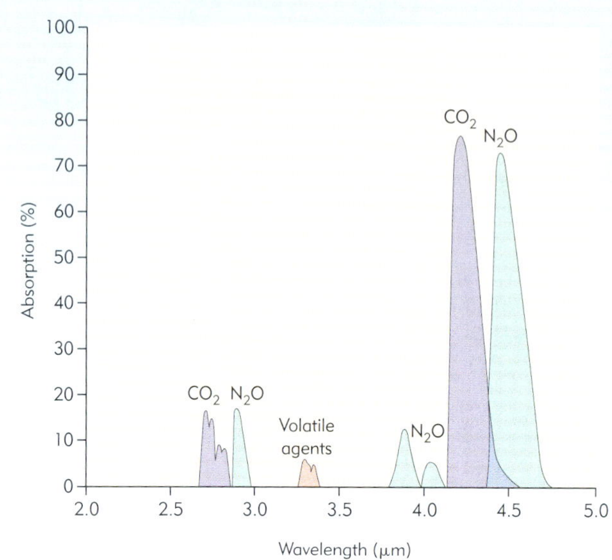

Figure 15.1 Absorption bands of respiratory gases in the infrared spectrum. (With permission from Raemer, 1992.)

Raman spectroscopy

Raman spectroscopy measures the energy of photons scattered when a laser beam strikes molecules of a gas. A portion of the energy of the laser photons is re-emitted at a longer wavelength, resulting in a spectrum shift that is used to calculate partial pressures. Unlike infrared spectrometry, Raman spectroscopy is not limited to dipolar compounds but measures all gases present in a mixture. Volumes are reported as partial pressures, which then can be converted to percentages. Disadvantages of this system include cost, the need for frequent calibration, and the limited life span of the laser.

Mass spectometry

When using mass spectometry, sampled gases are ionized and deflected by a magnetic field in a vacuum chamber onto collector cells, which identify the various components according to their particular mass/charge ratio, based on their trajectory through the magnetic field (Fig. 15.2). The mass spectrometer functions as a proportion system and assumes that all gases have been detected; therefore, an unidentified gas in the mixture will artificially elevate the concentration of the detected agents.

A magnetic sector respiratory mass spectrometer

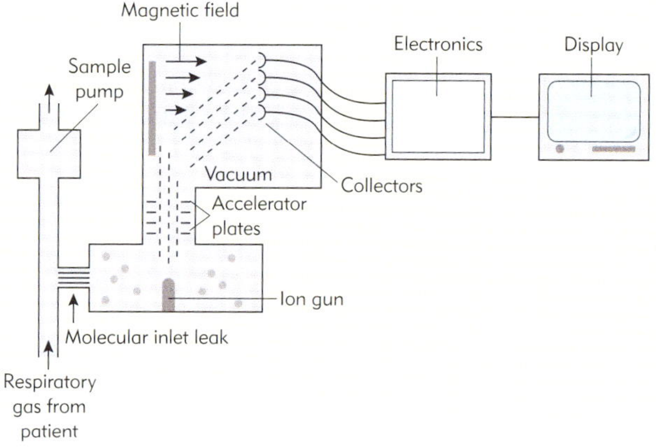

Figure 15.2 A magnetic sector respiratory mass spectrometer. Gas molecules enter a vacuum chamber (through the molecular inlet leak) where they are ionized and electrically accelerated. The mass and charge of the ions determine their trajectory in a deflecting magnetic field, and metal dish collectors are placed to detect them. The electrical currents produced by the ions impacting the collectors are processed and the results are displayed. (With permission from Raemer, 1992.)

Piezoelectric detection

A piezoelectric crystal changes its natural resonant frequency when exposed to volatile anesthetic agents. The magnitude of the frequency change is proportional to the partial pressure of the gas. Because this system lacks specificity, it cannot distinguish mixtures of agents and must be programmed manually. It cannot be used to measure CO_2 or other gases and is not in widespread use.

Limitations

The presence of *water vapor* can cause mechanical failure of Raman analyzers and mass spectrometers through condensation in the sampling cell and can interfere with infrared analyzers, particularly at the CO_2 absorption wavelengths, thus providing erroneous values. Some systems incorporate hydrophobic filters and/or tubing that are semipermeable to water vapor and are made of polymers of tetrafluoroethylene and fluorosulfonyl monomer to remove water vapor from the sample. This tubing does not remove water droplets and, therefore, must be positioned on the patient end of the gas-sampling line. If a heat and moisture exchanger is in use, placing it on the patient side of the gas-sampling site can protect the sampling line and analyzer from water vapor.

The presence of *propellant fluorocarbons* in inhaled aerosols (e.g. bronchodilators) can interfere with measurements by mass spectrometers, thus causing errors in measurements of the other gases.

Improper calibration is an obvious source of error. A simple test is to sample room air, which contains N_2 (79%), O_2 (21%), and minimal CO_2. After these values are displayed, exhale into the sampling site; this should produce an exhaled CO_2 of 33–42mmHg. An error in the room air check requires recalibration or servicing. An error in exhaled CO_2 may necessitate changing the sampling line (most commonly fractured tubing) or the unit.

Sampling line leaks are most common at the patient end of the sampling line. With a sidestream apparatus, a leak anywhere in the sampling line will dilute the sample since the sampling line has a negative pressure because it continuously aspirates gas (~150mL/min) from the circuit. For a spontaneously breathing patient, ambient air will be entrained primarily during inspiration, whereas with positive-pressure ventilation, entrainment will occur during exhalation when circuit pressure is lowest.

Oxygen analysis

Measurement of O_2 concentration in respired gas or within the anesthesia machine may be accomplished by using mass spectrometry, Raman spectroscopy, polarographic sensors (Fig 15.3), galvanic fuel cell sensors, or paramagnetic sensors. All but the galvanic fuel cell sensors are sufficiently rapid in their response time to allow real-time determination of inspired and expired O_2 concentration.

CAPNOGRAPHY: CARBON DIOXIDE ANALYSIS

The practice of measuring CO_2 in respiratory gases is called capnometry, and the instrument used is termed a capnometer. Capnography is the graphic representation of values of exhaled CO_2 over time (displayed by a capnograph) and is a standard monitor for general anesthesia. Both capnometers and capnographs report the minimal and maximal CO_2 values measured. These values are labeled inspired (P_Ico_2) and end-tidal ($P_{ET}co_2$) CO_2, respectively, and relate to the corresponding phases of the respiratory cycle. It is important not to confuse $P_{ET}co_2$ with mixed-expired CO_2 (P_Eco_2). The latter is the average concentration of exhaled CO_2 in a volume of expired gas collected over a period of time. It represents a mixture of alveolar and dead space gas and is used to calculate the physiologic dead space (V_dS) to tidal volume (VT) ratio by using the Bohr equation:

$$\frac{V_dS}{V_T} = Paco_2 - \left(\frac{P_Eco_2}{Paco_2}\right)$$

where $PaCO_2$ is the arterial Pco_2.

Several methods are available for detection and measurement of exhaled CO_2 (Fig. 15.3); infrared spectroscopy is the most common. Disposable devices that rely on a colorimetric pH change to document CO_2 can also be used to verify tracheal intubation. A semiquantitative color guide is used to estimate the CO_2 concentration. These devices lose their effectiveness when saturated with water vapor and do not have an alarm capability; therefore, they are not useful for continuous monitoring over longer periods of time.

Capnography provides significant advantages over a solely digital numerical value display. By examining the morphology of the trace (capnogram), one can diagnose inadvertent esophageal intubation, expiratory airway obstruction, rebreathing of CO_2, incompetent valves in the breathing circuit, insufficient fresh gas flow (FGF) with a Mapleson-type system, and dramatic changes in pulmonary blood flow.

A systematic examination of the capnogram allows the most information to be extracted (Fig. 15.4). One sequence is presented below:

1. Detection of exhaled CO_2;
2. Analysis of the four phases of the capnogram: inspiratory baseline, expiratory upstroke, expiratory plateau, and inspiratory downstroke;
3. Consideration of the $Paco_2 - P_{ET}co_2$ difference;
4. Determination of the etiology of hypercapnia or hypocapnia.

Techniques of gas analysis and their respiratory gas capabilities

Technique	Gases detected				
	O_2	CO_2	N_2O	VA	N_2
IR light spectroscopy		X	X	X	
IR photoacoustic		X	X	X	
Mass spectroscopy	X	X	X	X	X
Raman spectroscopy	X	X	X	X	X
Polarography	X				
Fuel cell	X				
Paramagnetic	X				
Magnetoacoustic	X				
Piezoelectric resonance	X				

VA, volatile anesthetic.

Figure 15.3 Techniques of gas analysis and their respiratory gas capabilities.

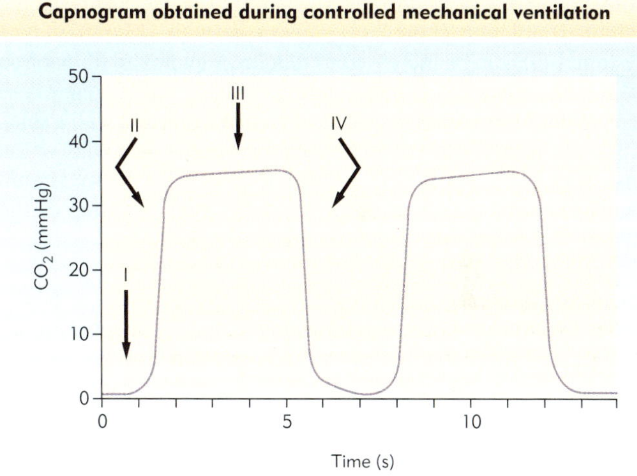

Figure 15.4 A typical capnogram obtained during controlled mechanical ventilation through a circle anesthesia breathing system. The capnogram is divided into four phases: (I, inspiratory baseline; II, expiratory upstroke; III, expiratory plateau, IV, inspiratory downstroke). The plateau contains alveolar gas; end-tidal CO_2 is obtained at the end of the expiratory plateau. (With permission from Good, 1991.)

Detection of exhaled carbon dioxide

Detection of exhaled CO_2 by capnography after tracheal intubation is the most sensitive method to detect ventilation of the lungs. Absence of exhaled CO_2 suggests apnea, esophageal intubation, or lack of pulmonary blood flow. Occasionally, low levels of exhaled CO_2 will be transiently detected following esophageal intubation because of the presence of CO_2 in the stomach; however, the capnogram is typically distorted and rapidly diminishes during the first six breaths. In anesthetized patients, particularly with spontaneous ventilation, the absence of a capnogram reading may be the first indication that a disconnection at the airway has occurred. Disappearance of the capnogram reading indicates failure of the mechanical ventilator or, in spontaneously breathing patients, either the absence of respiratory effort or complete airway obstruction. Delivery of CO_2 to the lungs parallels cardiac output and pulmonary blood flow. Cardiac arrest, pulmonary embolus, or other causes of low or absent pulmonary blood flow all diminish exhaled CO_2 (Fig. 15.5).

The four phases of the capnogram

The shape of the capnogram can vary depending on the breathing system used (circle versus Mapleson), the respiratory frequency and pattern, and the mode of ventilation (controlled versus spontaneous). The normal capnogram of a mechanically ventilated patient is ideally rectangular in shape with the four phases described in Figure 15.4.

Inspiratory baseline

The concentration of CO_2 during the inspiratory baseline phase is zero because there is no rebreathing with a normally functioning circle system. If the inspiratory baseline is elevated ($CO_2 > 0$), rebreathing of CO_2 may be taking place. This may represent an incompetent circuit valve (usually expiratory), exhausted CO_2 absorbent, or channeling of CO_2 through the absorbent. In patients breathing through a Mapleson (rebreathing) system, some inspired CO_2 is normal, unless the FGF exceeds twice the minute ventilation. If the P_ICO_2 is excessive with a Mapleson type system, FGF can be increased to reduce or eliminate it. Inspired CO_2 is also a common artifact during pediatric anesthesia, where a relatively high respiratory rate (>20), in conjunction with a small tidal volume and short inspiratory time exceeds the ability of the instrument to track the values back to zero or to the maximum (response time). This results in an artifactual elevation of the inspired CO_2 and artifactual depression of the $P_{ET}CO_2$.

Expiratory upslope

After inspiration ends, the lungs mechanically recoil and gas quickly exits through the trachea. The expiratory upslope appears after FGF from the equipment and anatomic dead space (without CO_2) is eliminated and replaced with alveolar gas. Under normal conditions, this results in a nearly vertical upstroke (see Fig. 15.4, phase II); if obstruction is present, the upslope becomes slanted. An obstruction can occur at the airway, the endotracheal tube, or the sampling site. A similar slanted upslope is observed if a sidestream analyzer is sampling gas too slowly or if the response time of the capnograph is too slow for the respiratory rate.

Expiratory plateau

As exhalation continues, the capnogram rapidly reaches a plateau. Under ideal conditions of ventilation and perfusion, this plateau is nearly horizontal (see Fig. 15.4, phase III). Since a degree of ventilation–perfusion ($\dot{V}/\dot{Q}$) mismatch occurs even in normal subjects, CO_2 from alveolar units with low $\dot{V}/\dot{Q}$ is last to reach the sampling site, therefore providing this phase with a gentle upward slope. In cases of expiratory airway obstruction, this phase manifests a steeper slope and may not reach the potential maximal value (i.e. plateau) before the next inspiration begins.

The expiratory plateau continues even after active exhalation is completed because exhaled CO_2 remains at the sampling site during the expiratory pause. Small dips may be seen in the terminal portion of the plateau caused by the pulsatile movement of blood through the pulmonary circulation. This draws gas in and out of the lungs and back and forth across the sampling site, causing the appearance of these so-called cardiogenic oscillations on the capnogram. At low respiratory rates, persistent sampling from a sidestream analyzer (usually 2–3mL/s) will cause the plateau to decline as fresh gas from the circuit is drawn into the analyzer. In patients receiving muscle relaxants, the regular appearance of small downward dips in the plateau phase often signifies inspiratory attempts caused by contraction of the diaphragm ('curare clefts').

The highest value near the end of the plateau is normally the maximum value and indicates the end of exhalation; hence, the term end-tidal. In cases of expiratory obstruction, terminal exhalation may be interrupted by the next inspiratory cycle and the true value of $P_{ET}CO_2$ is underestimated; thus P_ECO_2max may be more appropriate. Allowing for more prolonged expiration or introducing an expiratory pause enables a better determination of $P_{ET}CO_2$ in such circumstances.

Inspiratory downslope

Mechanical inspiration produces a steep decline in the CO_2 concentration at the sampling site. A slanted CO_2 inspiratory downslope suggests an incompetent inspiratory valve with accumulation of CO_2 in the inspiratory hose. A slanted downslope is evident with slow inspiration (e.g. partial obstruction), slow gas sampling, and partial rebreathing, as occurs with low FGF when using a Mapleson system.

Arterial to end-tidal carbon dioxide difference

The parameter $Paco_2$ best reflects the adequacy of ventilation. Under normal circumstances, the gradient between $Paco_2$ and $P_{ET}CO_2$ is only 3–5mmHg and is caused by regional differences in ventilation and perfusion. This gradient can increase slightly with changes in position or under anesthesia but, in general, is less than 10mmHg. Differences greater than 10mmHg suggest pulmonary disease, either acute or chronic. If it is important to know the $Paco_2$ precisely (e.g. hyperventilation to manage increased intracranial pressure), arterial blood gas analysis is needed. Differences between arterial and end-tidal values can result from several factors (Fig. 15.5).

Arterial to alveolar carbon dioxide gradient

Factors that increase the arterial to alveolar CO_2 gradient usually involve mismatching of $\dot{V}/\dot{Q}$ (e.g. pulmonary embolus, endobronchial intubation). In general, the gradient is much more affected by $\dot{V}/\dot{Q}$ values greater than 1 (increased dead space, occurring, for example, in pulmonary embolism) than those less than 1 (increased shunt, for example, from endobronchial intubation). With conditions of normal $\dot{V}/\dot{Q}$ in both lungs, a normal alveolar Pco_2 (P_ACO_2) is delivered to the capnometer (Fig 15.5b). In bronchial intubation (Fig. 15.5c), total ventilation occurs in one lung (with a P_ACO_2 of 40mmHg), while the P_ACO_2 from the other lung is essentially that of mixed venous blood (normally 46mmHg). An arterial sample demonstrates an increase of about 3mmHg after the blood from one lung containing a $Paco_2$ of 46mmHg mixes with the other lung with a $Paco_2$ of 40mmHg. The effects of increased dead space are more pronounced (Fig. 15.5d). Here ventilation of a lung with no blood flow rapidly exhausts alveolar CO_2, which will be approximate zero. When combined with alveolar CO_2 from the contralateral lung, the decline will be much more dramatic.

Alveolar to maximum mixed expired carbon dioxide gradient

The value of P_ECO_2max should reflect $P_{ET}CO_2$. Factors that influence delivery of alveolar CO_2 to the sampling site will be asso-

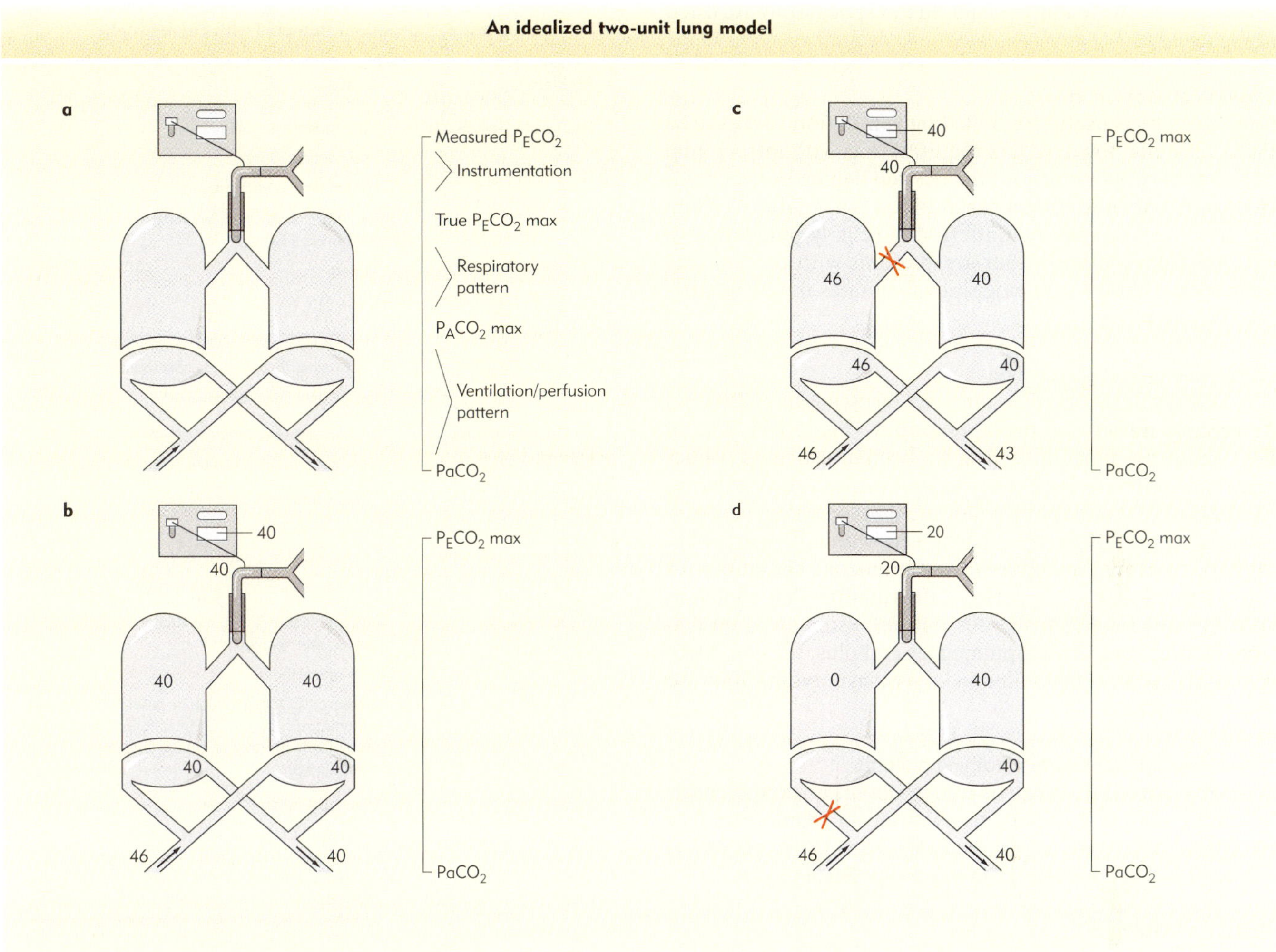

Figure 15.5 An idealized two-unit lung model. This demonstrates how ventilation-to-perfusion mismatching increases the difference between CO_2 in the arterial supply ($PaCO_2$) and that in the end-tidal gas ($PECO_2$max). (a) The components that can affect the difference between $PaCO_2$ and $PECO_2$max are shown. If there are no instrument problems, the measured end-tidal CO_2 should equal the true value. (b) In the normal lung with no faults in the measuring equipment, the gradient is zero. (c) If only one lung is ventilated (e.g. in bronchial intubation), CO_2 is removed only from this lung and a mismatch, of 3mmHg in this example, ensues. (d) If blood flow is restricted to one lung, as could occur in pulmonary embolism, only the perfused lung allows CO_2 movement and a greater gradient between $PaCO_2$ and $PECO_2$max occurs (20mmHg in this example). (With permission from Good, 1991.)

ciated with differences between exhaled CO_2 and alveolar CO_2 through the high dead space-to-tidal volume ratio. Some examples include high-frequency ventilation, rapid shallow breathing in infants and neonates, erratic breathing patterns, and incomplete exhalation with expiratory obstruction [chronic obstructive pulmonary disease (COPD), bronchospasm, kinked endotracheal tube].

Measured and true end-tidal carbon dioxide

Differences between the $P_ECO_2$max and true $P_{ET}CO_2$ (the measured value) occur when the capnograph is the source of error. Even if a true alveolar sample is delivered, factors such as water vapor, a slow response time, calibration errors, and leaks from the sampling catheter can result in a difference between the true and measured values.

Reverse gradient

Under normal circumstances, $PaCO_2$ values are greater than $P_ECO_2$max. In some patients, this gradient may be reversed. One explanation is that some lung units may have long time constants and a high P_ACO_2. These may continue to deliver CO_2 to the alveolar and exhaled gases even though $PaCO_2$ is low. A reverse gradient may also occur if arterial blood reflecting end-inspiration values, where $PaCO_2$ is at its lowest, is sampled. Calibration errors in the analyzer and the blood gas machine may also create an 'apparent' reverse gradient.

Clinical applications of capnography

Detection of untoward events

Capnography allows early recognition of events that, if undetected, may cause injury to the anesthetized patient. Some events that can be readily recognized by capnography are listed in Figure 15.6.

Titration of ventilation

Capnography is useful for adjusting ventilation to a desired $Pa{CO_2}$. When a low $Pa{CO_2}$ is required (e.g. with intracranial or pulmonary hypertension) the desired degree of hyperventilation is confirmed by arterial blood gas analysis. When hyperventilation may be undesirable (e.g. hypokalemia in patients taking digoxin therapy, patients with pre-existing metabolic alkalosis), capnography facilitates timely ventilator adjustments.

Cardiopulmonary resuscitation

The effectiveness of cardiopulmonary resuscitation (CPR) can be reliably monitored by capnography (Fig. 15.7). Use of $P_{ET}CO_2$ as a predictor of survival has been investigated. Values less than 10mmHg are not associated with survival, whereas values greater than 15mmHg indicate that some degree of pulmonary blood flow has been achieved, with a higher probability of returning the patient to spontaneous circulation. A persistently low $P_{ET}CO_2$ during CPR requires that clinicians consider several diagnostic possibilities: esophageal intubation, cardiac tamponade, pulmonary embolus, tension pneumothorax, severe hypovolemia, severe hyperventilation, or ineffective CPR.

Monitoring spontaneously breathing patients

A sidestream analyzer can be used to monitor spontaneously breathing, unintubated patients. A variety of adapters for face masks and nasal cannulae are available. Most give approximate values of $Pa{CO_2}$ and serve primarily as apnea monitors.

Untoward situations detected with capnography

Problem	Cause
No (or little) exhaled CO_2	Esophageal intubation
	Tracheal extubation
	Disconnection of capnograph or gas source
	Complete obstruction (equipment or pulmonary disease)
	Apnea
Elevated inspiratory baseline (phase I)	Open CO_2 bypass
	Partially exhausted CO_2 absorbent
	Channeling through CO_2 absorbent
	Incompetent expiratory valve
Prolonged expiratory upstroke (phase II)	Obstruction (equipment or pulmonary disease)
	Slow gas sampling or slow instrument response
Upsloping expiratory plateau (phase III)	Obstruction (equipment or pulmonary disease)
Prolonged inspiratory downstroke (phase IV)	Incompetent inspiratory valve
	Slow gas sampling or slow instrument response
Hypercapnia	Hypoventilation (leak, obstruction of air flow, inadequate ventilation)
	CO_2 rebreathing
	Increased CO_2 production or delivery (malignant hyperthermia, fever, CO_2 insufflation, bicarbonate administration, release of tourniquet or cross clamp)
Hypocapnia	Hyperventilation
	Decreased CO_2 production or delivery (hypothermia, decreased cardiac output) Increased gradient of arterial to maximum expired CO_2 [ventilation–perfusion mismatching, endobronchial intubation, pulmonary embolism (air, fat, thrombus, or amniotic fluid), shallow or rapid breathing, instrument or sampling problems, miscalibration]

Figure 15.6 Untoward situations detected with capnography. (With permission from Good, 1991.)

PULSE OXIMETRY

Principles

Pulse oximetry estimates arterial hemoglobin saturation ($Sp{O_2}$) by measuring the transmission of light at two wavelengths (660 and 940nm) through any pulsatile vascular tissue bed. Absorption of light at these wavelengths is different for oxyhemoglobin compared with deoxygenated hemoglobin. Pulse oximetry does not respond to nonpulsatile signals (e.g. from skin or venous blood) and is based on the assumption that arterial blood is the only pulsatile light absorber; the pulse oximeter algorithm separates the tissue (unvarying) or direct component from the pulsating–alternating component (Fig. 15.8). Any fluctuating influences other than arterial blood constitute sources of error. The oximeter calculates the ratio of the light absorbance at the two wavelengths during systole (maximum absorption) and uses an empirical calibration curve relating the O_2 saturation to the absorption ratio measured. The calibration curves are based on experimental data obtained from human volunteers (Fig. 15.9).

Regional oxygen saturation (rSO_2) can be measured noninvasively in the cerebral cortex by near infrared spectroscopy (transcranial cerebral oximetry) using similar principals as pulse oximetry. Light of wavelengths 600–1300nm penetrates human tissue to a depth of several centimeters. Positioning of light attenuated by oxyhemoglobin, deoxyhemoglobin and cytochrome a_3, and reflected in a parabolic path through the scalp, skull and brain tissue. Since the majority of blood in the brain is venous, values reflect the balance between oxygen supply and demand, as does jugular venous bulb oximetry (Chapter 20). An invasive technology using parenchymal probes sensitive to tissue oxygen, carbon dioxide and pH is also available. This technology also allows continuous oximetry using intravascular probes.

Limitations

Nail polish and synthetic nails may interfere with pulse oximetry. The reasons are not exactly known, but opaque nail polish diminishes the intensity of transmitted light and may result in an artifactual reading. Polishes with dark blue in them appear to be the worst offenders.

Dyes injected intravenously for diagnostic purposes can have significant effects on $Sp{O_2}$. Intravenous methylene blue can produce significant, transient decreases in $Sp{O_2}$ values. Indocyanine green has a lesser effect, and indigo carmine shows only minor decreases in $Sp{O_2}$. Bilirubin has no effect.

Insufficient signal strength may result from improper positioning of the light emitter and detector such that they are not directly opposite one another, or from inadequate light inten-

End-tidal carbon dioxide during cardiopulmonary resuscitation

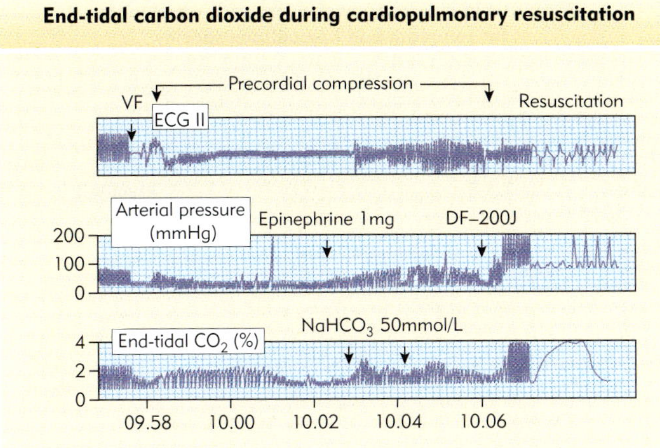

Figure 15.7 End-tidal carbon dioxide during pulmonary resuscitation. Note the fall in end-tidal CO_2 during the cardiac arrest and the transient increase after the administration of sodium bicarbonate. The original tracing has been modified because of space limitations. (With permission from Falk et al., 1988.)

sity to transilluminate the monitored site. In patients with vasoconstriction, reduced blood flow to the fingertips may result in the absence of signal. This problem can often be solved by using digital nerve blocks [1–2mL 1% lidocaine (lignocaine) without epinephrine (adrenaline), or topical application of nitroglycerin (glyceryl trinitrate)].

If the *probe position* is too distal on the fingertip, it may 'see' venous pulsations, thereby contaminating what is presumed to be a purely arterial signal. This artifact is most prominent in patients with warm fingers.

Noisy signals are commonly caused by ambient light such as warming lights, motion of the extremities, or interference by electromagnetic energy from an electrocautery device. Probe motion, in particular, causes incorrect readings by causing the light transmission at both wavelengths to be similar. This results in a change of ratio towards one that corresponds to an Spo_2 of 85% (Fig. 15.9).

Because the pulse oximeter measures light absorbance at only two wavelengths, it cannot measure *other hemoglobin species* such as carboxyhemoglobin and methemoglobin (Fig. 15.10). In their presence, Spo_2 values are overstated. For example, even when carboxyhemoglobin levels are >70%, the Spo_2 values remain >90%. The effect of methemoglobin on Spo_2 values is variable; at lower levels it reduces Spo_2 out of proportion to the Sao_2, but at 35% methemoglobin and above it elevates Spo_2 over Sao_2 values, with effects plateauing around 85% methemoglobin. Fetal hemoglobin appears to have little effect upon the accuracy of pulse oximetry because its light absorption at the two wavelengths used is similar to that of adult hemoglobin.

Clinical applications

Monitoring by pulse oximetry is a standard of care intraoperatively in the postoperative anesthesia care unit and during parenteral sedation. Critically ill patients are also usually monitored with continuous pulse oximetry as a noninvasive and inexpensive method for assessing arterial oxygenation. The

Tissue composite showing dynamic and static components that affect absorption during pulse oximetry

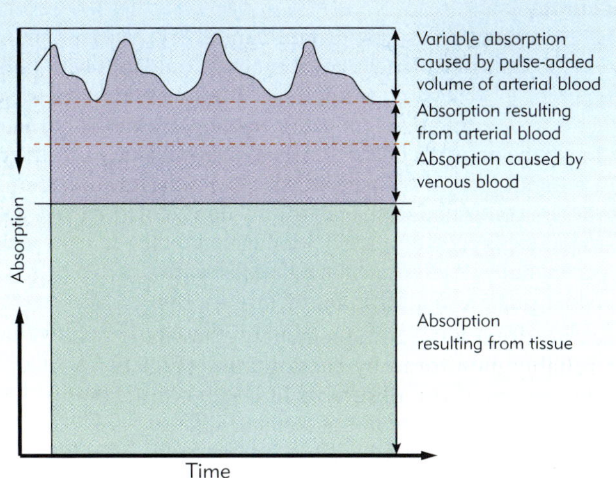

Figure 15.8 Tissue composite showing dynamic and static components that affect light absorption during pulse oximetry. (Adapted with permission from Ohmeda 3700, Pulse oximeter users manual, 1989.)

A typical pulse oximeter calibration algorithm

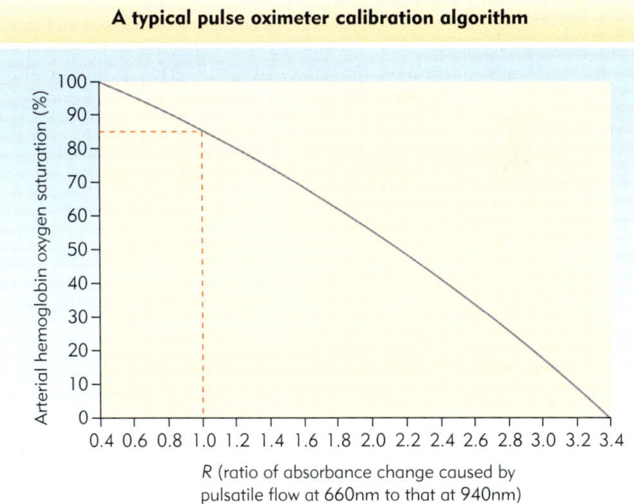

Figure 15.9 A typical pulse oximeter calibration algorithm. Arterial hemoglobin O_2 saturation is plotted against the ratio of the proportional increase in absorbance caused by pulsatile flow at 660nm to that at 940nm (*R*). The value of *R* varies from roughly 0.5 at 100% saturation to 3.4 at 0% saturation. An *R* value of 1.0 corresponds to 85%. Although a similar curve can be derived from the Lambert–Beer law, this curve is actually a composite of experimental data obtained on healthy adult volunteers. (Adapted with permission from Pologe, 1987.)

plethysmographic display on some oximeters has also been used to verify collateral circulation prior to arterial cannulation, or as an aid to estimate systolic blood pressure using loss or return of the signal associated with blood pressure cuff inflation and deflation, respectively.

Accuracy

The 'gold standard' for confirming clinical Spo_2 measurements is *in vitro* multiwavelength co-oximetry. Compared with pulse oximeters, laboratory co-oximeters utilize four additional wavelengths to determine functional or fractional hemoglobin saturation in the presence of abnormal hemoglobins such as carboxy- or methemoglobin. A suspiciously elevated saturation should always be confirmed with a laboratory determination. It is wise to request a direct saturation determination rather than the usual reported one, which is calculated based on Pao_2.

Most pulse oximeter manufacturers claim an accuracy of ±2% for Spo_2 values between 70 and 100% and ±3% for values between 50 and 70%. Accuracy progressively decreases for lower values. When functioning properly, and especially if set in the fast-response mode, the pulse oximeter efficiently warns of dangerous decreases in Pao_2. This is possible because of the nearly linear correlation between Pao_2 and Spo_2, when Pao_2 <60mmHg or less. A rule of thumb is that for Spo_2 below 90%, the $Pao_2 = Spo_2 - 30$. Importantly, at high Pao_2, a significant decrease in Pao_2 (e.g. 400 to 100mmHg) will not be obvious, as in both cases the Spo_2 is 100%.

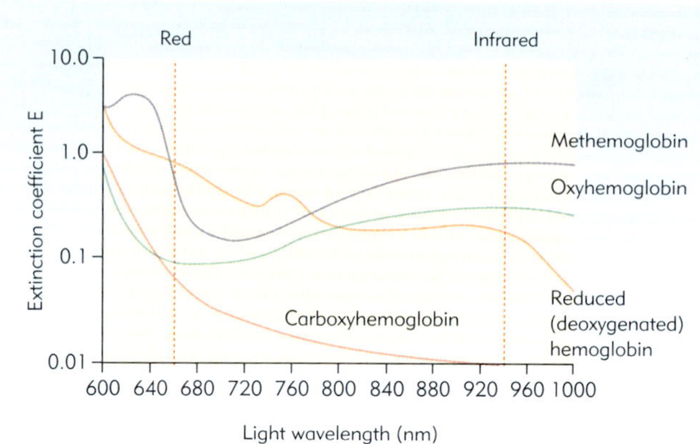

Figure 15.10 Variation in extinction coefficient with wavelength for four common hemoglobin species. The absorbance of carboxyhemoglobin is very similar to that of oxyhemoglobin in the visible red wavelengths. Methemoglobin has a high absorbance over a broad spectrum, giving it a characteristic brown color. (With permission from Tremper and Barker, 1987.)

Key References

Eichhorn JH. Prevention of intraoperative anesthesia accidents and related severe injury through safety monitoring. Anesthesiology. 1989; 70:572–7.

Eisenkraft JB, Raemer DB. Monitoring gases in the anesthesia delivery system. In: Ehrenworth J, Eisenkraft JB, eds. Anesthesia equipment. Principles and applications. St Louis, MO: Mosby;1993:201–3.

Good ML. Capnography: uses, interpretations, and pitfalls. In: Barash PG, Deutsch S, Tinker JH, eds. ASA refresher courses in anesthesiology, Vol. 18. Philadelphia, PA: Lippincott; 1991 179-90.

Moller JT, Johannessen NW, Expersen K, et al. Randomized evaluation of pulse oximetry in 20,802 patients. II. Perioperative events and postoperative complications. Anesthesiology. 1993; 78:445–53.

Raemer DB. Monitoring respiratory function. In: Rogers MC, Tinker JH, Covino BG, Longnecker DE, ed. Principles and practice of anesthesiology. St Louis, MO: Mosby; 1992.

Standards for Basic Anesthetic Monitoring. Park Ridge, IL: American Society of Anesthesiologists. 1998:439.

Tremper KK, Barker SJ. Pulse oximetry: applications and limitations. In: Tremper KK, Barker SJ, eds. International anesthesiology clinics. Advances in oxygen monitoring. Boston, MA: Little, Brown; 1987:155–175.

Westenskow DR, Smith KN, Coleman DL, Gregonis DL, van Wagenan RA. Clinical evaluation of a Raman scattering multiple gas analyzer for the operating room. Anesthesiology. 1989;70:350–3.

Further Reading

Barker SJ, Tremper KK, Hyatt J. Effects of methemoglobinemia on pulse oximetry and mixed venous oximetry. Anesthesiology. 1989;70:112–17.

Falk JL, Rackow EC, Weil MH. End-tidal carbon dioxide concentration during cardiopulmonary resuscitation. N Engl J Med. 1988;310:607–11.

Guyton DC, Gravenstein N. Infrared analysis of volatile anesthetics: Impact of monitor agent setting, volatile mixtures and alcohol. J Clin Monit. 1990; 6:203.

Matjasko MJ, Petrozza P, McKenzie CF. Sensitivity of end-tidal nitrogen in venous air embolism detection in dogs. Anesthesiology. 1985;63:418–23.

Ohmeda 3700. Pulse oximeter user's manual. Madison, WI: Ohmeda, BOC Group; 1989:22.

Pologe JA. Pulse oximetry: technical aspects of machine design. In: Tremper KK, Barker SJ, eds. International anesthesiology clinics. Advances in oxygen monitoring. Boston, MA: Little, Brown; 1987:142–54.

Sanders AB, Kern KB, Otto CW, Milander MM, Ewy GA. Carbon dioxide monitoring during cardiopulmonary resuscitation: a prognostic indicator for survival. J Am Med Assoc. 1989; 262:1347–51.

Scheller MS, Unger RJ, Kelner MJ. Effects of intravenously administered dyes on pulse oximeter readings. Anesthesiology. 1986;65:550–2.

Severinghaus JW, Spellman MJ Jr. Pulse oximeter failure thresholds in hypotension and vasoconstriction. Anesthesiology. 1990;73:532–7.

Chapter 16 Ultrasonography and other monitoring techniques

Nitin Shah

Topics covered in this chapter

Ultrasonography
Transcranial doppler
Transesophageal enchocardiography
Measurement of temperature
Measurement of humidity
Standards for basic anesthetic monitoring

ULTRASONOGRAPHY

Principles

Medical imaging in diagnostic ultrasound (US) utilizes the pulse–echo technique. This is different from other forms of medical imaging in that it uses information that is reflected back toward the source that generated the energy. In contrast, in X-ray (roentgenography) or computed tomography imaging, transmitted energy is imaged; that is the X-ray tube is on one side and the film or sensor is on the other side of the patient.

The reflected technique consists of a crystal that sends pulses of energy (sound waves) into the patient, which are reflected at different interfaces within the patient. Most of the energy passes through the various interfaces, but a small percentage of energy at each interface is reflected back toward the transducer. When this reflected wave reaches the transducer it is translated by the transducer into a very small voltage. Therefore, the US transducer acts as both a transmitter and a receiver of sound. This is possible because of piezoelectric properties of the transducer, which occur when the transducer is in the receiving mode.

Sound waves of frequencies in the range 1–30MHz are utilized by US. The pulse of electricity that generates a pulse of US is usually in the range 1–300V and lasts <1μsec. The time between pulses is long enough that all of the returning echoes, even those from the deepest part of the patient, have adequate time to return to the surface of the patient and reach the transducer while it is operating in its receiving mode.

Most US units pulse the transducer at 500–3000 times/second, which is called the pulse repetition frequency. It mechanically deforms and produces vibration of a crystal housed in a hand-held transducer or probe. The example of a transducer pulsing at 1000 times/second illustrates the long listening time used in diagnostic US. A transducer is pulsed for approximately two to three cycles, which lasts only 5–6μsec. After that time, the transducer is damped out and quietly listens for reflected echoes. For a unit that pulses at 1000 times/second, the time between each pulse is 1msec. Therefore, the transducer vibrates in the transmit mode for 5 or 6μsec and listens in the receive mode approximately 99.4% of the time. The short pulsing time (0.6%) means that very little energy enters the patient during the time the transducer is on the patient's skin. Because of the long listening period (99.4%), real-time scanning is possible.

Modes of scanning

The images formed from the echoes received by the transducer may be displayed in three ways – A-mode, B-mode, and C-mode.

The *A-mode* (amplitude mode) image was the earliest display form of US. It consists of an oscilloscope mapping of the received voltage on the y-axis and time on the x-axis. Since the velocity of sound in soft tissue is nearly uniform, the relationship between time and distance is linear. Therefore, the x-axis also represents distance. Figure 16.1a shows an A-mode display representing a vessel in the body surrounded by soft tissue with bone behind it.

The *B-mode* (brightness mode) image shows a two-dimensional, cross-sectional spatial representation of the examined tissue on the horizontal and vertical axes. Images are formed by assigning a degree of grayness to voltage amplitude values and displaying these gray levels on an image. For each A-line, the distance from the transducer can be computed from the time it takes for an echo to return. The amount of voltage generated in the transducer by the returning wave is read as a shade of gray and displayed on a television monitor in the position computed from the depth of the returning echo and position of the transducer when the echo was received. The transducer, constrained to move in a single plane, travels over the body of a patient, generating A-lines as it moves. Each pulse fills in another line of gray values. Most noncardiac imaging is B-mode imaging (Fig. 16.1b).

The *M-mode* (motion mode) technique is used in echocardiography, usually in conjunction with B-mode images; M-mode images are generated rapidly enough to image the heart, and are called real-time images. During the generation of M-mode images, the transducer is held against the body as the heart beats; movement in the body is imaged by recording the changes of reflecting surfaces over time (Fig. 16.1c). One axis of the image represents the distance of reflecting surfaces from the transducer and the other axis represents movement of these surfaces over time. If the surfaces do not move, M-mode imaging displays straight lines parallel to the face of the transducer. The strength

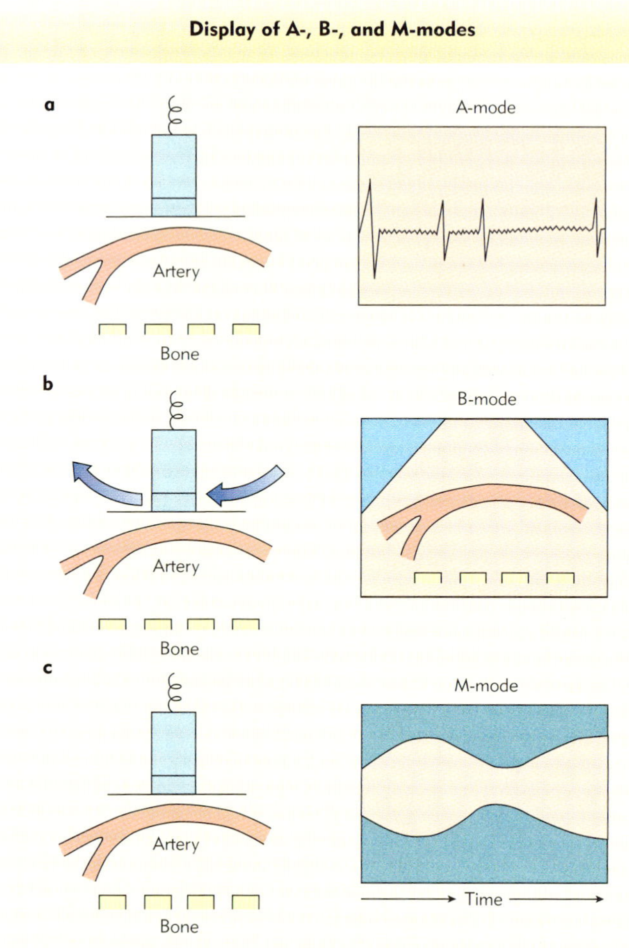

Figure 16.1 Display of A, B, and M modes. (a) A-mode imaging displays an artery as two amplitude spikes that separate slightly with each pulsation. (b) B-mode imaging creates a two-dimensional image of the artery on x and y axes. (c) M-mode imaging displays only one section of the artery over time. The pulsation of the walls of the artery is shown on the y-axis; time is shown on the x-axis. (Redrawn, with permission of Mosby, Inc., from Sarti DA. Diagnostic ultrasound: text and cases, 2nd edn. Chicago: Year Book Medical Publishers: 1987.)

of returning echoes is translated into voltage amplitudes, which are displayed as gray levels (as they are for B-mode images).

Visualization of adjacent tissues is improved when the difference between their acoustic textures is greatest. For example, differentiation of moving blood in the common carotid artery or internal jugular vein from the adjacent sternocleidomastoid musculature is clearer than differentiation of liver from adjacent kidney, given the smaller difference in echo texture of the latter.

As a general principle, the higher the frequency of the transducer, the higher the resolution of the image of superficial soft tissues, but the shallower the sound beam penetrates. Conversely, the lower the transducer's frequency, the deeper the sound beam penetrates. In the case of carotid US, a high-frequency transducer is optimal.

Advantages of US include relatively low cost, documented safety, and noninvasiveness. However, US sensitivity for lesion detection is operator dependent.

TRANSCRANIAL DOPPLER

Use of a low-frequency (2MHz) pulsed wave results in insonation through the temporal bone. The Doppler effect enables determination of blood flow and its direction based on Equation 16.1, in which v is the blood velocity, F_d the Doppler shift frequency, s the speed of sound, F_t the transducer frequency, and cos α the cosine of the angle between the sound beam and blood flow.

Equation 16.1

$$v = \frac{(F_d s)}{(2 F_t \cos \alpha)}$$

Equation 16.1 is used to calculate flow velocities from changes in Doppler frequencies. By evaluating the flow velocity spectrum of the cerebral arteries, it can provide information on cerebral hemodynamics, including direction of flow, patency of vessels, focal stenosis, and cerebrovascular reactivity. Spectral analysis of the Doppler signal is displayed on an oscilloscope as a wave of time versus velocity. Blood flow velocity varies proportionately with cerebral blood flow as long as the vessel diameter remains constant. Autoregulation of cerebral blood flow in response to changes in carbon dioxide or cerebral perfusion pressure occurs at the arteriolar level, which leaves the arteries measured by transcranial Doppler (TCD) relatively stable.

The strength of the signal is proportional to the cosine of the angle of insonation; therefore, a maximal velocity profile is attained when the angle of insonation is directly in line with the flow in the artery. The analysis that is generated contains peak systolic, end diastolic, and mean velocities along with a pulsatility index. Pulsatility index is considered an indirect measure of downstream resistance.

Examination of the cerebral vessels is performed through the use of transtemporal, transorbital, and posterior approaches or 'windows' (Fig. 16.2a). The transtemporal approach is usually used to assess cerebral arteries, as it allows visualization of the middle cerebral artery. Figure 16.2b represents a typical display of the signal. The transorbital approach reveals the flow from the ophthalmic artery and also identifies the carotid siphon. The posterior approaches (transforaminal and submandibular) visualize both vertebral arteries and the length of the basilar artery.

Hematocrit, arterial partial pressure of carbon dioxide, body temperature, regional brain activation, and level of consciousness affect TCD velocities. The absolute values determined by TCD are less valuable than the comparison of bilateral flows and changes in flow that occur over time.

TRANSESOPHAGEAL ENCHOCARDIOGRAPHY

Technical difficulty with transthoracic echocardiography in very obese patients or those who have extremely muscular chest walls led to the development of transesophageal echocardiography (TEE). The location of the esophagus immediately posterior to the heart permits a transducer position that circumvents US penetration through air, bone, fat, and muscle. Frazin in 1976

Transcranial Doppler ultrasonography

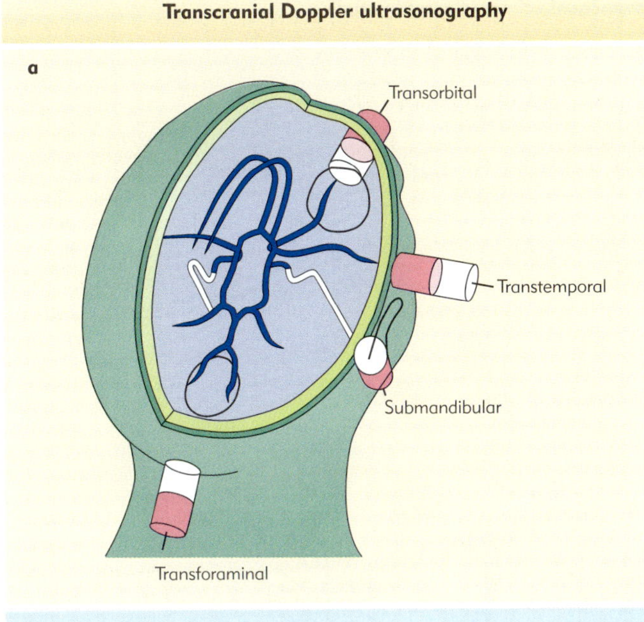

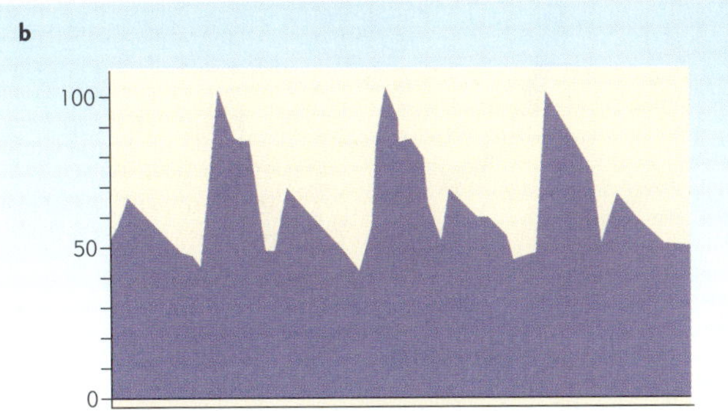

Figure 16.2 Transcranial Doppler ultrasonography. (a) Windows of the skull for transcranial Doppler ultrasonography – some natural acoustic windows through which ultrasonic beam penetration into the calvarium can occur with minimal beam attenuation. (b) Typical middle cerebral artery Doppler spectral display when the sample volume is centered on the straight segment of the vessel. [(a) Redrawn and (b) reproduced, with permission, from Fujioka KA, Douville CM. Anatomy and freehand examination techniques. In: Newell DW, Aaslid R, eds. Transcranial Doppler. New York: Raven; 1992.]

first used TEE, employing an M-mode transducer in patients in whom transthoracic echocardiography had been unsatisfactory. In 1980 Matsumo and colleagues reported intraoperative use of TEE. In 1987, color flow imaging was incorporated into the TEE imaging system which enabled the user to obtain information about blood flow in addition to cardiac morphology. In 1989, Omoto and colleagues reported the development of a biplane TEE probe, and in 1991 an omniplane probe became commercially available.

The transmitter and transducer are the two main components of TEE instruments. The transmitter is a complex device that controls the pulse repetition frequency and duration of the emitted US pulses, processes the returning signals, and displays the resultant image; the transducer physically contacts the patient to emit and receive the US signals.

The transmitter, known as an echocardiograph, emits an ultrasonic signal and manipulates the reflected signals to generate an image. The complex signal processing involves conversion of a radiofrequency signal into a video display.

Early echocardiograms were recorded simply to locate structures and to observe their motion, and so little variation in brightness was incorporated in the display. This permitted imaging within a relatively narrow dynamic range, that is the spectrum of signals (in decibels) that can be detected by the instrument, with those above and below the range discarded. The dynamic range required to record gray scale is much greater than the capacity of the instrument, a problem resolved by logarithmic compression of the range. Gray scale can be enhanced or accentuated by digital processing.

The system or master-gain control increases the intensity of all returning echoes, bringing more of them into the dynamic range. The time-gain compensation, on the other hand, selectively enhances echoes that are reflected by the deepest structures.

The primary component of the transducer is a piezoelectric element, a substance that expands and contracts in the presence of an electric field as the current changes polarity. The TEE transducers are miniaturized and affixed to the tip of a gastroscope for esophageal placement. M-mode echocardiography can be performed with a single crystal and is often recorded simultaneously with two-dimensional echocardiography by using one element of the two-dimensional array. The technologic evolution of TEE transducers has been rapid. In the newest instruments, with omniplane capability, the omniplane rotates from the horizontal plane at 0° to the vertical plane at 90° and then to a left–right reversed horizontal plane at 180°. This capability enables imaging of virtually any structure of the heart in multiple planes. Its only limitation remains the size of its tip, which must pass without difficulty into the esophagus of most adults.

Classically, transthoracic echocardiograms are made from various positions on or around the chest, known as 'windows'. The necessity of imaging through echocardiographic windows results from the very poor transmission of US through air and bone. Ribs, sternum, and lung tissue all must be avoided to produce a technically satisfactory transthoracic image. Hence the initial development of TEE was to circumvent these obstructions. Standard nomenclature has developed to describe the images obtained transthoracically, and has been adapted to describe TEE images. The major conventional two-dimensional views lie in one of three planes – basal short axis, four chamber or long axis, and transgastric short axis (Fig. 16.3). An image inversion switch, incorporated into the echocardiograph, allows the fan to be displayed with the apex at either the top or bottom of the monitor.

In patients undergoing cardiac and noncardiac surgery, TEE is used as an intraoperative monitor as well as a diagnostic tool. Intraoperative uses include:

- detection of air embolism;
- evaluation of signs of myocardial ischemia;
- determination of cardiac preload;
- assessment of ventricular function;
- assessment of valve structure and function;
- assessment of shunts and septal repairs; and
- diagnosis of intracardiac masses such as myxomas or thrombus.

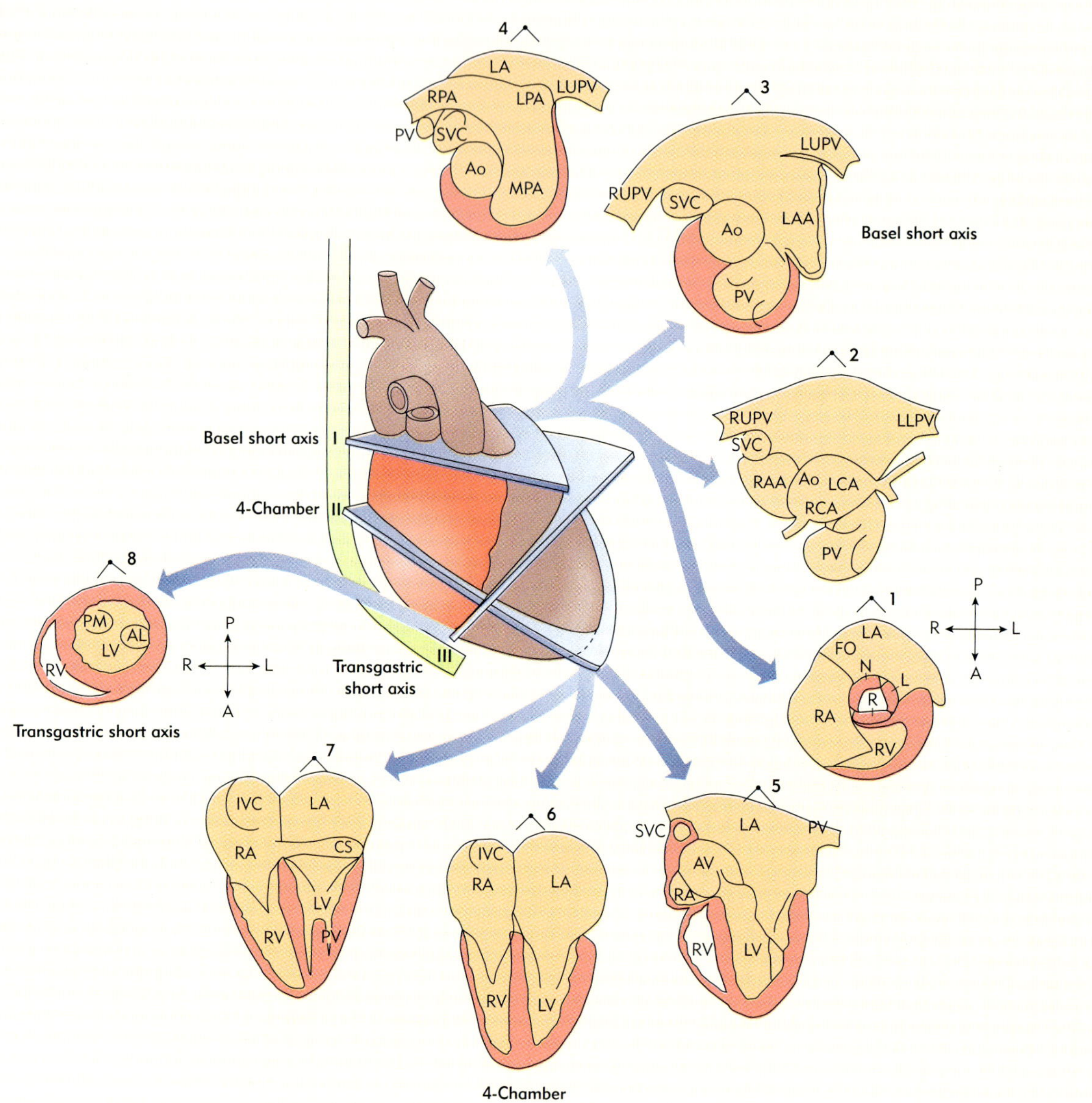

Figure 16.3 Common horizontal scan planes for transesophageal echocardiography studies. (I) Basal short-axis: (1) aortic root, (2) coronary arteries, (3) left atrial appendage, (4) pulmonary artery bifurcation. (II) Four-chamber (long-axis): (5) left ventricular outflow tract, (6) four-chamber view, (7) coronary sinus. (III) Transgastric short-axis: (8) ventricular short axis. (AL, anterolateral papillary muscle; Ao, aorta; AV, aortic valve; CS, coronary sinus; FO, fossa ovalis; IVC, inferior vena cava; L, left coronary cusp; LA, left atrium; LAA, left atrial appendage; LCA, left coronary artery; LLPV, left lower pulmonary vein; LPA, left pulmonary artery; LUPV, left upper pulmonary vein; LV, left ventricle; MPA, main pulmonary artery; N, noncoronary cusp; PM, posteriomedial papillary muscles; PV, pulmonary valve or pulmonary vein; R; right coronary cusp; RA, right atrium; RAA, right atrial appendage; RCA, right coronary artery; RLPV, right lower pulmonary vein; RPA, right pulmonary artery; RUPV, right upper pulmonary vein; RV, right ventricle; SVC, superior vena cava.) (Redrawn with permission from Seward, *et al.*)

Nonoperative uses include evaluation for:

- inadequate chest wall study;
- low cardiac output;
- tamponade;
- acute valve dysfunction;
- vegetations; and
- atral thrombus.

MEASUREMENT OF TEMPERATURE

Measurement of temperature was initiated by an English surgeon, John Hunter, in 1776 by using a mercury-in-glass thermometer placed under the tongue. Harvey Cushing in 1895 made temperature monitoring part of the anesthetic record.

Physiology

Usually an equilibrium exists between the amount of body heat generated by metabolism and the amount lost to the environment. Heat production occurs by means of cellular metabolism, which can be affected by basal metabolic rate, muscular activity, sympathetic arousal, hormonal activity, and heat administered exogenously. Heat loss occurs by radiation, conduction, convection, and evaporation. The majority of heat loss from a patient occurs by radiation (<60%), which is affected by cutaneous vasodilatation. Evaporation accounts for 25%, while convection accounts for 12%, and about 3% of heat is lost from the body by conduction (Chapter 64).

Control of the mechanisms of heat production and heat loss resides in the hypothalamus – warming or cooling the hypothalamus elicits the appropriate physiologic responses. Anesthesia upsets thermal control in two ways:

- direct inhibition of the hypothalamus results in less effective feedback control via this organ; and
- peripheral vasodilatation redistributes body heat and increases heat loss.

The sites for temperature monitoring are dictated by the procedure and patient considerations. The lower esophageal temperature approximates cerebral temperature in closed chest cases. Nasopharyngeal temperatures reflect the temperature of blood in the cartoid artery when properly placed, but precise placement is difficult. rectal temperature may not reflect core temperature, and rectal probes are easily dislodged. Skin temperature monitored by an axillary probe is convenient, but is typically 0.5°C less than oral and 1°C less than rectal temperature. With hypothermia induced during cardiopulmonary bypass, temperature mnitoring is critical, particularly during rewarming when hyperthermia must be avoided. Pulmonary artery and in-line blood temperatures are monitored, along with at least one other site, often the bladder, as an index of core temperature. Ischemic damage to the brain is greatly enhanced by hyperthermia during active rewarming, suggesting that nasopharyngeal temperature should be monitored as an index of cerebral temperature due to the marked regional temperature gradients, and that inflow temperature is kept below 39°C.

Technology

The two most commonly used electrical thermometers are the thermistor and the thermocouple. Electrical resistance of the thermistor varies as a function of temperature. The principle of a thermocouple is that if a circuit is made up of two dissimilar metal elements, the current in the circuit is directly proportional to the temperature difference between the two junctions of the dissimilar metals.

Infrared sensors are another type of thermometer, used to measure the temperature of the tympanic membrane. The response time of this type of thermometer is <5s. Two disadvantages of using this type of probe are:

- only intermittent spot checks can be made; and
- the probe must be accurately aimed at the tympanic membrane – false low readings off the sides of the ear canal can be a problem.

Liquid crystal thermometers employ a liquid crystal adhesive strip attached to the skin. Although the adhesive strip changes color with temperature, liquid crystal temperature correlates poorly with tympanic membrane temperature. Liquid crystal thermometry is an excellent example of how the novelty and convenience of a new technology often smothers its lack of usefulness in clinical care.

MEASUREMENT OF HUMIDITY

'Humidity' is a measure of the amount of water vapor present in a gas or a gas mixture, and may be expressed in a number of ways, such as dew point temperature or partial pressure. The definition of absolute humidity is 'mass of water vapor per unit volume of dry gas' (i.e. mg H_2O/L). Relative humidity is the ratio of the actual water vapor pressure to the saturation vapor pressure at a given temperature.

Most materials, whether natural or synthetic, react to the humidity of the atmosphere, as reflected by changes in physical, electrical, and chemical properties. Consequently, quantification of such changes may enable the humidity of the ambient atmosphere to be assessed. Measurement of humidity in respiratory or anesthetic gases has been carried out using a wide variety of measurement techniques and apparatus designs. The inherent difficulty is that the gases flow with continually changing velocities, which results in considerable variations in temperature and humidity during inspiration and expiration. A number of techniques can be used to measure humidity.

- Gravimetric hygrometer (weight of absorbed moisture) – a problem with the application of this principle to anesthetic gases is the impossibility of measuring gas volume exactly.
- Dew point hygrometry is based on measurement of the temperature at which moisture condenses out of the atmosphere, a condition commonly observed. At the dew point or frost point, the gas mixture is saturated with respect to water (or ice). Dynamic equilibrium occurs between the water (or ice) film on the cooled surface and water in the vapor phase. The saturation partial pressure of the condensate is equal to the water vapor partial pressure in the gas. One refinement of the technique is the photoelectric detection of dew formation on a mirror surface. Application of thermoelectric cooling to control the mirror temperature at the saturation temperature provides reliable and continuous measurement.
- Mass spectrometry is a complex and expensive technique; errors are introduced because of condensation of water vapor in the sampling system.
- Spectroscopic hygrometers – a number of absorption bands that characterize the water molecule fall into the infrared region (1–10μm). The response of these infrared analyzers is fast and sensitivity is high.

- Electrical hygrometry – variation in ambient relative humidity can produce a change of resistance in materials such as hygroscopic salts, carbon powder, ceramic materials, etc. The materials are usually applied as a film over an insulating substrate and are terminated by metal electrodes. Response time is slow, with a setting time of 5–10 minutes.

Measurement of water content of anesthetic gases is an appropriate approach to the assessment of airway climate. It does, however, require meticulous attention to avoid methodologic pitfalls. Clinically applicable techniques are scarce and a thorough understanding of their limitations is crucial for the interpretation of measured values. The use of reduced, fresh gas flow rates ('minimal flow') is a most appropriate means to improve airway climate. It offers a viable alternative to the use of heat and moisture exchangers in prolonged anesthesia and in patients who have respiratory complications. Significant damage to tracheobronchial epithelia is known to be caused by inadequate airway climatization and must be regarded as an avoidable complication of anesthesia.

STANDARDS FOR BASIC ANESTHETIC MONITORING

Until the past few years, major intraoperative anesthesia 'critical incidents' (such as an esophageal intubation or disconnection of the breathing system from the endotracheal tube connector underneath the drapes) often went unrecognized until marked cyanosis developed, followed quickly by arrhythmias and preterminal bradycardia. As the 'event' was well developed by the time it was recognized, very little time was left to diagnose and treat the problem before the patient injury occurred. Hence monitors were needed that gave early warning of problems. The original impetus for formal standards of practice grew out of a risk management committee at the Harvard Medical School, formed in response to a significant concern from Harvard's malpractice insurance company about the great expense of anesthesia-caused patient injury and death claims. They found the incidence of severe intraoperative events to be 1/75,700 between 1976 and 1984 in American Society of Anesthesiologists (ASA) class I and II patients, which is low compared with the widely believed mortality rate of 1/10,000. In early 1985, all nine Harvard teaching hospitals adopted the original standards. The original ASA *Standards for Basic Intraoperative Monitoring* were adopted unanimously by the ASA in 1986. Many amendments have been made to the original standards and the latest version is given below.

Given the nature of the complex technical environment in which anesthesia is administered today and the fallibility of humans who function in that environment, it is impossible to even suggest that critical incidents will be eliminated, or even dramatically decreased. In spite of all the advances, breathing system connectors will still become accidentally disconnected from endotracheal tubes, esophageal intubations will occur, breathing system tubing and endotracheal tubes will be kinked or internally obstructed, and oxygen supplies will occasionally fail. Monitoring does not prevent everything, but correct responses to a much earlier warning of an adverse development during anesthesia offered by monitoring can and do prevent severe intraoperative anesthesia accidents.

The monitoring standards have evolved as the most discussed and the best recognized element of the safety movement. To determine whether safety monitoring has made a difference, several different studies were carried out and the results published. The ASA Closed Claims Study is the most comprehensive retrospective analysis. In that study, among the adverse outcomes associated with respiratory events, 72% were judged by the reviewers as being preventable with better monitoring and nearly all of the 'inadequate ventilation' and 'esophageal intubation' cases would have been prevented. Predictably, the 'proper use' of the combination of pulse oximetry and capnography was 'deemed useful' in preventing the adverse outcome in over half the total cases. The British Confidential Enquiry into Perioperative Deaths is another such study. In this 1987 publication, the death rate solely attributable to anesthesia was 1/185,000; much lower than the long-accepted idea that anesthesia mortality was 1/10,000 to 1/20,000.

The only truly prospective trial of any part of the principles of safety monitoring is the Danish study of pulse oximetry in 20,802 patients. This effort focused specifically on pulse oximetry and any difference in outcome in approximately 10,000 who underwent pulse oximetry during and following their anesthesia versus 10,000 who did not. The rate of diagnosis of hypoxemia, of course, was much higher in the monitored group but, fundamentally, no major 'statistically significant' improvement in outcome was found in the monitored group. This does not mean that pulse oximetry should be abandoned; maybe an even larger population is required to find a statistically significant difference. While certainly provocative, the Danish study clearly reinforces the previously stated notion that it is physically impossible to execute a definitive prospective study to evaluate safety monitoring in traditional terms.

ASA standards for basic intraoperative monitoring

Under extenuating circumstances, the responsible anesthesiologist may waive the requirements marked with an asterisk (*).

Standard I

Qualified anesthesia personnel shall be present in the room throughout the conduct of all general anesthetics, regional anesthetics, and monitored anesthesia care.

Objective

As there are rapid changes in patient status during anesthesia, qualified anesthesia personnel shall be continuously present to monitor the patient and provide anesthesia care. In the event of a direct known hazard (e.g. radiation) to the anesthesia personnel that might require intermittent remote observation of the patient, some provision for monitoring the patient must be made. In the event that an emergency requires the temporary absence of the person primarily responsible for the anesthetic, the best judgment of the anesthesiologist will be exercised in comparing the emergency with the anesthetized patient's condition and in the selection of the person left responsible for the anesthetic during the temporary absence.

Standard II

During all anesthetics, the patient's oxygenation, ventilation, circulation, and temperature shall be continually evaluated

Oxygenation

Objective

To ensure adequate oxygen concentration in the inspired gas and the blood during all anesthetics.

Methods

- Inspired gas: during every administration of general anesthesia using an anesthesia machine, the concentration of oxygen in the patient breathing system shall be measured by an oxygen analyzer with a low oxygen concentration limit alarm in use.*
- Blood oxygenation: during all anesthetics, a quantitative method of assessing oxygenation such as pulse oximetry shall be employed.* Adequate illumination and exposure of the patient are necessary to assess color.*

Ventilation

Objective

To ensure adequate ventilation of the patient during all anesthetics.

Methods

- Every patient receiving general anesthesia shall have the adequacy of ventilation continually evaluated. While qualitative clinical signs such as chest excursion, observation of the reservoir breathing bag, and auscultation of breath sounds may be useful, quantitative monitoring of the carbon dioxide content and/or volume of expired gas is strongly encouraged.
- When an endotracheal tube or laryngeal mask is inserted, its correct positioning must be verified by clinical assessment and by identification of carbon dioxide in the expired gas. Continual end-tidal carbon dioxide analysis, in use from the time of endotracheal tube/laryngeal mask placement until extubation/removal or initiating transfer to a postoperative care location, shall be performed using a quantitative method such as capnography, capnometry, or mass spectroscopy.*
- When ventilation is controlled by a mechanical ventilator, there shall be in continuous use a device that is capable of detecting disconnection of components of the breathing system. The device must give an audible signal when its alarm threshold is exceeded.
- During regional anesthesia and monitored anesthesia care, the adequacy of ventilation shall be evaluated, at least, by continual observation of qualitative clinical signs.

Circulation

Objective

To ensure the adequacy of the patient's circulatory function during all anesthetics.

Methods

- Every patient receiving anesthesia shall have the electrocardiogram continuously displayed from the beginning of anesthesia until preparing to leave the anesthetizing location.*
- Every patient receiving anesthesia shall have arterial blood pressure and heart rate determined and evaluated at least every 5 minutes.*
- Every patient receiving general anesthesia shall have, in addition to the above, circulatory function continually evaluated by at least one of the following: palpation of a pulse, auscultation of heart sounds, monitoring of a tracing of intra-arterial pressure, US peripheral pulse monitoring, or pulse plethysmography or oximetry.

Body temperature

Objective

To aid in the maintenance of appropriate body temperature during all anesthetics.

Methods

There shall be readily available means to continuously measure the patient's temperature. When changes in body temperature are intended, anticipated, or suspected, the temperature shall be measured.

Key References

Bunegin L. Monitoring technology: capnography, intracranial pressure, precordial Doppler and transcranial Doppler. In: Albin MS, ed. Textbook of neuroanesthesia with neurosurgical and neuroscience perspectives. San Francisco: McGraw-Hill; 1997:277–324.

Cork RC. Temperature monitoring. In: Blitt CD, Hines RL, eds. Monitoring in anesthesia and critical care medicine. New York: Churchill Livingstone; 1995:543–56.

Cork RC, Vaughan RW, Humphrey LS. Precision and accuracy of intraoperative temperature monitoring. Anesth Analg. 1983;62:211–1020.

Eichhorn JH. Monitoring and patient safety. In: Blitt CD, Hines RL, eds. Monitoring in anesthesia and critical care medicine. New York: Churchill Livingstone; 1995:55–69.

Heitmiller ES, Lima JAC, Humphrey LS. Transesophageal echocardiography. In: Blitt CD, Hines RL, eds. Monitoring in anesthesia and critical care medicine. New York: Churchill Livingstone; 1995:261–314.

Manno EM. Transcranial Doppler ultrasonography in the neurocritical care unit. In: Critical care clinics – update on neurologic critical care. Philadelphia: WB Saunders; 1997:79–104.

Sarti DA, Kimme-Smith C. Physics of diagnostic ultrasound. In: Sarti DA, ed. Diagnostic ultrasound text and cases. Chicago: Year Book Medical Publishers; 1987:1–24.

Vaughan MS, Cork RC, Vaughan RW. Inaccuracy of liquid crystal thermometry to identify core temperature trends in postoperative adults. Anesth Analg. 1982;61:284–7.

Further Reading

Eichhorn JH, Cooper JB, Cullen DJ, et al. Standards for patient monitoring during anesthesia at Harvard Medical School. JAMA. 1986;256:1017–20.

Kleemann PP. Humidity of anesthetic gases with respect to low flow anesthesia. Anesth Intensive Care. 1994;22:396–408.

Moller JT, Pederson T, Rasmussen LS, et al. Randomized evaluation of pulse oximetry in 20,802 patients. II. Perioperative events and postoperative complications. Anesthesiology. 1993;79:445–53.

Muzzi DA, Lasasso TJ, Black S, et al. Comparison of a transesophageal and precordial ultrasonic Doppler sensor in the detection of venous air embolism. Anesth Analg. 1990;70:103–4.

Sessler DI. Temperature monitoring. In: Miller RD, ed. Anesthesia. New York: Churchill Livingstone; 1990:1227–42.

Seward JB, Khandheria BK, Oh JK, et al. Transesophageal echocardiography: technique, anatomic correlations, implementation, and clinical applications. Mayo Clin Proc. 1988;63:649–80.

Chapter 17 Statistics

Emery N Brown and Paul R Barach

Topics covered in this chapter

Paradigm for statistical inference
Clinical trials
Prospective observational studies
Retrospective observational studies
Meta-analysis
Bayesian statistics
Appendix: summary of statistical models and tests

To understand and apply correctly new medical information, an anesthesiologist must be able to analyze the medical literature critically. Such critical evaluations require a solid understanding of the basic concepts of statistics. Statistics is the branch of mathematics that uses the laws of probability theory to make decisions under uncertainty. In addition to their application in medical study design and evaluation of the medical literature, statistical principles are used daily in anesthesiology to make patient management decisions when data are incomplete and information is uncertain. Emphasis in this chapter is on demonstrating how statistical principles are used to quantify and control uncertainty in order to insure the scientific validity of inferences made from medical data.

PARADIGM FOR STATISTICAL INFERENCE

Because the practice of anesthesiology involves many uncertainties it is no surprise that statistics has the potential for extensive application in this field. Statistical principles are generally applied in two ways in anesthesiology. The first way in which anesthetists apply statistical principles is to make medical decisions with incomplete and uncertain information. These decisions may include determining if tests results or monitor readings are reliable; formulating differential diagnoses of diseases given symptoms; physical findings and laboratory tests; predicting the most successful course of therapy for a patient with a given diagnosis; and deciding if there has been improvement in a patient's condition under the current treatment regimen. For example, suppose that during surgery a patient's blood pressure suddenly decreases. Possible causes of the fall in pressure include hypovolemia from an acute bleed, an acute myocardial infarction, a pulmonary embolism, inadvertent administration of a vasoactive drug, or a monitor error. In evaluating the clinical scenario, the anesthetist must make a decision about the reliability of the information being collected, the most likely cause of the fall in blood pressure, and the most appropriate therapy given the best guess about the former two issues. The immediacy of the situation does not allow the anesthetist to perform a formal statistical analysis of the problem. However, using the principles of statistical decision theory, it is possible to demonstrate that until the cause of the hypotension is definitively established, the anesthetist reasons under uncertainty using well defined statistical strategies.

The second way in which statistical principles are applied in anesthesiology is in the design of medical studies and the evaluation of information in the medical literature. Medical studies use statistical analyses to characterize uncertainty and to assess how well the findings of the study have been established. The assessment of uncertainty addresses a number of questions: Is the information provided in a medical study reliable? Has the effect of a new therapy been established with sufficient certainty to accept it as an improvement over the standard therapy or placebo? Is the study sufficiently well designed to allow the investigator to make an inference? Does the use of a new monitoring device reduce the risk of an unfavorable outcome or undesirable side effect? How likely are side effects to occur with a new therapy? Do the findings of a study apply to my patients? To answer these queries, the anesthetist must use statistical principles to determine when and to what extent medical information is scientifically valid.

The use of statistics in a medical investigation follows a five-step paradigm (Fig. 17.1). The scientific question is formulated by the investigator as a testable hypothesis based on observations in daily medical practice, preliminary findings from laboratory research or information reported in the medical literature. The validity of the hypothesis is evaluated by conducting a study under

Paradigm for statistical inference

- Formulation of the question to be investigated as a testable hypothesis
- Design of study experiments
- Collection of experimental data
- Analysis of experimental data
- Making inferences based on findings of experimental analysis

Figure 17.1 Paradigm for statistical inference.

a *null hypothesis*. The null hypothesis is the assumption that the proposed hypothesis is incorrect and the objective of the study is disprove the null hypothesis. This process is termed proof by falsification. To study the hypothesis that pulse oximetry use in the operating room and the post-anesthesia care unit reduces the number of untoward perioperative events, the null hypothesis is that no reduction occurs. The objective of the study is to show that pulse oximetry is associated with a decrease in untoward perioperative events and to quantify the reduction in perioperative morbidity attributable to its use.

Experimental design entails the use of statistical principles to devise a study that will answer the scientific question. During the design of the experiment, the investigator works in close collaboration with a statistician to decide the population to be studied, the data to be collected, and the statistical models and tests that will used be to make inferences from the experimental data. Determination of the study sample size is one of the most crucial parts of the study design and depends on four factors:

- the magnitude of the average improvement of the treatment over the control that is medically important to detect;
- the degree of certainty the investigators would like to have about the findings;
- the level of type I error, i.e., the probability of rejecting the null hypothesis when it is true; and
- the variability in the outcome data.

The degree of certainty the investigator would like to have about the findings from the study defines the power or, the probability of detecting a medically important difference between the treatment and control groups if it exists. The smaller the medically important difference the study must detect, the greater the number of subjects the study will require. Most statisticians recommend that no study be undertaken unless the power is at least 0.8. One minus the power is the type II error probability. The type II error is the probability of not rejecting the null hypothesis when it is false. The smaller the type I error, the smaller the likelihood of falsely concluding that a treatment is effective when it is not, and the greater the number of subjects the study must impanel. By convention, a type I error of no more than 0.05 is typical for medical studies. Biological (inter- and intra-individual) and measurement variability are the two primary sources of variability in medical study data. Greater data variability means more noise or uncertainty; consequently, the study will need more subjects to detect the postulated difference. In practice, the statistician determines the sample size by using formulae or computer programs to estimate how many subjects are needed to have at least a 0.8 probability of detecting a medically important difference for a given probability of type I error and anticipated level of data variability.

The statistician is the one who principally performs the study data analysis by applying the statistical models and tests chosen during the experimental design step. Commonly used statistical methods include means, standard deviations, standard errors, odds ratios, relative risk ratios, confidence intervals, Kaplan-Meier estimates, linear and logistic regression methods, and analysis of variance (ANOVA) models. Some of the more commonly used tests are the t, z and χ^2 and F tests (see 'Appendix'). The tests are used to determine how probable the experimental findings are if the null hypothesis is true. If the findings are highly probable then the null hypothesis is not rejected and the investigator concludes that the data from the current study do not support the study hypothesis. If the findings are highly improbable, i.e., they would not be likely to occur if the null hypothesis were true, the investigator can reject the null hypothesis and conclude that the data support the hypothesis of the study. Findings, which are highly improbable, are termed statistically significant and probability of rejecting the null hypothesis is the p value. In the final step, the investigator and the statistician review the data analysis findings and decide what scientific inferences and conclusions may be drawn from the study.

CLINICAL TRIALS

A clinical trial investigates whether a new medical treatment is more effective than a standard therapy or placebo. A clinical trial may be performed with or without a control group, and with or without random assignment of study participants to treatment.

Nonrandomized clinical trials

In a nonrandomized treatment assignment with no controls, subjects are believed to have a well-defined response to standard therapy. Biological variability among patients makes this assumption untenable except in a limited set of circumstances. A nonrandomized design can also use historical controls, which are patients treated at another time, possibly by another physician and at another institution. Use of historical controls introduces dissimilarity between the control and treatment groups. Observed differences in outcome between the treatment and control groups may be due to this dissimilarity and not to a true treatment effect. A third nonrandomized design uses internal or concurrent controls, i.e., controls who are chosen non-randomly but at the same time as the treatment group. This approach is also biased as the physician and/or the patient participates in the assignment to treatment because one or the other has a prejudice as to effectiveness of the therapy to be tested.

Randomized clinical trials

A randomized clinical trial has at least two groups that are completely comparable on average in terms of pre-study characteristics. One group receives the new treatment and the second receives the standard treatment or placebo. The assignment to the two groups is determined objectively by a random mechanism such as flipping a coin, drawing a number from a random number table or with the aid of a computer. Randomized clinical trials are the gold standard for scientific investigation of a medical question.

Many randomized clinical trials are phase III trials which have been designed from phase I and phase II trials. A phase I trial is an initial uncontrolled administration in humans of a new treatment used to establish the dosage regimen, evaluate toxicities, establish indications, and determine if there is sufficient information to warrant further study. A Phase II trial is a small scale controlled or uncontrolled trial aimed to establish whether a randomized clinical trial should be undertaken. A Phase III trial is performed after the indications and therapeutic regimen have been decided but before the therapy has become widely used. If a new drug or therapeutic device does not have market approval from appropriate government agencies [e.g., the United States Food and Drug Administration (FDA)] then deciding the timing of the randomized control trial is straightforward. Difficulties arise in deciding when to conduct a randomized control trial if an existing therapy has market approval. In this case, if sufficiently many patients or physicians have prejudices about how well the therapy works, it may be perceived as unethical to study it in a randomized trial. For example, many anesthetists would deem it unethical to study in a randomized control trial the efficacy of pulmonary artery catheter use in the management of patients undergoing abdominal aortic aneurysm repairs.

The first steps in designing a randomized trial are formulating the question as a testable hypothesis, choosing the population to be studied, and deciding the study sample size and its projected power (see above). A power analysis should be reported with every clinical trial and is a must in a trial that reports a negative result such as no difference in the effect of therapy between the treatment and control groups. Without a power analysis, a correct interpretation of a study with negative findings is that the investigation failed to detect the expected difference due to a lack of power. The design of a clinical trial must not only ensure that the study is technically feasible but also that it is ethically sound. As just mentioned, a study may be considered unethical if the medical community or general public has a substantial bias about the efficacy of the therapy to be studied. It would also be unethical to give a placebo to a control group if a standard therapy exists. Similarly, it would be unethical to ask subjects to submit to substantial risk in a clinical study without realistic expectation of important benefit at least for the population of patients the subjects represent.

The strength of the randomized clinical trial lies in the random assignment of the study participants to either treatment or control. Randomization ensures that assignment to treatment groups is achieved by an objective mechanism. Under random assignment the portion of subjects with both known and unknown characteristics or covariates that may affect the study outcome will be evenly distributed across the control and treatment groups. That is, subjects who are extremely ill and those who are less ill will be evenly distributed between the two groups. In addition to state of health, other important pre-study covariates include smoking history, concurrent medical therapies, age, race and gender. Random treatment assignment also prevents seen and unseen biases such as placing subjects who will benefit from a therapy in the treatment group, paying more careful attention to the treatment group or unconsciously changing a therapy. Inglefinger and colleagues write:

'We feel that random allocation of treatment is almost always a prerequisite for a convincing study. Without randomization, results are at best "suggestive". Randomization is so important that the method of randomization should be briefly described ... to lend credence to statements that treatment is random.'

In large clinical trials the law of large numbers (commonly termed the law of averages) reduces the chance of serious imbalance in the study covariates due to randomization. In small studies, simple randomization may yield substantial covariate imbalance and unplanned imbalance in the size of the treatment groups themselves. If the sample size analysis suggests that a small number of subjects will be required to detect a medically important difference then, *stratification* and *blocking* should be used to guard against covariate and group size imbalance. To do so, the investigator identifies important covariates during the design of the experiment (stratification) and randomly assigns a fixed proportion within each stratum (blocking). Stratification can reduce bias at the cost of some decrease in the precision with which the treatment effect is estimated. Blocking should always accompany stratification and the method of stratification should be described. Statistical modeling of the effect of covariates on the outcome can be used to estimate the impact on study conclusions of covariate imbalance that was not corrected by stratification and blocking. Statistical modeling applied in this way can increase the precision of the treatment effect estimate and reduce bias.

The objective of the subject selection process is to create a homogeneous pool of study participants. If the study subjects are chosen by random sample from the population of patients with a given disease, then the subjects are representative of that population. In practice, subjects selected for a clinical trial are usually volunteers who meet defined inclusion and exclusion criteria. They provide informed consent, have potential harms explained and have the right to leave the study at any time. Some clinical trials may have a run in period, i.e., a period during which the subject's participation in the trial is conditionally accepted so that the investigator can evaluate the likelihood of compliance with the therapeutic regimen and follow-up schedule. The clinical trial should give detailed discussion about the subject selection, the target population, time frame, inclusion and exclusion criteria, number of subjects lost to follow-up, number of subjects eliminated from the analysis and the impact of the eliminated subjects on the findings.

Blinding or *masking*, is important for ensuring the integrity of the data collection and the validity of the inferences made from the study. Single blind means the subject is unaware of treatment assignment whereas double blind, means both the subject and the investigators are unaware of the treatment assignment. Double blinding eliminates bias due to patient response, ancillary care and investigator evaluation. Patients being followed closely may receive exemplary care for other medical problems. A study physician may unconsciously apply one set of criteria to patients receiving care and another set to those not receiving care. Investigators may ignore adverse outcomes that would be unfavorable to the treatment they personally prefer. Blinding helps to ensure the objectivity of the assessment process and helps to remove the possibility that differences in compliance, follow-up and assessment of outcome will be affected by knowledge of treatment assignment.

The anesthetist interested in applying the findings of a clinical trial to patient care must finally assess the *internal* and *external validity* of the study. If a clinical trial is well designed and well executed, the conclusions are internally valid, i.e., they are valid for the study group. The generalizability or external validity of the study refers to the population of patients to which the findings may be extrapolated. The recommendations of DerSimonian and colleagues provide an organized framework for evaluating the findings from a randomized clinical trial and a useful guide for determining its internal validity (Fig. 17.2). The anesthetist's assessment of a study's external validity should be based primarily on how comparable is the study sample to the patients in his/her practice and to what extent he/she can deliver the therapy as administered in the study.

PROSPECTIVE OBSERVATIONAL STUDIES

Observational studies are either prospective or retrospective. In a prospective observational study the investigator collects data on the subjects prospectively, moving forward in time from a defined starting point. The objective of the study is to relate an exposure to a specific outcome or set of outcomes. Unlike randomized control trials, there is no treatment allocation; rather, allocation is governed by nature. This design is commonly used in epidemiological investigations. For example, an

Summary of design and analysis of a clinical trial

Eligibility criteria: the criteria for admission of patients to the trial

Admission before allocation: eligibility criteria were applied before knowledge of the specific treatment assignment has been obtained

Random allocation: statement that assignment to treatment was random

Method of randomization: the mechanism used to generate the random assigment

Patients' blindness to treatment: whether patients knew which treatment they were receiving

Blind assessment of outcome: whether the person assessing the outcome knew which treatment had been given

Treatment complications: the presence or absence of side effects or complications after treatment

Loss to follow-up: the number of patients lost to follow-up and the reasons they were lost

Statistical analyses: takes assessment beyond reporting of simple mean summaries

Statistical methods: discussed together with citation of a readable reference

Power of the study: the probability of detecting a medically important difference between the treatment and control groups; a power of at least 0.8 is recommended

Figure 17.2 Summary of design and analysis of a clinical trial. (Modified with permission from Der Simonian et al., 1992.)

important epidemiological question in anesthesiology is, does exposure to anesthetic gases lead to a higher incidence of miscarriage in female anesthetists than women in the general population? A prospective investigation of this question requires an observational study because of the obvious ethical problems with conducting a randomized clinical trial. This statement of the question defines the population at risk (female anesthetists); the exposure (anesthetic gases); and the outcome (miscarriage). The population at risk is female anesthetists and nurse anesthetists in their childbearing years because they are the women with the greatest exposure to anesthetic gases. Another definitions of the population at risk might include all female operating room personnel. The control sample for this study is drawn not from the general population but from the population of hospital-based female physicians and nurses not working in the operating room.

Once the question has been defined, the population at risk has been identified, the exposure defined and the outcome has been clearly stated, the study design is completed by performing a power and sample size analysis. The study begins by collecting background data on the subjects. The background data might include information such as age, race socio-economic status, level of schooling, martial status, tobacco, drug and alcohol use. Additional background data for this study include history of infertility, pregnancies, miscarriages and abortions. These data are used to control for heterogeneity in the cohort or study sample and to identify other factors that may also be associated with the propensity to miscarry.

The exposure, contact with inhaled anesthetic gases, is one of the most difficult quantities to determine. Relevant historical information to define exposure includes length of time working as anesthetist, type of work environment, type of anesthetic technique, and the fraction of time spent directly delivering anesthesia compared with time supervising residents and/or nurses. The subjects may be asked to keep logs of anesthetic drugs use by case, and to agree to regular measurements of exposure using personal badges or ambient measuring device. If daily collection of exposure data is prohibitive because of time constraints, then the data may be collected by questionnaires administered at intervals. The follow-up frequency is determined and the outcome data are recorded. Of the women in both the exposure and control groups: only a fraction will become pregnant. Of the subgroup who become pregnant, the subjects will divide into two groups: those that miscarry and those who do not. Careful attention to confidentiality is essential if the investigator hopes to achieve accurate and reliable reporting of this very personal information.

Because there is no physical law that relates the propensity to miscarry to anesthetic gas exposure a statistical model has to be constructed to measure this association. Because the association may not be strong, many subjects may need to be impaneled in order to guarantee a reasonable likelihood of detecting the effect of the gases. As mentioned above, a sample size calculation should be used to estimate the projected number of subjects and the expected power of the study. The objective of the data analysis is to relate the anesthetic gas exposure to miscarriage propensity by using a statistical model that simultaneously corrects for the effects of background variables. The statistical analysis for this study answers the question, when background variables are controlled, do female anesthetists exposed inhalational anesthetics have a higher incidence of miscarriage than a cohort of hospital-based female physicians and nurses? Logistic regression methods would be the most likely statistical methods used to analyze these data (see 'Appendix'). Other commonly used statistical models used in prospective observational studies include, linear regression methods, survival models, and risk models.

Prospective observational studies have certain key features:

- the relation between and outcome and an exposure is analyzed in a specified population at risk and a control group;
- uniform data collection is conducted from a fixed point in time;
- subjects have nonuniform background characteristics and lengths of exposure; and
- statistical modeling is used to relate the exposure to the outcomes while controlling for the background variables.

The main advantage of this design is that the investigator can prospectively collect uniform information across a well-defined cohort. This helps to reduce bias. The major disadvantages of this type of study is that it requires a long time to complete, is often large scale and expensive, and often has high subject attrition.

RETROSPECTIVE OBSERVATIONAL STUDIES

A retrospective observational study is one in which a question is formulated and studied using data that have already been generated but not necessarily analyzed for the current study. Retrospective studies are used to:

- identify an effect of a drug, such as in a phase I trial;
- report a new unexpected finding; and
- to provide information from a series, such as a panel of patients receiving a certain type of anesthetic.

With the exception of uniform data collection from a fixed time point, retrospective studies with internal controls, i.e., controls for which the data are generated by the same investigator, have many of the same features of prospective observational studies. Therefore, they may be analyzed using many of the same principles as in prospective observational studies. A principal drawback of many retrospective studies is that the controls are often not part of the investigation and must be chosen from some external source. Bailar and colleagues have suggested five criteria to help evaluate a retrospective study with external controls (Fig. 17.3).

The use of these criteria are best illustrated with an example. Connolly and colleagues reported in a retrospective study that the drug Fenfluramine-Phenteramine (Fen-Phen) was associated with a significantly increased incidence of valvular heart disease and pulmonary hypertension in patients taking the medication to control appetite. Although both fenfluramine and phenteramine are amphetamines, the use of Fen-Phen was not expected to affect the cardiovascular conditions of patients except indirectly through reducing patients' weights. The possible association between the drug and heart disease was a compelling hypothesis with serious implications for many patients seeking therapy for obesity. Although some part of the data analysis had to done prior to formulating the hypothesis, the authors made clear that their intent to analyze and report their findings proceeded the generation of the complete body of data. This is a key point in evaluating this study. Because the study lacks a set of controls it is important to illustrate that the question was generated before a formal study was undertaken.

Did the authors show that they had a plausible rationale for their interpretation of the data before the data were inspected or the analysis undertaken? This criterion is similar to criterion 1. Would the results have been interesting, or publishable if they had been different in some important sense from those that were actually obtained? If it had been shown that there was no association between the use of Fen-Phen and valvular heart disease, then the study would have provided further evidence supporting the efficacy and safety of the therapy. While this information would be important, it is unlikely that this particular negative result by itself would have been published. Did the authors present reasonable grounds for generalizing their results? The response of the *New England Journal of Medicine* and the United States FDA suggests that they did. The incidence of valvular heart disease in the patients that used the drug compared to any reasonable cohort was remarkably high. This high correlation between the drug and heart disease suggested the possibility of a causal relation. The editors of *New England Journal of Medicine* forwent their standard embargo on prior release of information from articles in press and allowed the authors to announce their findings in a televised news conference several weeks ahead of the scheduled publication date of the report. As a result of the report by Connolly and colleagues, Fen-Phen has been removed from the market in the United States.

META-ANALYSIS

A meta-analysis is a statistical paradigm for systematically selecting, analyzing and combining information from different, independent investigations. One purpose of a meta-analysis is to address questions not answered in a single investigation by using the greater statistical power of the information combined across several studies. When several reports provide conflicting opinions about the efficacy of a therapy, such as the use of combined general and regional anesthesia, a meta-analysis can offer a quantitative synthesis of the information and thereby, provide the best possible summary of the findings from all sources. This summary not only helps the clinician understand the limits of the information in the literature it may suggest guidelines for safer and more effective use of the therapy as well as define directions for future research. A meta-analysis is superior to a literature review, which, because of its unsystematic and subjective nature, may give less accurate conclusions. Other uses of meta-analyses include improving estimates of the therapeutic effect, addressing questions not answerable at the start of the original studies, improving the quality of primary research, and contributing to medical technology assessment (Fig. 17.4).

One of the earliest meta-analyses in medicine was performed by the anesthesiologist Henry Beecher who in the 1950's combined results from 8 different studies to assess the medical importance of placebo therapies. His demonstration of an average improvement of 35% across a number of medical conditions

Criteria for evaluating a retrospective study without internal controls
An intent by the investigator, expressed before the study, that the treatment will affect the outcomes reported
Planning of the analysis before the data are generated
Articulation of a plausible hypothesis before the results are observed
A likelihood that the results would still have been of interest if they had been opposite in some sense
Reasonable grounds for generalizing the results from the study subjects to a substantially broader group of patients

Figure 17.3 Criteria for evaluating retrospective studies without internal controls. (Modified with permission from Bailar et al., 1992.)

Purposes of a meta-analysis
To increase statistical power for comparing primary end points and for subgroups
To resolve uncertainty when reports disagree
To improve estimates of the size of the effect
To answer new questions not posed at the start of individual trials
To bring about improvement in the quality of primary research
To contribute to medical technology assessment
To produce more objective summaries of the literature than unaided intellectual interpretation can supply

Figure17.4 Purposes of a meta-analysis. (Modified from Ingelfinger et al., 1993.)

for patients receiving placebo is responsible for making the regular use of placebo therapies a standard practice in clinical trials. Halvorsen and colleagues have suggested eight criteria for analyzing the findings from a meta-analysis (Fig. 17.5). Like other statistical investigations, a meta-analysis begins by posing the question of interest as a testable hypothesis. Identification of all relevant research should include data from both published and unpublished sources, such as doctoral dissertations, abstracts, grant reports, and registries of studies. The methods of search, the breadth of the search and the search time span are critical information that should be clearly stated. Stating the number and source of the studies identified in the search, and the number finally used in the meta-analysis, allows others to locate the same studies, avoids double counting, and helps the reader evaluate the scope of the research.

An important strength of a meta-analysis is the quality control it imposes on the information included in its evaluation. The inclusion and exclusion criteria for the studies in the meta-analysis are defined by the investigator and establish a large part of this quality control. These criteria may be based on the design of the studies, the types of outcomes used, the time frame of the study, the form of the therapy administered, and the statistical methods and analysis used in the study reporting. For example a meta-analysis may consider only randomized clinical trials or only studies performed within the last 10 years. The inclusion and exclusion criteria should reflect the investigator's understanding of the problem and what is necessary to define a scientifically valid study for that problem. The outcome variables used in the meta-analysis should be clearly stated, and should be the same or very similar to the ones extracted from the original studies.

The type of study design plays an important role in defining inclusion and exclusion criteria. It is preferable to combine information across studies of the same design, because different study designs reflect different scientific considerations. For example, the efficacy of a therapy may be established initially by a prospective observational study in a small cohort of patients (phase II trial), then followed by a randomized clinical trial. The prospective observational study and the randomized clinical trial carry related, yet different information about the therapy. It is possible to pool information across studies that have different designs, if they are of sufficiently good quality, target the same population and have reported the same outcome variables. One approach to conducting a meta-analysis is to include initially all studies, score each independently by two investigators in a double blind manner and arrive at a conclusion as to the quality of each. As part of this quality assessment the investigators must also evaluate the degree of data uniformity across the studies in terms of patients, treatments and outcomes. If any one of these is sufficiently diverse then a meta-analysis may not be possible. Reporting this finding is scientifically important. Finally, it may be possible with more recent studies to request the primary data from the investigators in the original studies and not rely solely on published statistical summaries.

The results used in combining the outcomes across various studies refer to the summary statistic used to combine the different information sources. Examples include the number of subjects, the means of the treatment and control groups, their respective variances, p values, confidence intervals, risk differences, risk ratios and odds ratios. If the studies report similar measures of variance for the same outcome, a statistically weighted summary can be computed across the studies. The homogeneity of the information across the studies describes the extent to which the information being combined is equivalent. This will depend on the study designs, the outcomes, and the results chosen in combining the information. The more homogeneous the information, the more reliable the subgroup and overall summaries. Well-designed studies of the same question may have differences in target populations, treatments and primary outcomes. These differences can sometimes be exploited by using statistical modeling to assess the effect of covariates on outcome (see 'Randomized clinical trials'). The effect size is one technique for combining information across different outcomes. The effect size expresses the difference between the treatment and control group means in units of the standard deviation of the individual measurements in the control group or average standard deviation of the control and treatment measurements. This 'rescaling' or 'normalization' expresses the mean differences in terms of the variability of the outcome under study. The statistical analysis used to combine the information in the meta-analysis should be clearly stated, and should include a readable reference to the statistical methods.

The Halvorsen criteria (Fig. 17.5) help the clinician assess the internal validity (how well the study was performed) and external validity (the cohort of patients to whom the results may be applied) of a meta-analysis. The more powerful subgroup and covariate adjustment analyses often possible with meta-analyses can help the clinician decide if a particular therapy is right for an individual patient and what is the actual likelihood of harmful side-effects. A frequently raised consideration when evaluating the findings from a meta-analysis is *publication bias*: the tendency to publish only studies with positive results and not ones that show negative results or have small numbers of subjects. Publication bias reflects more currently accepted practices about what is scientifically interesting or important to report than a problem of the meta-analysis paradigm. The structured review of information dictated by a meta-analysis simply makes publication bias more apparent.

Nevertheless, making a careful survey of published and unpublished sources in the initial information search may allay some concerns about publication bias. For a question about which several studies have been published, it is may be possible to estimate the degree of publication bias using funnel diagrams analysis. In other situations, a worse case analysis can be performed. Once the meta-analysis is complete, the investigator estimates how many well-designed studies demonstrating a result contrary to the current finding of the meta-analysis would

Criteria for assessing a meta-analysis
Method of search for the relevant articles
Eligibility criteria for the articles
Number of articles included
Outcome variables used
Study designs considered in the analysis
Results used in combining information
Homogeneity of studies
Statistical methods

Figure 17.5 Criteria for assessing a meta-analysis. (Modified with permission from Halvorsen et al., 1992.)

have to be missing in order to change the conclusion of the meta-analysis. This number is called the *fail-safe n*. A small fail-safe n suggests cause for concern, whereas a larger one offers more reassurance that publication bias is not a significant factor. A study which is an outlier in its outcome can be very helpful in interpreting the findings from a meta-analysis and should be paid special attention. This is especially important if this study has the same design and is of the same quality as the others included in the meta-analysis. The outlier study may indicate important science obscured by the other studies.

A meta-analysis can help identify deficiencies in medical knowledge about a therapy and more clearly define the direction for future investigations. It can also prevent continued study of issues about which there is already sufficient information to make a definitive statement about the efficacy of a given therapy. A meta-analysis provides more accurate measures of therapeutic effects, the factors that affect therapy outcome and safety. The use of meta-analysis can foster more uniform data and publishing standards. This paradigm necessarily obliges rethinking the way classical literature reviews are performed by requiring the same type of attention to quality of study design as any other study. Systematic selection, evaluation and pooling give more reliable and useful answers than casual intellectual synthesis unaided by protocols, careful records, reproducible materials, thorough searches and quantitative methods. Meta-analysis can contribute to improved delivery of patient care by assembling, organizing and disseminating information available about new treatments and keeping this information update.

BAYESIAN STATISTICS

Bayes' theorem is a basic law of elementary probability theory used to compute the probability of one event given that another event has occurred. The simple principle has been used to develop an entire branch of statistical theory that is widely applied in medicine and other fields of science. To illustrate the concept, if A and B are two events, then in the simplest form Bayes' theorem states that:

Equation 17.1

$$\Pr(B|A) = \frac{\Pr(B)\Pr(A|B)}{\Pr(A)}$$

where $\Pr(B)$ is the *prior probability* of B and describes how likely B is before A occurs. The probability of A given B, $\Pr(A|B)$, describes how likely A is to occur given that B has happened. $\Pr(A)$ is the *total* or *marginal probability* of the event A. $\Pr(B|A)$, the *posterior probability* of B given A defines how likely B is to occur once A has been observed.

The formula is best understood with a simple example. Suppose A is the event that a patient enters a hospital emergency room with chest pain and B is the event that the patient is having a myocardial infarction. The emergency room physician is interested in computing $\Pr(B|A)$, the probability that the patient is having a myocardial infarction given that he/she is having chest pain. In this case, $\Pr(B)$ is the prior probability of the myocardial infarction in an emergency room patient, $\Pr(A|B)$ is the probability of a myocardial infarction given chest pain and $\Pr(A)$ is the probability of chest pain for an emergency room patient considering all possible causes. Lee and colleagues have developed a protocol using Bayes' theorem for assessing the likelihood of a myocardial infarction in an emergency room patient whose chief complaint is chest pain. Even if actual quantitative calculations applying Bayes' rule are not carried out, the principle is often applied conceptually in the operating room and other medical settings.

As another example, suppose during a colectomy, a 45 years old patient has an acute onset of tachycardia. The acute onset of these symptoms warrants immediate attention by the anesthetist to diagnose its cause. Some of the possible causes include: hypoxia, decreased cardiac output, a light plane of anesthesia, hypovolemia or the administration of a vagolytic drug. Even if the anesthetist does not write down actual numbers for the prior probabilities of each of these events, and then compute a posterior probability for each one at this point in the operation, this is conceptually the calculus through which he/she proceeds in trying to determine the most probable cause. In fact, what he is really interested in is, given that the patient has an acute onset of tachycardia, what is the most likely cause? Bayes' rule is also part of the decision process in the example of the anesthetist diagnosing an intraoperative fall in blood pressure discussed in 'Paradigm for statistical inference'.

The formula above shows that if A and B are independent events, i.e., $\Pr(A \text{ and } B)=\Pr(A|B)\Pr(A) = \Pr(A)\Pr(B)$, then the probability of B given A is simply equal to the probability of B. The application of Bayes' rule only makes sense in situations when the two events are related. The Bayesian analysis allows assessment of how likely one event is given that information about a second relevant event has been received. The likelihood of the second event could increase or decrease depending upon how the information from the first event relates to the second. Returning to the chest pain example, suppose that the patient presenting with symptoms of chest pain was well known to the emergency room physician, and as a consequence, is known to have frequent anginal attacks. With this particular individual the prior probability of his having a myocardial infarction is relatively high and perhaps higher than that of a patient presenting to the emergency room with chest pain and no previous history of a myocardial infarction. After an electrocardiogram (ECG) is taken, the patient has an ECG pattern consistent with ischemia in the inferior aspect of the heart. As a consequence of this test, the chances that the patient is having chest pain due to a myocardial infarction increases, whereas, the probability that the subject is having chest pain due to gastric upset decreases.

Another way in which Bayes' rule is used in medical studies is to define the concepts of *positive* and *negative predictive values* and compute these quantities for specific diagnostic tests. When used in conjunction with the specificity and sensitivity of a test, these probabilities give predictions of how likely or unlikely a given disease is, once a positive or negative test result is received. For example, if B is the event that a patient has a specific disease and A is the event that a test for the disease is positive, then the right side of Bayes' rule (Equation 17.1) defines the positive predictive value of the test. Similarly, if B is the event that a patient does not have a specific disease and A is the event that a test for the disease is negative then the right side of Bayes' rule defines the negative predictive value of the test. In the last part of the chest pain example the emergency room physician assesses the positive predictive value of the ECG pattern of inferior ischemia as an indicator of a myocardial infarction.

The strong appeal of the Bayesian paradigm is the ability to represent uncertainty about knowledge available before study of a problem in terms of a prior probability density, and to use this representation as part of the formal investigation. Bayesian methods are being used to include prior knowledge about treatment effect in the analysis of randomized clinical trials and to provide a general framework for combining information across studies in meta-analyses.

APPENDIX: SUMMARY OF STATISTICAL MODELS AND TESTS

Figure 17.1 shows that statistical inference follows a five-step paradigm for statistical inference. The fourth step is the application of specific statistical methods for data analysis. Data analysis proceeds in four steps. The investigator chooses with the help of a consulting statistician, an appropriate probability model for the data to be collected in the study; the hypothesis of interest is formulated in terms of the parameters of the probability model; the model parameters are estimated from the experimental data using specific statistical techniques; and finally, the hypothesis is studied in terms of the estimated parameters. We summarize in this appendix some commonly used statistical models and tests.

Data and probability models

The data collected in a study are of two types: discrete and continuous. Discrete data are data that assume only discrete values. They can be either categorical, ordinal or cardinal. Categorical data separate into discrete groups whose descriptors have no numerical relationship, such as gender or eye color. The simplest categorical data are measurements that have only two values, such as yes or no, improved or not improved, true or false. For ordinal data, the discrete groups can be assigned numbers, whose order is meaningful but whose relationship in magnitude may or may not be quantitatively defined. For example, a pain rating scale may assign the numbers 0, 1, 2, and 3 to describe increasing severity of pain however, the difference between scores of 1 and 2 is not necessarily the same as the difference between scores 2 and 3. On the other hand, if the ordinal data are the number of cases per month an anesthetist performs then both order and magnitude are meaningful, and the data are termed cardinal data.

Continuous data are cardinal data that may assume any value between two end points. Those end points may be small as all the values in the interval from zero to one or long as the entire real line from negative to positive infinity. Examples of continuous data include blood pressure, height, weight and blood level of propofol. Truly discrete data may sometimes be modeled as continuous data if there are many ordinal groups and the numerical distance between the groups is small relative to the overall range of the data.

The probability model or probability distribution describes the frequency or likelihood with which data values occur. For discrete data it is termed the *probability mass function* and for continuous data it is termed the *probability density function*. Each probability model is defined by an explicit mathematical formula. A probability model can also be described by its *location* and *scale*. The mathematical formula defining the probability model includes parameters and the location and scale measures can often be expressed are functions of the parameters. Location describes where the central tendency or most of the mass of the probability model is situated. Three commonly used measures of location are the *mean* (arithmetic average), the *mode* (most likely value), and the *median* (middle number of the ordered data series or the data value at the 50th percentile). The most frequently used measures of scale are the *variance*, *standard deviation* and *interquartile range*. The variance is the average of the squared deviation of the data about the mean, the standard deviation is the square root of the variance and the interquartile range is the distance between the values at the 25th and 75th percentiles.

The most widely used probability model for the analysis of continuous data is the *Gaussian distribution*. This distribution is symmetric, unimodal and bell-shaped. The use of this distribution in analyses is often justified from empirical studies of preliminary samples of data. Theoretical justification for the use of this distribution comes from the central limit theorem which states that the sums of independent quantities have a Gaussian distribution as a number of terms being summed increases. Because the distribution is symmetric and unimodal its mean, median and mode are all the same. The Gaussian distribution can be characterized completely by two parameters: its mean and variance σ^2. The Gaussian distribution with mean 0 and variance 1 is termed the standard Gaussian or normal distribution. Any Gaussian distribution can be transformed into the standard Gaussian distribution with the z-transformation:

$$z = (x\text{-}\mu)/\sigma$$

where x is an observation for the Gaussian distribution with mean μ and variance σ^2.

The t-distribution is another widely used probability model for continuous data which, like the Gaussian distribution, is symmetric, unimodal and bell-shaped. The tails of the t-distribution are fatter and the mode is less prominent than the Gaussian distribution. As discussed below, the t-distribution is a sampling probability density used in statistical tests where the objective is to make an inference about the mean of a Gaussian distribution when the variance is also not known. The χ^2-distribution is frequently used to analyze both discrete and continuous data. The χ^2-distribution is a right-skewed probability density, which may be constructed by computing the distribution of the square of a quantity that has a standard Gaussian distribution. The χ^2-distribution is used also in many statistical tests, particularly those designed to measure association between two discrete variables or to assess agreement between a specific probability model and a set of experimental data.

The *binomial distribution* is the simplest and most frequently used discrete probability model. It describes the likelihood of a binary outcome, such as whether a patient improves or not, blood pressure decreases or not, etc. The binomial distribution is characterized by two parameters, the probability of success p – likelihood of one of the outcomes – and N, the number of trials generating the binomial sample. The mean of this probability model is Np, and the variance is $Np(1–p)$. A second commonly used discrete probability model is the Poisson distribution, which is characterized by a single parameter termed the rate, λ. The rate is both the mean and variance of the Poisson model. This probability model is defined on the counting of numbers and is used to describe the likelihood of a given number of events in a fixed unit of time or space. Examples of applications using the Poisson model include the number of patients admitted to the hospital per week following same day surgery, the number of monitor failures per month and the number of sick calls per week for the anesthesia staff.

Parameter estimation and sample statistics

Inferences about the population under study are made based on data sampled from the population and statistics computed from that sample. A *statistic* is any function of the sample data. Because tests of hypotheses are formulated in terms of parameters of the probability model, the parameters must be determined from experimental data. The most important statistics are the parameter estimates determined from the data. *Estimation* is the use of formal statistical methods to determine parameter values of the probability model from the experimental data. In the case of the Gaussian distribution, this means computing from experimental data the mean and variance, for the binomial, the probability of success, and for the Poisson, the rate parameter. Three commonly used methods of estimation in statistics are the method of moments, maximum likelihood, and least squares. In method of moments estimation the parameter value is determined by equating the moments of the probability model to the sample moments. The first moment is the mean and the second central moment is the variance. In general the kth population moment is the integral or sum of x^k with respect to the probability model and is given as:

$$\sigma^k = \sum x^k f(x)$$

if the data are discrete, and

$$\sigma^k = \int x^k f(x)dx$$

if the data are continuous and $f(x)$ is the probability model. The limits on the sum and integral are the range over which the probability model is defined. For example, to estimate the variance of a Gaussian distribution from a sample of data using the method of moments, one simply sets the population variance (population second central moment) equal to the sample variance (sample second central moment).

In maximum likelihood estimation the statistician specifies the probability model for the joint distribution of the data and then uses analytic formulae or numerical procedures to find the most likely value of the parameters given the data. Maximum likelihood is the most efficient method of statistical estimation because it uses all the information in the sample to determine the model parameter estimates. Least squares is an estimation method used when the objective is estimate the best lines or curve relation between two or more sets of numerical data. In simple least-squares a straight line is fit to a set of data – usually a collection of x's (independent variable) and y's (dependent variable) – by finding the parameters of the line which minimize the sum of squared vertical deviations of the data to the line. When fitting a straight line to data where the errors are assumed to be Gaussian and have a known variance, maximum likelihood and least squares estimation are identical.

Parameter estimates obtained by any estimation procedures are random quantities because they are statistics, i.e. functions of data. As a consequence, like the data from which they are derived statistics and parameter estimates have their own probability models. These models are related to the probability model of the data and are termed the *sampling probability distributions* of the statistics. The sampling distribution is the distribution of the statistic obtained over repeated draws of samples of the same size from the same population probability model. The sampling probability distribution is central to the process of hypothesis testing and statistical inference because it describes the properties of the estimated statistic under the null hypothesis. The hypothesis test about the parameter of interest is carried out in terms of this distribution. For example, given a sample of data, the method of moments and maximum likelihood estimates of the mean are both $\bar{x}$, the sample mean of the observations. This statistic is a random quantity and it has a probability distribution. The mean and variance of the distribution of $\bar{x}$ are μ and σ^2/n respectively. The quantity $\sigma/n^{1/2}$ is the *standard error of the mean* because it measures the uncertainty in the mean. That is, the variance of the sample mean is $n^{-1} \times$ the population variance and its standard deviation is $n^{-1/2} \times$ the population standard deviation. If the population probability model is Gaussian with mean μ, and variance σ^2/n, then the sampling probability distribution of $\bar{x}$ is also Gaussian and has mean μ, and variance σ^2/n. As another example of a sampling distribution, if s^2 is the sample variance computed from data arising from a Gaussian distribution with mean μ, and variance σ^2, then the sample distribution of s^2 is proportional to a χ^2-distribution with n–1 degrees of freedom. Similarly, the sampling distribution of the statistic:

$$t_n = (\bar{x}-\mu)s^{-1}$$

is a t-distribution with n–1 degrees of freedom.

Another important statistic used for measuring uncertainty and making inferences are confidence intervals. A 1–α confidence interval has probability 1–α of containing the true population value of the parameter where $0<\alpha<1$. For a sample from a Gaussian distribution with unknown mean μ, and known variance σ^2, if $\alpha=0.05$, then the 0.95 (commonly called the 95%) confidence interval from the population mean is:

$$\bar{x}\pm 1.96\sigma/n^{1/2}$$

where n is the sample size and 1.96 is the 97.5 percentile of a standard Gaussian distribution.

Common parametric statistical tests

Statistical tests defined in terms of specific model parameters are termed parametric tests. The estimated statistic related to the parameter of interest and the sampling distribution of that statistic are used to define the test of the hypothesis and measure the significance of the finding. The z-test is carried out on data assumed to be Gaussian when the hypothesis of interest is expressed in terms of the mean of the distribution and the variance is unknown. The significance of the finding is determined by the p-value computed from the standard Gaussian distribution. The z-test is based on the z-transformation, z-score, or z-statistics defined above as $z = (\bar{x}-\mu)\sigma^{-1}$. If the hypothesis is about the mean of a Gaussian distribution and the variance or equivalently the standard deviation is unknown, then the standard deviation in the z-test can be replaced by its estimate, the sample standard deviation. In this case, the z-test is converted into a t-test, the statistic is the t-statistic, $t_{n-1} = (\bar{x}-\mu)s^{-1}$, and the significance of the findings is measured in terms of the t-distribution. If the hypothesis is about the variance of a Gaussian distribution, the test statistic is s^2, the sample variance, the test is a χ^2-test, and significance is measured by a χ^2-distribution with n–1 degrees of freedom. If the hypothesis of interest is to compare the variance of two different Gaussian distributions, the test statistic is the ratio of the two sample variance estimates, the sampling distribution is the F-distribution and the test is the F-test. The F-test also forms the basis for hypothesis testing ANOVA models.

Regression models and measures of association

When the objective of a study is to relate one set of data (dependent variable) to another set of data (independent variables or covariates), the analysis can often be conducted with a *regression model*. Regression models for continuous outcomes can be either simple or multiple. In a simple linear regression model one independent variable is used to explain in a linear way the structure in a single dependent variable. In a multiple linear regression model several independent variables are used to describe the structure in a single independent variable. A *correlation coefficient* is a measure of association between two continuous variables that is constrained to lie between –1 and 1. It is straightforward to show that the correlation coefficient is a scaled version of the regression coefficient in a simple linear regression. The degree of association between the two variables is quantified by the sign and magnitude of the correlation coefficient; +1 is perfect positive correlation, –1 is perfect negative correlation, and 0 is no correlation. The degree of association between the dependent variable and the several independent variables in a multiple regression model is measured by the *squared multiple correlation coefficient* or R^2. The R^2 is constrained to lie between 0 and 1 and measures the fraction of variation in the dependent variable described by the independent variables. ANOVA is a regression analysis in which the independent variables are categorical, and the dependent variable is continuous. In a logistic regression model the dependent variable is binary and the independent variables can be either discrete or continuous. A logistic regression model expresses the binomial proportion as a function of the dependent variables. The linear relationship is expressed not between the binomial proportion and the dependent variables but between the logistic transform of the binomial proportion and these variables. The results of a logistic regression are often summarized in terms of the odds ratios and the relative risks.

Associations between two sets of categorical variables are often displayed in a *contingency table*, that shows the number of items or subjects falling in each different combination of the categories. For example, in a study comparing the incidence of sore throat following the use of two types of airway devices, patients in each group could be categorized according to whether they had no, mild, or severe sore throats. In this case, each patient would be counted in one of six cells of a 3×2 contingency table. A χ^2-test is used to assess the statistical significance of the association between the two variables provided the expected number of observations in each cell is not too small.

Nonparametric statistical tests

In the discussion to this point it has been assumed that a specific probability model could be formulated for the study data. In certain analyses it may not be possible to formulate a specific probability model, or the investigator may wish to test a hypothesis by making as few assumptions as possible about the statistical properties of the data. In both of these instances the alternative is to use a *nonparametric test*. While nonparametric tests require fewer assumptions and are more robust, i.e., are less dependent on the true distribution of the data, they often have less power. The three most widely used nonparametric tests in clinical studies are *Fisher's exact test* and the *Wilcoxon sign rank test* which are nonparametric analogs of the paired t-test and the *Wilcoxon rank sum test* (also termed the *Mann-Whitney U-test*) which is a nonparametric analog of the two sample *t*-tests.

Key References

Bailar III JC, Louis TA, Lavori PW, Polansky M. Studies without internal controls. In: Bailar III JC, Mosteller F, eds. Medical Uses of Statistics, 2nd edn. Boston: NEJM Books; 1992:99–110.

Bailar III JC, Mosteller F. Medical Uses of Statistics, 2nd edn. Boston: NEJM Books; 1992.

Der Simonian R, Charette LJ, McPeek B, Mosteller F. Reporting on methods in clinical trials. In: Bailar III JC, Mosteller F, eds. Medical Uses of Statistics, 2nd edn. Boston: NEJM Books; 1992:334–5.

Halvorsen KT, Burdick E, Colditz GA, Frazier HS, Mosteller F. Combining results from independent investigations: meta-analysis in clinics research. In: Bailar III JC, Mosteller F, eds. Medical Uses of Statistics, 2nd edn. Boston: NEJM Books; 1992:413–26.

Ingelfinger JA, Mosteller F, Thibodeau LA, Ware JH. Biostatistics in Clinical Medicine, 3rd edn. New York: McGraw-Hill; 1999.

Riegelman RK, Hirsch RP. Studying a Study and Testing a Test; How to Read the Health Science Literature, 3rd edn. Boston, MA: Little Brown; 1996.

Rosner, BA. Fundamentals of Biostatistics, 3rd edn. Belmont, CA: Duxbury Press; 1995.

Sackett DL, Haynes RB, Guyatt GH, Tugwell P. Clinical Epidemiology, 2nd edn. Boston, MA: Little Brown; 1991.

Sacks HS, Berrier J, Reitman D, Pagano D, Chalmers TC. Meta-analysis of randomized control trials: an update of the quality and methodology. In: Bailar III JC, Mosteller F, eds. Medical Uses of Statistics, 2nd edn. Boston: NEJM Books; 1992:427–44.

Further Reading

Beecher HK. The powerful placebo. J Am Med Assoc. 1955;159:1602–6.

Brophy JM, Joseph L. Placing trials in context using Bayesian analysis. J Am Med Assoc. 1995;273:871–5.

Connolly HM, Crary JL, McGoon MD, et al. Valvular heart disease associated with fenfluramine–phentermine. N Engl J Med. 1997;337:581–8.

Holland BK. Probability without Equations. Baltimore: Johns Hopkins University Press; 1998.

Hughes M. Reporting Bayesian analyses of clinical trials. Stat Med. 1993;12:1651–63.

Lee TH, Juarez G, Cook EP, et al. Ruling out acute myocardial infraction. a prospective multicenter validation of a 12-hour strategy for patients at low risk. N Engl J Med. 1991;324:1239–46.

Chapter 18 The structure and function of neurons

Robert E Study

Topics covered in this chapter

The structure of neurons
Membrane potential
Electrical properties of neurons
The action potential

Anesthesia, whether local, regional, or general, is essentially a neuronal phenomenon; effects of anesthetics on other tissues are side effects that are unimportant in the generation of anesthesia. An understanding of the nature of anesthesia, therefore, depends on understanding the functions and interactions of neurons. The actions of anesthetics have been defined increasingly by specific alterations of neuronal function and of proteins involved in the control of electrical activity that lead to alterations in excitability. Hence, the development of new anesthetic drugs is dependent on knowledge of the pharmacology and physiology of neurons.

Neurons and neuroglia (commonly called glia) are two principal classes of cell unique to the nervous system. Neurons are the fundamental structural and functional units of the nervous system in terms of its primary activity: information processing and storage. The functions of glia are less well understood. They participate in metabolic and structural support of neurons but probably have a role in information processing as well. Neurons are able to transmit and process information using electrical signaling, a property that allows much faster communication especially over long distances compared with chemical signaling. Neurons are electrically excitable; they are able to generate and propagate a stereotyped electrical impulse (the *action potential*). The action potential is the primary means of communication in the nervous system. Other cells, such as endocrine glands and muscle, also exhibit electrical excitability, but in neurons this property is highly developed for the purpose of information transfer and processing.

THE STRUCTURE OF NEURONS

Neurons have unique structural characteristics that enable them to perform their functions of information processing and transmission. Although there is wide structural variability, the basic structure is fairly consistent (Fig. 18.1). As in most cells, the cell body, or soma, contains the nucleus and most of the protein synthetic machinery for the cell. Extending out from the soma are processes called dendrites and axons. The dendrites receive information from other neurons, primarily via synapses. Synapses which are specialized structures that contain receptors for neurotransmitters released by other neurons in contact with the dendrite (Chapter 19). The activation of receptors at

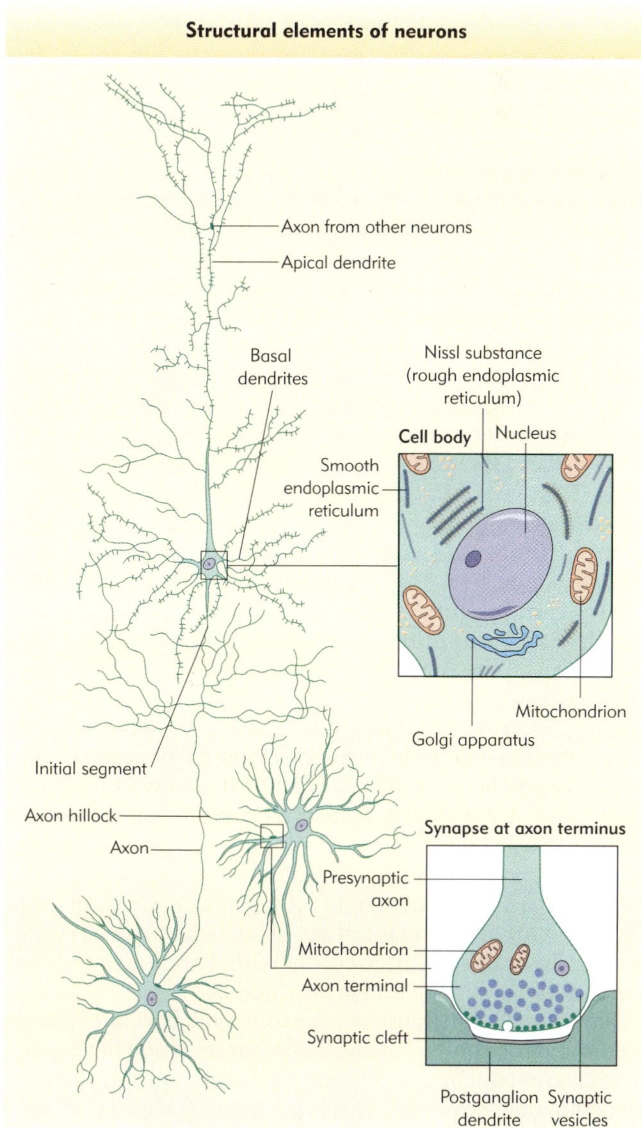

Figure 18.1 The basic structural elements of neurons. A typical CNS neuron exhibiting its major structural attributes, including dendrites (connections of many other neurons to dendrites not shown), a branching axon, and synapses onto other neurons.

the synapse can induce a change in ion current flow across the dendritic membrane that travels along the dendrite and converges with other dendritic signals on the cell soma. The combined signal, if large enough, triggers an action potential at the cell soma, which possesses a high degree of excitability. The action potential propagates away from the soma along the axon, which contacts another neuron or an end organ at a distance of a few micrometers to over a meter. Thus the information flow is from dendrite to axon.

Dendrites tend to have more extensive arborizations than axons, with multiple roots in most neurons. By comparison, the axon usually exits as a single fiber, although it may divide extensively along its course. The entire neuron may be electrically excitable, although not uniformly. Dendrites are generally less excitable, transmitting much of their electrical information passively (see below), but there are exceptions. The cell body is very excitable, especially at a specialized area at the root of the axon, the axon hillock, which is the trigger site for action potential generation. Although there are many exceptions to this basic model, such as dendro–dendritic and axo–axonic synapses and neurons that do not produce action potentials, it holds for the majority of neurons and provides a good starting point for understanding neuronal function.

Axoplasmic transport

A key characteristic of neurons is their length; a single cell may extend for a long distance, often more than a meter. However, the machinery for synthesizing proteins and the critical organelles such as mitochondria exists only in the cell body, synaptic terminals and some dendrites. To supply its axon with essential components over such a long distance, neurons have developed three transport systems: orthograde axoplasmic transport, retrograde axoplasmic transport, and axoplasmic flow. The first two are quite fast, moving organelles at a rate of up to 40cm/day away from and towards the cell soma, respectively. The third is slow, moving proteins and bulk cytoplasm at a rate of 1–10mm/day.

Both orthograde and retrograde axoplasmic transport involve adenosine triphosphate (ATP)-driven molecular motors, moving along a rail of microtubules that extends the length of the axon. Although the transport systems are similar processes, they involve different proteins, which are specific for transport in each direction. The principal proteins involved are kinesin for orthograde transport and dynein for retrograde transport. These proteins form links between transported organelles and the microtubule structure along which they move. Kinesin and dynein have many similarities to muscle myosin and presumably move using a similar ratchet-like mechanism, hydrolyzing ATP in the process. Also, like muscle fibers, axons are rich in actin, but its function in these fast transport processes is not as well understood as its role in muscle. Interestingly, transport in both directions can occur simultaneously along a single microtubule.

Slow axoplasmic transport, or axoplasmic flow, is responsible for the transport of many soluble proteins and other cytoplasmic components, such as microtubules, along the axon in an orthograde direction. This is presumably a means of supplying the axon and terminals with the wide range of substances required for basic metabolic functions.

The importance of transport away from the axon to the synapse or neuromuscular junction is obvious, but retrograde transport is more obscure. Two functions of retrograde transport are reasonably well established. First, components of used synaptic vesicles are transported back to the cell body, presumably for recycling. Second, endocytosis occurs at the nerve terminal, creating transport vesicles that travel back to the cell body. This phenomenon appears to be a form of communication, where information in the form of chemical signals, such as the presence of growth factors in the environment of the nerve terminal, is transported back to the soma. It is particularly important in development and repair of neurons, where connections may be established or eliminated based on such retrograde chemical signaling.

Glia

These cells were long thought to be simply structural support cells for neurons, but it is now becoming clear that they perform many essential, active roles in the function of the nervous system.

There are two main classes of glia: *microglia* and *macroglia*. Microglia participate in phagocytosis and repair after injury or disease and are essentially identical to tissue macrophages, although they appear to be permanent residents of the CNS. In the peripheral nervous system, this function is performed by the same blood and tissue macrophages that exist in other tissues. Macroglia, which are unique to the nervous system, are divided into two main classes: *astrocytes* and *oligodendroglia*. Astrocytes, which are larger, usually have a star-like shape with many fine processes and look remarkably like neurons. They have a wide variety of functions. Oligodendroglia, named for their less prominent arborizations, are more specialized in their role. They insulate and support axons by wrapping their cell processes. This covering may provide metabolic support and possibly some kind of communication with the axon. In many axons, the covering is wrapped in a spiral forming a tight insulating layer called myelin (Fig. 18.2). In the peripheral nervous system, the myelin-producing cells are called Schwann cells and are very similar to oligodendroglia. Myelin is a principal component of the nervous system, forming the bulk of white matter and many nerves.

The functions of glia are less well understood than those of neurons, but there is evidence for a variety of roles:

- Structural support and protection of neurons.
- Proliferation and repair after injury. Microglia perform the phagocytic duties, but other glia are also involved in this process. Glia also help guide and support the regrowth of axons back to their targets after injury.
- Formation of the blood–brain barrier. In the CNS, the appendages of astrocytes are linked by tight junctions to form the barrier around capillaries.
- Increasing the speed of impulse conduction along axons by myelination.
- Regulation of ionic gradients and metabolic interaction with neurons. Neurons release K^+ upon impulse generation and conduction, which can accumulate in the extracellular space and hamper further conduction (see below). Glia are permeable to K^+ and act as a pump for these ions, preventing large increases. Metabolic interactions with neurons are less well understood, but it is known that glia and neurons can exchange a variety of biochemical signals, even proteins. Schwann cells, for example, produce proteins that are important for neuronal differentiation and survival, and neurons produce growth factors that can induce proliferation of Schwann cells.
- Uptake and metabolism of neurotransmitters. Glia can remove neurotransmitters released by neurons and, thus, help to terminate their actions.

Myelin structure

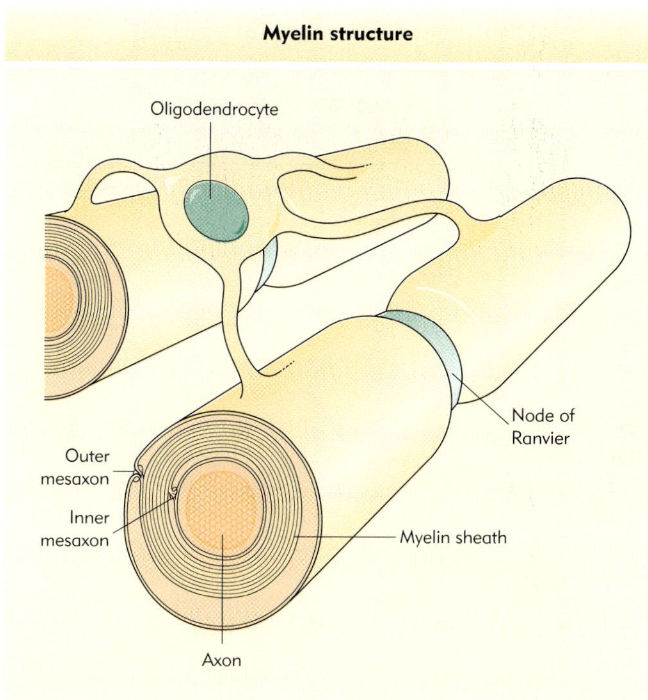

Figure 18.2 Myelin structure. Cross-section of a myelinated axon of the CNS, showing the oligodendroglia cell forming the myelin. The spiral wrapping of the glial cell membrane is shown in cross-section. Myelin is interrupted at regular intervals by a short unmyelinated segment called the node of Ranvier, where the axonal membrane is exposed to the extracellular environment and the current responsible for action potentials crosses.

- Information processing and memory. There is good evidence that glia have receptors for neurotransmitters and can respond electrically to them. The electrical response of glia differs from that of neurons. Instead of action potentials, glia have 'calcium waves', caused by the opening of Ca^{2+} channels that allow Ca^{2+} to enter the cell, subsequently activating the outward flow of K^+. This response is propagated both along a cell and between cells owing to electrically conductive gap junctions that connect the glia. These waves, which are over an order of magnitude slower than action potentials, may have an important role in information processing.

MEMBRANE POTENTIAL

The membrane potential is a fundamental property of all cells, a result of the difference in concentration of charged organic and inorganic molecules on the inside of a cell compared with the outside of a cell (Chapter 5). Membrane potential is essential to life; loss of membrane potential leads to loss of viability in neurons as well as in other cell types. Membrane potential is for many cells a basis for communication both within and between cells. The properties of membranes and of charge movement allow changes in potential to be propagated along membranes and integrated over time and space, which allows this electrical communication to be a form of computation. Regulation of membrane potential is, therefore, the essence of neuronal function.

Neuronal intra- and extracellular fluid composition

		Extracellular (CSF) (mmol/L)	Intracellular (mmol/L)
Cations	Na^+	138	10
	K^+	3	120
	Ca^{2+}	1.5	10^{-4}
	Mg^{2+}	2	6.5
	Total positive charge	148	143
Anions	Cl^-	122	2
	HCO_3^-	25	12
	Organic anions	0.7	94
	Others	0.3	35
	Total negative charge	148	143

Figure 18.3 Ionic composition of neuronal intra- and extracellular fluid in the brain. Extracellular fluid [cerebro-spinal fluid (CSF) in this case] is high in Na^+ and low in K^+ compared with intracellular fluid. Note that the positive and negative charges balance on each side of the membrane; the negative inside potential present at rest represents an extremely small surplus of negative ions at the inside face of the membrane. Free Ca^{2+} in cytoplasm is very low (~10^{-7}mol/L); it is higher in organelles that store Ca^{2+} such as mitochondria.

The ionic basis of the resting membrane potential

For most mammalian cells, the 'resting' membrane potential is negative inside relative to the outside, usually about –60 to –70mV. The predominant ions involved are K^+ and organic anions such as proteins and amino acids on the inside, and Na^+ and Cl^- on the outside (Fig. 18.3). The membrane potential is produced by ion pumps, which actively transport ions across membranes against their electrochemical gradients using the energy of ATP. The actual ionic concentration differences across the membrane are determined by the selective permeability of the membrane to specific ions. This selective permeability is imparted by specific ion channels: proteins that allow certain ions to cross the membrane and while excluding others. Such channels are called nongated or 'leak' channels, indicating that they are always open. This is in contrast to ion channels that are gated, meaning that they can open or close in response to a signal, usually a neurotransmitter or a change in membrane potential. Gated channels are critical to changing the membrane potential for the purposes of information processing, but are usually closed in the resting membrane. The relationship of ion distribution to membrane potential is a fundamental concept in neuroscience.

Ions move across a permeable membrane based on two forces: the relative concentrations of the ions on each side (the concentration gradient) and the relative charge on either side (the voltage gradient). Charged particles in solution are randomly moving and will tend to diffuse from areas where they are more concentrated to those where they are less concentrated; they will also move toward an opposite charge. The distribution of an ion across the membrane will reach equilibrium when the concentration forces exactly equal the electrical forces for that ion. The relationship of these electrical and chemical forces was first described in 1888 by Nernst:

Equation 18.1

$$E = \left(\frac{RT}{zF}\right)\ln\left(\frac{[\text{Ion}_{\text{out}}]}{[\text{Ion}_{\text{in}}]}\right)$$

where R is the universal gas constant, T is temperature (Kelvin), z is the valence of the ion, F is the Faraday constant, and E is the equilibrium potential (Nernst potential).

The Nernst equation gives the potential (in volts) across the membrane if the concentrations of the permeable species are known or, conversely, the concentrations of the species if the potential is known at equilibrium. Since neuronal membranes are permeable to many ions, the formulation of the Nernst equation must include all permeable ions factored in according to their relative permeabilities. This more complete equation is referred to as the constant-field equation, or the Goldman–Hodgkin–Katz equation after the investigators who developed it in the 1940s. An illustration of how these equations describe the relationship between membrane potential and the ionic concentrations can be clearly demonstrated with glial cells. Glia are almost exclusively permeable to K^+, so only this ion need be considered (other ions exist on both sides to nearly balance charge but the membrane is not permeable to these ions and, therefore, they do not enter into the equation). Most of the other values in the equation are constants under biologic conditions, so if one knows the concentration of K^+ on each side of the membrane, the membrane potential of the glial cell can be calculated using Equation 18.1 with K^+ as the ion. At normal temperature and pressure, with a monovalent cation:

Equation 18.2

$$E = 61\log\left[\frac{(K^+_{\text{out}})}{(K^+_{\text{in}})}\right]$$

If $[K^+_{\text{out}}]$ is 4mmol/L and $[K^+_{\text{in}}]$ is 120mmol/L, then E is –90mV.

As the concentration of K^+ outside the cell changes, the resting potential of the cell will change accordingly, as described by this equation; higher K^+ in the external solution results in a less negative potential (Fig. 18.4). This is also true of neurons, but to a lesser extent because the resting membrane potential of a neuron is determined by the relative permeabilities to several ions in addition to K^+. Ions with low membrane permeability, such as Na^+, are not necessarily at equilibrium and do not contribute significantly to the resting potential. However, while Na^+ is far from equilibrium at resting potential, the cell can rapidly increase permeability to Na^+ in response to a stimulus, causing these ions to flow across the membrane. This changes the membrane potential toward a value determined by the Nernst equation (or more properly, the Goldman–Hodgkin–Katz equation) using the values resulting from this greater permeability. Such changes in potential produced by changes in ion permeability are the basis of the action potential as well as for much of the electrical communication and integration among neurons.

Ion pumps and the generation of the resting potential

The Nernst and Goldman–Hodgkin–Katz equations describe the distribution of permeable ions at equilibrium at a given potential across the membrane, but they do not tell us how that potential was generated. In the example of a glial cell, a membrane permeable only to K^+ is at about –86mV at 'rest'. However, in most cells the membrane is not perfectly impermeable to all other ions; these will tend to cross the membrane down their electrochemical gradients, reducing the membrane potential toward zero (to –77mV in the case of glial cell). To counteract this tendency, neurons and other cells have ion pumps, proteins that utilize the energy of ATP hydrolysis to transport ions across membranes against their electrochemical gradients, thus maintaining the membrane potential (Chapter 5).

There are many types of ion pump, but the most important in maintaining neuronal membrane potential is the Na^+/K^+-ATPase. This protein spans the membrane and has the remarkable ability to move three Na^+ out of the cell and simultaneously move two K^+ into the cell powered by the hydrolysis of ATP. By moving more positive charges out than in, it causes a net separation of charge across the membrane and is, therefore, called an *electrogenic ion pump*. Not surprisingly, this pump is highly regulated by the metabolic needs of the cell, through second messenger cascades. The resting potential of most neurons is a dynamic balance between the active pumping of ions and the flow of ions back through ion channels down their electrochemical gradients, which tends to dissipate the potential. In

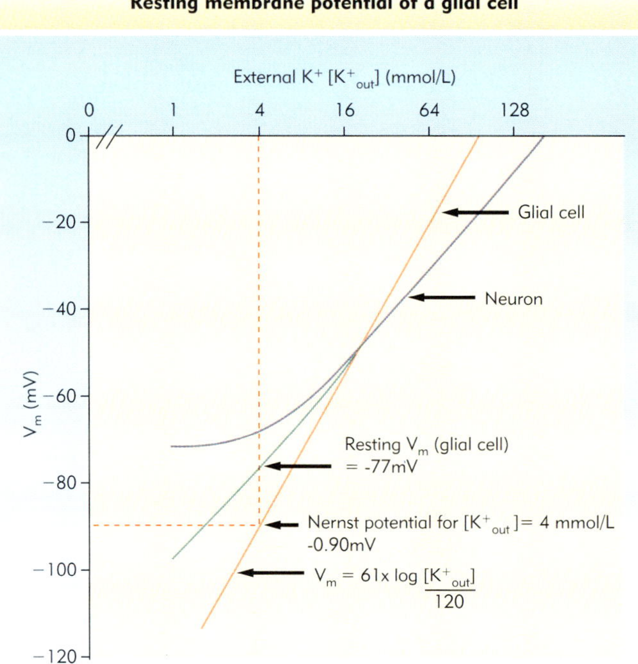

Figure 18.4 The resting membrane potential of a glial cell is dependent on K^+ concentration. Since the resting glial membrane is primarily permeable to K^+, manipulating the external concentration of K^+ alters the resting potential in a manner very close to that predicted by the Nernst equation, as seen by the close correspondence of its resting potential to the line that corresponds to the equation. Neurons, however, have additional ion channels contributing to permeability both at resting and at depolarized potentials, so these cells deviate more from this simple model, requiring other ions to be considered.

fact, many neurons have a resting potential that is just slightly greater (more negative) than that predicted by the Goldman–Hodgkin–Katz equation because of the active contribution of these electrogenic pumps.

ELECTRICAL PROPERTIES OF NEURONS

The ability of neurons to utilize membrane potential as a device for communication is determined by the neurons' underlying electrical properties. The electrical properties of nerves include passive properties, or the behavior of membranes with their pumps and nongated channels, and active properties, or the behavior of membranes as modified by the presence of gated channels, particularly those opened or closed in response to changes in membrane potential.

Electrical communication requires that membrane potential changes over time and that such changes are propagated along the membrane. The changes can be described using the same terminology and mathematics used to describe electrical circuits (Chapter 5). In fact, the cell membrane is a capacitor, with the lipid tails of the phospholipid bilayer acting as a dielectric (insulator) and the charged phosphate heads acting as a storage site for positive charges from the intra- and extracellular environments. Nongated channels in the membrane form a conduit for current flow in parallel with the capacitance, and the ion pumps provide the potential energy (voltage) for the flow of current. This situation can be represented schematically as an electrical circuit, as shown in Figure 18.5a. The membrane can be considered to act as a resistance–capacitance (RC) circuit. Both the active and passive behavior of the membrane can be described using this model.

When current flows across the membrane, as in the opening of a channel or with the injection of current from an electrode, current may flow almost instantly but membrane potential changes as an inverse exponential with time, as it would in an RC circuit. This occurs because much of the initial current (ion) flow goes to changing the charge on the capacitor before it changes the potential on the other side of the membrane (Fig. 18.5b). Therefore, very fast current flow results in slow, attenuated voltage changes. An important phenomenon that results from this property is temporal summation, in which a series of brief currents across the membrane of a neuron can be additive even though they are asynchronous, because the changes are spread out in time as a result of the membrane capacitance (Fig. 18.5c).

A phenomenon analogous to this occurs across space in propagation of voltage changes along the membrane. Potential changes are propagated passively along the membrane since electrical charge will travel to areas where there is less charge of that polarity. If the amount of charge is large enough, it can trigger an action potential at a distant point on the membrane surface. One can best understand this propagation by considering the case of a cylinder such as an axon or dendrite (Fig. 18.6). The circuit model still applies, but here there are many

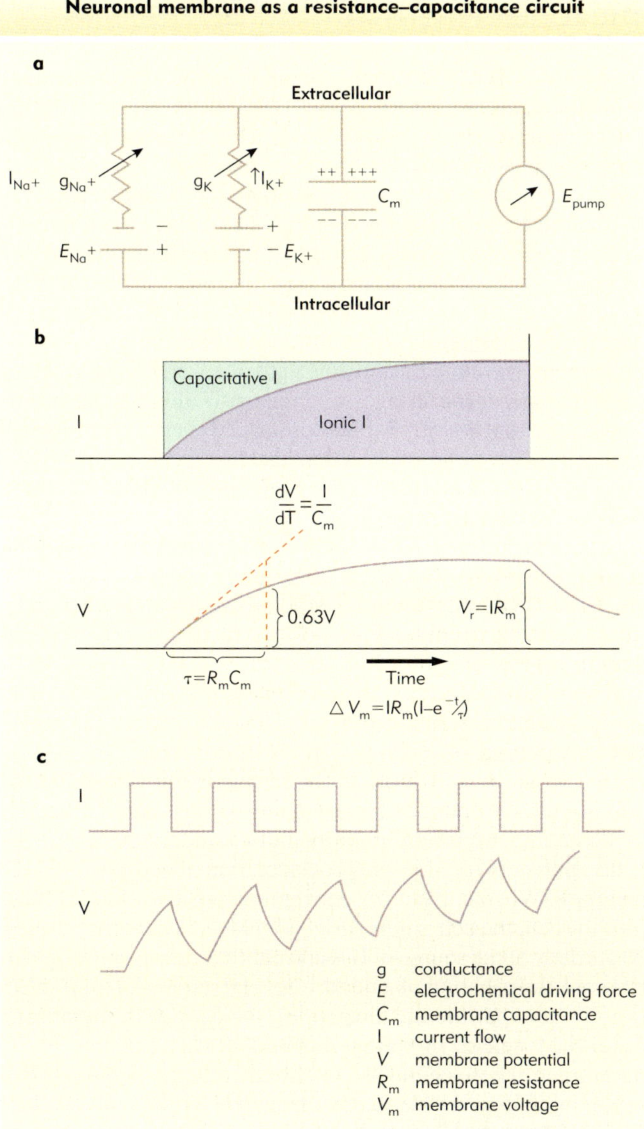

Figure 18.5 The neuronal membrane as a resistance–capacitance circuit. (a) Equivalent circuit representing the cell membrane with only gated ion channels in resting state: the electrochemical driving force (*E*) for ion flux across the membrane is shown for Na^+, K^+, and for the electrogenic Na^+/K^+ pump that creates the resting membrane potential. At rest, the conductances for Na^+ and K^+, represented by variable resistors, are nearly closed, so that the resting membrane potential depends mostly on the pump and on a small K^+ conductance. These Na^+ and K^+ conductances do not change in the resting membrane but are altered during the action potential (see Fig. 18.7). (b) The membrane potential changes with ion flow across a membrane, as described by the simple circuit in (a). The initial flow of charge is taken up by the membrane capacitance, so that the voltage across the membrane (the membrane potential) changes more slowly, according to an inverse first-order exponential relationship equivalent to that describing the potential across the capacitor in (a). The initial rate of change in potential is dependent upon the capacitance of the membrane; the final voltage change (V_r) is dependent upon the resistance. The membrane of the neuron, therefore, has a time constant τ, equal to the resistance across the membrane (R_m) multiplied by the capacitance (C_m), when the voltage has reached 63% of its value at the end of a long pulse of current. (c) This delay in voltage change across the cell membrane results in short pulses of current flow causing summating changes in membrane potential. This mechanism is found in neurons, where many short current fluxes from dendrites arriving apart may be partially additive.

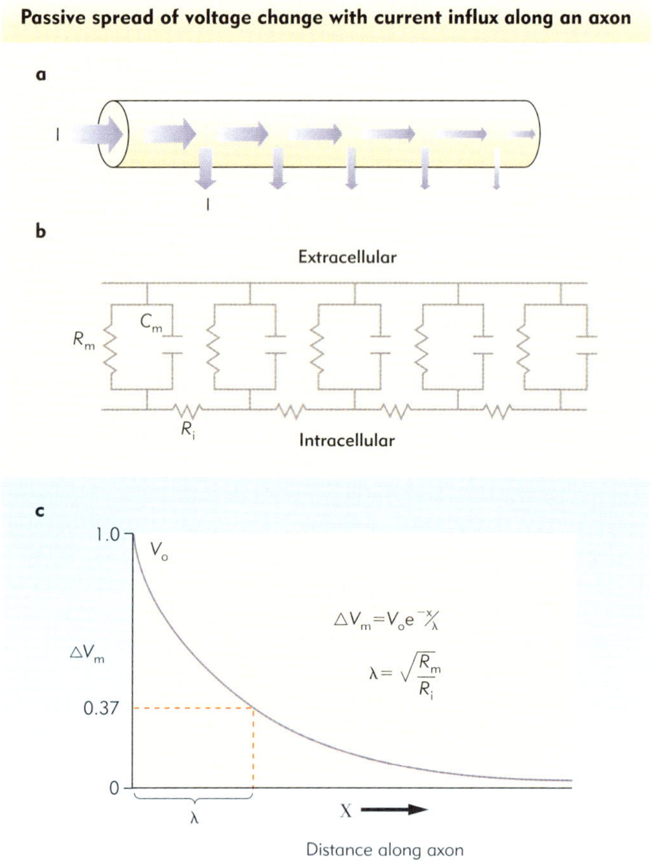

Passive spread of voltage change with current influx along an axon

Figure 18.6 Passive spread of voltage change with current influx along an axon. (a) Current flow along an axon, showing the flow across the membrane and within the cytoplasm gradually dissipating (arrow width is proportional to current flow). (b) In an equivalent circuit model of an axon, the resistance and capacitance of the membrane is shown as a series of resistances (R_m) and capacitances (C_m) in parallel. Extracellular fluid resistance is not shown since it is negligible compared with intracellular resistance (R_i). (c) Voltage change along the axon declines with distance as an inverse first-order exponential. The effective distance that the potential change travels is described by λ, the length constant (or space constant), which is the distance where the decrement is 1/e, or 37% of the initial voltage change. The length constant is dependent on the ratio of the resistance of the axonal membrane to the longitudinal resistance of the cytoplasm.

equivalent circuits linked in parallel, with a low resistance to current flow along the cylinder in the extracellular fluid and the cytoplasm, and a higher resistance across the membrane. If current enters at one end of the cylinder, there will be a change in membrane potential at that site (with the delay described above) representing a change in the distribution of charge across the membrane. The local change in charge across the membrane also means that there is a difference in charge between this site and adjacent sites on the same side of the membrane, such that current will flow along the membrane. As a result, the potential change will be propagated along the membrane as well. However, the change in potential will decrease with distance along the membrane since the cell membrane is not perfectly impermeable and will dissipate the charge difference. Consequently, the rate of voltage decrement is dependent not only on the capacitance of the membrane, which determines how much of the charge goes to the capacitor, but also on the relative resistance of the membrane, the cytoplasm, and extracellular fluid. This passive, or electrotonic, conduction is described by λ, the length constant (also called the space constant), which is the distance at which the potential charge has decreased to 1/e (or 37%) of its original value, since it declines as an inverse first-order exponential.

The capacitative properties of the cell membrane and the resistive properties of the cytoplasm and the extracellular fluid are quite constant in nearly all neurons. However, the resting resistance of the cell membrane may be quite variable from cell to cell. Length constants of over a hundred times the cell body diameter, or more than the length of some very long dendrites, have been measured. This suggests that much of the electrical communication within a neuron can take place with only the passive electrical properties of neurons taking part. Active properties are needed primarily for communication over very long distances.

THE ACTION POTENTIAL

All animal cells have a resting potential, ion pumps, and a membrane that acts like an RC circuit. What distinguishes neurons (and to a lesser extent muscle and endocrine cells) from other cells is their excitability. Excitability is the ability of a cell to generate and propagate a large, rapid potential change in response to a relatively small trigger stimulus. The central phenomenon of excitability is the action potential. It is the fundamental unit of information exchange over long distances in the nervous system, and often over very short distances as well. In contrast to passive conduction, the action potential conducts without decrement, traveling the entire length of an axon, up to meters, unchanging, regenerating itself constantly along its path. The action potential is a very rapid, stereotyped event: a coordinated sequence of several processes that lead to a specific, rapid depolarization (loss of negative intracellular potential), usually continuing to positive intracellular potentials then rapidly repolarizing back to negative potentials, all within a few milliseconds. It is a regenerative, all-or-none event set in motion when the membrane potential depolarizes to a level where adequate inward current begins a positive-feedback loop of depolarization (Fig. 18.7).

The action potential depends on the presence of voltage-gated ion channels that respond to changes in membrane potential by opening or closing. This is in contrast to nongated channels, which contribute to the resting membrane potential and are always open. There are many voltage-gated channels involved in neuronal excitability, but an understanding of the action potential requires only consideration of two: Na^+ and K^+ channels. When current (by convention, positive charge) flows into the cell, the cell is depolarized (made less negative inside). Regardless of the source of this current (neurotransmitter-gated channel, propagation of a nearby depolarization, current injection by an experimental electrode), the change in membrane potential is sensed by voltage-dependent Na^+ channels in the membrane. These channels are closed at the resting potential, but if the change in potential is adequately large (to above their threshold potential), they suddenly open. This allows Na^+ to

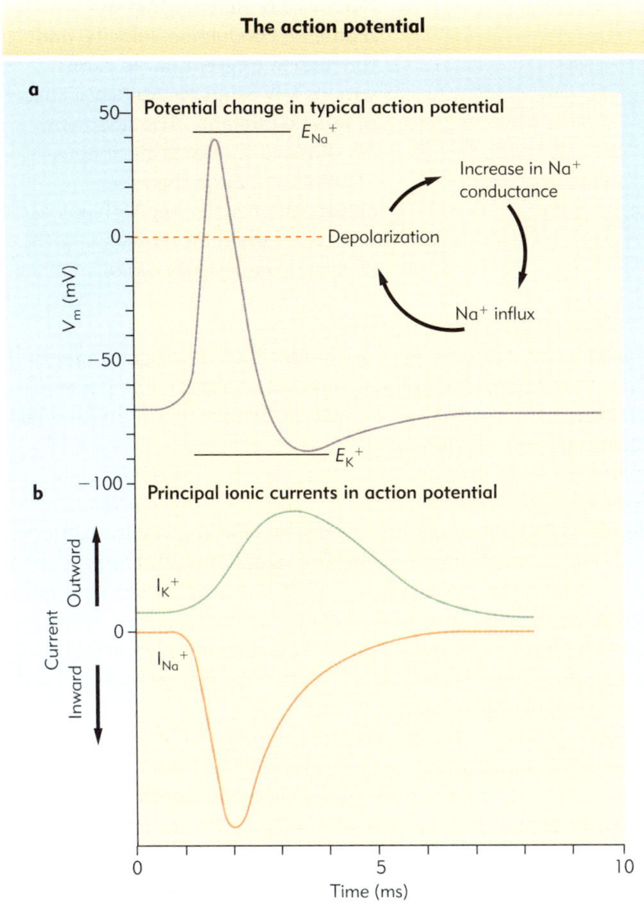

Figure 18.7 The action potential. (a) The potential change of a typical action potential rises from a resting potential of –70mV, reaching a maximum near the Nernst potential for Na^+ (E_{Na+}), then declining with a negative undershoot near the Nernst potential for K^+ (E_{K+}). The action potential is triggered by a positive feedback loop in which the initial depolarizing stimulus leads to opening of Na^+ channels, which leads to more depolarization. (b) Two principal ionic currents give rise to the action potential. Note that the outward K^+ current is slower and delayed in onset compared with the Na^+ current.

flow through into the cell, since at the resting potential Na^+ is not at equilibrium across the membrane; in fact it is far from it. The cell membrane at rest is quite impermeable to Na^+, and the electrogenic ion pumps make the intracellular concentration small relative to that outside the cell. As a result, the concentration gradient for Na^+ is toward the inside of the cell. Since the resting potential is about –70mV, there is also a substantial electrical gradient for Na^+ flow into the cell. The equilibrium potential (Nernst potential) for Na^+ is about +50mV, resulting in a net electrochemical gradient of 120mV. The initial ion flow through voltage-gated Na^+ channels with depolarization leads to more depolarization and then more channel opening, starting a positive-feedback loop until all the channels that can be opened are open and the membrane potential has approached the Nernst potential for Na^+. The membrane potential can go from a value of –50mV to as high as +40mV or more in less than a millisecond once this process is initiated.

Once the action potential is initiated, the process must be turned off for the membrane to return to its resting potential. The Na^+ channels, once open, spontaneously close after a very short period (a few milliseconds), a process called inactivation. Another type of voltage-gated channel, permeable to K^+, also opens in response to the depolarization produced by the action potential, but with a small delay compared with the Na^+ channels. As discussed above, the Nernst potential for K^+ is near the resting potential. When these K^+ channels open during an action potential, the membrane potential is positive, so there is a very strong gradient for K^+ to travel out of the cell, causing an outward current that tends to bring the membrane potential back to its resting state. In fact, there is a small overshoot to most action potentials, during which the membrane potential is more negative than the resting potential for several milliseconds; this is caused by the action of these K^+ channels. The opening of K^+ channels occurs a little slower than that of Na^+ channels; consequently, they do not oppose the action of Na^+ channels until after the action potential has been initiated, assisting primarily in resetting the potential back to the resting level. Because of this, they are referred to as delayed rectifier K^+ channels. The result of these two currents acting in this highly coordinated manner is a potential change, as shown in Figure 18.7. There are several other K^+ channels (not discussed here) that are involved in the regulation more than in the production of the action potential in various types of neuron.

The action potential has several characteristics that are important for its information-carrying function: threshold, all-or-none behavior, and the refractory period.

Threshold

The depolarization of the membrane must have enough speed and amplitude to activate an adequate number of Na^+ channels to initiate the positive-feedback mechanism that will cause the process to become regenerative. Otherwise, a small number of channels will be activated but not enough to depolarize the membrane further to start the positive feedback loop. The voltage at which the process becomes regenerative and self-sustaining is the action potential threshold. This is not a static value, but a dynamic phenomenon dependent on the initial resting potential, the rate of depolarization, the history of recent action potentials, and metabolic modulations.

All-or-none behavior

The second important characteristic of the action potential is that it is an all-or-none phenomenon and is essentially the same every time. This is particularly important in conduction, where an action potential propagates unchanged as long as there are enough voltage-gated Na^+ channels to support it. The two related phenomena of threshold and all-or-none behavior are key to information processing by the nervous system. One of the principal ways of processing information in neurons is the combination of graded excitatory (depolarizing) and inhibitory (hyperpolarizing) influences from synaptic and metabolic sources, which determine whether an action potential will be initiated. This is essentially a calculation at the level of the membrane; once the threshold is reached, it is encoded as an on/off signal that is propagated unchanged to the end of the axon.

Axon diameter and conduction velocity in afferent fibers

	Fiber type	Fiber diameter (μm)	Conduction velocity (m/s)	Function
Myelinated	Aα (group I)	12–20	75–120	Muscle stretch receptors, tendon afferents
	Aβ (group II)	5–12	30–75	Muscle stretch receptors, light touch
	Aδ (group III)	1–5	5–30	Fast pain (immediate, sharp)
Unmyelinated	C (group IV)	0.2–1.5	0.3–1.5	Slow pain (burning, ache)

Figure 18.8 Relationship of diameter, conduction velocity, and function in afferent nerve axons. Groups I–IV refers to the classification of muscle afferents. The fiber types Aβ, Aδ, and C refer to cutaneous afferents, although the latter classification, including Aα fibers, is often used when the classification is by conduction velocity alone.

Refractory period

The third important characteristic of the action potential is the refractory period. Once channels have opened to create an action potential, they cannot re-open immediately but require from a few milliseconds to several seconds to return to a fully activatable state. This has several consequences. First, it limits the rate at which action potentials can fire, which is an important aspect of neuronal signaling. Second, it allows conduction in only one direction at a time along a segment of axon. This is because two converging action potentials will collide and, since the membrane behind each action potential is refractory, conduction will terminate.

Propagation of the action potential

Propagation of action potentials involves the same process described above acting over space. The inward current caused by Na^+ influx depolarizes the membrane; this depolarization is easily propagated along the membrane toward areas with less charge by electrotonic conduction. As the depolarization spreads to other areas of the membrane, voltage-gated Na^+ channels nearby are opened and the action potential is propogated. Unlike electrotonic conduction, which decays with distance, action potentials maintain their size and shape and will conduct unchanged along a nerve for a theoretically infinite distance. The velocity of this conduction varies tremendously between nerves: depending on their physiologic function the velocity ranges from several centimeters per second to as much as 10m/s (Fig. 18.8). In some pathologic states, such as multiple sclerosis, nerve conduction is drastically affected so that it is slowed and may fail. The factors affecting conduction velocity can be derived from a mathematical analysis of the equivalent electrical circuit model of the membrane and knowledge of the nature of the action potential. The derivation is beyond the scope of this chapter, but the conclusions are quite simple and fit well with experimental observations.

Axon diameter

Bigger axons conduct faster. An increase in diameter increases the capacitance of a given length of axon linearly, which tends to slow conduction, but it decreases the resistance of the cytoplasm in proportion to the square of the radius, since this resistance is proportional to the cross-sectional area of cytoplasm. The result is an increase in conduction velocity proportional to the square root of the radius.

Channel kinetics

Channels that open faster will change the membrane potential faster and tend to open nearby Na^+ channels sooner, resulting in faster conduction. This also occurs with increased channel density. For example, the axons of neurons that conduct information about touch and movement have Na^+ channels that open faster than those of neurons that transmit some pain information or control autonomic function, which do not require fast information transmission.

Temperature

Temperature has complex effects. In general, cooling a nerve will slow conduction by slowing the rate that Na^+ channels open and close, as well as the rate that Na^+ traverses the channels. Substantial cooling can actually block conduction. Warming speeds conduction up to a point, but warming over about 40°C causes the channels to close too soon, reducing current flow and, thus, conduction velocity.

Membrane capacitance and resistance: myelination

The vertebrate nervous system can increase conduction velocity by wrapping the axon in an insulating layer of myelin over intermittent segments of the axon. This can increase conduction velocity up to 10-fold over that achieved in an unmyelinated nerve. Since myelination is so important in axonal conduction, it will be discussed in more detail.

Myelin and saltatory conduction

Invertebrates are limited to increasing axonal diameter to speed conduction for signals that must be conducted very fast, such as the signals for flight from danger. The squid, for instance, escapes quickly with signals that travel about 20m/s along a huge axon that is over 1mm in diameter. (A preparation of this giant axon was used to great advantage to characterize the electrophysiology of the axon.) This approach, however, is very inefficient in terms of space and metabolic requirements, since conduction velocity increases only as the square root of the radius. Myelination allows vertebrates to conduct signals along axons that are only a few micrometers in diameter at rates exceeding that achieved in the squid.

Myelin is a tight, spiral, multilayered wrapping of glial cell membranes around an axon (see Fig. 18.2). Since cell membranes are electrical insulators, they increase the effective resistance of the axon to current flow across its membrane. In addition, the myelin sheath, which is much thicker than the axonal membrane, increases the distance between the charges inside the cell and those in the extracellular fluid, which reduces the effective capacitance of the axon. In an ideal system, an action potential could then be conducted through the axoplasm of a myelinated nerve all the way to its end, where the current would escape into the extracellular fluid and complete the circuit in a similar manner to conductance through an insulated copper wire. However, axoplasm and extracellular fluid are not perfect conductors and myelin is not a perfect insulator, so signals need to be regenerated at regular intervals along the axon.

To do this, myelin is interrupted, usually every 1–2mm along the axon, for a very short distance (a few micrometers) and the axon membrane is exposed to the extracellular fluid. Essentially all the Na^+ channels in the axon are bunched in these zones, called nodes of Ranvier. Current traveling electrotonically in the axon from the nearby node causes a depolarization that is sufficient to trigger the opening of Na^+ channels in the next node, producing a full action potential that is then conducted to the next node. This node-to-node jump is called *saltatory conduction*. The ability of myelin to allow conduction through the axon with little need to charge the membrane capacitance along the way results in very high conduction velocity within relatively small axons. It is also energy efficient, because ions flow across the membrane only at the nodes. Myelinated axons also show improved gain from an increase in diameter: velocity increases directly with the axon diameter in myelinated axons, compared with changing with the square root of diameter in unmyelinated fibers.

Classification of nerves according to conduction velocity

Since different biologic functions necessitate different conduction velocities along axons, conduction velocity has been used to classify sensory axons (Fig. 18.8). This classification illustrates the relation between action potential conduction velocity and the two strategies used by the nervous system to alter it: axon diameter and myelination. It is also used clinically in the diagnosis of peripheral neuropathies. Most sensory nerves contain a mix of fiber types. When such a nerve is stimulated and the action potentials produced are recorded at a distance away, the record contains several impulse peaks (classically four) representing action potentials from hundreds to thousands of axons (compound action potential) arriving at different times according to their conduction velocities. The first peak to reach the recording electrode is that carried by the large-diameter, myelinated fibers, the fastest of which are the Aα axons (also called group I afferents), which exist only in nerves innervating muscle (Fig. 13.6). They are the sensory axons of the muscle spindle reflex arc. The next peak is from the small myelinated fiber, designated Aβ or group II axons, which carry sensory information about mechanical stimuli such as touch. The third peak is the Aδ or group III axons, which carry both mechanosensory information and also some types of pain information, typically that perceived as sharp or lancinating pain. These are even smaller myelinated fibers. The slowest fibers, often conducting at less than 1m/s, are small diameter unmyelinated sensory axons. They primarily carry information about temperature and pain, particularly pain that is perceived as burning or aching (Chapter 21).

The nature and function of voltage-gated ion channels

The existence of entities for conducting specific ions across membranes was demonstrated in the landmark studies of Hodgkin and Huxley in the 1950s in which they described the action potential in terms of specific ion currents. Since then we have gained detailed knowledge of the voltage-gated channels involved in excitability, advancing from theoretic concepts to increasingly well-understood molecular entities. This has been made possible by two experimental advances: the invention of the patch-clamp recording technique and the application of techniques of molecular biology to clone specific channels. In the mid 1970s, Neher and Sakmann succeeded in electrically isolating a single ion channel by sealing a tiny glass electrode around it on the surface of a muscle. These studies eventually led to a detailed knowledge of

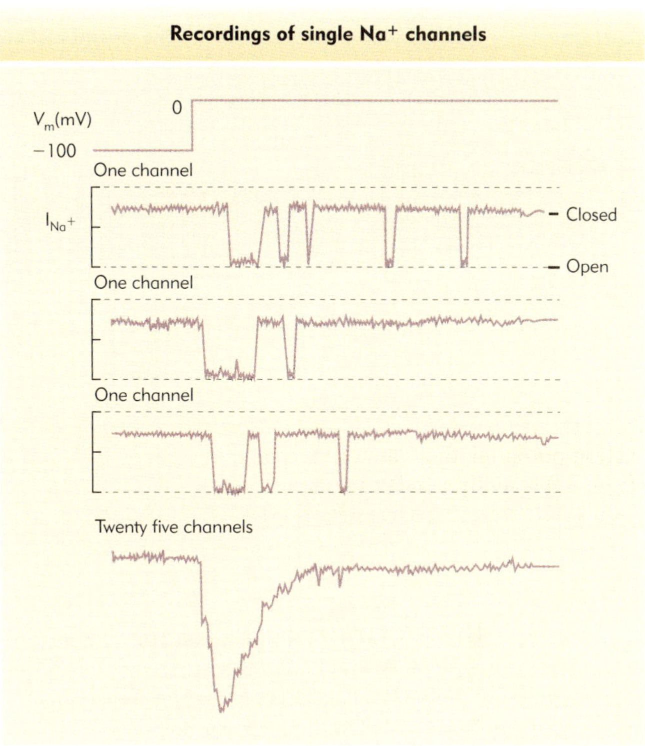

Figure 18.9 Recordings of single Na^+ channels. Schematic of patch clamp recordings of individual Na^+ channels activated by depolarization from a potential of −100 to 0mV. Note that channels open quickly to a uniform conductance with a more variable time course. Channels open with the initial depolarization then open less as the membrane is held at 0mV, representing channel inactivation. When many records of single channels are summed, the resulting trace reconstructs that seen with a whole cell recording (lowest trace).

the function of the individual channels that make up the action potential, as well as of many other channels. An example of single-channel recordings is shown in Figure 18.9.

Once ion channels were cloned and inserted into cells lacking such channels, both the molecular structure and the channel activity of these entities could be determined. For example, it has been found that there are several types of voltage-gated Na^+ channel involved in action potential generation, often with different properties depending on the tissue in which they are expressed (e.g. brain, peripheral neurons). This has become a recurrent theme with ion channels. As a result, there are more channels identified for each ion than could have been predicted with classical physiologic and pharmacologic approaches, leading to a tremendous opportunity for specific pharmacologic intervention. At the same time, it has been found that ion channels can be grouped into families based on their amino acid sequences. Voltage-gated channels for Na^+, K^+, and Ca^{2+} are all very similar in structure. They all have a subunit with a domain structure of six transmembrane segments. The Na^+ and Ca^{2+} channels are very similar in structure, with four subunits of this type. The K^+ channels, however, appear to have only one subunit. The structure of the pore-forming α-subunit of a typical Na^+ channel is shown in Figure 18.10. From knowledge of the amino acid sequence of these channels and studies of the effect of known mutations on channel function, certain inferences can be made about their structure. For

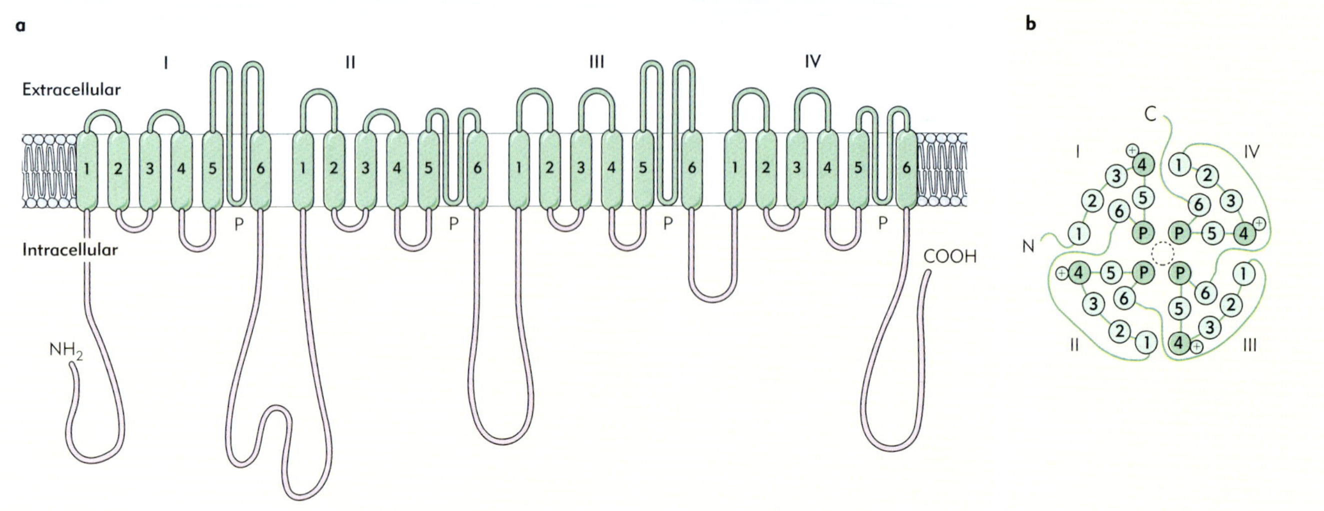

Figure 18.10 The structure of a voltage-gated Na^+ channel. (a) The tertiary structure of the α-subunit is based on maps of hydrophobicity of amino acids obtained by sequencing of the mRNA (cDNA). The channel has four similar domains, each consisting of six transmembrane segments. (b) The predicted structure of the channel as seen from outside the cell comprises a pore formed by the amino acid chain between segments 5 and 6 in each subunit. Segment 4 (indicated by positive charge symbols), having a preponderance of positive charges on the extracellular side, may be the voltage sensor that opens the channel in response to depolarization.

example, mutants of a type of voltage-gated K^+ channel have shown that a region of the channel protein called S4 (the fourth transmembrane segment of a subunit region) is probably responsible for the voltage-sensing properties of the channel. This same region probably confers voltage-sensitive opening of Ca^{2+} and Na^+ channels as well. In addition, a highly hydrophobic region, called the P segment, appears to be the pore or channel-forming area of the protein, and cytoplasmic segments appear to be involved in closing an open channel. They have positively charged amino acids at the ends of cytoplasmic segments. Following depolarization and channel opening, these amino acids may move and occlude the open channel like a drain plug on a chain. This conformational change may be the molecular mechanism underlying the phenomenon of channel inactivation. Such molecular descriptions of ion channel function are just beginning and may lead both to an understanding of the structure–function relationships of channels and to the design of drugs that act on specific functions to alter neuronal excitability (Chapters 5 and 28).

Key References

Hodgkin AL, Huxley AF. A quantitative description of membrane current and its application to conduction and excitation in nerve. J Physiol. 1952;117:500–44.

Hodgkin AL, Huxley AF. Currents carried by sodium and potassium ions through the membrane of the giant axon of Loligo. J Physiol. 1952;116:449–72.

Caterall WA. Structure and function of voltage-gated ion channels. Annu Rev Biochem. 1995;64:493–531.

Miller C. How ion channel proteins work. In: Kaczmarek LK, Levitan IB, eds. Neuromodulation: the biochemical control of neuronal excitability. New York: Oxford University Press; 1987:39–63.

Sheetz MP, Streuer ER, Shroer TA. The mechanism and regulation of fast axonal transport. Trends Neurosci. 1989;12:474–8.

Travis J. Glia: the brain's other cells. Science. 1994;266:970–2.

Dani JW, Chenjavsky A, Smith SJ. Neuronal activity triggers calcium waves in hippocampal astrocyte networks. Neuron. 1992;8:429–40.

Peters A, Palay SL, Webster HDF. The fine structure of the nervous system: the neurons and supporting cells. Philadelphia, PA: Saunders; 1976.

Further Reading

Hille B. Ion channels of excitable membranes, 2nd edn. Sunderland, MA: Sinauer; 1992.

Sakmann B, Neher E. Single-channel recording, 2nd edn. New York: Phenum Press;1995.

Levitan IB, Kaczmarek, LK. The neuron: cell and molecular biology, 2nd edn. New York: Oxford University Press; 1997.

Chapter 19 The synapse

Ken Mackie

Topics covered in this chapter

Presynaptic terminals
Fast and slow synaptic transmission
Peptide neurotransmitters
Neurotransmitter receptors
Neurotransmitter synthesis and metabolism
Synaptic transmission
Modulation of excitability and synaptic transmission
Neural plasticity

Synapses serve as the primary point of communication between neurons. Synapses are highly specialized neuronal structures at which most neurotransmitter release takes place. Their number in the human brain is immense; conservative estimates are that the human brain contains about 10^{11} neurons and $>10^{14}$ synapses. Both the large number of synapses and the ability of neurons to modulate the efficacy, or strength, of particular synaptic connections creates the complexity and flexibility of the human brain. In addition, the central role that synapses play in the functioning of the nervous system makes synaptic transmission an important target for many anesthetic drugs.

PRESYNAPTIC TERMINALS

Synaptic terminals may take many forms. These include the classic axodendritic type, but also dendrodendritic, dendroaxonal, axoaxonal, etc. While some of the more specialized synaptic structures occur in specific neuronal structures, it is useful to consider the classic axodendritic synapses as an example. As shown in Figure 19.1, the presynaptic terminal contains synaptic vesicles, mitochondria, and neurofilaments, and is a highly ordered structure.

Specialized structures opposite to presynaptic terminals are present in postsynaptic neurons (Fig. 19.1). In excitatory postsynaptic terminals, a band of electron dense material is present [the postsynaptic density (PSD)]. In addition, postsynaptic terminals contain receptors that bind released neurotransmitters as well as enzymes and ion channels that transduce the signal carried by the neurotransmitter into a physiologic response in the postsynaptic cell.

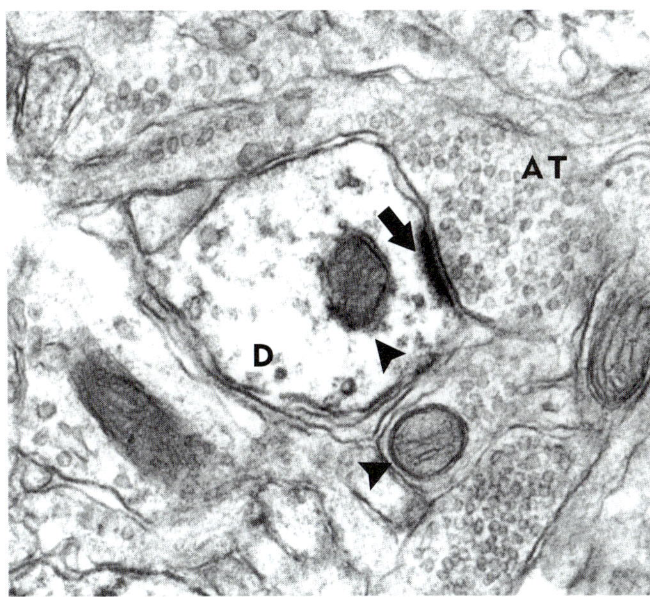

Figure 19.1 Ultrastructure of an excitatory synapse. Electron micrograph of an asymmetric synapse between an axon terminal (AT) and the dendrite (D) of a nonpyramidal cell in rat dorsal cortex. The terminal is packed with small vesicles that contain neurotransmitters. At the synaptic junction (arrow), the presynaptic and postsynaptic membranes are separated by a cleft (synapse), which contains extracellular matrix. The postsynaptic membrane has a prominent coat of dense material (PSD) on its cytoplasmic face. Note the mitochondria in the dendrite and an adjacent terminal (arrowhead). (Micrograph courtesy of Ruth Westenbroek.)

FAST AND SLOW SYNAPTIC TRANSMISSION

Neurotransmission can be conveniently, if simplistically, divided into two broad types – fast and slow (Fig. 19.2). Fast neurotransmission can be thought of as the point-to-point communication system in the brain. Slow neurotransmission can be thought of as setting the background tone for a group of synapses or brain region. A familiar example of fast neurotransmission is release of acetylcholine (ACh) at the neuromuscular junction (Chapter 31). Cation influx through the nicotinic ACh receptor (a ligand-gated ion channel) results in depolarization of the muscle cell membrane, which leads to Ca^{2+} release from the sarcoplasmic reticulum and muscle contraction. The action of ACh is terminated by its hydrolysis in the synaptic cleft by acetylcholinesterase. Fast neurotransmission by other transmitters in the CNS is also mediated by postsynaptic, ligand-gated ion channels. Examples include

Fast versus slow transmission in a submucous neuron

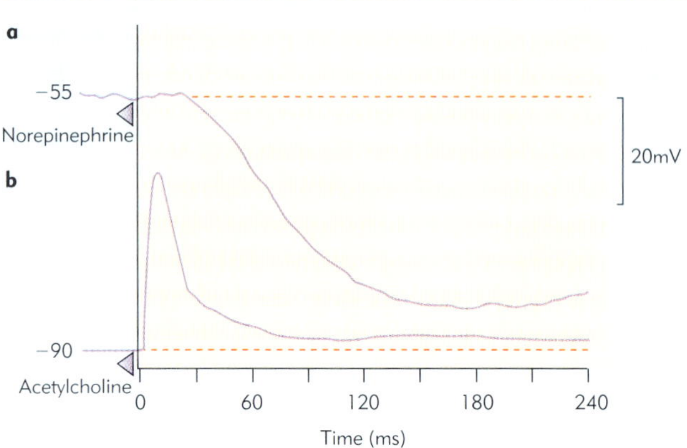

Figure 19.2 Fast versus slow neurotransmission in a guinea-pig submucous plexus neuron. (a) Norepinephrine induced hyperpolarization of membrane potential mediated by α_2-adrenergic receptors has a latency of approximately 30ms and reaches its maximum after approximately 180ms. (b) Acetylcholine (ACh)-induced depolarization mediated by the nicotinic ACh receptor in the same neuron has a very short latency and quickly reaches its peak and inactivates. In both cases a supramaximal amount of drug was applied for 0.5ms. (From North RA. Drug receptors and the inhibition of nerve cells. Br J Pharmacol. 1989;98:13–28.)

Fast neurotransmitter systems

Neurotransmitter	Receptor	Significantly permeant ions
Excitatory:		
Glutamate	NMDA	Na^+, K^+, (Ca^{2+})
	AMPA	Na^+, K^+
	Kainate	Na^+, K^+
ACh	Nicotinic	Na^+, K^+ > Ca^{2+}
Serotonin (5-hydroxytryptamine)	5-HT_3	Na^+, K^+, Ca^{2+}
ATP, ADP, UTP	P_{2X}	Na^+, K^+, $^{\pm}Ca^{2+}$
Vanillanoids, temperature	Capsaicin	Ca^{2+} > Na^+
Inhibitory:		
GABA	GABA	Cl^-
Glycine	Glycine	Cl^-

The receptors for these neurotransmitters belong to the superfamily of multimeric ligand-gated ion channels.

Figure 19.3 Fast neurotransmitter systems. (ADP, adenosine diphosphate; UTP, uridine triphosphate.)

glutamate [*N*-methyl-D-aspartate (NMDA), α-amino-3-hydroxy-5-methylisoxazole-4-propionic acid (AMPA), and kainate (KA) type receptors], γ-aminobutyric acid (GABA; $GABA_A$ receptors), glycine (glycine receptors), ACh (nicotinic ACh receptors), adenosine triphosphate [ATP; purinergic type 2X (P_{2X}) receptors], and serotonin [5-hydroxytryptamine (5-HT_3) receptors] (Fig. 19.3).

The other major class of neurotransmitters is the 'slow' neurotransmitters, often referred to as neuromodulators (Fig. 19.4). Their slowness is imparted by the type of receptors they interact with postsynaptically. These are often G-protein-coupled receptors (GPCRs). After the neurotransmitter binds to these receptors, they undergo a conformational change, which activates G proteins (Chapter 3). The activated G proteins dissociate and the α subunit and/or βγ subunits modulate the properties of specific enzymes and ion channels (effectors), setting in motion diverse cellular responses. Often a given neurotransmitter has both 'fast' and 'slow' effects. An example familiar to anesthesiologists is ACh, for which the fast effects (e.g. neurotransmission at the neuromuscular junction) are mediated by nicotinic ACh receptors and the slow effects (bronchoconstriction, salivation, gastrointestinal motility) by muscarinic ACh receptors. Other examples of neurotransmitters that have both fast and slow actions are GABA, serotonin, ATP, and glutamate. Many other neurotransmitters have only slow effects, and include the endogenous opioids, dopamine (DA), catecholamines, eicosanoids, etc. Many of these neurotransmitter systems are influenced by anesthetic drugs.

Another class of neuromodulators is that of free-radical messengers, which includes nitric oxide and carbon monoxide. While not stored in vesicles and released, as are most of the classic neurotransmitters mentioned above, they play important roles in neuronal signaling and neural plasticity.

NEUROTRANSMITTERS: EXCITATORY AND INHIBITORY

Another classification of neurotransmission is based on the effect of a neurotransmitter on a given neuron's membrane properties, termed excitatory or inhibitory. For fast neurotransmitters this distinction is fairly clear. Excitatory fast neurotransmitters open ligand-gated ion channels that are preferentially permeable to Na^+ and, often, Ca^{2+}. As these ions move down their electrochemical gradients, the membrane potential is displaced in a positive direction, which makes the cell more excitable (for example, more likely to fire an action potential). Inhibitory fast neurotransmitters, conversely, open ion channels that are more permeable to Cl^-, which keeps the membrane potential negative and makes the cell less excitable. Excitatory fast neurotransmitters include ACh, glutamate, ATP, and serotonin, while the inhibitory fast neurotransmitters in the mammalian CNS are GABA and glycine.

The major excitatory fast neurotransmitter is glutamate, which is integrally involved in neuronal function and plasticity. Activation of non-NMDA receptors (AMPA/kainate receptors) is thought to be responsible for most fast glutamatergic neurotransmission. The NMDA receptors only become fully activated by glutamate when their Mg^{2+} block has been relieved by depolarization of the neuron; also, their kinetics are much slower. Their activation results in a large Ca^{2+} influx, which has been linked to long-term metabolic and structural changes, which include synaptic plasticity (see below). These functional differences are reflected in their distinct subunit structures. *N*–methyl–D–aspartate receptors are heteromeric complexes (composed of four or five subunits) of NR1 and NR2 (subtypes A–D) subunits, while non-NMDA receptors

Slow neurotransmitter systems

Neurotransmitter	Receptor	Ion channels	Second messenger
Glutamate	Metabotropic	↓Ca^{2+}, ↑K^+	↑IP_3/DAG
GABA	$GABA_B$	↑K^+, ↓Ca^{2+}	↓cAMP ↑(IP_3/DAG) – minor
ACh	Muscarinic m_1, m_3, m_5	↓Ca^{2+}, ↓K^+ (M-current)	↑IP_3/DAG
	m_2, m_4	↓Ca^{2+}, ↑K^+	↓cAMP
Norepinephrine	α_1		↑IP_3/DAG
	α_2	↑K^+, ↓Ca^{2+}	↑IP_3/DAG
	β_1		↑cAMP
	β_2		↑cAMP
	β_3	↑Ca^{2+}	
Dopamine	D_1, D_5		↑cAMP
	D_2, D_3, D_4	↓Ca^{2+}, ↑K^+	↓cAMP
Serotonin (5-hydroxytryptamine)	$5\text{-}HT_1$	↑K^+, ↓Ca^{2+}	↓cAMP
	$5\text{-}HT_2$		↑IP_3/DAG
	$5\text{-}HT_4$		↑cAMP
	$5\text{-}HT_5$		↓cAMP
	$5\text{-}HT_6$		↑cAMP
	$5\text{-}HT_7$		↑cAMP
Substance P	NK_1	↓Ca^{2+}	↑IP_3/DAG
Histamine	H_1		↑IP_3/DAG
	H_2		↑cAMP
	H_3		↓cAMP, ?
ATP, ADP, UTP	P_{2Y}	↓Ca^{2+}, ↑K^+	↑IP_3/DAG
Adenosine	A_1		↓cAMP
	A_{2A}		↑cAMP
	A_{2B}		↑cAMP
	A_3		↓cAMP ↑IP_3/DAG
Opioids	μ	↓Ca^{2+}, ↑K^+	↓cAMP
	δ	↓Ca^{2+}, ↑K^+	↓cAMP
	κ	↓Ca^{2+}, ↑K^+	↓cAMP

The receptors for these neurotransmitters all belong to the superfamily of G-protein coupled receptors containing a predicted seven transmembrane domain structure. Different effects are seen with different subtypes. Not all effects are seen in all cells; net effect (e.g. on excitability) may be a complex balance of opposing effects. (IP_3, inositol trisphosphate; DAG, diacylglycerol; cAMP, cycline adenosine monophosphate.)

Figure 19.4 Slow neurotransmitter systems.

are composed of GluR (1–7) and KA (1–2) subunits. The major inhibitory fast transmitter is GABA, which is important in regulating neuronal excitability. Activation of pentameric $GABA_A$ receptors is responsible for fast GABAergic neurotransmission; these receptors are thought to be principal targets for anesthetic effects (Chapters 22–24). γ–Aminobutyric $acid_A$ receptors are made up at lease 17 different subunits classified as α (1–6), β (1–4), γ (1–3), δ, ϵ, and ρ (1–2), with additional diversity from alternative messenger ribonucleic acid (mRNA) splicing. The most common combination *in vivo* is two α, two β, and one γ subunit.

Slow neurotransmitters can be classified similarly, although often the distinctions are blurred as a single neuron may express multiple distinct receptors. This occurs because, although the receptors bind the same agonist, they couple to a different spectrum of G proteins that activate different effector systems and produce opposite effects on excitability (a good example of this is the muscarinic ACh receptor family). A related complicating factor in the interpretation of neurotransmitter action is that the same subtype of receptor can couple to different effectors in different cells. Thus, the examples given below are generalities only – specific exceptions exist. Examples of excitatory slow neurotransmitter receptors include substance P, bradykinin, metabotropic glutamate, and the odd numbered (m_1, m_3, and m_5) muscarinic receptors. As one of their actions, many of the excitatory slow neurotransmitter receptors activate phospholipase C (PLC). Specific polyphosphatide-containing membrane lipids are cleaved by PLC to release inositol trisphosphate (IP_3) and diacylglycerol (DAG). Release of Ca^{2+} from internal stores (endoplasmic reticulum) is mediated by IP_3, activating several cellular processes that tend to increase excitability. The DAG, in concert with IP_3-released Ca^{2+}, activates protein kinase C (PKC, see Chapter 3), which can also increase excitability. Furthermore, membrane depolarization by inhibition of a K^+ channel (the 'M-current') is another action of many of these receptors. All of these actions increase neuronal excitability.

Examples of inhibitory slow neurotransmitter receptors include opioid, even-numbered muscarinic (m_2 and m_4), and α_2 adrenergic receptors. Inhibitory slow neurotransmitters often inhibit adenylyl cyclase, activate K^+ channels (particularly inwardly rectifying K^+ channels), and inhibit N- and P/Q-type voltage-dependent Ca^{2+} channels, which are the Ca^{2+} channel in presynaptic terminals through which Ca^{2+} enters to cause synaptic vesicle fusion and neurotransmitter release (see below). These actions tend to decrease neuronal excitability.

PEPTIDE NEUROTRANSMITTERS

The neuropeptides form an important family of neurotransmitters. While the number of peptide neurotransmitters continues to expand, a list of the best-studied peptide neurotransmitters is shown in Figure 19.5. Those most relevant to the practice of anesthesiology include the endogenous opioids (enkephalins, endorphins, dynorphin, and their precursors and metabolites; Chapter 26), substance P, and bradykinin.

Peptides are slow neurotransmitters and typically exert their actions by binding to GPCRs (Chapter 3). While classic neurotransmitters, such as glutamate, ACh, GABA, etc., are released from small (40nm diameter) clear vesicles by the mechanisms outlined below, peptides are often released from large (100nm diameter) vesicles by less well understood pathway(s). Typically, these vesicles are not near active zones and it has been postulated that they fuse with the membrane and release their contents only during strong and prolonged increases in presynaptic Ca^{2+} concentration, as seen during repetitive depolarizations (peptide release is thus frequency dependent). A key difference between peptides and other neurotransmitters is that peptides are synthesized in the cell body and transported to the nerve terminal. Thus, replenishment of peptide-containing

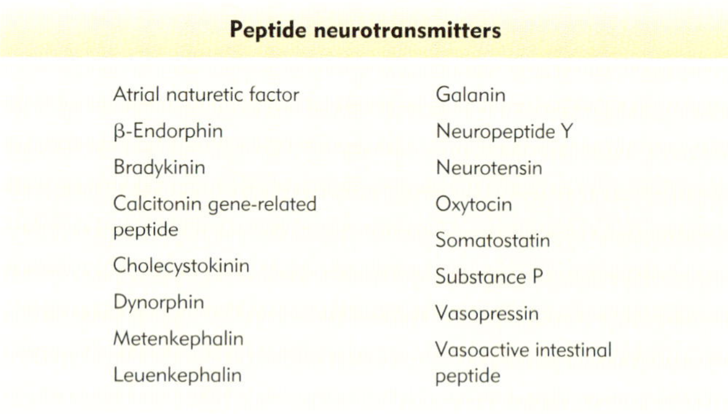
Peptide neurotransmitters

Atrial naturetic factor	Galanin
β-Endorphin	Neuropeptide Y
Bradykinin	Neurotensin
Calcitonin gene-related peptide	Oxytocin
Cholecystokinin	Somatostatin
Dynorphin	Substance P
Metenkephalin	Vasopressin
Leuenkephalin	Vasoactive intestinal peptide

Figure 19.5 Peptide neurotransmitters.

synaptic vesicles is much slower than that of other neurotransmitter-containing vesicles.

A once prevalent concept in neuropharmacology held that each neuron contained only a single transmitter. However, this concept has recently given way to the idea that neuropeptides coexist in many central and most, if not all, peripheral neurons with classic amino acid or monoamine transmitters. Peptides are thus positioned to increase the information transferred at a given synapse by regulating the amount of transmitter released with a given stimulus or modulating the response of a common target cell.

NEUROTRANSMITTER RECEPTORS

Neurotransmitter receptors can be conveniently divided into two classes. The first class contains the ligand-gated ion channels, which both bind the neurotransmitter and, when open, allow specific ions to pass through. These are the receptors that underlie fast neurotransmission discussed above (see Fig. 19.3). They consist of a large protein (an assembly of several smaller subunits, e.g. the nicotinic ACh receptor composed of two α subunits and β, γ, δ, and/or ϵ subunits) that both binds the neurotransmitter (usually with two binding sites per channel) and forms the ion pore. In addition, auxiliary subunits are often associated with the pore-forming and ligand-binding subunit. These subunits may convey specific pharmacologic properties (e.g. γ subunits of the $GABA_A$ channel contain the benzodiazepine binding site).

The second class of neurotransmitter receptor contains those that underlie slow neurotransmission (see Fig. 19.3). A classic example of a slow neurotransmitter receptor is GPCR; other examples include soluble guanylyl cyclase (the receptor for nitric oxide) and receptor tyrosine kinases (see Chapter 3). The effects of many neuromodulators are transduced by GPCRs, as briefly outlined above. Guanylyl cyclase is a 'receptor' for and activated by nitric oxide and related free-radical messengers. Receptor tyrosine kinases bind small peptides (e.g. cytokines and growth factors) in their extracellular domain, which leads to activation of the intracellular tyrosine kinase domain that phosphorylates specific target molecules in the cell. While these receptors have long been known to play a key role in regulating neuronal growth, differentiation, and survival, it is now clear that they also play an important role in regulating neuronal excitability through their effects on specific ion channels and G protein signaling pathways.

NEUROTRANSMITTER SYNTHESIS AND METABOLISM

The synthesis and metabolism of the small neurotransmitters [ACh, norepinephrine (noradrenaline), DA, epinephrine (adrenaline), glutamate, GABA, glycine, etc.] has been studied extensively. In addition to *de novo* synthesis, reuptake of released neurotransmitter from the synaptic cleft is an important mechanism used by neurons to recover released neurotransmitter or their metabolites.

Many neurotransmitters are synthesized *de novo* from amino acids or metabolic intermediates. Figure 19.6 shows the metabolic pathways for the synthesis of ACh, GABA, and the catecholamines (DA, norepinephrine, and epinephrine). Neurotransmitter synthesis is tightly regulated to enable the nerve terminal to adjust rapidly its rate of neurotransmitter synthesis over a wide range. This not only allows the nerve terminal to synthesize large amounts of neurotransmitter during periods of intense activity, but also allows it to slow metabolically costly synthesis during periods of relative inactivity. The best-studied example of regulated neurotransmitter synthesis is that of catecholamines. The rate-limiting step in catecholamine synthesis is the hydroxylation of tyrosine, a process catalyzed by the soluble enzyme tyrosine hydroxylase. Tyrosine hydroxylase activity is inhibited by norepinephrine through competition between it and the necessary cofactor, tetrahydropteridine. Thus, as the concentration of norepinephrine increases, enzyme activity declines. However, tyrosine hydroxylase activity increases during periods of nerve stimulation to compensate for the increased neurotransmitter release. This is likely a consequence of its phosphorylation by cAMP-dependent protein kinase, Ca^{2+}/calmodulin-dependent protein kinase II (Cam KII), and PKC. The activity of all three of these kinases is increased by repetitive depolarization, which results in increased phosphorylation and activation of tyrosine hydroxylase during periods of rapid synaptic transmission.

The synthesis of peptide neurotransmitters is quite different from that of small neurotransmitters. While the latter are synthesized in nerve terminals, peptide neurotransmitters are synthesized in the cell body and transported to the nerve terminal. Like other secreted proteins, peptide neurotransmitters are synthesized and modified in the rough endoplasmic reticulum and transported to the *cis*-Golgi, where they undergo further post-translational modifications (e.g. glycosylation) and are sorted based on their eventual destination. Neurotransmitter-containing vesicles bud off the Golgi stacks and are transported down to the nerve terminal by a specific transport process.

Most peptide neurotransmitters are synthesized as large prohormones that are proteolytically processed into smaller, biologically active peptides (Fig. 19.7). A typical example is the prohormone pro-opiomelanocortin (POMC), which is cleaved, in a tissue-specific fashion, to γ-melanocyte-stimulating hormone (γ-MSH), adrenocorticotropic hormone (or α-MSH and corticotropin-like intermediate lobe peptide), γ-lipotropin (γ-LPH), and β-endorphin. The other opioid peptides – enkephalins and dynorphins – are processed in a similar fashion (Chapter 26). Peptide diversity is increased at the level of transcription by alternative RNA processing (Fig. 19.8). The first example of mRNA processing delineated was for calcitonin and the calcitonin gene-related peptide (CGRP). Here a single gene gives rise to two distinct mRNAs through alternative splicing. These mRNAs are translated into two distinct prohormones that are processed to give calcitonin and CGRP.

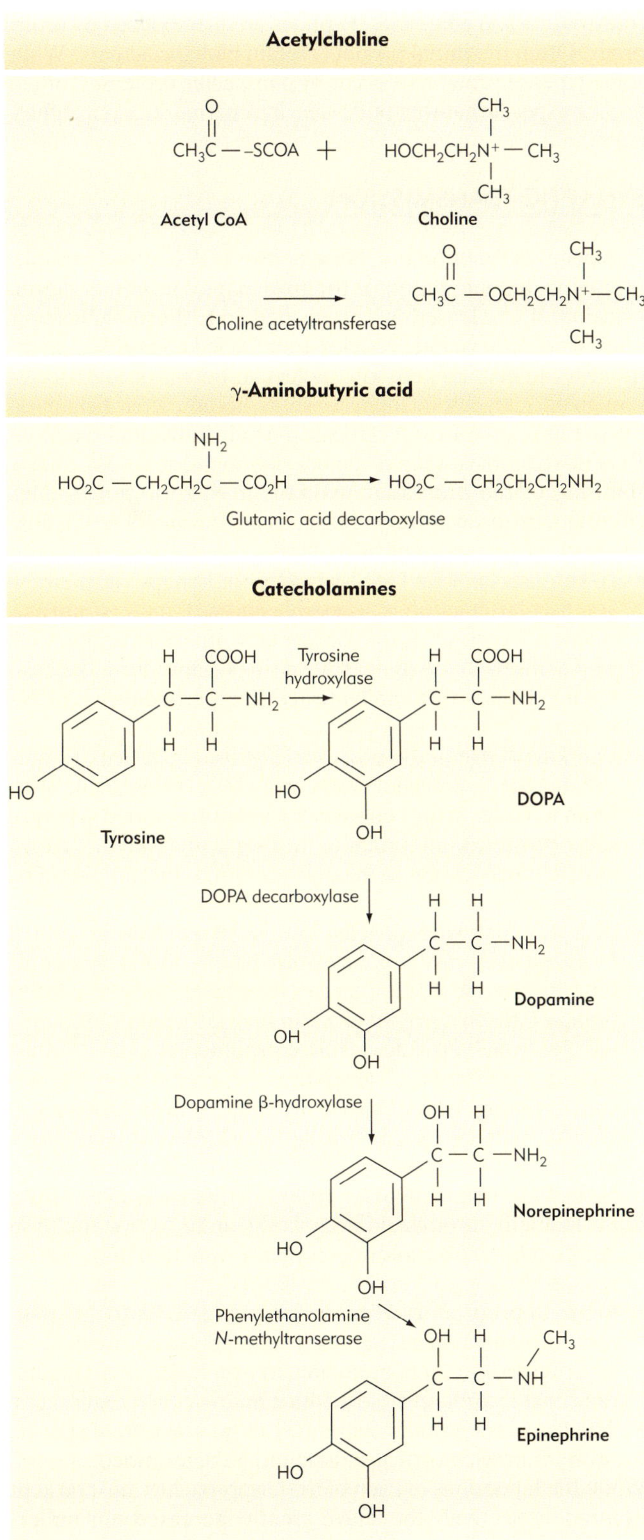

Figure 19.6 Synthetic pathways for small neurotransmitters. Small neurotransmitters, such as ACh, GABA, and the catecholamines, are synthesized in the nerve terminal. Activity of their synthetic enzymes is tightly regulated (see text).

Another class of neuromodulators are those derived from fatty acids, examples of which include the prostaglandins, platelet-activating factor, the endogenous sleep factor oleamide, and the

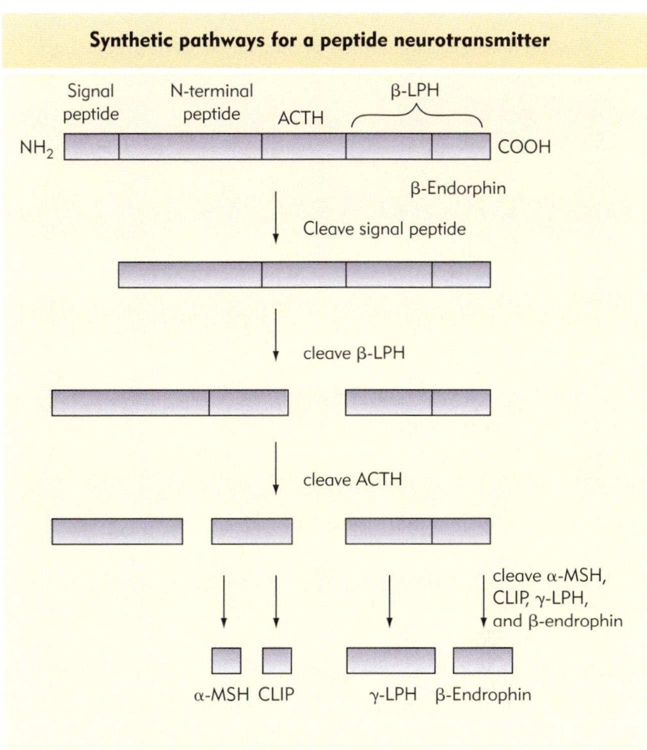

Figure 19.7 Synthetic pathways for a peptide neurotransmitter. Peptide neurotransmitters are often synthesized as a large precursor, cleaved into several biologically active fragments in the soma, packaged into vesicles, and transported to nerve terminals. Processing of the β-endorphin precursor, POMC is shown here. (ACTH, adrenocorticotropic hormone; LPH, lipotropin.)

endogenous cannabinoid anandamide. These compounds are derived from membrane lipids. Their synthesis or cleavage from preformed precursors is driven by specific enzymes (e.g. phospholipase A_2 and phospholipase D). Often these enzymes are activated by increases in nerve terminal cAMP or Ca^{2+}.

The activities of the small neurotransmitters are terminated by varying combinations of metabolism, reuptake, or diffusion away from the postsynaptic terminal. The relative importance of each of these processes varies between particular synapses and with the type and amount of neurotransmitter released (Fig. 19.9). Examples of metabolism include hydrolysis of ACh to acetate and choline by acetylcholinesterase (Chapter 31), transamination of GABA by GABA-glutamate transaminase to succinic semialdehyde, and modification of catecholamines by monoamine oxidase (in mitochondria) and by catecholamine-O-methyltransferase (in many tissues) to give rise to a number of metabolites that are ultimately excreted in the urine (and often measured as an assay of sympathetic nervous system activity; Chapter 63). Examples of reuptake include the monoamines DA, norepinephrine, epinephrine, and serotonin, as well as glutamate, GABA, glycine, and choline. Relatively specific transporters for each neurotransmitter on the presynaptic terminal take up neurotransmitter into the terminal.

In contrast to pumps (e.g. Na^+/K^+-ATPase), which directly couple transport to ATP hydrolysis, neurotransmitter transporters concentrate solutes against a concentration gradient by

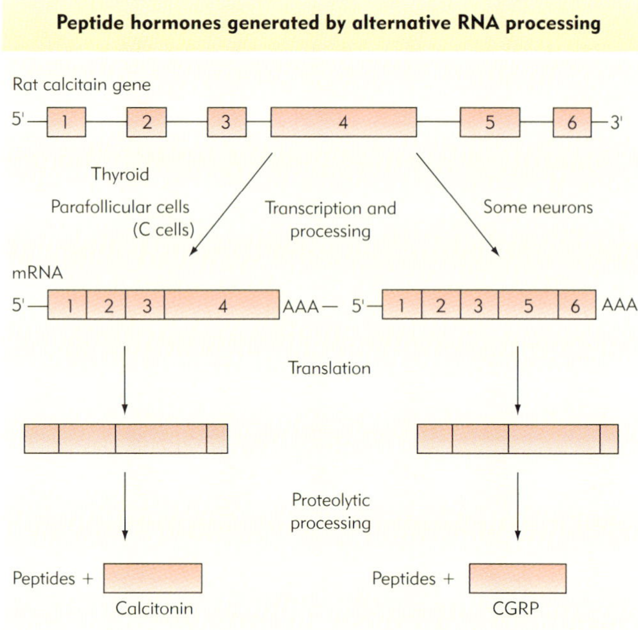

Figure 19.8 Distinct peptide hormones can be generated from a single DNA sequence by alternative RNA processing. Processing of the calcitonin gene to calcitonin and CGRP is shown here. Exons in the rat calcitonin gene are numbered 1–6. Exon 4 contains the sequence for calcitonin and exon 5 the sequence for CGRP. In the parafollicular cells of the thyroid, the mature RNA transcript contains exons 1–4. In CGRP-expressing neurons, the mature transcript contains exons 1–3, 5, and 6. Following translation and proteolytic cleavage, the final peptide products are produced.

a cotransport (with Na^+ or Cl^-) or antiport (with H^+ or K^+) mechanism that couples transport to the energy stored in transmembrane electrochemical potentials. Two plasma membrane neurotransmitter transporter families have been identified – Na^+/Cl^- dependent (DA, norepinephrine, serotonin, GABA, glycine, and choline) and Na^+/K^+ dependent (glutamate) (Chapter 25). A distinct H^+-dependent vesicular transporter family (monoamine, GABA and glycine, glutamate, ACh) mediates neurotransmitter transport from the cytoplasm into synaptic vesicles.

Important drugs that affect neurotransmitter transporters include antidepressants, amphetamines, and cocaine, which blocks the reuptake of norepinephrine, serotonin, and DA in addition to its local anesthetic and antimuscarinic effects. Pharmacologic evidence indicates the importance of reuptake for terminating synaptic transmission by most monoamines; for example, noradrenergic transmission is potentiated by inhibitors of norepinephrine reuptake, but not by inhibitors of its metabolism. General anesthetic effects on neurotransmitter transporters have been reported, but their role in the clinical effects of anesthetics is unclear. It is important to note that transporters can operate bidirectionally. Under certain conditions (e.g. anoxic depolarization), neurotransmitters can be transported out of the presynaptic terminal by these proteins, which allows a nonvesicular form of neurotransmitter release.

Examples of termination of neurotransmitter action by diffusion away from the synaptic cleft include the peptide neurotransmitters and glutamate. Peptides are metabolized by proteolysis. Often the initial products retain biologic activity. While some types of proteolysis occur by nonspecific proteases, others occur by specific neuropeptide cleaving enzymes (e.g. enkephalinase).

SYNAPTIC TRANSMISSION

The primary function of CNS synapses is deceptively simple: following depolarization of the presynaptic terminal, neurotransmitter is released in a controlled and adjustable fashion, after which the synaptic vesicles are recycled and refilled so the process can be repeated. The molecular details of this process remain unclear, despite intensive study, because their tight packing in the brain makes it difficult to study individual synapses. Recent years have seen a remarkable increase in our understanding of the processes involved in synaptic functioning, chiefly neurotransmitter release, as a consequence of a convergence of several fields of research.

- In comparison with CNS synapses, the synapse at the neuromuscular junction is accessible and well understood as a result of work by Katz, Eccles and others (Chapter 31). Mechanisms found to operate at this synapse form the basis for hypotheses that can be tested in experiments with CNS synapses.
- Our knowledge of the processes involved in vesicular transport between intracellular organelles (e.g. endoplasmic reticulum to Golgi to the cell surface) is well developed. Many of these processes are similar to the events involved in synaptic vesicle translocation to the plasma membrane and recycling (Chapter 2).
- Secretory pathways in yeast have been extensively studied (because of its easy genetic manipulation). Many of the proteins involved in these processes have homologs in the mammalian CNS that are involved in the trafficking of synaptic vesicles, which provides testable hypotheses.
- Simple organisms, such as squid and *Aplysia*, often have specialized large synapses that are amenable to biophysical measurements (e.g. electrophysiologic recording and dye-imaging of Ca^{2+} concentration). Recently, the large size of specialized mammalian synapses, such as the Calyx of Held in the median trapezoid body in the auditory system, have been exploited to explore presynaptic function in the mammalian CNS.
- When appropriately cultured for several weeks, CNS neurons form functional synapses. The dispersed nature of these synapses makes them accessible to experimental manipulations that are not possible in intact brain or even brain slices.
- The use of transgenic techniques allows the role of specific proteins in synaptic transmission to be determined.

While the limitations of each of these approaches must be kept in mind, collectively they have greatly increased our understanding of synaptic function.

Before considering the details of fast synaptic transmission, it is necessary to consider the steps involved in the process (Fig. 19.10). Following loading of a synaptic vesicle with neurotransmitter it is brought to the active zone in a process called docking. The active zone can be defined both morphologically and functionally. Morphologically, it corresponds to a thin band of electron-dense material just below the synaptic membrane, usually opposite the postsynaptic terminal (Fig. 19.1). Functionally, vesicles docked at the active zone are those that

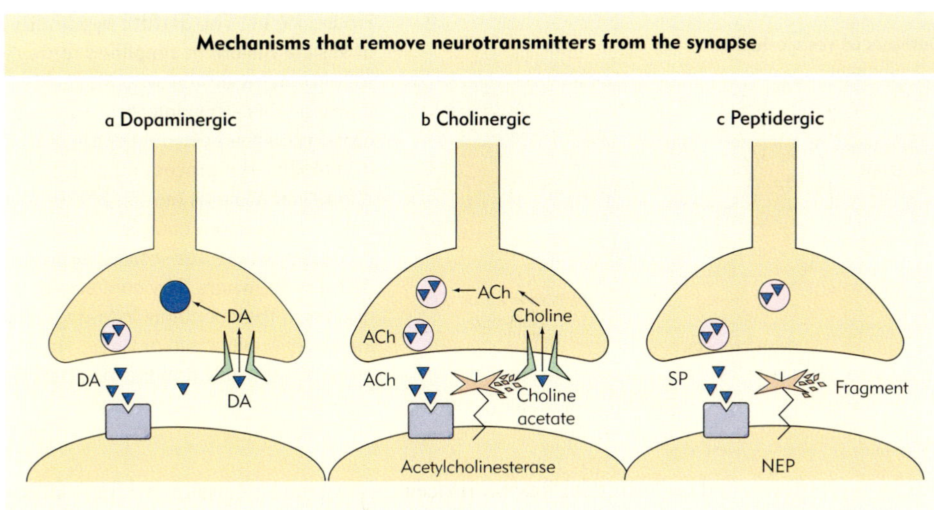

Figure 19.9 Mechanisms that remove neurotransmitters from the synapse. (a) Monoamines and modified amino acids, exemplified by DA, are removed by high-affinity transporters expressed by neurons and glial cells. (b) Acetylcholinesterase rapidly degrades ACh to inactive acetate and choline. Choline is taken up by a choline transporter to be reused for synthesis of ACh. (c) Neuropeptides, exemplified by substance P (SP), are degraded by ectoenzymes, such as neutral endopeptidase (NEP), to fragments that are usually devoid of biologic activity. (Adapted with permission from Böhm SK, Grady EF, Bunnett NW. Regulatory mechanisms that modulate signalling by G-protein-coupled receptors. Biochem J. 1997;322:1–18.)

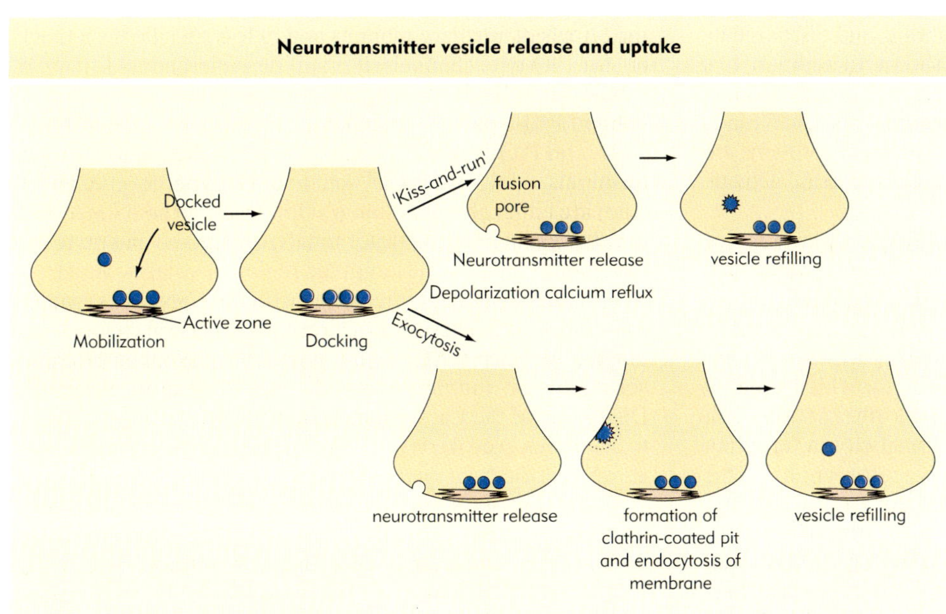

Figure 19.10 Two theories of neurotransmitter vesicle release and reuptake. The upper pathway, termed 'kiss-and-run', involves the transient formation of a fusion pore. This pore opens only briefly, to allow discharge of its contents, closes again, and the vesicle returns to the interior of the synaptic terminal where it is refilled with neurotransmitter. In the lower pathway, the entire vesicle fuses with the membrane of the synaptic terminal, discharging its contents. The synaptic vesicle membrane is directed to clathrin-coated pits, from which it is retrieved as an intact vesicle and refilled with neurotransmitter.

are immediately ready to fuse with the membrane and discharge their contents. There are currently two main, competing hypotheses for vesicle fusion (Fig. 19.10).

Recent research focused on the complex and highly regulated mechanisms involved in synaptic vesicle release, because of the central role this process plays in neurotransmission. The polar nature of the vesicle and plasma membranes leads to mutual repulsion, which creates a considerable energy barrier that must be overcome to allow fusion and exocytosis. The current hypothesis with the most experimental support holds that specific proteins on discrete sites of vesicles interact with complementary proteins on the synaptic membrane (the SNARE hypothesis), and this interaction is modulated by a third set of proteins. These interactions are strengthened by conditions that promote neurotransmitter release (i.e. elevation in intracellular Ca^{2+}). The energy (ATP)-dependent formation and breakdown of a fusion-core complex regulates vesicle fusion and exocytosis, as illustrated in Figure 19.11.

The term 'SNARE' has its origins in experiments that investigated the shuttling of vesicles from the endoplasmic reticulum to the Golgi, and presumably also underlies the transport of vesicles to target membranes. The proteins and mechanisms involved in vesicular transport, whether between organelles or for exocytosis, are remarkably similar. The vesicle-fusion process was found to be disrupted by alkylation of a protein [*N*-ethylmaleimide (NEM)-sensitive factor (NSF)] by NEM. A family of proteins crucial in the process interacted with NSF and were designated SNAPs (soluble NSF attachment proteins). It was found that NSF and SNAPs interact with proteins of both the vesicle being transported, designated v-SNAREs (vesicle SNAP receptors), and the membrane to which it was targeted, designated t-SNAREs (target SNAP receptors). Our current understanding suggests that in the

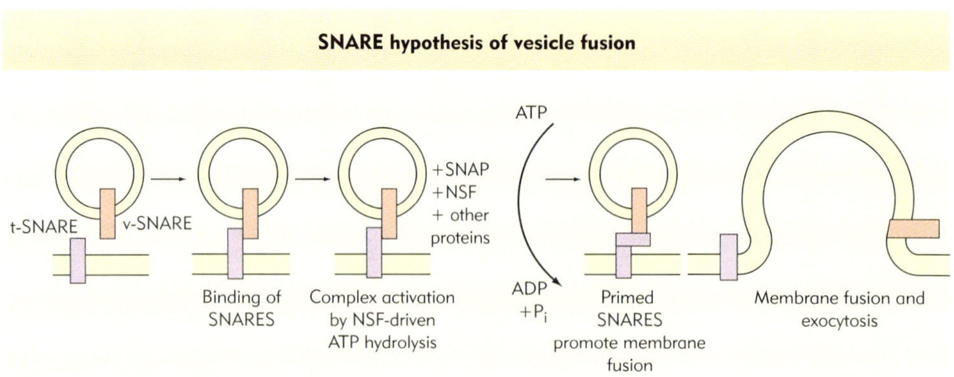

Figure 19.11 The SNARE hypothesis of vesicle fusion, in simplified form. A set of proteins on the synaptic vesicle (termed v-SNAREs) interacts with proteins on the presynaptic terminal (t-SNAREs) in a process mediated by a family of proteins termed SNAPs to form a fusion-core complex. This process positions the vesicles in the active zone, where they can readily discharge their contents following increases in intracellular Ca^{2+}. The order of assembly remains unclear.

nerve terminal there is one major v-SNARE (synaptobrevin) and two major t-SNAREs {syntaxin 1 and SNAP-25 [synaptosome-associated protein of 25 kDa (not to be confused with SNAP)]}. These three proteins spontaneously form a tight complex in a 1:1:1 stoichiometry. While it is thought that these three proteins serve to anchor the synaptic vesicle close to the membrane (the active zone) in a position to fuse with the membrane and discharge its contents, this has not been conclusively shown. In addition, it is likely that interactions between other synaptic vesicles and terminal proteins play a major role. For example, SNAP-25 binds directly to synaptotagmin (see below). The SNARE proteins are cleaved by clostridial and tetanus toxin metalloprotease activity, which disrupts neurotransmitter release.

While synaptobrevin, syntaxin, and SNAP-25 play a major role in neurotransmitter release, other proteins have critical roles, two of which are briefly discussed here. Small guanosine triphosphate (GTP)-binding proteins are important in providing direction to a number of vesicular pathways. A similar situation seems to hold in the neuron, for which small G proteins, particularly rab3a, through its interaction with rabphilin and other proteins, provide specificity in targeting of synaptic vesicles. Also important is synaptotagmin 1. This abundant synaptic vesicle-associated protein binds Ca^{2+}, and thus has been proposed as the Ca^{2+} sensor that drives exocytosis after increases in Ca^{2+} in the presynaptic terminal. Experimental results to support this hypothesis are the observations that moderate (about 2.2mmol/L) Ca^{2+} levels increase the binding of synaptotagmin to both membrane phospholipids and the presynaptic membrane protein syntaxin 1, and that targeted deletion of synaptotagmin in mice eliminated fast Ca^{2+}-dependent exocytosis.

MODULATION OF EXCITABILITY AND SYNAPTIC TRANSMISSION

Neuronal excitability and synaptic transmission are controlled by many factors, such as the dendritic integration of small synaptic potentials (miniature postsynaptic potentials) that arise from each synaptic contact, events at the cell soma (most notably resting membrane potential), and factors that affect neurotransmitter release. Here the focus is on the factors that affect neurotransmitter release.

In most terminals neurotransmitter release is supported by the entry of Ca^{2+} through two main families of Ca^{2+} channel, designated N-type and P/Q-type, based on their sensitivity to peptide toxins. The pore-forming α_1 subunit of the N-type Ca^{2+} channel has been cloned (designated class B), which enables substantial structure–function relationships to be established. It is likely that the α_1 subunit clone designated as class A corresponds to the electrophysiologically defined P/Q-type Ca^{2+} channel. However, because of the heterogeneity of responses that results from alternative splicing, species differences, and the effects of auxiliary subunits and of less specific toxin blockers for P/Q type channels, it is still possible that additional α_1 subunits may be discovered that correspond to the functionally defined P/Q-type Ca^{2+} channel.

N- and P/Q-type Ca^{2+} channel are enriched in presynaptic terminals, while other Ca^{2+} channel (L-type, R-type, and T-type) are either absent or found at low levels. In addition to their localization in presynaptic terminals, evidence is emerging that the channels tend to cluster in the region of synaptic vesicles as a consequence of their interaction with the t-SNAREs syntaxin 1 and SNAP-25. These interactions position Ca^{2+} channels in a domain in which the Ca^{2+} that passes through them promotes vesicle fusion and neurotransmitter release most efficiently. Disruption of the Ca^{2+} channel and t-SNARE interaction leads to decreases in evoked (Ca^{2+} channel dependent), but not asynchronous (Ca^{2+} channel independent), release.

Reduction of Ca^{2+} influx into the presynaptic terminal after its depolarization by an action potential reduces neurotransmitter release and is termed presynaptic inhibition. Both N- and P/Q-type Ca^{2+} channels are inhibited by a wide range of neuromodulators that act through GPCRs. The largest, and best studied, group of neuromodulators act through a membrane-delimited pathway using G proteins that can be identified based on their sensitivity to pertussis toxin. Neuromodulators that use this pathway include adenosine, GABA ($GABA_B$), and opioids. In this case, for both N- and P/Q-type Ca^{2+} channels it is likely that the direct interaction of G protein β/γ-subunits with the Ca^{2+} channel α_1 subunit makes the channel less likely to open for a given degree of depolarization (voltage-dependent inhibition; Fig. 19.12). Since the probability of vesicle fusion and neurotransmitter release increases as a power function of Ca^{2+} concentration in the nerve terminal (i.e. probability of release is proportional to $[Ca^{2+}]^n$, n = 2–4), even small changes in Ca^{2+} influx can profoundly affect neurotransmitter release. The membrane-delimited pathway has its strongest influence in neurons that fire at slow rates (<5Hz). Presumably, during faster firing more than enough Ca^{2+} for vesicle fusion enters, and even decreases in Ca^{2+} influx of about 50% have little affect on the total number of vesicles released. In addition to the membrane-delimited pathway of Ca^{2+} channel inhibition, another pathway

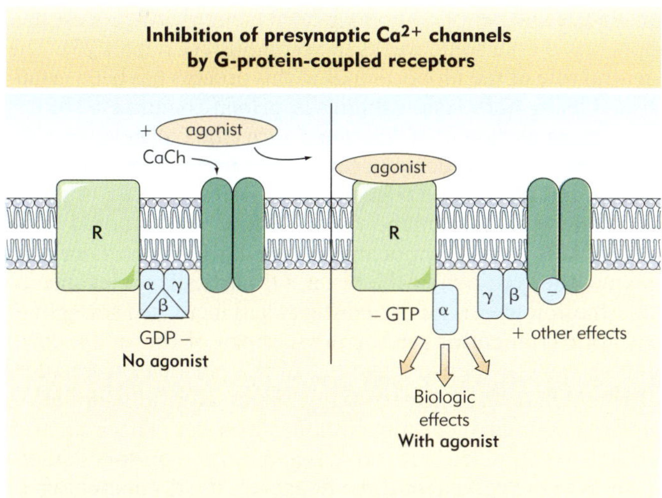

Figure 19.12 Inhibition of presynaptic Ca^{2+} channels by G-protein coupled receptors. In the absence of agonist, voltage-gated Ca^{2+} channels (CaCh) open as the nerve terminal depolarizes. The Ca^{2+} that enters through these channels enables synaptic vesicles to fuse with the presynaptic membrane and release their contents. Following binding of agonist to receptor, G proteins are activated and dissociate into α and β/γ subunits. The β/γ complex binds to the Ca^{2+} channels, which decreases its probability of opening for a given degree of depolarization. This results in less Ca^{2+} influx into the terminal, and thus fewer vesicles fuse and less neurotransmitter is released. In addition to inhibition of Ca^{2+} channel, the activated G-protein subunits also modulate other processes in the terminal.(GDP, guanosine diphosphate; GTP, guanosine triphosphate.)

(understood less well) is used by a number of neurotransmitter receptors coupled to PLC, which increases intracellular Ca^{2+}, and phosphatidylinositol turnover. While signaling through this pathway can decrease currents through Ca^{2+} channels, the net effect on neurotransmitter release is more difficult to predict as these receptors often activate PKC (which tends to increase flux through Ca^{2+} channels) and inhibit K^+ currents (which tends to make the neuron more excitable).

It is likely that GPCRs that operate through the membrane-delimited pathway inhibit neurotransmitter release by additional mechanisms. This hypothesis is supported by the observation that, even in the absence of nerve terminal depolarization, spontaneous vesicle fusion and neurotransmitter release occurs. This release is Ca^{2+} independent, yet can be inhibited by activation of the membrane-delimited pathway in a pertussis toxin-sensitive fashion. One explanation for this observation is that activated G proteins or downstream effectors may interact directly with and inhibit some aspect(s) of the release machinery.

In addition to presynaptic inhibition, other mechanisms serve to modulate neurotransmitter release. One well-known example of protein phosphorylation that stimulates neurotransmitter release is synapsin I phosphorylation by cAMP-dependent protein kinase and Cam KII during periods of intense neurotransmission. Synapsin I is highly enriched in presynaptic terminals, and serves as a link between cytoskeleton and synaptic vesicles, binding to both in its dephosphorylated form. Following its phosphorylation by cAMP-dependent protein kinase or Cam KII, its affinity for vesicles is reduced. This decrease in affinity of the vesicles for the cytoskeleton may allow them to dock at the active zone, from which they are readily released. In addition to the well-defined role of synapsin I phosphorylation in neurotransmission, many of the other proteins involved in synaptic vesicle docking and fusion are also substrates for protein kinases (Chapter 3). However, the functional role of phosphorylation of these proteins remains unclear.

General anesthetics affect excitatory and inhibitory synaptic transmission both presynaptically, by altering neurotransmitter release, and postsynaptically, by altering the responses of neurons to neurotransmitters. Electrophysiologic studies in the CNS indicate that clinically relevant concentrations of general anesthetics affect synaptic transmission rather than axonal conduction or neuronal excitability by enhancing inhibitory (GABA-mediated) and depressing excitatory (glutamate-mediated) transmission. Many volatile and intravenous general anesthetics potentiate postsynaptic $GABA_A$ receptors and inhibit Na^+ and Ca^{2+} channels (Chapters 23, 24). Inhibition of presynaptic Na^+ and/or Ca^{2+} channels may underlie the anesthetic inhibition of neurotransmitter release.

NEURAL PLASTICITY

Neural plasticity refers to the ability of neurons and particular neuronal networks to change the number and efficacy of their connections. It is commonly believed that plasticity underlies the process of learning as well as the development of several states of chronic pain after tissue injury (Chapter 21). The modulation of neurotransmitter release discussed above is a simple form of neuronal plasticity. Other forms of plasticity last for some time and persist long after removal of the triggering event. Much of what is understood about neural plasticity relies on studies in invertebrates with relatively simple nervous systems and relatively large neurons that facilitate experimental design and execution. Studies with invertebrates, notably *Aplysia californica*, show that the brief stimulation of one neuron can strengthen or weaken the communication between two other neurons and that this effect can last for days. Typically, if the change is to be long-lasting, it requires new protein synthesis, protein phosphorylation, and often changes in gene transcription.

In the mammalian CNS, the neural structure that has been the most extensively studied in terms of neural plasticity is the hippocampus, since the pathways between groups of neurons are preserved in the thin sections (brain slices) that are necessary for *in vitro* work and since it plays a role in several learning states. The phenomenon most often studied is long-term potentiation (LTP) – the strengthening of synaptic connection(s) following an experimental maneuver (ideally one that reflects an event in the intact, behaving animal during a learning task). The phenomenon of LTP was first observed by Bliss and Lomo, who found that brief, high-frequency stimulation of any of the three afferent pathways in the rabbit hippocampus (see below) increased the response to subsequent low-frequency stimulation in the postsynaptic cell. Interestingly, this enhancement of neurotransmission persisted for weeks after a single, brief stimulation. Several of the paradigms used to elicit LTP in the hippocampus mirror the patterns of neuronal firing seen in animals during the learning of a task.

Anatomy of the hippocampus and long-term potentiation

a Anatomy of hippocampus

b Long-term potentiation

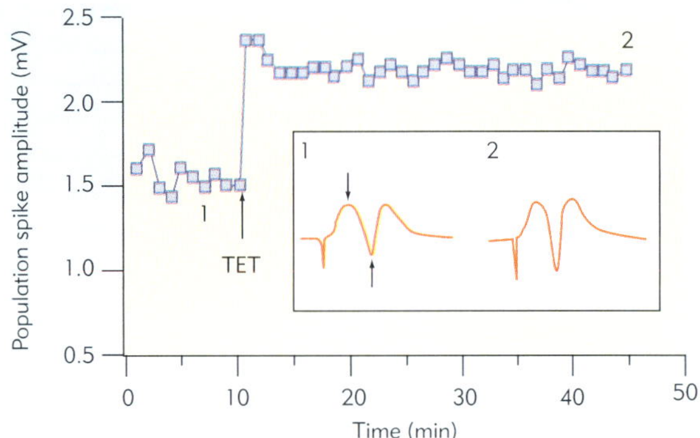

Figure 19.13 Anatomy of the hippocampus and demonstration of the phenomenon of LTP. (a) A thin slice of rat hippocampus illustrates the three sets of excitatory synaptic connections (perforant path, mossy fibers, and Schaeffer collaterals). [DG, dentate gyrus; pp, perforant path from the entorhinal cortex to the dentate granule cells; mf, mossy fiber projection from the granule cells to the CA3 pyramidal cells; Sch, Schaeffer collaterals, the projection of CA3 pyramidal cells to ipsilateral CA1 pyramidal cells; comm, the commissural pathway, the projection of contralateral CA3 pyramidal cells to CA1 pyramidal cells through the fimbria (fim)]. (Modified with permission from Nature 361:31–9.) (b) A typical example of LTP in the perforant path recorded extracellularly from a guinea-pig hippocampal slice. The population spike increases approximately 40% following tetanus stimulation (TET). The inset shows representative population spikes before (1) and after (2) tetanic. Amplitude was measured as the voltage between the arrows. (Courtesy of Greg Terman, MD, PhD.)

The hippocampal formation (Fig. 19.13) consists primarily of three excitatory synapses that use glutamate as the neurotransmitter. In the first, the perforant path (projecting from the subiculum and entorhinal cortex) enters the dentate gyrus, synapsing on the granule cells. The axons of the dentate granule cells project to the CA3 region of the hippocampus, and synapse on the dendrites of the pyramidal cells. These large, distinctive terminals are termed mossy fibers. The axons of the CA3 pyramidal cells project to the dendrites of the CA1 pyramidal cells as the Schaeffer collateral pathway. Finally, the axons of the CA1 pyramidal cells project out of the hippocampus back to the subiculum. The hippocampus plays a key role in the consolidation of short-term memories (particularly of objects and people) into long-term memories, a process that appears to take some weeks to accomplish (Chapter 25). The central role of the hippocampus in this process has been established using both lesion studies in primates and case studies in humans. Ischemia of Ammon's horn (the CA fields) results in severe anterograde amnesia, despite intact recall of distant events and unchanged cognitive abilities.

While the phenomenon of LTP has been studied most extensively in the hippocampus, similar processes occur in many other regions of the brain. Of particular relevance to anesthesiologists is neural plasticity and increased strength of synaptic connections in the dorsal horn of the spinal cord. Increasingly, evidence suggests that this plasticity may underlie the deleterious affects of prolonged painful stimulation and the genesis of certain chronic pain states. This is an area of active basic-science research that may have profound implications in the clinical practice of anesthesia. A counterpart of LTP is long-term depression (LTD), which has been particularly studied in the hippocampus and cerebellum. As its name suggests, LTD is a long-lasting inhibition of neurotransmission, and may also contribute to neural plasticity by providing a mechanism to decrease the strength of 'unwanted' synaptic connections.

Two forms of LTP occur in the hippocampus – associative and nonassociative. Associative LTP is observed at the perforant path and dentate granule cell synapse and the CA3–CA1 pyramidal cell synapse. Nonassociative LTP is found at the mossy fiber–CA3 pyramidal cell synapse. Both forms are produced by high-frequency stimulation of the appropriate afferent path. However, in associative LTP concomitant depolarization of the postsynaptic neuron is required. Interestingly, associative LTP offers a cellular mechanism to encode coincidences between two different events. That is, a synaptic connection is strengthened only if two events, binding of glutamate to AMPA receptors on the postsynaptic cell and depolarization of the postsynaptic cell, occur simultaneously. This is a feature of a 'Hebbian' synapse, an important building block in several theories of neural networks.

The mechanisms that underlie associative LTP have been extensively studied and, although some aspects remain unclear, the following outline is emerging. The central feature of associative LTP, that concurrent depolarization of the postsynaptic cell is required, is provided by the NMDA-type of glutamate receptor (Fig. 19.14). This receptor is found on dendritic spines and opens after binding of the excitatory amino acid glutamate. Under resting physiologic conditions, ions cannot pass through the NMDA receptor, even if glutamate is bound, because its pore is blocked by physiologic concentrations of external Mg^{2+}. However, if the postsynaptic cell is depolarized simultaneously with glutamate binding, Mg^{2+} is displaced from the mouth of the NMDA receptor, allowing passage of Na^+, K^+, and, most importantly, Ca^{2+} through the channel pore.

The necessity of Ca^{2+} entry through NMDA receptors in the establishment, or induction, of associative LTP is firmly established, but its mechanisms of action are less clear. The role of protein phosphorylation in the expression of LTP is highlighted by the observation that the introduction of inhibitors of Ca^{2+}/Cam KII or PKC into the postsynaptic cell blocks the induction of LTP. It has been proposed that one or both of these kinases might phosphorylate AMPA receptors, increasing their conductance and strengthening synaptic

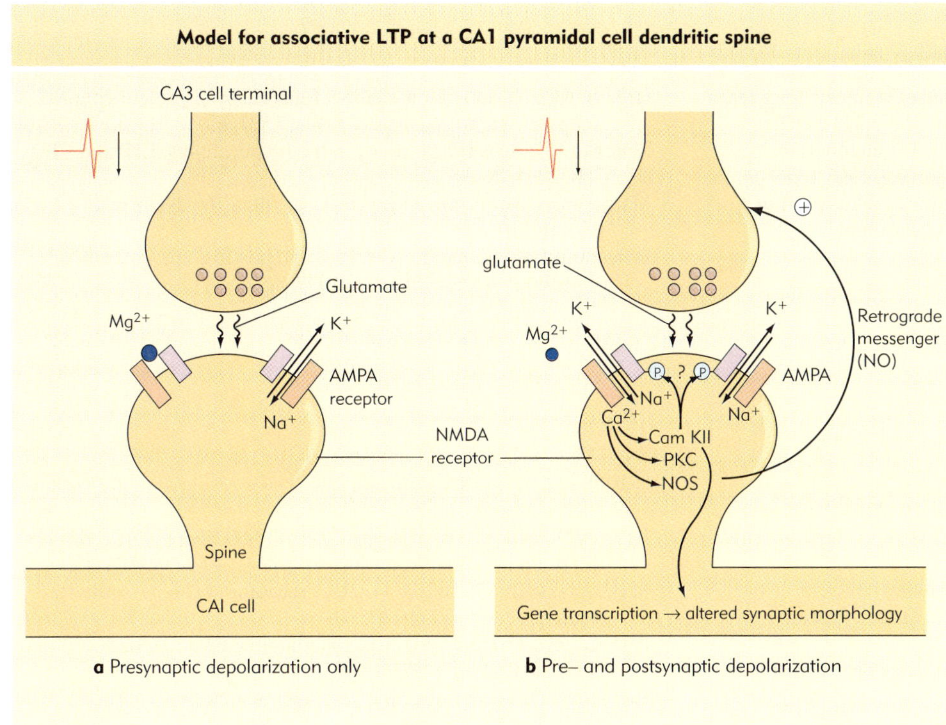

Figure 19.14 Model for associative LTP at a CA1 pyramidal cell dendritic spine. (a) During periods of slow stimulation, glutamate released from the presynaptic terminal only activates AMPA receptors because of the block of NMDA receptors by Mg^{2+}. (b) During periods of intense activity (e.g. synchronous activation of many excitatory synapses on the same dendrite) spine depolarization displaces Mg^{2+}, which allows influx of Na^+ and Ca^{2+} through the NMDA receptor channels. Increased intracellular Ca^{2+} sets in motion several biochemical cascades, resulting in activation of effectors such as PKC, Cam KII, and nitric oxide synthase (NOS). These and other enzymes act to enhance postsynaptic functions (e.g. to increase the conductance of AMPA receptors). Presynaptic effects, possibly mediated by nitric oxide, are also present, leading to increased neurotransmitter release.

transmission. In addition, associative LTP may also involve presynaptic events (e.g. increased neurotransmitter release). To link the well-established role of postsynaptic NMDA receptors to presynaptic responses it has been proposed that a retrograde messenger is produced postsynaptically that diffuses to the presynaptic terminal. Experimental support exists that both nitric oxide (or related molecules) and arachidonic acid metabolites may be retrograde messengers. There are several ways that nitric oxide might act. Stimulation of guanylyl cyclase by nitric oxide would increase presynaptic cyclic guanosine monophosphate (cGMP) levels which might stimulate cGMP-dependent protein kinase or activate cGMP-gated cation channels. Alternatively, nitric oxide might increase the level of ADP ribosylation of certain presynaptic proteins, enhancing neurotransmitter release.

Since most LTP found in the CNS is of the associative type, this is the type most extensively studied, but we also have a partial understanding of the mechanism of nonassociative LTP. Nonassociative LTP appears to be primarily mediated presynaptically, and NMDA receptors are not involved. Rather, it seems that increased presynaptic Cam KII, which arises during the induction of nonassociative LTP, mediates this process. In addition, this form of LTP is blocked by inhibitors of cAMP-dependent protein kinase, which suggests a role of protein phosphorylation by this kinase. Both Ca^{2+} and cAMP signaling pathways converge at the level of type I adenylyl cyclase (type I AC). Interestingly, mossy fiber LTP is deficient in mice with a targeted disruption of the type I AC gene, which suggests activation of this isoform of adenylyl cyclase is necessary for nonassociative LTP.

Key References

Bliss TVP, Collingridge GL. A synaptic model of memory: long-term potentiation in the hippocampus. Nature. 1993;371:31–9.
Dunlap K, Luebke JI, Turner TJ. Exocytotic Ca^{2+} channels in mammalian central neurons. Trends Neurosci. 1995;18:89–98.
Hanson PI, Heuser JE, Jahn R. Neurotransmitter release – four years of SNARE complexes. Curr Opin Neurobiol. 1997;7:310–15.
Hille B. Modulation of ion-channel function by G protein-coupled receptors. Trends Neurosci. 1994;17:531–6.
Malenka RC. Synaptic plasticity in the hippocampus: LTP and LTD. Cell. 1994;78:535–8.
Matthews G. Neurotransmitter release. Annu Rev Neurosci. 1996;19:219–33.
Rahamimoff R, Fernandez JM. Pre- and postfusion regulation of transmitter release. Neuron. 1997;18:17–27.

Further Reading

Amara S, Kuhar MJ. Neurotransmitter transporters: recent progress. Annu Rev Neurosci. 1993;16:73–93.
Cooper JR, Bloom FE, Roth RH. The biochemical basis of neuropharmacology, 7th edn. New York: Oxford University Press; 1996.
Cremona O, De Camilli P. Synaptic vesicle endocytosis. Curr Opin Neurobiol. 1997;7:323–30.
Hudspith MJ. Glutamate: a role in normal brain function, anaesthesia, analgesia and CNS injury. Br J Anaesth. 1997;78:731–47.
Jaber M, Robinson SW, Missale C, Caron MG. Dopamine receptors and brain function. Neuropharmacology. 1996;35:1503–19.
MacDonald RL, Olsen RW. $GABA_A$ receptor channels. Annu Rev Neurosci. 1994;17:569–602.
Pertwee RG. Pharmacology of cannabinoid CB1 and CB2 receptors. Pharmacol Ther. 1997;74:1–52.
Richards CD. The synaptic basis of general anaesthesia. Eur J Anaesth. 12:5–19, 1995.
Zhang J, Snyder SH. Nitric oxide in the nervous system. Annu Rev Pharmacol Toxicol. 1995;35:213.

Chapter 20 Neurophysiology

Patricia Fogarty Mack and William L Young

Topics covered in this chapter

Circulation
Cerebrospinal fluid dynamics
Cerebral Edema
Intracranial pressure
Seizures and anticonvulsants
Cerebral ischemia and stroke
Neurotoxicity
Jugular venous oxygen saturation

CIRCULATION

The primary arterial supply to the brain consists of the anterior circulation, which comprises the paired carotid arteries and their branches, and the posterior circulation, which comprises the paired vertebral arteries and the basilar artery and their branches (Fig. 20.1). Collateral arterial inflow channels are integral for compensatory cerebral blood flow (CBF) changes during ischemia. The circle of Willis, a ring of vessels that encircles the pituitary gland in the subarachnoid space, forms the cornerstone of collateral circulation, although it is incomplete in many patients. The anterior communicating artery connects the carotid circulations, and two posterior communicating arteries join the carotid and vertebral circulations. If the arterial supply is compromised and collateral flow via the circle of Willis is inadequate, other potential collateral pathways may be recruited. These include leptomeningeal communications that bridge 'watershed' areas (i.e. surface connections between the anterior and middle cerebral arteries), pathways from the external to internal carotid (i.e. via facial arteries to the ophthalmic artery), and (rarely) meningeal collaterals.

Venous drainage of the brain is complex and variable. Intracerebral veins are thin walled and valveless. They terminate in thick walled venous sinuses, which are noncompliant and noncollapsible because of their bony connections. The confluence of larger venous sinuses results in significant admixture of blood. Often venous drainage is predominantly unilateral, which may be evident on angiograms.

Circle of Willis with collateral pathways

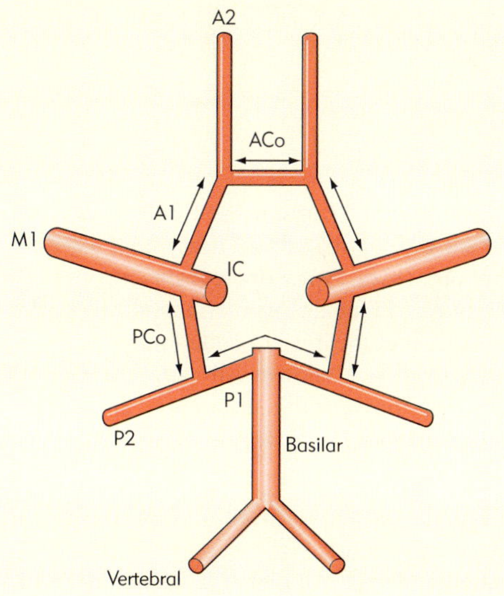

Figure 20.1 Circle of Willis with collateral pathways. The principal pathways for collateral flow are marked by arrows. Not shown are potential pathways from the extracranial circulation. ACo, anterior communicating artery; PCo, posterior communicating artery; A1, A2, M1, P1, P2, anterior, middle and posterior branches; IC, internal cortoid artery.

CEREBROSPINAL FLUID DYNAMICS

Cerebrospinal fluid (CSF) is contained in the two lateral ventricles, the third (cerebral) ventricle, the aqueduct of Sylvius, the fourth (cerebellar) ventricle, the spinal cord central canal, and the subarachnoid space. The total volume of these spaces is approximately 50mL in infants, 80mL in small children, 100mL in large children, and 150mL in adults. Ventricular volume comprises approximately 17% of this volume in adults. Total volume of extracellular fluid (ECF; interstitial fluid plus CSF) in the brain is 350mL in adults.

Production of CSF is by the choroid plexus and the ependymal lining of the ventricles, and extrachoroidally by cerebral capillary endothelium. At the level of cerebral capillaries, little exchange occurs between CSF and ECF because of the impermeability of the blood–brain barrier (BBB). The BBB comprises tight junctions (zonae occludens) that join cells of the capillary endothelium and restrict movement of molecules with a diameter greater than 20Å (Fig. 20.2). In addition, capillaries throughout the brain, with the exception of

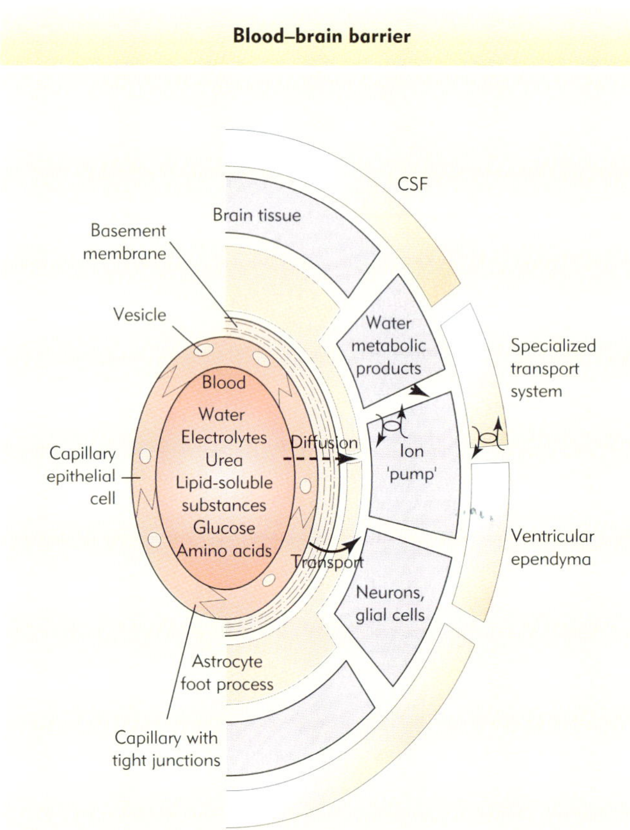

Figure 20.2 Blood–brain barrier. The BBB consists of capillary endothelial cells with tight junctions, basement membrane, and astrocyte foot processes. Water and constituents of plasma cross the BBB into brain ECF by diffusion or active transport. Water and other cellular metabolites are added to the ECF from neurons and glial cells. (Redrawn with permission from Cottrell JE, Smith DS. Anesthesia and neurosurgery. St Louis: Mosby–Yearbook; 1994.)

Composition of human cerebrospinal fluid and plasma

	Mean cerebrospinal fluid value	Mean plasma value
Specific gravity	1.007	1.025
Osmolality (mOsm/kg H_2O)	289	289
pH	7.31	7.41
Partial pressure of carbon dioxide (mmHg)	50.5	41.1
Sodium (mEq/L)	141	140
Potassium (mEq/L)	2.9	4.6
Calcium (mEq/L)	2.5	5.0
Magnesium (mEq/L)	2.4	1.7
Chloride (mEq/L)	124	101
Bicarbonate (mEq/L)	21	23
Glucose (mg/dL)	61	92
Protein (mg/dL):	28	7000
Albumin	23	4430
Globulin	5	2270
Fibrinogen	0	300

Figure 20.3 Composition of cerebrospinal fluid and plasma in humans. (Reprinted with permission from Cottrell JE, Smith DS. Anesthesia and neurosurgery. St Louis: Mosby–Yearbook; 1994.)

the choroid plexus and several small regions, are surrounded by astrocyte foot processes.

Characteristic of CSF are higher concentrations of Na^+, Cl^-, and Mg^{2+}, and lower concentrations of glucose, proteins, amino acids, uric acid, K^+, bicarbonate, and phosphate than found in plasma, with which it is isotonic (Fig. 20.3). The normal concentration of protein in CSF is extremely low, pH = 7.3, and the partial pressure of carbon dioxide (P_{CO_2}) is about 50mmHg (6.7kPa).

Comparisons with plasma indicate that active secretion occurs in CSF formation. Regional differences in CSF composition (i.e. higher protein and lower K^+ content in lumbar versus intracerebral CSF) support the hypothesis that sites other than the choroid plexus are involved in the transport of solutes into the CSF. (Movement of Ca^{2+} in and out of CSF occurs via a concentration-independent transport mechanism.)

Formation of CSF is at a rate of 0.35–0.40mL/min (500–600mL/day); the total CSF volume is replaced 3–4 times per day. Between 40 and 70% of CSF is produced by the choroid plexus, whereas 30–60% is produced by the ependyma and pia.

The capillary endothelium of the choroid plexus is fenestrated and lacks tight junctions (Fig. 20.4). Thus, blood entering these capillaries is filtered and forms a protein-rich fluid, similar in composition to interstitial fluid elsewhere in the body, within the stroma of the choroid plexus. The choroid plexus interstitium is separated from the macroscopic CSF spaces by epithelial cells that contain apical tight junctions, which restrict passive solute exchange. First, Na^+ is moved from the interstitial fluid into the epithelial cell and from there into the CSF. Whether this occurs via diffusion or via membrane pumps dependent on adenosine triphosphate (ATP) is unclear. Water follows the resultant osmotic gradient, both into the epithelial cell and out to the CSF. From epithelial cells, Cl^- is coupled to Na^+ transport and enters the CSF passively, as does bicarbonate, along an electrochemical gradient. Water, Ca^{2+}, and Mg^{2+} may also enter the CSF via 'leaky' epithelial tight junctions. Extrachoroidal CSF formation results from water produced by the oxidative metabolism of glucose (60%) and through ultrafiltration from cerebral capillaries (40%).

Glucose concentration in CSF is 60% that of blood (when blood glucose is <270mg/dL). Glucose enters the CSF by facilitated transport; at normal blood-glucose levels diffusion of glucose into the CSF is insignificant. Glucose is removed from the CSF into the blood via several mechanisms – ouabain-sensitive and -insensitive fluxes, diffusion, and metabolism by periventricular tissue.

Protein concentrations in CSF are usually 0.5% those of serum levels because of the inability of protein to cross the BBB. Of CSF protein, 60% enters at the choroid plexus, where the epithelial apical tight junctions are less restrictive than those in other cerebrovascular sites. In addition, vesicular transport across the choroid plexus endothelium may play a role.

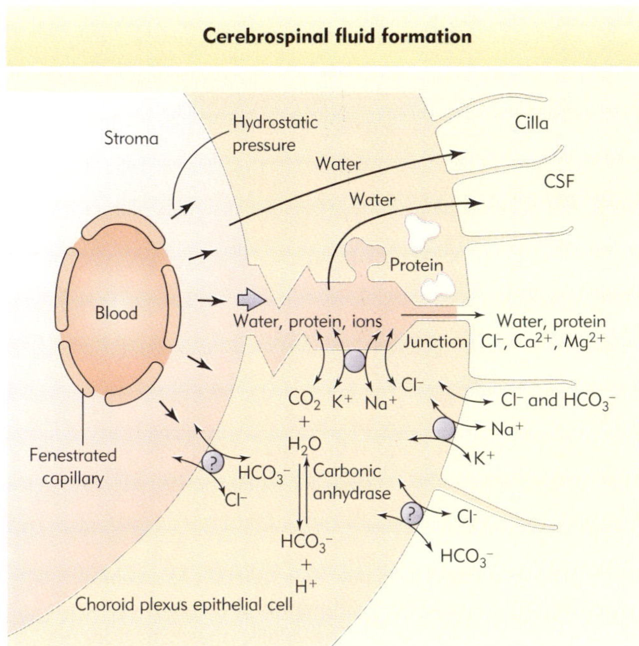

Figure 20.4 Cerebrospinal fluid formation. Some of the processes in CSF formation. The ATP-dependent membrane pumps transport Na^+ across the abluminal surface to within the choroid plexus cell and across the secretory surface, into the macroscopic CSF space, in exchange for K^+ and H^+. Water moves from the stroma to the CSF as it follows the concentration gradient produced by the ionic pumps. (Redrawn with permission from Cucchiara RF, Michenfelder JD, eds. Clinical neuroanesthesia. New York: Churchill Livingstone; 1990.)

A decrease in cerebral perfusion pressure (CPP) reduces CSF formation, especially if the decrease results from a combination of arterial hypotension and increased intracranial pressure (ICP). If CPP remains above 70mmHg (9.3kPa), an increase in ICP to 20mmHg (2.7kPa) does not reduce CSF formation. Reduced CSF production because of arterial hypotension is caused by both a reduction in choroid plexus blood flow, which is further diminished by increased ICP, and a decrease in hydrostatic pressure in the choroid plexus vasculature.

Various routes are taken by CSF from areas of production to areas of reabsorption. From the lateral ventricles, CSF moves through the foramina of Monro to the third ventricle, and then through the aqueduct of Sylvius into the fourth ventricle. From the fourth ventricle it may pass through the foramina of Luschka into the cerebellopontine angle and prepontine cisterns, or through the foramen of Magendie to the cisterna magna. After leaving the cisterna magna, CSF passes into the subarachnoid space that surrounds the cerebellum, or flows inferiorly along the dorsal surface of the spinal cord to return along the ventral surface of the cord to the basilar cisterns. CSF flow is determined by:

- hydrostatic pressure of 15cmH_2O (1.5kPa) at the site of CSF formation;
- cilia on ependymal cells directing flow toward the fourth ventricle and its foramina; and
- respiratory variations and vascular pulsations.

Reabsorption of CSF occurs via arachnoid villi and arachnoid granulations, which consist of arachnoid cells protruding into the subarachnoid space through the wall of an adjacent venous sinus, and are located in dural walls that border the superior sagittal sinus and venous lacunae intracranially (85–90% of reabsorption) and that border the spinal dural sinusoids on dorsal nerve roots (10–15%). The endothelium of the villus acts as a barrier that limits the rate of passage of CSF and solute into venous blood. Flow through the subarachnoid villi is determined by the transvillus hydrostatic pressure gradient [6cmH_2O (0.6kPa)], which is equal to CSF pressure [15cmH_2O (1.5kPa)] minus venous sinus pressure [9cmH_2O (0.9kPa)].

Pharmacologic effects on cerebrospinal fluid dynamics

Anesthetics and other drugs affect CSF dynamics by changing the rate of formation or the rate of reabsorption of CSF. The mechanisms by which anesthetics alter CSF dynamics are unclear. Enflurane may increase choroid plexus metabolism, and so increase CSF formation, and halothane may decrease formation secondary to stimulation of vasopressin receptors. Hypocapnia may also affect CSF dynamics. The effects of volatile anesthetics and intravenous agents on CSF dynamics are summarized in Figure 20.5. The clinical implication of these effects is probably minimal for all but the most prolonged anesthetic times.

Diuretics usually decrease the formation of CSF. Acetazolamide, a carbonic anhydrase inhibitor, decreases the hydrogen ions available for exchange with Na^+ on the abluminal side. It may also decrease formation by changing ion transport via an effect on bicarbonate and may constrict the choroid plexus, which results in decreased blood flow. Furosemide (frusemide) decreases formation by reducing the transport of Na^+ and Cl^-. Mannitol reduces both choroid plexus output and ECF flow from cerebral tissue to the CSF compartment. Corticosteroids may affect both rate of formation and resistance to absorption (RA). In situations where RA is increased, such as meningitis and pseudotumor cerebri, methylprednisolone and prednisone return RA toward normal values. Dexamethasone decreases formation by up to 50% by inhibiting the Na^+,K^+-ATPase pump at the choroid plexus epithelial membrane.

Metabolism – cerebral metabolic rate for oxygen

Neuronal function is usually completely dependent on the oxidative metabolism of glucose to provide ATP, except in certain states such as chronic starvation in which the brain can utilize ketone bodies. The brain accounts for 20% of total resting oxygen consumption; a lack of energy substrate storage and high metabolic rate account for its sensitivity to oxygen deprivation. Brain metabolism can be divided into basal metabolism and activation metabolism. Basal metabolism involves basic cellular functions, protein and neurotransmitter synthesis, and primarily maintenance of transmembrane ionic gradients. Activation metabolism is that which is necessary for neuronal activity and synaptic transmission. Metabolic rates differ between different brain regions and is fourfold more in gray matter than in white matter. Positron emission tomography studies suggest that neuronal activation also may involve nonoxidative metabolism, but this remains controversial.

The coupling of CBF to brain metabolism is preserved under physiologic conditions as well as under general anesthesia (Fig. 20.6). Increases in metabolic demand are instantaneously met by local increases in CBF. Thus, regional CBF increases in contralateral motor areas following hand movement and posterior cerebral artery blood flow velocity increases during visual stimulation.

Effects of volatile anesthetics and intravenous agents on CSF dynamics

Inhaled anesthetics	VF	RA
Desflurane	0, +#	0
Enflurane		
Low concentration	0	+
High concentration	+	0
Halothane	–	+
Isoflurane		
Low concentration	0	0, +#
High concentration	0	–
Nitrous oxide	0	0
Sevoflurane	–	+
Sedative-hypnotic and related intravenous drugs		
Etomidate		
Low dose	0	0
High dose	–	0, –*
Flumazenil		
Low dose	0	0
High dose	0	–
Midazolam		
Low dose	0	+, 0*
High dose	–	0, +*
Pentobarbital (phenobarbitone)	0	0
Propofol	0	0
Thiopental (thiopentone)		
Low dose	0	+, 0*
High dose	–	0, –*
Opioids and other intravenous drugs		
Alfentanil		
Low dose	0	–
High dose	0	0
Fentanyl		
Low dose	0	–
High dose	–	0, +*
Sufentanil		
Low dose	0	–
High dose	0	+, 0*
Ketamine	0	+
Lidocaine (lignocaine)	–*	0

Figure 20.5 Effects of volatile anesthetics and intravenous agents on cerebrospinal fluid dynamics. (+, increase; 0, no change; –, decrease; *, effect dependent on dose; #, effect occurs only during hypocapnea.) (Redrawn with permission from Albin MS, ed. Textbook of neuroanesthesia with neurosurgical and neuroscience perspectives. New York: McGraw Hill; 1997.)

The cerebral metabolic rate for oxygen ($CMRO_2$) is normally 3.5–5.5mL/100g per minute, but it is higher in children. Regional differences occur throughout the brain, with cortical regions having the highest $CMRO_2$. Brain metabolism decreases with decreasing temperature. For each 1°C decrease in body temperature, $CMRO_2$ decreases by about 7%. The metabolic temperature Q_{10} is defined as the ratio of $CMRO_2$ at a given temperature (T) divided by the $CMRO_2$ at temperature $T - 10$°C. The cerebral Q_{10} from 37 to 27°C is between 2.0 and 3.0. Below 27°C, Q_{10} increases to 4.5. Between 37 and 27°C most of the effect is thought to result from slowing of biochemical processes, whereas the larger Q_{10} below 27°C is thought to be caused by reduced cellular function. As CBF is coupled to metabolism, reduction in temperature leads to a decrease in CBF; this effect is most prominent in the cerebral and cerebellar cortex, less apparent in the thalamus, and insignificant in the hypothalamus and brain stem.

CBF as a function of $CMRO_2$

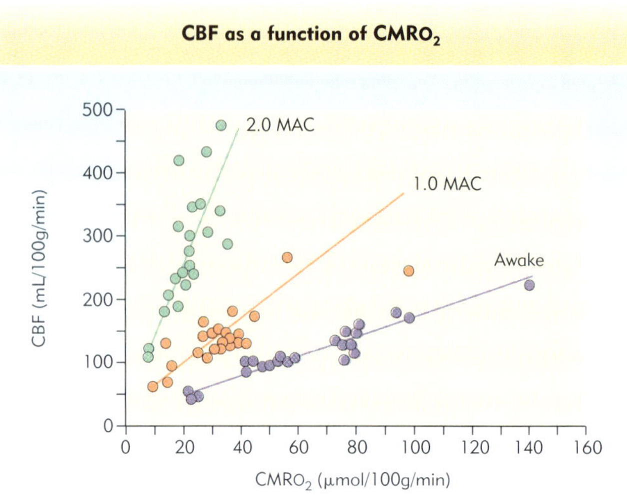

Figure 20.6 Cerebral blood flow as a function of cerebral metabolic rate for oxygen in different brain regions of the rat during isoflurane anesthesia. The volatile anesthetic does not uncouple flow and metabolism, rather it is 'reset' along a different line. (Redrawn with permission from Cottrell JE, Smith DS. Anesthesia and neurosurgery. St Louis: Mosby–Yearbook; 1994.)

Cerebral blood flow and autoregulation

Autoregulation is the hemodynamic response of blood flow to changes in perfusion pressure without regard to flow–metabolism coupling (Chapter 38). Active vasomotion in response to changes in perfusion pressure and flow–metabolism coupling may or may not be mechanistically related. The prevailing influences in this coupling are thought to be local metabolic factors. Specific factors possibly involved include H^+, K^+, adenosine, glycolytic intermediates, phospholipid metabolites, and endothelium-derived factors [e.g. nitric oxide (NO)]. The myogenic response of vascular smooth muscle to changes in perfusion pressure (the Bayliss effect) may actually consist of two mechanisms, one sensitive to mean pressure and the other sensitive to pulsatile pressure. In addition, there is evidence that flow, irrespective of pressure, may affect vascular resistance.

Cerebral vessels have sympathetic and parasympathetic innervation, which is more dense in the anterior than in the posterior circulation, as well as nonadrenergic noncholinergic innervation. Norepinephrine (noradrenaline), acetylcholine, neuropeptide Y, vasoactive intestinal peptide, calcitonin gene-related peptide, and substance P are some of the amines and peptides that may serve as neurotransmitters. The function of the perivascular innervation of the cerebral vasculature remains obscure. While not thought to be essential for hemodynamic autoregulation, it may modify, or in some cases initiate, regulatory responses.

It appears that NO influences basal arterial tone, including the endothelium-dependent response to acetylcholine in cerebral arteries and vasogenic dilatation because of stimulation of nonadrenergic, noncholinergic nerves. A direct role for NO in CO_2-mediated vasodilatation has not been consistently demonstrated, but a permissive role has been suggested. Although NO does not appear to be important in hypoxia-induced vasodilatation, it may play a role in the cerebral vasodilatory effects of halothane and isoflurane, and is also involved with many aspects of neuronal transmission.

Regulation of cerebral vascular resistance (CVR) occurs primarily in smaller arteries and arterioles (muscular), not in larger conductance (elastic) vessels, although the contribution of larger conductance arteries, capillaries, and venules is unclear. Ohm's Law is applied as a model to describe the cerebral circulation (Equation 20.1); CPP is given by Equation 20.2, in which MAP is the mean arterial pressure and CVP is central venous pressure.

Equation 20.1

$$CBF = \frac{CPP}{CVR}$$

Equation 20.2

$$CPP = MAP - \text{outflow pressure (the greater of CVP or ICP)}$$

Cerebrovascular resistance (CVR) can be modeled, though not entirely accurately, by the Hagen–Poiseuille model (Equation 20.3).

Equation 20.3

$$CVR = \frac{(8 \times \text{length of conduit})(\text{viscosity})}{\pi(\text{radius})^4}$$

In normal individuals CBF is constant (autoregulation) when CPP is 50–150mmHg (6.7–20kPa; Fig. 20.7). At the extremes, CBF passively follows changes in CPP, although resistance may not stay fixed and vessel collapse and passive dilatation may potentiate the predicted decline or increase in CBF. The lower limit of autoregulation may be higher in patients who have hypertension, and is probably >50mmHg (6.7kPa) even in normal individuals [e.g. 60–70mmHg (8.0–9.3kPa)].

Increases in CBF by arteriolar vasodilation lead to increases in cerebral blood volume (CBV). However, at a constant CBF an increase in CPP results in a decrease in CBV as CVR increases to maintain CBF. The physiology of CBV is less well understood than that of CBF. The role of the venous system in autoregulation is unclear; some investigators believe that the venous system is merely a passive recipient of arterial inflow. However, since most CBV is contained within the venous system, a slight change in vessel diameter might have a profound effect on CBV.

Blood viscosity has a major influence on CVR, and hematocrit is the major determinant of blood viscosity. At the microcirculatory level, the Hagen–Poiseuille model does not accurately describe the behavior of flow, because the red blood cells that flow near vessel walls create shearing forces, which increase resistance. Therefore, the blood flow is faster in the center of the vessel than in the periphery. In small

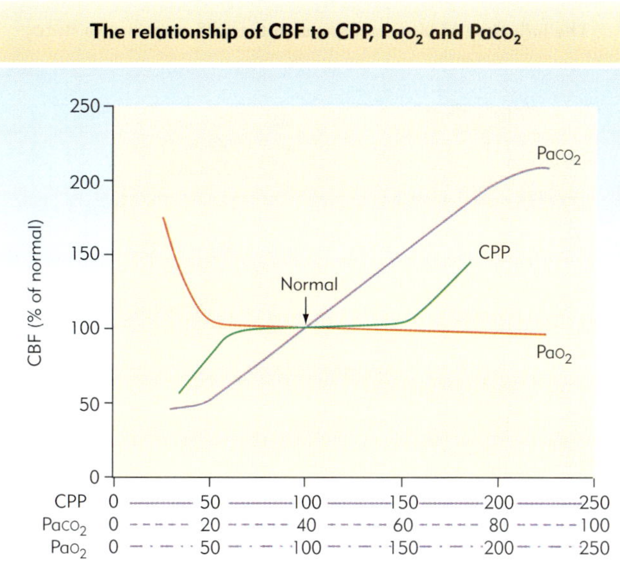

Figure 20.7 The relationship of cerebral blood flow to cerebral perfusion pressure, and to the arterial partial pressures of oxygen and carbon dioxide. (Redrawn with permission from Michenfelder JD. Anesthesia and the brain: clinical, functional, metabolic, and vascular correlations. New York: Churchill Livingstone; 1988.)

vessels, cells move faster than the plasma (Fahraeus effect), which reduces microvascular hematocrit (Chapter 38). Carbon dioxide is a powerful modulator of CVR. Rapid diffusion across the BBB allows carbon dioxide to modulate arteriolar resistance by its effects on extracellular pH. Systemic pH changes in the presence of an intact BBB do not affect cerebral arteriolar resistance, but H^+ ions released directly into the CSF or the ECF secondary to lactic acidosis reduce CVR. The CSF, via active exchange of HCO_3^-, buffers alterations in pH because of carbon dioxide diffusion. Although usually assumed to occur over a period of 6–10 hours, this may vary widely in individual patients. Sudden normalization in arterial PCO_2 ($PaCO_2$) in patients who have been chronically hypocapneic or hypercapneic may result in relative hyperperfusion or hypoperfusion, respectively.

At normotension, the response of CBF to $PaCO_2$ is almost linear from 20 to 80mmHg (2.7–10.5kPa). Doubling $PaCO_2$ from 40 (2.7) to 80mmHg (10.5kPa) roughly doubles CBF, and halving $PaCO_2$ from 40 (5.3) to 20mmHg (2.7kPa) halves CBF. Values quoted for the percentage change in CBF secondary to a change in $PaCO_2$ depend on the method of CBF measurement, but generally range from 3 to 5% change in CBF per mmHg CO_2, but there is interindividual variation.

The response of CBF to CO_2 is limited by maximal vasodilatation at extreme hypercapnia or maximal vasoconstriction at extreme hypocapnia, similar to blood pressure autoregulation. Hypocapnia may adversely affect cellular metabolism and shift the oxyhemoglobin dissociation curve to the left (Chapter 45). Thus, extreme hypocapnia leads to anaerobic metabolism and lactate production, such that $PaCO_2$ values <25mmHg (3.3kPa) are best avoided.

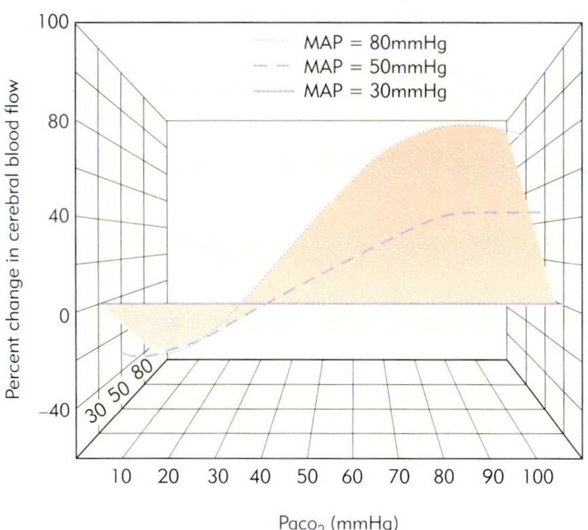

Figure 20.8 The influence of blood pressure on the cerebral blood flow response to arterial partial pressure of carbon dioxide. The effects of alteration of $Paco_2$ on cortical blood flow in dogs with normotenson [MAP, 80mmHg (10.6kPa)], moderate hypotension [MAP, 50mmHg (6.7kPa)], and severe hypotension [MAP, 30mmHg (4.0kPa)]. (Redrawn with permission from Cottrell JE, Smith DS. Anesthesia and neurosurgery. St Louis: Mosby–Yearbook; 1994.)

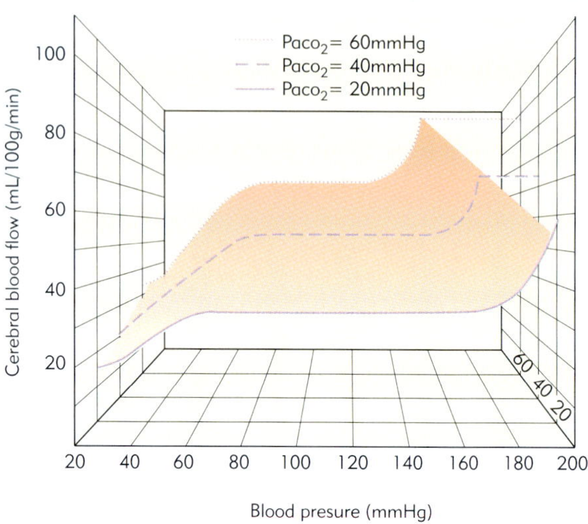

Figure 20.9 The influence of partial pressure of carbon dioxide on pressure autoregulation of cerebral blood flow. The effects of an alteration of blood pressure on CBF at hypocapnea [$Paco_2$, 20mmHg (2.7kPa)], normocapnea [$Paco_2$, 40mmHg (5.3kPa)], and hypercapnea [$Paco_2$, 60mmHg)]. Note the reduction in the autoregulatory plateau with increasing $Paco_2$. (Redrawn with permission from Cottrell JE, Smith DS. Anesthesia and neurosurgery. St Louis: Mosby–Yearbook; 1994.)

Arteriolar tone, determined by mean arterial blood pressure, modulates the effect of $Paco_2$ on CBF. Moderate hypotension blunts the ability of the cerebral circulation to respond to changes in $Paco_2$ and severe hypotension abolishes it (Fig. 20.8). Conversely, $Paco_2$ modifies pressure autoregulation, with hypocapnia widening the autoregulatory plateau and hypercapnia narrowing it (Fig. 20.9). Carbon dioxide responsiveness varies by region by unknown mechanisms.

Within physiologic ranges, Pao_2 does not affect CBF. However, at Pao_2 50mmHg (6.7kPa) CBF begins to increase, and it doubles at Pao_2 30mmHg (4.0kPa). Hyperoxia decreases CBF by 10–15% at 1 atmosphere (100kPa), and hyperbaric oxygenation may decrease CBF further.

Autoregulation and CO_2 reactivity are preserved at moderate hypothermia during cardiopulmonary bypass. Autoregulation may become impaired under pH-stat blood gas management, in which exogenous CO_2 is added to the bypass circuit to maintain 'normal' pH at the patient's actual temperature (Chapter 41).

Effects of anesthetics on cerebral metabolic rate for oxygen and cerebral blood flow

Most general anesthetics reduce $CMRo_2$; however, some anesthetics (i.e. enflurane) increase metabolic rate in certain brain structures, with coupling of CBF maintained. With most volatile anesthetics, however, CBF increases while $CMRo_2$ decreases. There is a positive correlation between multiples of minimal alveolar concentration (MAC) and the CBF:$CMRo_2$ ratio, which indicates that the CBF:$CMRo_2$ ratio is reset as anesthetic depth increases.

Halothane causes a dose-dependent reduction in $CMRo_2$ (up to 50%). At low doses (<0.5 volume %), this response predominates and CBF is diminished. At higher concentrations, halothane has a vasodilatory effect and increases CBF if MAP is maintained. The vasodilatation in cerebral tissue that surrounds brain tumors is more pronounced with halothane than with equipotent doses of enflurane or isoflurane.

Enflurane causes a dose-dependent increase in $CMRo_2$. At high concentrations (3.5 volume %) it produces frequent spiking on an electroencephalogram (EEG) and causes an increase in CBF and an increase in CMR for glucose (CMRGLU) in intercortical and corticothalamic pathways.

In animal studies, isoflurane increases CBF to a lesser extent than does halothane. Also, $CMRo_2$ decreases with increasing concentrations of isoflurane up to 2 MAC, after which no further decrease occurs. In humans who receive nitrous oxide, no change in CBF was noted with isoflurane, while $CMRo_2$ decreased (associated with EEG burst suppression). Desflurane and sevoflurane effects on $CMRo_2$ and CBF are similar to those of isoflurane. With desflurane at 1 MAC and hypocapnia, CBF was lower, but at 1.5 MAC, CBF was not different from that with isoflurane. Some evidence indicates that cerebral pressure autoregulation is better maintained with sevoflurane than with other volatile anesthetic agents.

The effects of nitrous oxide on $CMRo_2$ and CBF vary widely between species. In dogs, both CBF and $CMRo_2$ increase with a substantial elevation in CBF. In rodents, no change in CBF or $CMRo_2$ occurs. The interaction between nitrous oxide and volatile or intravenous agents is complex. In humans, the addition of nitrous oxide to volatile anesthetics appears to produce an increase in CBF without any change or only a slight increase in $CMRO_2$. With intravenous agents, the results vary widely among species and intravenous agents. In humans, the addition of nitrous oxide to intravenous agents does not alter CBF and causes a slight decrease in $CMRO_2$, although baseline vascular tone, other anesthetic agents, and body temperature may affect these results.

Intravenous anesthetics reduce $CMRO_2$, which leads to a decrease in CBF because of flow–metabolism coupling. Thiopental reduces $CMRO_2$ by 55–60% at the point of EEG isoelectricity, after which no further decrease occurs. In isolated cerebral arteries, thiopental is a cerebral vasodilator. Barbiturates also attenuate the cerebral vasodilatation produced by ketamine and nitrous oxide. Etomidate also decreases $CMRO_2$ and CBF (by 30–50%). The CBF decrease occurs prior to a reduction in $CMRO_2$, which suggests a component of direct vasoconstriction. As with thiopental, no further decrease in $CMRO_2$ or CBF occurs beyond EEG silence. Propofol decreases CBF and $CMRO_2$ in a dose-dependent manner and, like barbiturates, it dilates isolated cerebral arteries.

Ketamine increases CBF and $CMRO_2$ as the result of a direct metabolic stimulating effect, a direct vasodilating effect, and perhaps a cholinergic effect (ketamine-induced CBF increases can be blocked by scopolamine). In humans, ketamine (3mg/kg) increases CBF by 60%, without a significant change in $CMRO_2$.

In humans, midazolam decreases CBF and $CMRO_2$ by about 30%, an effect reversed by flumazenil.

The effects of opioids on CBF and $CMRO_2$ are influenced by the background anesthetic. In unanesthetized humans and animals, up to 1mg/kg of morphine or 4.4μg/kg of fentanyl have no effect on $CMRO_2$ or CBF. If a nitrous oxide background anesthetic is used, opioids decrease CBF and $CMRO_2$. At very high doses, synthetic opioids may induce seizures, in which case $CMRO_2$ and CBF increase.

Lidocaine (lignocaine), often used during anesthesia to attenuate the sympathetic response to intubation or to avoid coughing, produces a dose-related decrease (up to 30%) in CBF and $CMRO_2$. However, at high doses seizures may be induced and result in increases in $CMRO_2$ and CBF.

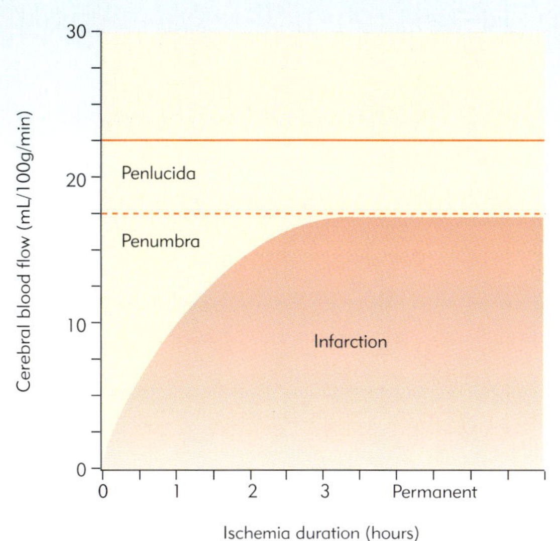

Figure 20.10 Interaction of degree and duration of flow reductions with neurologic function. Tissue that receives blood flow between approximately 18 and 23mL/100g per minute is functionally inactive, but function can be restored at anytime with reinstitution of increased perfusion (penlucida). For tissue perfused at lower blood pressure, the development of infarction is a function of time. If tissue is restored to adequate perfusion before the time limit of infarction it will recover function (penumbra).

CEREBRAL EDEMA

Cerebral edema is defined as an increase in brain intracellular fluid (ICF) and/or extracellular fluid (ECF) volume, which is usually associated with an increase in brain tissue volume and ICP. Several types of edema lead to cerebral edema – vasogenic, ischemic, osmotic, hydrocephalic (interstitial), cytotoxic, edema caused by metabolic storage diseases, and edema caused by increased CBV.

Vasogenic edema is the most frequent type of cerebral edema, and is characterized by increased ECF volume (by up to 50%) secondary to increased permeability of the BBB. Dysfunction of the BBB, whether from tumor, infection, inflammation, or traumatic injury, results in extravasation of a protein-rich fluid under the force of systemic pressure, which accumulates mainly in the white matter. Dysfunction of the BBB appears to be related to opening of tight junctions, increased pinocytosis, and disruption of cells, but can be seen even in cells that appear structurally normal.

Ischemic edema (cytotoxic) occurs following failure of the Na^+,K^+-ATPase pump because of the lack of energy substrate following a prolonged decrease in CBF below the ischemic threshold (Fig. 20.10). Na^+, Cl^-, and H_2O move into the intracellular space. In contrast to vasogenic edema, ischemic edema is more pronounced in gray matter.

Hydrocephalic edema is similar to lymphedema in other tissues, in which the tissue proximal to an obstruction accumulates fluid in the ECF space. In acute hydrocephalus, this occurs in periventricular tissue. Astrocytes are particularly susceptible to this form of edema and undergo cell swelling and eventually cell death.

INTRACRANIAL PRESSURE

The intracranial space contains three components – brain tissue (80–85%), CSF (7–10%), and CBV (5–8%). The pressure caused by the total volume within the nondistensible intracranial space is the ICP. The Monro–Kellie hypothesis states that for ICP to remain normal, an increase in any one of the volumes must be matched by a decrease in another volume. Brain tissue volume comprises mainly ECF and ICF; CSF volume is determined by the ratio of production to absorption; and CBV is the sum of arterial and venous blood volumes. The presence of an intracranial mass lesion, be it tumor or hematoma, may increase ICP because of a volume effect and/or the position of the lesion (it may obstruct CSF outflow pathways).

Cerebral or intracranial elastance is the change in ICP (ΔP) divided by the change in intracranial volume (ΔV), while intracranial compliance is given by $\Delta V/\Delta P$ (Fig. 20.11). The pressure– volume response (PVR) is defined as the change in ICP after the injection or withdrawal of 1mL of CSF over 1

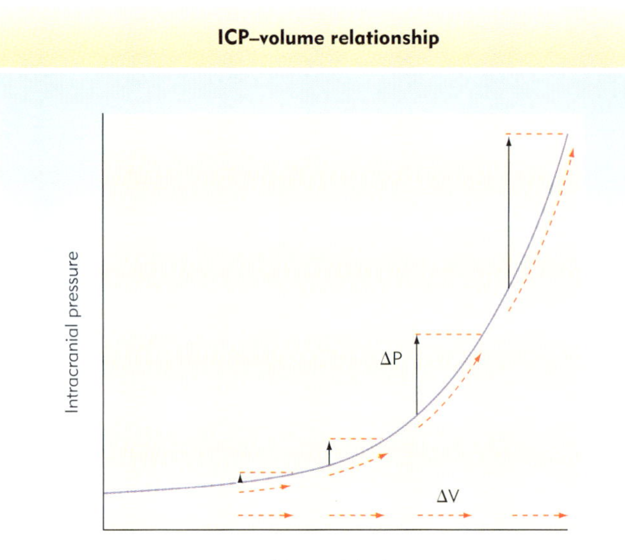

Figure 20.11 The intracranial pressure–volume relationship. The dotted lines and arrows indicate the point to which the volume additions shift the system along the pressure–volume curve. Although for each individual the curve undergoes minor changes in response to therapeutic measures or physiologic changes, the general exponential nature of the curve is retained. (Reprinted with permission from Cottrell JE, Smith DS. Anesthesia and neurosurgery. St Louis: Mosby–Yearbook; 1994.)

second. A normal PVR is less than 2mmHg/mL, whereas a PVR >5mmHg/mL signifies decreased intracranial compliance. Although PVR is a sensitive indicator of elastance and/or compliance, it has not been shown to predict outcome in patients who have intracranial hypertension.

Anesthetics alter ICP via effects on production and reabsorption of CSF; however, these effects are small compared with the effects of anesthetics on CBV. The change in CBV is determined mainly by the degree of vasodilatation caused by the anesthetic and the concomitant increase in CBF. Also, CBV may be affected by changes in $Paco_2$ and MAP if autoregulation is not intact. Patient positioning, increased CVP and intrathoracic pressure, positive end-expiratory pressure, and coughing may all affect ICP as well. Acute changes in CVP are blunted by venous valves at the thoracic inlet.

Halothane appears to be the most potent of the volatile anesthetics in increasing ICP, an increase that can be avoided if hypocapnia is induced prior to administration of halothane. With enflurane, increases in ICP are minimal in subjects who have normal ICP, but are severe in patients who have space-occupying lesions. In animals, isoflurane alone minimally increases ICP, but increases ICP when used in high inspired concentrations or in conjunction with nitrous oxide. The increase in ICP with isoflurane lasts only 30 minutes, as compared with increases by halothane or enflurane, which last approximately 3 hours. The increase in ICP is attenuated or blocked completely by the institution of hypocapnia (even after introduction of isoflurane) or thiopental. With space-occupying lesions, ICP may increase when isoflurane concentration is above 1.5%. In animals, sevoflurane produces a minimal increase in ICP and desflurane has no significant effect. Desflurane increases lumbar CSF pressure at 1 MAC, whereas isoflurane does not, but 0.5 MAC desflurane does not affect lumbar CSF pressure in patients who have supratentorial mass lesions. Desflurane has no effect on CSF pressure in patients without mass lesions. Studies of the effect of nitrous oxide on ICP have produced conflicting results. In patients who have decreased intracranial compliance, nitrous oxide may increase ICP.

As a result of reduction in CBF and CBV, ICP is reduced by barbiturates. Etomidate decreases ICP without decreasing CPP. Propofol either decreases or does not change ICP; however, CPP may also decrease because of a decrease in MAP. Ketamine causes a substantial increase in ICP. Benzodiazepines produce either no change or a decrease in ICP, which can be reversed by flumazenil. Although opioids produce no effect or small increases in ICP [(<10mmHg (<1.3kPa)], with decreased intracranial compliance opioids may increase ICP secondary to a vasodilatory response to a decrease in MAP. Vasodilatory responses may occur in patients who are not on mechanical ventilation because of an increase in $Paco_2$ that results from opioid-induced respiratory depression.

Succinylcholine increases ICP in lightly anesthetized humans. This effect, which is diminished by pretreatment with intravenous lidocaine (lignocaine) or nondepolarizing muscle relaxants, may result from increased muscle spindle afferent activity, which leads to increased CBF as well as fasciculation of neck muscles, causing stasis in the jugular veins. In neurologically injured patients, however, succinylcholine causes no change in ICP.

SEIZURES AND ANTICONVULSANTS

A seizure is the manifestation of the excessive discharge of an aggregate of neurons that depolarize synchronously. Seizures are commonly categorized as *partial* (focal), in which a focal area of neuronal hyperexcitability is surrounded by neurons that remain polarized and unexcited, or *generalized*, in which depolarization spreads throughout the brain with EEG involvement of both cerebral hemispheres. A simple partial seizure produces no alteration in consciousness, while complex partial seizures involve automatism with variable degrees of responsiveness. A seizure may be partial in onset with generalization, in which a focal electrical disturbance spreads to involve much of the brain and brain stem in producing convulsive seizures. Generalized seizures may be inhibitory (absence or atonic) or excitatory seizures (myotonic, tonic, and clonic). A partial (focal) seizure can cause a postictal focal neurologic deficit (Todd's paralysis). An extensive scheme based on epileptic syndromes, rather than type of seizure, has been developed by the International League Against Epilepsy.

Seizure disorder (chronic) affects 0.5–1.0% of the population, while 2–5% of people experience at least one nonfebrile seizure during their lifetime. Epidemiologic studies suggest a genetic link, with a 2.5-fold increased risk of epilepsy among first-degree relatives, and a multifactorial mode of inheritance involving a number of genes. Common causes of seizures include structural brain lesions and drugs; however, many causative factors exist. The EEG is the most important test in making a diagnosis (Chapter 13). Magnetic resonance imaging is useful in detecting focal areas of atrophy that may be associated with seizure disorder. Examination of the CSF may be useful if infection is contributory.

The many theories regarding the molecular and cellular causes of epilepsy all address the disruption of the delicate balance between cellular depression and excitation. Theories of macrocircuit dysfunction involve the substantia nigra and hippocampus. The substantia nigra is thought to act as a gating mechanism, modulating excitation in other brain structures via γ-aminobutyric acid (GABA)-ergic efferents. Hippocampal (medial temporal) sclerosis is often associated with epilepsy and resection of this area can reduce seizures. Damage to the hippocampus from an initial seizure may predispose to further seizures, which creates a vicious cycle. Microcircuit theories address the excitation–inhibition imbalance on a cellular level. The dormant basket cell hypothesis purports that temporal lobe seizures cause loss of excitatory hippocampal neurons that excite GABAergic interneurons (Basket cells), which in turn modulate the effects of the excitatory afferent and other cells in the hippocampus. The mossy fiber sprouting hypothesis involves increased dentate granule cell excitability as a result of loss of mossy cells secondary to damage from seizures, which forces granule cells to synapse on themselves and so increases their response to excitatory stimuli.

Enhanced excitatory amino acid receptor function and diminished number and function of GABA and benzodiazepine receptors have been reported as molecular mechanisms of epilepsy. Increased levels of extracellular K^+ have been linked to excitatory events in several ways:

- shifting membrane potential closer to spike threshold by partial depolarization;
- increasing the risk of repetitive firing by decreasing postburst hyperpolarization;
- reducing K^+ efflux from cells, thus reducing the $GABA_A$ and $GABA_B$ components of the inhibitory postsynaptic potential; and
- enhanced *N*-methyl-D-aspartate (NMDA) receptor activation.

Kindling is a phenomenon in which subconvulsive stimuli lead to progressive increases in seizure activity until a generalized convulsion occurs. This process results in increased sensitivity to stimuli despite long stimulus-free periods. Kindling is used extensively as an experimental model of epilepsy in animals.

Treatment of idiopathic seizure disorder is primarily via antiepileptic drugs (AEDs). Mechanisms of action of AEDs include:

- inhibition of repetitive firing by blockade of Na^+ channels [carbamazepine, phenytoin, valproate, lamotrigine, and possibly felbamate (felbate)];
- blockade of slow Ca^{2+} channels (valproate, ethosuximide);
- prolonging $GABA_A$ Cl^- channel opening (phenobarbital, clonazepam);
- inhibition of glutamate and aspartate release (lamotrigine);
- blockade of the glycine co-agonist site on NMDA receptors (felbamate); and
- increasing GABA concentration (gabapentin, vigabatrin).

Treatment with AEDs is often monitored by drug levels, although clinical response is more important.

Anesthetic management is affected by AEDs in several ways. Most are metabolized by the liver and induce the cytochrome P450 system, altering the metabolism of other drugs. Increased requirements for fentanyl and nondepolarizing neuromuscular blocking agents in patients chronically treated with phenytoin, carbamazepine, or phenobarbital is secondary to hepatic enzyme induction. Phenytoin-induced increase in hepatic oxidative and reductive metabolism of halothane may be linked to post-halothane hepatitis. Conversely, sedating AEDs, such as phenobarbital, clonazepam, and gabapentin, may potentiate general anesthetics, so reducing the dosages required. This interaction is consistent with the facilitory actions of most volatile (Chapter 24) and intravenous (Chapter 23) general anesthetics at the $GABA_A$ receptor.

The effects of AEDs on other organ systems are varied. The immune system may be affected adversely by carbamazepine- and phenytoin-induced leukopenia. Lymphadenopathy, systemic lupus erythematosus, and vasculitis have been noted in patients on AEDs. Valproate affects the hematologic system by an intrinsic system coagulopathy and a dose-related thrombocytopenia. Since abnormal hemostasis may be present despite a normal platelet count, prothrombin time, and partial thromboplastin time, a bleeding time test is recommended prior to surgery. Thrombocytopenia is also associated with felbamate, as is aplastic anemia. Anemia may occur with lamotrigine. Liver function tests are usually elevated by 25–75%, usually without clinical significance, although liver failure has been reported with felbamate. Valproate can cause pancreatitis, especially in young patients, in combination with other AEDs. Corticosteroid, thyroxine (T_4), and vitamin D_3 metabolism and function may be altered by phenytoin, carbamazepine, and barbiturates. Protein binding of T_4 and sex hormones may be changed and release of calcitonin, insulin, and clotting factors dependent on vitamin K may be impaired. Most patients appear euthyroid because of reduced binding of T_4 to plasma proteins secondary to the extensive protein binding of AEDs.

Carbamazepine metabolism (by CYP3A4) is inhibited by erythromycin and cimetidine, both of which may be used preoperatively. Increased blood levels may lead to toxicity and heart block. Blood levels of AEDs may fluctuate for as long as 1 week after general anesthesia and surgery; therefore, it may be useful to check levels postoperatively.

Certain drugs are known to lower the seizure threshold or activate epileptogenic foci and thus should be avoided in patients who have seizure disorder. For example, methohexital can activate seizure foci and has been used in mapping for surgical resection. Ketamine and propofol have been reported to elicit seizures in patients who have seizure disorder, but their epileptogenic potential is unclear. Although propofol can successfully treat status epilepticus, both seizures and opisthotonos have been reported in patients with and without previously diagnosed seizure disorder. Propofol is an effective anticonvulsant for bupivacaine-, picrotoxin-, and pentylenetetrazol-induced seizures in animals and in seizures produced by GABAergic inhibition; however, seizures produced by a glutamatergic mechanism have been augmented by propofol. Antagonism of glycine in subcortical structures has been proposed as a mechanism to explain the seizure-like activity associated with propofol. Inhalational anesthetics exhibit both anticonvulsant and proconvulsant properties in various studies in both humans and animals, with isoflurane and desflurane having the least proconvulsant activity. Generally, clinical use of potent agents is anticonvulsant. In fact, isoflurane has been used to treat status epilepticus.

CEREBRAL ISCHEMIA AND STROKE

The assessment of specific anesthetics as cerebral protectants is complicated by several factors. In most studies the anesthetic is added to a standard background anesthetic, such that few studies employ a control group that is not anesthetized. In addition, many models of ischemia are used in different species – global versus focal models and, within focal models, permanent versus temporary ischemia, with variable duration and magnitude of temporary ischemia. In general, no single anesthetic agent is unequivocally and uniquely cerebroprotective in all settings.

Barbiturates decrease $CMRO_2$, theoretically via enhanced $GABA_A$-receptor activity that leads to increased Cl^- flux. The $CMRO_2$–CBF linkage is preserved such that CBF is decreased. There is no additional benefit to barbiturate administration beyond that required for EEG silence. The reduction in $CMRO_2$ is not unequivocally cerebroprotective however. Other possible mechanisms of cerebroprotection by barbiturates include decreased production of free fatty acids during ischemia, and reduced excitatory amino acid release and/or receptor activation following ischemia. A reduction in brain temperature by reducing heat delivery (decreased CBF) might also play a role. Although one primate study found thiopental to be protective after global ischemia, the results could not be repeated, and a randomized trial of thiopental loading in comatose survivors of cardiac arrest showed no benefit. In focal ischemia, barbiturates are more effective cerebroprotectants in temporary as opposed to permanent vascular occlusion in animal models. Results from clinical studies that involve middle cerebral artery occlusion, acute stroke, and carotid endarterectomy are conflicting.

Ketamine, which noncompetitively antagonizes glutamate activation of NMDA receptors (Chapter 23), has been studied in models of focal ischemia. No consistent neuroprotective effect was observed, but lack of temperature control may have affected the results. In a recent study of rat axonal transection, (*S*)(+)-ketamine was comparable with the NMDA receptor antagonist MK-801 in producing neuroprotection. Racemic ketamine was somewhat effective, but (*S*)(–)-ketamine was ineffective, indicating stereospecificity.

Etomidate reduces $CMRO_2$ and CBF while maintaining systemic blood pressure. In a dog model of global incomplete ischemia (residual EEG activity), etomidate preserved cerebral high-energy phosphates (ATP and phosphocreatinine) and reduced lactic acid accumulation. In doses that achieved EEG silence, etomidate was equally neuroprotective with thiopental in severe forebrain ischemia in rats. Recent studies suggest, however, that etomidate may potentiate ischemic neuronal injury. In addition, in patients undergoing aneurysm clipping cerebral tissue PO_2 decreased after a dose of etomidate, causing burst suppression.

α_2-Adrenoreceptor agonists, such as clonidine and dexmedetomidine, may be protective via decreased norepinephrine release following cerebral ischemia. In animal models of focal and global ischemia, they protect against immediate and delayed neuronal death.

Volatile anesthetics have been evaluated as potential cerebroprotectants in both global and focal models of ischemia. The mechanism of protection is not known, but may involve cerebral vasodilatation. Most volatile agents produce a sustained increase in CBF in primates. There is a decrease in $CMRO_2$ (linked to EEG activity) and CMRGLU with preserved high-energy (e.g. ATP) phosphate metabolism. The mechanism of vasodilatation by volatile anesthetics may be related to NO because NO synthase (NOS) inhibition blocks increases in CBF secondary to inhaled agents. The role of NO in brain injury is controversial and may be dependent on which NOS isoform (neuronal versus endothelial versus inducible) is inhibited. Therefore, volatile anesthetics may exert a cerebroprotective effect via the NO pathway. Vasodilatation as a result of volatile agents may also be mediated via a prostanoid pathway, as isoflurane-induced vasodilatation is attenuated by indomethacin.

Another potential mechanism for neuroprotection by volatile anesthetics is inhibition of glutamate binding at the NMDA receptor. Isoflurane reduces NMDA receptor and L-glutamate mediated Ca^{2+} fluxes. However, neither halothane nor isoflurane reduce the amount of glutamate or glycine released following global ischemia.

In primates subjected to severe temporary focal ischemia, isoflurane provided the same degree of neuroprotection as thiopental. Data from retrospective, uncontrolled studies suggest that EEG threshold for minimal CBF is lower in patients anesthetized with isoflurane (10mL/100mg per minute) and sevoflurane (11.5mL/100mg per minute) compared with enflurane (15mL/100mg per minute) or halothane (20mL/100mg per minute) for carotid endarterectomy. However, well-controlled animal studies suggest that cerebroprotection is similar between halothane, enflurane, isoflurane, and sevoflurane.

The effect of nitrous oxide on cerebral ischemia has not been directly evaluated. Studies of the use of nitrous oxide as a sole anesthetic agent would be associated with increases in systemic catecholamines, which may themselves worsen outcome following an ischemic insult. In a rat model, nitrous oxide diminished isoflurane-induced neuroprotection; however, the protective effects of barbiturates were not attenuated.

Other pharmacologic agents under investigation as neuroprotectants include Mg^{2+}, lamotrigine, and dextromethorphan. Mg^{2+} competes with Ca^{2+} for entry into neuronal cells and blocks NMDA receptors. Lamotrigine, a Na^+ channel blocker, inhibits glutamate release during transient global ischemia in rabbits. Dextromethorphan, an antitussive opioid with no respiratory depression and no addiction potential, is a functional NMDA receptor antagonist that presynaptically inhibits evoked release of glutamate secondary to ischemia.

A confounding factor in studies on neuroprotective effects of anesthetics is the lack of controlled temperature. Deliberate mild hypothermia, a reduction of 2–3°C, which provides more protection than the volatile agents, is frequently employed by neuroanesthesiologists for neuronal protection. These small decreases in temperature have relatively minimal effect on $CMRO_2$. Hypothermia may provide protection in part via a decrease in release of excitatory neurotransmitters following ischemia. In patients who have closed head trauma, deliberate hypothermia appears to improve outcome. In neurosurgical patients, studies of deliberate mild hypothermia in aneurysm clipping demonstrated neither improved outcome nor increased morbidity and mortality. A much larger number of patients will need to be studied to detect a difference in outcome.

NEUROTOXICITY

As anesthetic agents interfere with normal neuronal function, the possibility of neurotoxicity is a concern. Sufentanil, alfentanil, and morphine have been studied in a dog model with chronic intrathecal or epidural catheters and intermittent daily injections over 15–28 days. No morphologic or histopathologic evidence of neurotoxicity was found compared with vehicle controls over a range of doses and concentrations, which were greater than would be used clinically. Ketamine is not itself neurotoxic, but the preservative, chlorobutanol, induced severe spinal cord lesions in a rabbit model. No evidence of neurotoxicity has been reported for propofol, barbiturates, or volatile anesthetics.

Although nondepolarizing neuromuscular blocking agents are highly ionized and normally do not cross the BBB, these agents and their metabolites have been found in the CSF of patients who have neurologic disease or who are critically ill and in whom the BBB may not be intact. In rat brain cortical slices, pancuronium and vecuronium increased intracellular Ca^{2+} via prolonged activation (rather than inhibition) of nicotinic acetylcholine receptors; atracurium and laudanosine did not have this effect. The clinical relevance of this finding has yet to be established.

JUGULAR VENOUS OXYGEN SATURATION

The CMR for oxygen can be expressed as in Equation 20.4, otherwise expressed as in Equation 20.5, in which $Cao_2 - Cjvo_2$ is the difference in oxygen content in simultaneous arterial and jugular bulb blood samples.

Equation 20.4

$$CMRo_2 = CBF \times (Cao_2 - Cjvo_2)$$

Equation 20.5

$$Cao_2 - Cjvo_2 = \frac{CMRo_2}{CBF}$$

Arterial oxygen content minus $Cjvo_2$ is constant (7–8mL oxygen/100mL blood) as long as flow–metabolism coupling is intact, although hypothermia, hyperthermia, and anesthetic states may change baseline values. In head trauma, which disrupts flow–metabolism coupling, $Cao_2 - Cjvo_2$ reflects the adequacy of oxygen delivery for metabolic demand; levels of 4mL oxygen/100mL blood indicate increased supply (decreased extraction) relative to demand, whereas levels >9mL oxygen/100mL blood indicate global ischemia (increased extraction). Further decreases in oxygen delivery at this point exceed the brain's ability to compensate for hypoperfusion, and infarction may occur. After ischemia and/or infarction, $Cao_2 - Cjvo_2$ decreases, since infarcted tissue does not extract oxygen.

The oxygen content of blood (Co_2 in mL/dL) depends primarily on hemoglobin concentration (Hb), the amount of oxygen dissolved in plasma (to a much lesser extent), and the oxygen saturation of hemoglobin (So_2; Chapter 45), as in Equation 20.6.

Equation 20.6

$$Co_2 = (Hb \times 1.34 \times So_2) + [0.003 \times Po_2\ (mmHg)]$$

If the hemoglobin concentration and the amount of dissolved oxygen remain constant, $Cao_2 - Cjvo_2$ is primarily dependent on the oxygen saturation of the jugular venous blood (Equation 20.7).

Equation 20.7

$$Cao_2 - Cjvo_2 \propto (1 - Sjvo_2) \text{ and } Sjvo_2 \propto CBF/CMRo_2$$

Fiberoptic intravascular catheters are available which allow continuous measurement of $Sjvo_2$. Normal $Sjvo_2$ is 66–70%; a saturation >75% indicates either cerebral hyperemia (oxygen supply exceeding demand) or global cerebral infarction. Conversely, decreases in $Sjvo_2$ to <54% indicate 'compensated cerebral hypoperfusion' but not ischemia, whereas a value <40% indicates global cerebral ischemia. If there are fluctuations in the arterial oxygen saturation, cerebral oxygen extraction ratio (OER) may be calculated as in Equation 20.8.

Equation 20.8

$$OER = Sao_2 - \frac{Sjvo_2}{Sao_2}$$

Although $Cao_2 - Cjvo_2$ or $Sjvo_2$ may be useful in identifying patients who have impending cerebral ischemia in spite of adequate CPP and aid in maximizing therapy in those who have intracranial hypertension, $Sjvo_2$ monitoring reflects global cerebral oxygenation and may falsely reassure in the setting of focal ischemia.

Key References

Artru AA. Cerebrospinal fluid. In: Cottrell JE, Smith DS, eds. Anesthesia and neurosurgery. St Louis: Mosby–Yearbook; 1994:93–116.

Brian JE Jr. Carbon dioxide and the cerebral circulation. Anesthesiology. 1998;88:1365–86.

Cheng MA, Theard MA, Tempelhoff R. Intravenous agents and intraoperative neuroprotection: beyond barbiturates. Crit Care Clin. 1997;13:185–99.

Cucchaiara RF, Michenfelder JD. Clinical neuroanesthesia. New York: Churchill Livingstone; 1990.

Edvinsson L, MacKenzie ET, McCulloch J. Cerebral blood flow and metabolism. New York: Raven Press; 1993.

Iadecola C. Bright and dark sides of nitric oxide in ischemic brain injury. Trends Neurosci. 1997;20:132–9.

KofkeWA, Templehoff R, Dasheiff RM. Anesthetic implications of epilepsy, status epilepsies and epilepsy surgery. J Neurosurg Anesth. 1997;9:349–72.

Michenfelder JD. Anesthesia and the brain: clinical, functional, metabolic and vascular correlates. New York: Churchill Livingstone; 1988.

Sakabe T, Nakatumura K. Effects of anesthetic agents on cerebral blood flow, metabolism and intracranial pressure. In: Cottrell ME, Smith DS, eds. Anesthesia and neurosurgery. St Louis: Mosby–Yearbook; 1994:149–74.

Werner C, Kochs B, Hoffman WE. Cerebral blood flow and metabolism. In: Albin M, ed. Textbook of neuroanesthesia: with neurosurgical and neuroscience perspectives. New York: McGraw Hill; 1997:21–59.

Young WL, Ornstein E. Cerebral and spinal cord blood flow. In: Cottrell JE, Smith DS, eds. Anesthesia and neurosurgery. St Louis: Mosby–Yearbook; 1994:17–57.

Further Reading

Bell BA. A history of the study of the cerebral circulation and the measurement of cerebral blood flow. Neurosurgery. 1984;14:238–46.

Brian JE Jr, Faraci FM, Heistad DD. Recent insights into the regulation of cerebral circulation. Clin Exp Pharmacol Physiol. 1996;23:449–57.

Hansen TD, Warner DS, Todd MM, et al. The role of cerebral metabolism in determining the local cerebral blood flow effects of volatile anesthetics: evidence for persistent flow–metabolism coupling. J Cereb Blood Flow Metab. 1989;9:323–8.

Illievich UM, Zornow MH, Choi KT, Strnat MA, Scheller MS. Effects of hypothermia or anesthetics on hippocampus glutamate and glycine concentrations after repeated transient global cerebral ischemia. Anesthesiology. 1994;80:177–86.

Karibe H, Zarow GJ, Graham SH, Weinstein PR. Mild intraischemic hypothermia reduces post-ischemic hyperperfusion, delayed hypoperfusion, blood–brain barrier disruption, brain edema, and neuronal damage after temporary focal cerebral ischemia in rats. J Cereb Blood Flow Metab. 1994;14:620–7.

Minamisawa H, Nordstrom CH, Smith ML, Siesjo BK. The influence of mild body and brain hypothermia on ischemic damage. J Cereb Blood Flow Metab. 1990;10:365–74.

Paulson OB, Standgaard S, Edmusson L. Cerebral autoregulation. Cerebrovasc Brain Metab Rev. 1990;2:161–92.

Siesjo BK. Pathophysiology and treatment of focal cerebral ischemia. Part I: Pathophysiology. J Neurosurg. 1992; 77:169–84

Siesjo BK: Pathophysiology and treatment of focal cerebral ischemia: Part II. Mechanisms of damage and treatment. J Neurosurg. 1992;77:337–54.

Chapter 21 Sensory systems and pain

Philip J Siddall, Michael J Hudspith and Rajesh Munglani

Topics covered in this chapter

Peripheral pain mechanisms
Dorsal horn mechanisms
Spinal mechanisms following nerve injury and inflammation
Modulation at a spinal level
Ascending spinal tracts
Supraspinal structures
Clinical significance of inflammation and nerve injury

Sensory systems have evolved to provide organisms with information regarding the state(s) of both the internal and external milieu. Normal human sensory systems can discriminate a spectrum of physical and chemical stimuli with high spatial and temporal resolution. They comprise means of transducing specific aspects of physical stimuli into neurally encoded information relayed to appropriate integrative higher centers. At these higher centers sensory information may reach conscious perception, and neural activity at the level of consciousness is, therefore, many synapses distant from the initial sensory transduction.

Sensory perception and the experience of pain are fundamental to the practice of anesthesia. This discipline grew out of the desire to suppress or abolish the perception of pain during surgical procedures and has continued and expanded to include the management of pain itself in many settings from acute postoperative pain to chronic pain conditions.

In the past, pain was often regarded as a simple response by the brain to a noxious stimulus in the periphery; this nociceptive information was then transmitted along well-defined 'pain' pathways. The biologic processes involved in pain perception are no longer viewed as a simple 'hard-wired' system with a pure 'stimulus–response' relationship. The International Association for the Study of Pain has defined pain as '... an unpleasant sensory and emotional experience associated with actual or potential tissue damage, or described in terms of such damage'. In consequence, the perception of pain and its threshold are the result of complex interactions between sensory, emotional, and behavioral factors. Inflammation and nerve injury can decrease pain thresholds and increase sensitivity to sensory stimuli. Conversely, 'battlefield analgesia' in which soldiers receive severe injuries with little immediate awareness of pain is a situation in which thresholds can increase. This chapter emphasizes the dynamic nature of sensory perception with specific reference to pain and analgesia. Such changes of gain in pain perception can occur over a wide range of time scales: from milliseconds determined by a balance of ion-channel and receptor-operated channel function, through longer-term processes initiated by tropic factors over minutes to hours, leading ultimately to altered gene expression and altered neuronal phenotype and synaptic architecture within the CNS.

What is the purpose or function of acute physiologic pain? A withdrawal reflex response to an acute noxious stimulus is an understandable and necessary reaction that has an obvious protective function. Experiences of pain lead to avoidance of potentially harmful situations and possible injury. The severe deformities often seen in those with congenital insensitivity to pain illustrate the useful protective function provided by the sensation of pain. The immobility and withdrawal of those in pain may also serve to provide an environment in which healing and restoration of function can occur.

The usefulness of chronic pain, for example that following nerve injury and the pain associated with migraine, is more difficult to understand. Unfortunately, chronic pain states are most difficult to treat; this appears to be related to the pathophysiologic processes that occur following inflammation and nerve injury, which are quite different from those seen following acute, 'physiologic' pain. Current research efforts are directed toward understanding the pathophysiologic processes associated with chronic pain conditions, which are relevant to our understanding and management of pain in the clinical setting.

Psychologic factors, which include emotional and behavioral responses, are important components in the perception and expression of pain; the person in pain should always be considered in the context of the interactions between biologic and psychosocial processes. Attempts to manage pain that fail to take these interactions into account will inevitably lead to frustration and failure. Nevertheless, this chapter focuses upon those neurobiologic (as opposed to the neuropsychologic) processes in the peripheral nervous system, spinal cord, and higher centers initiated by a variety of noxious insults that are the key to appropriate pharmacologic pain management. A concise overview of the anatomy and physiology of sensory pathways will provide a background for more detailed discussions of central and peripheral adaptive processes pertinent to pain transduction.

PERIPHERAL PAIN MECHANISMS

Primary afferent nociceptors

Stimuli that have the potential to cause damage (e.g. thermal, mechanical, or chemical stimuli) produce cutaneous pain by acting on primary afferent nociceptors; these are generally the initial structures involved in nociceptive processes. Nociceptors are widespread in skin, muscle, connective tissues, blood vessels, and thoracic and abdominal viscera.

Primary afferent nociceptors are pseudounipolar neurons with the cell body located in the dorsal root ganglion (DRG). The peripheral processes of these neurons ramify profusely and innervate a wide variety of tissues where they lose their perineural sheath. Their central process projects to the spinal cord dorsal horn (Fig. 21.1). While large-diameter myelinated afferents serving low-intensity mechanical stimulus transduction may develop specialized terminal structures (e.g. Pacinian corpuscles), nociceptive afferents lack specialized terminal structures and are morphologically 'free' nerve endings. The peripheral axon terminal is not only a transducer of mechanical, thermal or chemical energy into series of action potentials relayed to the spinal cord; it also releases peptides in response to injury [such as substance P, calcitonin gene-related peptide (CGRP), and neurokinin A] that contribute to peripheral inflammatory processes (Fig. 21.2).

There are two main categories of cutaneous receptors associated with noxious stimulation. The majority of nociceptors are C fiber polymodal nociceptors, which means that they respond to different modes of stimuli: noxious thermal (generally above approximately 45°C), noxious mechanical, and noxious chemical. C fibers of less than 2μm diameter are unmyelinated with a conduction velocity of less than 2m/s. Not all unmyelinated fibers are nociceptors; some respond to heat in the non-noxious range and some are activated by non-noxious mechanical stimuli. The other major group of nociceptors are thinly myelinated Aδ fibers, which have a diameter of 2–5μm and conduction velocity of 6–30m/s. The ratio of myelinated to unmyelinated fibers in cutaneous nerves is about 1:4. Most small-diameter primary afferents are mechanically sensitive, although some are sensitive to thermal stimuli. Approximately 10% of cutaneous myelinated fibers and 90% of unmyelinated fibers are nociceptive.

Brief cutaneous stimuli can result in separate and distinct sensations, which are sometimes referred to as 'fast' and 'slow' pains. Fast pain is thought to be caused by activation of faster conducting cutaneous Aδ fibers and is perceived as a short-lasting, pricking type of pain. Slow pain is believed to be caused by activation of slower conducting cutaneous C fibers and is perceived as a dull, poorly localized, burning type of pain.

Trigeminal system

In contrast to the spinal segmental nerves of the trunk and limbs, the face, head, and parts of the mouth are innervated by the ophthalmic, mandibular, and maxillary divisions of the trigeminal nerve (see Fig. 21.1). Analogous to the DRG of spinal nerves, the cell bodies of trigeminal sensory neurons are located in the trigeminal or Gasserian ganglion. Central terminals of these nerves enter the trigeminal sensory nucleus (the equivalent of the spinal dorsal horn), which is located within the rostral segments of the cervical spinal cord. Neurons that are responsive to noxious stimuli are located in the nucleus caudalis of the spinal trigeminal complex, which becomes contiguous with the cervical spinal dorsal horn. Second-order neurons in the trigeminal nucleus project to the contralateral ventroposterior region of the thalamus. Convergence of input from both cervical spinal and trigeminal afferents onto second-order neurons of cervical segments of the spinal cord may lead to cervical pathology being perceived as referred facial or oral pain.

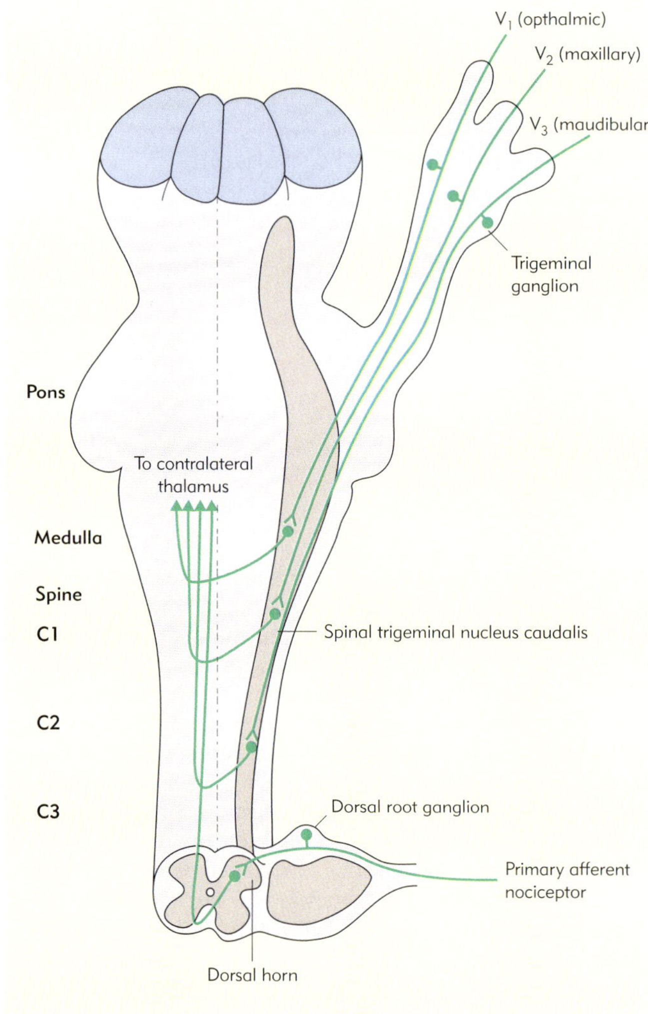

Figure 21.1 Nociceptor input to spinal cord and brainstem. The dorsal aspect shows spinal primary afferent nociceptor input via dorsal root ganglion and trigeminal nociceptor input via trigeminal ganglion. Trigeminal nociceptive afferents course ipsilaterally and caudal to synapse with second-order projection neurons within the pars caudalis of the spinal trigeminal nucleus located in the upper cervical segments. Note that the pars caudalis of the spinal trigeminal nucleus is contiguous with the superficial dorsal horn of the spinal cord, where spinal nociceptive primary afferents similarly synapse with projection neurons.

Visceral afferents

Information from nociceptors is transmitted by visceral afferents from visceral organs to the spinal cord and then in the spinothalamic tracts to the brain (Fig. 21.3). The cell bodies are located in the dorsal root ganglia and fibers travel with sympathetic and parasympathetic axons. Stimuli that are usually painful when applied to the skin, such as thermal and mechanical stimuli, are not usually painful when applied to the viscera. For example, the brain can be cut without any sensation of pain. Visceral pain commonly results from distension of a hollow organ or prolonged contraction of the smooth muscle making up its wall.

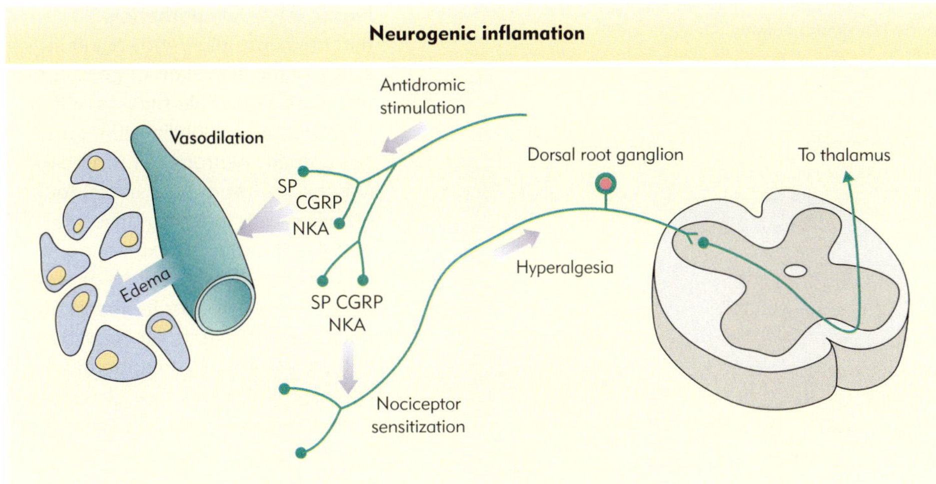

Figure 21.2 Neurogenic inflammation. Antidromic stimulation of nociceptive primary afferents results in the release of neuropeptides from primary afferent peripheral terminals; these neuropeptides bind to peripheral tachykinin receptors to produce vasodilatation, edema, and hyperalgesia (triple response of Lewis). Substance P, SP; calcitonin gene-related peptide, CGRP; neurokinin A, NKA.

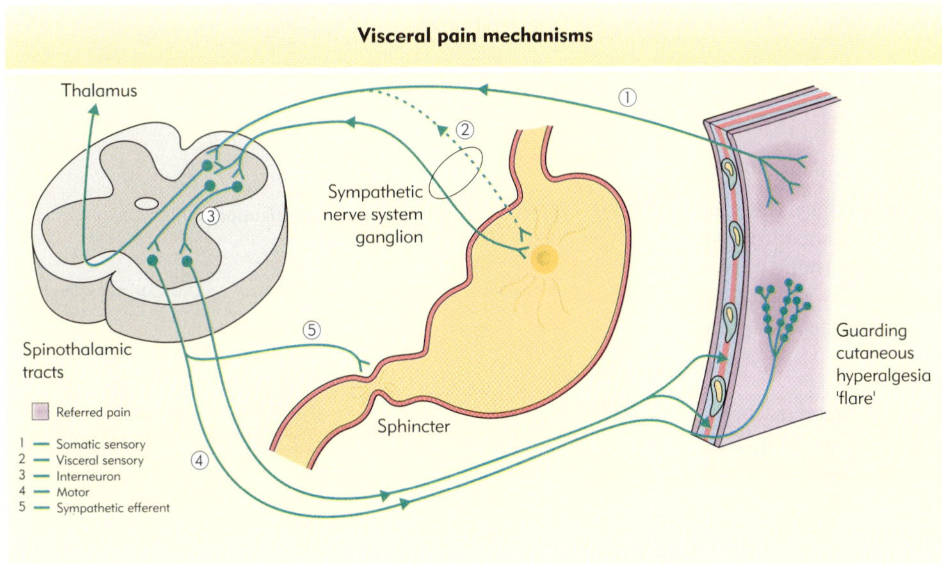

Figure 21.3 Visceral pain mechanisms: convergence of visceral and somatic nociceptive afferents on the same dorsal horn neuron. A small number of somatic nociceptive afferents may dually innervate both visceral and somatic structures. Reflex somatic motor activity results in muscle spasm and 'guarding'. Reflex sympathetic activity may result in altered visceral motility, sphincter spasm, and visceral ischemia, further exacerbating pain.

In contrast to cutaneous pain, which is usually well localized to the area of stimulation, visceral pain is poorly localized, dull, and may be perceived as a sensation of fullness or nausea. The poor localization may be a consequence of the low number of afferent fibers compared with the size of the surface that is innervated; these fibers converge on dorsal horn neurons over a wide number of segments. Visceral afferents converge onto second-order dorsal horn cells that also receive cutaneous spinal segmental input. This may give rise to the phenomenon of referred pain in dermatomal segments corresponding to their cutaneous innervation and may result in allodynia and hyperalgesia in this skin area. Cutaneous referral may also be a consequence of considerable branching of peripheral visceral afferents such that a single DRG cell may have axonal branches supplying both deep and superficial structures.

Sympathetic nervous system

Although visceral nociceptive afferents colocalize with sympathetic efferent nerves and are clearly involved in pelvic, abdominal, and thoracic visceral nociception described above, the sympathetic nervous system (SNS) is best considered as an efferent neuroeffector system modulating cardiovascular, bronchial, visceral, metabolic, and sudomotor function. The role of efferent sympathetic neurons in pain and nociception is considerably more complex. The SNS plays a central role in global behavioral responses to noxious input such as confrontational defense or flight mediated by hypothalamic and suprahypothalamic networks. Of greater relevance to anesthesia is the potential role of SNS dysfunction in the generation of diffuse burning pain and hyperalgesia following injury. Formerly classified as *reflex sympathetic dystrophy* and *causalgia*, dependent upon the absence or presence of macroscopic nerve injury, the current terminology is complex regional pain syndromes (CRPS) I and II, respectively. Simplistically, these pain syndromes have been ascribed to the development of sensitivity of peripheral nociceptive afferents to norepinephrine (noradrenaline) or other products of the efferent SNS (hence sympathetically maintained pain).

The clinical features of CRPS reflect autonomic dysfunction. Vasomotor and sudomotor changes, abnormalities of hair and nail growth, and osteoporosis are accompanied by sensory symptoms of spontaneous burning pain, hyperalgesia, and allodynia. There is frequently an associated disturbance of motor function.

Basic science studies have demonstrated a number of complex and incompletely understood changes involving the SNS

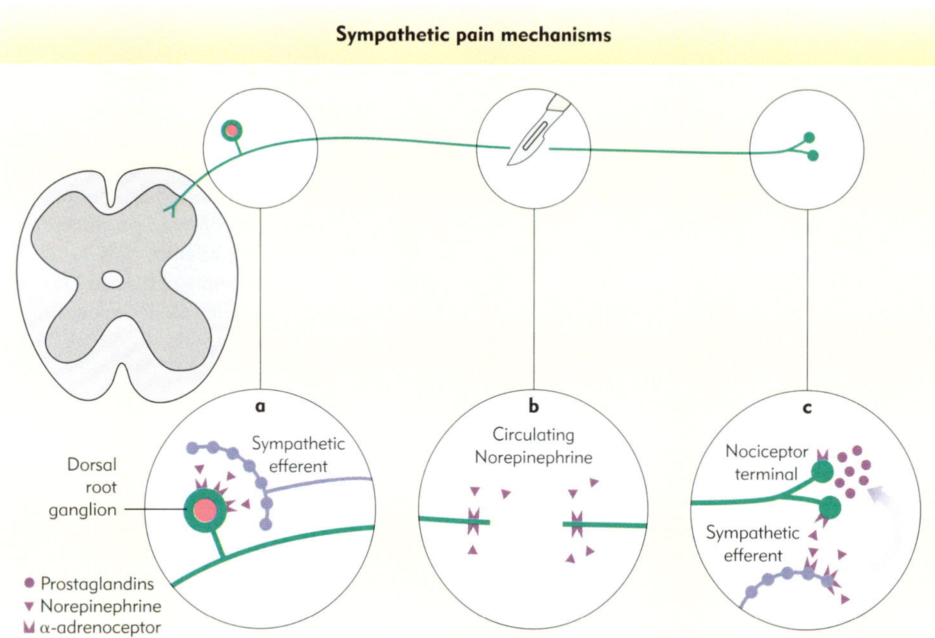

Figure 21.4 Sympathetic pain mechanisms. Injury may result in sympathetic activation of nociceptive afferents at multiple sites. (a) Altered tropic factor availability stimulates sympathetic neurons to form basket-like outgrowths around dorsal root ganglion cells that may drive ganglion activity. (b) Expression of functional α-adrenoceptors at the site of nerve injury results in activation of nociceptive afferents via circulation catecholamines. (c) Peripheral nociceptor afferents may also express α-adrenoceptors and be activated by locally released or circulating catecholamines. Peripheral inflammation results in α-adrenergic-mediated release of prostaglandins from sympathetic terminals with resultant sensitization.

that may be responsible for the development of these features (Fig. 21.4). These include the expression of adrenoceptors on nociceptive afferents and the sprouting of sympathetic nerves into the DRG following nerve injury, which may provide an anatomic basis for sympathetically maintained pain syndromes.

Peripheral sensitization/inflammation

Thermal, mechanical, and chemical stimuli activate high-threshold nociceptors that signal this information to the first relay in the spinal cord. Many forms of pain arise from direct activation or sensitization of primary afferent neurons, especially C fiber polymodal nociceptors. This is a dynamic process. Nociceptor activation sets in train processes that modify responses to further stimuli; for example, a relatively benign noxious stimulus such as a scratch to the skin initiates peripheral inflammation that reduces the threshold for response of the nociceptor to subsequent sensory stimuli (Fig. 21.5). It is essential to appreciate that surgical or traumatic noxious stimuli are usually prolonged and associated with tissue damage of variable degree. Clinical pain is, therefore, almost universally associated with peripheral sensitization.

Part of the inflammatory response is the release of intracellular contents from damaged cells and inflammatory cells such as macrophages, lymphocytes, and mast cells. Nociceptive stimulation also results in a neurogenic inflammatory response, with the release of compounds such as substance P, neurokinin A, and CGRP from the peripheral terminals of nociceptive afferent fibers. These peptides modify the excitability of sensory and sympathetic nerve fibers, induce vasodilatation and extravasation of plasma proteins, and promote release of further chemical mediators by inflammatory cells (see Fig. 21.2). These interactions result in a 'soup' of inflammatory mediators including K^+ and H^+, serotonin, bradykinin, substance P, histamine, cytokines, nitric oxide, and products from the cyclooxygenase and lipoxygenase pathways of arachidonic acid metabolism (see Fig. 21.5). These chemicals then act to sensitize high-threshold nociceptors and produce the phenomenon of peripheral

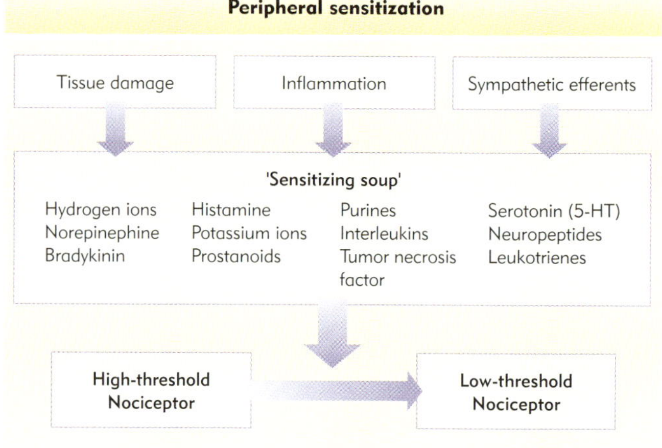

Figure 21.5 Peripheral sensitization. The gain of high-threshold nociceptors can be modified in the periphery by a combination of chemical mediators. Tissue damage and inflammatory cell mediator release is supplemented by neuropeptide and catecholamine release from peripheral nociceptive afferent and sympathetic efferent terminals. (Modified and redrawn from Woolf and Chong, 1993.)

sensitization. Following sensitization, low-intensity mechanical stimuli that would not normally cause pain are now perceived as painful. There is also an increased responsiveness to thermal stimuli at the site of injury. This zone of 'primary hyperalgesia' surrounding the site of injury is a consequence of peripheral changes and is commonly observed following surgery and other forms of trauma.

Peripheral sensitization may encompass the SNS and there is evidence that sympathetic nerve terminals may themselves release prostanoids and products of arachidonic acid metabolism after peripheral injury. This provides a potential link

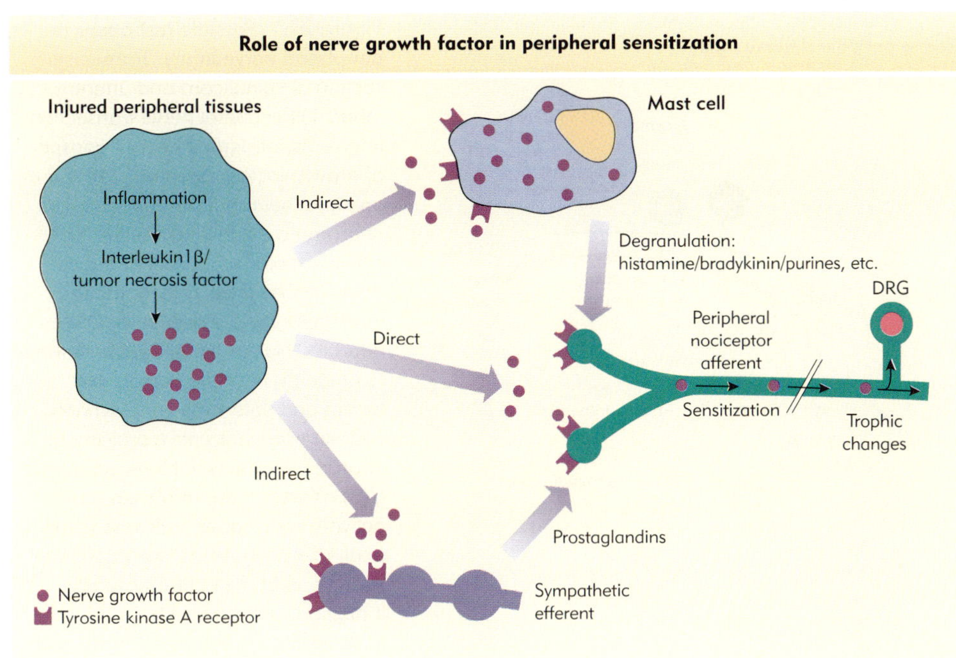

Figure 21.6 Role of nerve growth factor in peripheral sensitization. Nerve growth factor acts both directly and indirectly.

between the peripheral sympathetic efferent and the peripheral nociceptor in CRPS, where pain complaints may vary with sympathetic efferent activity.

Role of nerve growth factor in peripheral sensitization

Recent research indicates a central role for nerve growth factor (NGF) in the etiology of inflammatory pain. Nerve growth factor belongs to the family of neurotropic peptides including brain-derived neurotropic factor, neurotropins 3, 4/5, and 6, which specify the phenotypic development of central and peripheral neurons. Neurotropins interact with a low affinity p75 receptor, which may modulate the expression and function of specific high-affinity tyrosine kinase (Trk) receptors for each neurotropin. The biologic effects of NGF are mediated via the TrkA receptor.

The TrkA receptor is expressed on small unmyelinated afferents that coexpress the nociceptive peptide CGRP on a wide variety of tissues constitutively expressing NGF at low levels. This constitutive production of NGF may determine nociceptor phenotype: 'neurotropin hypothesis'. However, inflammation (possibly via the cytokines interleukin-1β and tumor necrosis factor) is associated with increased NGF expression and synthesis in peripheral tissues (Fig. 21.6). The rapid onset of hyperalgesia following experimental subcutaneous administration of NGF strongly suggests a direct peripheral action mediating peripheral sensitization. Tyrosine kinase A receptors are not restricted to nociceptive afferents but are expressed by both mast cells and postganglionic efferents. Nerve growth factor plays a central role in peripheral sensitization mediated by both direct and indirect actions of inflammatory mediators on nociceptive afferents. Furthermore, growth factors may mediate upregulation of various types of Na^+ channel that are more likely to fire spontaneously (e.g. pacemaker cells in the myocardium) but also are more sensitive to Na^+ channel blockers such as lidocaine (lignocaine). The development of such Na^+ channels may contribute to the features of spontaneous pain and extreme mechanosensitivity seen in many pain states. Axonal transport of NGF taken up by nerve terminals has tropic effects within the spinal cord dorsal horn, contributing to central sensitization (see below).

Silent nociceptors

Silent or 'sleeping' nociceptors are inactive under most circumstances but become active following inflammation and sensitization by NGF. They have been described in joints and in cutaneous and visceral nerves. Following sensitization, they become responsive and discharge vigorously even during ordinary movement; they also display changes in receptive fields. This class of nociceptor may contribute to mechanical allodynia and hyperalgesia associated with peripheral inflammation.

Peripheral nerve injury

Peripheral nerve injury results in a number of biochemical, physiologic, and morphologic changes at the peripheral and spinal level that reflect altered afferent sensory input and that may act as a focus of pain in themselves (Fig. 21.7). Nerve damage results in an inflammatory response around the site of injury, with increased production of compounds, including NGF and other tropic factors, that normally modulate neuronal growth. Normal sensory processing and primary afferent phenotype is critically dependent upon a balance of both retrograde and anterograde axonal transport of tropic factors typified by NGF. For example, following nerve injury there is a loss of the primary afferent peptide transmitters substance P and CGRP, and corresponding upregulation of neuropeptide Y and galanin within the DRG and dorsal horn of the spinal cord. This complex pattern of neuropeptide changes reflects altered tropic factor availability; exogenous application of NGF after experimental nerve injury can partially reverse such phenotypic changes. Although altered neuronal phenotype within the DRG and dorsal horn may contribute to the development of pathologic pain states, certain changes such as upregulation of neuropeptide Y may also represent adaptive analgesic responses to injury.

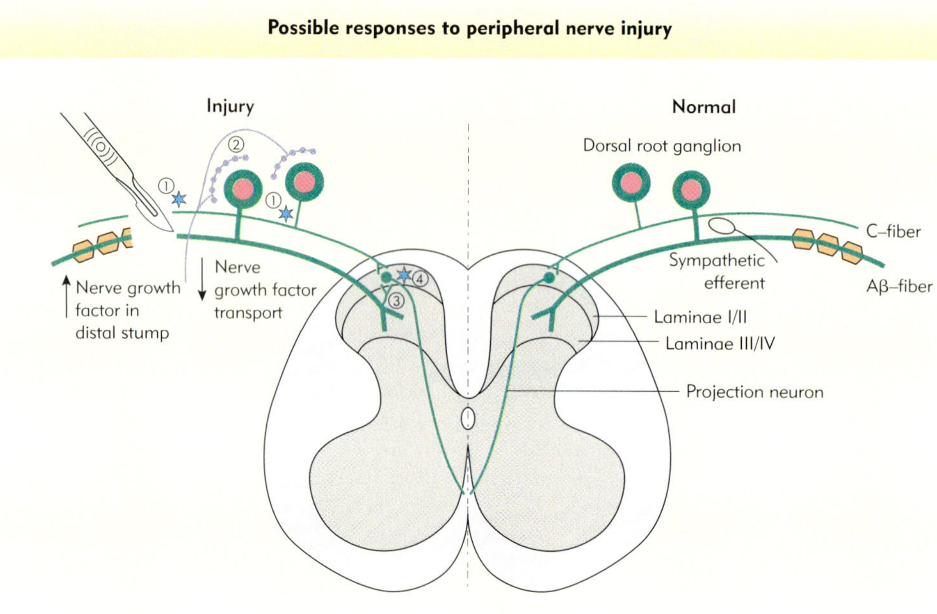

Figure 21.7 Possible responses to peripheral nerve injury. Transverse section of spinal cord and afferent input. 1) Peripheral nerve transection interrupts retrograde axonal transport of growth factors. Sprouting of proximal neuronal stumps produces neuromata expressing altered Na^+ channel isoforms; similar changes occur in the DRG. 2) Sympthatic innervation and activation of DRG neurons (Fig. 21.4). 3) Aβ fibres within laminae III, IV of the dorsal horn sprout and potentially form synaptic contact with nociceptive projection neurons of lamina II. Non-nociceptive (Aβ) afferent input may therefore activate nociceptive pathways resulting in allodynia. 4) Altered neuropeptide expression and loss of GABAergic inhibition within dorsal horn may result in spontaneous activity of dorsal horn projection neurons.

Furthermore, there is a loss of γ-aminobutyric acid (GABA) interneurons within the spinal cord after peripheral nerve injury. GABA is the major inhibitory transmitter within the spinal cord and reduction in the population of GABAergic neurons in the spinal cord may contribute to the hyperalgesia and allodynia seen in chronic pain. The vulnerability of the nervous system through loss of inhibitory control may be accentuated by the increased input from the periphery, as described above, as well as by increased activation of sympathetic nerves, which may 'fire up' the somatosensory system.

Nerve injury involving loss of axonal integrity typically results in tropic factor-mediated sprouting of the peripheral end of the damaged fibers, which may result in neuroma formation. Neuromata express heterogeneous populations of spontaneously and repetitively active Na^+ channels, which may contribute to spontaneous action potential generation after nerve injury. Furthermore, neuromata are typically mechanosensitive and may be sensitive to norepinephrine and sympathetic nerve activity. Damage to the vasa nervorum causes a reduction in the blood supply to myelinated fibers with resultant demyelination and the production of ectopic impulses.

Similar changes occur within the DRG. Partial ligation of a peripheral nerve results in spontaneous firing of these cells, at least in part as a consequence of altered synthesis and expression of Na^+ channels, as described above. Peripheral nerve injury also induces the formation of abnormal basket-like terminations of sympathetic neurons around primary afferent cell bodies in the DRG that may contribute to SNS-mediated pain. Together, changes at the site of nerve injury and in the DRG may give rise to the perception of sharp, shooting, or burning pain in conditions such as diabetic neuropathy, postherpetic neuralgia, and peripheral nerve trauma. Contributing to this state of excitability is the feature of cross-excitation in which DRG neuron discharges may excite otherwise inactive neurons, further contributing to the hyperalgesic and allodynic state.

Clinical implications for peripheral analgesic action

Nonsteroidal anti-inflammatory drugs

Nonsteroidal anti-inflammatory drugs (NSAIDs) are commonly used for 'peripheral' analgesia and have as one of their actions a reduction in the peripheral inflammatory response. Agents such as aspirin, acetominophen (paracetamol), and other NSAIDs provide their anti-inflammatory action by blocking the cyclooxygenase pathway (see Chapter 27). It is now apparent that cyclooxygenase exists in two forms, COX-1 and COX-2. While COX-1 is always present in tissues, including the gastric mucosa, COX-2 is induced by inflammation. This presents an opportunity for the development of agents that have a selective anti-inflammatory effect without gastric side effects. To date, only meloxicam with partial COX-2 selectivity and a good gastric side-effect profile has been licensed for clinical use in the UK. As well as the peripheral action of NSAIDs, there is increasing evidence that they exert their analgesic effect through central mechanisms involved in the development and maintenance of spinal cord sensitization. This observation has led to the successful use of intrathecal and epidural NSAIDS in experimental animal pain models.

Opioids

Opioids have traditionally been considered centrally acting drugs (see Chapter 26). However, there is evidence for action of endogenous opioids on peripheral nociceptor terminals following tissue damage (Fig. 21.8). Opioid receptors are synthesized in the cell body (DRG) and transported toward the central terminal in the dorsal horn and toward the periphery. Peripheral receptors become active within hours following local tissue damage. This occurs with unmasking of opioid receptors and the arrival of immunocompetent cells that possess opioid receptors and have the ability to synthesize opioid peptides. This finding has led to an interest in the peripheral administration of opioids for postoperative analgesia, both at the site of surgery and as supplements to local anesthetics

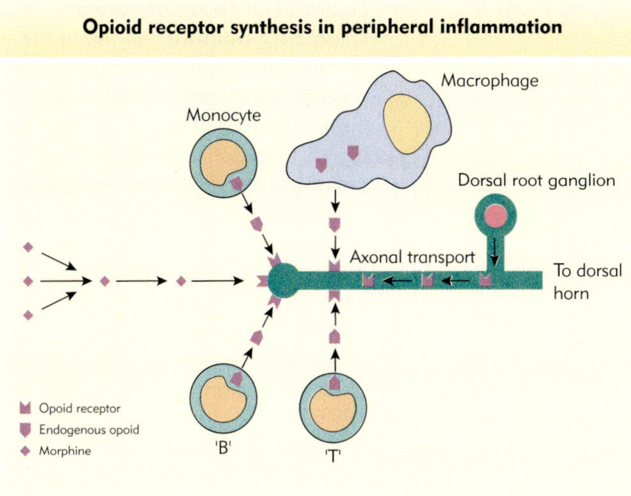

Figure 21.8 Opioid receptor synthesis in peripheral inflammation. Synthesis occurs within the dorsal root ganglia and receptors are transported to the periphery. Peripheral opioid receptors are activated by the release of endogenous opioid peptides from inflammatory cells at the site of injury. Local application of exogenous opioids, therefore, attenuates firing of sensitized nociceptors. (Redrawn with permission from Stein, 1995.)

in nerve and plexus blocks. Systematic review of these techniques demonstrates that intra-articular administration of opioids following knee surgery or arthroscopy may be efficacious, although clinically relevant analgesia has not been obtained by opioid supplementation of regional anesthetic blocks. Nevertheless, opioids with physicochemical properties that favor peripheral action are under development and may be useful for regional application.

Local anesthetics

Systemic administration of local anesthetic agents such as lidocaine can result in a marked reduction in pain following peripheral nerve injury and is a useful diagnostic tool in determining the etiology of pain syndromes. Relatively low concentrations of local anesthetic can reduce ectopic activity in specific populations of Na^+ channels in damaged nerves at concentrations below those required to produce conduction block at classical 'tetrodotoxin-sensitive' voltage-dependent Na^+ channels. Although intravenous or subcutaneous lidocaine may be used as an analgesic adjunct in neuropathic malignant pain, oral congeners of local anesthetics such as mexiletine or flecainide and the anticonvulsant lamotrigine are more commonly used for long-term analgesia in neuropathic pain of nonmalignant origin.

Sympathetic blockade

Complex regional pain syndromes have been divided into those that are sympathetically maintained or those that are sympathetically independent. Pain problems that are sympathetically maintained may respond to sympathetic blockade by agents administered systemically, regionally, or around the sympathetic ganglion. It is well established that the analgesia provided by sympathetic blocks may permit the mobilization and physiotherapy essential to the treatment of the condition. However, there is considerable dispute over the long-term efficacy of repeated sympathetic blocks, whether performed with local anesthetic, neurolytic solutions, or by radiofrequency thermocoagulation.

DORSAL HORN MECHANISMS

Termination sites of primary afferents

The dorsal horns of the medulla and spinal cord are the major sites of termination of nearly all sensory afferents irrespective of peripheral origin. Small myelinated and unmyelinated fibers tend to aggregate in the lateral aspect of the dorsal root and enter the dorsal horn laterally; larger fibers tend to travel medially. While the principal route of entry for primary afferents is through the dorsal root, a significant number of primarily unmyelinated afferent neurons enter via the ventral root.

In transverse section, the spinal cord gray matter is divided into 10 laminae according to Rexed's classification of their light microscopic morphology. The most superficial of these is lamina I and the dorsal horn extends to lamina VI. The ventral horn comprises laminae VII–IX with lamina X being the region surrounding the central canal. The architecture of these laminae is of considerable significance when considering differing modalities of afferent sensory input to the spinal cord.

Unmyelinated C fiber nociceptors terminate principally in lamina II (the substantia gelatinosa). Some unmyelinated fibers also ascend and descend several segments in Lissauer's tract before terminating on neurons that project to higher centers. Small myelinated Aδ nociceptors terminate principally in the superficial dorsal horn (lamina I) and deeper in lamina V. Nociceptors from joints terminate in lamina I as well as more deeply in laminae VI and VII. Large fiber low-threshold mechanoceptors, which transmit non-noxious information regarding fine touch, proprioception, and vibration, terminate mainly in lamina III and IV or more rostrally in the dorsal column nuclei of the medulla oblongata.

The terminations of primary afferent nociceptors transmit information to the first relay of neurons in the dorsal horn, sometimes known as second-order neurons. These are often divided into two main classes ('nociceptive specific' or 'high threshold' and 'wide dynamic range' or 'convergent') that have different response properties to afferent input and are located in different regions of the dorsal horn. Nociceptive specific neurons are located within the superficial laminae of the dorsal horn and respond selectively to noxious stimuli. Neurons with wide dynamic range are generally located in deeper laminae and respond to both noxious and non-noxious inputs. Neurons normally do not signal pain in response to a tactile stimulus at a non-noxious level. However, if they become sensitized and hyper-responsive, they may discharge at a high rate following a tactile stimulus. If the activity of the neuron exceeds a threshold level following this stimulus then the non-noxious tactile stimulus will be perceived as painful and give rise to the phenomenon of allodynia.

Outputs from primary afferents

There is a polysynaptic, intraspinal pathway that connects primary afferents to motoneurons. This is a basic pathway that underlies the withdrawal reflex and can occur even in the absence of pain perception, such as under anesthesia or following spinal cord injury. It is heavily modified by local and descending inhibitory influences; when descending controls are lost (as happens following complete spinal cord injury), the pathway can be activated by non-nociceptive afferents

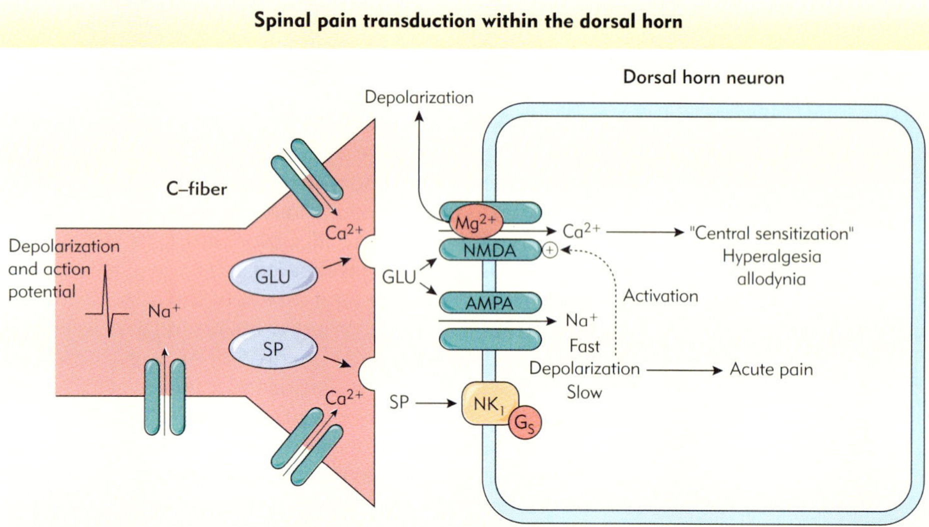

Figure 21.9 The pharmacology of spinal pain transduction within the dorsal horn. Acute pain causes brief postsynaptic depolarization of dorsal horn neurons and activation of central pain pathways. More prolonged afferent input via Aδ and C fibers causes NMDA receptor activation. NMDA, *N*-methyl D-aspartate; Glu, glutamate; NK_1, neurokin 1; SP, substance P; AMPA, α-amino-3-hydroxy-5-methyl-4-isoxazolepropionate; G_s, G_s protein. (With permission from Hudspith, 1997.)

such that even innocuous stimuli will result in a flexor withdrawal response.

An acute noxious stimulus will also result in autonomic responses such as a rise or fall in blood pressure and a change in respiration. Responses appear to be related to the structures involved; nociceptive stimuli from viscera frequently result in a fall in blood pressure, whereas cutaneous stimuli usually lead to increases in blood pressure. These changes occur as a result of spinal and supraspinal activation of regions involved in autonomic regulation following nociceptor stimulation.

The sensation and interpretation of pain requires activation of those brain regions associated with spatial discriminative and affective components of pain perception. This is clearly a potential (but not inevitable) consequence of activity of the primary afferent nociceptor and involves integration of the polysynaptic output from the primary afferent through multiple ascending pathways. The exact location of specific supraspinal regions associated with pain perception is complex and incompletely understood and will be discussed further below. Current research has focused upon spinal mechanisms of pain transduction and these will be reviewed in some detail.

Neurotransmitters and neuromodulators

The dorsal horn contains a host of peptide and amino acid neurotransmitters, neuromodulators, and their respective receptors. Neurotransmission within the dorsal horn encompasses:

- excitatory transmitters released from the central terminals of primary afferent nociceptors;
- excitatory transmission between neurons of the spinal cord;
- inhibitory transmitters released by interneurons within the spinal cord;
- inhibitory transmitters released from supraspinal sources.

The concept of a single neuron releasing a single transmitter within the synaptic cleft clearly does not apply within the dorsal horn. Although exocytotic release of individual peptide or amino acid transmitters may occur, experimental data suggest that this rarely happens under physiologic conditions and two or more compounds are commonly released at the same time (corelease). Differing ratios of cotransmitter release may occur depending upon stimulus intensity. Neurotransmitters may be released in close proximity to pre- or postsynaptic receptors within the dorsal horn; however, it is clear that 'volume transmission' also occurs within the dorsal horn where spatially distant receptors may be activated by transmitters outside of a classical synapse.

Excitatory nociceptor transmission

Excitatory amino acids

Glutamate is the major neurotransmitter within the CNS and plays a major role in nociceptive transmission in the dorsal horn. Glutamate acts at α-amino-3-hydroxy-5-methyl-4-isoxazolepropionic acid (AMPA) receptors, *N*-methyl D-aspartate (NMDA) receptors, kainate (KA), and metabotropic glutamate receptors (see Chapter 19). Multiple variants of each glutamate receptor subtype are expressed throughout the CNS, depending upon subunit composition, and can be identified by molecular biologic techniques.

AMPA receptors are ligand-operated ion channels; the channel is not voltage dependent and permits the selective entry of Na^+ under physiologic conditions. The result is a short-latency excitatory postsynaptic potential (EPSP), and AMPA receptors are responsible for 'fast' transmission of impulses in nociceptive pathways (Fig. 21.9). This information may encode the onset, offset, and intensity of a noxious stimulus. AMPA receptors are not selectively localized to regions of the nervous system involved in nociception and antagonists at the AMPA receptor may, therefore, have limited use as analgesics because of their widespread presence and function in the CNS.

AMPA receptors may mediate responses in the 'physiologic' processing of sensory information. However, prolonged release of glutamate or concurrent activation of neurokinin receptors results in sustained activation of AMPA and/or neurokinin receptors. This appears to be crucial in the development of abnormal responses to further sensory stimuli by priming the NMDA receptor so that it reaches a state ready for activation.

The NMDA receptor complex is a multimeric channel permeable to Na^+ and Ca^{2+} that is both voltage and ligand gated (see Chapter 19). At a normal resting potential (–70mV), the ion pore of the NMDA receptor is blocked by Mg^{2+} and binding of glutamate in the presence of its co-agonist glycine does not result in channel opening. Priming of the NMDA receptor occurs with

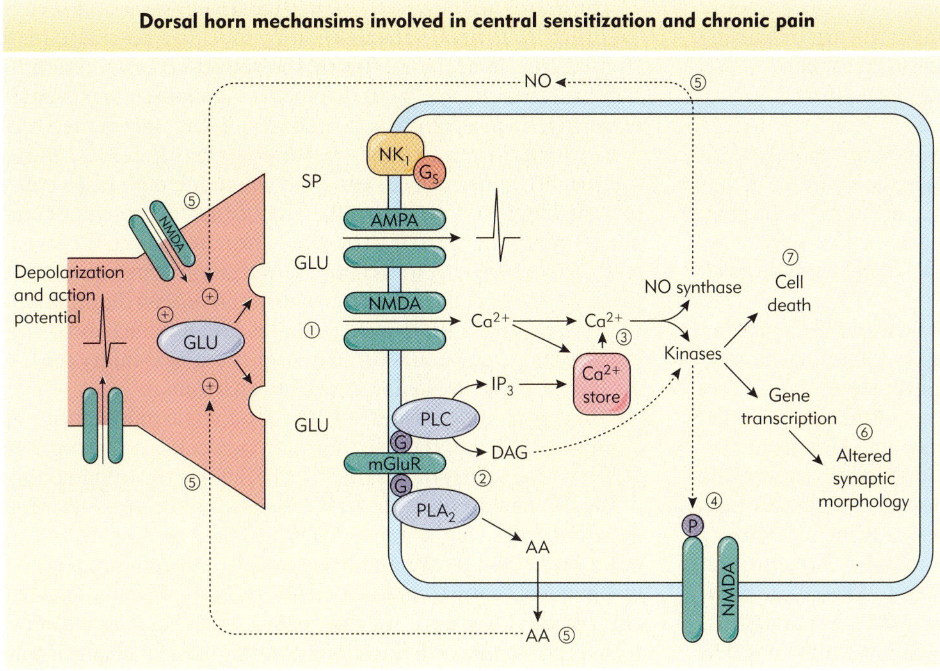

Figure 21.10 Dorsal horn mechanisms involved in central sensitization and chronic pain. There are at least seven places at which changes causing central pain can occur. GLU, glutamate; NMDA, *N*-methyl D-aspartate; AMPA, α-amino-3-hydroxy-5-methyl-4-isoxazolepropionate; mGluR, metabotropic glutamate receptor; PIP, phosphatidylinositol 4,5-bisphosphate; NO, nitric oxide; PLC, phospholipase C; IP_3, inositol 1,4,5-trisphosphate; IP_3R, IP_3 receptor; PLA_2, phospholipase 2; G, GTP-binding protein; P, phosphorylation site; DAG, diacylglycerol; SP, substance P; NK1, neurokinin 1 receptor.
1. Enhanced Ca^{2+} entry into the postsynaptic neuron follows GLU release and NMDA receptor activation. Presynaptic NMDA receptors may mediate similar enhancement of Ca^{2+} availability and potentiate glutamate release.
2. The Ca^{2+} signal may be supplemented by Ca^{2+} release from IP_3-gated stores as a consequence of coactivation of mGlu receptors.
3. The rise in Ca^{2+} concentration in the postsynaptic cell initiates a chain of events secondary to the activation of numerous Ca^{2+}-dependent enzymes.
4. Postsynaptic hyperexcitability follows phosphorylation of NMDA receptors, which alters their voltage-gating characteristics.
5. Postsynaptic hyperexcitability may be augmented by release of retrograde transmitter(s) (NO and arachidonic acid?), causing the presynaptic nerve terminal to enhance its release of GLU and SP. Enhanced transmission occurs at the affected synapses.
6. Within the postsynaptic cell, protein kinase activation may lead to gene transcription, altered neuronal phenotype, and changes in synaptic morphology.
7. Within the postsynaptic cell, protein kinase activation may lead to neuronal death, which may be immediate or delayed.
(Modified with permission from Hudspith, 1997.)

depolarization of the membrane to –30mV, which enables Mg^{2+} to leave the channel (see Fig 21.9). This degree of depolarization will occur when glutamate and peptides are co-released after intense afferent activation and act on AMPA and neurokinin receptors within the dorsal horn. Activation of the NMDA receptor causes large and prolonged depolarization associated with Ca^{2+} mobilization in neurons that are already partly depolarized. Activation of NMDA receptors at pre- and postsynaptic loci initiates processes that contribute to the medium- or long-term changes observed in chronic pain states, including central sensitization, changes in peripheral receptive fields, induction of gene transcription, and long-term potentiation (LTP). The last refers to the changes in synaptic efficacy identified as a synaptic correlate of memory in the hippocampus and cerebral cortex and may play a role in the development of a cellular 'memory' for pain or enhanced responsiveness to noxious inputs.

Metabotropic glutamate receptors are coupled to G proteins and are linked to both phosphoinositide and cAMP signaling pathways (see Chapters 3 & 19). Their role in nociception is currently poorly defined. Although there is little evidence for a role in acute pain transduction, they may act in concert with NMDA-mediated systems inducing longer-term changes in dorsal horn function.

Peptides

Small-diameter nociceptive primary afferent fibers are characterized by a variety of peptide transmitters, including substance P, neurokinin A, and CGRP. Release of substance P, which coexists in primary afferents with glutamate, occurs following cutaneous thermal, mechanical, or chemical noxious stimuli and is potentiated by peripheral inflammation. Although historically substance P was considered the major neurotransmitter involved in spinal mechanisms of nociception, experimental data from animals lacking the substance P receptor (NK-1 receptor 'knock-out' mice) demonstrate that acute nociception persists in animals lacking substance P-mediated neurotransmission. Rather, substance P plays a modulatory role in nociception, modifying the gain of afferent transmission. Animal data demonstrate that it may play an important role in the transmission of prolonged or highly noxious stimuli. The actions of substance P may be potentiated by neurokinin A and CGRP within the dorsal horn, although the role of these peptides is less well understood. Disruption of the preprotachykinin A gene, which encodes for substance P and neurokinin A, significantly reduces the response to moderate-to-intense pain and abolishes neurogenic inflammation without affecting responses to mild pain. The release of these tachykinins from primary afferent nociceptors is, therefore, required to produce intense pain. Neurokinin A or substance P antagonists are promising targets for the development of new drugs to treat pain.

Intracellular events

N-methyl D-asparate receptor activation and Ca^{2+} mobilization set in train a cascade of secondary events in the neuron that has been activated by prolonged and intense afferent input (Fig. 21.10). Subsequent changes within the neuron increase its responsiveness to further afferent input and lead to some or all of the phenomena described above.

Influx of Ca^{2+} into the neuron leads to activation of a number of pathways involving second messengers including inositol trisphosphate (IP_3), cGMP, eicosanoid, nitric oxide, and protein kinase C (see Chapter 3). The exact role of nitric oxide in nociceptive processing is unclear and it does not appear to be important in acute nociception. However, production of nitric oxide is implicated in the induction and maintenance of chronic pain states. Nitric oxide may act as a positive feedback mechanism acting in conjunction with presynaptic NMDA receptors to upregulate afferent input further and thereby potentiate nociceptive input. Inhibition of nitric oxide synthesis results in a decrease in the behavioral correlates of pain in animal models of neuropathic pain.

Immediate early gene induction and altered protein synthesis are key steps that follow Ca^{2+} mobilization within the dorsal horn and manifest as longer-term changes in neuronal excitability and ultimately in altered pain behavior. Uncontrolled release of glutamate (as may occur after major nerve or CNS injury) may induce cell death within the CNS. This may be immediate (excitotoxicity); however, more significantly, neuronal and glial death may occur by programmed mechanisms involving protein synthesis (apoptosis) for periods long after the initial injury. Small GABAergic inhibitory interneurons appear to be particularly susceptible, with a net loss of inhibitory tone within the dorsal horn after nerve injury.

SPINAL MECHANISMS FOLLOWING NERVE INJURY AND INFLAMMATION

Central sensitization and synaptic plasticity

NMDA-mediated mechanisms underlying central sensitization may occur at both pre- and postsynaptic sites within the dorsal horn. Presynaptic sensitization may (in conjunction with retrograde transmission by nitric oxide) further enhance glutamate release from the primary afferent. At the postsynaptic site, NMDA receptor activation in second-order neurons results in phosphorylation of the NMDA receptor such that the voltage gating of the receptor for subsequent stimuli is removed (see Fig. 21.10). Functionally this is manifest as increased gain of transmission for a given afferent input and the earliest stages in this process are demonstrable electrophysiologically within the dorsal horn as 'wind-up'. Wind-up is a progressive increase in the frequency of firing of second-order spinal neurons elicited by a peripheral stimulus sufficient to excite C fibers at a frequency above 0.5Hz. A key observation is that low doses of conventional analgesics such as μ-opioids administered prior to such stimulation prevent wind-up but do not reverse the established sensitized state. This has had a major impact on the current view of pain and has led to a surge of interest in approaches such as pre-emptive analgesia.

The rationale behind pre-emptive analgesia is to prevent 'wind-up' or central sensitization by blocking the acute pain stimulus and thereby inhibiting the supposed progression to 'sub-acute' or chronic pain. Attempts to demonstrate pre-emptive analgesia in a clinical setting have met with only limited success, which, in part, reflect methodologic difficulties. More significantly, postsurgical and post-traumatic pain has a complex etiology involving both inflammatory and neuropathic components and will result in prolonged afferent input to the spinal cord. While 'wind-up' and central sensitization demonstrate that the response of cells in the dorsal horn can outlast the stimulus, they are relatively short-lived (minutes) phenomena and ongoing afferent input hours or days after the initial injury probably have a key role in clinical pain mechanisms.

Chronic pain necessitates pathophysiologic modulations of synaptic efficacy that persist for days or weeks, an example of which is long term potentiation (LTP), a form of strengthening of the efficacy of synaptic transmission that occurs following activity across that synapse. LTP has been demonstrated to occur in the spinal cord and shares many of the physiologic and biochemical features implicated above in the development of chronic pain. Indeed, we may now talk of 'memory traces' within the spinal cord. Such long-term functional changes may coexist with physical changes in synaptic architecture exemplified by sprouting within the dorsal horn.

Sprouting

Peripheral nerve injury induces morphologic changes within the laminae of the dorsal horn (see Fig. 21.7). The sprouting of central terminals of myelinated afferents with sprouting from lamina IV into lamina II results in a reorganization of the normal synaptic architecture, possibly as a result of altered NGF availability. Functional contact between Aδ fiber terminals (which normally transmit non-noxious information) and second-order neurons of superficial laminae that normally receive nociceptive input would provide a mechanism for the pain and hypersensitivity to light touch (allodynia) that is seen following nerve injury.

Sensory and physiologic changes

Changes occur in the periphery following trauma that lead to peripheral sensitization and primary hyperalgesia. However, the sensitization that occurs can only be partly explained by the changes in the periphery. Following injury, there is increased responsiveness to normally innocuous mechanical stimuli (allodynia) in a zone of 'secondary hyperalgesia' in uninjured tissue surrounding the site of injury. In contrast to the zone of primary hyperalgesia, there is no change in the threshold to thermal stimuli and these changes are the behavioral manifestation of central sensitization. Central sensitization is associated with an expansion in receptive field size so that a spinal neuron responds to stimuli outside the region of cutaneous innervation that responds to nociceptive stimuli in the nonsensitized state. In addition, there is an increase in the magnitude and duration of the response to stimuli that are above threshold in strength. Lastly, there is a reduction in threshold; consequently, stimuli that are non-noxious activate neurons that normally transmit nociceptive information. These changes underlie the enhancement of postoperative pain by movement and coughing and the perception of pain in dermatomes distant from the incision site; if unresolved, they will result in the development of chronic pain.

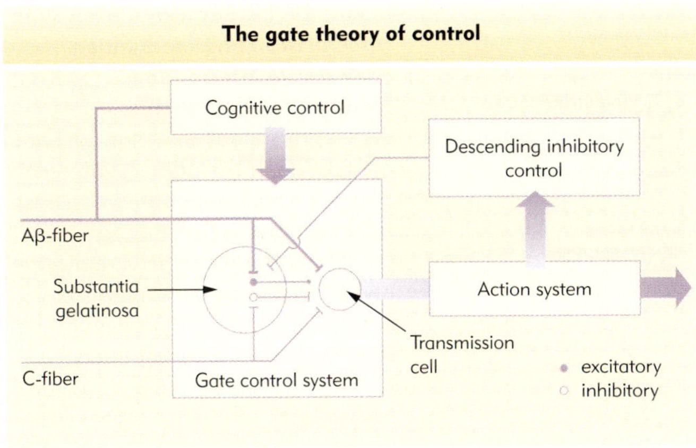

Figure 21.11 The gate theory of control. The activity of transmission cells is modulated by both excitatory and inhibitory links from the substantia gelatinosa and by descending inhibitory controls from the brainstem. The inhibitory link may involve both pre- and postsynaptic inhibition. All other connections are excitatory. (Redrawn with permission from Melzack, 1998.)

MODULATION AT A SPINAL LEVEL

The gate theory

Transmission of nociceptive information is subject to modulation at several levels of the neuraxis including the dorsal horn. Afferent impulses arriving in the dorsal horn initiate inhibitory mechanisms that limit the effect of subsequent impulses. Inhibition occurs through local inhibitory interneurons and descending pathways from the brain. A model of how this interaction occurs in relation to pain processing was proposed by Melzack and Wall in 1965 and has been termed the 'gate theory' (Fig. 21.11).

They proposed that transmission or T cells located in the dorsal horn project to the brain, that the output from these cells depends on information entering the dorsal horn in different types of primary afferent, and that the cells could be activated by noxious input from small-diameter primary afferents and by non-noxious information in large-diameter primary afferents. The output from transmission cells is regulated or modulated by inhibitory cells in the substantia gelatinosa, which also receive information from the primary afferents, but the effect on the inhibitory cell is dependent on whether it is non-noxious information in large-diameter afferents or noxious information in small-diameter afferents. Non-noxious input along large-diameter afferents will primarily activate inhibitory cells and, therefore, reduce output from transmission neurons. Noxious input along small-diameter afferents will primarily act to inhibit the inhibitory cells and, therefore, increase the output from transmission cells. Thus, the output from transmission cells to the brain is determined by the relative balance in activity in small- and large-diameter fiber afferents arriving at the dorsal horn. Another component of the gate theory is that descending pathways from the brain can also act to inhibit transmission of information by transmission cells.

The gate theory has had a significant impact on concepts of pain and has helped to explain why pain may occur in some conditions and why some treatments (such as transcutaneous nerve stimulation and dorsal column stimulation) may be effective. However, it has been difficult experimentally to demonstrate some of the specific circuitry suggested in the original proposal. While descending inhibitory controls have been demonstrated, most cells in the spinal cord respond to noxious and non-noxious stimuli and do not fit the proposed characteristics of transmission cells. Clinically, people with selective large-fiber loss often experience pain that is contrary to what is predicted by the gate theory. It also does not help to explain why some people have pain following complete loss of afferent input, as occurs, for example, following complete spinal cord transection. While an important and helpful advance in our understanding of pain, the gate theory does not completely resolve the specific mechanisms responsible for pain processing.

γ-aminobutyric adid and glycine

Both GABAergic and glycinergic interneurons are involved in tonic inhibition of nociceptive input; downregulation or loss of these neurons can result in features of neuropathic pain such as allodynia. Although both $GABA_A$ and $GABA_B$ receptors have been implicated at both pre- and postsynaptic sites, $GABA_A$ receptor-mediated inhibition occurs through largely postsynaptic mechanisms. In contrast, $GABA_B$ mechanisms may be preferentially involved in presynaptic inhibition through suppression of excitatory amino acid release from primary afferent terminals. This finding may help to explain the disparity between laboratory findings, which demonstrate that $GABA_B$ receptor agonists such as baclofen have an antinociceptive action, and clinical experience, which has found that intrathecal baclofen is of limited use in the management of chronic pain. Particularly in neuropathic pain, where there is increased excitability of second-order neurons with no direct relationship to the amount of excitatory amino acids released by primary afferents, intrathecal administration of $GABA_A$ agonists may be more effective.

Clinical implications for modulation of spinal sensitization

Reduction of excitory amino acid release

Central sensitization is dependent upon NMDA receptor activation by endogenous glutamate. Riluzole (currently licensed for use in motor neuron disease) and the anticonvulsant lamotrigine attenuate glutamate release and have analgesic properties in experimental pain models. Lamotrigine is increasingly used for the management of refractory neuropathic pain such as trigeminal neuralgia.

N-methyl D-aspartate antagonists

The NMDA receptor complex provides many potential targets for modulation of the initial stages of central sensitization, including open channel blockers, competitive NMDA antagonists, and glycine and polyamine site allosteric modulators. Ketamine and dextromethorphan both bind to the open channel site. Recent evidence suggests that methadone also produces NMDA antagonist-mediated analgesia in addition to μ-opioid actions. Therapeutic manipulation of Mg^{2+} concentration may influence NMDA receptor function and Mg^{2+} infusions have been reported to reduce postoperative pain. Psychotomimetic side effects limit the usage of ketamine and other experimental NMDA antagonists, even if administered epidurally or intrathecally. Concerns have also been raised over potential neurotoxicity, particularly with intrathecal administration. There remains the potential for the development of NMDA receptor antagonists with a more acceptable side-effect profile, and several agents are being investigated either for analgesia or neuroprotection.

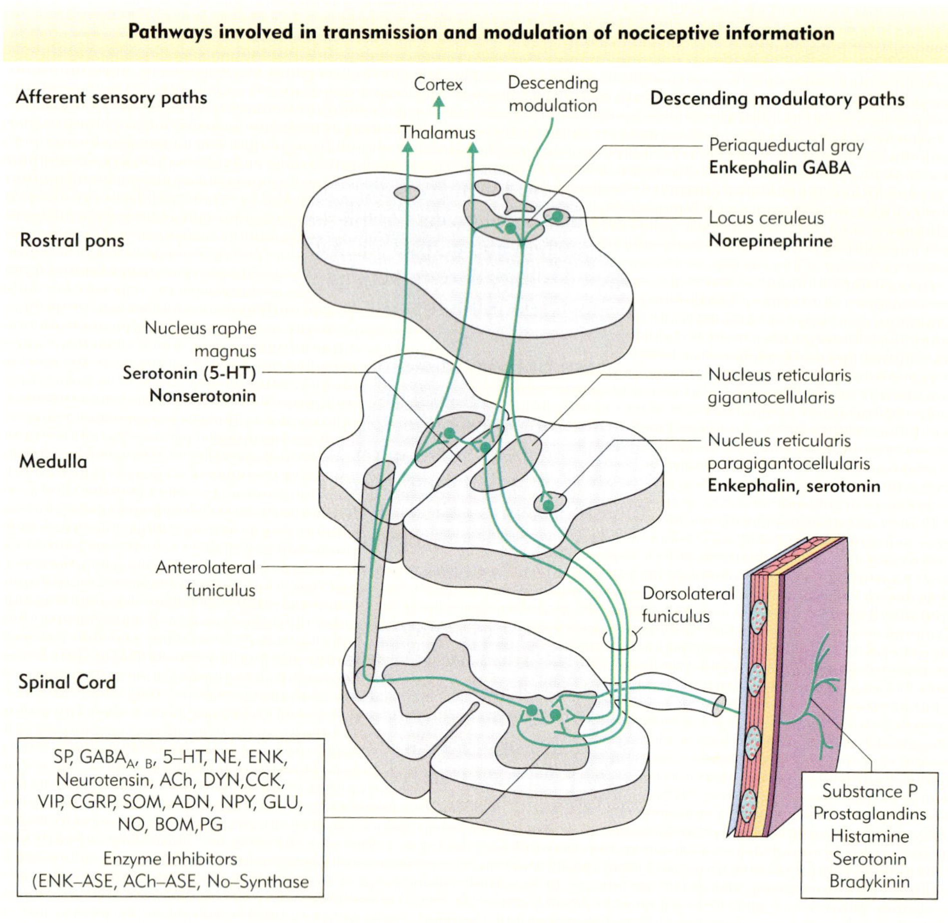

Figure 21.12 Pathways involved in transmission and modulation of nociceptive information. Stimulation of cutaneous nociceptors leads to action potential generation in the primary afferent and concomitant peripheral release of neurogenic inflammatory mediators. Information is relayed to and from a number of brainstem sites (see text). Neurotransmitters are released by afferent fibers, descending terminations, or local interneurons in the dorsal horn and modulate peripheral nociceptive input. SP, substance P; GABA; 5-HT serotonin; NE, norepinephrine; ENK, enkephalin; ACh, acetylcholine; DYN, dynorphin; CCK, cholecystokinin; VIP, vasoactive intestinal peptide; CGRP, calcitonin gene-related peptide; SOM, somatostatin; ADN, adenosine; NPY, neuropeptide Y; GLU, glutamate; NO, nitric oxide; BOM, bombesin; PG, prostaglandin E. (With permission from Siddall and Cousins, 1998.)

Nonsteroidal anti-inflammatory agents

The production of arachidonic acid metabolites is part of the cascade that follows NMDA receptor activation. Although the peripheral effects of NSAIDs have been emphasized in the past (see Chapter 27), it appears that there are also spinal cord targets for NSAID action. Spinally, NSAIDs inhibit cyclooxygenase-mediated processes involved in the maintenance of central sensitization and may also interact at the strychnine-insensitive glycine site of the NMDA receptor complex. Concerns regarding potential neurotoxicity preclude intrathecal or epidural administration of currently available NSAIDs.

Molecular approaches

Traditional approaches to analgesia have focused on classical ligand–receptor blockade as a means to reduce nociceptive input. The rapid progress in our understanding of the molecular and genetic mechanisms involved in nociception provides the potential for a new and powerful approach to pain management. Using agents that modify tropic factor function, or antisense strategies to limit gene expression selectively, it may be possible to target selectively factors that are involved in the transmission of nociceptive and neuropathic messages.

ASCENDING SPINAL TRACTS

Target structures

Fibers associated with the transmission of noxious information may ascend one or two segments from their point of origin before crossing in the dorsal commissure (Fig. 21.12). Primary afferent nociceptors relay to projection neurons within the dorsal horn, which ascend in the anterolateral funiculus to terminate in the thalamus. En route, collaterals of the projection neurons activate multiple higher centers, including the nucleus reticularis gigantocellularis. Neurons project from here to the thalamus and also activate the nucleus raphe magnus and periaqueductal gray (PAG) of the midbrain. Descending fibers from the last project also to the nucleus raphe magnus and adjacent reticular formation. These neurons activate descending inhibitory neurons that are located in these regions and travel via the dorsolateral funiculus to terminate in the dorsal horn of the spinal cord. Descending projections also arise from a number of brainstem sites including the locus ceruleus. Several other sites within what is often referred to as the limbic system receive projections from the spinal cord such as the amygdaloid and septal nuclei. These projections to supraspinal sites are contained within the ventrolateral funiculus in the contralateral anterolateral quadrant of the spinal cord, comprising the spinothalamic, spinoreticular, spinomesencephalic, and spinolimbic tracts. The spinocervicothalamic tracts and the postsynaptic dorsal column pathway provide additional pathways for nociceptive input.

Spinothalamic tract

The spinothalamic tract is regarded as having a central role in pain perception and transmits information regarding pain, cold, warmth, and touch. The cells of origin of the spinothalamic tract are located predominantly within laminae I and IV–VI of the dorsal horn with some in lamina X and the ventral horn. These cells project mainly to the contralateral thalamus with some projecting ipsilaterally. The nuclei in the thalamus that receive these projections are located either laterally (ventral posterior lateral and ventral posterior inferior nuclei and medial posterior complex) or medially in the central lateral nucleus and other intralaminar nuclei.

There appears to be a somatotopic organization within the spinothalamic tract and spinothalamic projection neurons have restricted receptive fields. Fibers arising from more caudal segments tend to be located laterally and those entering from more rostral segments tend to be located in the more medial and ventral part of the tract. They respond well to noxious mechanical and thermal stimuli but many also respond to non-noxious mechanical stimuli.

Spinoreticular tract

The cells of origin of the spinoreticular tract are located in the deep layers of the dorsal horn and in laminae VII and VIII of the ventral horn. These cells send projections to several nuclei within the reticular formation of the brainstem including the lateral reticular nucleus, nucleus gigantocellularis, nucleus paragigantocellularis lateralis in the medulla, the pontine nuclei oralis and caudalis, and parabrachial region. There is no clear somatotopic organization of the spinoreticular tracts. These projections terminate in close apposition to regions that are involved in blood pressure and motor control and the descending inhibition of pain. Therefore, it appears that this pathway is involved in the basic autonomic, motor, and endogenous analgesic responses to nociceptive input.

Spinomesencephalic tract

The cells of origin of the spinomesencephalic tract are predominantly located in laminae I and IV–VI of the dorsal horn, with some found in lamina X and the ventral horn. These cells project to several nuclei in the midbrain including the PAG, cuneiform nucleus, red nucleus, superior colliculus, pretectal nuclei and Edinger–Westphal nucleus. In contrast to the spinoreticular tract, the spinomesencephalic tract appears to be somatotopically organized, with projections from caudal body regions terminating in the caudal midbrain and projections from rostral body regions terminating in more rostral regions of the midbrain. In contrast to the spinothalamic tract, cells in this tract have large and complex receptive fields. The sites of termination of this tract suggest that some of its components are involved in a range of more organized and integrated motor, autonomic, and antinociceptive responses to noxious input, such as orienting, quiescence, defense, and confrontation.

Spinolimbic pathway

Ascending projections from the brainstem relay information from the spinoreticular tract to the medial thalamus, hypothalamus, and other structures in the limbic system. As well as this multisynaptic pathway, there are direct projections from the spinal cord to the hypothalamus, nucleus accumbens, septal nuclei, and amygdala. Projections to the hypothalamus arise chiefly from cells in the deep dorsal horn and lateral spinal nucleus as well as from cells in laminae I, VII, and X. Projections to the amygdala arise from cells in the deep dorsal horn and lamina X. These projections may be responsible for the motivational or affective responses associated with pain perception.

Spinocervicothalamic pathway

The spinocervicothalamic pathway comprises neurons that have their cells of origin in lamina IV of the spinal dorsal horn and fibers that ascend in the dorsal part of the lateral funiculus. The fibers terminate in the lateral cervical nucleus at the level of C1 and C2 before crossing and ascending with the medial lemniscus to terminate in the contralateral ventral posterior lateral nucleus and medial part of the posterior complex of the thalamus. Most cells in this tract respond to light touch and do not appear to have a primary role in nociception. However, some do respond to nociceptive stimuli and, therefore, it may serve as a potential pathway for the transmission of nociceptive information.

Postsynaptic dorsal column pathway

The dorsal columns and nuclei (gracile and cuneate nuclei) are generally considered to be the pathway for information regarding the non-noxious sensations of fine touch, proprioception, and vibration. Stimulation of the dorsal columns is normally reported to produce a sensation of vibration rather than pain, although there are reports that mechanical stimulation of the medial aspect of the nucleus gracilis may result in pain. It has also been demonstrated that cells in the gracile nucleus respond to noxious stimulation of the viscera. The pathway that supplies this information is referred to as the postsynaptic dorsal column pathway. This pathway has cells of origin in lamina III of the dorsal horn as well as just lateral to lamina X.

Further evidence for a role for the dorsal column nuclei in pain perception comes from the demonstration that a phenotypic change occurs in neurons projecting the dorsal column following nerve injury. Damage to large myelinated fibers results in the *de novo* synthesis of substance P within these neurons and may be part of the mechanism responsible for the hypersensitivity to light touch that occurs following peripheral nerve injury.

Clinical implications

Many surgical and percutaneous procedures have been employed to disrupt specific tracts within the spinal cord. These include cordotomy, extralemniscal myelotomy, and commissural myelotomy. The distribution of fibers associated with pain transmission within the anterolateral quadrant would suggest that section of these tracts using an anterolateral cordotomy should be a useful procedure in abolishing or relieving pain. This concept is based on the Cartesian or 'private line' model of pain perception and results are variable and often transient. Sometimes, excellent relief can be obtained in the short term but long-term results are usually disappointing and complications include return of pain, motor weakness, and loss of bladder and bowel function. Consequently, these procedures are usually limited to treatment of cancer pain.

SUPRASPINAL STRUCTURES

Thalamus

Axons within the spinothalamic pathway are divided into two main groups depending on their terminations. One group travels in the anterolateral funiculus, together with projections from the medulla, pons, and midbrain, terminates more laterally in the ventroposterior nuclei and posterior complex of the thalamus, and is believed to be involved in the sensory discriminative component of pain (Fig. 21.13). Another group terminates more medially in the intralaminar nuclei, including the centrolateral, ventroposterolateral, and submedian nuclei, which project to the

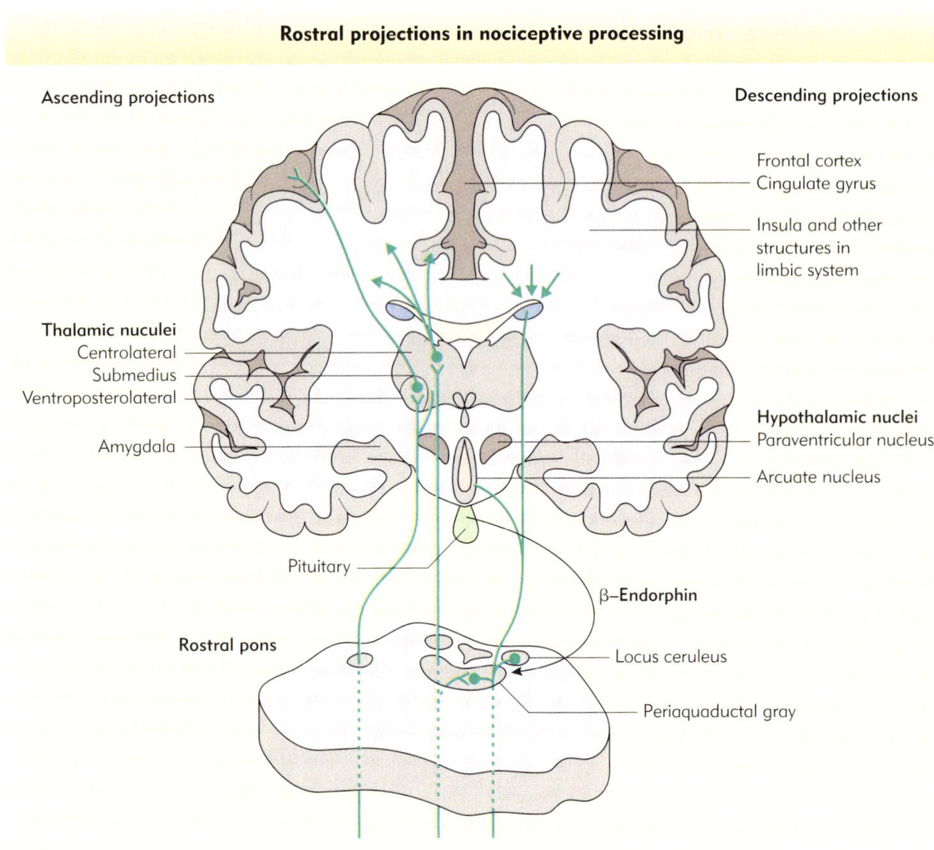

Figure 21.13 Rostral projections of nociceptive progressing. Ascending projections terminate in the thalamic nuclear complex. The descending fibers inhibit transmission of nociceptive information between primary afferents and projection neurons in the dorsal horn. In addition to direct neural connections, endorphins are released into the cerebrospinal fluid and blood where they can exert an inhibitory effects at multiple centers. (With permission from Siddall, 1998.)

somatosensory cortex. The centromedian nuclei project more diffusely, including projections to the limbic system, and are believed to be involved in the affective–motivational aspects of pain. The medial thalamus also receives projections from the spinoreticular and spinomesencephalic tracts. Projections from the spinocervical and postsynaptic dorsal column pathways terminate in the ventral posterior lateral nucleus and posterior complex.

Animal studies indicate that there is a spinothalamic projection with terminations within the ventral posterior thalamic nucleus. Neurons within this region have restricted receptive fields and respond to noxious stimuli. These findings suggest that nuclei within this region have a role in the discriminative aspects of pain processing. However, it is interesting that stimulation of the ventrocaudal nucleus (analogous to the ventral posterior nucleus in animals and supposedly part of the 'pain' pathway) in awake humans rarely results in pain except in those people who have central deafferentation pain. In contrast to cells in the lateral thalamus, cells in the medial thalamus have large, often bilateral receptive fields, suggesting a minor role in discriminative aspects of pain perception. It has been reported that a nucleus within the medial thalamus is specific for pain and temperature sensation.

Positron emission tomography (PET) studies have identified a number of subcortical structures that are presumed to be involved in nociceptive transmission and pain perception. These include the thalamus, putamen, caudate nucleus, hypothalamus, amygdala, PAG, hippocampus, and cerebellum. While previous physiologic and anatomic experiments have suggested that some of these structures are responsible for pain transmission, the role of others is unclear. The activation of these subcortical structures may vary with differing pain complaints: studies indicate that while an acute experimental painful stimulus results in increased activity in the thalamus, chronic pain caused by cancer and chronic neuropathic pain are associated with a decrease in activity in the thalamus.

Cortical structures

The effect of cortical stimulation and lesions on pain perception is confusing and intriguing. Patients who have had a complete hemispherectomy can have almost normal pain sensation. In the awake human, stimulation of the primary somatosensory cortex typically evokes nonpainful sensations. Neurosurgical lesions of cortical regions produce varying effects depending on the region ablated. Lesions of the frontal lobe and cingulate cortex result in a condition in which pain perception remains. However, the suffering component of pain appears to be reduced, the person only reports pain when queried and spontaneous requests for analgesia are reduced. These effects contrast with those seen following lesions of the medial thalamus and hypothalamus, in which there is pain relief but without demonstrable analgesia.

Both PET and functional magnetic resonance imaging have been helpful in elucidating cortical regions involved in pain processing, although there is some inconsistency in results. This may be because of the differing stimuli used in various studies. Painful stimuli result in activation of somatosensory, motor, premotor, parietal, frontal, occipital, insular, and anterior cingulate regions of the cortex. While it is by no means clear, it has been suggested on the basis of PET findings that the parietal regions of the cortex are responsible for evaluation of the temporal and spa-

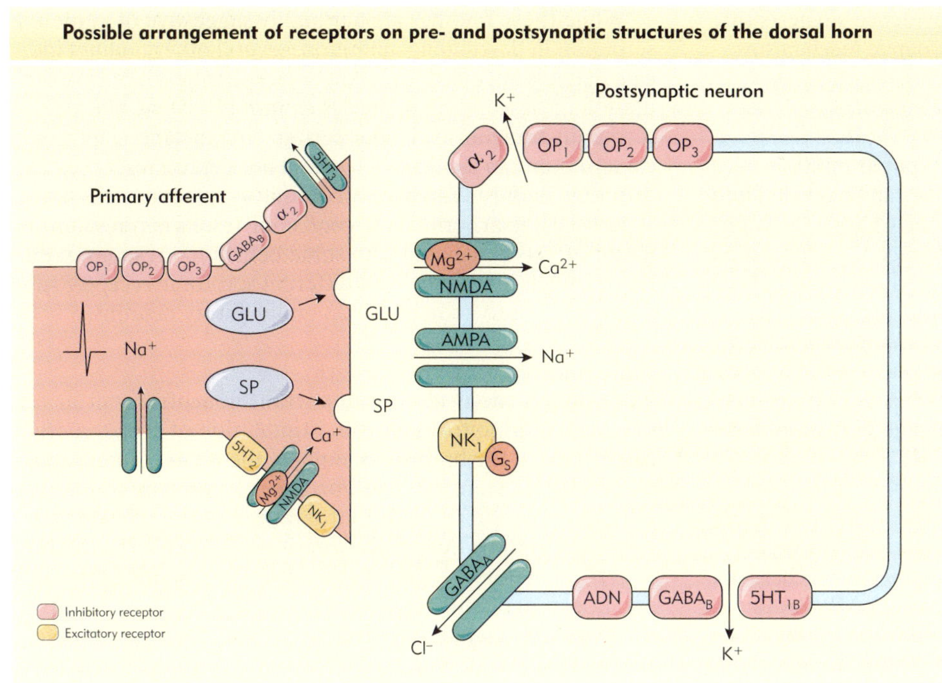

Figure 21.14 Possible arrangement of receptors on pre- and postsynaptic structures of the dorsal horn of the spinal cord.

tial features of pain and the frontal cortex, including anterior cingulate, is responsible for the emotional response to pain.

Descending inhibition

There are powerful inhibitory influences arising from the brain that descend in the spinal cord to modulate spinal reflexes. Interest from those studying pain strengthened with the demonstration in the late 1960s that electrical stimulation of the PAG of the midbrain enabled abdominal surgery to be performed on animals with little evidence of discomfort. It is now known that there are powerful inhibitory (as well as facilitatory) influences on nociceptive transmission acting at many levels of the neuraxis. The PAG receives projections from a number of brain regions including the amygdala, frontal and insular cortex, and hypothalamus. In addition to direct neural connections, endorphins synthesized in the pituitary are released into the cerebrospinal fluid and blood where they can exert an inhibitory effects at multiple centers including the PAG. Descending inhibition may be activated by external factors such as stress (stress-induced analgesia) and noxious input (diffuse noxious inhibitory controls) or can be induced by peripheral or central nervous stimulation.

Although the role of descending systems has been emphasized, there is also evidence for ascending modulation of 'higher' structures. For example, stimulation in the PAG can produce inhibition of the responses of neurons in the medial thalamus. Although it is possible that this inhibition may occur through the activation of descending pathways, it indicates that there are multiple interactions at many levels of the nervous system.

Brain structures involved in descending inhibition

Descending inhibitory influences arise from a number of supraspinal structures including hypothalamus, PAG, locus ceruleus, nucleus raphe magnus, and nucleus paragigantocellularis lateralis. Electrical stimulation of and microinjection of excitatory amino acids into these regions inhibits nociceptive responses. Descending inhibition does not require 'turning on'. Even though descending inhibition is activated by external stimuli, it is also tonically active and maintains a resting level of inhibitory function. This is demonstrated by reversible spinal cord block, which results in an increased responsiveness of spinal cord neurons.

The midbrain PAG appears to have a major role in descending inhibition. Stimulation in this region results in antinociception; although the PAG does not project directly to the spinal cord, descending fibers from the PAG relay in several structures that are also implicated in descending inhibition. These structures include the midline medullary nucleus raphe magnus and the paragigantocellular nucleus situated lateral to it. The PAG also appears to be highly organized. It has been demonstrated that analgesia obtained from the lateral PAG is nonopioid in nature, whereas opioid analgesia is obtained from stimulation of the medial PAG.

As with the PAG, electrical or chemical stimulation of the midline nucleus raphe magnus or ventrolateral (paragigantocellular nucleus) medulla results in antinociception. Fibers descend directly from these regions to the dorsal horn of the spinal cord, suggesting a role in descending inhibition and relaying information from the PAG. Tracts from these structures descend predominantly in the dorsolateral funiculus of the spinal cord and terminate in laminae I, II, and V. Stimulation of the locus ceruleus also results in inhibition of nociceptive-evoked dorsal horn activity. This nucleus receives inputs from a number of brain structures and provides descending inputs to the spinal dorsal horn. These descending fibers travel ipsilaterally in the ventrolateral funiculus.

Terminations of descending pathways interact with several different neural elements in the dorsal horn. These include projection neurons that transmit information from spinal cord to the brain, local interneurons within the spinal cord, and primary afferent terminals. Inhibition may occur presynaptically by modulation of transmitter release or postsynaptically by either excitation of local inhibitory interneurons or direct inhibition of second-order projection neurons. The bulk of evidence suggests that descending inhibition is exerted via postsynaptic mechanisms.

Neurotransmitter mechanisms

Opioids

Opioid receptors modulate nociceptive input at multiple sites within the CNS, although functionally these can be divided into supraspinal and spinal sites of analgesia (see Chapter 26 & Fig. 21.14). The μ, δ, and κ opioid receptors (recently reclassified as OP_1, OP_2, and OP_3) are differentially distributed throughout the CNS together with the orphan opioid receptor ORL-1. Endogenous opioid ligands include β-endorphin and the newly described endomorphins 1 and 2, which are μ-opioid ligands, together with enkephalin and dynorphin, which act on κ- and δ-receptors, respectively. Nociceptin (or orphanin FQ), an endogenous ligand for the ORL-1 receptor, has been isolated, although its role in nociceptive and analgesic mechanisms remains obscure. Opioid receptors are members of the G protein-coupled receptor superfamily and their analgesic actions are a consequence of G protein-mediated inhibition of voltage-gated Ca^{2+} channels, activation of K^+ currents, and a reduction in cAMP. Paradoxic excitatory effects involving cAMP stimulation, phosphoinositide breakdown, and Ca^{2+} mobilization may contribute to opioid tolerance and hyperalgesia with prolonged administration.

Supraspinally, there is a high density of opioid receptors in the PAG, nucleus raphe magnus, and locus ceruleus. The profound analgesia produced by electrical stimulation of these regions is reversed by the opioid antagonist naloxone, which confirms the importance of endogenous opioid agonists in nociceptive behavior. However, microinjection of opioid agonists into these regions results in complex alterations in pain behavior reflecting both inhibition and disinhibition (the inhibition of an inhibitory interneuron) of pathways involved in nociception. Subregional differences, dose dependence, and action at specific opioid receptor subtypes further increase the complexity of supraspinal analgesia. For example, high doses of morphine in the clinical setting have occasionally been reported to result in hyperalgesia rather than analgesia.

Opioids act at a spinal level in the dorsal horn by activation of presynaptic opioid receptors, which inhibit glutamate and neurokinin release from primary afferent terminals, and postsynaptic receptors, which inhibit second-order neuron depolarization. Particularly within the spinal cord dorsal horn, opioid receptor density and distribution is dynamic: inflammation may enhance and nerve injury markedly reduce opioid-mediated spinal analgesia. Changes in presynaptic opioid receptor number and function at least in part underlie these effects.

Opioid analgesic mechanisms are themselves modulated by release of cholecystokinin within the dorsal horn. Pathologic upregulation of this system has been proposed as a mechanism contributing to opioid-resistant chronic pain states.

Serotonin

Serotonin has been long suggested as a major neurotransmitter in descending controls. Serotonin is contained within a high proportion of nucleus raphe magnus cells, and in terminals of descending fibers in the dorsal horn. Electrical stimulation of the nucleus raphe magnus increases release of serotonin in the spinal cord. Agents that block serotonin synthesis attenuate stimulation-produced analgesia, and application of some serotonin agonists in the spinal cord inhibits cells responsive to nociceptive stimuli.

While these findings appear highly suggestive of a role for serotonin in descending inhibition, several other findings indicate that it is not conclusive. Antinociception produced by stimulation of descending pathways cannot always be blocked by serotonin antagonists. Under certain circumstances, intrathecal serotonin can facilitate behavioral nociceptive responses and serotonin agonists can have an excitatory effect on cells in the superficial dorsal horn. These conflicting results may result from motor effects associated with some behavioral responses, differing effects associated with different serotonin receptor subtypes, and observation of effects on inhibitory neurons.

Norepinephrine

Norepinephrine is also an important neurotransmitter for descending inhibitory controls. Stimulation of noradrenergic cell groups in the brainstem, notably the locus ceruleus, produces antinociception, and norepinephrine-containing terminals are found in the upper laminae of the spinal dorsal horn. Iontophoretic application of norepinephrine inhibits activation of dorsal horn neurons by noxious stimuli; intrathecal norepinephrine results in inhibition of nociceptive responses, and α_2-adrenoceptor antagonists and compounds that reduce the amount of norepinephrine in the spinal cord increase nociceptive responses.

Other neurotransmitters

Other transmitters that appear to be important in descending inhibition are acetylcholine, GABA, thyrotropin-releasing hormone, and somatostatin.

Clinical implications

Antidepressants

Tricyclic antidepressants, typified by amitriptyline, produce spinally and supraspinally mediated analgesia in chronic pain states by mechanisms distinct from those enhancing mood. Tricyclic antidepressants have multiple actions; they inhibit the uptake of both norepinephrine and serotonin and have muscarinic anticholinergic effects (see Chapter 25). The selective serotonin-reuptake inhibitors are a class of antidepressant that have weaker analgesic actions than traditional tricyclic antidepressants, which implicates noradrenergic mechanisms as the most significant mode of analgesia.

Opioids

Opioids remain the primary analgesics for the management of acute, severe nociceptive pain. Respiratory depression and sedation are supraspinally mediated and limit maximally tolerated systemic doses. Selective targeting of opioid receptors in the dorsal horn via epidural or intrathecal administration is, therefore, a logical means to achieve analgesia and reduce supraspinally mediated side effects.

Opioid tolerance results in a requirement for increasing dose to achieve a given degree of analgesia for a constant nociceptive stimulus. The mechanisms include opioid-mediated enhancement of cAMP levels, protein phosphorylation, and subsequent upregulation of NMDA receptor mechanisms within the dorsal horn and supraspinal sites. In addition, accumulation of the morphine metabolite morphine 3-glucuronide, which may antagonize the analgesic action normally produced by opioid receptor activation, may play a supplementary role. Tolerance is rarely of clinical significance in acute pain management, and while frequently described in the context of chronic pain, it is not an inevitable consequence of long-term opioid administration. Neuropathic pain states with pre-existing NMDA receptor activation may predispose to the development of opioid tolerance or insensitivity. Animal studies indicate that administration of an NMDA antagonist can prevent both development of tolerance to morphine and the withdrawal syndrome in morphine-dependent rats. Therefore, coadministration of NMDA antagonists such as dextromethorphan or ketamine with opioids may attenuate the development of opioid tolerance and potentiate opioid analgesic mechanisms. The observation that methadone enantiomers are analgesic as a result of NMDA receptor antagonism in addition to μ-opioid receptor activation provides a logical basis for its long-term administration.

Nitrous oxide

Nitrous oxide produces analgesia via complex mechanisms involving supraspinal opioid-mediated activation of descending noradrenergic pathways and direct activation of spinal α_2-adrenoceptors. In addition, recent evidence suggests that nitrous oxide may also inhibit NMDA receptor function.

Clonidine

The α_2-adrenergic agonist clonidine is analgesic when administered epidurally or intrathecally: activation of pre- and postsynaptic α_2-adrenoceptors inhibits primary afferent transmitter release and second-order neuronal depolarization. Clonidine potentiates spinal opioid analgesia, and combination therapy may be efficacious in neuropathic pain. Epidural and intrathecal clonidine provide analgesia in CRPS states that are opioid insensitive.

Stimulation-produced analgesia

The demonstration that powerful inhibition of nociceptive responses can be obtained by activation of descending pathways led to a resurgence of interest in techniques such as acupuncture and transcutaneous electrical nerve stimulation. It also led to the development and investigation of new techniques such as dorsal column stimulation and deep brain stimulation. Although not widely used, deep brain stimulation involves the insertion of fine electrodes into brain regions where inhibition can be obtained. Initial studies focused on the PAG and periventricular gray matter, but other sites such as thalamus are also used and provide significant analgesia in selected patients.

CLINICAL SIGNIFICANCE OF INFLAMMATION AND NERVE INJURY

Peripheral and central sensitization that result from inflammation or nerve injury are a common consequence of surgical or traumatic injury. In most individuals, acute postoperative pain is amenable to 'conventional' therapy with combinations of opioids, NSAIDs, and local anesthetics and is self-limiting. The resolution of the injury is generally associated with resolution of pain, indicating that, at least at the behavioral level, the manifestations of central sensitization are reversible. Experimental evidence indicating that phenotypic changes outlast behavioral changes in pain models suggests that adaptive analgesic mechanisms usually compensate within the spinal cord.

Pre-emptive analgesia

There is evidence that severe postoperative pain may be a significant predictor of long-term pain and that steps which reduce or abolish noxious input to the spinal cord during a painful event such as surgery may reduce or minimize spinal cord changes and thereby lead to a reduction of postoperative, and possibly chronic, pain. However, what duration or degree of noxious input is required before these long-term changes occur remains unclear. Furthermore, it is uncertain how much these long-term changes depend on the afferent barrage during surgery and how much they depend on continuing inputs from the wound after surgery. At both stages, there will be sustained noxious input and, therefore, the potential to produce central sensitization; however, it would be expected that interventions that pre-empt central sensitization and seek to prevent it occurring, rather than attempts to treat it after it has occurred, should be more successful.

The pre-emptive effects of local anesthetics, opioids, and NSAIDs (alone or in combination) administered locally, epidurally, intrathecally, or systemically at a variety of time points before, during, or after surgery have been studied. A number of trials have purported to show that pre-emptive analgesia results in reduced pain, decreased analgesic requirements, improved morbidity, and decreased hospital stay. However, these are balanced by a similar number that have failed to show benefit. The variability in agent, timing, and method of administration, as well as differences in the type of surgery and anesthetic procedure, have made it difficult to compare many studies of pre-emptive analgesia. Furthermore, many studies have been flawed methodologically. As examples, nitrous oxide and volatile agents may influence central sensitization and the increased anesthetic requirement in patients not receiving pre- or intraoperative analgesia may influence outcome. Similarly, basic science studies suggest that NSAIDs are equally effective at attenuating sensitization whether administered pre- or poststimulus: postoperative administration of NSAID may mask or minimize opioid pre-emptive effects. Therefore, despite the logical appeal of pre-emptive analgesia and its ready clinical application, further trials are necessary before a definitive statement can be made regarding its benefits and advantages.

Much of the focus of pre-emptive analgesia has been on reducing acute pain in the early postoperative period. Pre-emptive analgesia may also be important in reducing chronic pain; this has not been systematically evaluated. The study that has generated most interest was the finding by Bach and colleagues that preoperative epidural blockade of patients undergoing lower limb amputation resulted in a lower incidence of phantom limb pain at 6 and 12 months following surgery than seen in a control group that had intraoperative block alone. Although there are several inadequacies in the study design and not all subsequent studies have confirmed their findings, it demonstrates that pre-emptive analgesia may have the potential to prevent the development of chronic pain states. Further studies are urgently required to address this important question.

Chronic pain

Ongoing nociceptive input

Perhaps the simplest explanation of chronic pain is that of pure ongoing peripheral nocigenic input. This is typified by chronic inflammatory degenerative conditions (e.g. rheumatoid arthritis or degenerative osteoarthritis). Ongoing activation of peripheral nociceptors with or without the presence of inflammatory mediators results in ongoing peripheral sensitization. However, this is commonly supplemented by central sensitization. Clinical manifestations include ongoing peripheral mechanothermal hyperalgesia and allodynia. Peripheral nociceptor sensitization may respond to NSAIDs, while opioids will attenuate primary

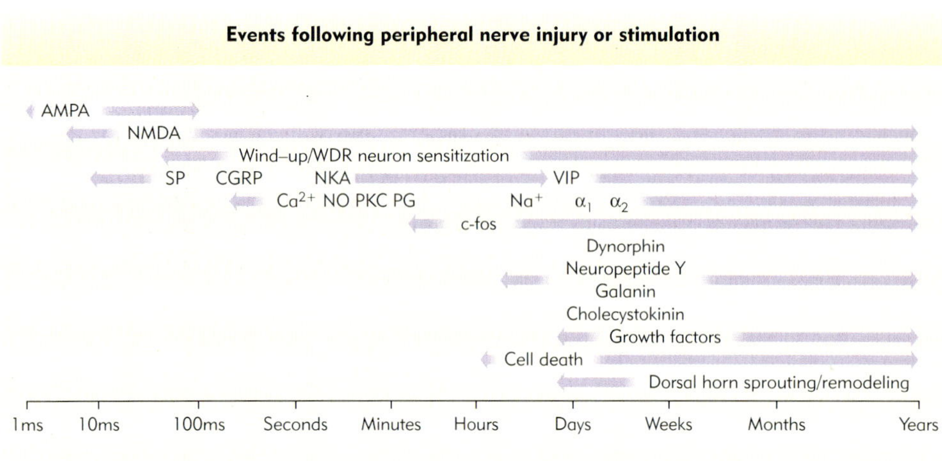

Figure 21.15 The cascade of molecular events that may occur in the spinal cord following peripheral nerve injury or stimulation. Many of the changes are common to both acute and chronic pain stages but may then be followed by more permanent changes in the nervous system, which may be the basis of pain memories (see text). Inhibiting the earlier events may delay and perhaps prevent some of the later events. AMPA, α-amino-3-hydroxy-5-methyl-isoxazole; NMDA, *N*-methyl D-aspartate; SP, substance P; CGRP, calcitonin gene-related peptide; NKA, neurokinin A; NO, nitric oxide; PKC, protein kinase C; PG, prostaglandins; VIP, vasoactive intestinal polypeptide. (With permission from Munglani, 1998.)

afferent transmitter release in the dorsal horn. Conditions of pure peripheral nociceptor activation should respond to conventional analgesics. Opioid resistance suggests the involvement of central sensitization mechanisms.

Peripheral maintenance of central sensitization

Central sensitization, once established, can clearly be maintained by ongoing peripheral activation of nociceptive afferents where a peripheral inflammatory or nocigenic stimulus persists. Following nerve injury, spontaneously discharging neuromata and spontaneously active DRG cells provide an alternative mechanism for the maintenance of central sensitization. Sympathetic efferent activity may play a similar role in CRPS pain states, where sprouting of sympathetic neurons results in activation of primary afferent cell bodies within the DRG. Furthermore, sensitized dorsal horn neurons with enlarged receptive fields can be activated by non-noxious input; this effect may be potentiated by sprouting of Aβ fibers. Non-noxious mechanical and proprioceptive afferent input may thereby maintain central sensitization after resolution of the initial injury. These mechanisms underlie zygapophysial facet joint-generated spinal pain and possibly myofascial pain. Specific blockade of the neuronal mechanisms maintaining sensitization (e.g. local anesthetic blockade of neuroma, facet joint, or efferent SNS innervation) may markedly attenuate spontaneous pain, allodynia, and hyperalgesia and provide insight into the etiology of the pain complaint.

Ongoing central sensitization

Pain perception requires activity only in cortical and associated supraspinal regions many synapses distant from the peripheral nociceptor. Therefore, ongoing afferent input into the spinal cord is not a prerequisite for ongoing pain. If the normal spinal inhibitory mechanisms are overwhelmed by the magnitude of the initial stimulus (e.g. massive loss of inhibitory interneurons), and there is a failure in adaptive analgesic mechanisms that might oppose otherwise uncontrolled excitation in pain pathways, then a self-maintaining state of central sensitization may be established. The determinants leading to 'centralization' of pain are imprecisely understood, but severity and chronicity of noxious stimulus in individuals with genetically determined 'vulnerable neurochemistry' are proposed as key factors.

The concept of a balance between excitation and inhibition is of prime importance in the pathophysiology of pain; for example, cerebrovascular accident, head injury, and spinal cord injury are frequently associated with 'central' pain syndromes (e.g. 'thalamic pain') that reflect aberrant excitatory activity in central neurons involved in pain transduction, resulting in spontaneous pain. Furthermore, a spontaneous loss of spinal and/or supraspinal inhibitory tone and consequent disinhibition of projection neurons should result in spontaneous pain, hyperalgesia, and allodynia. Fibromyalgia and similar diffuse pain syndromes that are not clearly linked to an initial nocigenic event could, at least in part, be explained by such mechanisms.

Centrally mediated and maintained pain will be 'referred' to dermatomes representative of pathologically activated central neurons. Peripheral neural blockade of afferent input from these dermatomes will not abolish spontaneous pain sensation, although hyperalgesia and allodynia may be relieved and quality of pain altered. Such 'central' pain states rarely respond to conventional analgesic strategies. They are associated with downregulation of opioid receptor number and function and pain is likely to be independent of primary afferent excitory amino acid transmitter release, which is a primary target of opioid analgesia. Potentiation of spinal and supraspinal noradrenergic and GABAergic systems together with suppression of ectopic Na^+ channel activation may provide significant analgesia, necessitating combination therapy with tricyclic antidepressants, anticonvulsants, and membrane-stabilizing drugs.

Peripheral nerve blockade in chronic pain

Peripheral nerve blockade is often used as a diagnostic procedure to predict outcome for nerve section or neuroablative procedures. However, isolated, uncontrolled nerve blocks have little diagnostic or predictive value in the assessment of sciatic pain caused by lumbosacral disease. The recent evidence for physiologic and morphologic changes within the spinal cord following sustained peripheral input suggests that there are pitfalls in diagnostic neural blockade. First, chronic pain caused by peripheral nerve damage may no longer be dependent on peripheral input, and there is no evidence that treatments aimed at the periphery modify established central sensitization. For example, a long-standing intercostal neuralgia will not be expected to respond to intercostal neurectomy; indeed the pain may increase as the processes of central sensitization may be enhanced. Second, diagnostic nerve blocks seek to identify a 'pain' source and can isolate the person from the disease process that is thought to be responsible for the pain. Using diagnostic nerve blocks in this way can mean that little recognition is made of the complex psychologic issues that can underlie the chronic pain presentation. It may even mean that a psychologic 'diagnosis' is made on the basis of the person's response to a diagnostic procedure. Therefore, diagnostic procedures must be done in the context of a multidisciplinary assessment with an understanding of the complex biologic and psychologic components of chronic pain and placebo response to interventions.

Transitions from acute to chronic pain

The development of chronic pain represents a cascade of molecular events that are initiated at the time of peripheral stimulation or injury (Fig. 21.15). Many of the changes are common to both acute and chronic pain stages (e.g. the activation of the NMDA channel, increase in intracellular Ca^{2+}, involvement and upregulation of neuronal nitric oxide synthase, and increase in *c*-fos expression). These changes in ion channel function, second messengers, immediate early genes, and neuropeptides may then be followed by more permanent changes in the nervous system consisting of changes in synaptic efficacy of preexisting synapses, nerve sprouting, and formation of novel synapses via growth factors. These latter changes may be the basis of pain memories in the spinal cord and brain. Particular changes may be prominent in certain conditions (e.g. changes in α_1- and α_2-adrenoreceptor function may contirbute to sympathetically maintained pain). There is evidence that inhibiting the earlier events may delay and perhaps prevent some of the later events, that is, prevent the occurrence of long-term changes that are associated with persistent pain.

The persistence of pain may be a result of plastic changes within the nervous system both in the periphery and centrally within the spinal cord, with or without persistence of the original stimulus. Yet it is clear that a group of individuals who have identical injuries will not all develop chronic pain symptoms. Genetic variations between individuals may account for such varying outcome. Failure to increase the levels of analgesic peptides such as neuropeptide Y, marked declines in GABAergic function, or even accentuated sympathetic responses may predispose to chronic pain in some individuals. Since the early 1980s, a rapid increase has occurred in our understanding of chronic pain mechanisms. The translation of this understanding to the introduction of novel therapies and elucidating the genetic basis of the predisposition to chronic pain are the challenges for the early 21st century.

Key References

Bach S, Noreng MF, Tjellden NU. Phantom pain in amputees during the first 12 months following limb amputation. Pain. 1988;33:297–301.

Cao YQ, Mantyh PW, Carlson EJ, et al. Primary afferent tachykinins are required to experience moderate to intense pain. Nature. 1998;392:390–4.

Hudspith MJ. Glutamate: a role in normal brain function, anesthesia, analgesia and CNS injury. Br J Anaesth. 1997;78:731–47.

Lambert DG (ed.). Recent advances in opioid pharmaology [various authors]. Br J Anaesth. 1998;81:1–84.

Mao J, Price DD, Mayer DJ. Mechanisms of hyperalgesia and morphine tolerance: a current view of their possible interactions. Pain. 1995;62:259–74.

Melzack R. Psychological aspects of pain. In: Cousins MJ, Bridenbaugh PO, eds. Neural blockade in clinical anesthesia and management of pain. Philadelphia: Lippincott-Raven; 1998:781–91.

Siddall PJ, Cousins MJ. Introduction to pain mechanisms. In: Cousins MJ, Bridenbaugh PO, eds. Neural blockade in clinical anesthesia and management of pain. Philadelphia: Lippincott-Raven; 1998:675–713.

Stein C. Morphine – local analgesic. Pain: clinical updates. 1995;3:1.

Strunin L (ed.). Inflammatory and neurogenic pain: new molecules, new mechanisms [various authors]. Br J Anaesth. 1995;75:123–227.

Woolf CJ, Chong MS. Pre-emptive analgesia: treating postoperative pain by preventing the establishment of central sensitization. Anesth Analg. 1993;77:362–79.

Woolf CJ, Shortland P, Coggleshall RE. Peripheral nerve injury triggers central sprouting of mylelinated afferents. Nature. 1992;355:75–8.

Further Reading

Borsook D. Molecular biology of pain. Progress in pain research and management, Vol. 9. Seattle: IASP Press; 1997.

Brodal P. The central nervous system: structure and function, 2nd edn. Oxford: Oxford University Press, 1998.

Dickenson A, Besson JM. The pharmacology of pain. Handbook of experimental pharmacology. Berlin: Springer. 1997.

Molloy AR, Power I. Acute and chronic pain. Int Anesthesiol Clin. 1997;35.

Munglani R. Advances in chronic pain therapy with special reference to low back pain. In: Kaufman L, Ginsburg R, eds. Anaesthetic review, Vol. 14. Edinburgh: Churchill Livingstone; 1998:153–74.

Munglani R, Hunt SP, Jones GJ. Spinal cord and chronic pain. In: Kaufman L, Ginsburg R, eds. Anaesthetic review, Vol. 12. Edinburgh: Churchill Livingstone; 1996:53–76.

Willis WD Jr, Coggleshaw RE. Sensory mechanisms of the spinal cord, 2nd edn. London: Plenum Press; 1991.

Chapter 22 Mechanisms of anesthesia

Philip M Hopkins and William Winlow

Topics covered in this chapter

The mechanism of action of general anesthetic drugs is not only of intellectual interest but also is of relevance to the design and production of new general anesthetics. Several new anesthetics have been introduced into clinical practice in recent years, but none is ideal. As well as the desired anesthetic action, all have a wide profile of side effects, which commonly include cardiovascular and respiratory depression; in certain patient groups, these are major contributors to anesthetic morbidity and mortality. The goal of new anesthetic drug development is, therefore, to produce drugs that target specifically those cellular and molecular processes that produce anesthesia while avoiding those effects that produce the unwanted actions. Clearly the first stage in this process is to determine which effects contribute to anesthesia. However, general anesthetics tend to have a great variety of cellular and molecular effects on different cell systems and, sometimes, in different species (Fig. 22.1). Different properties of cellular anesthetic actions have been proposed to indicate the relevance of the effects to anesthesia. Currently, the most popular view is that general anesthesia results from an action directly on proteins that form postsynaptic ligand-gated inhibitory ion channels in the CNS. Other hypotheses will also be discussed, since these currently less popular theories may soon become more logical explanations for general anesthetic effects.

DEFINITION OF GENERAL ANESTHESIA

The first problem in anesthesia research is to define the term. In the early part of the 20th century, anesthesia was defined as a combination of unconsciousness/amnesia, analgesia, and muscle relaxation (immobility). All these components of anesthesia can be produced by volatile anesthetics, but with differing dose dependencies. As the concentration of volatile anesthetic is increased, patients first lose consciousness and become amnesic. As the concentration is increased further, analgesia is produced with muscle relaxation or immobility developing only at high concentrations of anesthetic. This dose–response relationship is complicated by the effects of surgical stimulation. With increasing surgical stimulus, the concentration of anesthetic required to ensure unconsciousness and lack of response (immobility) increases. Great care must be taken, therefore, in defining anesthesia in absolute terms, as the depth of anesthesia must always be expressed relative to the degree of stimulus imposed. With the advent of more specific analgesic and muscle relaxant drugs, balanced anesthetic techniques have become popular. In these techniques, the principal use of the anesthetic drug is to produce hypnosis, which can be achieved with either a volatile or an intravenous anesthetic. Intravenous anesthetics are good hypnotic drugs, but most have only weak, if any, analgesic properties, while none produce muscle relaxation sufficient for body cavity surgery. A crucial question is whether the complete spectrum of anesthetic effects, as produced by volatile anesthetics, results from an ever increasing effect at a single site of action or from recruitment of different effects or sites of action at increasing dosage of anesthetic.

We must be careful when interpreting studies on the mechanisms of general anesthetics that the drug under investigation can truly produce at least hypnosis and lack of response to a surgical stimulus. For example, benzodiazepines (see Chapter 25) are good sedative drugs, good amnesics, and (if used in high-enough dose) can produce hypnosis. They are not good drugs, however, for preventing responses to surgical stimuli. The commonly used intravenous induction agents thiopental (thiopentone), propofol, and etomidate are also principally hypnotic drugs but if given in high-enough dose can obtund responses to mild surgical stimuli. If a single cellular process is responsible for anesthesia, it is to the volatile anesthetic drugs that we must look.

ANESTHETIC ACTION ON THE BRAIN AND SPINAL CORD

It is possible that anesthetics could act solely on the brain, solely on the spinal cord, or globally on the CNS. It may be difficult to envisage a mechanism that does not involve the brain, the seat of consciousness, but it is well recognized that afferent block at the level of the spinal cord can induce drowsiness or even sleep. This is said to indicate that consciousness is dependent on the brain being able to receive sensory input. Furthermore, in animal preparations in which the brain has been removed and cardiorespiratory function maintained artificially, anesthetic requirements to prevent response to surgical stimulation is little affected. However, in patients with chronic transection of the cervical spinal cord there is adaptation by the brain to reduced sensory input, consciousness is normal, and anesthesia is

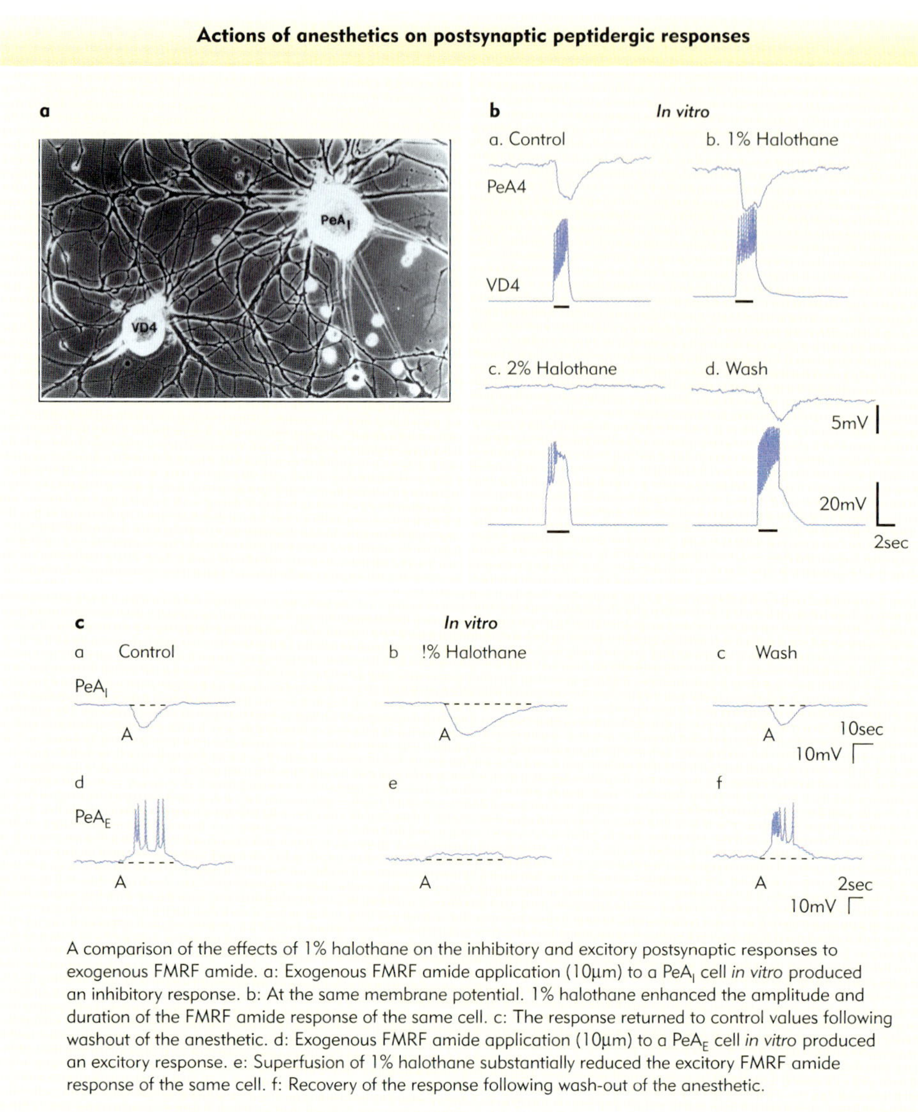

Figure 22.1 Actions of anesthetics on postsynaptic peptidergic responses. The pond snail *Lymnaea* is a gastropod mollusk used as a model system for neuron research. The neurons are large and pigmented and are easily identified and manipulated. They can be studied in the anesthetized animal or in culture. (a) Neurons can reform synapses in culture. The peptidergic neuron VD4 makes monosynaptic inhibitory connections with pedal A cluster neurons (PeA$_I$) after 24–48 hours in culture. (In about 50% of cases, VD4 will make excitatory connections.) (b) Halothane-induced depression of synaptic transmission *in vitro* between identified neurons VD4 and PeA4. Simultaneous intracellular recordings revealed an inhibitory effect of VD4 stimulation on PeA4 that was unaffected by halothane 1%. In the presence of 2% halothane, a paroxysmal depolarization shift-like activity was seen in VD4 and, despite the presence of these action potentials, the postsynaptic response was blocked. Wash-out of the anesthetic allowed recovery of both the firing of VD4 and the normal postsynaptic inhibitory response, an important observation in anesthetic studies *in vitro*. (c) VD4 contains a cocktail of RF amides and its postsynaptic actions can be mimicked by the molluscan peptide FMRF amide in both excitatory and inhibitory synapses. Halothane 1% enhanced the amplitude and duration of the inhibitory response of FMRF amide (10μmol/L), applied exogenously by a puffer pipette, and substantially reduced the excitatory response. The response returned to control values following wash-out of the anesthetic. Addition of FMR amide is indicated by A in the sequence of a–f. PEA$_I$ = inhibitory; PEA$_E$ = exhibitory.

required for surgical procedures. Recent evidence suggests that the hypnotic effect of anesthetics is caused by actions in the brain, while actions at the spinal cord prevent movement in response to surgical stimulation.

It is now well accepted that, unlike local anesthetics, general anesthetics at concentrations achieved clinically do not markedly affect conduction of electrical impulses along nerve axons. Attention has consequently focused on synaptic transmission. It is clear that anesthetics diminish many types of excitatory chemical synaptic transmission and facilitiate inhibitory synaptic transmission, although their precise pre- and postsynaptic actions have yet to be clearly determined. Given the complexity of the mammalian nervous system, slices of the brain and spinal cord are tending to yield the valuable evidence in this area, as are invertebrate preparations (Fig. 22.1).

HOW DO GENERAL ANESTHETICS AFFECT MEMBRANES?

General anesthetics may affect membranes by perturbation of the lipid component of the membrane or by binding directly to membrane proteins. The classic view proposed by Meyer and Overton at the beginning of the 20th century was that anesthetics had a lipid site of action. This theory was based on the linear relationships of anesthetic potency to lipid solubility. The reversal of anesthesia in animals exposed to high atmospheric pressures led to the suggestion that anesthetics enter the cell membrane and cause expansion of the lipid component; high pressure would compress the membrane, thereby reducing the effects of the anesthetics. Further work, however, suggested that rather than reversing the depressant effects of anesthetics, high

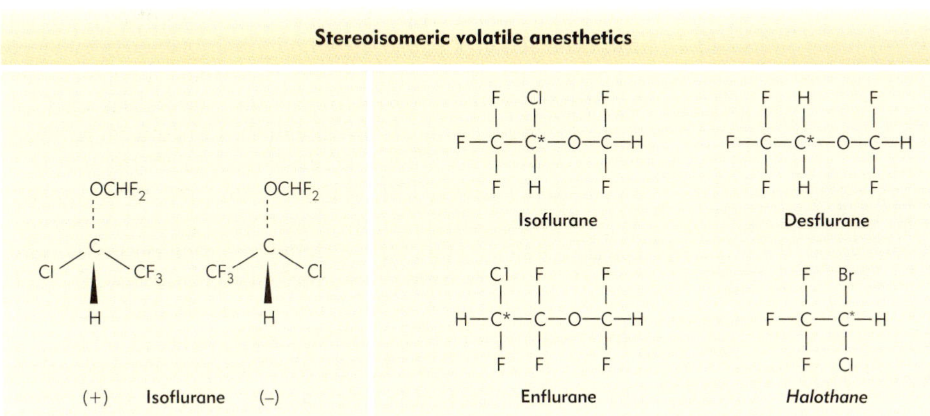

Figure 22.2 Some stereoisomeric volatile anesthetics. Stereoisomers of isoflurane and chiral centers (*) of isoflurane, desflurane, enflurane, and halothane.

pressure increases the excitatory pathways in the brain and, thus, produces a physiologic rather than a pharmacologic reversal of anesthesia (see Chapter 24). A further argument against a lipid site of action has come from the study of cyclobutanes and long-chain hydrocarbons, which, from their lipid solubility, might be predicted to be anesthetic but which actually are not complete anesthetics (they can produce amnesia but not immobility).

To support the notion that general anesthetics may act by binding to proteins directly, it is necessary to demonstrate that anesthetics can indeed bind to soluble proteins in a lipid-free environment. This has been demonstrated for hemoglobin, albumin, and luciferases (which are light-emitting proteins produced, for example, by fireflies).

Drug molecules are three-dimensional structures and many exist as stereoisomers (see Chapter 1 and Fig. 22.2). The different spatial organization of atoms around the chiral center affects the three-dimensional structure of the molecule. In addition, the electron field distribution around the molecule is altered and this influences its ability to form hydrogen bonds and van der Waals interactions. As hydrogen and van der Waals bonds are of crucial importance in the reaction of a drug with a protein, which is itself composed of chiral amino acids, it is anticipated that if the drug–protein interaction is responsible for the effect of the drug then the two stereoisomers of that drug would have differing efficacy and/or potency. The effects of stereoisomers of barbiturates and isoflurane have been studied by several groups. Stereoselectivity for their actions at the γ-aminobutyric acid type A ($GABA_A$) receptor has been reported. However, differential anesthetic effects of the stereoisomers of isoflurane have not been consistently demonstrated (see Chapter 24).

It is now realized that the lipid membrane of cells has a far more complex structure than previously thought. The bilayer structure is well known, but interface interactions are now considered to be of crucial importance, including that between the outermost and innermost parts of the membrane and those between the membrane and the extracellular and intracellular aqueous solutions in contact with it. The interaction of the lipid with the water-based solution results in solubility characteristics for the interfacial parts of the cell membrane that are quite different to those of the central portion of the cell membrane, which is sandwiched by the outer and inner interfacial parts. Biophysical studies demonstrate that anesthetic drug molecules dissolve preferentially in the interfacial parts of the lipid membrane, with much less solubility in the central part of the membrane (Fig. 22.3). This preferential solubility for the interfacial region of the cell membrane is not found with compounds that would be expected to be anesthetic from the simple Meyer–Overton hypothesis, although, in fact, are not. The presence of anesthetic molecules in these regions of the membrane is thought to induce intense lateral pressure within the outermost and innermost parts of the membrane. It has been predicted that this pressure is able to distort the structure of proteins within the membrane, such as ion channel subunits (Fig. 22.3).

EFFECTS OF ANESTHETICS ON MEMBRANE ION CHANNELS

Ligand-gated ion channels

The ligand-gated ion channel superfamily, including the inhibitory $GABA_A$ and glycine receptors, and the nicotinic cholinergic excitatory receptor, has been the focus of much attention in recent years. This followed the discovery that benzodiazepines amplify the Cl^- current at the $GABA_A$ receptor in response to the endogenous neurotransmitter GABA. An increase in Cl^- current hyperpolarizes the cell membrane, which leads to a reduction in excitability of that neuron (see Chapter 5). Barbiturates, etomidate, propofol, and the volatile anesthetics all have a similar effect. Such amplification of an inhibitory system in the CNS is certainly a plausible candidate for the mechanism of anesthetic action of these drugs. Effects of the anesthetics *in vitro* are observed at concentrations that are comparable with concentrations of intravenous agents found clinically and concentrations of volatile anesthetics that, if used as the sole anesthetic agent, would produce anesthesia sufficient to permit only a relatively mild surgical stimulus without invoking movement in response.

Herein lies the problem in proposing that effects on $GABA_A$ receptor Cl^- channels explain the anesthetic action of volatile anesthetics. First, the maximum effect on the $GABA_A$ receptor Cl^- current achievable with volatile anesthetics is about five times less than the maximum effect achievable with pentobarbital (pentobarbitone), but one would expect the greatest effect to be achieved with the drugs that can achieve the greatest depth of anesthesia, that is the volatile agents. The second problem relates to the concentration of volatile anesthetic that achieves maximal amplification of the effect of GABA. For example, the concentration of halothane that achieves maximal effect at $GABA_A$ is equivalent to about 0.85% v/v, while the depth of anesthesia can be increased much beyond the level achievable at that concentration of halothane. Similar results are emerging in the study of the effects of anesthetics on the inhibitory glycine-induced Cl^- current. Such results are consistent with the possibility that inhibitory Cl^- channel current amplification by $GABA_A$ and glycine receptors contributes to

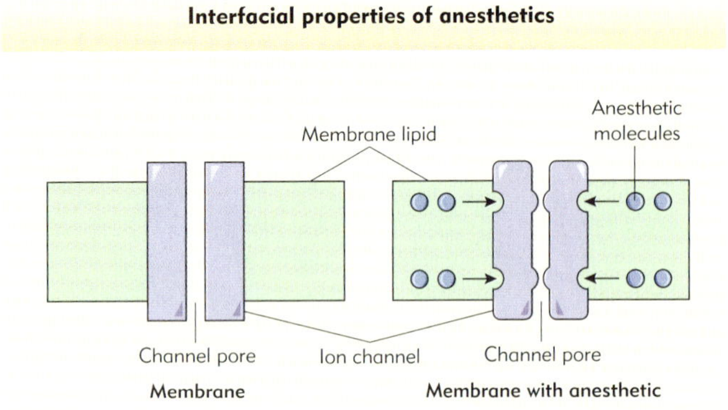

Figure 22.3 Interfacial properties of anesthetics. The solubility of anesthetics in lipid membranes is much greater where the membrane interfaces with an aqueous medium. Sufficient numbers of anesthetic molecules can partition in these regions to, in theory, distort membrane proteins such as ion channels.

the hypnotic effect of general anesthesia, but it seems unlikely that this mechanism contributes greatly to inhibition of the autonomic and movement responses to surgical stimulation. The actions of barbiturates and isoflurane on $GABA_A$ receptor-mediated Cl^- currents are stereoselective. The idea that $GABA_A$ receptor-mediated effects may only contribute partially to anesthesia may explain the inconsistency in results obtained on the potencies of stereoisomers of isoflurane in inducing anesthesia in whole animals.

Depressant effects of volatile anesthetic drugs have also been demonstrated on excitatory ligand-gated ion channels. The effects on CNS nicotinic cholinergic channels suggest that these are possibly the most sensitive channels to the effects of anesthetics. These effects and those on glutamate receptors are discussed further below in the section on presynaptic versus postsynaptic actions of anesthetics.

Peptide receptors

Until recently, little research had been carried out on the actions of general anesthetics on peptidergic synapses. At identified, reconstructed molluscan synapses, inhibitory responses to the octapeptide FMRF amide are enhanced by halothane (1%) even though transmitter release is blocked (see Fig. 22.1c). This is in line with findings on conventional transmitter systems in which inhibition is enhanced. However, at other peptidergic synapses, the inhibitory effect of met-enkephalin is irreversibly abolished and replaced with a novel excitatory response that only appears in the presence of halothane. Therefore, postsynaptic peptide receptors are substantially modified by halothane at clinical concentrations.

Voltage-gated ion channels

Investigation of the effects of general anesthetics on voltage-gated ion channels has focused on Ca^{2+}, Na^+, and K^+ channels. Volatile and barbiturate anesthetics abolish the Ca^{2+} components of action potentials of identified neurons of the molluscan brain (Fig. 22.4a), which suggests that Ca^{2+} channels may be sensitive to these anesthetics. However, it should not be assumed that anesthetics always block or partially inactivate channels, since in some of these neurons an anesthetic-induced K^+ current causes hyperpolarization. Some of the observed effects on action potential shape could be explained by enhancement of K^+ currents, which would cause an early action potential repolarization. Effects of volatile anesthetics on Ca^{2+} currents have also been investigated in various mammalian tissue preparations. Studies on cardiac muscle cells demonstrate a dose-dependent reduction in Ca^{2+} currents. Similar results were obtained using various neural cell lines and dorsal root ganglion cells. Some of these studies also demonstrated minimal effects on Na^+ and K^+ channels at clinical doses of volatile anesthetic. However, recent studies of purified or cloned and expressed human Na^+ channels indicate that volatile anesthetics have potent voltage-dependent effects that are enhanced by physiologic membrane potentials.

One problem in determining whether voltage-gated channel effects are relevant to general anesthesia is heterogeneity among the different ion channel subtypes. Isoflurane depresses at least four types of Ca^{2+} current in hippocampal pyramidal cells, three of which were identified as T, L, and N type channels. The fourth type could be the P-type Ca^{2+} channel, but another study has shown these to have a low sensitivity to isoflurane. It seems likely that novel Ca^{2+} channels are involved, possibly the Q and R type or even Ca^{2+} channel subtypes that have yet to be characterized and named (Fig. 22.4b).

The diversity of K^+ channel subtypes may be even greater, and assumptions about the effects of general anesthetics have been made on the basis of studies of very few different types. In this area, anesthesia research is dependent on progress in ion channel neuroscience research. Both volatile and barbiturate anesthetics diminish delayed rectifier, ATP-dependent, and Ca^{2+}-dependent K^+ currents in cultured molluscan neurons (Fig. 22.4c). It is also apparent that there is much variation in Na^+ channel properties between different tissues, which must be considered when evaluating anesthetic effects on Na^+ channels.

The major argument against a role for voltage-gated ion channels in anesthetic action is their relative insensitivity to the depressant effects of anesthetics compared with the effects of anesthetics on ligand-gated ion channels. It is vital to consider both the potency and the efficacy of the drug effects on the different channel types. Furthermore, considerable confusion is apparent in the literature because of a lack of understanding of the difference between quantal and graded dose–response curves.

Volatile anesthetics, on the whole, are more potent in their actions at ligand-gated ion channels compared with voltage-gated ion channels. However, the effects on ligand-gated channels tend to have a ceiling at relatively low concentrations of anesthetic (i.e. their efficacy is low). Within the the major groups of voltage-gated Ca^{2+}, Na^+, and K^+ channels studied so far, volatile anesthetics have increasing depressant effects as anesthetic concentration is increased through the range relevant to clinical anesthesia. In fact, volatile anesthetics at supraclinical concentrations appear to have the potential to inhibit voltage-gated ion channel function completely. We can summarize these findings with the generalization that volatile anesthetics have high-potency but low-efficacy effects on ligand-gated ion channels, whereas they have relatively low-potency and high-efficacy effects on voltage-gated ion channels.

In laboratory experiments, it is standard pharmacologic practice for graded dose–response or concentration–effect curves of drugs to be constructed. In the present context, such relationships have been described, for example, for the depressant effects of volatile anesthetics on Ca^{2+} conductance. In such

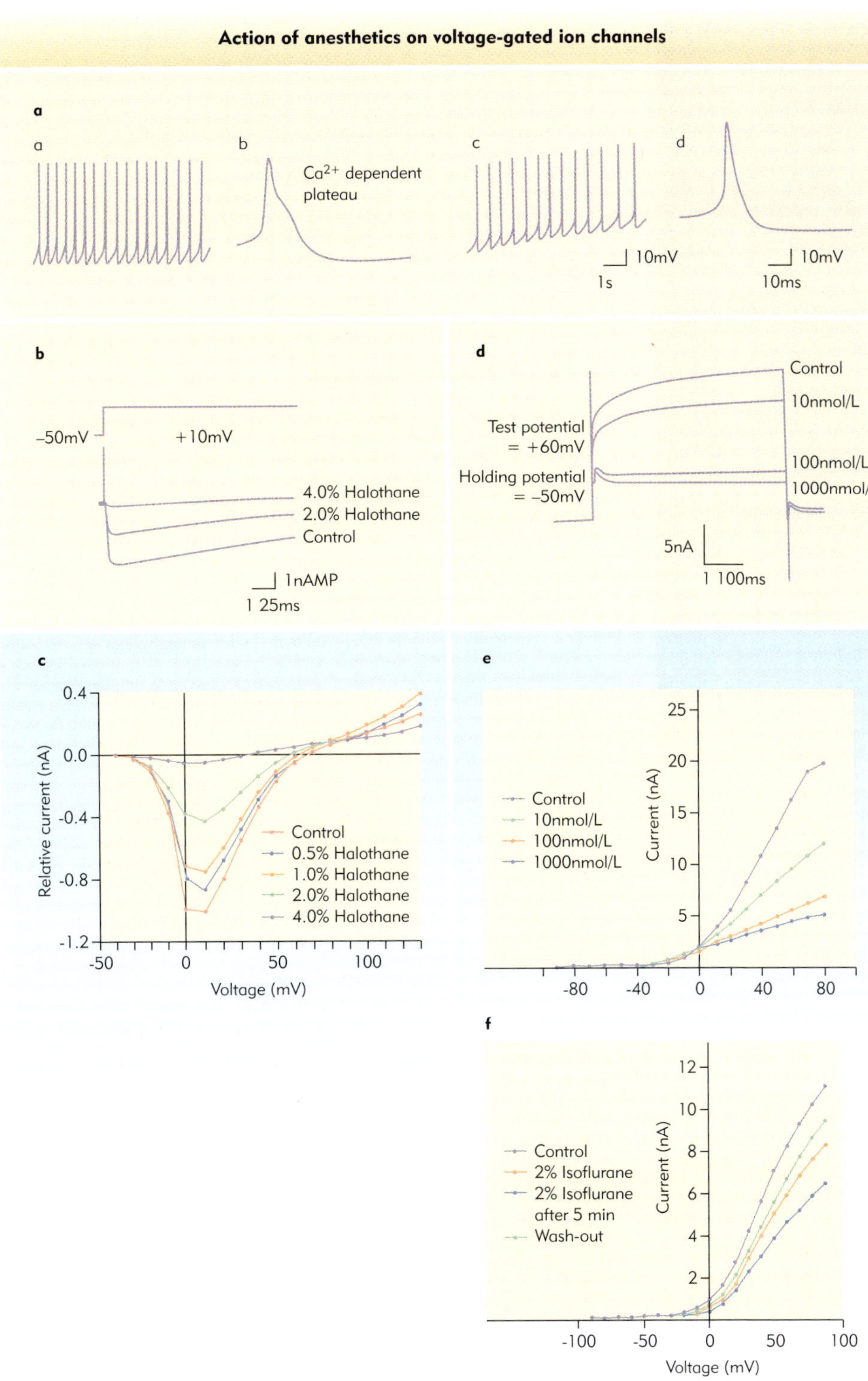

Figure 22.4 Actions of anesthetics on action potentials and voltage-gated Ca^{2+} and K^+ currents. (a) The action potentials of *Lymnaea* nerve cell bodies and nerve terminals often have a Ca^{2+}-dependent plateau associated with the repolarization phase and this increases in width as frequency increases. A train of *Lymnaea* action potentials recorded from an identified cell body grown for 2 days in culture are shown plus a single spike from this spike train. In halothane 1% this cell became quiescent, but a train of spikes at a similar frequency to those in the control solution was generated by a depolarizing ramp stimulus. The spikes had lost their Ca^{2+} plateaus, which demonstrates that the voltage-gated Ca^{2+} current generating the plateau is much more sensitive to the anesthetics than the Na^+ currents generating depolarization or the K^+ currents generating repolarization. (b) Patch-clamp analysis of L-type Ca^{2+} currents in cultured neurons. Halothane decreases currents in a dose-dependent manner. (c) This dose dependency is more clearly demonstrated by the current–voltage relationship of the Ca^{2+} current. (d) Patch-clamp analysis in cultured neurons showed K^+ current reduced in a dose-dependent manner by sodium pentobarbital. (e) The current–voltage relationship for the K^+ current is characteristically different from that for Ca^{2+} currents. (f) The K^+ current is also reduced by isoflurane. It takes several minutes for the maximum effect to occur and it is partially reversible within 5 minutes of wash-out of the anesthetic saline.

experiments, the percentage of the maximal achievable response for the drug is plotted against drug concentration. Such a curve is more difficult to construct when the drug effect under question is clinical anesthesia, because no method of grading the clinical anesthetic response is widely accepted. One of the major difficulties in doing this is that the anesthetic response is intimately dependent on the degree of surgical stimulus.

What has been done to produce a measure of comparative potency of different anesthetics is to use a quantal dose–response curve for a single standardized stimulus. It is with these methods that minimum alveolar concentration (MAC) values have been determined (see Chapter 24). Quantal dose–response curves are produced by determining the proportion of patients who respond to the standard surgical stimulus at each concentration of anesthetic. The nature of these experiments makes it more practical and ethically feasible for the standardized surgical stimulus to be relatively mild. Similar experiments carried out using more

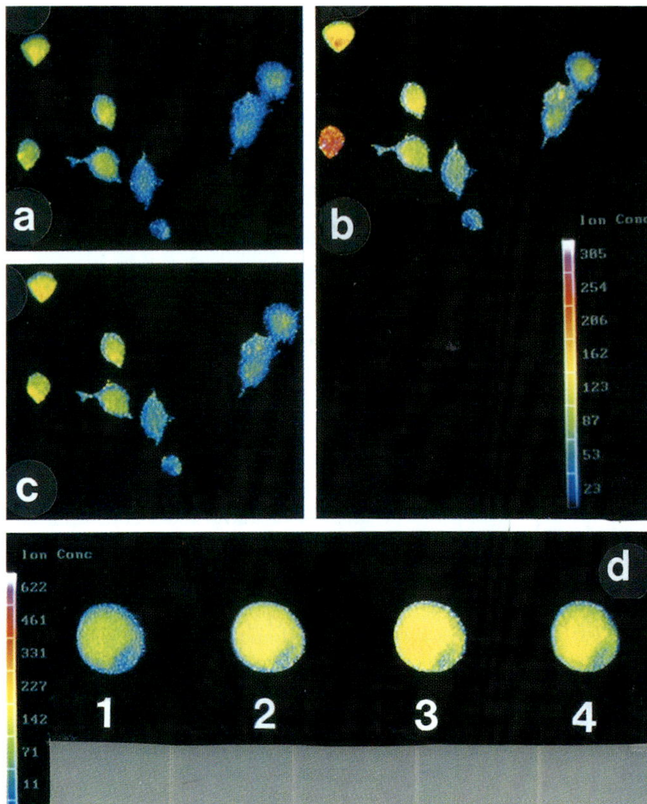

The effects of halothane on intracellular Ca2+ concentration in cultured neurons

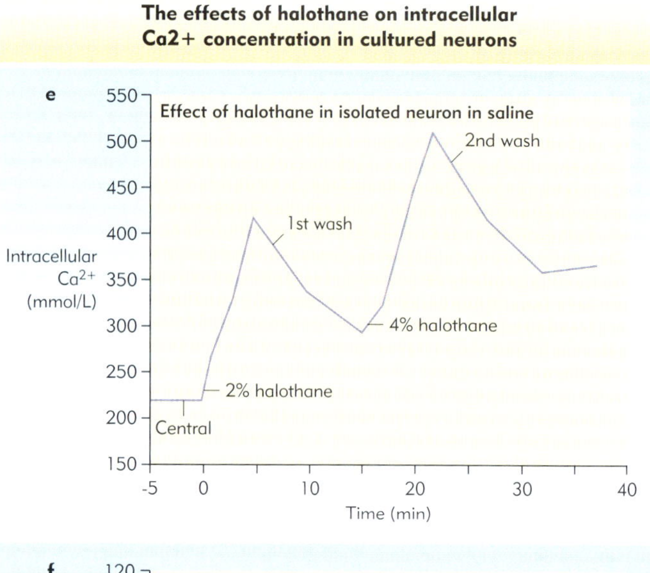

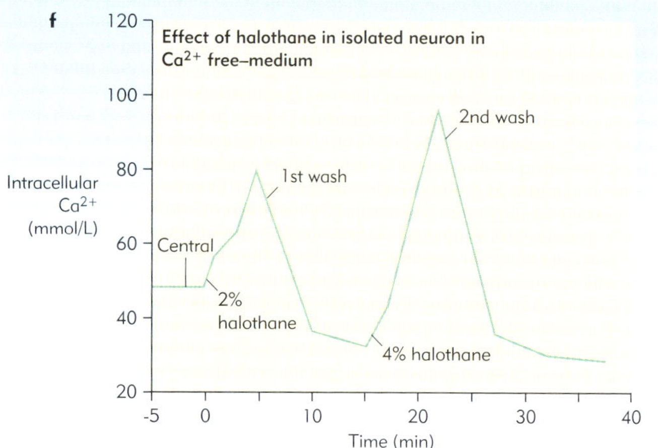

Figure 22.5 The effects of halothane on intracellular Ca^{2+} concentration in cultured neurons. Rat hippocampal neurons (a) before, (b) during, and (c) after exposure to halothane 2%. (d) A single snail neuron is shown at four time points, each separated by a 5-minute interval. Halothane 2% was applied between points 1 and 2, and washed from the preparation between points 2 and 3. (e) The effect of halothane on intracellular Ca^{2+} in the presence and absence of extracellular Ca^{2+}. This indicates that halothane releases Ca^{2+} from intracellular stores. (Part (e) with permission from Winslow et al., 1996.)

noxious stimuli produce very different curves, shifted to the right with increasing severity of stimulus. The slope of these curves is merely an indication of the variability in response to anesthetics between individual subjects. This point is best illustrated by considering the results of these experiments if they were carried out with genetically identical individuals. In this instance, we would anticipate that all the subjects would fail to respond to the stimulus at an identical concentration of anesthetic and the slope of the curve would be infinity. It is, therefore, nonsensical to compare the quantal dose–response curve for anesthesia with graded dose–response curves for the effects of anesthetics on ion channels and use these comparisons as the basis for predicting whether ion channel effects are likely to be clinically relevant or not.

INTRACELLULAR SECOND MESSENGER SYSTEMS

Second messenger, or intracellular signaling, systems are described in detail in Chapter 3. Various second messenger systems are obvious potential targets for anesthetic action, such as the cyclic nucleotides (especially cAMP and cGMP), the inositol trisphosphate system, and intracellular Ca^{2+}. Of these, effects of anesthetics on intracellular Ca^{2+} are the most studied (Fig. 22.5). Volatile anesthetics produce a rise in intracellular Ca^{2+} in various tissues, including neural cell lines, hippocampal cells, hepatocytes, and striated muscle cells, which is probably mediated by a reversible Ca^{2+} efflux from the sarcoplasmic or endoplasmic reticulum. If anesthetics act by increasing intracellular Ca^{2+}, it is logical to suppose that the increase should be maintained in the continuing presence of the drug. Not all of these studies demonstrate this characteristic, but experiments using molluscan and mammalian neurons in culture suggest that halothane, at least, produces an increase in intracellular Ca^{2+} at clinically relevant concentrations (Fig. 22.5). General anesthetics have also been found to potentiate protein kinase C activation and to inhibit the cGMP/nitric oxide pathway (see Chapter 3).

PRESYNAPTIC VERSUS POSTSYNAPTIC ACTIONS

Of the various potential sites for anesthetic effects, most could be relevant either to a presynaptic or postsynaptic action (Fig. 22.6). Research has tended to focus on postsynaptic receptors and their corresponding ion channels (e.g. see Fig. 22.1), but this is more a reflection of the relative difficulty of investigating presynaptic mechanisms than anything else. A reduction in release of neurotransmitter from the presynaptic terminal, as

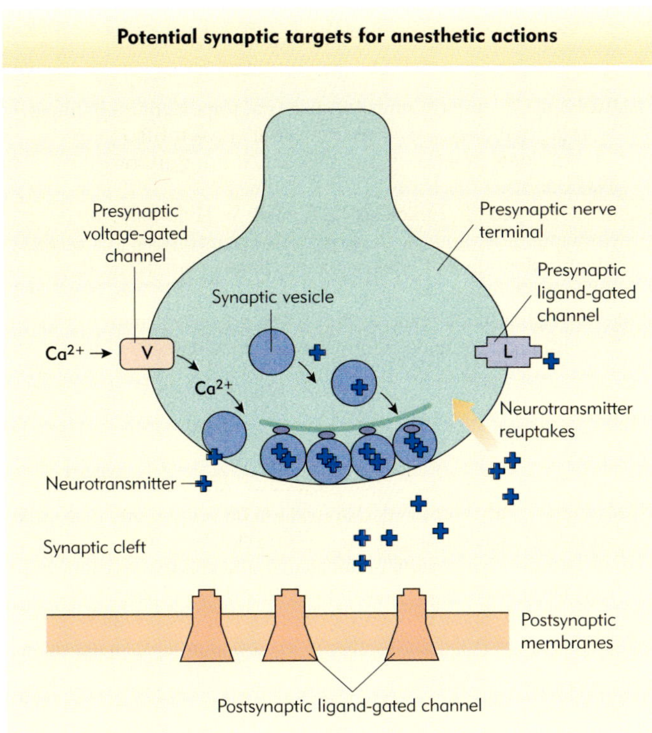

Figure 22.6 Potential synaptic targets for anesthetic actions.

shown in Figure 22.1b, would seem an obvious mechanism by which anesthetic drugs have their actions. This could be mediated by prevention of terminal depolarization by Na^+ channel inhibition, by inhibition of Ca^{2+} influx by blocking presynaptic voltage-gated Ca^{2+} channels, or by activation of K^+ channels (K^+ current is responsible for repolarization and termination of the opening of presynaptic voltage-activated Ca^{2+} channels). Anesthetics could also act by reducing the effect of Ca^{2+} that has entered the presynaptic terminal (e.g. by altering the affinity of Ca^{2+} for its effector protein or by some other action on the manufacture, storage, or processing of neurotransmitter in synaptic vesicles). Alternatively, or in addition, actions on other presynaptic ion channels, which include both ligand-gated and voltage-gated channels or receptors, could modulate the release of neurotransmitter. For example, barbiturates, propofol, halothane, and isoflurane inhibit glutamate release from nerve terminal preparations through a mechanism that appears to involve voltage-gated Na^+ channels. The presynaptic membrane could also be the location of neuronal nicotinic cholinergic receptors, which have been shown to be inhibited by some anesthetic drugs (ketamine, propofol). Finally, reuptake of neurotransmitter into the presynaptic terminal could be influenced by anesthetics; volatile anesthetics may increase glutamate uptake in mammalian nerve terminal preparations.

CONCLUSIONS

It is difficult to explain the anesthetic actions of drugs that can be used as sole anesthetic agents by implying a single, common target site of action. Rather, most studies support a multiple-site and agent-specific basis for general anesthetic effects. We provide here an outline of potential target sites and an account of some theories of the mechanisms that underlie the anesthetic effects. The ability to draw firm conclusions is limited by our knowledge of the functioning of the brain, by the technical difficulties associated with the laboratory use of volatile anesthetics, and by a lack of studies that attempt to relate drug effects observed at subcellular levels to effects on single synapses, single neurons, simple neuronal networks, more complex neuronal networks, and finally intact animal models. It is possible that several of the effects of anesthetic drugs outlined in this chapter contribute to anesthetic action. For example, it could be that the hypnotic and 'light' anesthetic effects arise predominantly through increased inhibitory actions in the brain, such as by increasing the Cl^- currents induced by $GABA_A$ and glycine receptors postsynaptically. 'Deeper' anesthesia, and specifically inhibition of motor responses and depression of autonomic responses to noxious stimuli, might depend on a general reduction in excitatory mechanisms, perhaps through presynaptic effects on voltage-gated ion channels. These latter effects may occur in both the brain and the spinal cord.

Key References

Franks NP, Lieb WR. Stereospecific effects of inhalational general anesthetic optical isomers on nerve ion channels. Science. 1991;254:427–30.

Jones MV, Brooks PA, Harrison NL. Enhancement of γ-aminobutyric acid-activated Cl^- currents in cultured rat hippocampal neurones by three volatile anaesthetics. J Physiol. 1992;449:279–93.

Mody I, Tanelian DL, Maciver MB. Halothane enhances tonic neuronal inhibition by elevating intracellular calcium. Brain Res. 1991;538:319–23.

Prys-Roberts C. A philosophy of anesthesia; some definitions and a working hypothesis. In: Prys-Roberts C, Brown BR Jr, eds. International practice of anesthesia. Oxford: Butterworth-Heinemann; 1996:1/4/1–14.

Spencer GE, Syed NI, Lukowiak K, Winlow W. Halothane affects both inhibitory and excitatory synaptic transmission at a single identified molluscan synapse, *in vivo* and *in vitro*. Brain Res. 1996;714:38–48.

Study RE. Isoflurane inhibits multiple voltage-gated calcium currents in hippocampal pyramidal neurons. Anesthesiology. 1994;81:104–16.

Further Reading

Franks NP, Lieb WR. Molecular and cellular mechanisms of general anaesthesia. Nature. 1994;367:607–14.

Krnjevic K. Cellular and synaptic actions of general anaesthetics. Gen Pharmacol. 1992;23:965–76.

Moody EJ, Harris BD, Skolnick P. The potential for safer anaesthesia using stereoselective anaesthetics. Trends Pharmacol Sci. 1994;15:387–91.

Prys-Roberts C, Strunin L, eds. Symposium on cellular and molecular aspects of anaesthesia. Br J Anaesth. 1993;71:1–163.

Various authors. Symposium on molecular and cellular mechanisms of general anesthesia. Toxicol Lett. 1998;100/101:1–470

Winlow W, Yar T, Spencer T, Girdlestone D, Hancox J. Differential effects of general anaesthetics on identified molluscan neurones *in situ* and in culture. Gen Pharmacol. 1992;23:985–92.

Chapter 23 Intravenous anesthetic agents

Hugh C Hemmings Jr

Topics covered in this chapter

Barbiturates
Propofol
Etomidate
Ketamine
Neurosteroids
Hypnotics

Induction of general anesthesia by the administration of intravenous agents is usually employed regardless of the technique used for maintenance of anesthesia; it can be combined with inhalation, opioid, balanced, or total intravenous anesthesia (TIVA). This chapter covers the intravenous anesthetic agents that are primarily used for the induction of general anesthesia. Other uses of intravenous anesthetics include maintenance of general anesthesia, conscious sedation (defined as minimally depressed level of consciousness with continuous retention of spontaneous airway control and verbal responsiveness), and brain protection.

Appropriate use of intravenous anesthetics requires an understanding of their pharmacokinetic (Chapter 7) and pharmacodynamic properties. Elimination half-time ($t_{1/2}$), a useful clinical parameter, is directly proportional to the volume of distribution (V_d) and inversely proportional to the clearance (Cl); it is approximately $0.693V_d$ /Cl. Many intravenous anesthetics have very large volumes of distribution at steady state (V_{dss}>100L) because of high tissue:plasma partition coefficients and/or protein binding, which are reflected in a large apparent compartment volume. The potency of intravenous anesthetics has been defined as the plasma concentration required to prevent a response in 50% of subjects (Cp_{50}) to a specific stimulus, analogous to the use of the minimum alveolar concentration (MAC) to prevent a response in 50% of subjects for potent volatile anesthetics (Chapter 24). Computer-controlled drug infusion systems are being developed 'based on derived pharmacokinetic models' to allow targeting of blood concentration more effectively (target controlled infusion; TCI).

There is no ideal intravenous anesthetic agent. The ideal agent would be water-soluble, stable, nonirritating, rapid in onset, short-acting with inactive and nontoxic metabolites, and lacking excitatory effects, cardiorespiratory depression, histamine release, neuromuscular-blocking effects, or hypersensitivity reactions. A variety of drugs of diverse molecular structure are available with differing pharmacologic profiles and side effects. Appropriate drugs are selected based on the anesthetic goals for each individual patient, which are dictated by the procedure to be performed and the pathophysiologic state of the patient.

BARBITURATES

Chemistry and formulation

The barbiturates are weak acids and are poorly soluble in water. The most commonly used barbiturates, which include thiopental (thiopentone), thiamylal (thioseconal), and methohexital (methohexitone) (Fig. 23.1), are formulated as racemic mixtures of their water-soluble sodium salts. Sodium carbonate is included to maintain an alkaline pH of 10–11, which prevents precipitation of the free acids through acidification by atmospheric carbon dioxide. The alkalinity of these solutions can result in severe tissue damage if they are injected extravascularly or intra-arterially. They will also induce precipitation of drugs that are weak bases, such as pancuronium, vecuronium, lidocaine (lignocaine), and morphine sulfate. As acidic lipophilic compounds, most barbiturates bind to plasma albumin.

The barbiturates are broadly classified as thiobarbiturates (sulfur at C2: thiopental, thiamylal) and oxybarbiturates (oxygen at C2: methohexital). Substitution of sulfur for oxygen at C2 increases lipophilicity, which results in increased potency, a more rapid onset, and a shorter duration of action [compare pentobarbital (pentobarbitone) with thiopental, its thio-analog]. Alkylation of N1 also increases lipophilicity and thereby speeds onset, but it also increases excitatory side effects, such as spontaneous involuntary movements (e.g. as seen with methohexital, a methylated oxybarbiturate). The L-isomers of thiopental and thiamylal are more than twice as potent as the D-isomers as anesthetics, although both are used as racemic mixtures. Methohexital has two asymmetric carbons, yielding four enantiomers, and is marketed as a racemic mixture of the two α-enantiomers. The β-enantiomers are proconvulsant.

Pharmacokinetics

The short duration of action of thiopental, thiamylal, and methohexital can be explained by their pharmacokinetic behavior. Following rapid bolus intravenous administration, these agents distribute rapidly within the intravascular space and to the highly perfused (vessel-rich) tissues, such as the brain (Fig. 23.2), resulting in induction of anesthesia within one arm–brain circulation time or about 60 seconds, depending on

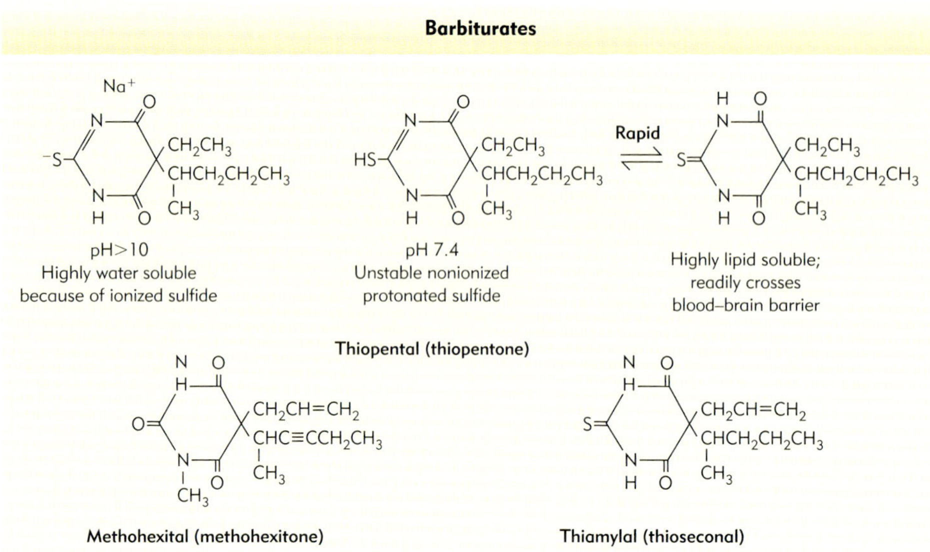

Figure 23.1 Chemical structures of intravenous barbiturates. The water-soluble sodium salts are formed by association of Na^+ with an unstable structural isomer (tautomer) in alkaline solution, as illustrated for thiopental. At physiologic pH (7.4), the sulfide is protonated, forming an unstable un-ionized structure that rapidly isomerizes to form a highly lipid-soluble tautomer that readily crosses the blood–brain barrier. Analogous tautomerism occurs for thiamylal and methohexital.

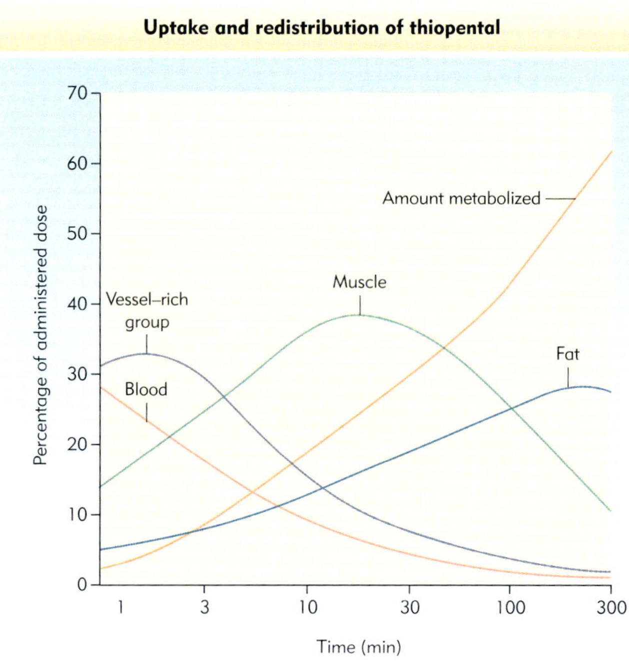

Figure 23.2 Uptake and redistribution of an intravenous bolus of thiopental. The amount of thiopental in the blood rapidly decreases as drug moves from blood to body tissues. The time to peak tissue levels is a direct function of the tissue capacity for barbituate uptake relative to blood flow. Redistribution between tissues and metabolism results in removal of tissue contents. (Modified with permission from Saidman, 1974.)

the cardiac output. Subsequently, thiopental is redistributed to muscle and to a lesser extent to fat. Throughout this period, small but substantial amounts of thiopental are removed by the liver and metabolized. Unlike removal by redistribution to the tissues, this removal is cumulative. The rate of metabolism equals the early rate of removal by fat. The sum of this early removal by fat and metabolism is comparable to the removal by muscle. Data for thiopental and methohexital (Fig. 23.3) indicate that the central V_d values (equivalent to the central compartment) exceed the intravascular volume, consistent with their rapid distribution to brain and other highly perfused tissues. The action of a single bolus injection is terminated primarily by redistribution to the much larger apparent V_{dss}, which includes lean vessel-rich tissues such as muscle. Therefore, the appropriate induction dose should be calculated based on lean body mass. This phenomenon may underlie the increased sensitivity to barbiturates of women and the elderly. The high fat:plasma partition coefficient of the lipophilic barbiturates has little effect on their initial distribution because of the poor perfusion of adipose tissue but provides a large reservoir for delayed drug uptake.

The pharmacokinetic properties of the barbiturates also help to explain the mechanism of delayed recovery observed after large or repeated doses or after prolonged infusions. Their short duration depends on a redistribution mechanism, which is limited by the mass of lean tissue and is easily overwhelmed by a large cumulative dose that saturates this reservoir. The marked prolongation of recovery time with increasing duration of thiopental infusion is reflected in its context-sensitive half-time (Fig. 23.4). At this point, the duration of action is no longer related to the initial redistribution half-time but to the terminal half-time, which is relatively slow given its high V_{dss} and low clearance (Fig. 23.3). Under these conditions of zero-order elimination (rate is constant and independent of plasma concentration), methohexital is eliminated more quickly than thiopental because of its higher clearance (despite a similar V_{dss}). Recovery is also hastened by methohexital's lack of active metabolites. The ultimate elimination of barbiturates, which is very slow relative to drug uptake by lean tissue and makes little contribution to terminating their effects acutely, is primarily through hepatic extraction and metabolism.

Mechanism of action

Electrophysiologic evidence suggests that the anesthetic barbiturates inhibit excitatory synaptic transmission, possibly by blocking postsynaptic glutamate receptors, and facilitate inhibitory synaptic transmission by both enhancing and mimicking γ-aminobutyric acid (GABA)-mediated Cl^- influx at the

Pharmacokinetic properties of intravenous anesthetic agents

	Thiopental	Methohexital (methohexitone)	Propofol	Etomidate	Ketamine
Water solubility	Yes (sodium salt)	Yes (sodium salt)	No	No	Yes
pK_a	7.6	7.9	11	4.2	7.5
Half-time ($t_{1/2}$)					
Initial (min)	8.5	5.6	2	1	16
Intermediate (min)	62	58	50	12	–
Terminal (h)	12	3.9	4.8	5.4	3.0
Volume of distribution (L/kg)	2.4	2.4	4.6	5.4	3.0
Clearance (mL/min per kg)	3.4	11	25	18	19
Protein binding (%)	80	85	98	75	12
Induction dose (mg/kg i.v.) adult	2.5–4.5	1–1.5 (30 p.r.)	1.5–2.5	0.2–0.4 (6–7 p.r.)	0.5–2.0 (4–6 i.m.)
children	5–6	1–2	2–3		
infants	7–8	2–3	3–4.5		
Active metabolites	No	No	No	No	Yes (minimal)

Figure 23.3 Pharmacokinetic properties of intravenous anesthetic agents. Data obtained after a single intravenous dose were analyzed using a three-compartment model for all but ketamine, which were analyzed using a two-compartment model (Modified with permission from Hull, 1989.)

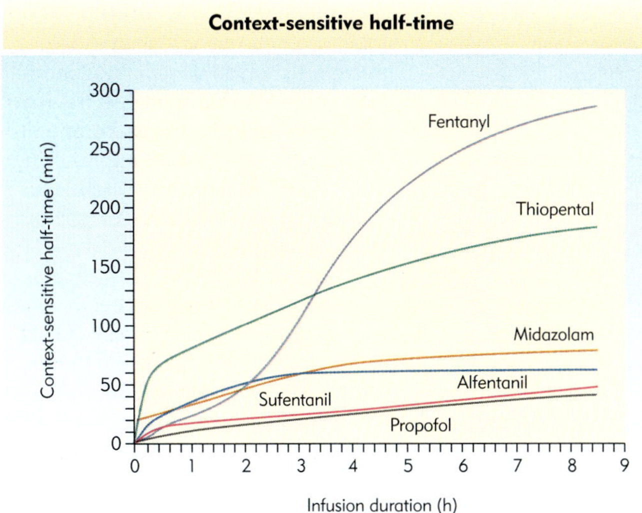

Figure 23.4 Context-sensitive half-times as a function of infusion duration for various drugs used in anesthesia. Context-sensitive half-time is the time required for the central compartment drug concentration to decrease by 50% at the end of infusion as predicted by agent-specific multicompartment pharmacokinetic models, where context refers to the duration of the infusion. This index is more useful in predicting the time course of recovery of many agents than is elimination half-life. Note the early steep increase in context-sensitive half-time for thiopental compared with propofol. (With permission from Hughes, 1992.)

$GABA_A$ receptor (Fig. 23.5). Barbiturates also block voltage-dependent Na^+ channels and can scavenge free radicals, effects that may contribute to their neuroprotective actions. Effects have also been reported at K^+ channels and nicotinic acetylcholine receptors. A variety of pharmacologic evidence suggests that effects at the $GABA_A$ receptor are important for the anesthetic effects of barbiturates.

Clinical use

Until the 1990s, barbiturates were the most popular anesthetic induction agents, a role that is being challenged by propofol, especially in ambulatory anesthesia. Following intravenous injection, thiopental, thiamylal, and methohexital induce anesthesia rapidly and effectively within one arm–brain circulation time (peak effect in approximately 60 seconds), with a duration of 4–8 minutes. Dose requirements are reduced by pharmacodynamic interactions (opioid or benzodiazepine premedication, acute ethanol intoxication), and by pharmacokinetic effects (anemia, malnutrition, uremia, shock, or severe systemic disease). Reduced cardiac output prolongs induction and allows higher peak blood drug levels to develop, which decreases the dose requirement. Thiamylal is slightly more potent than thiopental; methohexital is about 2.7 times more potent than thiopental.

Barbiturates are used by anesthesiologists as anticonvulsants in acute situations; for brain protection during neurosurgery, cardiac valvular surgery or circulatory arrest; and for reduction of intracranial pressure in patients who have intracranial hypertension. The cerebroprotective effect of barbiturates has been attributed to a reduction in cerebral metabolism as a result of a dose-related reduction in neuronal activity. However, recent studies indicate that equivalent reductions in cerebral metabolism by hypothermia are more effective in neuroprotection. Reduced neuronal activity is reflected in a dose-dependent depression of the EEG (Chapter 13 and Fig. 23.6a), which progresses from an awake pattern of alpha activity through high amplitude and low frequency delta and theta activity to burst suppression and subsequently electrical silence (isoelectric EEG; at a thiopental dose of about 4mg/kg body weight per hour), at which point there is a maximal decrease of 55% in the cerebral metabolic rate for oxygen ($CMRO_2$). These EEG changes correlate with serum thiopental concentrations. However, the biphasic nature of the relationship

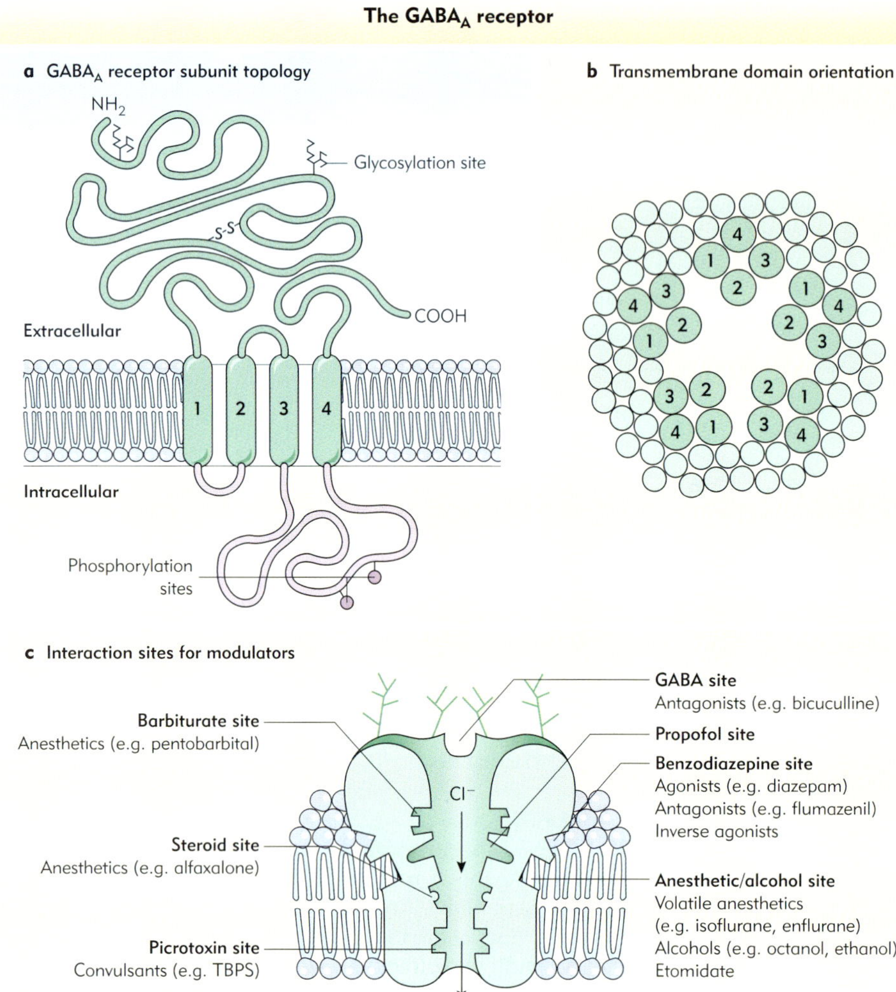

Figure 23.5 The GABA$_A$ receptor. (a) The generic GABA$_A$ receptor subunit has four hydrophobic transmembrane segments that are thought to form amphipathic α-helices. The N-terminal domain contains *N*-glycosylation sites and a conserved cystine bridge; it forms the agonist-binding site. The large intracellular loop undergoes phosphorylation in several isoforms. (b) Plane view of the transmembrane hydrophobic segments showing interactions to form a central ion-conducting pore lined by the second transmembrane domains. The hetero-oligomeric structure consists of five subunits, with each subunit contributing to the ion channel pore. (c) The GABA$_A$ receptor gates an anion channel permeable to Cl^- and HCO_3^-. The general anesthetics are distinguished from the benzodiazepines (which allosterically modulate GABA binding to potentiate GABA responses) by their ability to activate/gate the GABA$_A$ receptor channel directly. A separate site at the interface between the third and fourth transmembrane segments appears to interact with volatile anesthetics, alcohols and etomidate, as demonstrated by site-directed mutagenesis studies.

of EEG frequency to thiopental serum concentration makes EEG inadequate for monitoring depth of anesthesia (Fig. 23.6b).

Although thiopental is a vasodilator *in vitro*, there is a dose-dependent reduction in cerebral blood flow and intracranial pressure *in vivo* that preserves cerebral perfusion pressure despite a reduction in mean arterial pressure. Cerebral blood flow decreases with anesthetic depth until the EEG becomes isoelectric, after which there is no further decrease (up to approximately 50% reduction). The normal coupling between cerebral blood flow and $CMRO_2$ (autoregulation) and arterial partial pressure of carbon dioxide ($PaCO_2$) is not affected. Barbiturates may be useful in reducing temporary *focal* or regional cerebral ischemia by suppressing oxygen consumption in the ischemic zones and by reducing perfusion to normal zones. However, thiopental was ineffective in cerebral resuscitation after *global* ischemia (cardiac arrest) when administered 10–50 minutes after restoration of spontaneous circulation. Vasoconstriction in normal zones as a result of decreased $CMRO_2$ may lead to increased perfusion of ischemic zones ('inverse steal'). By reducing cerebral blood volume, barbiturates can reduce intracranial pressure, although this action may be lost with severe brain injury. Thiopental can reduce intracranial pressure refractory to mannitol or hyperventilation. These properties make the barbiturates particularly useful in neurosurgical patients.

The use of barbiturates administered by continuous infusion for maintenance of anesthesia has been largely supplanted by propofol, which allows for more rapid recovery (see below). However, barbiturates are occasionally used as infusions to treat intracranial hypertension. Continuous infusion of barbiturates leads to drug accumulation, as the lean tissue reservoir for redistribution becomes saturated. Drug elimination from plasma then depends on hepatic metabolism, which is also saturated at high plasma concentrations. Of the barbiturates, methohexital, with a terminal elimination half-time of about 4 hours, is most suitable for continuous infusion; by comparison, thiopental has a terminal elimination half-time of almost 12 hours because of its 30% lower clearance.

Cardiovascular and respiratory effects

The principal hemodynamic effects of barbiturates administered by bolus intravenous injection for induction of anesthesia in healthy, normovolemic patients are transient reductions in systemic arterial pressure and cardiac output and an increase in heart rate, with no change or an increase in systemic vascular resistance (Fig. 23.7). Hypotension results from marked venodilatation, with peripheral pooling of blood and decreased cardiac filling pressures; these reduce cardiac output and arterial pressure. Usual doses of thiopental produce minimal

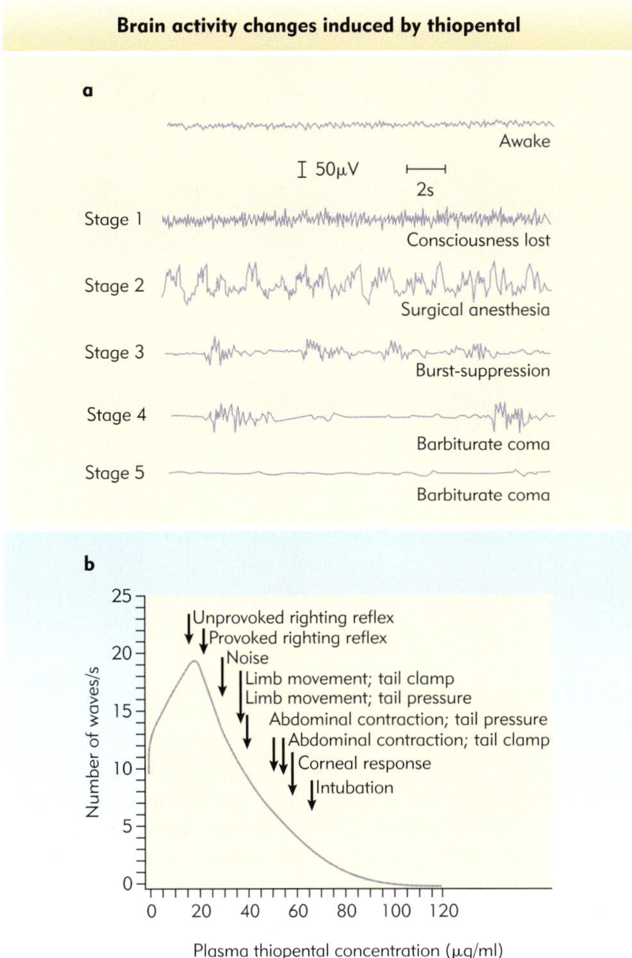

Figure 23.6 Brain activity changes induced by thiopental. (a) EEG shows the changes induced by thiopental. As consciousness is lost in stage 1, there is an increase in frequency and amplitude. Amplitude increases further and frequency is markedly reduced in stage 2, while stage 3 is characterized by bursts of electrical activity interspersed between isoelectric periods (burst-suppression). Progressive prolongation of isoelectric periods ensues through stage 4 until a continuously isoelectric EEG is obtained in stage 5. (b) EEG effect versus pseudosteady-state plasma thiopental concentration in rats. Modeled values required to suppress response to various stimuli are also shown. Note that the EEG returns to baseline frequency at 40μg/ml. The biphasic response has also been shown in humans and confounds efforts to relate clinical effect measures to the EEG. [Modified with permission from (a) Kiersey et al., 1951; (b) Gustafsson et al., 1996.)

myocardial depression, although higher doses reduce contractility. The increased heart rate, which is more marked with methohexital than with thiopental, results from baroreceptor reflex sympathetic stimulation of the heart and may partially mask the negative inotropic effects. Thiopental and thiamylal, but not methohexital, can induce histamine release, which exacerbates their cardiovascular effects.

The hypotensive effects of barbiturates are more pronounced in patients who have treated or untreated hypertension and in conditions in which compensatory mechanisms are impaired, such as hypovolemia, valvular or ischemic heart disease, or shock. The hemodynamic effects of barbiturates can be particularly deleterious in conditions that are worsened by reduced preload or tachycardia, such as myocardial ischemia, congestive heart failure, pericardial tamponade, and valvular heart disease. Barbiturates are not arrhythmogenic but can sensitize the heart to catecholamines (in dogs).

Anesthetic barbiturates are potent central respiratory depressants. They produce dose-dependent decreases in both minute volume and tidal volume; respiratory rate may increase slightly at lower doses but is reduced by higher doses, which lead ultimately to apnea. The medullary center ventilatory responses to both hypercarpnia and hypoxia are depressed. Laryngospasm and, rarely, bronchospasm can occur on induction of anesthesia with the barbiturates, especially with upper airway stimulation by secretions, artificial airways, or laryngoscopy, since laryngeal and tracheal reflexes are not depressed by usual doses. Cough and hiccup are not uncommon, especially with methohexital.

Effects of intravenous induction agents

Function	Thiopental	Propofol	Etomidate	Ketamine
Heart rate	↑	−/↓	−	↑↑
Systemic vascular resistance	−/↓	↓↓	−	−/↑
Cardiac contractility	−/↓	↓	−	↑
Histamine release	↑	−/↑	−	−
Mean arterial pressure	↓	↓↓	−	↑
Respiration	↓↓	↓↓	−/↓	−/↓
Cerebral blood flow	↓	↓	↓	↑
Cerebral metabolic rate of O_2 consumption	↓	↓	↓	↑
Intracranial pressure (ICP)	↓	↓	↓	↑/−
CNS excitation	−/+	+	++	++

Figure 23.7 Cardiovascular, respiratory, and CNS effects of intravenous induction agents.

Other effects

Pain on intravenous injection is rare with thiopental but is more common with methohexital. Venous thrombosis and phlebitis may occur up to several days postoperatively. Intra-arterial or subcutaneous injection can cause tissue irritation or necrosis, depending on the amount and site of injection.

Barbiturates do not acutely affect gastrointestinal or hepatic function. There is a low incidence of postoperative nausea and vomiting. Chronic administration can lead to hepatic enzyme induction, resulting in accelerated metabolism of the barbiturates as well as of other drugs. Stimulation of the mitochondrial enzyme δ-aminolevulinic acid (δ-ALA) reductase, the rate-limiting enzyme in porphyrin biosynthesis, can exacerbate acute intermittent porphyria in susceptible patients; barbiturates are, therefore, contraindicated in porphyria.

Barbiturates can contribute to intraoperative oliguria by reducing renal blood flow and glomerular filtration, an effect that is effectively managed by treating hypotension and providing adequate intravenous fluid. In contrast to etomidate, barbiturates do not suppress adrenocortical stimulation.

Thiopental can be safely used for anesthetic induction for cesarean section; however, doses greater than 8mg/kg may cause neonatal depression as a result of its placental transfer. This effect can be minimized by delivering the baby within 10 minutes of induction. Thiopental has little effect on uterine contractions.

Undesirable CNS effects observed with barbiturates include paradoxic excitement with small doses (possibly owing to central disinhibition or an antalgesic effect, especially in the presence of pain) and involuntary skeletal muscle movements (myoclonus, a central excitatory effect). Methohexital (40–50mg) can trigger seizure foci in susceptible patients, an effect which can be used to advantage in epilepsy surgery and for anesthesia for electroconvulsive therapy. Prolonged neurobehavioral effects can be observed for several hours after induction with large or repeated doses. Significant effects on neuromuscular transmission or skeletal muscle function do not occur with barbiturates. Barbiturates have minimal effects on somatosensory or motor evoked potential, but cause dose-dependent reductions in brain stem auditory evoked potentials.

PROPOFOL

Chemistry and formulation

Propofol (2,6-di-isopropylphenol) is an achiral, lipophilic, sterically hindered alkylated phenol (Fig. 23.8). It is a very weak acid (pK_a=11) that is un-ionized at physiologic pH. It exists as an oil at room temperature and is very insoluble in water. Because of its poor water solubility, propofol is formulated at 1% in an oil/water emulsion containing 10% soy bean oil, 1.2% egg lecithin, and 2.25% glycerol (as an osmotic agent) with a pH of 6–8.5. A previous formulation, in Cremophor EL, was withdrawn owing to anaphylactic reactions. The oil/water emulsion is an excellent medium for microbial growth and care must be taken to avoid contamination and to minimize the time between withdrawal from the ampule and administration (not greater than 6 hours). Recent formulations include the metal chelator ethylenediamine tetraacetic acid (EDTA) or sodium metabisulfite to impede microbial growth. Propofol is extensively bound to plasma albumin.

Pharmacokinetics

Like the intravenous barbiturates, propofol is a rapidly acting intravenous anesthetic that induces anesthesia within one arm–brain circulation time following intravenous injection. Following bolus intravenous injection, plasma concentration decreases rapidly owing to the combined effects of redistribution and elimination. When plasma concentrations are fitted to a three-compartment pharmacokinetic model, the initial and terminal half-times are less than those of thiopental (Fig. 23.3). The V_{dss} of propofol is extremely large compared with that of thiopental. However, in contrast to thiopental, the clearance of propofol is also extremely high and exceeds hepatic blood flow, which suggests extrahepatic metabolism. Propofol is rapidly and completely metabolized by the liver to inactive compounds that are eliminated by the kidney. Despite its hepatic metabolism, the clearance of propofol is not impaired in patients who have cirrhosis. Clearance is also unaffected by renal failure. Although the terminal half-time is long, recovery is rapid since the terminal half-time, which is influenced primarily by the slow elimination from lipophilic tissue compartments (e.g. fat), does not reflect its rapid clearance from the central compartment (i.e. propofol has a short context-sensitive half-time). The high lipophilicity of propofol contributes to its rapid uptake into the brain; redistribution and a very high clearance result in a short duration of action. Children have an increased central compartment volume and clearance rate, which requires a larger induction dose (about 1.5 times) and maintenance infusion rate, respectively.

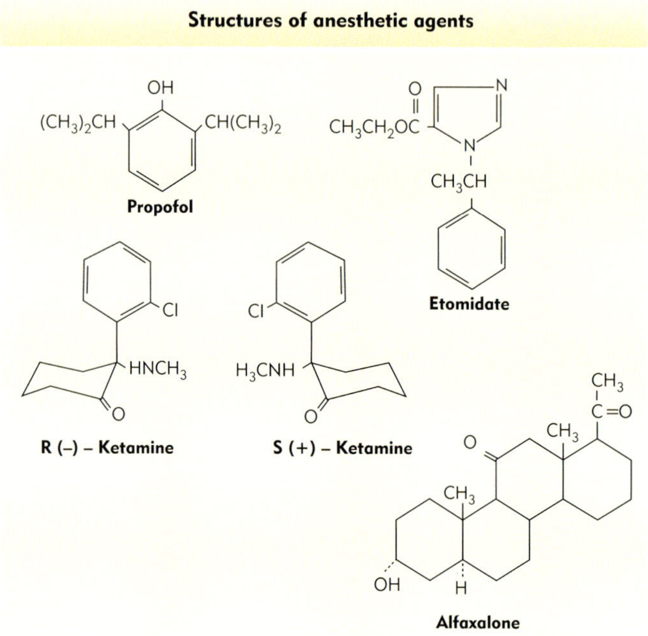

Structures of anesthetic agents

Figure 23.8 Chemical structures of propofol, etomidate, ketamine, and alfaxalone.

Mechanism of action

As is the case with a number of other general anesthetics, propofol facilitates inhibitory synaptic transmission by potentiating and directly gating $GABA_A$ receptors at both spinal and supraspinal synapses (Fig. 23.5). Propofol can also block voltage-dependent Na^+ and Ca^{2+} channels and potentiate glycine receptors, which may also contribute to its CNS effects. In contrast to other anesthetics, propofol appears to have marked subcortical effects, which may underlie some of its atypical actions (see below).

Clinical use

Rapid redistribution and elimination, which result in a rapid return to consciousness with minimal residual effects, and a low incidence of nausea and vomiting make propofol particularly useful for short procedures and ambulatory surgery. The rapid clearance and short context-sensitive half-time of propofol make it useful for maintenance of anesthesia by continuous infusion without significant cumulative effects; plasma concentrations decrease rapidly when the infusion is terminated. Infusion of propofol can be combined with infusions of other short-acting drugs (e.g. remifentanil, alfentanil, sufentanil, mivacurium) for total intravenous anesthesia and is widely used as a sedative technique and as an adjunct to regional anesthesia.

Propofol possesses a number of unique characteristics, including antiemetic and antipruritic properties, that may result from its effects at subcortical sites. Its marked anxiolytic and euphorogenic properties are useful in sedation. Subhypnotic doses of propofol do not cause an increased sensitivity to somatic pain and may even provide analgesia, in contrast to thiopental, which can be antalgesic. Propofol also acts as an anticonvulsant and can be used for treating refractory epilepsy. The rapid titratibility of propofol is very useful for neurosurgical procedures, including awake craniotomy, stereotactic biopsy, and neuroradiology. Propofol exhibits pharmacodynamic synergism with midazolam, fentanyl, or alfentanil in anesthesia induction (hypnotic effect), allowing a reduction in propofol induction dose (Chapter 9).

Cardiovascular and respiratory effects

An intravenous injection of propofol (2mg/kg) in healthy patients decreases arterial blood pressure by 15–40%; reductions in blood pressure are generally greater with propofol than with comparable doses of thiopental (Fig. 23.7). Propofol produces significant reductions in systemic vascular resistance and venous return to the heart, with little or no direct effect on myocardial contractility. The effect of propofol on heart rate is variable, but in general it produces less tachycardia than thiopental. Propofol resets baroreceptor reflex control of heart rate, resulting in an unchanged heart rate despite lower levels of blood pressure compared with baseline. This mechanism may explain the greater hypotensive effect of propofol compared with thiopental. The pressor response to tracheal intubation is less marked with propofol than with the barbiturates. Propofol produces a minimal increase in plasma histamine levels.

The hemodynamic effects of propofol may be magnified in hypovolemic or elderly patients and in patients who have impaired left ventricular function. These patients benefit from a reduced dose of propofol in conjunction with an intravenous opioid or benzodiazepine to reduce the propofol requirement and minimize cardiovascular effects. Patients should be adequately hydrated before induction to minimize hypotension. Propofol is not arrhythmogenic and does not sensitize the heart to catecholamines.

Propofol is a potent respiratory depressant and often produces an apneic period of 30–60 seconds following a normal induction dose. Hiccup, cough, and laryngospasm are less common than with barbiturates, possibly because of greater depression of laryngeal reflexes. Propofol also causes some bronchodilatation, in contrast to thiopental or etomidate, which makes it a useful agent for asthmatic patients.

Other effects

Pain on injection remains a significant problem with intravenous propofol. This may be minimized by using larger veins with a rapid carrier infusion rate, by injecting lidocaine (lignocaine) before or with the propofol emulsion, or by injecting a synthetic opioid before the propofol emulsion. The incidence of venous thrombosis and phlebitis following propofol injection is low.

Propofol does not have adverse gastrointestinal or hepatic effects. Even high doses produce no significant changes in hepatic transaminases, alkaline phosphatase, or bilirubin. Coagulation and fibrinolytic activities are also unaffected. Propofol has significant antiemetic activity, even at subanesthetic doses (10mg i.v.). Propofol is also an effective antipruritic and can be used to relieve pruritus associated with neuraxial opioids. Propofol is more effective in reducing intraocular pressure than thiopental or etomidate.

Propofol has no significant direct effects on renal function and does not interfere with cortisol secretion. If used as a prolonged infusion (days), it can lead to hypertriglyceridemia. As with other intravenous anaesthetics, propofol does not trigger malignant hyperthermia. Propofol does increase δ-ALA reductase activity *in vitro* and is, therefore, potentially porphyrinogenic, but its use has been described in patients who have acute intermittent porphyria without producing a porphyric attack. Propofol has no direct effect on neuromuscular transmission, nor are there significant interactions between propofol and neuromuscular blocking agents. Propofol has been used successfully in pregnancy and obstetrics but may cause neonatal depression after prolonged infusion.

Excitatory phenomena such as tremor, hypertonus, opisthotonos, and spontaneous or dystonic movements can occur with induction or at emergence from anesthesia induced by propofol. Propofol induces dose-related changes in the electroencephalogram (EEG) from increased beta activity with sedation, to increased delta activity with unconsciousness, and burst suppression at higher doses. Propofol does not induce EEG seizure activity in normal patients but can be epileptogenic in patients who have seizure disorders. In fact, propofol has anticonvulsant properties similar to thiopental in animal models. Proconvulsant effects of propofol have not been clearly demonstrated; the majority of apparent propofol-induced 'seizures' are likely to be caused by spontaneous excitatory movements secondary to selective disinhibition of subcortical centers, which may be avoidable by using adequate doses. Propofol can shorten the duration of convulsions following electroconvulsive therapy, which may be a therapeutic disadvantage. Propofol depresses somatosensory and motor evoked potentials but does not appear to affect brain stem auditory evoked potentials (Chapter 13).

Cerebral blood flow (more than $CMRO_2$), $CMRO_2$, and intracranial pressure (normal or elevated) are reduced by propofol. In contrast, propofol causes direct cerebral arterial and venous dilatation *in vitro*. Cerebrovascular reactivity to carbon dioxide and autoregulation are preserved. Its marked potential for reducing mean arterial pressure often results in greater reductions in cerebral perfusion pressure than do other agents. Propofol appears to have cerebral protective properties similar to those of barbiturates. These properties, together with its rapid recovery and antiemetic effect, make propofol a useful drug in neuroanesthesia.

ETOMIDATE

Chemistry and formulation

Etomidate is a carboxylated imidazole derivative that is chemically unrelated to other general anesthetics (see Figs 23.3 & 23.8). It is a weak base that is poorly water soluble and is currently formulated as a hyperosmotic solution in 35% propylene glycol. Etomidate is about 75% bound to both albumin and α_1-acidic glycoprotein in plasma. (*R*)(+)-Etomidate is synthesized and used as a single isomer.

Pharmacokinetics

The onset of unconsciousness following intravenous injection of etomidate is rapid, occurring in one arm–brain circulation time, as a result of its lipophilicity, which facilitates penetration of the blood–brain barrier. Duration is dose dependent but is usually 3–5 minutes with an average dose (0.3mg/kg).

Awakening after a single injection of etomidate is rapid because of the drug's rapid and extensive redistribution to peripheral tissue, which is reflected in a large but variable V_{dss} (see Fig. 23.3). Pharmacokinetic investigations of plasma etomidate concentrations after rapid bolus intravenous injection reveal its rapid distribution (half-time 1 minute) and slower elimination (half-time 5.4 hours). Etomidate is rapidly and essentially completely metabolized in plasma and liver by ester hydrolysis to the inactive carboxylic acid derivative. Etomidate clearance is relatively high (18–24mL/min per kg), similar to propofol clearance. The larger terminal half-time of etomidate compared with propofol results primarily from the larger V_{dss} of etomidate. Although etomidate has been used by continuous infusion without evidence of accumulation, large doses will result in cumulative effects. Limited pharmacokinetic data suggest that in hepatic cirrhosis V_{dss} and terminal half-time are approximately twice normal.

Mechanism of action

The general anesthetic properties of etomidate result from the facilitation of inhibitory synaptic transmission at GABAergic synapses through potentiation of $GABA_A$ receptor function (Fig. 23.5). A single amino acid residue change in the β_3-subunit of the receptor can eliminate the normal allosteric effect of etomidate. (*R*)(+)-Etomidate is much more potent as an anesthetic than (*S*)(–)-etomidate *in vivo* and is also more potent at $GABA_A$ receptors *in vitro*.

Clinical use

A number of troublesome side effects and its cost have limited the widespread use of etomidate as an intravenous induction agent despite its rapid onset and short duration of action. Etomidate has found a niche as an induction agent with less cardiovascular and respiratory depressant actions than thiopental. It is, therefore, particularly useful in the induction of anesthesia in patients who have impaired ventricular function, with cardiac tamponade, or in hypovolemic patients who require emergency surgery in the absence of adequate fluid resuscitation. A short duration of action makes it useful as a sole anesthetic agent in short, painless procedures such as electroconvulsive therapy or cardioversion in patients who have ventricular dysfunction or hypovolemia.

Etomidate has effects on the CNS similar to those of barbiturate anesthetics. Dose-dependent changes occur in the EEG from an awake alpha pattern to delta and theta activity, and changes culminate in burst suppression at doses greater than 0.3mg/kg; in contrast to thiopental, beta activity is not seen initially. Etomidate also decreases $CMRO_2$ (by about 45%) and cerebral blood flow (by about 35%) to a similar extent as thiopental and reduces elevated intracranial pressure without reducing arterial blood pressure or cerebral perfusion pressure, thereby producing an increase in the cerebral oxygen supply/demand ratio. This results from direct vasoconstriction and coupled reductions in $CMRO_2$ and cerebral blood volume. Carbon dioxide reactivity is preserved. These properties make it attractive for use in neurosurgical procedures, where its short duration is advantageous. Although etomidate has anticonvulsant activity, it can also activate seizure foci in patients who have focal seizure disorders, and grand mal seizures can occur. Although this property limits its use in these patients, it may be used to facilitate the identification of seizure foci in patients undergoing resection of epileptogenic tissue.

Cardiovascular and respiratory effects

Etomidate is remarkable for its relative lack of cardiovascular effects (see Fig. 23.7). In normal patients or in patients who have mild cardiovascular disease, etomidate (0.15–0.3mg/kg) has minimal effects on heart rate, stroke volume, cardiac output, and ventricular filling pressures; arterial blood pressure is also minimally affected, although decreases of up to 20% can occur in patients who have valvular heart disease. The hemodynamic stability of etomidate appears to be related to its lack of effects on the sympathetic nervous system and baroreceptor reflex responses. Etomidate produces a smaller change than thiopental or ketamine in the balance of myocardial oxygen supply and demand, and has a twofold lower negative inotropic effect than equianesthetic doses of thiopental. Studies *in vitro* suggest that the negative inotropic effect of etomidate may result from the propylene glycol vehicle and not from etomidate itself. Etomidate does not evoke histamine release and has a low incidence of allergic reactions.

Etomidate causes less respiratory depression than the barbiturates, which makes it a useful induction agent for patients when maintenance of spontaneous ventilation is desirable. Transient apnea may occur, especially in geriatric patients, an effect that may be reduced by premedication. Etomidate does depress the sensitivity of the medullary respiratory center to carbon dioxide, but ventilation is usually greater at a given $PaCO_2$ than with barbiturates. In most patients, minute ventilation and tidal volume are decreased, while respiratory rate is increased.

Other effects

Pain on injection and myoclonus are the most frequent undesirable effects of etomidate. Pain on injection occurs in up to 80% of patients, but its incidence varies with the size and location of the vein used, the vehicle, the speed of injection, and premedication. Use of large veins, a rapid carrier infusion, or opioid premedication decreases the incidence.

Induction of anesthesia with etomidate is accompanied by a high incidence of excitatory phenomena (up to 87% of unpremedicated patients), including spontaneous muscle movement, hypertonus, and myoclonus. Although these effects may resemble seizure activity, they are associated with epileptiform EEG activity in only about 20% of patients. As with propofol, excitatory phenomena probably result from disinhibition of subcortical extrapyramidal pathways. The incidence of myoclonus associated with etomidate is reduced by prior administration of opioids or benzodiazepines. Etomidate causes less depression of evoked potentials than thiopental or propofol. Brain stem auditory evoked responses are unaffected, while somatosensory evoked potentials show minimally increased latency and increased amplitude, which can improve poor signals in procedures that employ this monitor (Chapter 13).

Etomidate administered by single injection or by continuous infusion directly suppresses adrenal cortical function. Although the clinical significance of this effect following single injections is unclear, increased mortality has been observed in critically ill patients receiving long-term etomidate infusions. Etomidate reversibly inhibits the activity of 11β-hydroxylase, a key enzyme in steroid biosynthesis. This effect persists 6–8 hours after an induction dose and is unresponsive to adrenocorticotropic hormone (ACTH). Etomidate has no significant effects on hepatic and renal function. In contrast to other intravenous anesthetics and volatile anesthetics, there is no reduction in renal blood flow.

Nausea and vomiting are more common following induction of anesthesia with etomidate than with other induction agents. Etomidate is potentially porphyrinogenic and should be avoided in patients with porphyria. There are insufficient data to support the use of etomidate in pregnancy and obstetrics. Etomidate is an inhibitor of plasma cholinesterase and may prolong the action of succinylcholine (suxamethonium) in patients who have plasma cholinesterase deficiency; it may also potentiate the action of nondepolarizing neuromuscular blockers.

KETAMINE

Chemistry and formulation

Ketamine is a partially water-soluble arylcyclohexylamine derivative with a pK_a of 7.5 (Figs 23.3 & 23.8). It is currently formulated as a racemic mixture of two enantiomers in aqueous solution with sodium chloride and benzethonium chloride. The (*S*)(+)-enantiomer is three to four times more potent than the (*R*)(–)-enantiomer in producing anesthesia and is associated with fewer psychoactive side effects; it therefore, has a higher therapeutic index. There are no apparent differences between the enantiomers in their cardiovascular effects in humans, although some differences have been detected *in vitro*.

Pharmacokinetics

Following an intravenous injection of ketamine, its plasma concentration shows rapid distribution (half-time 16 minutes) and elimination (half-time 3 hours). Ketamine is extremely lipophilic (5–10 times more lipid soluble than thiopental), which leads to a moderate V_{dss}. As a result of its high lipophilicity and its pK_a near physiologic pH, it is rapidly taken up into the brain and has a fast onset of action. The rapid elimination of ketamine is a result of its high clearance, which is roughly equal to hepatic blood flow. Ketamine is metabolized by hepatic microsomal enzymes by *N*-demethylation (to norketamine) and hydroxylation to derivatives that are glucuronidated and excreted in the urine. Norketamine has significantly less pharmacologic activity than the parent compound but may be clinically significant. The (*S*)(+)-enantiomer is cleared more rapidly than the (*R*)(–)-enantiomer, leading to a shorter duration of action for the same dose. Redistribution from highly perfused tissues to lean tissue is responsible for its short duration of action, which is unaffected by hepatic or renal dysfunction following a single dose. With repeated doses or continuous infusion, cumulative drug effects can occur since ketamine is ultimately dependent on hepatic metabolism for clearance. Chronic administration of ketamine can induce the hepatic enzymes involved in its metabolism, which may lead to tolerance on repeated exposures; pharmacodynamic tolerance may also occur. Ketamine is not extensively bound to plasma proteins.

Mechanism of action

The general anesthetic effects of ketamine result from inhibition of excitatory synaptic transmission by noncompetitive antagonism of the *N*-methyl-D-aspartate (NMDA) receptor, an excitatory ionotropic glutamate receptor subtype (Fig. 23.9; see Chapter 19). Ketamine is relatively selective for inhibition of NMDA receptors, although it also interacts with opioid receptors, muscarinic and nicotinic cholinergic receptors, monoaminergic receptors, and voltage-dependent Ca^{2+} and Na^{+} channels. Its stereoselectivity in producing anesthesia is also observed in its effects at NMDA receptors and at μ and κ opioid receptors. N-methyl-D-aspartate receptor inhibition would be of theoretic benefit in treating glutamate-mediated neurotoxicity. However, ketamine and other noncompetitive NMDA receptor antagonists have neurotoxic effects in several limbic structures when given continuously for several days to rats.

Ketamine may be unique among anesthetics in not producing its effects primarily through interactions with the $GABA_A$ receptor. The anesthetic effects of ketamine also differ from other agents clinically and have been described as 'dissociative anesthesia' because of electroencephalographic evidence of dissociation between the thalamocortical and limbic systems. Electroencephalographic activity in the thalamus and cortex exhibit marked synchronous delta wave bursts, while the ventral hippocampus and amygdala exhibit theta waves characteristic of arousal. Dissociative anesthesia is characterized by intense analgesia, amnesia, and a cataleptic-like state of unresponsiveness with occasional purposeful movements. The analgesic effects of ketamine, which occur at subanesthetic doses, result from inhibition of excitatory glutamatergic transmission at both spinal and supraspinal sites. Ketamine possesses only modest affinity for opioid receptors ($\mu > \delta$ and κ), and its central analgesic effects are not antagonized by naloxone.

Clinical use

Ketamine possesses a number of properties that limit its routine clinical use, although some can be advantageous in specific situations. The psychedelic effects of ketamine, which is structurally similar to phencyclidine (PCP, angel dust), are therapeutically undesirable and a source for potential abuse. Emergence reactions, including excitement, confusion, euphoria, fear, vivid dreaming, and hallucinations, occur most frequently during the first hour of emergence. The incidence of emergence reactions (10–30% in adult patients) is lower in children and elderly patients and with use of the (S)(+)- enantiomer, and can be reduced by coadministration of benzodiazepines with a lower dose of ketamine.

The sympathomimetic properties of ketamine give it an important role in the induction of anesthesia under specific conditions. Ketamine is useful in the rapid induction of anesthesia in hemodynamically unstable patients who have acute hypovolemia, hypotension, cardiomyopathy, constrictive pericarditis, or cardiac tamponade and in patients who have congenital heart disease (with the potential for right-to-left shunting) or bronchospastic disease. Indeed, ketamine may be the agent of choice for rapid induction of anesthesia in patients who have acute asthma or cardiac tamponade. Ketamine is also effective by intramuscular injection and can be used for the induction of anesthesia in children and uncooperative patients without necessitating intravenous access. A unique advantage of ketamine is the ability to administer it by the intravenous, intramuscular, oral, or rectal routes. The efficacy of epidural or intrathecal ketamine is controversial.

Subanesthetic doses of ketamine by intermittent bolus (0.1–0.5mg/kg i.v.) or by continuous infusion (10–20μg/min per kg body weight) can be used to provide intravenous sedation and intense analgesia. These properties are beneficial in short painful procedures (e.g. debridement, dressing changes, skin grafting, closed reduction of bone fractures, biopsies, etc.) and as a supplement to regional anesthesia, both during placement of painful blocks and for inadequate or resolving blocks. Ketamine combined with a benzodiazepine is also useful for sedation of pediatric patients for procedures outside the operating room (e.g.

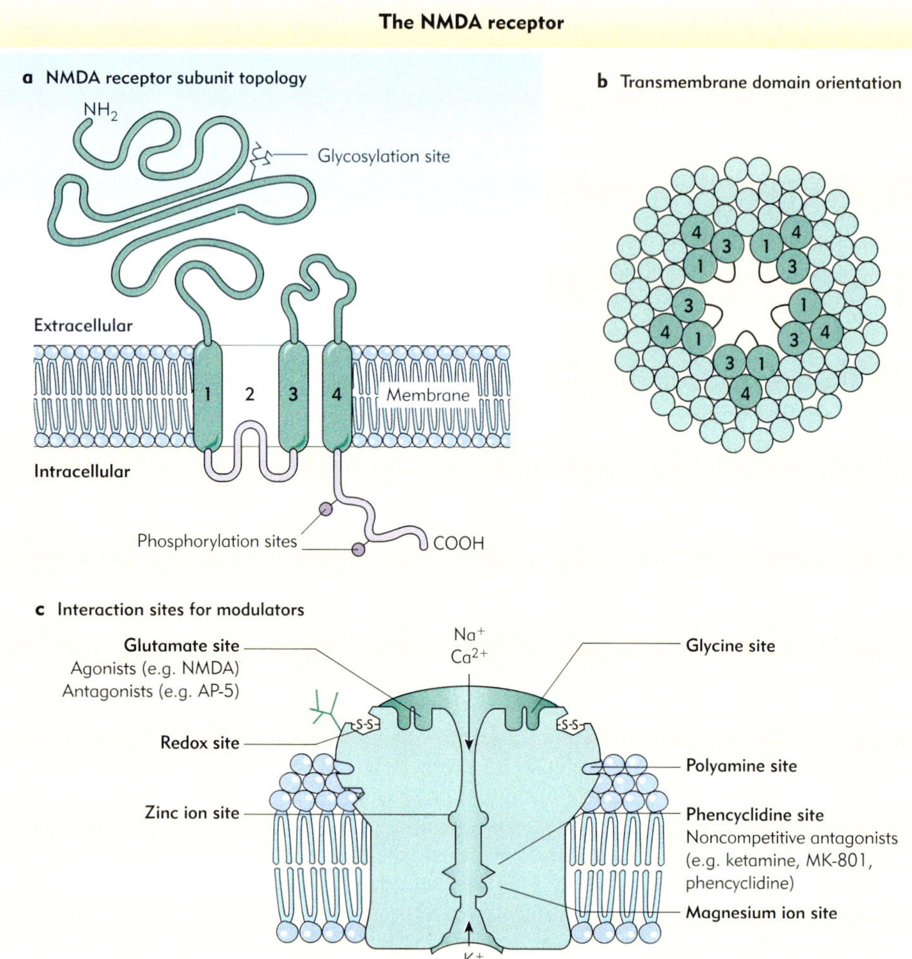

Figure 23.9 The NMDA receptor. (a) The NMDA NR1 receptor has three transmembrane segments and a fourth hydrophobic segment (designated 2) that loops into the membrane without traversing it. Mutation studies suggest that this loop is the putative channel-lining segment and that blockade by dizocilpine (MK-801), phencyclidine, and ketamine occurs through binding to a site that overlaps the Mg^{2+} site in the pore. The C-terminal domain undergoes phosphorylation, which regulates channel activity and mediates interactions with intracellular anchoring proteins. (b) Transmembrane hydrophobic segments interact to form a central ion-conducting pore lined by the second hydrophobic segments. The stoichiometry of the hetero-oligomer is not known but may be four or five (as shown), by analogy with the homologous nicotinic cholinergic receptor. (c) The NMDA receptor gates a cation channel that is permeable to Na^+, Ca^{2+}, and K^+ and is gated by Mg^{2+} in a voltage-dependent fashion. Agonists (glutamate, NMDA) and the coagonist glycine, required for full activation, bind to the extracellular domain.

cardiac catheterization, dressing changes, radiation therapy, diagnostic radiology, etc.). Ketamine has been used in clinical situations requiring high inspired oxygen concentrations (e.g. one-lung anesthesia) and in combination with propofol by infusion with minimal cardiorespiratory depression or psychedelic effects. Despite its disturbing psychoactive properties, ketamine possesses several clinically useful characteristics that promote its use including analgesia, bronchodilatation, and reduced cardiorespiratory depression.

Cardiovascular and respiratory effects

The cardiovascular effects of ketamine result primarily from stimulation of the sympathetic nervous system by a direct effect on the CNS, resulting in tachycardia and hypertension (Fig. 23.7). Ketamine increases A-V conduction time and has a direct myocardial depressant effect; these effects are usually masked by the sympathomimetic effect. In patients who have depletion of catecholamine stores or exhausted sympathetic nervous system compensatory mechanisms (i.e. critically ill patients or patients in shock), ketamine may have significant hypotensive effects. Ketamine inhibits catecholamine reuptake by both neuronal and extraneuronal sites and potentiates norepinephrine (noradrenaline) release from sympathetic ganglia, which may contribute to stimulation of the sympathetic nervous system. Both enantiomers of ketamine are potent m_1 muscarinic receptor antagonists, which may contribute to its tachycardic effects.

The stimulatory cardiovascular effects of ketamine include increases in systemic and pulmonary arterial vascular resistance and pressure, heart rate, cardiac output, myocardial oxygen consumption ($M\dot{V}O_2$), coronary blood flow, and cardiac work. These effects are in contrast to the effects of other anesthetic drugs, which produce either no change or hypotension and myocardial depression. The hemodynamic effects of ketamine are not related to dose and are usually less pronounced following a second dose. The cardiac stimulation produced by ketamine can be blocked by a number of pharmacologic methods including α- and β-adrenoceptor antagonists, clonidine, benzodiazepines, and volatile anesthetics. Ketamine is relatively contraindicated in patients who have coronary artery disease (it increases myocardial work and $M\dot{V}O_2$) or pulmonary hypertension (it increases pulmonary vascular resistance). Equianesthetic doses of the (*S*)(+)-enantiomer may allow for decreased cardiovascular side effects as well as a quicker recovery (because of the reduced dose and more rapid metabolism).

Ketamine does not appreciably depress the ventilatory response to carbon dioxide. Respiratory rate may decrease transiently immediately following induction of anesthesia; apnea rarely occurs following rapid administration. Upper airway reflexes and muscle tone are maintained, which is beneficial during deep sedation. However, ketamine stimulates salivary and tracheobronchial secretions, which can lead to cough and laryngospasm. For this reason, an antisialagogue is recommended in conjunction with ketamine; glycopyrrolate (glyopyrronium) is preferred to atropine or scopolamine (hyoscine) because of its lack of CNS effects.

The bronchodilatory effect of ketamine makes it extremely useful in patients who have reactive airway disease or active bronchospasm. The mechanism of this effect is uncertain but may involve inhibition of catecholamine uptake, anticholinergic effects (muscarinic and/or nicotinic), and/or direct smooth muscle relaxation. Ketamine can stimulate uterine contraction in the first trimester of pregnancy but has variable effects in the third trimester.

Other effects

Ketamine is a potent cerebral vasodilator that increases cerebral blood flow (more than $CMRO_2$), $CMRO_2$, and intracranial pressure in spontaneously breathing patients, which has made it relatively contraindicated in neurosurgical procedures. However, recent studies indicate that the increase in intracranial pressure can be attenuated by controlled ventilation, hypocapnia, or prior administration of diazepam, thiopental or propofol. The cerebrovascular effects appear to be direct. Ketamine also produces mydriasis, nystagmus, and excitatory CNS effects, evident in the development of slow wave theta activity on EEG. However, ketamine does not appear to decrease the seizure threshold in patients who have seizure disorders and has anticonvulsant efficacy in animals. Ketamine in low doses may control neurogenic pain and reverse the 'wind-up' phenomenon (Chapter 21). Ketamine enhances the amplitude of somatosensory evoked potentials but suppresses the amplitudes of auditory and visual evoked potentials.

Ketamine does not impair hepatic or renal function and its elimination is not significantly altered by hepatic or renal dysfunction. It does not evoke histamine release, and allergic reactions are rare, although a transient erythematous rash is not uncommon. Ketamine enhances the action of nondepolarizing neuromuscular blockers possibly by blocking nicotinic receptors. In contrast to phencyclidine, it does not significantly prolong the action of succinylcholine by inhibition of plasma cholinesterase. Ketamine can increase muscle tone but does not trigger malignant hyperthermia.

NEUROSTEROIDS

A number of other compounds with general anesthetic properties have been used as induction agents but are not currently available for clinical use. Of these, the neurosteroid anesthetics are of particular interest. Althesin, a proprietary mixture of alfaxalone (alphaxalone) (the active anesthetic) and alfadone (alphadolone), is poorly soluble in water (Fig. 23.8). A formulation in Cremophor EL was withdrawn from the market because of a high incidence of hypersensitivity reactions. Minaxolone and 2-aminosteroids have been developed as water-soluble steroid anesthetics but are associated with a high incidence of excitatory phenomena. 5β-Pregnenolone (Eltanolone) was under development until recently as an intravenous induction agent. It is a water-insoluble enantiomeric pair and is formulated in a lipid emulsion. Advantages of this agent include minimal hemodynamic side effects, reduced respiratory depression, a short duration of action, and a low incidence of venous irritation. However, involuntary excitatory movements and urticaria are problems. The mechanism of action of steroid anesthetics appears to be through facilitation of $GABA_A$ receptors (see Fig. 23.5).

HYPNOTICS

The natural state of sleep and the induced state of anesthesia share many characteristics, but they are clearly distinct. This is discussed in more detail in Chapter 13. Both are characterized by unconsciousness, impaired thermoregulation, analgesia, amnesia, and atonia. The effects of anesthetics on the EEG vary with the agent (above and Chapter 13) and are dose dependent but can resemble patterns observed in certain stages of sleep (e.g. the spindles observed with barbiturates). Natural sleep is characterized by autonomic variability, while most anesthetics produce autonomic stability, even in the face of painful stimuli.

The most widely used hypnotics (sleep-promoting drugs) are benzodiazepines (Chapter 25) and barbiturates (which are now rarely used), both of which enhance inhibitory GABAergic transmission by modulating $GABA_A$ receptors. The mechanisms of action of paraldehyde and chloral hydrate (which is metabolized to the active compound trichloroethanol) may also involve effects on the $GABA_A$ receptor. Muscarinic cholinergic antagonists (e.g. scopolamine) and antihistamines (e.g. diphenhydramine) also promote sleep. All hypnotics alter the normal sleep cycle to suppress rapid eye movement (REM) and decrease stages III and IV non-REM sleep; they produce tolerance with continued use. Rapid eye movement rebound with intense dreaming and nightmares is common on drug withdrawal. Consequently, hyponotics should only be used over the short term. Opioids also inhibit REM sleep and can cause REM rebound on withdrawal.

Key References

Biebuyck JF. Propofol: a new intravenous anesthetic. Anesthesiology. 1989;71:260–77.

Franks NP, Lieb WR. Molecular and cellular mechanisms of general anesthesia. Nature. 1994;367:607–14.

Hughes MA, Glass PSA, Jacobs JR. Context-sensitive half-time in multicompartment models for anesthetic drugs. Anesthesiology. 1992;76:334–41.

Olsen RW. Barbiturates. Int Anesth Clin. 1988;26:254–61.

Olsen RW, de Lorey TM. GABA and glycine. In: Siegel GJ, Agranoff BW, Albers RW, Fisher SK, Uhler MD, eds. Basic neurochemistry: molecular, cellular and medical aspects, 6th edn. Philadelphia: Lippincott-Raven; 1999:335–46.

Peoples RW, Weight FW. Anesthetic actions on excitatory amino acid receptors. In: Yaksh TL, Lynch C III, Zapol WM, Maze M, Biebuyck JF, Saidman LJ, eds. Anesthesia: biologic foundations. Philadelphia: Lippincott-Raven; 1998:239–58.

Saidman LJ. Uptake, distribution and elimination of barbiturates. In: Eger EJ, ed. Anesthetic uptake and action. Baltimore, MD: Williams & Wilkins; 1974:264–84.

Sear JW. New induction agents. Can J Anaesth. 1997;44:R3–7.

Smith I, White PF, Nathanson M, Gouldson R. Propofol. An update on its clinical use. Anesthesiology. 1994;81:1005–43.

White PF, Way WL, Trevor AJ. Ketamine: its pharmacology and therapeutic uses. Anesthesiology. 1982;56:119–36.

Further Reading

Albanèse J, Arnaud S, Rey M, et al. Ketamine decreases intracranial pressure and electroencephalographic activity in traumatic brain injury patients during propofol sedation. Anesthesiology. 1997;87:1328–34.

Brain Resuscitation Clinical Trial Study Group. Randomized clinical study of thiopental loading in comatose survivors of cardiac arrest. N Engl J Med. 1986;314:397–403.

Borgeat A, Wilder-Smith OHG, Suter PM. The nonhypnotic therapeutic applications of propofol. Anesthesiology. 1994;80:642–56.

Gustafsson LL, Ebling WF, Osaki E, Stanski DR. Quantitation of depth of thiopental anesthesia in the rat. Anesthesiology. 1996;84:415–27.

Hirota K, Lambert DG. Ketamine: its mechanism(s) of action and unusual clinical uses. Br J Anaesth. 1996;77:441–4.

Hull CJ. Pharmacokinetics and pharmacodynamics, with particular reference to intravenous anesthetic agents. In: Nunn JF, Utting JE, Brown Jr BR, eds. General Anesthesia, 5th edn. London: Butterworths; 1989:96–114.

Kiersey DK, Bickford RG, Faulconer A Jr. Electroencephalographic patterns produced by thiopental sodium during surgical operations: description and classification. Br J Anaesth. 1951;23:141–52.

Kohrs R, Durieux ME. Ketamine: teaching an old drug new tricks. Anesh Analg. 1998;87:1186–93.

Lydic R, Biebuyck JF. Sleep neurobiology: relevance for mechanistic studies of anesthesia. Br J Anaesth. 1994;72:506–8.

Nakashima K, Todd MM, Warner DS The relation between cerebral metabolic rate and ischemic depolarization. A comparison of the effects of hypothermia, pentobarbital, and isoflurane. Anesthesiology. 1995;82:1199–208.

Pagel PS, Kampine JP, Schmeling WT, Warltier DC. Ketamine depresses myocardial contractility as evaluated by the preload recruitable stroke work relationship in chronically instrumented dogs with autonomic nervous system blockade. Anesthesiology. 1992;76:564–72.

Reddy RV, Moorthy SS, Dierdorf SF, Deitch RD Jr, Link L. Excitatory effects and electroencephalographic correlation of etomidate, thiopental, methohexital and propofol. Anesth Analg. 1993;77:1008–11.

White PF, Schütter J, Shafer A, et al. Comparative pharmacology of the ketamine isomers. Br J Anaesth. 1985;57:197–203.

Chapter 24 Inhalational anesthetic agents

Eric J Moody

Topics covered in this chapter

Physical properties
Potency determination
Volatile anesthetics
Nitrous oxide
Xenon
Pressure reversal

The first demonstration of general anesthesia with ether, just over 150 years ago, marked the beginning of the modern era of surgery and anesthesia. Since that time, inhalational anesthetics have been the most commonly used agents for general anesthesia and remain the backbone of anesthetic practice.

PHYSICAL PROPERTIES

The term inhalational anesthetic refers to anesthetics administered in a gaseous form. This includes nitrous oxide, a gas at room temperature, and the volatile anesthetics, which exist in liquid form at room temperature (Fig. 24.1).

Lipid solubility

At the turn of the 20th century, it was noted that the potency of general anesthetics correlates with their lipid solubility (Fig. 24.2). This relationship, termed the Meyer–Overton correlation, has been interpreted to mean that general anesthetics act at hydrophobic targets. It holds true for a broad range of compounds and potencies, even when different end points of anesthesia are used. Data from various species also fit the correlation well. Recent findings indicate a closer correlation between anesthetic potency and solubility at the water–membrane interface, consistent with an amphiphilic site of action. A more complete discussion of anesthetic targets is found in the chapter on anesthetic mechanisms (Chapter 22).

Stereoselectivity

The structures of the commonly used volatile anesthetics are shown in Fig. 24.3. Isoflurane, enflurane, desflurane, and halothane have chiral centers and exist as stereoisomers. Some of the actions of the anesthetics are affected by the stereochemistry of the molecule; this stereoselectivity is an important factor in understanding the mechanisms of action of anesthetics. Many

Physical properties of volatile anesthetics

Physical property	Halothane	Isoflurane	Desflurane	Sevoflurane	Enflurane	Nitrous Oxide
MAC [EC_{50}] (% atmosphere)	0.77	1.15	6	2	1.7	110
Blood: gas partition coefficient	2.5	1.43	0.42	0.60	1.82	0.47
Specific gravity (g/ml)	1.87	1.50	1.47	1.50	1.52	NA
Boiling point (°C)	50	48.5	22.8	58.5	56.5	-88.5
Vapor pressure (mmHg, 20°C)	243	238	669	120	175	Gas
Molecular weight (daltons)	197.4	184.5	168	200	184.5	44.0
Metabolism	+++	–	–	++	++	–
Specific toxicity	Hepatitis	–	–	? compound A	Seizures	Bone marrow depression, neuropathy
Degrades in soda lime	–	–	–	+	–	+
Releases fluoride	–	+	–	+	++	+

+ Presence of effect
– No effect

Figure 24.1 Physical properties of the currently used volatile anesthetics.

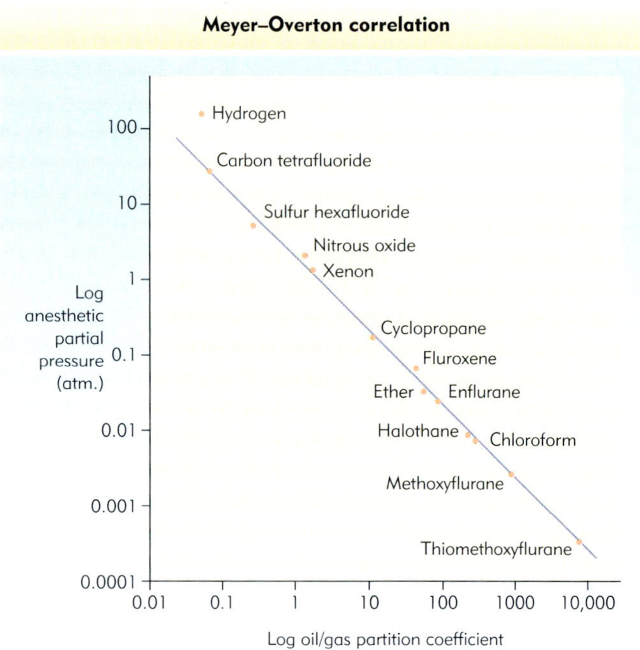

Figure 24.2 Meyer–Overton correlation. Anesthetic potency is robustly correlated with lipid solubility. Note that the axes are log–log, which tends to minimize small variations from the norm.

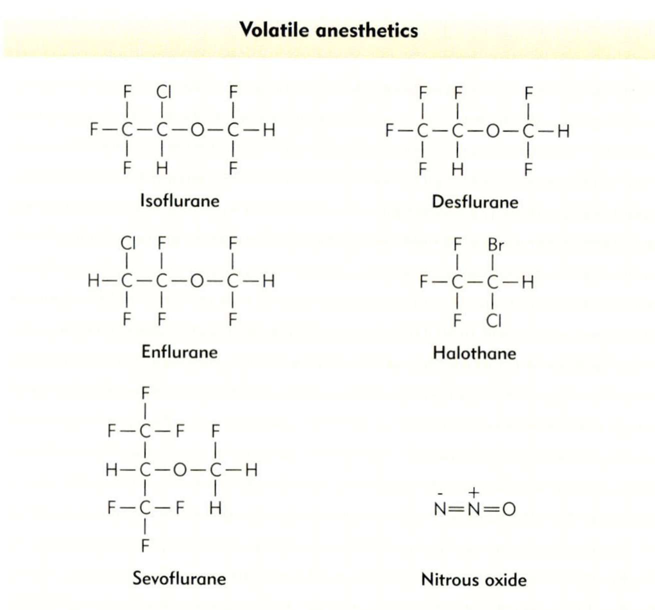

Figure 24.3 Structures of the currently used volatile anesthetics. Isoflurane and enflurane are isomers while desflurane is identical to isoflurane except for a F substituted for the Cl. All three of these compounds as well as halothane have chiral centers and exist as stereoisomers. The clinically used compounds are racemic mixtures of those enantiomers containing equal amounts of each isomer.

organic chemical compounds contain a center of asymmetry (chiral center) where four different chemical groups are attached to the same carbon and can be arranged in two different patterns. The two resulting compounds are identical in all respects except that they are mirror images of each other and rotate polarized light in opposite directions (Chapter 1). Drugs that are produced naturally by enzymes are typically a single stereoisomer, while drugs produced by chemical means are usually an equal mixture of stereoisomers because routine chemical reactions do not distinguish between the two forms. Many drugs in clinical use are single stereoisomers, including the opioids, which are derived from poppy oil and contain a number of chiral centers. The availability of stereoisomers provides the opportunity to determine the specificity of interactions between drugs and their targets or receptors. The presence of stereoselectivity is considered strong evidence of a receptor-mediated event and, indeed, is frequently cited as a requirement for defining a receptor interaction. In the case of opioids, a series of stereoisomers with the opposite chirality to the native molecules have been produced. These compounds are essentially inactive at opioid receptors, indicating that they do not bind to the site where the natural active form acts.

The clinically used volatile anesthetics are chemically produced and are racemic mixtures of enantiomers containing equal amounts of each isomer. The stereoisomers of a number of these drugs have been purified in an effort to determine whether their effects differ. Very limited amounts are available so extensive testing has not been performed. *In vitro* studies indicate that there are differences in potency between the stereoisomers of isoflurane at some, but not all, receptors. In neurochemical and electrophysiologic measures at γ-aminobutyric acid ($GABA_A$) receptors, the (+)-isomer is two to four times more potent than the (–)-isomer, indicating a modest difference between the two forms. The small amounts of drug available limit *in vivo* assays, but two independent groups found that (+)-isoflurane was more active in mice and rats, which is consistent with the *in vitro* studies (Fig. 24.4). These data are consistent with the stereoselective difference seen in neurochemical and electrophysiologic assays and strongly suggest that isoflurane has specific requirements for interacting with its targets. However, a more recent study failed to find evidence of differences in anesthetic potency, but the reasons for these discrepancies may be methodologic.

Partial pressures

Volatile anesthetics are liquids at room temperature and are administered as a gas via vaporizers. Because the partial pressure of these agents increases with temperature, modern vaporizers are temperature compensated to ensure a constant delivery of gas over a range of environmental conditions (Chapter 8). The partial pressure of volatile anesthetics greatly exceeds their anesthetic potency. For example, the vapor pressure of halothane at room temperature is approximately 30% and its minimum alveolar concentration (MAC), a measure of potency, is 0.77%, indicating that delivery of oxygen saturated with halothane would result in a massive overdose. Given the low therapeutic index of halothane (2–4), this would rapidly be lethal. Consequently, most modern vaporizers are of a variable bypass design, which dilutes the saturated vapor with gas that has not been in contact with the liquid anesthetic to achieve the desired concentration. Because of the different vapor pressures of the anesthetics, vaporizers are agent specific and use with agents of a different vapor pressure will result in delivery of concentrations other than those indicated. If two agents are in the same vaporizer, an overdosage will result because each of the agents will be vaporized independently. Similarly, if three agents are in the same vaporizer all three will

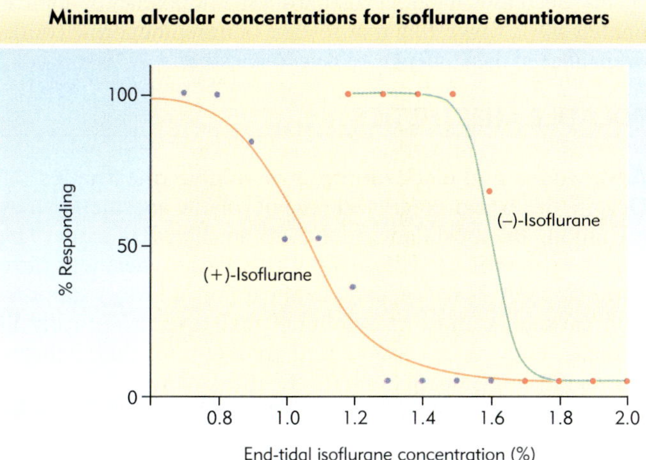

Figure 24.4 The stereoselectivity of isoflurane minimum alveolar concentration (MAC). Anesthetic potency (MAC) was determined in a group of rats in which individual rats were exposed to various concentrations of single enantiomers of isoflurane to determine the points at which they responded. (+)-Isoflurane was more potent (MAC=1.06%) than (−)-isoflurane (MAC=1.62%) or the racemic mixture (MAC=1.32%). (Modified from Lysko et al., 1994.)

be delivered. The use of key-indexed vaporizer filling keys significantly reduces the chances of this sort of error. The current infrared agent analyzers typically in use are not able to distinguish between agents or determine whether more than one agent is present in the exhaled gas.

While volatile anesthetics are poorly soluble in aqueous media, a variety of techniques exist that could create anesthetic solutions or emulsions. In this form, it is theoretically possible to administer them intravenously. If storage and delivery issues are overcome, this might be of value in unusual circumstances (e.g. military or hyperbaric conditions).

POTENCY DETERMINATION

The basic principles of potency and efficacy for drugs are discussed in Chapter 6. The unique pharmacokinetic properties of inhalational agents make the determination of their potency problematic. Thus, the setting of the vaporizer dial and the inspired concentration do not necessarily reflect blood and brain concentration of inhaled drugs, except under equilibrium conditions. In order to compare the potencies of inhalational drugs, the concept of MAC was developed in the 1960s. It is a 50% effective dose (ED_{50}) measurement of potency to produce immobility in response to a painful stimulus under defined conditions. Consequently, fractions or multiples of MAC have no intrinsic meaning without knowledge of the slope of the dose–response curve. It is determined only at equilibrium such that there are no concentration gradients and there is the same partial pressure of anesthetic throughout the body. Minimum alveolar concentration is defined as the partial pressure of anesthetic required to produce lack of response to a painful stimulus in half of a population. In humans, the stimulus is usually surgical incision and the response is termed gross purposeful movement. Dose–response relationships for volatile anesthetics are very steep. Values of MAC show little variation between species of higher vertebrates, suggesting that anesthetic mechanisms are conserved. Figure 24.4 shows a typical dose–response relationship that is used to generate a potency value in a group of animals. Because MAC is determined by anesthetic as partial pressure, it is independent of atmospheric pressure and altitude.

Limitations of minimum alveolar concentration

While MAC has been useful in comparing equally effective concentrations of anesthetics and determining the relative frequency of side effects, it has some limitations. One is in the quantitation of the gross purposeful movement response. This is a quantal response and each subject is scored as either responding or not; there can be discrepancies in determining whether a subject actually responded. However, is a small movement in response to the stimulus really equal to a large movement? Likewise, there are issues raised by the stimulus used. After determining that values obtained for MAC increased with increasing stimulus intensity, the concept of supramaximal stimulus was developed. Briefly stated, further increases in intensity of a painful stimulus after the supramaximal point do not lead to any further decrease in apparent potency. Not surprisingly when different stimulus or experimental paradigms are used to determine anesthetic potency, different values are obtained. In animal studies, tail clamping for rats yields different results than loss of righting reflex, which is more sensitive to anesthetics. Other end points have also been used including responsiveness to commands and lack of hemodynamic response to stimuli. While these have sometimes been referred to by terms such as MAC-awake or MAC-BAR, it may be more appropriate to term them EC_{50} measurements under conditions used in the determination. Importantly, the results obtained from various measures closely correlate with one another, indicating that MAC correlates with physiologically significant phenomena.

Recently, it has been reported that spinal transection does not significantly alter MAC as measured by painful stimuli to the lower extremity. This suggests that this measurement of MAC is determining volatile anesthetic effects on a spinal reflex. While there is abundant evidence that MAC correlates with clinically observed anesthetic potency, it is very likely that MAC is an epiphenomenon that reflects changes in the spinal cord, which are occurring in parallel with changes in consciousness mediated at other unknown supraspinal CNS loci. It is not surprising that different loci in the CNS modulate different aspects of anesthesia; a single site of action is not expected to account for all properties of general anesthetics, and many side effects of these drugs are mediated outside the CNS. For example, the decrease in cardiac contractility produced by volatile anesthetics is attributed to direct actions at the heart and occurs in isolated heart preparations (Chapter 34). Therefore, it is impossible to define the multiple actions of these agents in terms of a single mechanism. The finding that the motor reflexes measured with MAC are independent of forebrain structures has led to the realization that different CNS structures (pathways, receptors, etc.) are responsible for different anesthetic actions (multisite hypothesis). The important question is which general anesthetic actions are relevant to the clinical state of anesthesia; this depends to some extent on the definition of the anesthetic state.

Ablation of consciousness is, of course, a clinically relevant property of anesthetics. The absence of autonomic responses to stimulation while under anesthesia is also an important component of anesthesia. This is sometimes termed the analgesic component of anesthesia and indeed the coadminstration of opioids with inhalational anesthetics is a common practice. Nonetheless, inhalational anesthetics clearly block many hemodynamic responses and are routinely used for this purpose. Viewed on a continuum, consciousness is disrupted at low concentrations, while movement is blocked at MAC and autonomic actions are inhibited in a concentration-dependent fashion over the entire range. At very high concentrations, stress responses can still be detected, implying that there is a ceiling effect for the inhalational anesthetics. The unconsciousness properties of inhalational anesthetics are most relevant to their clinical use, followed by their autonomic blocking actions and their actions on movement.

Advantages of minimum alveolar concentration

MAC is useful in that it provides a means of directly comparing anesthetic potency independent of pharmacokinetic issues. This has allowed determination of the effects of various physiologic states on anesthetic potency and the evaluation of side effects of inhalational anesthetics at equipotent doses rather than at arbitrary concentrations. It has also served as an important tool in drug development as a screening tool and in mechanistic studies. Some alterations in apparent anesthetic potency result from altered pharmacokinetic parameters such as cardiac output, respiratory rate, body fat content, etc. These are not true alterations in anesthetic potency, which must be determined at equilibrium. Generally, states that are characterized by debility result in greater sensitivity to anesthetics. Conversely, states of excitation (pain, stress, hyperthermia) probably result in increased anesthetic requirements. A wide variety of variables have been studied in both humans and animals to determine their effects on MAC as a measure of anesthetic potency. Factors that have no significant effects on MAC include gender, time of day, and metabolic acid–base balance.

Hypoxia results in increased sensitivity to anesthetics, which may be a function of the altered consciousness associated with severe hypoxia. Coadministration of sedative hypnotics, opioids, and other anesthetics also results in reduced volatile anesthetic requirements – a fact routinely utilized in clinical practice. Hypothermia results in a significant decrease in anesthetic requirements, which is also likely to result from the decreased consciousness that results from hypothermia. This is consistent with the clinical observation that recall rarely occurs in patients on hypothermic cardiopulmonary bypass. Hypotension to a mean blood pressure below 40mmHg is also associated with a significant decrease in anesthetic requirement, which may be related to decreased CNS function at reduced perfusion pressures. Increased anesthetic potency is observed in pregnancy; this may relate to the anesthetic properties of circulating progesterone-like steroids. Anesthetic requirement decreases with age (Chapter 8); patients at age 80 years are approximately 20% more sensitive to isoflurane than young adults.

Hyperthermia is associated with increased anesthetic requirements in animal studies. Tolerance to alcohol also causes increased MAC in animal studies, which is likely caused by a downregulation of CNS receptors, since volatile anesthetics are poorly metabolized under most conditions. Tolerance to other sedative hypnotics results in cross-tolerance to volatile anesthetics as well. For example, mice selectively bred for resistance to alcohol demonstrate resistance to intravenous and volatile anesthetics. Administration of ephedrine (but not other adrenergic agents) decreases apparent volatile anesthetic potency by approximately 50%, suggesting that release of norepinephrine (noradrenaline) in the CNS plays a role in anesthesia.

VOLATILE ANESTHETICS

Advantages and disadvantages of volatile anesthetics

Despite the extraordinary wide use of volatile anesthetics, they are among the most dangerous drugs in clinical practice. The therapeutic indices (LD_{50}/ED_{50}) of volatile anesthetics are approximately 2–4. The significant cardiorespiratory suppression caused by these drugs limits their use in critically ill patients. They require specialized apparatus for their delivery and significant training in their safe/effective use.

Despite these limitations, volatile anesthetics enjoy wide usage since there is great clinical experience and comfort with them, albeit gained with several years of training. In addition, there is the widespread availability of end-tidal agent analyzers, which provide on-line values that approximate blood concentrations (Chapter 15). Since these drugs have very little metabolism and are administered via the lungs, the inspired concentration equals the blood and brain concentrations at equilibrium. Even after prolonged periods of anesthesia, a practitioner can be assured that there is not undue accumulation of drug. This is in contrast to intravenous anesthetics, where fixed infusions may lead to much higher or lower blood levels if the infusion does not equal the removal of the drug via redistribution and metabolism. While much is made of the importance of end-tidal measurements of volatile agents, they are nearly unique in that regard. With no other drugs do we have the capability, or feel that we need, continuous measurement of blood concentrations.

Volatile anesthetics also have a particular niche in anesthetic practice in that significant tolerance is rare. Therefore, patients maintained on a background of volatile anesthesia are very unlikely to have recall even if usual signs for determining the level of anesthesia are unavailable. Even with refinements in intravenous anesthesia, induction of anesthesia with volatile anesthetics will be used quite commonly in young children where it is less traumatic than intravenous cannulation. Breathdown inductions will continue to be used occasionally in adults where spontaneous ventilation is needed. Epiglottitis and mediastinal masses, where there is fear of dynamic obstruction of the trachea, are examples.

Cardiovascular effects

Volatile anesthetics are not very potent drugs and have low therapeutic indices. Cardiac toxicity limits their use in compromised patients. Volatile anesthetics decrease blood pressure through suppressing both vascular tone and cardiac contractility. These actions are mediated via distinct mechanisms and individual drugs differ in their relative ratios of cardiac suppression to vasodilation. As in other organ systems, volatile anesthetics have many effects on the heart, which makes identification of pharmacologically relevant actions difficult. There are a number of different Ca^{2+} channels in the heart that mediate aspects of contraction and relaxation (Chapter 34). Figure 24.5 shows the effects of volatile anesthetics on cardiac output. The L-type voltage-dependent Ca^{2+} channel is intimately involved in cardiac contractility and is inhibited by relevant concentrations of volatile anesthetics. Inhibition of L-type Ca^{2+} channels is the most important factor in the negative inotropic effect, but depletion of sarcoplasmic reticulum Ca^{2+} and reduction in myofilament Ca^{2+} sensitivity also contribute, especially for halothane. Of the modern inhaled anesthetics, halothane

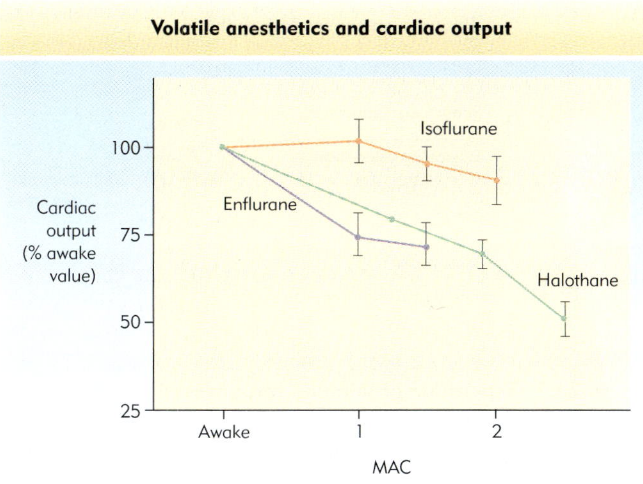

Figure 24.5 The effect of volatile anesthetics on cardiac output. Suppression of cardiac output and blood pressure is concentration dependent but the degree of suppression varies with different drugs.

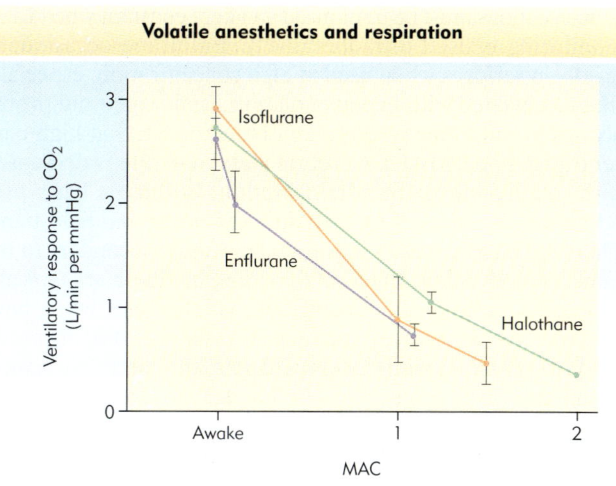

Figure 24.6 The effects of volatile anesthetics on respiration. Volatile anesthetics decrease the normal ventilatory response to CO_2 in a concentration-dependent manner; consequently, in the presence of a volatile anesthetic a spontaneously breathing patient will have a higher arterial partial pressure of CO_2 than normal.

produces more depression of cardiac contractility than other agents, while isoflurane lowers blood pressure predominately via vasodilation. The mechanisms of anesthetic-induced vasodilation are also likely to be mediated through inhibition of L-type Ca^{2+} channels. Differences between anesthetics in their relative potency on heart and vascular Ca^{2+} channels are a consequence of the existence of different isoforms of the channel in the two tissues.

The volatile anesthetics suppress heart rate at high concentrations. However, at lower concentrations, isoflurane and desflurane may increase heart rate. With rapid increases in blood concentration, desflurane and, to a lesser extent, isoflurane can produce clinically significant tachycardia. Baroreceptor function is also suppressed by the volatile anesthetics; as a result normal compensatory mechanisms to support blood pressure are deficient and may be exacerbated by hypovolemia (Chapter 29).

Respiratory effects

A normal physiologic response to increased arterial partial pressure of CO_2($Paco_2$) is an increase in minute ventilation. Volatile anesthetics suppress the CO_2 response in a concentration-dependent manner (Fig. 24.6). As volatile anesthetics are administered to the spontaneously breathing patient, $Paco_2$ increases, indicating that a higher $Paco_2$ is required to stimulate a given minute ventilation. This is analogous to the situation observed in patients with chronic obstructive pulmonary disease, who also have suppressed CO_2 responsiveness and increased $Paco_2$. There is also a hypoxic respiratory response that normally results in increased minute ventilation as a consequence of decreased arterial O_2 partial pressure. This phenomenon is suppressed by volatile anesthetics at quite small doses (e.g. 10% of an anesthetic dose) and completely abolished by anesthetic doses. This accounts for the significant respiratory depression that can result postoperatively in patients who have residual volatile anesthetic in their blood. While some volatile anesthetics, such as ether, cause increases in minute ventilation, the volatile anesthetics in current use all suppress ventilation (Chapter 47). All cause a decrease in tidal volume but have varied actions on respiratory rate. Halothane and isoflurane cause an increase in respiratory rate (but still a decrease in minute ventilation), while enflurane and the newer agents result in less tachypnea.

Airway reactivity represents a significant clinical issue in anesthesia because of the potential for exacerbation of underlying asthma and the intrinsic stimulation of instrumentation of the airway. Contraction of smooth muscle associated with the airway dramatically increases airway resistance. Just as volatile anesthetics cause vasodilation via relaxation of smooth muscle in the vasculature, they also decrease airway resistance by dilating smooth muscle in the airway. In a variety of *in vitro* measures, halothane is the most efficacious anesthetic in decreasing airway resistance. However, clinical experience indicates that isoflurane and enflurane are also very effective. Another important action of inhaled anesthetics is their effect on hypoxic vasoconstriction. Normally this response optimizes ventilation/perfusion relationships to avoid systemic hypoxia. Volatile anesthetics inhibit hypoxic pulmonary vasoconstriction which may contribute to pulmonary shunting during anesthesia (Chapter 44).

Halothane has been the traditional drug of choice for inhalation inductions and is still extensively utilized in pediatrics. However, its use in adults has been limited because of concerns of halothane hepatitis (see below). Isoflurane is relatively difficult to use because of its smell and tendency to cause coughing. Desflurane has been associated with a high incidence of laryngospasm during inhalation induction and is, therefore, not recommended. Enflurane was used extensively for inhalation induction in adults before the introduction of sevoflurane and is satisfactory but somewhat slower than halothane. Sevoflurane is currently the drug of choice in adults and has rapid onset and suppresses airway reflexes well.

Neurologic effects

All volatile anesthetics result in electroencephalographic (EEG) changes in a concentration-dependent manner (Chapter 13). This effect is typically characterized by decreases in amplitude and frequency (slowing). Importantly these effects are indistinguishable from those of ischemia and hypothermia, so anesthetic concentrations must be minimized and kept constant when EEG monitoring is used intraoperatively. Enflurane occasionally results in seizures when used in high concentration, especially when associated with hyperventilation. Isoflurane (and probably desflurane) may result in an isoelectric EEG at high concentrations (>2 MAC). Cerebral metabolic rate is decreased with volatile anesthetic administration. Isoflurane has a proportionally greater effect than does enflurane and halothane. There are also decreases in cerebral perfusion secondary to the direct hemodynamic effects of the drugs, but these are typically counterbalanced by the vasodilation. Volatile anesthetics have the potential to increase intracranial pressure because of vasodilation of cerebral blood vessels (Chapter 20). This effect is most pronounced with drugs such as isoflurane that have more vasodilating properties. Volatile anesthetic-induced cerebral vasodilation is reversed or prevented by hyperventilation.

Metabolism and toxicity

Anesthetics are metabolized much less than most other drugs in clinical use. Estimations of the extent to which volatile anesthetics are metabolized are difficult because it is not possible to extrapolate from known conditions to other circumstances. For example, halothane metabolism may undergo zero-order kinetics under some clinical circumstances where it saturates its metabolizing enzymes. Of the inhaled anesthetics in current clinical use, halothane has the most extensive metabolism (10–20%). Sevoflurane (2–5%) and enflurane (2%) are metabolized less, while only about 0.2% of an isoflurane dose is degraded. Desflurane is even more unreactive and probably undergoes <10% the metabolism of its isomer isoflurane. Some biotransformation results in F^- release, which has renal toxicity (discussed below). Halothane is subjected to oxidative metabolism in the liver where trifluoroacetic acid, Cl^-, and Br^- are produced. A smaller amount may also undergo reductive metabolism yielding 1,1-difluoro-2-chloroethylene and 1,1,1-trifluoro-2-chloroethane as well as other intermediates.

Halothane is associated with acute hepatic necrosis in approximately 1/35,000 administrations. This disorder does not occur in children. Risk factors seem to be repeated administration, obesity, and intraoperative hypotension. The exact mechanism is unclear; its rarity complicates its study. It is likely that immune-mediated reactions to a metabolite cause liver damage, and antibodies directed against hepatic cellular constituents have been identified. It has been hypothesized that anitbodies are directed against a product of halothane metobolism and that this antibody cross-reacts with hepatocytes resulting in liver damage (Fig. 24.7). There may also be a component of direct toxic damage because hypoxia, hypotension, and poor liver perfusion are frequently implicated. The mortality rate for patients who develop massive hepatic necrosis is high. There are a few case reports of massive liver injury where other volatile anesthetics have been implicated, including a handful for enflurane and one for isoflurane. The disease essentially occurs only with halothane and seems to be related to the proportion of drug that is metabolized.

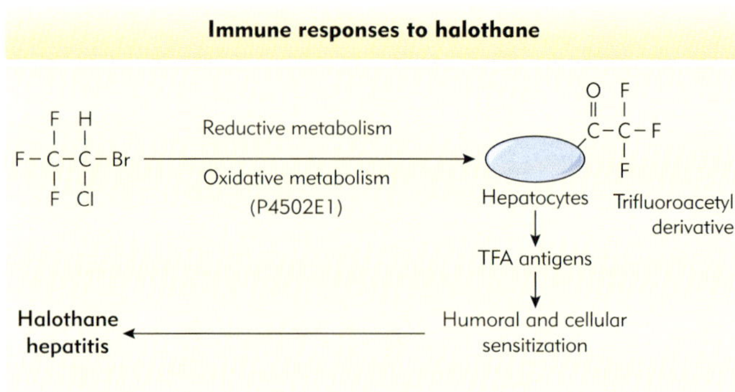

Figure 24.7 Generation of immune responses to halothane. Oxidative metabolism gives rise to a trifluoroacetyl product that binds to liver proteins and generates an immune response in susceptible individuals. When exposure is repeated, antibodies may lead to hepatic toxicity. (Figure courtesy of D Njuko, 1997.)

Renal effects

There is some decrement in kidney function with administration of all volatile anesthetics. This results primarily from hemodynamic alterations that decrease renal blood flow and depress glomerular filtration rate (Chapter 54). Metabolism of some volatile anesthetics results in F^- release, which under some circumstances reaches high enough concentrations to result in direct nephrotoxicity. The use of methoxyflurane first highlighted this problem as its metabolism resulted in much higher concentrations of F^- than that of other anesthetics. The generation of F^- is a dose-dependent effect, and its accumulation correlates with the cumulative dose. Symptoms generally begin with 3 MAC-hours of exposure when serum F^- is over 50μmol/L. Initial symptoms are impaired urine-concentrating ability followed by polyuria and hypernatremia. Halothane does not yield significant F^- on its metabolism but enflurane occasionally results in F^- levels of over 50μmol/L after a prolonged anesthetic (>10 MAC-hours of exposure). Isoflurane and desflurane result in much lower F^- release and have not been associated with renal toxicity. Sevoflurane undergoes more defluorination than enflurane but less than methoxyflurane. Exposures of 2–7 MAC-hours result in F^- concentrations of 20–40μmol/L, which decrease significantly by the next day. It is now recognized that nephrotoxicity is not associated with high serum F^- levels *per se* as cases of F^- poisoning from other sources that resulted in concentrations in excess of 500mmol/L were not associated with renal impairment. The problem with methoxyflurane appears to be that the drug undergoes defluorination in the kidney itself. Sevoflurane and enflurane are not metabolized in the kidney.

Sevoflurane reacts with soda lime to produce compound A, which may have some renal toxicity in rats at concentrations of 50–100ppm (Chapter 8). Compound A may accumulate in breathing circuits when there is low fresh gas flow, which did result in the recommendation (subsequently withdrawn) that sevoflurane should not be used in closed-circuit or low-flow situations. However, even under low-flow conditions, compound A concentrations are less than 15ppm. Halothane is subject to similar degradation with soda lime and neither drug has been implicated in significant renal failure. Compound A is metabolized through different pathways in humans to those in rats; consequently the toxic metabolite is not generated in humans.

Other toxicities

Unlike nitrous oxide, the volatile anesthetics have no significant action on folate metabolism, blood cell formation, or sperm production. Volatile anesthetics are not mutagenic in *in vitro* tests. A number of large-scale epidemiologic studies have examined the risk of carcinogenesis among personnel exposed to volatile anesthetics. Several studies showed a one- to threefold increase in the incidence of cancer among exposed women, but most studies showed no effect. Some early studies were performed before effective scavenging of anesthetic waste gases and may not be applicable today. Animal studies have failed to demonstrate any carcinogenic effect of volatile agents. In contrast to nitrous oxide, volatile anesthetics are not teratogenic in animal studies. While a number of studies have demonstrated increased incidence of spontaneous abortions or congenital anomalies in operating room personnel, it is difficult to separate anesthetic gas exposure from other factors. All volatile anesthetics, but not nitrous oxide, act as triggers for malignant hyperthermia (Chapter 30).

NITROUS OXIDE

Nitrous oxide (N_2O)is delivered as a gas via calibrated flow meters and mixed with oxygen. It is stored as liquid in cylinders with a pressure of 750psi (60atm.). Because of its liquid state, the pressure in the cylinder will not fall until the liquid is exhausted and only gas remains. At that point there are about 200L of nitrous oxide remaining in an E cylinder and the pressure will fall in proportion to the gas used. A full nitrous oxide cylinder contains approximately 1500L of gas. Nitrous oxide is relatively insoluble in aqueous solutions; consequently its blood concentration rises and falls rapidly with changes in inspired concentrations. Its advantages clinically are that it can achieve rapid changes in anesthetic depth and can ensure amnesia until the very end of a procedure and still allow a rapid emergence from anesthesia. However, its potency is quite low and greater than 1atm. is required to achieve effective anesthesia alone. Since this is impractical except under hyperbaric conditions, it is more frequently used in combination with other drugs as a method of decreasing the required doses of the more potent volatile anesthetics with less-favorable pharmacokinetics. It is considered preferable to volatile anesthetics by many practitioners because it results in less cardiovascular depression and more rapid changes in blood concentrations.

Nitrous oxide likely works in a different manner from volatile anesthetics and most intravenous anesthetics since it does not affect *in vitro* assays of $GABA_A$ receptors. Some of its actions are reversed stereospecifically by naloxone, which suggests that it has opioid receptor-mediated actions. However, this is unlikely to be a direct effect, since it does not affect opioid radioligand binding *in vitro*. It is more likely that it indirectly modulates secretion of endogenous opioids, which results in the clinically observed analgesia. Recent evidence also suggests that it antagonizes *N*-methyl-D-aspartate (NMDA) receptors, which may contribute to its anesthetic and analgesic properties.

Long-term administration of nitrous oxide may result in polyneuropathy as well as anemia because of its inhibition of vitamin B_{12} synthesis. Of greater importance in its acute use is its ability to expand existing air pockets or bubbles in the body. For example, air emboli are increased in size by the administration of nitrous oxide, and the amount of air that is lethal is much smaller in the presence of nitrous oxide. Therefore, its use is contraindicated in situations where air emboli are likely (e.g. cardiopulmonary bypass, sitting-position craniotomy). Nitrous oxide also increases the volume of other gas pockets, including pneumothorax and bowel gas. It is often avoided in extensive bowel surgery as it may lead to distension of the intestines. It may contribute to postoperative nausea, perhaps via changes in middle-ear air volume. Perhaps its greatest risk is that it may contribute to hypoxia because it must be given in relatively high concentrations (>50%) in order to contribute to the anesthetic effect. Modern anesthesia apparatus incorporates devices to prevent accidental hypoxic mixtures by limiting the ratio of nitrous oxide to oxygen that can be administered.

Respiratory effects

In common with the volatile anesthetics, nitrous oxide depresses normal ventilatory responses to hypoxia. It has little effect on CO_2 responsiveness at concentrations typically used clinically (<70%). At higher concentrations, it blunts physiologic increases in minute ventilation in response to increases in $Paco_2$, although this depression of respiratory drive is much less profound than that of the volatile anesthetics. In the absence of volatile anesthetics, administration of nitrous oxide does not lead to significant alterations in $Paco_2$. Tidal volume decreases somewhat but this is compensated by increases in the respiratory rate to keep the minute ventilation approximately normal. Airway reflexes are depressed in a similar fashion to that seen with volatile anesthetics at equipotent doses. Nitrous oxide is well tolerated and does not produce coughing or bronchospasm; it has no odor that would limit its delivery via mask.

Cardiovascular effects

Nitrous oxide mildly suppresses cardiac contractility, but the effect is less pronounced than that occurring with the volatile agents. For example, 40% nitrous oxide produces approximately a 10% decrease in cardiac output in human subjects. Under some circumstances, these changes will not be observed because there is a modest sympathetic stimulation that counters the direct depressant effects of nitrous oxide, assuming that the cardiovascular system is able to respond. In some animal studies, nitrous oxide results in a small decrease in stroke volume with a concomitant increase in heart rate, resulting in a stable cardiac output. While these circumstances are probably not clinically significant, increases in heart rate may predispose at-risk patients to the development of cardiac ischemia. Systemic vascular resistance is sustained or slightly increased up to 1atm., resulting in a stable blood pressure over the clinically relevant range. Clinical studies in adults have found that pulmonary vascular resistance may increase, but the results are highly variable and depend on the anesthetic technique and pre-existing conditions. Nitrous oxide is usually avoided in patients who have known increased pulmonary vascular resistance. If pulmonary pressures are being monitored, nitrous oxide can always be discontinued if pulmonary artery hypertension occurs. In pediatric patients with congenital heart conditions and pulmonary artery hypertension, nitrous oxide may have much more profound effects and may result in reversal of shunting.

Neurologic effects

In the highest dose typically used clinically (70%), nitrous oxide causes amnesia and frequently unconsciousness in the absence of stimulation. Minimum alveolar concentration for response to painful stimuli is greater than 1atm. Many studies on the CNS effects of nitrous oxide have yielded conflicting results because of variations in anesthetic technique. Generally, clinically significant doses (40–70% inspired) result in some increase in intracranial pressure through vasodilation. However, these changes are reversed by hyperventilation. Nitrous oxide has little effect on cerebral metabolic rate. Nitrous oxide has complicated effects on the EEG. At low doses (20–30%), it results in an increase in frequency and a decrease in voltage, while at higher concentrations the voltage increases. At concentrations above 1atm., there is slowing of the EEG. In a number of animal studies, there have been seizures after hyperbaric concentrations of nitrous oxide have been discontinued, although the clinical significance of this is unclear. Nitrous oxide appears to have potent analgesic properties at concentrations below the anesthetic range. Release of endogenous opioids has been implicated in this effect, which may contribute to its abuse potential.

Metabolism and toxicity

Nitrous oxide is not significantly metabolized or retained in the body. *In vitro* studies with liver homogenates have failed to detect metabolites, and liver uptake in rodents was less than 0.05%. Intestinal bacteria may metabolize minute quantities of nitrous oxide but there is no evidence linking this to any toxicity. Nitrous oxide inactivates the enzyme methionine synthetase by inhibiting the vitamin B_{12} cofactor. This results in inhibition of folate metabolism, which can result in megaloblastic anemia. Toxicity is unlikely if exposure is less than 24 hours in duration but has been observed where nitrous oxide is used for long-term sedation in an intensive-care situation and when patients undergo repeated lengthy anesthetics within a week. This latter observation suggests that there are cumulative effects and that recovery of enzyme action is slow. The polyneuropathy observed with chronic exposure is also likely a manifestation of inhibition of this enzyme. In addition, nitrous oxide depresses macrophage activity and production, which may predispose patients to wound infections. However, separation of these effects *in vivo* from the stress effects of surgery is difficult.

Nitrous oxide has not been shown to be mutagenic by *in vitro* assays such as the Ames test. There are no convincing data that this drug is carcinogenic in humans based on retrospective surveys of operating room personnel. Nitrous oxide has been observed to be teratogenic in some rodent studies but, generally, exposure must continuous.

XENON

The inert gas xenon is currently under evaluation for use as an anasthetic. It is anesthetic with a MAC of approximately 70%. It has a very low blood/gas solubility coefficient of 0.114 and, therefore, equilibrates rapidly. It appears to have minimal effects on the cardiovascular system. Xenon is currently expensive to produce.

PRESSURE REVERSAL

The reversal of anesthesia by hyperbaric pressure is an important issue in understanding the mechanisms of anesthetics. The application of increased hydrostatic pressure has been observed to reverse the effects of a number of anesthetics. This finding has been used to support the critical volume hypothesis of general anesthesia: the application of pressure forces anesthetic molecules out of their binding pocket(s) and restores the site to its original volume. The application of pressure results in a 2 fold rightwards shift in the dose–response curve for anesthetics. In addition, the pressures required are quite large, typically of the order of 50–100atm. Pressure reversal of anesthesia has been suggested as a necessary criterion for assessing the validity of putative sites of anesthetic action, but the significant question is whether pressure reversal is a specific phenomenon. If high pressure reverses anesthesia by directly antagonizing the effects of anesthetic molecules at their loci of action, then this phenomenon would be useful in identifying loci that are modulated by both anesthetics and pressure. However, pressure may reverse anesthetic actions *in vivo* via a locus distinct from that where the anesthetic acts. For example, if pressure exposure resulted in generalized neural hyperactivity, it might account for the left shift of anesthetic action but not provide useful mechanistic information on general anesthetic action. Recent evidence suggests that elevated pressure exposure is more likely to do the latter. Exposure to high pressures causes the high-pressure neurologic syndrome characterized by agitation and seizures. Electrophysiologic and neurochemical studies indicate that pressure *per se* has a stimulating effect through inhibition of inhibitory glycine receptors. Therefore, it is quite possible that elevated pressure results in a nonspecific excitatory state that modulates anesthetic potency.

Key References

Various authors. The clinical pharmacology of sevoflurane. Anesth Analg. 1995;81:S1–72.

Eger II E I. Anesthetic uptake and action. Baltimore: Williams & Wilkins; 1974.

Eger II E I. Nitrous oxide, N2O. New York: Elesevier; 1985.

Eger II E I. Desflurane. a compendium and reference. Rutherford NJ: Anaquest. Healthpress Publishing; 1993.

Lysko GS, Robinson JL, Casto R, Ferrone RA. The stereospecific effects of isoflurane isomers in vivo. Eur J Pharmacol. 1994;263:25–9.

Njoku D, Laster MJ, Gong DH. Biotransformation of halothane, enflurane, isoflurane and desflurane to trifluoroacetylated liver proteins: association between protein acylation and hepatic injury. Anesth Analg. 1997:84;173–8.

Further Reading

Eger II EI, Saidman LJ, Brandstate B. Minimum alveolar anesthetic concentration: a standard of anesthetic potency. Anesthesiology. 1965;26:756–81.

Moody E. Prospects for the development of new volatile anaesthetics. Exp Opin Invest Drugs. 1995;4:971–83.

Tanelian DL, Kosek P, Mody I, MacIver MB. The role of the GABA receptor/chloride channel complex in anesthesia. Anesthesiology. 1993;78:757–76.

Chapter 25 Anesthetic adjuvants and other CNS drugs

Robert A Veselis

Topics covered in this chapter

Anesthetic adjuvants can be defined as drugs active within the CNS that, no matter how high the concentration, do not induce general anesthesia when used alone. Some drugs discussed in this chapter (e.g. dexmedetomidine) may not quite fit this definition, but clinically they are used as adjuvants. Most commonly, these drugs are used to induce sedative states or to modify the effects of general anesthesia. Some of these drugs are used for their antipsychotic and mood effects [treatment of patients in the intensive-care unit (ICU) with psychosis, delirium, depression, etc.]. This chapter will review various drug classes , including benzodiazepines, α_2-agonists, antidepressants, and dopaminergic agents, used or encountered clinically by the anesthesiologist. Many of these drugs affect memory and attention mechanisms, and the normal physiology of these cognitive mechanisms will be discussed. This will allow the reader a better grasp of literature relating to sedative and memory effects of anesthetic agents. Emphasis is placed on mechanisms of action and clinically relevant information that may be difficult to find in other texts.

From a scientific point of view, the most interesting question is how these agents work on the CNS to produce their effects. Unfortunately, knowing which receptors a drug acts on and the receptor distribution in the CNS is often not sufficient. For example, the observation that benzodiazepines increase the action of γ-aminobutyric acid (GABA) at $GABA_A$ receptors does not explain how amnesia is produced or why amnesia produced by benzodiazepines differs from that produce by barbiturates, which also act at $GABA_A$ receptors. Knowledge of drug–receptor interactions alone is not sufficient to explain clinical effects for several reasons: drugs are rarely 'pure' agonists or antagonists; most drugs have actions at multiple receptors; most receptors belong to families that are classified into subtypes, often based on molecular biology (e.g. GABA has many possible receptors of which three to ten may have clinical significance); it is frequently unclear which receptor subtypes are responsible for particular effects; functional neuroimaging studies indicate that the distribution of drug receptors often does not overlap the distribution of drug effects in the CNS.

Understanding the functional neuroanatomy of drug effects can help to illuminate how these drugs work and can serve as a link between receptor physiology and clinical effects. Until recently, most anatomic information regarding CNS function was obtained from pathologic analysis (e.g. the famous case of Phineas Gage). However, in the 1990s, physiologic effects associated with neural activity in the brain can be imaged in real time. Examples include changes in cerebral blood flow as imaged by ^{15}O positron emission tomography (^{15}O-PET), changes in glucose metabolism as imaged by ^{18}F-labeled deoxyglucose PET (FDG-PET), or changes in oxyhemoglobin as imaged by functional magnetic resonance imaging (fMRI) (Fig. 25.1). The underlying principle of these imaging techniques is that within 200–1000 milliseconds of a change in neuronal activity, changes in regional physiology occur that can serve to locate specific areas of activation or deactivation in the brain. The ability to image changes in neural activity occurring with various memory, auditory, visual, and other tasks is rapidly advancing our understanding of how the brain operates. Examining drug effects on the CNS using these techniques will complement receptor physiology in explaining drug mechanisms of action.

MEMORY

Anesthesiologists directly manipulate memory mechanisms to provide profound, reversible amnesia and anxiolysis during sedation and to ensure that no recall occurs after general anesthesia. Consequently, anesthesiologists need to have some concept of what memory is and why certain phenomena, such as awareness during general anesthesia, can occur. Current memory research has two areas of emphasis: describing memory in a pure cognitive sense and localization of various aspects of the cognitive memory model to discrete anatomic locations using techniques such as PET, fMRI, or electrophysiology [electroencephalography (EEG) and event related potentials (ERP)].

The advantage of the cognitive approach is that it allows research pertaining to memory mechanisms to proceed without the need to identify specific neuroanatomic structures, which until recently was a difficult task. It remains unclear whether various aspects of memory are localized to a specific cerebral structure or whether they are embodied diffusely in

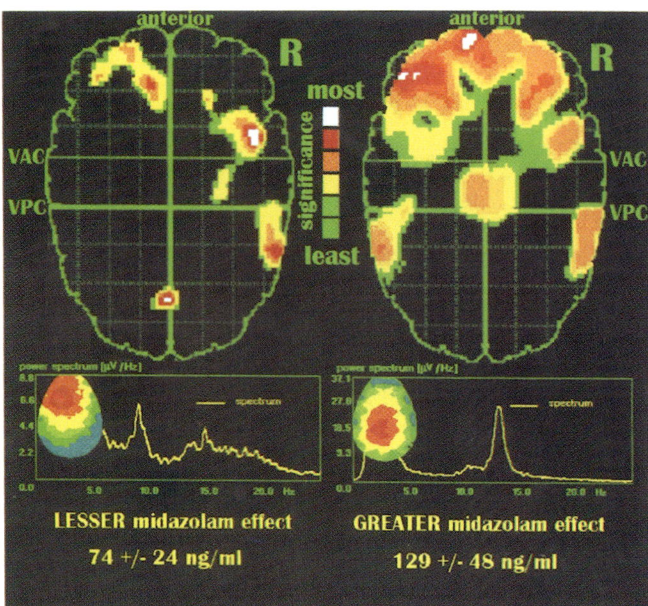

Figure 25.1 Functional neuroimaging of cerebral blood flow changes with midazolam. The top images indicate regions of statistically significant decreases in regional cerebral blood flow (rCBF) beyond any global changes in CBF. Midazolam decreases global CBF about 12% from resting baseline. Two groups of subjects were imaged: those receiving a low dose of midazolam (74ng/mL) and those receiving a high dose of midazolam (129ng/mL). Changes occurring in the low-dose group are a subset of those in the high dose group. The areas demonstrating differential decreases in blood flow correspond to areas in the brain involved with memory and attention processing (e.g. prefrontal cortex and thalamus). Therefore, it is likely that midazolam affects certain areas of the brain preferentially, and these correspond to its clinical effects. These blood flow changes are different from benzodiazepine receptor distribution, which is much more widespread throughout the cortex. Below each statistical image is a corresponding electroencephalography (EEG) power spectrum and map of the topographic distribution over the head of EEG beta power (10–20Hz). Midazolam causes high-frequency EEG activity primarily over the anterior cortex at lower doses (left). As concentration increases to the hypnotic effect (unresponsiveness to verbal commands), rhythmical activity occurs in the EEG, mainly over the central cortex (right; note the change in the scaling of the EEG power axis because of the power present in 'sleep spindles' occurring at this concentration of midazolam). VAC, vertical anterior commissure line; VPC, vertical posterior commissure line.

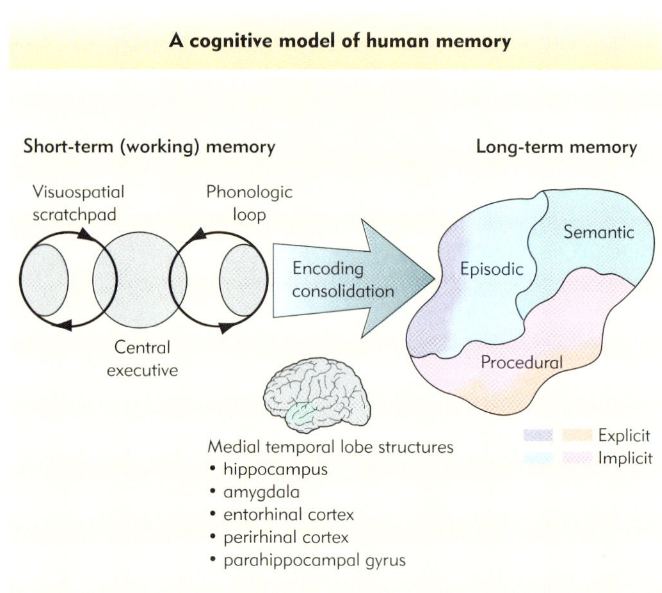

Figure 25.2 A cognitive model of human memory. The model represents an amalgam of various theories on how memory is organized. Sensory information is processed first as working memory, where it is held and manipulated for a certain period of time. This area has a small working capacity (according to some psychologists 'seven plus or minus two words'). For long-term storage, events are encoded into long-term memory, which depends on medial temporal lobe structures. Using the technique of double dissociation, long-term memory has been shown to have distinct components: episodic, semantic, procedural, and explicit and implicit memory (see text).

the brain. Considerable amounts of cortex can be removed from an experimental animal without abolishing a specific memory, yet lesions to a very small structure such as the hippocampus can profoundly affect memory. Memory has multiple components that can be conceptually divided on the basis of time (short and long term; anterograde and retrograde) and/or content (knowledge of the world, remembrance of specific events, procedural skills) (Fig. 25.2). Anterograde refers to 'after the event', in this case administration of drug, and retrograde refers to 'before the event'.

'Double dissociation' is a fundamental concept in memory research that is important to understand. Double dissociation constitutes necessary, but not sufficient, evidence of a unique form of memory. For this, two memory systems are postulated: for example, remembering a name and remembering how to skate. It is unclear if remembering a name is distinct from remembering how to skate, or if they are different manifestations of a single memory system. A double dissociation means that remembering names and how to skate can be manipulated or affected independently of each other. Double dissociations can be found in the following circumstances:

Anatomic–pathologic lesions (stroke, surgery, brain injury). These can selectively affect a certain type of memory. For example, patients who can remember their names but have forgotten skating can be compared with patients with intact skating ability who cannot remember their names.

Developmental changes. Children demonstrate adult behavior in certain memory systems as early as 3 years of age, and elderly patients loose certain forms of memory out of proportion to others.

Drug-induced changes. Many drugs, such as anticholinergics, alcohol, and benzodiazepines, affect one form of memory and leave others intact.

Manipulation of testing procedures in normal subjects.

Multiple lines of evidence from different fields are required before the existence of independent memory systems is generally accepted.

Short-term and long-term memory

Short-term memory, now termed *'working memory'*, represents transient storage of sensory information that is held and manipulated as part of other cognitive functions, such as speech or attention, under the direction of a 'central executive' control system. Working memory comprises two slave systems: a 'visuospatial scratchpad' for temporary storage of visual images and the 'phonologic loop' for articulatory rehearsal of verbal material.

Transfer of information from working memory to *long-term memory* appears to be critically dependent on the integrity of medial temporal lobe structures. However, it can also be affected by various conditions, including head injury, electric shock, extreme stress, and certain drugs that inhibit protein synthesis or REM sleep.

Long-term memory can be further divided into a number of categories. *Episodic memory* involves specific events, people, places, and so on, and can be tested by memorizing a list of words for later recall. Episodic memory can be further divided into explicit and implicit memory. *Explicit memory* (also referred to as event, declarative or explicit memory, though these are not entirely interchangeable) is memory as we normally think of it (e.g. conscious recollection of how and where events occurred). *Implicit memory* does not require conscious recollection; it is manifested as a subtle, unconscious influence on behavior by stimuli that were previously presented but which are not consciously remembered.

Semantic memory (also known as knowledge systems) is formed from unrecalled events: knowledge such as geography, the working rules of a language, etc. *Procedural memory* (also known as associative memory) represents memory for tasks such as mirror writing, skating, bicycle riding, etc. This form of memory is dissociable from explicit episodic memory.

Implicit memory is of particular interest to anesthesiologists because it has been implicated as a mechanism for memory formation during anesthesia. Implicit memory can be dissociated from explicit memory; this dissociation can occur with pharmacologic agents, including diazepam, midazolam, and scopolamine (hyosine). Implicit memory can be demonstrated using various types of priming test. Priming is defined as increasing the probability of a correct response by the occurrence of some prior event that is not consciously recollected (this forms the basis of the now-banned subliminal advertising). Examples include faster relearning of information that had been encountered before, completion of word stems or word fragments with words from a previously presented list, and 'perceptual priming' or enhanced perception of visually degraded words or pictures.

An anatomic model of memory

Memory depends on many neural structures, but specifically which ones and how they interact is still very much a mystery. Though a few structures are critically involved with memory (e.g. the hippocampus), many memory mechanisms depend on a number of highly interconnected regions. Structural division based on type of memory is somewhat artificial. The emerging concept of memory (and CNS function in general) is that many neural networks subserve the memory process, and that areas of activation coexist with corresponding areas of deactivation during a given task. A number of important regions have been identified repeatedly in various studies using different methods (Fig. 25.3).

Medial temporal lobe, hippocampus, and amygdala

Patients with lesions in the medial temporal lobe, hippocampus, and amygdala have severe memory loss for episodic or context-sensitive events, such as where one lives, the time of day, etc. Animal models of amnesia have identified the medial temporal lobe, diencephalon (thalamus and mammillary nuclei), and basal forebrain as essential structures for memory. Both the hippocampus and amygdala are important in episodic memory formation, and the destruction of both is needed for severe and lasting amnesia. The surrounding cortical masses, which include the entorhinal cortex and perirhinal cortex, are critical for the transfer of episodic information to long-term memory, the location of which is still unclear but is probably spread throughout the cortex.

Frontal lobes: prefrontal cortex

The dorsolateral prefrontal cortex appears critical for working memory. Patients with lesions in the prefrontal cortex have difficulty making estimates or inferences from everyday experiences. They have severe problems when irrelevant information must be ignored and are particularly disrupted by irrelevant or extraneous details. Often socially inappropriate behavior is present. These patients have difficulty in shifting between different strategies and often persevere with an inappropriate response.

Basal forebrain, medial diencephalon, and basal ganglia

The basal forebrain, medial diencephalon, and basal ganglia areas appear to operate in parallel with the medial temporal system, and there is some indication that these two systems are dissociable. Critical components of the implicit memory system may reside here, for instance in the dorsomedial nucleus of the thalamus. Patients with lesions in the basal ganglia have poor procedural memories and demonstrate no priming for these memories. For example, patients with Huntington's chorea (basal ganglia degeneration) have normal episodic memory and episodic priming but poor skill and skill-priming memories. The opposite occurs with patients in Alzheimer's disease, where the pathology is primarily cortical with normal basal ganglia. This provides a double dissociation between implicit memory elicited by priming for episodic memories and implicit memory elicited in procedural tasks.

Cerebellum

The cerebellum makes a far more important contribution to cognition than was previously thought. Far from being exclusively a motor organ, the cerebellum appears to be involved in some cognitive, linguistic, and emotional functions through links to the limbic system and the prefrontal cortex. Lesions in frontal or parietal cortex are often associated with depressed metabolism in the contralateral cerebellar hemisphere.

ANESTHESIA AND MEMORY

There is little doubt that sufficient general anesthesia will completely ablate explicit memory; no careful study to date has demonstrated the existence of explicit memory during adequate levels of general anesthesia. However, awareness during anesthesia can and does occur at a rate of 0.2%. The occurrence of explicit recall/awareness is probably related to administration of insufficient anesthetic. The preservation of other forms of memory, in particular implicit memory, during general anesthesia is more controversial. It is well documented that patients can follow commands intraoperatively but usu-

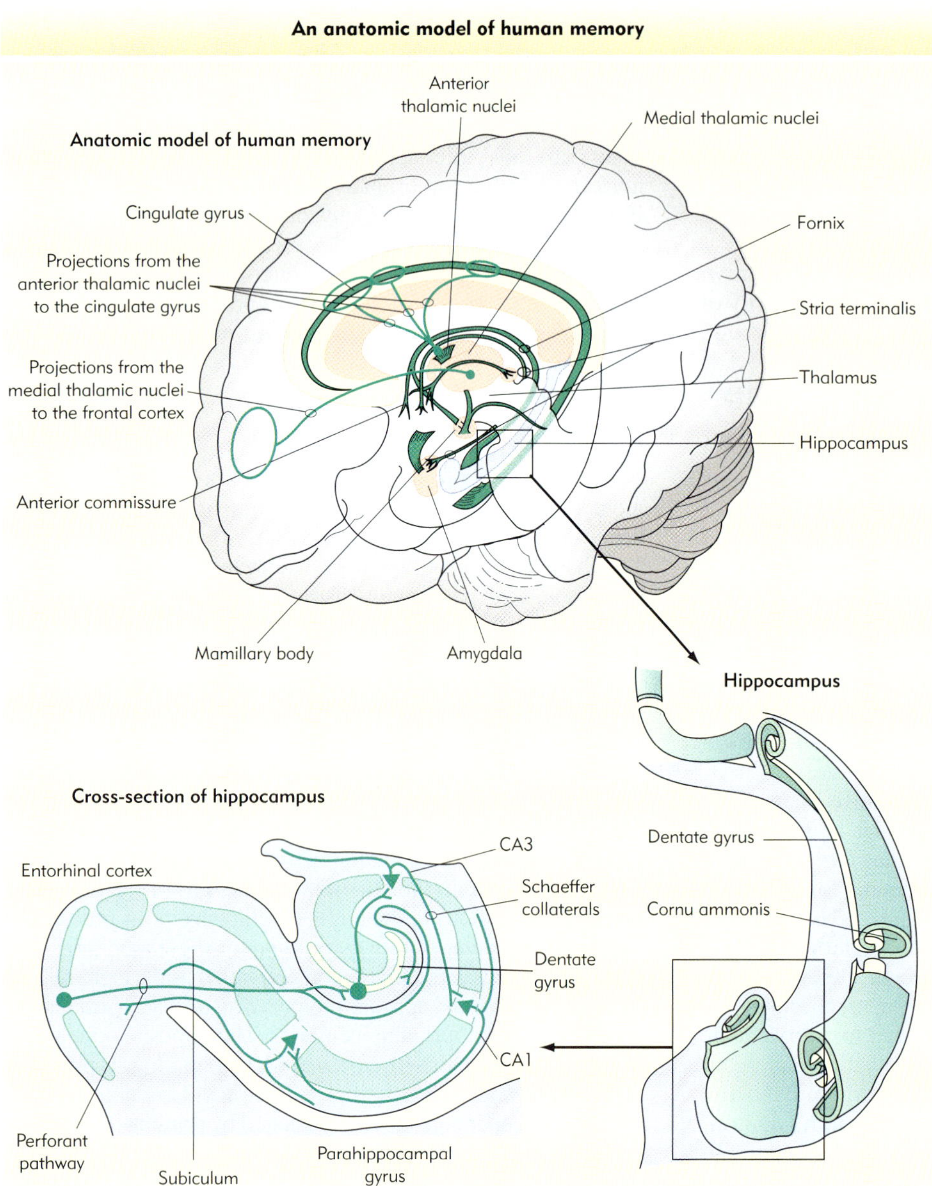

Figure 25.3 An anatomic model of human memory. The various components of memory are widely distributed (e.g. semantic memory), but key structures are involved in certain processing steps (such as the medial temporal lobe structures in encoding and retrieving information or the hippocampus in encoding and retrieval of episodic memory). The microscopic diagram (bottom left) shows the flow of information from the entorhinal cortex and subicular region to the dentate gyrus via perforant fibers to synapse onto granule cells. The axons from these form a bundle, the mossy fiber pathway, that runs to the pyramidal cells in the CA3 region. These cells send excitatory input to the CA1 region via the Schaeffer collaterals. The efferents from the hippocampus travel through the fornix to the septal nuclei, the hypothalamus, the mamillary bodies, and the anterior nuclei of the thalamus, which in turn projects to the cingulate gyrus. Some of these structures (e.g. cingulate gyrus and septal nuclei) also provide afferents to the hippocampus. In this way, the arrangement of neurons in the hippocampus and tracts to and from the hippocampus form a recurrent network. This system has been extensively studied as a model of synaptic plasticity – the modification of synaptic interactions that have the ability to store information. For example, the CA1 and CA3 fields exhibit long-term potentiation to form spatial memories.

ally have no recollection of these events, even in the presence of pain. Electrophysiologic studies indicate that fairly high levels of cognitive processing of auditory stimuli can occur under general anesthesia. Thus, the encoding requirement for learning/memory during anesthesia is met. Whether these stimuli can be processed and stored and subsequently retrieved by implicit memory testing is controversial. Most investigators now feel that some form of memory can be formed during adequate levels of general anesthesia, which is distinct from the explicit recall of awareness. However, the implications of this type of memory are far from clear. Much of the difficulty in this field is related to methodologic considerations, and much previous work can be faulted on this basis.

BENZODIAZEPINES

Until the introduction of propofol, benzodiazepines were the most commonly used drugs to produce sedation and amnesia in surgical or critically ill patients. Until recently, the choice of benzodiazepine for clinical use has been largely driven by pharmacokinetic considerations, such as short half-life and water solubility, with midazolam being the most appropriate drug for these considerations (Figs 25.4 & 25.5). Now the overriding concern is cost, and lorazepam is being used extensively because of its low cost, even though it has a significantly longer half-life than midazolam.

Pharmacokinetics

Diazepam is the prototypical benzodiazepine but has some undesirable properties subsequently eliminated in newer drugs. It is highly lipid soluble and thus insoluble in water. The solvent for the parenteral preparation of diazepam (a mixture of ethanol and propylene glycol) is highly irritating when given intravenously. An emulsified form (Dizac, Diazemuls) that is not as irritating in intravenous injection is recently available in some countries. Diazepam has an exceedingly long half-life and active metabolites, which may

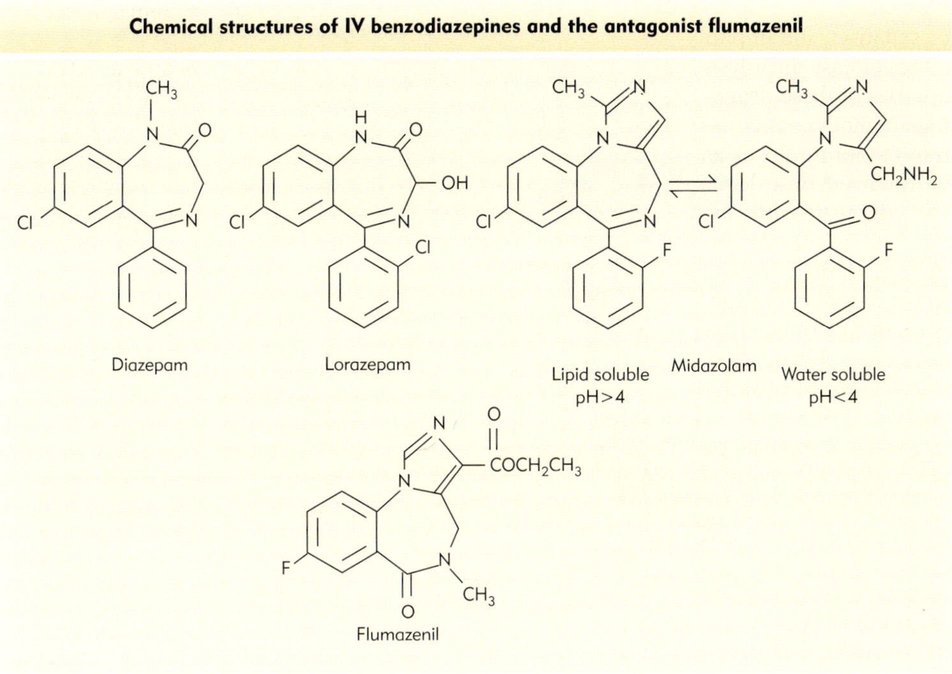

Chemical structures of IV benzodiazepines and the antagonist flumazenil

Figure 25.4 Chemical structures of intravenous benzodiazepines and the antagonist flumazenil. The reversible pH-dependent ring opening of midazolam is shown.

Pharmocokinetic properties of benzodiazepines

Drug	Terminal half-life (h)	Equivalent IV/IM dose or total daily PO dose	Potency relative to midazolam ([MDZ]:[drug])
Diazepam (Valium)	25–40	0.3mg/kg, 4–40mg/day	1:7
Lorazepam (Ativan)	10–20	0.05mg/kg, 2–6mg/day	1:0.5
Midazolam[a] [Versed (USA); Hypnoval (UK)]	2–6 (15–26)[b]	0.15mg/kg	–
Chlordiazepoxide [Librium (USA); Librium, Tropium (UK)]	5–30	15–100mg/day	–
Alprazolam (Xanax)	10–15	0.75–4.0mg/day	1:1
Clonazepam [Klonopin (USA); Rivotril (UK)]	18–50	0.5–4.0mg/day	–
Triazolam (Halcion)	2.5	0.125–0.25mg/day	–
Temapzepam (Restoril)	10–40	15–30mg/day	–
Oxazepam (Serax)	5–20	30–120mg/day	–
Clorazepate (Tranxene)	50–100 (metabolite)	15–60mg/day	–

[a]Serum concentrations at which 50% of subjects show an effect (Cp50): loss of memory, 35–80ng/mL; loss of response to command, 400–600ng/mL. Subjects awaken at about 200ng/mL.
[b]Value in patients in intensive-care unit (h)

Figure 25.5 Pharmacokinetic properties of benzodiazepines. As these drugs are frequently referred to by their trade names, some of these are also included. If pharmacodynamic equivalency data are available [e.g. electroencephalography (EEG) effects], relative potency is indicated referenced to midazolam.

be of benefit in long-term therapy or in withdrawal situations. Though the newer drugs (e.g. midazolam) are purported to have inactive metabolites, thorough investigation of all metabolites has not been carried out, and it is likely that some metabolites will be found to be active (as recently shown with the EEG effects of midazolam and α-hydroxymidazolam).

In general, the pharmacokinetics (see Fig. 25.4) of these drugs are age dependent, with increasing elimination half-life in elderly patients. Critically ill patients or even otherwise healthy patients recovering from major surgery can have significantly prolonged drug elimination half-lives, which must be taken into consideration, especially if these drugs are administered by continuous intravenous infusion.

A specific antagonist, flumazenil (bolus dose 8–15μg/kg intravenous; infusion of 0.1–0.4mg/h; maximum cumulative dose 5mg) is now available. It works well to reverse the effects of benzodiazepines given acutely, though when benzodiazepines have been given chronically (e.g. continuous intravenous infusion in the ICU), the reversal effect is much less pronounced and of brief duration.

Pharmacodynamics

Benzodiazepines reduce anxiety, induce sedation, and impair memory to various degrees. For the anesthesiologist, anxiolysis and amnesia are the most desirable properties of these drugs.

Benzodiazepines have relatively benign hemodynamic/respiratory effects, especially when given in moderate doses as a continuous infusion. Respiration is impaired in a dose-dependent manner; as a result, action is synergistic with respiratory depression by volatile anesthetics and opioids. When these drugs are given acutely by the intravenous route, hypotension may occur. This is most likely related to a reduction in sympathetic tone, though there is some evidence that midazolam causes direct vasodilatation. Cerebral bood flow is decreased to a degree that is related to the extent of sedation present.

Benzodiazepines result in dependence when administered for prolonged periods (months). Acute withdrawal produces agitation, anxiety, dysphoria, increased awareness of sensory stimuli, perceptual distortion, and depersonalization. Severe withdrawal can include confusion, delirium, and seizures.

The effects of benzodiazepines on memory are very specific and do not result from general brain depression (i.e. amnesia is not a result of the sedative effect). As with other drugs affecting memory, benzodiazepines produce an anterograde amnesia in both adults and children (Fig. 25.6). This results from a specific impairment of acquisition and encoding of novel information. There is no convincing evidence of retrograde amnesia with benzodiazepines or any other drug. The benzodiazepines generally do not impair short-term memory (e.g. digit span) but do impair immediate free recall. Information learned during benzodiazepine administration is easily forgotten. This effect is seen during sedation when a patient repeatedly asks the same question or starts a statement and cannot finish it because the beginning of the sentence has been forgotten.

Though benzodiazepines produce a profound selective impairment of new learning, access to previously learned material or to the semantic or procedural knowledge system is unaffected. The benzodiazepines have specific effects on implicit perceptual priming, depending on the drug studied. For example, diazepam leaves priming effects intact while explicit memory is impaired. In contrast, lorazepam abolishes the priming effect. The literature regarding midazolam and implicit memory is insufficient to draw any conclusions.

Respiratory effects

The respiratory effects of benzodiazepines are rather insubstantial by themselves. However, as with any powerful sedative given intravenously, respiration can be substantially depressed when large doses are administered and profound sedation occurs. The most detailed investigation of respiratory effects has occurred with midazolam, for which a number of deaths have been reported in situations with inadequate monitoring. The primary effect on the respiratory system is upper airway obstruction and altered breathing mechanics. Premedication doses of midazolam do not seem to predispose patients to respiratory depression beyond that which normally occurs with natural sleep. Midazolam alone has little effect on the response to carbon dioxide or hypoxia. Midazolam can have a synergistic effect with the respiratory depression caused by opioids.

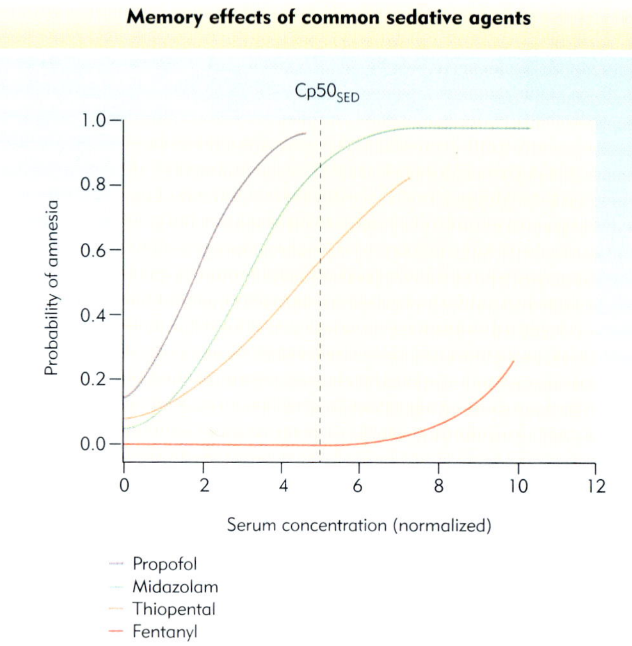

Figure 25.6 Memory effects of common sedative agents. Explicit recall of episodic memory was tested using a word list where amnesia was defined as forgetting 50% of the list. Agents active at the $GABA_A$ receptor have significant memory effects, whereas fentanyl does not. Serum concentrations have been normalized so that 5 represents the serum concentration at which sedation occurs in 50% of subjects ($Cp50_{SED}$): midazolam 65ng/mL (190nmol/L), propofol 0.7μg/mL (4μmol/L), thiopental 2.9μg/mL (12μmol/L), and fentanyl 0.9μg/mL (2.7μmol/L). (Unpublished data from R A Veselis.)

THE α_2-AGONISTS

Originally introduced into clinical practice as antihypertensive agents, the effects of α_2-agonists on nociception, sedation, and hypnosis also make them useful to the anesthesiologist. These agents have much greater activity at α_2- than at α_1-adrenoceptors and produce a characteristic spectrum of effects (Figs 25.7 & 25.8). The sympatholytic effects are utilized in situations where high sympathetic tone may be expected, such as open-heart surgery during relatively light anesthesia.

The α_2-adrenoceptors

The α_2-adrenoceptors are present at various central and peripheral sites, including primary sensory afferent terminals (spinal and peripheral), the superficial laminae of the spinal cord (mediating analgesia), and various brainstem nuclei, in particular the locus coeruleus (Fig. 25.9). Activation of presynaptic α_2-adrenoceptors inhibits norepinephrine (noradrenaline) release from the nerve terminal, hence the inhibitory effect of α_2-agonists on noradrenergic transmission and their consequent sympatholytic effects. Presynaptic α_2-adrenoceptor activation probably also inhibits acetylcholine release, accounting for some side effects of clonidine, such as dry mouth, constipation, and blurred vision.

Effects of α_2-adrenoceptor agonists

Effect	Central	Peripheral
Hypotension/sympatholysis (α_{2A})	X	X
Hypertension (α_{2B})	–	X
Bradycardia/increase vagal tone	X	–
Sensitize baroreceptors	X	–
Antinociception	X	–
Sedation (locus coeruleus)	X	–
Enhanced memory/learning (?)	X	–
Suppress renin secretion	X	X
Diuresis (block vasopressin, increase glomerular filtration rate)	–	X
Dry mouth	–	X
Attenuation of stress response	X	–
Hyperglycemia (decreased insulin release)	–	X
Enhanced growth hormone secretion	X	
Decreased postoperative shivering	X	

Figure 25.7 Effects of α_2-adrenoceptor agonists. The effects of these drugs are mediated by both central and peripheral mechanisms.

Molecular cloning of α_2-adrenoceptors has revealed three subtypes: α_{2A}, α_{2B}, and α_{2C}. The sedative, analgesic, and hypotensive effects are mediated by α_{2C}-adrenoceptors, the hypertensive effects and vasoconstriction by α_{2B}, and the function of the α_{2C}-adrenoceptors is unknown. Current efforts are focused on the development of selective α_{2A}-agonists to eliminate the undesired hypertensive effects of current agonists.

Locus coeruleus

There are two central noradrenergic nuclei, the locus coeruleus and the lateral tegmental nuclei. The locus coeruleus is a bilateral nucleus located in the floor of the fourth ventricle underneath the cerebellar peduncles. It has a bluish color from the presence of neuromelanin, hence its name. It has few neurons, but there are morphologically distinct subdivisions. The locus coeruleus receives input from probably all sensory modalities; many of the inputs are, in turn, influenced by autonomic pathways. The locus coeruleus is activated by 'threatening' stimuli, including pain, blood loss, and cardiovascular collapse. The locus coeruleus has the largest efferent network originating from any nucleus in the brain and is the origin of virtually all noradrenergic tracts in the brain. These diffusely innervate many structures, including the reticular formation, cranial nerve nuclei, spinal cord, thalamus, hypothalamus, hippocampus, Meynert's nucleus, and other forebrain structures. Meynert's nucleus contains cholinergic fibers that seem to be selectively lost in Alzheimer's disease and may be the locus for the memory-enhancing effects seen with anticholinergic drugs in this disease. The locus coeruleus is involved in sleep–wakefulness, attention, learning–memory, stress response, nociception, and autonomic–endocrine functions. Opioids (via μ-receptors) and α_2-agonists inhibit locus coeruleus neurons by hyperpolarization, which leads to a reduction in central sympathetic nervous system activity.

Drugs

Clonidine

Clonidine has moderate specificity as an agonist for α_2-adrenoceptors (α_2:α_1 200:1), but also has effects at imidazoline receptors, a novel class of receptor. Therefore, complete α_2-blockade does not interfere with some of the effects of clonidine, such as hypotension. Imadazoline receptors interact with endogenous substances, including agmatine and clonidine displacing substance (CDS). Imidazole-binding sites are located in the rostral ventrolateral medullary area. Various ligands can act at these sites to produce an increase in blood pressure and, therefore, clonidine can be

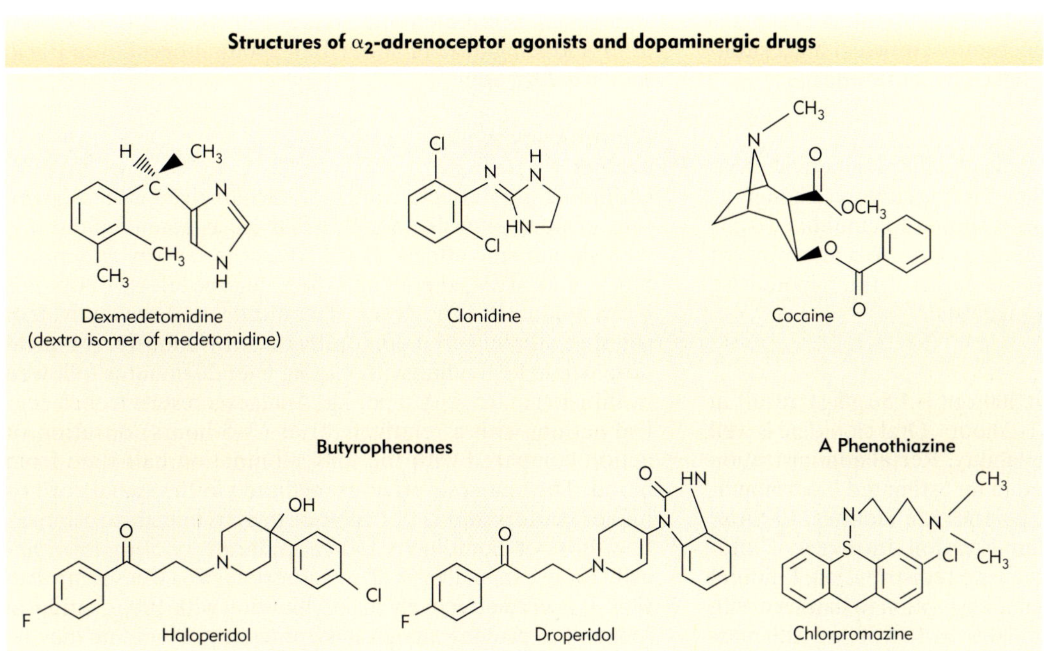

Figure 25.8 Structures of α_2-adrenoceptor agonists and dopaminergic drugs.

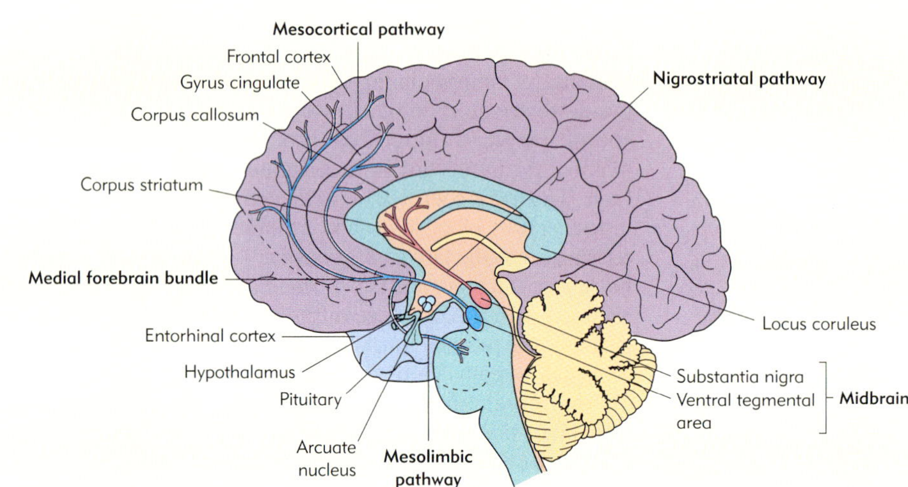

Figure 25.9 Dopaminergic reward system of the brain and the locus coeruleus. The mesolimbic dopaminergic system originating in the ventral tegmental area and projecting to many structures in the limbic system and prefrontal cortex plays a key role in drug addiction. The locus coeruleus, which is the origin of most of the noradrenergic fibers in the CNS, is closely related to the dopamine reward system. The locus coeruleus is located just below the floor of the rhomboid fossa at the rostal end just under the cerebellar peduncles and is inhibited by α_2-agonists, which explains their usefulness in withdrawal syndromes.

regarded as an antagonist of these endogenous substances, producing a hypotensive effect. Though α_2-adrenoceptors mediate many of the effects of clonidine, other neurotransmitter systems (cholinergic, serotonergic) are also affected. Effects on other neurotransmitters result from either actions on presynaptic α_2-adrenoceptors or effects on different receptors. Clonidine is available for clinical use in Europe for epidural/intrathecal use and should soon be available for clinical use in the USA.

Dexmedetomidine

Dexmedetomidine is much more specific for α_2-adrenoceptors than clonidine (α_2:α_1 1600:1). It is a full agonist, whereas clonidine is considered a partial agonist. Dexmedetomidine is the dextro isomer of medetomidine (the levo isomer is without effect), suggesting that dexmedetomidine acts specifically at a protein-receptor site. However, dexmedetomidine also binds with modest affinity to α_1-adrenoceptors, which at higher concentrations antagonizes the α_2-linked hypnotic effects.

Mivazerol

Mivazerol is a new agent being evaluated for perioperative sympatholysis in patients undergoing cardiac surgery. Though its selectivity for α_2-adrenoceptors is similar to clonidine (α_2:α_1 119:1), it binds to the imidazoline receptor to a lesser extent than clonidine. This may mitigate some of the hypotensive effects associated with other α_2-agonists.

Pharmacokinetics

Oral doses of clonidine, about 300μg (3–4.5μg/kg), result in peak serum concentrations in 1–2 hours. Oral clonidine is well absorbed with 75–95% bioavailability. Rectal administration of 2.5μg/kg in children resulted in an estimated bioavailability of 95%. After absorption, kinetics are identical to those obtained with intravenous administration. Intravenous infusion demonstrates rapid and extensive redistribution. Epidural clonidine results in similar systemic absorption to that seen with oral administration. The epidural dose is 150–500μg with maximum concentration in the CSF occurring 30–60 minutes after injection. The degree of analgesia is directly related to the CSF concentration, with poor correlation with blood concentrations. Clonidine is highly lipid soluble and rapidly crosses the placental barrier. It is present in maternal milk at about twice the concentration of blood.

The major route of excretion of clonidine is as unchanged drug in the urine, with metabolism forming a minor portion (10–50%) of elimination. There is little first-pass metabolism through the liver after oral administration. There is significant enterohepatic circulation, with a subsequently relatively long mean terminal half-life of 8–13 hours.

There is less literature on dexmedetomidine. Peak concentrations after intramuscular administration of 2μg/kg occur after 10–30 minutes, with 85% bioavailability. The terminal elimination half-life is 4–10 hours. Most hemodynamic changescan be avoided with an infusion rate of 0.4–0.6μg/min after a loading dose of about 100–200μg infused over 10–30 min in a 70kg adult.

Pharmacodynamics

Analgesia

Clonidine is an effective analgesic when given either epidurally or intravenously, though it is twice as potent epidurally, with similar side effects. It enhances the sensory and motor block of local anesthetics and the analgesic effects of opioids given epidurally. The doses of clonidine used are equivalent whether administered epidurally or intravenously. A typical dose would be loading with 4μg/kg over 20 minutes followed by infusion at 0.5–2μg/h per kg. Analgesia results from a central action, with a relatively brief (3–5 hours) duration of action compared with the long elimination half-time from blood. The analgesic effect is mediated in the spinal cord or higher centers and is not related to systemic absorption. A 'low' dose of clonidine is 150μg epidurally or 50μg intrathecally for use in analgesia after surgery such as Caesarean section. It is used effectively in combination with 100μg epidural fentanyl to prolong analgesia significantly. Clonidine may be more useful for neuropathic pain (e.g. cancer pain) than for acute pain relief. Clonidine's analgesic effects may, in part, be mediated by cholinergic mechanisms, which may be more important in neuropathic pain. Patients should be closely monitored for 2–4 hours following bolus administration of epidural clonidine, especially when large (>300μg) doses are given.

Hemodynamic effects

The hemodynamic effects of clonidine are complex, partly because the opposing effects of central sympatholysis and a direct peripheral vasoconstrictive effect from activation of presynaptic α_2-adrenoceptors. Clonidine may produce greater hypotensive effects than other α_2-agonists that do not act on imidazoline receptors. The dose response is biphasic, with maximum hypotension occurring at about 200μg epidural clonidine with little blood pressure effect at 800μg. More profound hypotension occurs when clonidine is injected at thoracic levels. Hypotensive effects depend, in part, on the level of pre-existing sympathetic tone. Clonidine reduces heart rate, cardiac output, and systemic vascular resistance, more so in the upright than in the supine position. Decreased cardiac output results from decreased cardiac filling owing to systemic venodilatation and from concomitant bradycardia. If clonidine is administered chronically (longer than 6 days), there is danger of rebound hypertension.

Dexmedetomidine has similar effects to those of clonidine: 2.0μg/kg causes a transient, mild increase in blood pressure that is larger with intravenous (20% above baseline) than with intramuscular administration. Following this short-lived hypertension, a 20% decrease in blood pressure ensues. Following intravenous administration, a transient 30% decrease in heart rate occurs, which returns to a value of 10% below baseline as found with intramuscular administration. Bolus intravenous administration of dexmedetomidine is contraindicated by these hemodynamic changes.

The high incidence of bradycardia and/or hypotension with dexmedetomidine may preclude its routine use in anesthesia. Patients receiving dexmedetomidine premedication require more fluids and interventions for hypotension intraoperatively. Premedication doses of about 1μg/kg are relatively well tolerated, whereas 2–4μg/kg results in a high incidence of bradycardia or hypotension that requires treatment. However, in situations where hypertension/sympathetic outflow predominates, such as cardiovascular surgery, it may be useful.

Sedation and hypnosis

Anesthetic requirements are related to central noradrenergic activity. Therefore, agents such as reserpine that deplete central norepinephrine stores cause a reduction in inhalational anesthetic requirements. Conversely, increases in central norepinephrine activity with stimulant agents (amphetamines) increase anesthetic requirements.The α_2-agonists decrease anesthetic requirements by 40–50% by inhibition of central noradrenergic transmission. Dexmedetomidine is more potent than clonidine, and at high enough doses dexmedetomidine may itself be sufficient as an anesthetic.

Clonidine has been used as an oral premedicant in doses of about 5μg/kg to reduce anesthetic requirements, to provide preoperative sedation, and decrease blood pressure response to stressful events during surgery. Dexmedetomidine 1–2μg/kg can produce profound sedation in volunteer subjects, and 0.6μg/kg intravenously 10 minutes before induction reduces isoflurane requirements by approximately 25%. If dexmedetomidine is given as a continuous infusion, isoflurane requirements can be reduced by 90%. Except for the lack of anterograde amnesia, the psychomotor effects of 1.5–2.5μg/kg are equivalent and longer lasting than 0.08μg/kg midazolam. Dexmedetomidine decreases fentanyl requirements by 60%. An antagonist, atipamezole, is available.

Interactions with other drugs

Clonidine, 4–5μg/kg, may blunt the heart rate response to atropine and may enhance the pressor response to ephedrine by about 10%. There are significant pharmacokinetic interactions of dexmedetomidine with other drugs. The dose reduction with thiopental (thiopentone) results from changes in pharmacokinetics (a decrease in distribution volume) rather than a pharmacodynamic effect on the CNS, in contrast to the synergistic effects seen with inhalational agents. This effect may also explain the higher plasma concentrations seen when alfentanil is administered in conjunction with clonidine. The decrease in distribution volume probably reflects changes in cardiac output as a result of the bradycardia and hypotension associated with dexmedetomidine. This effect may be present for other drugs that depend on rapid redistribution for termination of effect (e.g. propofol and other lipophilic, hypnotic, or analgesic agents).

Respiratory effects

Clonidine has few respiratory effects. Neither change in respiratory control nor potentiation of opioid effects with either morphine or alfentanil are found. Intravenous dexmedetomidine at 2μg/kg can impair ventilation secondary to deep sedation, with obstructive respiratory patterns. Otherwise, there is little effect on resting ventilation, P_{CO_2}, or hypoxic ventilatory response.

Stress hormone effects

Clonidine partially inhibits the neurohormonal reaction to stress. The α_2-agonists induce hyperglycemia. Clonidine (75–150μg) can stop shivering by resetting the central threshold. However, intraoperatively, clonidine promotes ongoing temperature loss after 2 hours of anesthesia.

Addiction/poisoning

The locus coeruleus is also an important site for the action of addictive substances. It has a high concentration of opioid receptors as well as α_2-adrenoceptors. In opioid addiction, the locus coeruleus as well as cholinergic neurons are chronically inhibited. When the addictive substance is rapidly removed (e.g. by the use of naloxone) a state of locus coeruleus hyperexcitability exists, with profound noradrenergic outflow and high cholinergic activity (diarrhea, sweating, etc.) Therefore, α_2-agonists, which inhibit this outflow, are useful in treating withdrawal symptoms. However, treatment of the noradrenergic symptoms does not mean all withdrawal symptoms are equally affected. Behavioral effects such as craving can still be present. There are probably some spinal interactions involved with opioid addiction, owing to the high concentration of opioid receptors in the spinal cord. Though clonidine has been most studied in opioid withdrawal, it may have similar effects on alcohol withdrawal.

Learning/memory

There may be some beneficial effect of α_2-agonists in patients with Korsakoff's syndrome (where central noradrenergic

Antidepressant drugs				
Generic name	**Trade name(s)**	**Uptake inhibition**		**Comments**
		Norepinephrine	**Serotonin**	
First generation: tricycle antidepressants (TCA)				
Amitriptyline	Elavil, Endep, Lentizol, Tryptizol	Moderate	High	–
Clomipramine	Anafranil	Moderate	High	–
Desipramine	Norpramin, Pertofrane	High	Low	Fewer anticholinergic side effects
Doxepin	Sinequan, Adapin	Low	Moderate	–
Imipramine	Tofranil, Janimine	Moderate	Moderate	Prototypical tricyclic compound
Nortriptyline	Aventyl, Pamelor, Allegron	Moderate	Low	–
Protriptyline	Vivactil, Concordin	Moderate	Low	–
Trimipramine	Surmontil	Low	Low	–
Amoxapine	Ascendin, Ascendis	Moderate	Low	Second generation: dopamine D2 receptor-blocking properties
First generation: monoamine oxidase inhibitors (MAOIs)				
Phenelzine	Nardil	Depresses plasma cholinesterase		
Tranylcypromine	Parnate			
Moclobemide	Aurorix, Manerix, Moclamine	Reversible MAOI: may be better tolerated than other MAOIs		
Selegiline	Eldepryl, Denepryl	Type 'B' inhibitor: used to treat Parkinson's disease; inhibits metabolism of dopamine		
Second generation or atypical antidepressants				
Maprotiline	Ludiomil	Moderate	Low	Tetracyclic
Trazodone	Desyrel, Molipaxin	Very low	Moderate	–
Bupropion	Wellbutrin, Wellbatrin, Zyban	Very low	Very low	Inhibits dopamine reuptake
Selective serotonin reuptake inhibitors (SSRIs)				
Fluoxetine	Prozac	Very low	High	–
Fluvoxamine	Luvox	Very low	Very high	–
Paroxetine	Paxil, Seroxat	Very low	Very high	–
Sertraline	Zoloft, Lustral	Very low	Very high	–
Serotonin/norepinephrine-reuptake inhibitors				
Nefazodone	Serzone, Dutonin	Very high	Very high	–
Venlafaxine	Effexor	Very high	Very high	–

Figure 25.10 Antidepressants. These agents are active on the norepinephrine and serotonin systems, though very effective agents are available that are 'atypical' and do not work directly on these neurotransmitter systems. (From Lacey et al. with permission 1997.)

depletion is present) through improved cholinergic function from presynaptic α_2-actions. Though these drugs should help in Alzheimer's disease, studies have indicated little effect.

DOPAMINERGIC AGENTS

The dopamine system plays a key role in motor and reward activities. There are two main CNS dopaminergic pathways (Fig. 25.9). One originates in the substantia nigra and projects to the caudate-putamen (striatum) and is related to movement control, particularly in planning or organization of movement sequences. Loss of dopamine in the substantia nigra results in Parkinson's disease, and blockade of dopamine receptors by major tranquilizers can result in tardive dyskinesias.

The other pathway originates in the ventral tegmental area of the mesencephalon and projects to areas in the limbic system (amygdala, septal area, nucleus accumbens) and the prefrontal cortex. Projections to the prefrontal cortex may modulate executive control behaviors. Damage to, or dopamine deficiency in, this area of the cortex produces increased perseveration (inappropriate repetition of a previously rewarded response) and abnormalities in working memory, behavioral inhibition, affect, attention, planning, drive, and social interactions. This mesolimbic system rewards the organism for behavior that responds to cues which signal the availability of incentives or reinforcers. Exogenous stimulation of this system by various drugs (marijuana, cocaine, alcohol, etc.) can result in addictive behaviors.

Dopamine receptors have been classified pharmacologically and biochemically into two classes: D_1 receptors (D_1 and D_5 subtypes) and D_2 receptors (D_2, D_3, and D_4 subtypes), which have distinct cellular locations and intracellular signaling mechanisms. Dopamine D_1 receptors may be particularly important in the reinforcing effects of addictive drugs.

Dopaminergic drugs

Haloperidol

Haloperidol is the drug of choice for treatment of severe agitation in the ICU or in the postoperative period. There is a large body of literature on the use of haloperidol in the ICU setting. It has been administered in a doubling dose fashion, as a continuous intravenous infusion, and used in large doses if necessary. Initially 1–2mg is administered, and if agitation is severe the dose is doubled (4, 8, 16mg, etc.) until the agitation is controlled. Patients requiring doses of 300–1200mg/day have been reported. Once the initial agitation is controlled, a maintenance dose is given every 6 hours or an infusion of 1–20mg/h can be used. Serious complications are rare. Tardive dyskinesia can occur but is infrequent with acute intravenous administration. The QT_C interval should be monitored, as torsades de pointe has been reported. When combined with a benzodiazepine, smaller doses of haloperidol are effective to treat severe agitation. Consequently, a combination of agents is prefered to treat major delirium or in prophylaxis of acute drug withdrawal.

One complication of large and prolonged doses of haloperidol is the neuroleptic malignant syndrome (NMS). It is more common with oral administration than with acute intravenous administration. This syndrome results from central effects of chronic administration of haloperidol and other psychoactive drugs [e.g. other butyrophenones, phenothiazines, monoamine oxidase (MAO) inhibitors, lithium, or combinations]. The patient usually develops an impairment of motor function with generalized rigidity, akinesis, and/or extrapyramidal disturbances. Deterioration in mental status occurs, with coma, stupor, and/or delirium. Most notably, hyperpyrexia develops, with diaphoresis, blood pressure and heart rate fluctuations, and tachypnea. The picture may be quite similar to that of acute malignant hyperthermia, but their etiologies are distinct and the onset of NMS generally requires several days to several weeks. Treatment involves discontinuation of the drugs and symptomatic control of temperature, acid–base balance, intravenous fluid balance, and muscle tone. Recovery is slow because the drug effects dissipate very slowly. Dantrolene can aid in therapy of NMS by lowering muscle heat production and thereby reducing body temperature.

ADDICTIVE DRUGS

The reasons for addiction with certain drugs is a current area of much research with huge socioeconomic implications. Compared with drug enforcement, research in this area is vastly underfunded. Although 20–50% of trauma patients that present to large city emergency rooms in the USA have positive blood/urine tests for cocaine or its metabolites, there is almost no research or literature regarding the administration of anesthesia in these circumstances.

Cocaine

The therapeutic uses of cocaine as a local anesthetic will not be discussed here. Cocaine is an inhibitor of catecholamine (principally norepinephrine) reuptake at nerve terminals. The resultant synaptic catecholamine excess results in central stimulant effects and peripheral vasoconstrictive effects. The addictive properties of cocaine are related to its dopaminergic effects. Cocaine, as well as amphetamines, bind to the dopamine transporter, which clears dopamine from the synaptic cleft. A key site for addictive drug action is the nucleus accumbens, the projection site of the mesolimbic dopaminergic pathway.

Acute intoxication with cocaine can result in seizures, focal neurologic symptoms or signs, headache, transient loss of consciousness, hyperthermia, and hyperglycemia. Other signs of peripheral catecholamine release include diaphoresis and pupillary dilatation. Psychiatric disturbances include agitation, anxiety or depression, psychosis and paranoia, and suicidal ideation. The agitation can be severe and responds poorly to normal doses of sedatives. Hemodynamic instability is to be expected. Arrhythmias frequently occur and are the presumed cause of sudden death from cocaine. The combination of ethanol with cocaine is particularly toxic.

Depending on the time course of drug administration and the chronic patterns of stimulant use, a variety of hemodynamic responses can be seen during anesthesia. These range from severe hypertension, tachycardia, and profound vasoconstriction to hypotension unresponsive to indirect sympathomimetics (e.g. ephedrine). Vasoconstriction can result in cerebral aneurysm rupture or acute myocardial infarction and can be so severe that peripheral pulses are not palpable. This has lead to the erroneous administration of vasopressors. The vasoconstriction persists past the acute hemodynamic effects of cocaine administration. In fact, coronary vasoconstriction can occur for up to 6 weeks after the last use of cocaine, resulting in anginal symptoms or electrocardiograph changes. The hemodynamic response depends on whether cocaine is acutely preventing catecholamine reuptake or whether these stores are already depleted. For instance, there are reports indicating either no response or a severe hypertensive response to ephedrine.

Chronic use of cocaine impairs cognitive function, even when no drug is present. It can also lead to thrombocytopenia. Pulmonary changes occur in chronic users, especially with inhalation. These patients are particularly vulnerable to pulmonary edema, pulmonary hemorrhage, pneumothorax, and bronchospasm and can develop interstitial fibrosis.

Ethanol

Ethanol is itself a sedative agent: acute ingestion will decrease anesthetic requirements. In fact, ethanol has been used as a standardized control for sedative effects of various anesthetic drugs. Acute intoxication results in delayed gastric emptying. It also depresses left ventricular function with autonomic compensation, resulting in tachycardia and a reduced ejection fraction. Preload should be maintained at higher levels to maintain normal cardiac function.

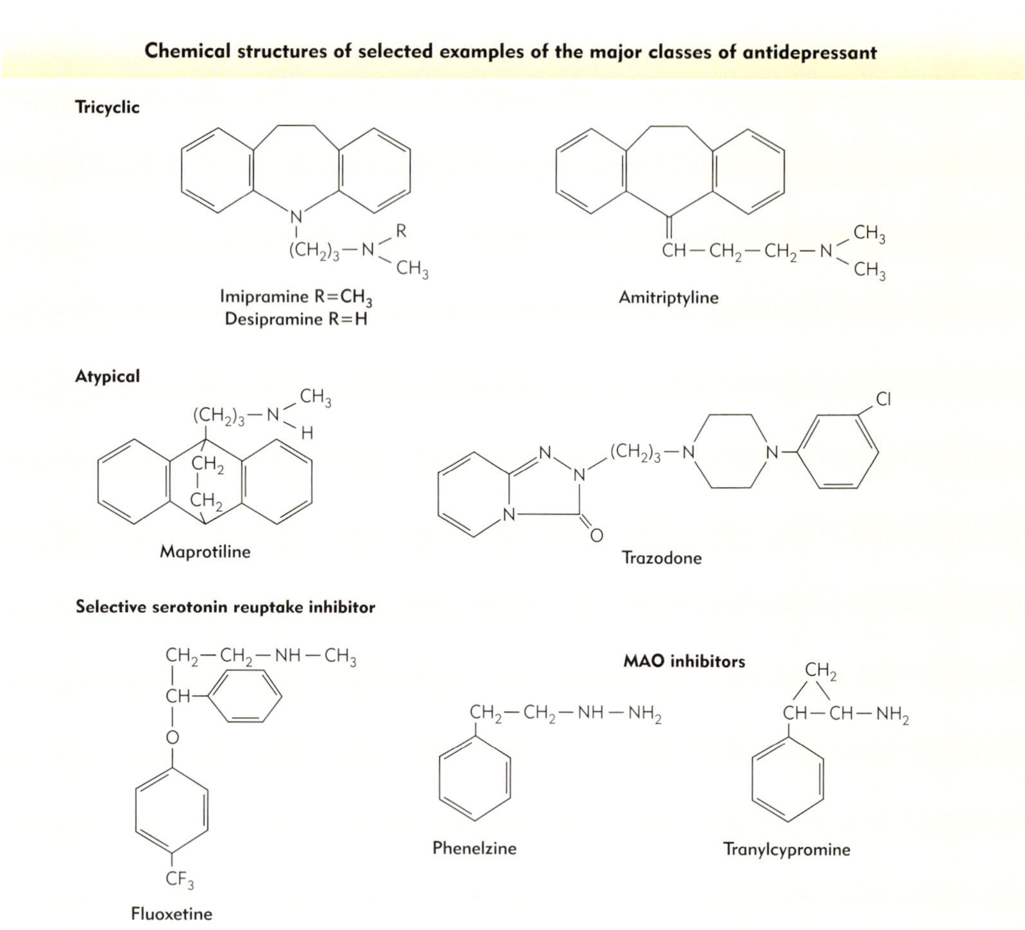
Chemical structures of selected examples of the major classes of antidepressant
Tricyclic
N
(CH2)3—N
R
CH3
Imipramine R=CH3
Desipramine R=H
CH—CH2—CH2—N
CH3
CH3
Amitriptyline
Atypical
(CH2)3—N
CH3
H
CH2
CH2
Maprotiline
N
N
(CH2)3—N
N
N
O
Cl
Trazodone
Selective serotonin reuptake inhibitor
CH2—CH2—NH—CH3
CH
O
CF3
Fluoxetine
MAO inhibitors
CH2—CH2—NH—NH2
Phenelzine
CH2
CH—CH—NH2
Tranylcypromine

Figure 25.11 Structures of selected antidepressants.

Chronic alcohol abuse may have varying effects on anesthetic requirements; most evidence indicates that more anesthetic drug is needed. The larger required doses may just reflect altered pharmacokinetic parameters, with no change in CNS sensitivity. Consequently, the anesthetic requirements in this patient population will be more variable than for the average patient and will depend on the degree of chronic consumption, any acute ingestion (which the patient may not reveal), and various physiologic changes accompanying chronic alcohol abuse. Careful titration of anesthetic drugs is required in this situation. A difficult problem occurs postoperatively when patients can develop withdrawal symptoms.

Withdrawal

Acute withdrawal from various addictive substances, particularly that precipitated by the administration of an antagonist, can be lethal, with pulmonary edema, seizures, arrhythmias, or myocardial infarction. A common component of withdrawal is the stress response, marked by release of corticotropin-releasing factor particularly in the amygdala. A major problem is how to manage patients requiring surgery who chronically abuse addictive substances. The intraoperative course may be stormy, but the use of general anesthetics masks many withdrawal symptoms, and indeed can be used as a means to allow rapid detoxification. The more difficult management problem occurs in the postoperative acute care unit or the ICU after surgery, where usual sedation regimens may be ineffective. Various regimens have been suggested that involve administration of benzodiazepines, major tranquilizers, or the substance itself (e.g. intravenous ethanol), which seem to be equally effective. The administration of sympatholytic agents (β blockers, central α_2-agonists) may be effective in ameliorating some of the peripheral (hypertension, tachycardia) symptoms but not the central (craving, hallucinations) withdrawal symptoms. The use of β blockers may exacerbate coronary vasospasm, which can occurr with acute cocaine use.

ANTIDEPRESSANTS

Depression is an under-reported and undertreated disease. With the advent of newer, more effective, and better tolerated agents, much greater use of antidepressants is expected in the general population. A plethora of antidepressants are now available, and anesthesiologists will frequently encounter patients receiving these medications (Fig. 25.10 & 25.11).

The most important interactions of antidepressants with anesthetics in the perioperative period occur with MAO inhibitors. There are numerous case reports of severe hemodynamic alterations under general anesthesia in patients treated with MAO inhibitors. Unfortunately, MAO inhibitors are used when other therapies fail, and discontinuation of these drugs before surgery is not without risk. Other antidepressant drugs seem to have few interactions with anesthesia, but most are relatively new. Even though tricyclic antidepressants and MAO inhibitors have been in use for decades, only recently have blunted responses to catecholamines been reported in patients taking chronic therapy with tricyclic antidepressants or MAO inhibitors.

In addition to the older and tricyclic and tetracyclic antidepressants, serotonin (5-HT) reuptake inhibitors (fluoxetine, sertraline, and paroxetine) and antidepressants with atypical mechanisms of action (bupropion, trazodone, venlafaxine, and nefazodone) are now available. Antagonism of monoamine transport is the primary cellular action of many antidepressant medications. However, an increased synaptic concentration of monoamines, which occurs minutes after administration, does not explain the antidepressant response, which is often delayed a matter of weeks. Furthermore, antidepressants have widely different effects on norepinephrine and serotonin reuptake, but all have comparable efficacy. Other drugs that increase norepinephrine at the synapse [e.g. levodopa and amphetamine (amfetamine)] have no clinical effect in depression. A common effect is that chronic administration of any of the antidepressants increases the efficiency of serotonergic transmission, albeit by different mechanisms. Serotonergic pathways are broadly distributed in the CNS, including the limbic forebrain (see Fig. 25.9), which is implicated in affective illness.

Most newer antidepressants are associated with a risk of clinically significant drug interactions. A rapidly growing body of literature provides evidence for a distinct profile of cytochrome P450 (CPY) inhibition and drug interaction risks with individual antidepressants. It is likely that administration of antidepressants will affect the metabolism of at least some anesthetic agents (e.g. alfentanil).

Tricyclic antidepressants

Tricyclic antidepressants, the most commonly used antidepressants, were originally synthesized from the phenothiazines. In common with phenothiazine, side effects include sedation, anticholinergic and sympatholytic effects, cardiotoxicity (orthostatic hypotension, flattened T waves, prolonged PR and QRS intervals), and increased sensitivity to catecholamines. A few animal experiments and some case reports indicate that long-term treatment with these substances can lead to intraoperative blood pressure fluctuations, tachycardia, and arrhythmias. Acute administration of tricyclic antidepressants may exaggerate the blood pressure response to catecholamines; long-term therapy may result in downregulation of receptors, depletion of endogenous stores, and a decrease in the response to catecholamines.

Monoamine oxidase inhibitors

Monoamine oxidase inhibitors are used as treatment for depression not responsive to initial drug therapy. In contrast to the irreversible blockade produced by many MAO inhibitors, moclobemide produces a reversible blockade and this results in fewer side effects. MAO inhibitors are the antidepressants associated with the highest incidence of adverse interactions with anesthesia, though it is likely that moclobemide will have fewer anesthetic interactions than previous MAO inhibitors.

Meperidine (pethidine), in particular, has been associated with severe interactions with MAO inhibitors. A syndrome of coma, hyperpyrexia, and hypertension can occur. A similar interaction with other opioids does not occur or is very rare. The mechanism appears to be an inhibition of neuronal serotonin uptake by meperidine, which results in toxic central serotonergic effects. Monoamine oxidase inhibitors may modify the response to catecholamines, with potentiation of catecholamine effects or hypertensive reactions. Anesthetic interactions with MAO inhibitors seem to be idiosyncratic, as meperidine, ketamine, and various catecholamines have been administered without incident to patients receiving MAO inhibitors. Treatment for this idiosyncratic reaction is supportive. Use of steroids and phenothiazines can be considered, though phenothiazines have themselves induced adverse reactions in patients taking MAO inhibitors. For patients taking long-term MAO inhibitor therapy, it takes some time for normal adrenergic responsiveness to return following discontinuation of the drug. Refractory hypotension may occur in this situation, possibly as a result of receptor downregulation.

Selective serotonin-reuptake inhibitors

Selective serotonin-reuptake inhibitors (SSRIs) apparently have very few side effects, and no significant adverse interactions with anesthetics have been reported. Drugs of this class differ substantially in their pharmacokinetics and effects on P450 enzymes. Most have a half-life of approximately 1 day. Fluoxetine, however, has a half-life of 2–4 days, and its active metabolite, norfluoxetine, has an extended half-life of 7–15 days. A discontinuation syndrome can occur with cessation of therapy and is most evident with drugs with short half-lives (paroxetine, venlafaxine, and fluvoxamine). The syndrome includes nausea, lethargy, insomnia, and headache; it also occurs with abrupt discontinuation of tricyclic antidepressants. The similarity may be related to cholinergic rebound. Although generally mild and short lived, discontinuation symptoms can be severe and chronic. Consequently, discontinuation of SSRIs before anesthesia is not recommended.

Selective serotonin-reuptake inhibitors can be associated with hyponatremia from the syndrome of inappropriate vasopressin (antidiuretic hormone) release (SIADH), especially in elderly patients. In a large series, hyponatremia and SIADH was associated with fluoxetine in 75%, paroxetine in 12%, sertraline in 11.7%, and fluvoxamine in 1%. The median time to onset of hyponatremia was 13 days (range 3–120 days).

Lithium

Lithium was the first effective drug used to treat psychiatric disorders. At the end of the 1990s, it has a major role in the treatment of bipolar affective disorder, with particular efficacy in the manic phase. It also has a role in treating recurrent depression. The major toxicity is renal, which is rare if therapeutic levels are adequately monitored. Lithium may potentiate the action of neuromuscular blocking drugs and may theoretically decrease anesthetic requirements. It can affect the T waves in the ECG.

Key References

Frackowiak RS, Friston KJ. Functional neuroanatomy of the human brain: positron emission tomography – a new neuroanatomical technique. J Anat. 1994;184:211–25.
Ghoneim MM, Ali MA, Block RI. Appraisal of the quality of assessment of memory in anesthesia and psychopharmacology literature. Anesthesiology. 1990;73:815–20.
Ghoneim MM, Block RI. Learning and memory during general anesthesia. Anesthesiology. 1997;87:387–410.
Ghoneim MM, Mewaldt SP. Benzodiazepines and human memory: a review. Anesthesiology. 1990;72:926–38.
Koob GF. Drug addiction: the yin and yang of hedonic homeostasis. Neuron. 1996;16:893–6.
Lacey CL, Armstrong LL, Ingrim NB, Lance LL. Drug information handbook, 5th edn. Lexi-Comp Inc: 1997;1393-4.
Maze M, Tranquilli W. Alpha-2 adrenoceptor agonists: defining the role in clinical anesthesia. Anesthesiology. 1991;74:581–605.
McFarlane HJ. Anaesthesia and the new generation monoamine oxidase inhibitors. Anaesthesia. 1994;49:597–9.
McKernan RM, Whiting PJ. Which GABA-A receptor subtypes really occur in the brain? Trend Neurosci. 1996;19:139–43.
Pich EM, Pagliusi SR, Tessari M, et al. Common neural substrates for the addictive properties of nicotine and cocaine. Science. 1997;275:83–6.
Prichard JW, Rosen BR. Functional study of the brain by NMR. J Cereb Blood Flow Metab. 1994;14:365–72.
Scheinin M, Schwinn DA. The locus coeruleus. Site of hypnotic actions of alpha-2 adrenoceptor agonists? Anesthesiology. 1992;76:873–5.
Thapar P, Zacny JP, Choi M, Apfelbaum JL. Objective and subjective impairment from often-used sedative/analgesic combinations in ambulatory surgery, using alcohol as a benchmark. Anesth Analg. 1995;80:1092–8.
Ungerleider LG. Functional brain imaging studies of cortical mechanisms for memory. Science. 1995;270:769–75.

Further Reading

Alkire MT, Haier RJ, Barker SJ, et al. Cerebral metabolism during propofol anesthesia in humans studied with positron emission tomography. Anesthesiology. 1995;82:393–403.
Andrade J. Learning during anaesthesia: a review. Br J Psychol. 1995;86:479–506.
Bruce DL. Alcoholism and anesthesia. Anesth Analg. 1983;62:84–96.
Eisenach JC, de Kock M, Klimscha W. Alpha(2)-adrenergic agonists for regional anesthesia. A clinical review of clonidine (1984–1995). Anesthesiology. 1996;85:655–74.
Ghoneim MM, Block RI. Learning and consciousness during general anesthesia. Anesthesiology. 1992;76:279–305.
Gold MS. Opiate addiction and the locus coeruleus. The clinical utility of clonidine, naltrexone, methadone, and buprenorphine. Psychiatr Clin North Am. 1993;16:61–73.
Jones JG. Perception and memory during general anaesthesia. Br J Anaesth. 1994;73:31–7.
McSPI–Europe Research Group. Perioperative sympatholysis. Beneficial effects of the alpha 2-adrenoceptor agonist mivazerol on hemodynamic stability and myocardial ischemia. Anesthesiology. 1997;86:346–63.
Robbins TW, Everitt BJ. Drug addiction: bad habits add up. Nature. 1999;398:567–70.
Schacter DL, Chiu C-YP, Ochsner KN. Implicit memory: a selective review. Annu Rev Neurosci. 1993;16:159–82.
Sprung J, Schoenwald PK, Levy P, et al. Treating intraoperative hypotension in a patient on long-term tricyclic antidepressants: a case of aborted aortic surgery. Anesthesiology. 1997;86:990–2.
Tulving E, Schacter DL. Priming and human memory systems. Science. 1990;247:301–6.
Veselis RA, Reinsel RA, Beattie B, et al. Midazolam changes cerebral blood flow in discrete brain regions: an $H_2^{15}O$ positron emission tomography study. Anesthesiology. 1997;87:1106–117.
Zola-Morgan S, Squire LR. Neuroanatomy of memory. Annu Rev Neurosci. 1993;16:547–63.

Chapter 26 Opioids

Gavril W Pasternak

Topics covered in this chapter

Endogenous pain-modulatory systems
Opioid drugs
Pharmacokinetics
Opioid receptors
Opioid analgesia
Other opioid actions
Clinical pharmacology

Opioids have long been used in the relief of pain. The search for nonaddicting agents and for analgesics that avoid many of the side effects encountered with current drugs has led to the synthesis of thousands of analogs, which, in turn, has provided important tools in our understanding of opioid actions. We now know that the opioids act through a complex system of receptors and opioid peptides, components of the endogenous opioid systems.

Opioids have unique actions in the relief of pain. Unlike local anesthetics, which interfere with all sensation, opioids act upon pain without interfering with objective sensations such as touch and temperature. Pain is made up of two components (Chapter 21). The first component, fast pain, is carried through the neospinothalamic pathways and conducts the well-localized 'objective' aspect of painful sensations. Neurons in the dorsal horn of the spinal cord receive input from sensory nerves, cross the midline of the cord, and then ascend to the thalamus. The thalamic neurons then project directly to the sensory cortex. Damage to the sensory cortex, such as seen in stroke, leads to the loss of these sensations.

The second component of pain, slow pain, is transmitted rostrally more slowly because of extensive synaptic interactions with the brainstem and limbic structures. Unlike fast pain, slow pain is poorly localized and is responsible for the 'hurt', or suffering, component of pain. Opioids specifically target 'slow pain', relieving the 'hurt' of pain. Indeed, patients often comment after receiving an opioid that the pain is still there but it does not hurt.

ENDOGENOUS PAIN-MODULATORY SYSTEMS

Pain is an essential, although unpleasant, sensation that protects the individual by warning of potential injury or damage. Yet, it is easy to think of situations in which pain must be suppressed. A wounded soldier, for example, must still defend himself. Therefore, it is not surprising that the sensory nervous system is able to filter nociceptive stimuli, modulating the perception of pain. The first clinical study implying such a system came from studies comparing the morphine needs of wounded soldiers in the Second World War to those of civilians undergoing elective surgery. Despite their far more serious wounds, the soldiers required less analgesics than the civilians. The first experimental evidence emerged from studies looking at direct brain stimulation. These studies found that stimulating specific brain regions induced a potent analgesic action both in experimental animals and in humans. Only certain brain regions were capable of producing these actions, and the analgesic activity could be prevented by naloxone, a very specific opioid antagonist. This provided the first evidence for an endogenous pain-modulatory system that could be activated by opioids.

The endogenous opioid system comprises a family of peptides and their receptors. Pharmacologically, opioid peptides share many characteristics including the ability to produce analgesia. However, their mechanisms of action are very different. The enkephalins were the first opioid peptides identified, followed soon after by the dynorphins and β-endorphin. Structurally, all the opioid peptides have striking similarities. Two – Met^5-enkephalin and Leu^5-enkephalin – are highly related pentapeptides differing only in their C-terminal amino acid (Fig. 26.1). Enkephalins are the endogenous ligands for the δ-class of opioid receptors. Peptides within the dynorphin family are longer than the enkephalins. Dynorphin A, the most intensely studied member of this family, contains 17 amino acid residues and is the endogenous ligand for the κ_1-opioid receptor. Like other members of this opioid peptide family, dynorphin A contains the sequence of Leu^5- enkephalin at its N-terminus. Less is known about other members of this family, such as dynorphin B or α-neoendorphin. Beta-endorphin represents the third member of the opioid peptide family. It is far larger than the other opioid peptides, containing 31 amino acid residues. Although its precursor, pro-opiomelanocortin, encodes only one opioid peptide, it also generates several other physiologically important peptides, including adrenocorticotropic hormone (ACTH), which is co-released from the pituitary with β-endorphin (Chapter 63).

The presence of an enkephalin sequence within the dynorphin series and in β-endorphin suggested that the enkephalins might be breakdown products of these larger peptides. However, this is clearly not the case. Three major families of opioid peptides have been established and the genes encoding their precursors have been cloned (Fig. 26.2). The opioid peptides are derived from larger precursors through extensive

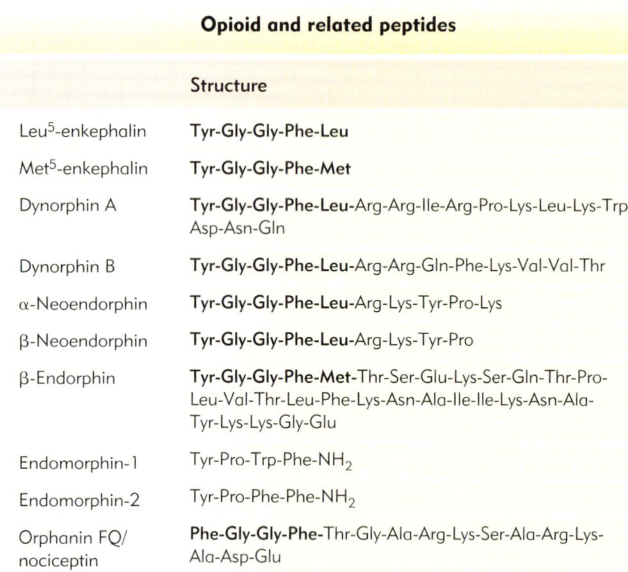

Opioid and related peptides

	Structure
Leu⁵-enkephalin	**Tyr-Gly-Gly-Phe-Leu**
Met⁵-enkephalin	**Tyr-Gly-Gly-Phe-Met**
Dynorphin A	**Tyr-Gly-Gly-Phe-Leu**-Arg-Arg-Ile-Arg-Pro-Lys-Leu-Lys-Trp-Asp-Asn-Gln
Dynorphin B	**Tyr-Gly-Gly-Phe-Leu**-Arg-Arg-Gln-Phe-Lys-Val-Val-Thr
α-Neoendorphin	**Tyr-Gly-Gly-Phe-Leu**-Arg-Lys-Tyr-Pro-Lys
β-Neoendorphin	**Tyr-Gly-Gly-Phe-Leu**-Arg-Lys-Tyr-Pro
β-Endorphin	**Tyr-Gly-Gly-Phe-Met**-Thr-Ser-Glu-Lys-Ser-Gln-Thr-Pro-Leu-Val-Thr-Leu-Phe-Lys-Asn-Ala-Ile-Ile-Lys-Asn-Ala-Tyr-Lys-Lys-Gly-Glu
Endomorphin-1	Tyr-Pro-Trp-Phe-NH_2
Endomorphin-2	Tyr-Pro-Phe-Phe-NH_2
Orphanin FQ/ nociceptin	**Phe-Gly-Gly-Phe**-Thr-Gly-Ala-Arg-Lys-Ser-Ala-Arg-Lys-Ala-Asp-Glu

Figure 26.1 Opioid and related peptides.

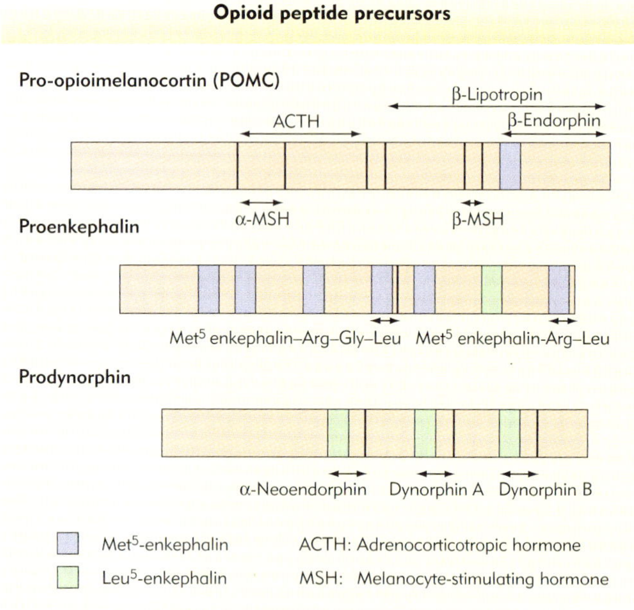

Figure 26.2 The opioid peptide precursors.

proteolytic processing. Although prepro-opiomelanocortin contains only β-endorphin, the other precursor peptides contain multiple copies of opioid peptides. The isolation and cloning of all three precursors unequivocally established that each generates distinct neurotransmitters (Fig. 26.2).

Regional differences have been documented in the distribution of the various opioid peptides within the CNS. The enkephalins are widely distributed, implying a wide range of actions beyond simple analgesia. In contrast, β-endorphin is limited to the pituitary and the arcuate region of the hypothalamus, although these areas do have extensive projections.

A major difficulty faced in early studies of the enkephalins was their instability because of rapid enzymatic degradation *in vivo*. The development of metabolically stable derivatives has greatly facilitated the evaluation of these compounds. In addition to enhancing their stability, variations in structure have led to extraordinary differences in selectivity for the various opioid receptors. For example, the synthetic opioid D-Ala²–MePhe⁴–Gly(ol)⁵-enkephalin (DAMGO) is a very selective morphine-like drug with properties quite different from the natural enkephalins. These synthetic opioid peptides have become a major resource for investigations of these systems, providing highly selective agonists and antagonists for most opioid receptors.

Another pair of opioid peptides, the endomorphins, has recently been isolated. Endomorphin-1 and endomorphin-2 are tetrapeptides that are structurally distinct from other members of the opioid peptide family. The major difference between the endomorphins and other opioid peptides is their high selectivity for μ-receptors, which suggests that they may represent endogenous ligands for these receptors. Our knowledge of the endomorphins is quite limited, but it is likely to open new areas in drug development and provide insights into the μ-opioid system.

The recent cloning of the opioid receptors has identified a receptor within the opioid family that has poor affinity for traditional opioids. Although this receptor is related to the opioid κ_3-receptor, they are not the same. The endogenous ligand for this receptor is orphanin FQ or nociceptin, a heptadecapeptide (see Fig. 26.1) with some similarities to dynorphin A. The pharmacology of this peptide is quite complex and will require further study. For example, it was originally proposed to be hyperalgesic. More recent studies have demonstrated that it can functionally reverse the analgesic actions of a number of opioids, but it can elicit analgesia in other paradigms.

OPIOID DRUGS

Morphine-related compounds

Morphine and codeine were first isolated from opium, which contains a mixture of alkaloids (Fig. 26.3). Structurally, they differ only in the presence of a methyl group at the 3-position. Codeine must be metabolized by 3-*O*-demethylation to morphine for a full analgesic effect. This reaction is catalyzed by the genetically polymorphic P450, isozyme CYP 2D6, which is absent in about 8% of the British population, and which is inhibited by tricyclic antidepressants, selective serotonin reuptake inhibitors, neuroleptics, quinidine, etc. These individuals are unable to convert codeine to morphine and do not experience codeine hypoalgesia (i.e. codeine acts through metabolically formed morphine). Morphine 6β-glucuronide (M6G) is a potent morphine metabolite with pharmacologic properties that are distinct from those of morphine. Heroin (diacetylmorphine, diamorphine) is not used for therapeutic purposes in the USA but is used in the UK and remains the major opioid of abuse. It is synthesized from morphine by acetylation at both the 3- and 6-positions. When administered, the 3-acetyl group is rapidly removed enzymatically to form 6-acetylmorphine, the active component of heroin. Nalorphine (Fig. 26.4) was the first opioid antagonist identified and reverses the actions of morphine. It differs structurally from morphine only in the replacement of the *N*-methyl group with an *N*-allyl moiety. It is not used clinically

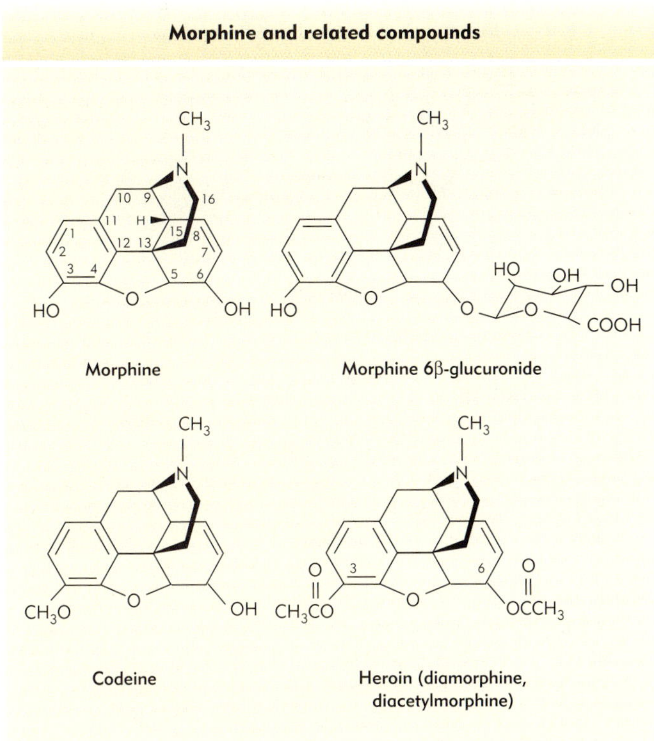

Figure 26.3 Structure of morphine and related compounds.

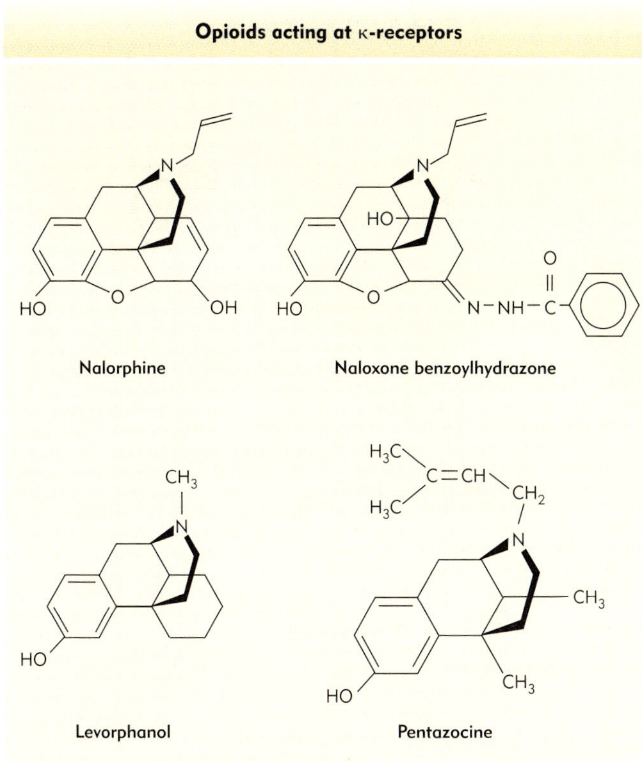

Figure 26.4 Structure of opioids acting at κ-receptors.

since it also has activity at κ-receptors and produces severe dysphorias and psychotomimetic actions.

Opium also contains thebaine, which has been used to make a number of additional opioid compounds, many of which are important clinically (Fig. 26.5). Hydromorphone is a potent analgesic, as is oxymorphone. Oxycodone is widely used in combination with acetominophen (paracetamol) or aspirin. Naloxone and naltrexone (Fig. 26.6) are both pure opioid antagonists and are used clinically. It is interesting that the simple replacement of the *N*-methyl group of oxymorphone converts this potent analgesic to a pure antagonist.

A number of these agents are now available in slow-release formulations, including morphine and oxycodone. The ability to increase the dosing interval to up to 12 hours has been a major advantage clinically, although care must be taken with dose titration since it may take several days to reach steady-state levels of drug.

Phenylpiperidines

The first phenylpiperidine used was meperidine (pethidine) (see Fig. 26.5), one of the most widely used opioids for many years. Loperamide is a structurally similar compound which is peripherally acting μ-opioid agonist. A number of additional useful compounds have been synthesized, particularly the fentanyl series (Fig. 26.7). Fentanyl and its analogs are highly potent opioids that act predominantly through μ-receptors. However, they differ pharmacologically from morphine in a number of ways, as discussed below. Their short half-lives and rapid onset and offset have led to their extensive use in anesthesiology. Fentanyl is now also available as a transdermal patch, which has major advantages particularly for patients who cannot take medications orally.

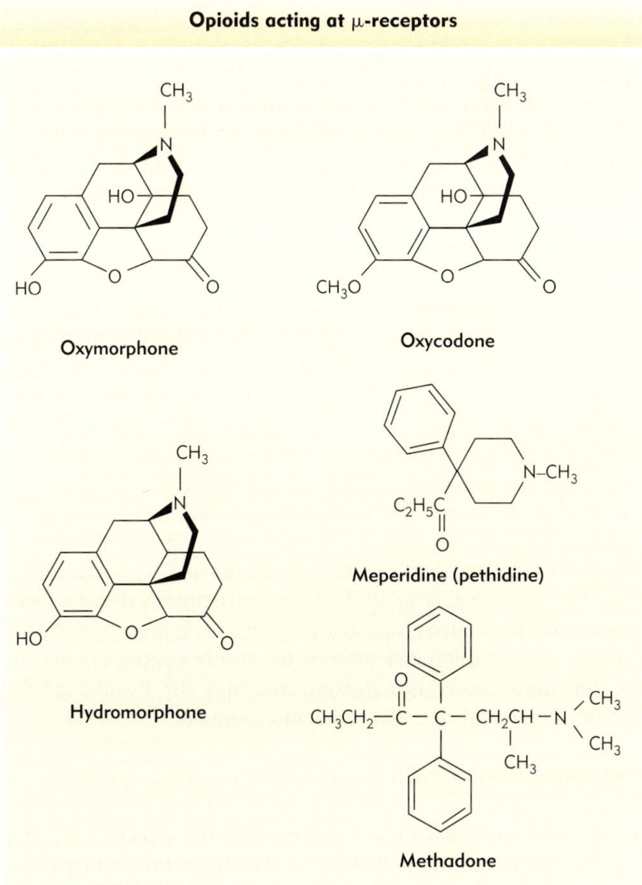

Figure 26.5 Structures of opioids acting at μ-receptors.

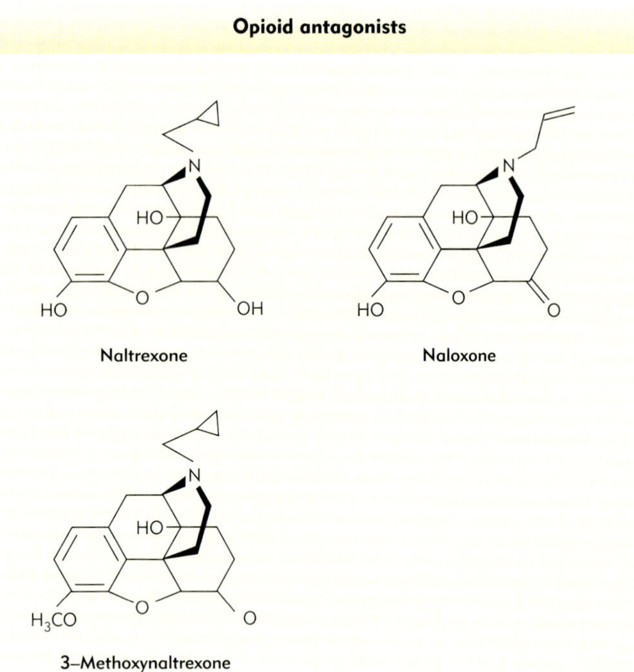

Figure 26.6 Structure of opioid antagonists.

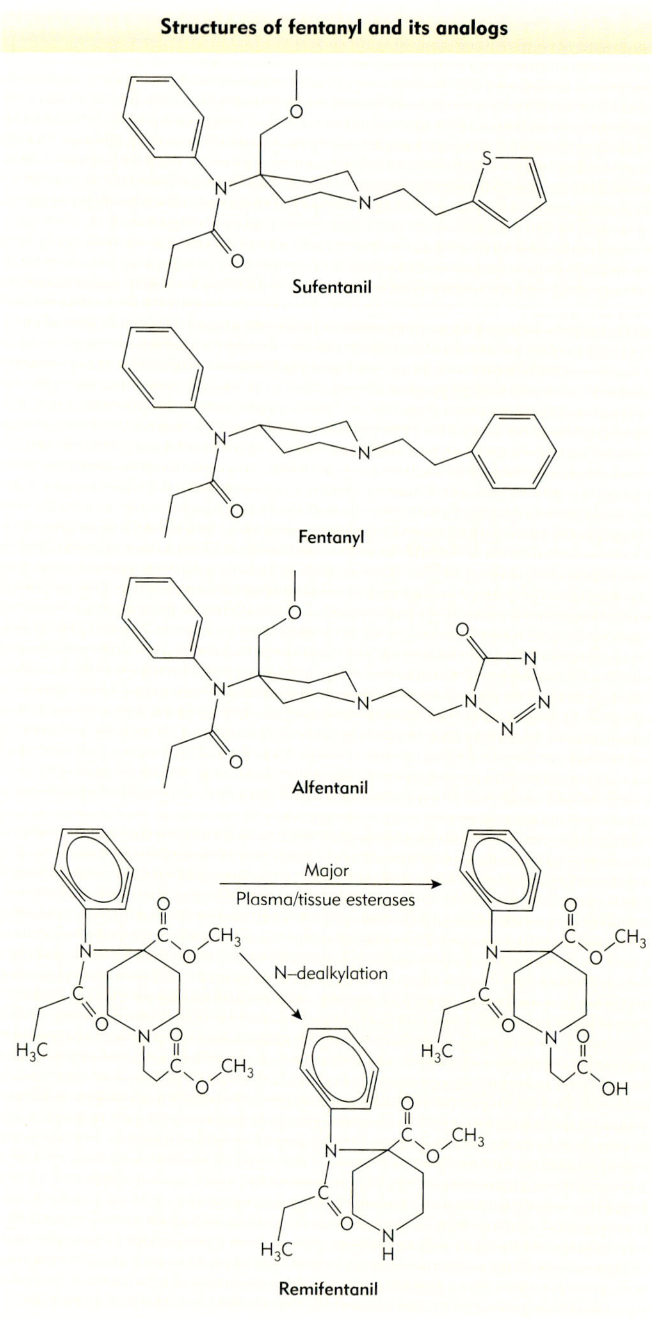

Figure 26.7 Structures of fentanyl and its analogs. The metabolic pathway of remifentanil is also shown. Its major metabolite is <0.001% as potent as remifentanil.

Methadone and propoxyphene (dextropropoxyphene)

Methadone (Fig. 26.5) is a μ-opioid with actions similar to those of morphine. One of the first synthetic opioids, methadone is used extensively in the management of opiate abuse, but it is also a valuable analgesic. It has a long half-life, permitting less frequent dosing. Propoxyphene (dextropropoxyphene), which is structurally related to methadone, is a weak opioid widely used in conjuction with either acetominophen or aspirin.

Mixed agonist/antagonists

Pentazocine (Fig. 26.4) is the most widely used drug with mixed agonist/antagonist properties. It has analgesic actions mediated primarily through κ_1-receptors but also has antagonist activity at μ-receptors. In general, the use of pentazocine should be limited to opioid-naive patients. Nalbuphine and butorphanol are also mixed agonist/antagonists. Their analgesic actions are mediated through κ-receptors, while they have antagonist actions at μ-receptors. These drugs may more accurately be described as partial agonists at both κ and μ receptors, which show antagonist activity toward full μ agonists. Buprenorphine has a similar profile, but dissociates slowly from μ receptors and is poorly antagonized by naloxone. Tramadol, which is structurally distinct from other opioids, is either a partial μ agonist or a full agonist with low potency and minimal κ affinity. Its antinociceptive effects are not fully antagonized by naloxone, and may also involve inhibition of norepinephrine and serotonin reuptake.

PHARMACOKINETICS

In addition to their widely varying receptor selectivities, the various opioid analgesics also can be differentiated by their durations of action (Fig. 26.8). In general, the duration of analgesia corresponds to the elimination half-time of the drug. However, many of the drugs need to be given more frequently than anticipated to maintain analgesic activity. Half-times vary depending upon the route of administration and mechanism of clearance.

Some physicochemical and pharmacokinetic properties of the fentanyl family of opioids are summarized in Figures 26.9–26.10. Simple comparison of their elimination half-times does not predict the rates of decrease in effect-site concentration detected by pharmacokinetic studies. An intravenous bolus of fentanyl undergoes rapid distribution to highly perfused tissues; peak concentrations occur in brain in 2–3 minutes, with peak analgesia about 2 minutes later. Brain levels rapidly decline through redistribution into the high volume of distribution (V_d), followed by a slower elimination through hepatic metabolism (by *N*-dealkylation) as the drug re-enters the central compartment. This slow elimination phase can result in prolonged and cumulative effects with repeated or large doses, as reflected in the steep increase in the context-sensitive half-time [the time to a 50% decrease in effect-site concentration after termination of an infusion, which depends on the rates of distribution and elimination ($t_{1/2\beta}$) *and* on the duration of infusion] (Fig. 26.10). Alfentanil exhibits similar pharmacokinetics, but its reduced lipophilicity results in less protein and lipid binding, a lower V_d, and more rapid clearance (by cytochrome P450 CYP3 A4). Consequently, alfentanil is much less likely to produce cumulative effects (Fig. 26.10). Despite its lower lipid solubility, the onset of alfentanil action is much faster than fentanyl: the initial plasma concentration is higher because of its lower central V_d, and its acidic pK_a means that it is 90% non-ionized at blood pH and is, therefore, diffusible across the blood–brain barrier. Sufentanil has the highest lipid solubility, with a large V_d and high clearance (by hepatic *N*- and *O*-dealkylation) compared with alfentanil. Its context-sensitive half-time demonstrates its utility in short procedures compared with alfentanil and fentanyl (Fig. 26.9). Remifentanil, a 4-anilidopiperidine, has a unique metabolic and pharmacokinetic profile. It undergoes rapid methyl ester hydrolysis by tissue and plasma esterases (not plasma cholinesterase) to relatively inactive metabolites; as a result, its effect is terminated by rapid metabolic clearance rather than redistribution (Fig. 26.10). This results in rapid reduction in plasma concentration after bolus or prolonged infusion independent of age, weight, sex, or hepatic and renal function. It is a potent, fast-acting μ-opioid with a rapid recovery, which is useful for infusions or short, painful procedures. Is short-duration analgesic effect requires pre-emptive use of longer-acting analgesics at discontinuation of infusion to prevent postoperative pain.

Elimination half-times of opioids

Drug	Approximate half-life
Remifentanil	10min
Naloxone	75min[a]
Alfentanil	90min
Morphine	120min
Hydromorphone	150min
Oxymorphone	150min
Nalbuphine	150min
Sufentanil	150min
Butorphanol	180min
Codeine	180min
Meperidine (pethidine)	200min
Fentanyl	220min
Propoxyphene (dextroproproxyphene)	8h
Levorphanol	15h
Methadone	24h

[a]Note that the half-time of the μ-receptor antagonist naloxone is far shorter than that of most clinically used opioids.

Figure 26.8 Elimination half-times of opioids.

OPIOID RECEPTORS

Opioid receptors are members of the G protein-coupled receptor family (Chapter 3). Despite major advances in our understanding of these receptors, many questions remain. There are three major classes of opioid receptor: μ, δ, and κ. Although they share the ability to elicit analgesia, their pharmacologic properties differ. The μ-agonists are far more potent respiratory depressants and constipating agents than the others, for example. Even their ability to modulate the perception of pain is mediated through distinct mechanisms. As a result, they display no cross-tolerance and highly selective antagonists can reverse the actions of one class without blocking others. This makes each opioid receptor class a potential therapeutic target. However, the relationships between the subtypes defined pharmacologically and those identified at the molecular level are not entirely clear. More subtypes have been identified by binding and pharmacologic studies than have been identified by molecular cloning, which has yielded four genes: encoding μ (*MOR-1*), δ (*DOR*-1), κ_1 (*KOR-1*), and

Properties of the fentanyl family opioids

Parameter	Remifentanil	Alfentanil	Fentanyl	Sufentanil
Lipid solubility (octanol: water solubility coefficient)	17.9	129	816	1727
pK_a	7.1	6.5	8.4	8.0
Non-ionized fraction at blood pH	67	89	8.5	20
Volume of distribution (L/kg)	0.47	0.75	4.0	2.9
Elimination half-time (min)	9–11	94	219	164
Clearance (L/h per kg)	2.48	0.48	0.78	0.76
Relative potency	1	0.014	1	9

Figure 26.9 Physicochemical and pharmacokinetic properties of the fentanyl family opioids

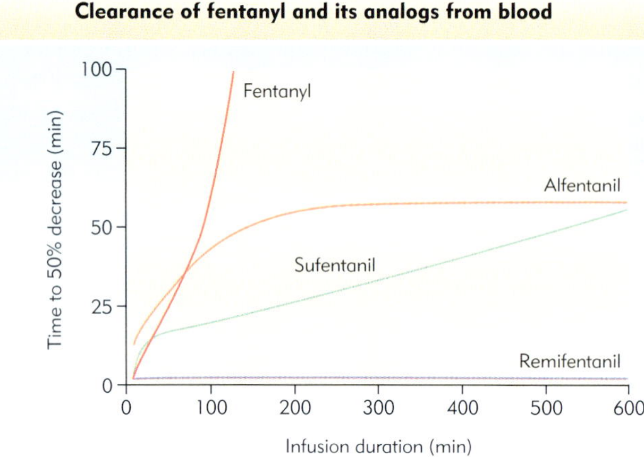

Figure 26.10 Clearance of fentanyl and its analogs from blood. A simulation of the time necessary to achieve a 50% decrease in drug concentration in the blood (or plasma) after variable times of intravenous infusions of remifentanil, fentanyl, alfentanil, and sufentanil. Note that alfentanil has a longer context-sensitive half-time than sufentanil despite having a shorter elimination half-life. (With permission from Egan et al., 1993.)

a related orphan opioid clone (*KOR-3/ORL1*) that binds the novel peptide orphanin FQ/nociceptin.

The μ-receptors

Morphine and related alkaloids act primarily through μ-receptors to produce their classical actions, foremost of which is analgesia (Fig. 26.11). Most clinically used analgesics act at μ-receptors, including morphine, oxymorphone, methadone, and the fentanyl series. Many opioid side effects are also produced through μ-receptors, such as constipation and respiratory depression.The μ-receptors are antagonized by a number of drugs. Some are highly selective and only block μ-receptors (β-funaltrexamine). Others reverse the actions of a variety of opioids and show only slight selectivity for μ-receptors (e.g. naloxone, which is extensively used clinically).

As with other G protein-coupled receptors, the *MOR-1*-encoded receptor has seven transmembrane domains that are arranged to form a donut-like structure spanning the membrane, with the binding pocket for the drug located in the center. Morphine and other μ-acting drugs bind to this site with high affinity, confirming that it represents a μ-receptor. *MOR-1* contains four exons, and several splice variants have been identified, indicating that various molecular forms of this receptor exist.

Pharmacologic evidence now suggests three subtypes of μ-receptors. The initial characterization of μ-receptor subtypes was based on the opioid antagonist naloxonazine and indicated μ_1 and μ_2 sites (Fig. 26.11). Both types elicit analgesia but at different sites within the CNS. The μ_1 sites are important for supraspinal and peripheral analgesia, while μ_2 sites act at the spinal level. The respiratory depressant actions of morphine and many of the signs of dependence are mediated through μ_2-receptors, raising the possibility of producing analgesics lacking gastrointestinal or respiratory depressant activity. Conversely, a μ_2-antagonist might prove useful to reverse the respiratory and gastrointestinal actions of morphine and related compounds. In animal studies, an antagonist has been reported that selectively blocks the gastrointestinal effects of morphine at doses that do not interfere with analgesia.

The third member of the μ-receptor family is perhaps the most intriguing. It mediates the actions of M6G, a very potent morphine metabolite. When administered directly into the CNS to avoid the blood–brain barrier, M6G is over 100-fold more potent than morphine. The importance of the M6G receptor was recently demonstrated by its involvement in mediating the actions of heroin. Evidence for this third μ-receptor subtype comes from a variety of sources. The CXBK strain of mouse is insensitive to morphine. Yet, M6G and heroin retain their analgesic activity. A new antagonist, 3-methoxynaltrexone, unlike the other μ-antagonists, is selective for the M6G site and blocks both M6G and heroin analgesia at doses that are inactive against morphine.

Antisense mapping studies provide a method for decreasing mRNA levels for a specific protein with a selectivity and specificity far greater than any of the available antagonists. In antisense mapping, probes are designed to examine different mRNA sequences corresponding to various exons, which provides the opportunity to attribute functional activity to specific splice variants. Antisense mapping analysis of the four exons of *MOR-1* revealed dramatic differences between the actions of morphine and M6G. Probes targeting exon 1 effectively block morphine analgesia without interfering with M6G analgesia. Conversely, probes targeting exon 2 are inactive against morphine but block M6G analgesia. These studies imply that the μ- and M6G receptors are related to *MOR-1* but are distinct from each other and might represent splice variants of *MOR-1*.

The relationship of these two receptors to each other and to *MOR-1* at the molecular level is still uncertain. However, two sets of knock-out mice (Chapter 4) provide interesting insights. In knock-out mice in which the first exon of the *MOR-1* has been eliminated, morphine lacks analgesic actions, while M6G and heroin are active; this is consistent with the antisense mapping studies above. In knock-out mice in which exon 2 was inactivated, both morphine and M6G are completely inactive. This suggests that the M6G receptor is a product of *MOR-1* and that it is distinct from the μ_1- or μ_2-receptor. It remains to be cloned.

The *MOR-1* exon 1 knock-out mice also have proven valuable in assessing many traditional opioid analgesics. For example, fentanyl has been classified as a drug acting upon μ-receptors based upon extensive pharmacologic testing. Yet, fentanyl is active in the *MOR-1* exon knock-out mice, implying that it can act through M6G mechanisms distinct from those of morphine and, therefore, has a different pharmacology to morphine. The availability of these genetic models will yield new insights into the pharmacology of many analgesics, including those already widely used.

The δ-receptors

The δ-receptors are highly selective for enkephalins. They were first identified in mouse vas deferens bioassays and subsequently in brain by binding studies. Like μ-receptors, δ-receptors produce analgesia both spinally and supraspinally. A δ-receptor, encoded by *DOR-1*, has been cloned and demonstrates the anticipated selectivity for enkephalins and related

Opioid receptor classification and localization of analgesic actions

Receptor	Clone	Analgesia	Other actions
μ-Receptors	MOR-1		
μ_1	–	Supraspinal	Prolactin release, acetylcholine release in the hippocampus, feeding
μ_2	–	Spinal	Respiratory depression, gastrointestinal transit, dopamine release by nigrostriatal neurons, guinea pig ileum bioassay, feeding
	M6G	Spinal and supraspinal	–
κ-Receptors			
κ_1	KOR-1	Spinal and supraspinal	Psychotomimetic, sedation
κ_2	–	Unknown	Diuresis, feeding
κ_3	KOR-3/ORL1 (?)	Supraspinal	Unknown
δ-Receptors			Mouse vas deferens bioassay, dopamine turnover in the striatum, feeding
δ_1	–	Supraspinal	–
δ_2	DOR-1	Spinal and supraspinal	–

Some of the actions attributed to a general family of receptor have not yet been associated with a specific subtype. The correlations in this table are based on animal studies, which can show species differences.

Figure 26.11 Opioid receptor classification and localization of analgesic actions.

compounds. Two δ-receptors have been proposed pharmacologically, δ_1 and δ_2, which can be differentiated by both agonists and antagonists. Spinally, δ_2-receptors mediate analgesia while both δ subtypes are active supraspinally. The cloned δ-receptor appears to correspond to the δ_2 subtype. Although δ-receptors remain a viable therapeutic target, no agents acting at δ-receptors are yet available clinically.

The κ-receptors

The κ-receptors were identified based on the pharmacology of opioid analogs such as ketocyclazocine, but their existence was firmly established with the discovery of dynorphin A, the endogenous ligand for the κ_1-receptor, and the development of highly selective agonists such as U50,488 and U69,593 and the antagonist norbinaltorphimine. Many of the mixed agonist/antagonist opioids act at the κ_1-receptor, including pentazocine. Although several of the highly selective κ_1-agonists were analgesic in clinical trials, unpleasant side effects prevented further development. In addition to a significant diuretic action, these drugs produce psychotomimetic effects and dysphoria. The suggestion of subtypes within the κ_1-receptor group has raised the possibility of selective analgesic agents lacking these side effects.

The κ_2-receptor was identified in binding studies. By using nonselective agents that label most opioid receptors, binding to established receptors could be displaced, leaving binding to the κ_2 site. Although easily demonstrated biochemically, the pharmacology of these sites remains unclear, primarily because of the absence of selective drugs. The approach used in the binding studies is not applicable to *in vivo* pharmacology.

The κ_3-receptor was first proposed based on binding and pharmacologic actions of naloxone benzoylhydrazone (Fig. 26.4). Subsequent studies suggest that the κ_3-receptor corresponds to the nalorphine receptor. A number of clinical analgesics act, in part, through κ_3-receptors, including levorphanol and nalbuphine.

With the isolation of clones encoding the traditional opioid receptors, an additional member of the family was cloned by several groups from mouse (*KOR-3*), rat, and human (*ORL1*). Several lines of evidence associated this gene with the κ_3-receptor. First, a monoclonal antibody that selectively labeled the κ_3-receptor recognized the new receptor. Second, antisense probes designed from this clone blocked κ_3-mediated analgesia. Despite this close association, this receptor differed from the κ_3-receptor: the κ_3-receptors bind many traditional opioids with high affinity, but the new receptor does not. Furthermore, an endogenous ligand for the new clone, orphanin FQ/nociceptin, does not compete for κ_3-receptor binding. The relationship between the two receptors is still not established. It will be interesting to see if they represent splice variants of a single gene or totally distinct entities. A number of splice variants have been identified and several have unique pharmacologic profiles.

Opioid receptor transduction mechanisms

In general, the opioid receptors are inhibitory, acting primarily through the $G_i\alpha$ and $G_o\alpha$ classes of G proteins. They have been associated with inhibitory effects on adenylyl cyclase (μ, δ, and κ), and can also stimulate K^+ channel activity (μ and δ) and inhibit Ca^{2+} channel activity (κ) (Fig. 26.12). Chronic opioid exposure can lead to molecular adaptations including upregulation of the cAMP pathway, with increased expression of specific subtypes of adenylyl cyclase and cAMP-dependent protein kinase (PKA) involving the CREB transcription factor. Drug induced regulation of this and other transcription factors may represent molecular mechanisms underlying persistent alterations of brain function characteristic of addiction and tolerance.

OPIOID ANALGESIA

Opioid pharmacology is quite complex, extending far beyond the utility of opiods as analgesics. Opioids suppress the hurt,

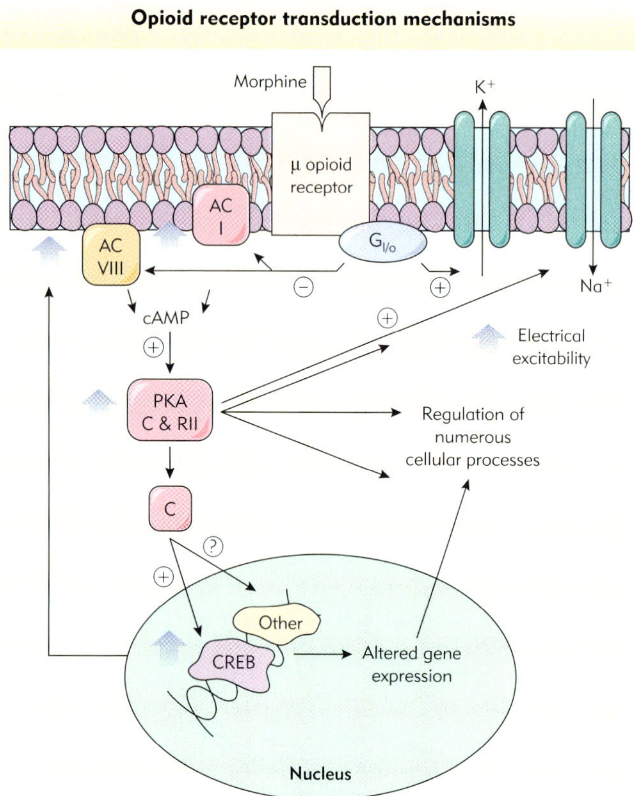

Figure 26.12 Opioid receptor transduction mechanisms. Opioids acutely inhibit neurons by increasing the conductance of an inwardly rectifying K^+ channel through coupling with $G_{i/o}$, as well as by decreasing a Na^+ current through coupling with $G_{i/o}$ and the consequent inhibition of adenylyl cyclase. Reduced concentrations of cAMP decrease PKA activity and the phosphorylation of the responsible channel or pump. Inhibition of the cAMP pathway also decreases phosphorylation of numerous other proteins and thereby affects many additional processes. It reduces the phosphorylation state of CREB, which may initiate some of the longer-term changes. Upward bold arrows summarize effects of chronic morphine administration in the locus coeruleus, the major nonadrenergic nucleus in the brain which is involved in opioid withdrawal. Chronic morphine increases concentrations of adenylyl cyclase types I and VIII (AC I and VIII), PKA catalytic (C) and regulatory type II (RII) subunits, and several phosphoproteins, including CREB. These changes contribute to the altered phenotype of the drug-addicted state. The intrinsic excitability of locus coeruleus neurons is increased by enhanced activity of the cAMP pathway and Na^+-dependent inward current, which contributes to the tolerance, dependence, and withdrawal exhibited by these neurons. (With permission from Nestler and Aghajanian, 1997.)

or subjective, component of pain, with each opioid receptor class acting through distinct receptor mechanisms in different locations within the CNS. The complexity of the system is markedly increased by extensive synergistic interactions between various regions, the development of tolerance, and the existence of anti-opioid systems. Finally, there are wide ranges in genetic sensitivity towards different classes of opioid; this is attributed to a number of factors, including opioid receptors themselves and the activity of anti-opioid systems.

Opioids exert both central and peripheral analgesic actions. Morphine analgesia has been most widely studied. Despite the extensive information regarding the clinical pharmacology of morphine, our understanding of the receptor systems rests predominantly on animal models. Systemic morphine analgesia is mediated primarily through supraspinal μ_1-systems, which also are important when the morphine is given intracerebroventricularly. A number of brainstem regions mediate morphine analgesia, including the periaqueductal gray, nucleus raphe magnus, and locus coeruleus. At the spinal level, μ_2-receptors in the dorsal horn are responsible for morphine analgesia. Morphine also acts peripherally on sensory neurons, primarily through a μ_1-receptor mechanism. This is illustrated by the antihyperalgesic effect of loperamide, a μ agonist that does not cross the blood-brain barrier and is locally active.

Although all the locations are active alone, they are more effective in combination, displaying profound synergistic interactions. Synergy was first demonstrated between spinal and supraspinal systems. Although morphine is active when given either supraspinally or spinally alone, its potency is markedly increased by giving divided doses into both regions. Synergy is not limited to spinal/supraspinal interactions. Within the brainstem, synergy has been demonstrated between the periaqueductal gray and locus coeruleus and between the periaqueductal gray and nucleus raphe magnus. Peripheral mechanisms also synergize with central ones. These interactions are most pronounced between peripheral and spinal systems, although peripheral/supraspinal interactions also are present. The importance of these interactions cannot be overstated. Small spinal doses of morphine, for example, can shift the ED_{50} (median effective dose) for systemic morphine in mice by as much as 100-fold. This may explain the utility of epidural morphine. When given epidurally, morphine concentrations at the spinal level are very high. However, there also is significant systemic absorption, leading to blood concentrations similar to those seen with intramuscular injections. Although spinal morphine alone is active, it is likely that the overall efficacy of this approach is enhanced by spinal/systemic synergy. These interactions also suggest that the utility of epidural drugs can be enhanced with the concomitant administration of systemic drugs.

Although most opioids are quite similar in their ability to relieve pain, they are not exactly the same and patient responses can vary. The mixed agonist/antagonists are easily distinguished from morphine. Differences also exist among μ-receptor drugs, as illustrated above by the distinct activities of morphine, M6G, fentanyl, and heroin. Unfortunately, it is not yet possible to predict which agent will be most effective for a particular patient or a particular type of pain, and clinicians are encouraged to switch medications as needed. Also, opioids are not completely cross-tolerant. Patients tolerant to one agent may not be as tolerant to another, which must be considered when changing agents.

Tolerance and dependence

Tolerance is the progressive decline in efficacy of a drug with prolonged use. Although it is frequently encountered with opioids, tolerance can usually be overcome by increasing the dose, by switching to a different drug, or both. Opioid tolerance can be quite profound, resulting in a requirement for doses 100-fold higher than those used in naive patients. Tolerance usually is not a problem unless dose-limiting side effects prevent further escalation of dose. The need to escalate opioid doses may result from other factors, such as progressive disease in cancer patients.

Tolerance involves a number of mechanisms. Early studies focused on receptor transduction mechanisms, which are affected by chronic exposure to opioids. The most intriguing system associated with tolerance involves the *N*-methyl-D-aspartate (NMDA)/nitric oxide cascade (Chapters 19 & 21). Blockade of NMDA glutamate receptors has no effect on the analgesic activity of opioids such as morphine. Yet, NMDA antagonists can effectively block the progressive tolerance seen with opioids in animal models, which demonstrates that the mechanisms responsible for analgesia and tolerance can be dissociated. This system may offer important targets in the treatment of pain.

Dependence invariably develops with continued opioid use; however, this should not interfere with their appropriate use. Dependence is a physiologic response to opioids and does not imply addiction, which involves drug-seeking behavior. Very few patients given opioids for management of pain ever become addicted, although patients with a prior history of drug abuse have a greater likelihood of abuse.

Dependence does, however, raise several issues. First, patients taking opioids long term should not be given mixed agonist/antagonists since they precipitate withdrawal. Withdrawal is also a concern when stopping opioids abruptly, although patients who are drug dependent can be easily tapered off opioids without evidence of withdrawal. The severity of withdrawal signs and symptoms, which include nausea, diarrhea, yawning, rhinorhea, piloerection, sweating, increases in temperature and blood pressure, coughing and insomnia, may vary depending on the degree of dependence and the rate of elimination of the drug. Agents such as methadone that are long-lasting may have a more mild, but protracted withdrawal period. The dose can usually be decreased by 50% every 2 days without manifestations of withdrawal.

Antiopioid systems

There is extraordinary variability in the response of patients to nociceptive stimuli and to analgesics. While cultural issues clearly play a role, recent work has identified genetic factors that also may prove important. Investigators have identified marked differences in sensitivity to opioid analgesics among various strains of mice. Sensitivities of the various opioid receptor subtypes vary independently of each other. Some strains respond well to morphine and related μ-receptor drugs but not to κ-acting agents. Others display a reduced sensitivity to all opioid classes. These differences in analgesic sensitivity can correspond to levels of receptors, but in most situations they do not.

Pain and the analgesic effectiveness of endogenous opioid systems are modulated by antiopioid transmitter systems that have recently been identified. These systems including cholecystokinin, the newly isolated neuropeptide orphanin FQ/nociceptin, and the σ system. The σ-receptors were first identified based on the pharmacology of benzomorphan opioids, but it has become obvious that σ-receptors do not belong in the opioid receptor classification. This conclusion has recently been bolstered by the cloning of the guinea pig, human, and mouse σ-receptors. Unlike the opioid receptors, which belong to the G protein-coupled family of receptors, σ-receptors do not have the same distinguishing structures, such as seven transmembrane-spanning domains. Structurally σ-receptors have little similarity to any known membrane receptor and their functions remain to be elucidated.

Despite our limited understanding of σ-receptor functions at the biochemical level, a wide number of σ-agonists and antagonists have been identified. (+)-Pentazocine is a potent agonist at σ_1-receptors. Unlike its optical isomer, (–)-pentazocine, which is a potent opioid analgesic, (+)-pentazocine has little affinity for opioid receptors. One of the most useful σ-antagonists is haloperidol, which binds σ-receptors as potently as dopamine receptors. (+)-Pentazocine blocks opioid analgesia regardless of which opioid receptor system is involved, whereas (–)-pentazocine is a clinically useful analgesic. Blockade of σ-receptors with haloperidol reverses the actions of (+)-pentazocine. Opioid systems typically show little tonic activity, as demonstrated by naloxone's inactivity in measures of pain sensitivity. In contrast, σ-systems appear to have important tonic activities, which may help to explain the varying analgesic sensitivity of some mouse strains, particularly for the κ-systems. Haloperidol shifts the dose response for morphine almost twofold in a number of strains of mice. Similarly, it enhances the analgesic actions of δ- and κ-acting drugs. However, in a mouse strain that is not very sensitive to κ-drugs, haloperidol increased the κ-receptor sensitivity over 10–fold, indicating tonic activity of the σ-system. This and other anti-opioid systems may prove important in the future understanding of the sensitivity of patients to opioids and nociceptive input.

OTHER OPIOID ACTIONS

Opioids have a number of actions other than analgesia. Some, such as nausea, are mediated through unknown mechanisms. However, a number of undesirable side effects are mediated by opioid receptors. The two most problematic effects are respiratory depression and constipation.

Respiratory depression

Respiratory depression is often seen with μ-opioids. It is rarely a problem in the outpatient setting in the absence of underlying pulmonary disease, but problems may be more common in the perioperative setting. Morphine and related opioids reduce respiratory drive by shifting the ventilation–arterial carbon dioxide partial pressure ($PaCO_2$) response curve down and to the right. Therefore, patients who retain carbon dioxide are most sensitive to the respiratory depressant actions of opioids. Respiratory depression is mediated predominantly through opioid μ_2-receptors and can be readily reversed by naloxone. The difficulty with current antagonists is that they also reverse analgesia and, in patients who are drug dependent, can precipitate withdrawal. Although lower doses can be used to reduce respiratory depression without completely antagonizing analgesia, κ-acting drugs have less respiratory depressant activity and their use should be considered in patients with respiratory compromise. However, most of the κ-acting agents currently available also have antagonist activity at μ-receptors and can precipitate withdrawal in patients who are drug dependent.

Gastrointestinal transit

Morphine and other μ-acting opioids act both centrally and through receptors located in the myenteric plexus to impede gastrointestinal transit, which can lead to constipation. Like respiratory depression, the constipating actions of opioids are mediated through a subpopulation of μ-receptors and can be difficult to avoid. Theoretically, oral opioids should present a greater problem than parenteral ones, but constipation remains a frequent issue even in patients on parenteral drugs. Since the receptors responsible for these actions are a distinct subtype within the μ-opioid receptor family, the potential of using selective antagonists to reverse constipation without interfering with analgesia remains. One agent capable of blocking the gastrointestinal effects of morphine without interfering with analgesia has been described.

Other effects

Opioids also have a number of additional actions, including causing bradycardia, hypothermia, and miosis. All are naloxone sensitive, implying a role for opioid receptors. In addition, the fentanyl series of agents has been associated with rigidity, but the receptor mechanisms associated with this action are incompletely understood. Opioids can also alter after the function of the immune system by suppressing cytokine production and perhaps by inducing apoptosis in lymphocytes.

CLINICAL PHARMACOLOGY

Treatment of pain depends on the nature of the pain and the patient and must be individualized for each patient and situation. Assessing the intensity of pain can be difficult. Painful stimuli are not perceived equally by everyone, owing to both genetic and situational factors. For example, an acute episode of excruciating back pain in a patient with a remote history of cancer may dramatically subside if the patient is assured that it does not imply tumor recurrence. Pain has meaning, and understanding its meaning to the patient is essential in assessing its severity. In any event, the only accurate measure of pain is the patient's report. Acute pain is often associated with well-recognized autonomic signs. However, these signs are typically lost in chronic pain syndromes despite the persistence of pain.

Treatment of pain should focus on the simplest regimen with the fewest side effects. Treating pain requires an understanding of the type of pain involved and the utility of various drugs for specific types of pain. Somatic pain is well treated by opioids while other types, such as neuropathic pain, are far less responsive. For many neuropathic pain syndromes, other classes of drug are useful, including antidepressants such as amitriptyline and anticonvulsants such as carbamazepine and gabapentin (Chapter 25).

Pain should be treated aggressively with the goal of keeping the patient pain free. Patients should not wait until pain returns before taking their next analgesic dose. It is easier to prevent pain than to take it away, and patients on around-the-clock dosing typically require less opioid over 24 hours than those taking opioids on an as-needed basis.

Key References

Pasternak GW. Pharmacological mechanisms of opioid analgesics. Clin Neuropharmacol. 1993;16:1–18.

Payne R, Pasternak GW. Pain. In: Johnston MV, Macdonald RL, Young AB, eds. Principles of drug therapy in neurology. Philadelphia, PA: Davis; 1992:268–301.

Reisine T, Bell GI. Molecular biology of opioid receptors. Trend Neurosci. 1993;16:506–10.

Reisine T, Pasternak GW. Opioid analgesics and antagonists. In: Hardman JG, Limbird LE, eds. Goodman & Gilman's pharmacological basis of therapeutics, Vol. 9. New York: McGraw-Hill; 1995:521–55.

Further Reading

Burkle H, Dunbar S, van Aken H. Remifentanil: a novel, short-acting μ opioid. Anesth Analg. 1996;83:646–51.

Egan TD, Lemmens HJM, Fiset P, et al. The pharmacokinetics of the new short-acting opioid remifentanil (G187084B) in healthy adult male volunteers. Anesthesiology. 1993;79:881–92.

Evans CJ, Keith DE Jr, Morrison H, Magendzo K, Edwards RH. Cloning of a delta opioid receptor by functional expression. Science. 1992;258:1952–5.

Lord JAH, Waterfield AA, Hughes J, Kosterlitz HW. Endogenous opioid peptides: multiple agonists and receptors. Nature. 1977;267:495–9.

Nestler EJ, Aghajanian GK. Molecular and cellular basis of addiction. Science. 1997;278:58–63.

Pasternak GW, Standifer KM. Mapping of opioid receptors using antisense oligodeoxynucleotides: correlating their molecular biology and pharmacology. Trend Pharmacol Sci. 1995;16:344–50.

Pleuvry BJ. Opioid receptors and their relevance to anaesthesia. Br J Anesth. 1993;71:119–26.

Rosow C. Altentanil. Semin Anesth. 1988;VII:107–12.

Shafer SL, Varvel JR. Pharmacokinetics, pharmacodynamics, and rational opioid selection. Anesthesiology. 1991;74:53–63.

Standifer KM, Pasternak GW. G proteins and opioid receptor-mediated signalling. Cell Signal. 1997;9:237–48.

Yeung JC, Rudy TA. Multiplicative interaction between narcotic agonisms expressed at spinal and supraspinal sites of antinociceptive action as revealed by concurrent intrathecal and intracerebroventricular injections of morphine. J Pharmacol Exp Ther. 1980;215:633–42.

Chapter 27 Nonopioid analgesics

R Andrew Moore and Henry J McQuay

Topics covered in this chapter

Currently there are three major classes of nonopioid analgesics:

- nonsteroidal anti-inflammatory drugs (NSAIDs);
- centrally acting nonopioid analgesics (e.g. acetaminophen, tramadol); and
- adjuvant analgesics (e.g. tricyclic antidepressants).

The nonopioid analgesics are a cornerstone of pain management. They are highly effective and can be administered by both oral and parenteral routes. Although NSAIDs are used most often to treat mild-to-moderate pain associated with inflammation, parenteral NSAIDs are also used for moderate-to-severe postoperative pain, but are ineffective in treating neuropathic pain and more severe nociceptive pain (Chapter 21). The centrally acting non-narcotic agent acetaminophen is used for mild to moderately severe pain. Adjuvant analgesics are commonly used for neuropathic pain (Chapter 21). A number of structurally distinct NSAIDs share a common mechanism of action and side-effect profiles, but differ primarily in their pharmacokinetic properties.

NONSTEROIDAL ANTI-INFLAMMATORY DRUGS

Cyclo-oxygenase (COX) activity is inhibited by NSAIDs, and this reduces the production of prostaglandins (PGs) – members of a large family of endogenous compounds known as eicosanoids, a diverse group of oxygenated, unsaturated 20 carbon fatty acids. These compounds exert profound effects on practically all cells and tissues and therefore are important targets for pharmacologic intervention in a variety of diseases. The structures and biosynthesis of PGs are summarized in Figure 27.1.

In the body, PGs are not stored in tissues, but are synthesized in response to diverse stimuli and enter the extracellular space. They act primarily as local hormones – their biologic activities are usually restricted to the tissue in which they are synthesized. They are rapidly inactivated through oxidation of the 15-hydroxyl group by 15-hydroxy-PG dehydrogenases, which are widely distributed.

The PGs act by binding to specific G protein-coupled receptors (Chapter 3). A variety of PG receptor subtypes have been identified; these are coupled to diverse signal transduction pathways, including adenylyl cyclase and phospholipase. Many cells possess more than one PG receptor subtype, and respond in a variety of ways to different PGs.

The analgesic and antipyretic effects of NSAIDs appear to be produced through inhibition of PG synthesis. Intravenous administration of certain PGs can induce headache, pain, and hyperalgesia in humans. The antipyretic effect of NSAIDs depends on inhibition of PGE_2 biosynthesis within the thermoregulatory preoptic hypothalmic nucleus (Chapter 64). The analgesic effects of NSAIDs result primarily from local actions (as opposed to the principally central analgesic actions of opioids) to inhibit PG endoperoxide formation (PGG_2 and PGH_2) by COX. The anti-inflammatory actions of NSAIDs are also potent, because PGs are major contributors to inflammation – PGE_2 and PGI_2 enhance edema and leukocyte infiltration and the pain-producing properties of bradykinin. Certain NSAIDs, such as diclofenac and indomethacin, but not salicylate, also inhibit the lipoxygenase pathway that converts arachidonic acids into leukotrienes, which are also major contributors to inflammation. Also, NSAIDs may have effects unrelated to the inhibition of PG biosynthesis, particularly at higher concentrations; some of these other effects may also be involved in their anti-inflammatory and analgesic effects. Significant risks associated with NSAIDs include gastrointestinal bleeding and hepatic and renal toxicity (Fig. 27.2).

CYCLO-OXYGENASE-1 AND CYCLO-OXYGENASE-2

It is now appreciated that there are two isoforms of COX responsible for the breakdown of arachidonic acid via the unstable endoperoxide intermediates PGG_2 and PGH_2 to PGs and thromboxanes (see Fig. 27.1). From the effects of different NSAIDs on PG formation it was suspected in the 1970s that different isoforms of COX might be in the cell, and this was confirmed when a second isoform of COX (COX-2) was discovered in 1991. The isoform COX-1 is a 'constitutive' isoform (it is present for normal functions). For example, its activation leads to the formation of prostacyclin, which is cytoprotective in the gastric mucosa. It is found in most cell types, including blood vessels, stomach, and kidney, mainly in the endoplasmic reticulum. The isoform COX-2 is induced by inflammation, and is called up to synthesize more prostanoids, but is also constitutively expressed (i.e. under normal conditions) in the brain, renal cortex, testis, and lung.

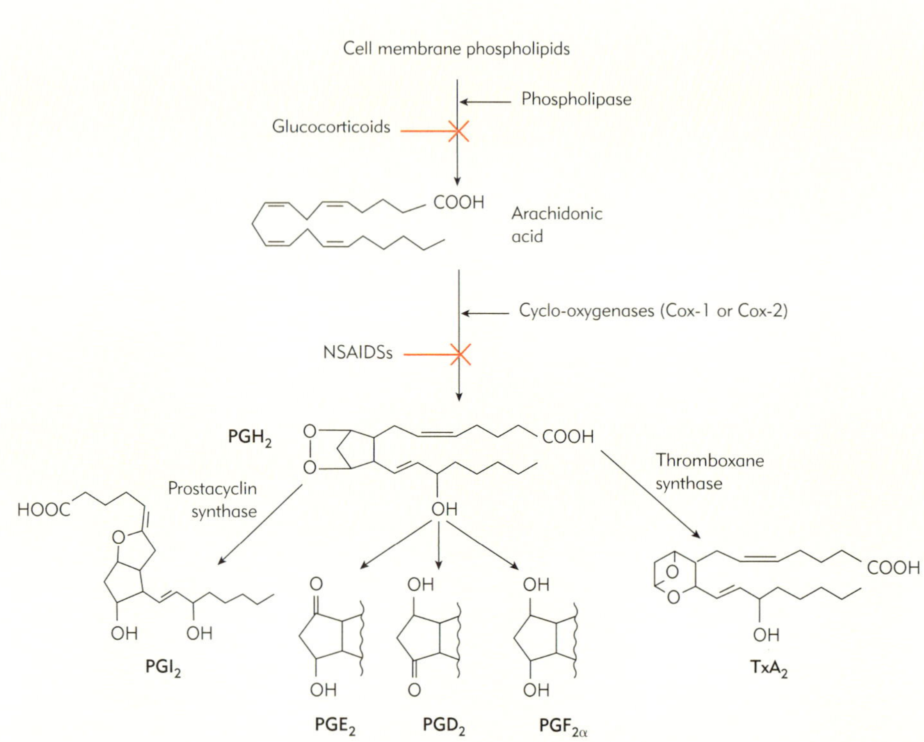

Figure 27.1 Chemical structures and biosynthesis of principal prostaglandins. Endoperoxide PGH_2 differs from PGI_2 (prostacyclin), PGE_2, PGD_2, and $PGF_{2\alpha}$. (TX, thromboxane.)

Side effects shared by NSAIDs

- Gastrointestinal ulceration and intolerance[a]
- Blockade of platelet aggregation (inhibition of thromboxane synthesis)
- Inhibition of uterine motility (prolongation of gestation)
- Inhibition of prostaglandin-mediated renal function[b]
- Hypersensitivity reactions[c]

[a]Lesser side effects with nonacetylated salicylates or *p*-aminophenol derivatives

[b]Of special importance for patients who have decreased renal blood flow; retention of Na^+, K^+, and water (edema) can reduce effectiveness of antihypertensive regimens

[c]Most pronounced with aspirin than with nonacetylated salicylates

Figure 27.2 Side effects shared by NSAIDs.

The activity of COX-2 is mostly localized to the nucleus, whereas COX-1 is involved in the constitutive synthesis of cytoprotective PGs in the stomach, in maintaining blood flow in the compromised kidney (e.g. in congestive heart failure, liver cirrhosis, or renal insufficiency), and in platelet function, where it is the only COX expressed. Inhibition of COX is therefore responsible for the principal side effects of NSAIDs (see Fig. 27.2). Thus, COX-1 occurs normally to organize prostanoid synthesis and COX-2 is triggered by inflammation to make more. Both COX-1 and COX-2 are encoded by distinct genes, but are clearly homologous with similar three-dimensional structures and active sites as determined by X-ray crystallography.

In most cells and tissues, expression of COX-2 is transient and tightly controlled with peak levels occurring 4–6 hours after stimulation and returning to baseline by 24 hours. Normal levels are low, but it can be induced by a number of cytokines and intracellular messengers. Importantly, the induction of COX-2 expression can be prevented by anti-inflammatory glucocorticoids such as dexamethasone. This suggests that some of the anti-inflammatory actions of glucocorticoids may result from inhibition of COX-2 expression.

Aspirin covalently modifies both COX-1 (by acetylation of serine-530) and COX-2, with a resultant irreversible inhibition of COX activity by preventing access of arachidonic acid to the active site. This is a unique property of aspirin, and the duration of its effects depends on the turnover rate of COX in different tissues. Platelets are especially susceptible to this effect, since they have little or no capacity for protein biosynthesis. In contrast to aspirin, most NSAIDs are reversible competitive inhibitors of COX activity, but also act by competing with the substrate arachidonic acid for the active site.

Most currently available NSAIDs inhibit both the COX-1 and COX-2 isoforms or have modest selectivity for the constitutive COX-1 isoform (Fig. 27.3). Indeed, aspirin, indomethacin, and ibuprofen are much less active against COX-2 than against COX-1, and also cause the most damage to the stomach. Thus, the variations in the side effects of current NSAIDs (Fig. 27.4) can be explained by their COX-2:COX-1 activity ratios (i.e. the higher the ratio, the fewer the gastric and renal side effects at anti-inflammatory doses).

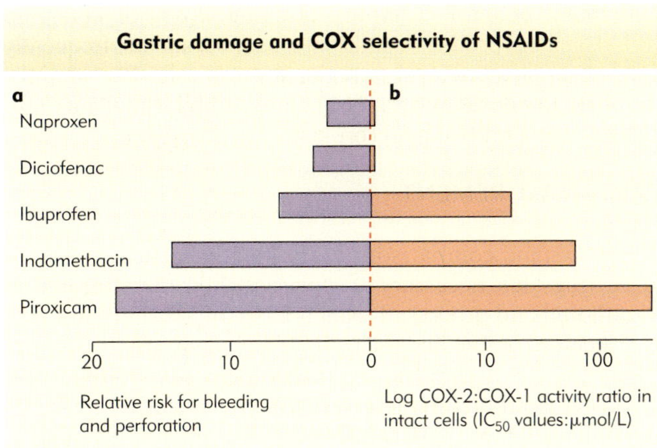

Figure 27.3 Comparisons of gastric damage and COX selectivity of NSAIDs. (a) Adjusted relative risk for bleeding and perforation of the upper gastrointestinal tract; values for anti-inflammatory doses of NSAIDs are shown. (b) Log COX-2:COX-1 activity ratios (ratio of COX-2:COX-1 IC_{50} values, μmol/L) for these NSAIDs.

Compounds that selectively inhibit COX-2 may have anti-inflammatory and analgesic activities but not the gastrointestinal toxicity of conventional NSAIDs, since most gastrointestinal toxicity seen with NSAIDs results from inhibition of COX-1-mediated PG production in the gastric mucosa. Compounds have been developed that are several hundred fold more potent against COX-2 as against COX-1 (Fig. 27.4). Selectivity of the COX-2 inhibitors depends on subtle differences in the structure of the active site. Celecoxib (rofexicob) and an analogue of L-745,337 lacking the sulfonyl group, were recently released for clinical use in the US, while meloxicam and nimesulide are in use in several countries (Fig. 27.5). Dual COX-2–lipoxygenase inhibitors are also being developed for improved anti-inflammatory action. The use of selective COX-2 inhibitors should enable relatively higher doses with fewer side effects than those of currently available NSAIDs (Fig. 27.6). The association of COX-2 with colon cancer indicates a potential future use for these drugs as well.

Enantiomeric *R* and *S* forms – separating analgesia and anti-inflammatory actions

Separation of analgesic and anti-inflammatory actions has been shown with the *R* and *S* enantiomers of flurbiprofen. The *S* form has both anti-inflammatory and analgesic action. The *R* form blocks nociception, but has little effect on PG formation and inflammation. In addition, while the *S* form is ulcerogenic the *R* form is reported to have negligible effect. These findings suggest that the anti-inflammatory and analgesic actions of the NSAIDs may involve distinct molecular targets, which may allow development of more specific and possibly safer agents.

CENTRALLY ACTING NONOPIOID DRUGS

Acetaminophen

Acetaminophen (*N*-acetyl-*p*-aminophenol; paracetamol) is an effective analgesic–antipyretic with weak anti-inflammatory actions. It is well tolerated, but can cause fatal hepatic damage with acute overdosage (Chapter 61). The mechanisms for the analgesic–antipyretic actions of acetaminophen are unclear, but it appears to synergize with NSAIDs in the treatment of pain.

The standard explanation is that it acts as a PG synthetase inhibitor, which would explain both the analgesic and the antipyretic actions. That acetaminophen is not anti-inflammatory may be because it does not act on peripheral COX – perhaps there is a parallel with the flurbiprofen *R* enantiomer mentioned above.

Tramadol

Tramadol is a centrally acting analgesic with a unique, dual mechanism of action – it exerts agonistic properties at opioid receptors

Comparison of nonsteroidal anti-inflammatory drugs for their selectivity toward cyclo-oxygenases 1 and 2

Drug	IC_{50} COX-1 (mmol/L)	IC_{50} COX-2 (mmol/L)	Ratio IC_{50} COX-2/COX-1
Nonselective for cyclo-oxygenase 2			
Piroxicam	0.0005	0.3	600.0
Aspirin	1.67	278.0	166.0
Indomethacin	0.028	1.68	60.0
Diclofenac	1.57	1.1	0.7
Selective for cyclo-oxygenase 2			
Etodolac	34.0	3.4	0.1
Meloxicam	4.8	0.43	0.09
Nimesulide	9.2	0.52	0.06
L-745, 337	369.0	1.5	0.004
Celecoxib	15	0.04	0.003

Figure 27.4 Comparison of NSAIDs for their selectivity toward COX-1 and COX-2.

Chemical structures of some selective COX-2 inhibitors

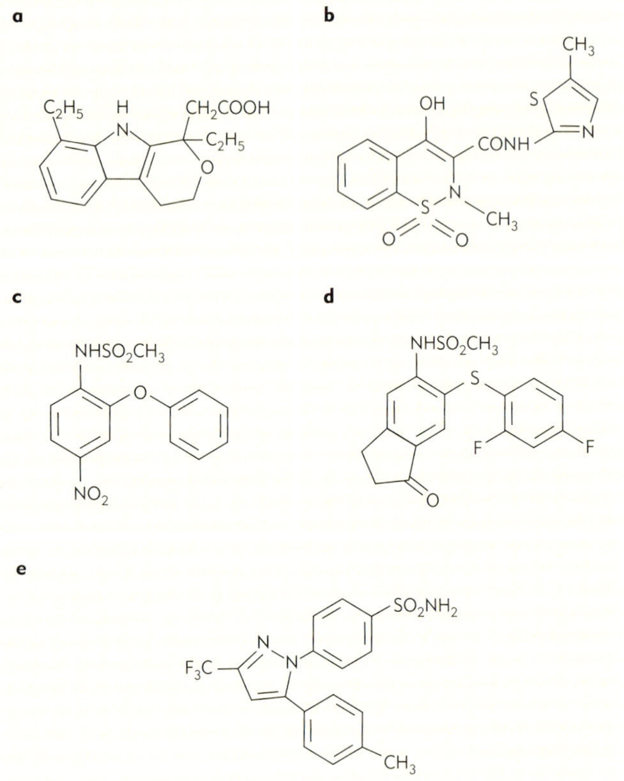

Figure 27.5 Chemical structures of some selective COX-2 inhibitors. (a) Etodolac, (b) meloxicam, (c) nimesulide, (d) L-745,337, and (e) celecoxib.

and interferes with neurotransmitter reuptake. Tramadol inhibits the reuptake of the natural neurotransmitters norepinephrine (noradrenaline) and serotonin, and also binds weakly to μ-opioid receptors, blocking the transmission of pain signals to the brain. Tramadol's only active metabolite, *O*-demethyltramadol has greater affinity for μ-opioid receptors than does tramadol. The The μ-opioid receptor antagonist naloxone only partially blocks the effect of tramadol on nociceptive activity.

Ziconotide

Ziconotide is a novel analgesic derived from the N-type Ca^{2+} channel blocking ω-conotoxin GVIA. Ziconotide is a 15 amino acid peptide derivative of the parent toxin that specifically blocks a subtype of neuronal voltage-dependent Ca^{2+} channel that is involved in the release of various neurotransmitters, including glutamate, and also blocks the transmission of nociceptive neurons in the spinal cord. Early evidence suggests that intrathecal administration of the peptide reduces neuropathic pain, with no tolerance development, in patients who have chronic malignant pain.

Ketamine

Ketamine is a potent analgesic that acts primarily as a noncompetitive antagonist of the *N*-methyl-D-asparate (NMDA) glutamate receptor (Chapter 23). Low doses of ketamine (0.1–0.5mg/kg) produce significant analgesia, and are frequently used to supplement local or regional anesthesia. The administration of low doses of ketamine before painful stimuli may also reduce postoperative pain (pre-emptive analgesia).

PAIN MEASUREMENT

To understand comparisons of the relative efficacy of analgesic drugs, it is necessary to appreciate how the information is gathered and processed. Pain is a personal experience that is difficult to define and measure. It includes both the sensory input and its modulation by physiologic, psychologic, and environmental factors. Not surprisingly, objective measures are not available – pain cannot be measured directly by sampling blood or urine or by performing neurophysiologic tests. Measurement of pain must therefore rely on the patient's report. It is often assumed that because the measurement is subjective it must be of little value. However, if the measurements are carried out properly, remarkably sensitive and consistent results can be obtained. The most important rule is that if pain is not of moderate or severe intensity, then measuring an analgesic effect is likely to be unreliable. There are contexts, however, in which it is not possible to measure pain at all or patient reports are likely to be unreliable. These include impaired consciousness, young children, psychiatric pathology, severe anxiety, unwillingness to cooperate, and inability to understand the measurements. Such problems are deliberately avoided in trials.

Measurement scales

Most analgesic studies include measurements of pain intensity and/or pain relief. The most common tools used are categoric and visual analog scales.

Categoric scales use words to describe the magnitude of pain, for which most research groups use four words (none, mild, moderate, and severe). Scales to measure pain relief were developed later, the most common of which is the five category scale (none, slight, moderate, good or lots, and complete). For analysis numbers are given to the verbal categories (for pain intensity, none = 0, mild = 1, moderate = 2, and severe =3, and for relief none = 0, slight = 1, moderate = 2, good or lots = 3, and complete = 4). Few studies present results as discrete data, but give the number of participants who report a certain level of pain intensity or relief at any given assessment point. The main advantages of the categoric scales are that they are quick and simple, but the small number of descriptors may force the scorer to choose a particular category when none describes the pain satisfactorily.

The visual analog scale (VAS), which uses a line with the left end labeled 'no relief of pain' and right end labeled 'complete relief of pain', seems to overcome this limitation. Patients mark the line at the point that corresponds to their pain. Scores are obtained by measuring the distance between the no relief end and the patient's mark, usually in millimeters. The main advantages of the VAS are that it is simple and quick to score, avoids imprecise descriptive terms, and provides many points from which to choose.

Pain relief scales are perceived as more convenient than pain intensity scales, probably because patients have the same baseline relief (zero), whereas they could start with different baseline intensity (usually moderate or severe). Relief scale results are thus easier to compare. They may also be more sensitive

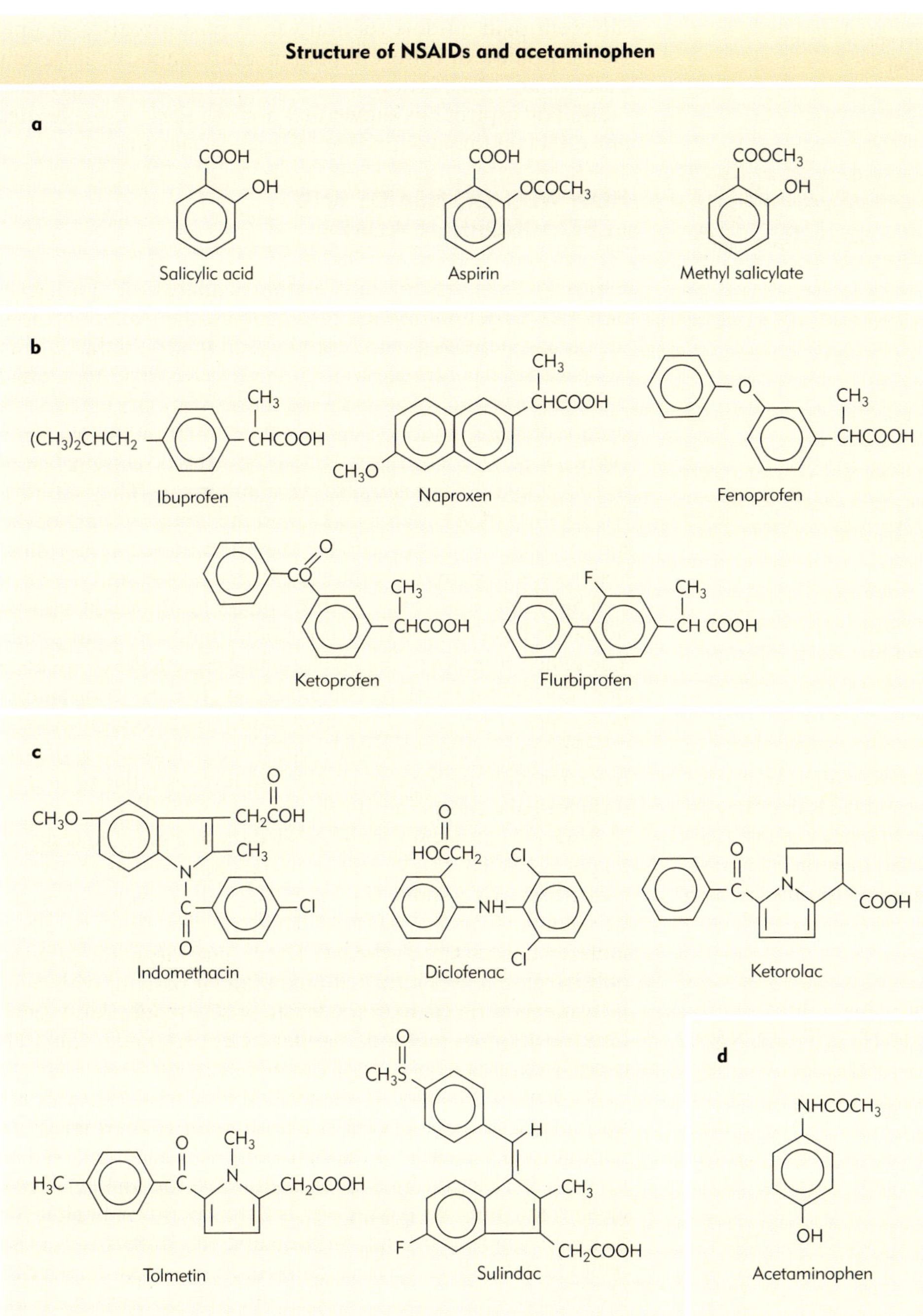

Figure 27.6 Chemical structures of NSAIDs and acetaminophen. (a) Salicylates, (b) arylpropionic acids, (c) acetic acids, and (d) acetaminophen.

than intensity scales. A theoretic drawback of relief scales is that the patient has to remember what the pain was like to begin with.

Analysis of scale results – summary measures

In the research context, pain is usually assessed before the intervention is made and subsequently on multiple occasions. Ideally, the area under the time–analgesic effect curve for the intensity (sum of pain intensity differences; SPID) or relief (total pain relief; TOTPAR) measures is derived (Equations 27.1 & 27.2), in which at assessment point t ($t = 0, 1, 2, \ldots n$), P_t and PR_t are the pain intensity and pain relief measured at that point, respectively; P_0 is pain intensity at $t = 0$; and PID_t is the pain intensity difference calculated as $(P_0 - P_t)$.

Equation 27.1

$$\text{SPID} = \sum_{t=0\text{–}6}^{n} \text{PID}_t$$

Equation 27.2

$$\text{TOTPAR} = \sum_{t=0\text{–}6}^{n} \text{PR}_t$$

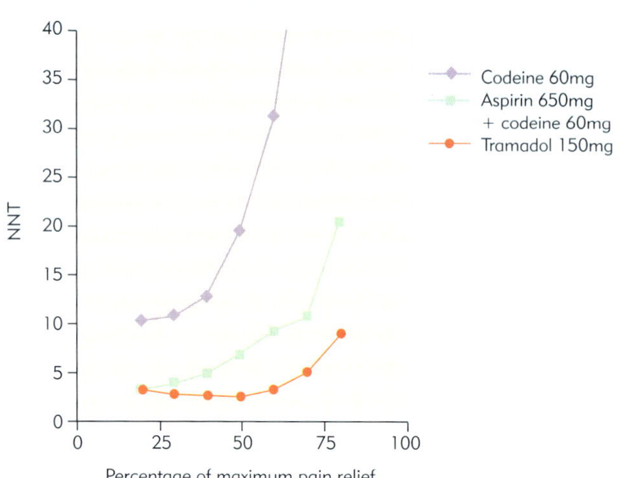

Figure 27.7 Numbers needed to treat and the use of different cut points for maximum pain relief.

The summary Equations 27.1 & 27.2 reflect the cumulative response to the intervention. Their disadvantage is that they do not provide information about the onset and peak of the analgesic effect. If onset or peak are important, then time to maximum pain relief (or reduction in pain intensity) or time for pain to return to baseline are necessary.

Efficacy

Increasingly, a common method of expressing treatment efficacy is the number needed to treat (NNT). The NNT is defined as 1/(proportion of patients with at least 50% pain relief with analgesic – proportion of patients with at least 50% pain relief with placebo). The best NNT is obviously 1, when every patient treated benefits, and no patient given placebo does. Generally, NNT values between 2 and 5 are indicative of effective analgesic treatments.

The NNT for pain relief in postoperative pain is relatively insensitive to the magnitude of the pain relief between about 20 and 60% pain relief (Fig. 27.7). Where the NNT is good, as for tramadol 150mg, the NNT does not change very much with the use of different cut points. Where the NNT is poor, as with codeine 60mg, the NNT rises (becomes worse) rapidly as the quality of pain relief required increases. At 50% pain relief we obtain a point at which there is excellent sensitivity to distinguish between effective and less effective analgesics, and, of course, the concept of half pain relief is one easily understood.

Questions have been raised in the past about the wisdom of combining information gathered in analgesic trials using different pain models (dental versus postoperative or episiotomy pain), or different pain measurements, or different durations of observation. Analysis of the great mass of information on aspirin has shown that none of these variables has any effect on the magnitude of the analgesic effect.

HOW WELL DO NSAIDS AND ACETAMINOPHEN WORK?

Figure 27.8a shows the information available on oral acetaminophen, acetaminophen plus codeine, aspirin, ibuprofen, diclofenac, naproxen, and bromfenac from systematic reviews of randomized controlled trials of single-doses in postoperative pain. It shows the dose with the most information for each drug – for acetaminophen significant information was available for two doses. It is clear that the four NSAIDs do extremely well in this single-dose postoperative comparison. They all have NNT values of between 2 and 3, and the point estimate of the mean is below that of (i.e. better than) intramuscular morphine 10mg, even though the confidence intervals overlap.

The simple analgesics aspirin and acetaminophen are significantly less effective than 10mg of intramuscular morphine. The point estimates of the NNT are higher, and the confidence intervals do not overlap. The analgesic efficacy of the simple analgesics is improved by combination with weak opioids. Combination of acetaminophen 600/650mg with codeine or dextropropoxyphene lowers the NNT to levels similar to that of intramuscular morphine 10mg.

Figure 27.8b presents the NNT data in a graphic form. A league table like this is easy to understand, and as more systematic reviews compile similar data on other analgesics, it can be extended to make comparison and choice of drugs based on more evidence-based efficacy. The league table is legitimate only because it uses information on similar patients with valid inclusion criteria (pain of moderate or severe intensity), similar measurement methods, similar outcomes, and a common comparator, placebo.

We have not produced a league table of analgesic efficacy for injected or rectal NSAIDs in postoperative or other acute pain states. The reason is that in almost all trials of injected or rectal NSAIDs that have been conducted the analgesic was given when there is no pain – before the operation begins, for instance. This has become fashionable partly because of the belief that if pain can be pre-empted, the need for analgesics postoperatively is reduced (Chapter 21), but reviews both questioned the methodologic validity of most trials that have been conducted and showed that analysis of valid studies does not support the theory. Certainly, most randomized trials that compare the same intervention given before or after pain begins do not show clinical advantage of pre-emptive analgesia. The injectable form of paracetamol, proparacetamol, undoubtedly works, but as yet there are too few published 'modern' trials to allow meta-analysis.

Pooled information for randomized, double-blind trials in patients who have moderate-to-severe pain

a

Analgesic (oral except morphine)	Dose (mg)	Number of patients studied	NNT (95% confidence interval)
Bromfenac	25	370	2.2 (1.9 to 2.6)
Diclofenac	50	636	2.3 (2.0 to 2.7)
Naproxen	440	257	2.3 (2.0 to 2.9)
Ketorolac	10	790	2.5 (2.2 to 3.0)
Ibuprofen	400	2898	2.7 (2.5 to 3.0)
Morphine (i.m.)	10	946	2.9 (2.6 to 3.6)
Acetaminophen plus codeine	600/650 + 60	816	3.1 (2.6 to 3.9)
Acetaminophen plus dextropropoxyphene	650 + 65	963	4.4 (3.5 to 5.6)
Aspirin	600/650	5061	4.4 (4.0 to 4.9)
Acetaminophen	1000	2283	4.6 (3.9 to 5.4)
Acetaminophen	600/650	1167	5.3 (4.1 to 7.2)

b

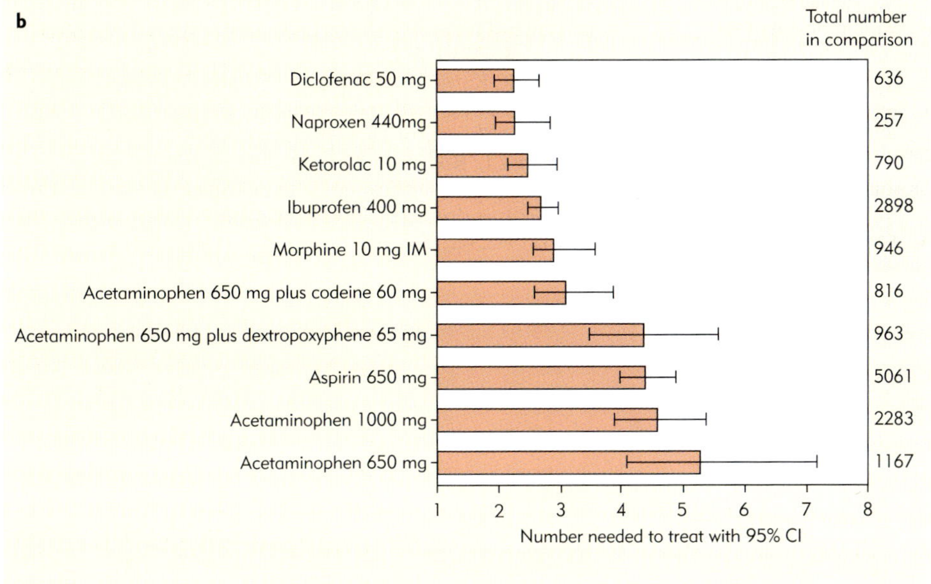

Figure 27.8 Pooled information for randomized, double-blind trials in patients who have moderate-to-severe pain. (a) Analgesic efficacy of simple analgesics and NSAIDs. (b) Comparison of number needed to treat.

Key References

Appleton I. Non-steroidal anti-inflammatory drugs and pain. In: Dickenson AH, Besson J, eds. The pharmacology of pain (Handbook of Experimental Pharmacology). Berlin: Springer Verlag. 1997;130:43–60.

Cook RJ, Sackett DL. The number needed to treat: a clinically useful measure of treatment effect. Br Med J. 1995;310:452–4.

McQuay HJ, Moore RA. Using numerical results from systematic reviews in clinical practice. Ann Intern Med. 1997;126:712–20.

Tramèr M, Williams J, Carroll D, Wiffen PJ, McQuay HJ, Moore RA. Systematic review of direct comparisons of non-steroidal anti-inflammatory drugs given by different routes for acute pain. Acta Anaesth Scand. 1998;42:71–9.

Vane JR. Inhibition of prostaglandin synthesis as a mechanism of action for the aspirin-like drugs. Nature New Biol. 1971;231:232–5.

Vane JR, Bakhle YS, Botting RM. Cyclooxygenases 1 and 2. Annu Rev Pharmacol Toxicol. 1998;38:97–120.

Further Reading

Littman GS, Walker BR, Schneider BE. Reassessment of verbal and visual analogue ratings in analgesic studies. Clin Pharmacol Ther. 1985;38:16–23.

McQuay H, Carroll D, Moore A. Variation in the placebo effect in randomized controlled trials of analgesics: all is as blind as it seems. Pain. 1996;64:331–5.

McQuay HJ, Moore RA. An evidence-based resource for pain relief. Oxford: Oxford University Press; 1998.

Schulz KF, Chalmers I, Hayes RJ, Altman DG. Empirical evidence of bias: dimensions of methodological quality associated with estimates of treatment effects in controlled trials. J Am Med Assoc. 1995;273:408–12.

Sriwatanakul K, Kelvie W, Lasagna L. The quantification of pain: an analysis of words used to describe pain and analgesia in clinical trials. Clin Pharmacol Ther. 1982;32:141–8.

Henry D, Lim LL, Rodriguez LAG, et al. Variability in risk of gastrointestinal complications with individual non-steroidal anti-inflammatory drugs: results of a collaborative meta-analysis. Br Med J. 1996;312:1563–6.

Chapter 28 Local anesthetics and regional anesthesia

John F Butterworth IV

Topics covered in this chapter

Local anesthetics
Regional anesthesia

This chapter considers the mechanisms by which local anesthetics produce both their desired and their toxic effects, as well as the physiology and application of several of the major clinical regional anesthetic procedures. Although cocaine-induced local anesthesia was first described by Koller in 1884, the mechanisms by which local anesthetics inhibit the excitability of nerves have become well understood only within the past generation.

Local anesthetics reversibly inhibit excitability in nerves and muscle cells. At concentrations below those that completely 'block' nerve conduction, local anesthetics serve as antiarrhythmic agents, supplement general anesthesia, and provide therapy for central pain syndromes. When applied to peripheral nerves, local anesthetics produce reversible voltage-, frequency-, and state-dependent inhibition of Na^+ channels. These actions can be exploited to produce the many forms of regional anesthesia.

LOCAL ANESTHETICS

Local anesthetics and their structures

The clinically used local anesthetics all contain an aromatic (benzene ring) moiety connected through either an ester or an amide bond to an aliphatic (hydrocarbon) chain, at the end of which all [except benzocaine (ethyl aminobenzoate)] contain a tertiary amino group (Fig. 28.1). The aromatic region of the molecule contributes to the high degree of lipid solubility of local anesthetics. At physiologic pH, tertiary amines can exist as either the neutral free base or, after binding a proton, as a positively charged form. Increasing pH favors free-base forms over positively charged (cationic) forms. The neutral free-base forms are considerably more lipid soluble and membrane permeable than the positively charged ones. This property results in a pronounced pH dependence of local anesthetic potency and speed of onset (Fig 28.2).

Specific local anesthetics

Esters

Cocaine is the only naturally occurring local anesthetic and was the first to be given to patients. Its addictive properties and toxicity limit its usefulness; however, it is an excellent topical anesthetic. Cocaine is also the only local anesthetic that releases norepinephrine from nerve terminals, the only local anesthetic that consistently produces vasoconstriction after local application, and the only local anesthetic with addictive properties.

Procaine, the first synthetic local anesthetic, has limited potency and duration but a relatively low systemic toxicity. It is hydrolyzed to PABA, which may elicit anaphylaxis. It is most commonly used for infiltration or spinal anesthesia.

2-Chloroprocaine is used mainly for short-duration epidural anesthesia. It has a rapid onset and a short duration of action. Its rapid hydrolysis in blood limits its potential for systemic toxicity. Epidural 2-chloroprocaine may cause more postoperative backache than lidocaine. 2-Chloroprocaine is useful for regional blocks in ambulatory patients when surgery will last less than 1 hour. The use of 2-chloroprocaine for intravenous regional anesthesia has been criticized based on a single report of vascular complications after use of a high concentration; nevertheless, low concentrations of this agent are commonly used for intravenous regional anesthesia in European centers without adverse effects.

Tetracaine is used primarily for prolonged spinal and topical anesthesia.

Benzocaine is used only for topical anesthesia. As with procaine, benzocaine is metabolized to PABA and may produce anaphylaxis.

Amides

Among the amides, *lidocaine* is the most versatile, being used for infiltration, topical anesthesia, intravenous regional anesthesia, peripheral nerve blocks, and spinal and epidural anesthesia. Lidocaine is also used intravenously to inhibit ventricular arrhythmias, supplement general anesthesia, and inhibit neuropathic pain.

Prilocaine has similar potency to lidocaine but less tendency to produce CNS toxicity. It has been widely used outside the USA for intravenous regional anesthesia, because it produces fewer toxic CNS side effects after release of the tourniquet than an equivalent dose of lidocaine. Some European centers have used hyperbaric prilocaine as an alternative to hyperbaric lidocaine.

Etidocaine, another lidocaine analog, has the most rapid onset of all local anesthetics and an extremely prolonged duration of action, particularly of motor block. Etidocaine is used for infiltration, peripheral nerve blocks, and epidural anesthesia for long operations requiring muscle relaxation.

Mepivacaine, ropivacaine, and *bupivacaine* are structurally similar. Mepivacaine is used for infiltration, peripheral nerve blocks, epidural anesthesia, and in some centers for isobaric

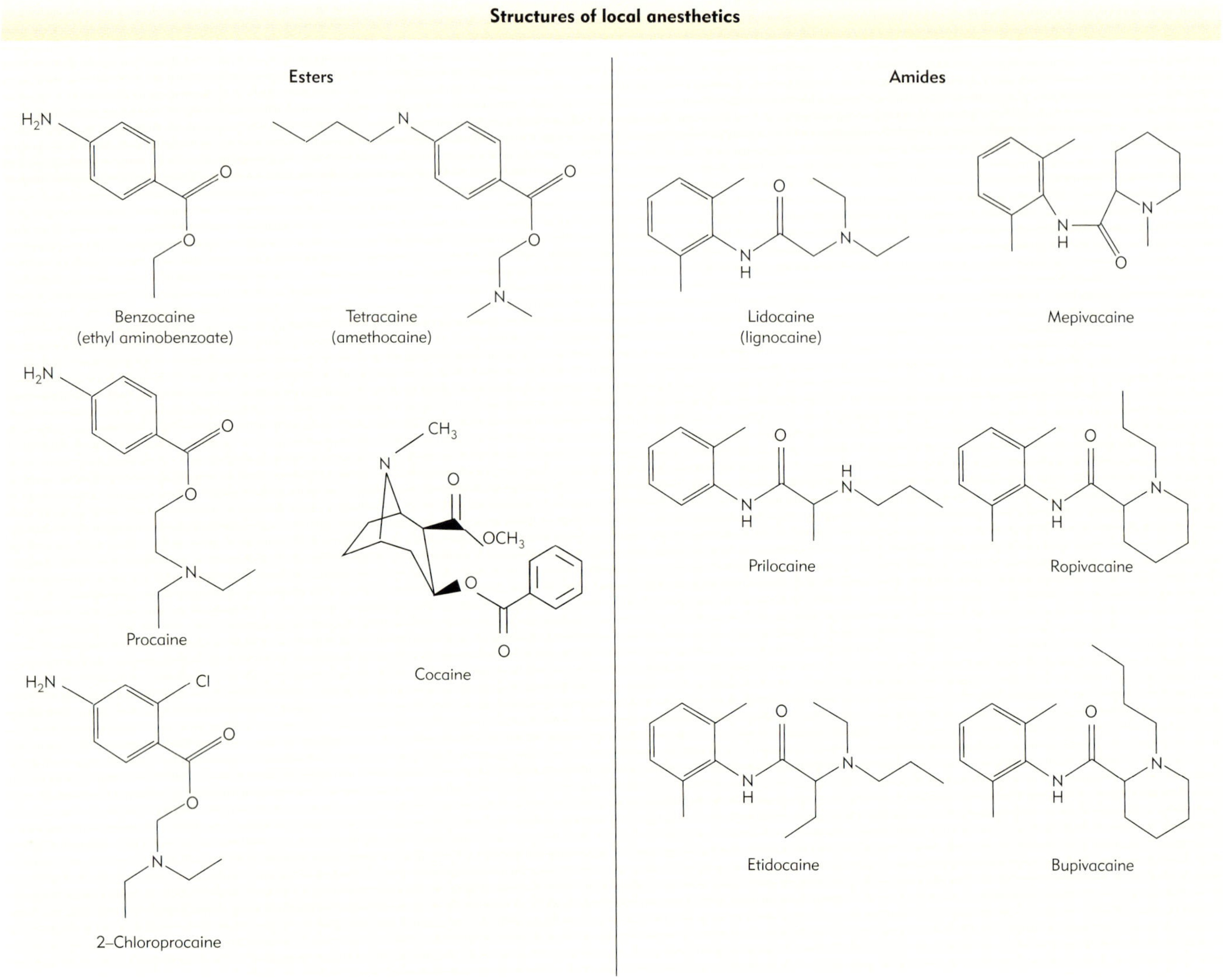

Structures of local anesthetics

Esters: Benzocaine (ethyl aminobenzoate); Tetracaine (amethocaine); Procaine; Cocaine; 2-Chloroprocaine

Amides: Lidocaine (lignocaine); Mepivacaine; Prilocaine; Ropivacaine; Etidocaine; Bupivacaine

Figure 28.1 Local anesthetic chemical structures. The fundamental difference between amides and esters lies in the bond connecting the aromatic region of the molecule to the aliphatic region. The aromatic portion has lipophilic properties while the aliphatic region confers water solublity.

spinal anesthesia. It produces slightly longer durations of anesthesia than lidocaine. Ropivacaine has an analgesic profile similar to bupivacaine but may be less potent and less cardiotoxic. In most respects, ropivacaine resembles bupivacaine in onset and duration. Bupivacaine, used for infiltration, peripheral nerve blocks, epidural, and spinal anesthesia has a long duration of action and prolonged delay of onset. Like ropivacaine, bupivacaine seems to be relatively selective for sensory fibers over motor fibers, particularly with dilute local anesthetic concentrations, making it especially attractive for postoperative analgesia, as epidural analgesia for the pain of labor, and for chronic pain states. Bupivacaine shares with etidocaine and tetracaine a propensity for producing cardiovascular toxicity from which resuscitation is difficult. Bupivacaine has recently become available as the single S(–)-isomer (levobupivacaine) with reduced cardiotoxicity and neurotoxicity compared to the racemic mixture.

The eutectic mixture of local anesthetics (*EMLA*) is a cream formulation of 2.5% lidocaine and 2.5% prilocaine used on intact skin. EMLA cream provides satisfactory anesthesia for venous cannulation if applied under an occlusive dressing for at least 30–40 minutes.

Cellular electrophysiology

Excitable cells have the special ability to produce action potentials, which are brief, propagating waves of membrane depolarization (Chapter 18). In most nerves, action potentials are initiated by voltage-gated Na^+ channels, which are heavily glycosylated integral membrane proteins containing up to three different types of subunit. The Na^+ channels from mammalian neurons contain a larger subunit of about 260 kDa with four membrane-spanning regions (I–IV) and varying numbers of secondary β-subunits (Fig. 28.3). Channels from rat brain contain one β_1-subunit of approximately 36kDa and another smaller β_2-subunit of approximately 33kDa. The β_1-subunits are noncovalently associated with the α-subunit; β_2-subunits are bonded to the α-subunit through disulfide links. Na^+ channel α-subunits have been cloned from the electric eel electric organ, rat brain

Physicochemical and pharmacologic properties of local anesthetic agents

Agent	Physicochemical properties				Pharmacologic properties		
Esters	**Molecular weight (base)**	**pK_a (25°C)**	**Partition coefficient[a]**	**Protein binding (%)**	**Onset**	**Relative potency**	**Duration of action**
Procaine	236	9.1	1.7	6	Slow	1	Short
Tetracaine (amethocaine)	264	8.6	221	76	Slow	8	Long
Chloroprocaine	271	9.3	9.0	–	Fast	1	Short
Amides							
Prilocaine	220	8.0	25.0	55	Fast	2	Moderate
Lidocaine (lignocaine)	234	7.9	43.0	64	Fast	2	Moderate
Mepivacaine	246	7.9	21.0	78	Fast	2	Moderate
Bupivacaine	288	8.2	346	96	Moderate	8	Long
Etidocaine	276	8.1	800	94	Fast	6	Long
Ropivacaine	274	8.2	115	94	Moderate	6	Long

[a]Octanol/buffer partition coefficients expressed as (total drug/mL octanol)/(total drug/mL buffer) at pH 7.4 and 25°C.

Figure 28.2 Physiochemical and pharmacologic properties of local anesthetic agents. (Modified with permission from Strichartz et al., 1995.)

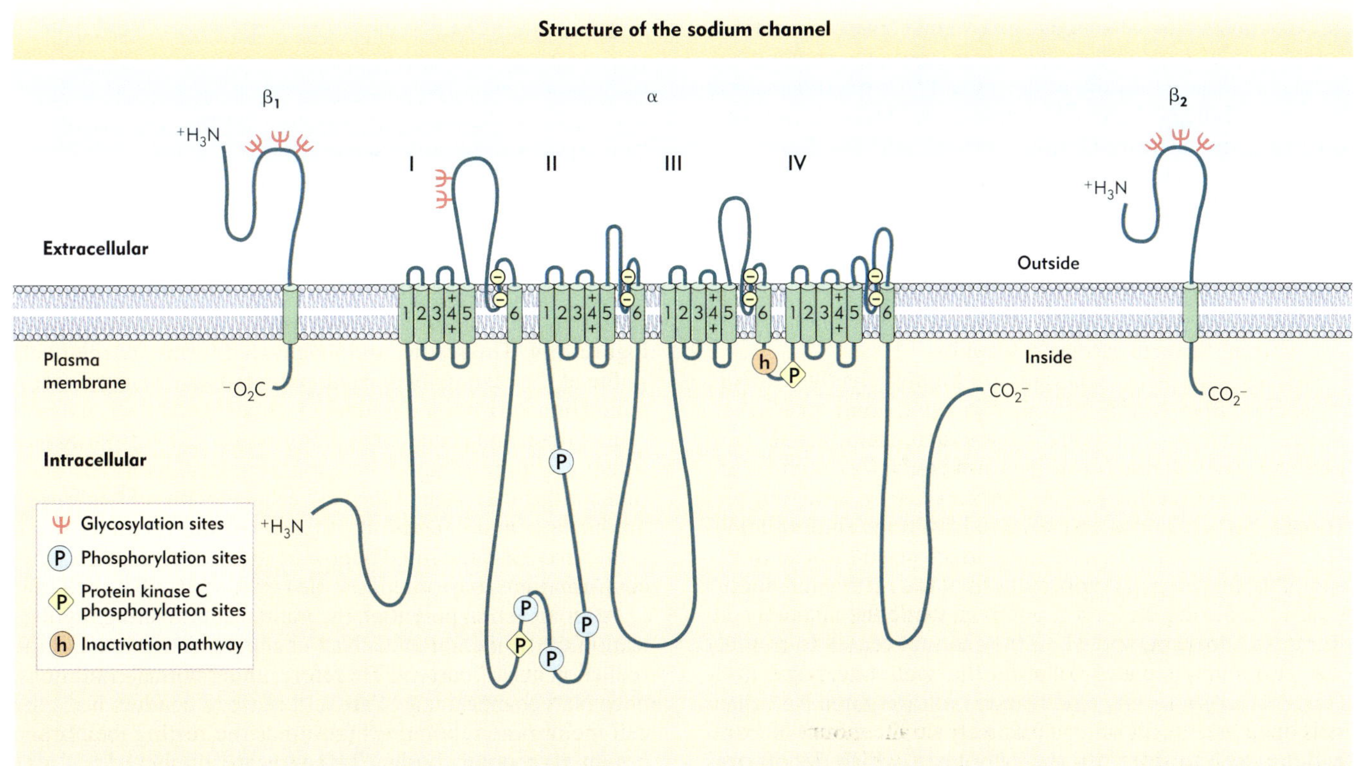

Figure 28.3 Structure of the sodium channel. The Na^+ channels from mammalian neurons contain one larger subunit (α) and varying numbers of smaller subunits (β) (see text for details). Local anesthetic binding and ion conduction occurs in the α subunit; however, the β_1-subunit can inhibit local anesthetic association with the α-subunit. The short span between III and IV denotes the region responsible for inactivation. The Na^+ conducting pore is lined by segments 5 and 6 of the four transmembrane spanning regions of the α-subunit. (With permission from Caterall, 1995.)

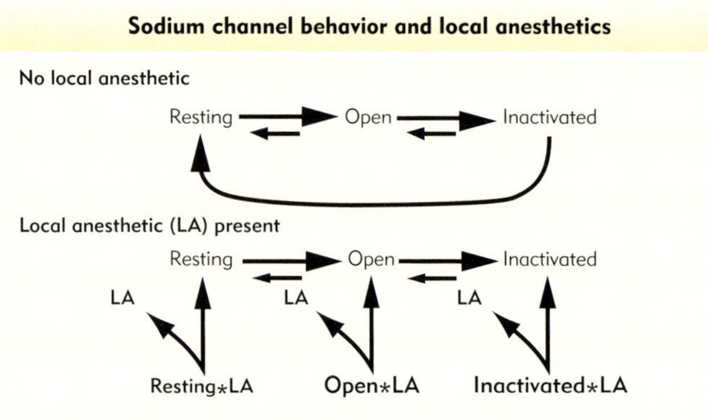

Figure 28.4 Simplified model for sodium channel behavior in the presence and absence of local anesthetics. The likelihood of a Na^+ channel being inactivated increases with the duration of depolarization; similarly, upon repolarization, channels increasingly tend to assume the resting conformation. Other conformations likely exist; only open channels that have not bound local anesthetic will conduct ionic current. The dependence of local anesthetic binding to the Na^+ channel on its conformational state (inactivated > open > resting) is known as the modified receptor hypothesis.

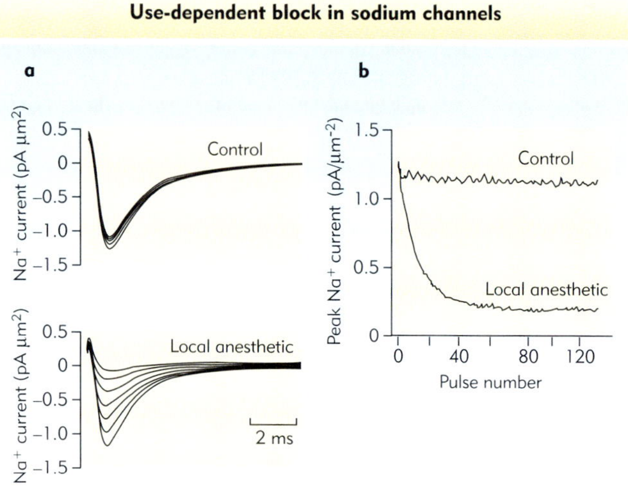

Figure 28.5 Use-dependent block in sodium channels from cardiac muscle. (a) Pulse depolarization of canine cardiac Purkinje fibers, which were subjected to voltage-clamp at –150mV, then depolarized to 0mV for 10 milliseconds. In the absence of local anesthetic, depolarization causes Na^+ channels to shift from resting to open conformations, eliciting inward (downward on the figure) Na^+ current. The Na^+ channels rapidly inactivate and the Na^+ current declines despite continued depolarization. The overlapping control traces represent the currents recorded during depolarization numbers 1, 2, 4, 8, 16, 32, 64, and 128 in a 130-pulse train. When a local aneshetic, QX222 [an obligatory positively charged lidocaine (lignocaine) derivative (0.5mmol/L)] was introduced, repetitive depolarizations elicited sequentially diminished Na^+ current, indicative of use-dependent (also known as phasic or frequency-dependent) block. (b) The peak inward (Na^+) current measured after the indicated sequential depolarizations. With increasing numbers of depolarizations, the Na^+ current declined to a minimal value. (With permission from Hanck et al., 1994.)

(where there are three distinct subtypes), rat skeletal muscle, and rat ventricle. These various Na^+ channel forms demonstrate great homology in segments S1 to S6 (occurring in all four membrane-spanning regions). The β_1- and β_2-subunits in rat brain Na^+ channels have also been cloned and consist of relatively small cytoplasmic domains, a single membrane-spanning segment, and large extracellular domains. The three-dimensional structure of the Na^+ channel, particularly that of the ion-conducting pore in the α-subunit, is not known. The β-subunits influence peak current, activation, and inactivation. Isolated α-subunits from mammalian brain and skeletal muscle have slower decay of Na^+ currents than native (complete) Na^+ channels. Cardiac Na^+ channel α-subunits produce Na^+ currents that resemble those from native (complete) channels. By comparison, the β_1-subunit inhibits lidocaine (lignocaine) block of Na^+ current through cardiac α-subunits.

Voltage-gated Na^+ channels are highly selective for Na^+ relative to other cations prevalent in living organisms; nevertheless, other ions of similar atomic size, including H^+, will permeate Na^+ channels readily. Conversely, Ca^{2+} and K^+ are very nearly impermeant. As formulated by Hodgkin and Huxley, Na^+ channels can exist in at least three conformations (or states): 'resting,' 'open', and 'inactivated'. These correspond to the channel conformations at the resting membrane potential, during the action potential while the channel conducts Na^+ current, and when the channel ceases to conduct Na^+ current immediately following the open state, respectively (Fig. 28.4). As a result of 'activation,' voltage-gated Na^+ channels open briefly, allowing a relatively small amount of extracellular Na^+ to flow into the cytoplasm, which depolarizes adjacent regions of the plasma membrane (driving the membrane potential toward a positive value). Conduction through open Na^+ channels ceases spontaneously after only a brief time because of 'inactivation' of the channel. The relative likelihood that a channel will be in any conformation is determined by the current value and recent history of the membrane potential, as is shown on the simplified scheme in Figure 28.4. The resting and inactivated forms are relatively stable at the resting membrane potential and during a maintained depolarization, respectively. Inactivated Na^+ channels cannot open and conduct Na^+ in response to a depolarization without first returning to the resting conformation. The open (ion-conducting) form of the Na^+ channel is present only early on during a depolarization; it converts into the inactivated form during a maintained depolarization. Other Na^+ channel conformations may (and likely do) exist.

After an action potential, the main factor favoring repolarization of the membrane is Na^+ channel inactivation and the reduction in Na^+ current. Therefore, under normal conditions, once Na^+ channels inactivate and cease to conduct Na^+, the cell membrane repolarizes (resumes the resting membrane potential) spontaneously. The aggregate number of Na^+ions that enters the cell during an action potential is minuscule relative to the concentration of Na^+ in extracellular fluid. Although an outward flow of K^+ makes a contribution to nerve repolarization in studies of lower organisms, there are very few K^+ channels present in human or other mammalian nodes of Ranvier, and repolarization of nerve fibers *in vitro* proceeds uneventfully even when all K^+ channels have been pharmacologically blocked.

Mechanisms of local anesthetic action

Local anesthetics increase the firing threshold of muscle cells and neurons, rendering them less excitable, by binding and inhibiting voltage-gated Na^+ channels. Although many details of the mechanism are unresolved, Na^+ channels that have bound a local anesthetic will not conduct Na^+. Local anesthetics bind open and inactivated channels more avidly than resting channels (see Fig. 28.4). When membranes depolarize frequently, Na^+ channels spend more time in open and inactivated conformations and are, therefore, more likely to bind local anesthetics. This phenomenon is called use-dependent, frequency-dependent, or phasic block to distinguish it from the lesser degree of inhibition obtained with infrequent depolarizations (tonic block) (Fig. 28.5). Which Na^+ channel conformation has the greatest affinity for local anesthetics? In cardiac tissue, inactivated channels are thought to bind local anesthetics more avidly, while in neuronal tissue open channels are thought to be more avid. In all tissues, resting Na^+ channels have relatively low affinity for local anesthetics. Use-dependent block almost certainly underlies the ability of lidocaine and similar agents to inhibit ventricular arrhythmias (Chapter 35). It may also explain the increased potency of local anesthetics in inhibiting ongoing pain (e.g. after surgery and during labor) than in inhibiting new incisional pain. The significance of other local anesthetic actions, such as their ability to inhibit K^+ and Ca^{2+} channels, nicotinic acetylcholine receptors, and β-adrenoceptors, is unclear.

The location of the receptors for local anesthetics on the Na^+ channel is currently being defined with molecular genetic techniques. How local anesthetics interact with the Na^+ channel depends on pH, charge, and the specific local anesthetic species. At physiologic pH, local anesthetics (with pK_a values ranging from 7.8 to 9.2) exist in an equilibrium between protonated and neutral base forms (see Fig. 28.2). Permanently charged local anesthetic derivatives have almost no membrane permeability and inhibit Na^+ channels only when applied within the cytoplasm. Similarly, extracellular local anesthetics 'leashed' to large, membrane-impermeant macromolecules show no ability to inhibit Na^+ channels if the 'leash' lengths are 1.5nm or shorter, confirming the lack of a binding site on the external surface of the plasma membrane and the importance of membrane permeability for efficacy of local anesthetics applied extracellularly. The permanently neutral local anesthetic (benzocaine) freely permeates the plasma membrane and inhibits Na^+ channels whether applied intracellularly or extracellularly. Once within the cytoplasm, tertiary amine local anesthetics bind Na^+ channels more avidly if positively charged. Local anesthetics show a moderate degree of stereospecificity: generally the $R(+)$-isomers have greater potency than the $S(-)$-isomers. Differences between optical isomers are greater for local anesthetic binding to inactivated cardiac Na^+ and K^+ channels than for binding to open neuronal Na^+ channels. These enantiomeric differences underlie the decisions to formulate ropivacaine and bupivacaine as the single $S(-)$-isomers rather than as racemic mixtures: to reduce their potential cardiac toxicity without markedly reducing potency at nerve block. Tetrodotoxin and many other neurotoxins inhibit Na^+ channels more potently than do local anesthetics. In general, these agents bind to receptors (sites) other

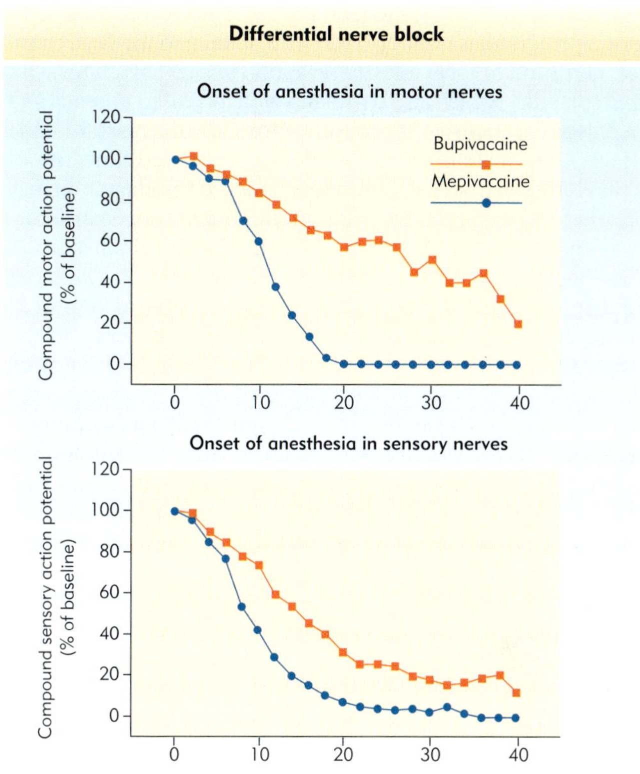

Figure 28.6 Differential nerve block. Human volunteers underwent bilateral median nerve block with mepivacaine (1%) or bupivacaine (0.33%). Onset of anesthesia in sensory nerves (assessed with the compound sensory nerve action potential) and motor nerves (assessed with the compound motor action potential) was monitored. Onset of motor and sensory block was faster with mepivacaine in general and significantly slower with motor than with sensory nerves. During the onset of block, a motor-sparing effect could be observed. Such effects during the onset of anesthesia underlie most differential blocking with local anesthetics used for clinical anesthesia. (With permission from Butterworth et al., 1998.)

than those to which local anesthetics bind and do not demonstrate the voltage-, frequency-, and state-dependent block characteristic of local anesthetics.

Factors influencing local anesthetic activity

The greater the length of nerve exposed to a given local anesthetic concentration, the more complete will be the inhibition of nerve conduction. Inhibition can also depend on the size of the nerve, its conduction velocity, whether the nerve is myelinated, and the function of the nerve. Certain physical properties of local anesthetics have been correlated with their rate of onset, potency, and duration. The more lipophilic local anesthetics [e.g. bupivacaine, etidocaine, ropivacaine, and tetracaine (amethocaine)] permeate membranes more readily and bind the local anesthetic receptor site on Na^+ channels with greater affinity, resulting in a good correlation between the octanol:water partition coefficient (lipophilicity) and ester or amide local anesthetic potency *in vitro*.

Local anesthetic duration is often said, erroneously, to be determined by protein binding. More lipophilic anesthetics are more highly protein bound (see Fig 28.2); however, binding to serum proteins has nothing to do with binding to the Na^+ channel. Duration of local anesthetic action *in vivo* correlates with lipid solubility (which also correlates with increased potency and increased propensity to produce toxic cardiovascular side effects). During clinical nerve blocks, shortened duration of action resulting from local anesthetic-induced vasodilatation may be offset by mixing the local anesthetic with a vasoconstrictor.

With the sole exception of etidocaine, all local anesthetics with long duration also have a longer delay of onset. The more lipid-soluble, membrane-permeable agents may also bind to myelin and other lipid-rich membranes in preference to the local anesthetic-binding site on the Na^+ channel. It is often claimed that local anesthetic speed of onset increases with decreasing pK_a, reasoning that at a given pH agents with lower pK_a values have a greater percentage of local anesthetic drug molecules in the uncharged (neutral) form than agents with higher values. However, of the two local anesthetics of fastest onset, etidocaine and chloroprocaine, one has a low and the other a high pK_a (see Fig.28.2).

Selective inhibition of sensory nerves with preservation of motor function (differential block) is an unfulfilled goal of regional anesthesia. Local anesthetics inhibit smaller nerves in a given class before larger nerves (e.g. among myelinated fibers, Aδ before Aα). Although smaller than most myelinated nerve fibers, unmyelinated C fibers are more resistant to block than the smaller Aδ nerve fibers. Nevertheless, using current drugs, there is considerable overlap among nerve fiber types in their susceptibility to local anesthesics (Fig. 28.6). During clinical anesthesia, bupivacaine and ropivacaine show relatively greater selectivity for sensory fibers over motor fibers than do other local anesthetics.

For nearly any nerve block procedure, increasing the local anesthetic dose will increase the speed of onset, adequacy, and duration of anesthesia. The site of injection also influences local anesthetic pharmacokinetics. The most rapid onset and shortest duration are seen with spinal anesthesia and subcutaneous injection. The slowest onset and longest duration are seen with brachial plexus blocks. These differences likely relate, in part, to the anatomy of the injection site, the relative rate of absorption from the site of injection, and the amount of drug injected.

Local anesthetics are often administered with vasoconstrictors [typically epinephrine (adrenaline) at 2–10μg/mL] to decrease the rate of local anesthetic absorption, reduce the peak concentration in blood, and prolong the duration of action (see below). The ability of epinephrine to prolong anesthesia depends on the injection site and the drug. Epinephrine can also serve as a marker for accidental intravenous injection of local anesthetic. Other common local anesthetic additives include sodium bicarbonate and, in ophthalmologic practice, hyaluronidase. This enzyme is extracted from bull testicles; it metabolizes hyaluronic acid in connective tissue and is added to local anesthetic solutions to increase their spread. Cholinergic agents (neostigmine) (e.g. clonidine, α-adrenergic agents, epinephrine) and opioids are also added to local anesthetic solutions used for spinal or epidural analgesia techniques for their own analgesic actions.

Most clinically used local anesthetics are prepared as hydrochloride (HCl) salts. Lidocaine carbonate solution (not available in USA) may have more rapid onset of brachial plexus and epidural blockade than lidocaine HCl solutions. The mechanism for this difference is unclear; however, carbon dioxide is known to readily permeate the nerve plasma membrane and to acidify the pH within the cytoplasm, favoring protonated local anesthetic forms. More alkaline local anesthetic solutions generally have increased local anesthetic potency *in vivo*. Alkaline pH increases the percentage of local anesthetic molecules in the uncharged base form and increases local anesthetic potency at tonic block; therefore, clinicians commonly add bicarbonate to local anesthetic solutions. The effects of alkaline conditions during onset of block do not continue once the local anesthetic is on or near the Na^+ channel, where extracellular hydrogen ions (acidic pH) potentiate use-dependent block. This effect of extracellular pH may be clinically significant: acidemia enhances the ability of lidocaine to reduce impulse conduction velocity and delays recovery from lidocaine-induced Na^+ current depression. Sodium bicarbonate appears most effective at speeding the onset of nerve blocks when added to local anesthetic solutions mixed with epinephrine by the manufacturer. These local anesthetic solutions prepackaged with epinephrine have acidic pH (4.5) to retard oxidation of epinephrine and show a relatively large increase in pH with bicarbonate. Addition of bicarbonate to local anesthetic solution not mixed with epinephrine by the manufacturer produces little change in solution pH or in rate of onset of anesthesia.

Temperature can influence local anesthetic action and cooling per se can produce conduction block. The *in vitro* potency of local anesthetics increases with cooling. The *in vivo* results are mixed, with studies showing no consistent action of cooling during clinical local anesthesia, with the exception of an increase in the pain of injection. Pregnancy increases the spread of epidural and spinal anesthesia (Chapter 65). This may partly result from an increased sensitivity to local anesthetics, probably mediated by progesterone, in nerves in the pregnant compared with the nonpregnant state, as demonstrated by a greater median sensory nerve block produced by 1% lidocaine in pregnant (third-trimester) women compared with women who are not pregnant.

Local anesthetic pharmacokinetics

Local anesthetics are applied directly on or near their target site through regional administration; most other drugs are carried by the blood to their sites of action.Therefore, blood concentrations of local anesthetics bear little relationship to their desired effects. Local anesthetic concentrations in blood depend on the dose of local anesthetic injected, whether or not a vasoconstrictor was included with the local anesthetic, and the site of injection. For a given local anesthetic dose, the highest local anesthetic blood concentrations are obtained after intercostal blocks, particularly when epinephrine-free local anesthetics are used. Most local anesthetics are subject to considerable first-pass absorption by the lung. The lack of lung binding in patients with right-to-left cardiac shunts can lead to toxic reactions from otherwise appropriate intravenous doses of lidocaine.

All local anesthetics in clinical use are lipid soluble; consequently, all local anesthetics are at least partially protein bound in blood, primarily to α_1-acidic glycoprotein and secondarily to albumin. The proteins that bind local anesthetics have a high binding capacity, and the extent of local anesthetic protein binding depends on the local anesthetic concentration in blood only at very high (and very toxic) concentrations. Conditions in which concentrations of α_1-acidic glycoprotein and local anesthetic protein binding decrease include pregnancy, oral contraceptive use, and in newborns. Concentrations of α_1-acidic glycoprotein increase (and the extent of local anesthetic binding increases) with trauma, myocardial infarction, or uremia. The ratio of whole blood-to-plasma concentrations is highest for the least potent, shortest-acting local anesthetics (e.g. lidocaine) and lowest for more potent, longer-acting agents (e.g. etidocaine) (see Fig. 28.2).

Local anesthetic metabolism

Local anesthetics are metabolized into smaller compounds that can be excreted in urine or bile. For local anesthetics that are esters, the primary step is ester hydrolysis by pseudocholinesterase in blood. The rate of ester hydrolysis is rapid: half-lives of elimination are measured in seconds for procaine and chloroprocaine. Procaine and benzocaine are metabolized to *para*-aminobenzoic acid (PABA), a species that can produce anaphylactic reactions. Chloroprocaine and tetracaine are metabolized similarly, but not to PABA. Cocaine undergoes ester hydrolysis or *N*-demethylation followed by ester hydrolysis.

The amides are metabolized in the liver; less than 5% of a dose of these agents is excreted unchanged in urine. Lidocaine undergoes oxidative *N*-dealkylation (by cytochrome P450 CYP3A4) to monoethylglycine xylidide and glycine xylidide. These compounds are further metabolized to 4-hydroxy-2,6-xylidine. Bupivacaine, mepivacaine, etidocaine, and ropivacaine undergo oxidative *N*-dealkylation and hydroxylation. Prilocaine undergoes hydrolysis to *ortho*-toluidine, a metabolic product unique among local anesthetics. This compound causes a degree of methemoglobinemia proportional to the dose of prilocaine used. Amide local anesthetic clearance is highly dependent on hepatic blood flow, hepatic extraction, and hepatic enzyme function. Amide clearance is reduced by treatments that decrease hepatic blood flow, including β-adrenoceptor or histamine H_2-receptor blockers, heart failure (reduced cardiac output), and hepatic cirrhosis.

Toxic side effects of local anesthetics

Systemic local anesthetic toxicity results from local anesthetic interaction with Na^+, K^+, and Ca^{2+} channels in brain, vascular tissue, or heart, or from allergy. In the CNS, side effects of local anesthetics reflect 'disinhibition', progressive excitation, then depression of function as the concentration in blood increases. Humans receiving intravenous infusions of local anesthetics may report or exhibit circumoral numbness and paresthesia of the tongue or extremities. The following side effects increase as the local anesthetic concentration in blood increases: tinnitus, visual abnormalities, ominous feelings, garrulousness, muscular twitching, tremors, and seizures (excitatory effects). In animal experiments when local anesthetic dosing continues above the dose that produces seizures, CNS excitation will progress to respiratory depression and cardiac arrest. The specific cardiac effects of local anesthetics are discussed in Chapter 35. The convulsive local anesthetic potency correlates with potency at nerve block. More-potent agents, (bupivacaine, ropivacaine, amethocaine, and etidocaine) produce CNS side effects (including seizures) at lower blood concentrations and doses than less-potent local anesthetics (lidocaine, procaine, mepivacaine, and prilocaine). Both respiratory and metabolic acidosis decrease the local anesthetic convulsive dose.

Cardiovascular toxicity requires higher local anesthetic concentrations in blood than does CNS toxicity. Local anesthetics inhibit cardiac excitation and conduction by inhibiting Na^+ channels. The more-potent anesthetics inhibit conduction at lower concentrations than the less-potent agents. Bupivacaine binds Na^+ channels more avidly (and with a longer duration) than lidocaine. For local anesthetics with asymmetric carbons, *R*(+)-enantiomers bind cardiac Na^+ channels at lower concentrations than *S*(−)-enantiomers. Local anesthetics produce dose-dependent depression of myocardial contractility with a rank order of potency consistent with that for producing nerve block.

Experimentally, the vascular smooth muscle effects of local anesthetics depend on whether the endothelium remains intact or not, the agent used to preconstrict the vessel, and local anesthetic concentration. In general, local anesthetics cause vasoconstriction at low concentrations by inhibiting nitric oxide production; nevertheless, all local anesthetics except cocaine cause vasodilatation by inhibiting tonic sympathetic nerve-mediated vasoconstriction at concentrations relevant to regional nerve block. Intravenous local anesthetics produce dose-dependent increases in systemic vascular resistance during CNS excitation, followed at higher concentrations by dose-dependent decreases in systemic vascular resistance. CNS mediated effects have also been implicated in the cardiotoxicity of bupivacaine.

Local anesthetics also bind and inhibit cardiac Ca^{2+} and K^+ channels and β-adrenoceptors, and inhibit cAMP formation. These effects require concentrations greater than those which inhibit Na^+ channels. It is unclear whether any of these actions cause or contribute to toxic side effects and/or impede resuscitation from cardiotoxic effects.

Allergic reactions to local anesthetics

Patients rarely experience true allergic reactions to local anesthetics but often report untoward reactions from accidental intravenous injection of local anesthetic, epinephrine, or both. True allergic reactions have been reported more commonly for ester local anesthetics, particularly those metabolized to PABA (procaine and benzocaine), than for amides. Skin testing of subjects without previous history of local anesthetic allergy elicits a relatively high incidence of reactions to esters. Anaphylactic reactions (and positive skin tests) to amide anesthetics are less common and may reflect allergy to preservatives. Suspected local anesthetic allergy can be evaluated with skin testing; one study identified at least one local anesthetic as safe for each of 90 patients referred after an apparent allergic local anesthetic reaction. In the absence of skin testing, the prudent approach would be to use a structurally dissimilar agent when a patient presents with a history suggesting allergy to a particular local anesthetic.

Neurotoxic effects of local anesthetics

In the 1980s, there were several reports of cauda equina syndrome when large doses of 2-chloroprocaine were injected (accidentally) into spinal fluid during attempted lumbar epidural or caudal anesthesia. Animal studies demonstrated that 2-chloroprocaine caused neurotoxicity only when formulated with sodium metabisulfite at an acidic pH. Reports of neurotoxicity virtually disappeared after 2-chloroprocaine was reformulated. More recently, there have been reports of persisting sacral nerve root deficits after single-shot or (more often) continuous spinal anesthesia, particularly with hyperbaric 5% lidocaine administered through miniature (>30gauge) continuous spinal catheters. *In vitro*, 5% lidocaine (unlike other clinical local anesthetic formulations including 2% lidocaine) irreversibly interrupted nerve conduction (was neurotoxic) in isolated nerves; it also produced neurologic deficits after subarachnoid administration in animals. The long record of safety of 5% lidocaine probably results from the usual mixing of the agent within spinal fluid. The rare, persistent deficits after use of 5% lidocaine in patients may relate to restricted drug distribution, which might occur after injection into a nerve root sleeve. The issue may be avoided by using a different agent or a less-concentrated lidocaine solution for spinal anesthesia.

Treatment of local anesthetic toxicity

Reactions of less severity than a generalized seizure require only that no further local anesthetic be given. If a seizure should occur, the essential treatment consists of maintaining airway patency, ventilation, and providing oxygen. Seizures may be terminated (if judged necessary) with small intravenous doses of thiopental (thiopentone) (1–2mg/kg), diazepam (0.1–0.2mg/kg), or midazolam (0.05–0.10mg/kg). Succinylcholine (suxamethonium) (0.5–1mg/kg) and tracheal intubation may facilitate oxygenation and ventilation. If local anesthetic intoxication produces hypotension (without cardiac arrest), treatment may include intravenous fluids and vasopressors [phenylephrine (0.5–5μg/min per kg) or norepinephrine (0.02–0.2μg/min per kg)]. Intravenous epinephrine (1–15μg/kg per intravenous bolus) may be required if cardiovascular toxicity progresses to cardiac arrest. Based on animal studies, bretylium was considered useful for bupivacaine arrhythmias; however, it was ineffective in patients. Rodent studies indicated that coadministration of epinephrine or phenylephrine with bupivacaine reduced the local anesthetic dose required for lethality; conversely, β-adrenoceptor blockers increased the local anesthetic dose required for lethality. There is experimental evidence that bupivacaine inhibits binding to the β-adrenoceptor and inhibits cAMP production; consequently, resuscitation drugs that bypass the β-adrenoceptor system (such as amrinone or milrinone) may be more effective than β-adrenoceptor agonists (such as epinephrine). Although epinephrine potentiates bupivacaine toxicity, perhaps by enhancing its arrhythmogenicity, once bupivacaine has produced cardiac arrest, epinephrine is an essential therapy to increase coronary perfusion pressure. Treatment of local anesthetic allergic reactions includes antihistamines (H_1 and H_2 blockers) and corticosteroids. Severe anaphylactic reactions may require resuscitation with intravenous fluids and epinephrine and tracheal intubation.

REGIONAL ANESTHESIA

Spinal anesthesia

Spinal anesthesia is an old and reliable anesthetic technique with a very rapid onset. Block of both motor function and sensation is usually complete. Nevertheless, how local anesthetics produce spinal anesthesia remains unclear. It is commonly assumed that local anesthetics act where they bind most avidly after subarachnoid injection: to myelinated regions of nerve roots, spinal cord, and dorsal root ganglia. Nevertheless, the mechanistic significance of this local anesthetic binding is unknown. Differential block appears at the upper dermatomal margins of spinal anesthesia: inhibition of kinesthetic sensibility exceeds that of light touch, which, in turn, exceeds that of pinprick sensibility. Similarly, inhibition of sensation extends above that of motor block on a dermatomal basis. Sympathetic block exceeds pinprick sensory block. Differential spinal anesthesia, in which injection of dilute local anesthetic concentrations inhibits sympathetically mediated but not somatic pain, is

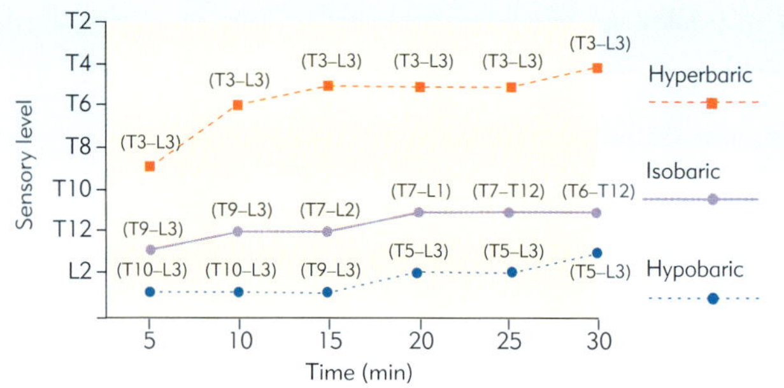

Figure 28.7 Greater dermatomal spread of hyperbaric compared with isobaric or hypobaric bupivacaine spinal anesthesia. Bupivacaine (0.5%) was mixed with an equal volume of 10% dextrose, 0.9% saline, or water and 3mL (7.5mg) was injected into patients to produce hypobaric, isobaric, or hyperbaric spinal anesthesia. The median and range (in parentheses) of pinprick anesthesia measured 30 minutes after local anesthesic injection at L2–L4 is plotted. The median dermatomal levels of pinprick anesthesia varied with technique: the hyperbaric technique produced the highest levels; the isobaric technique produced significantly greater spread of anesthesia than the hypobaric technique. (With permission from van Gessel et al., 1991.)

a useful diagnostic tool; however, sufficient spinal analgesia for a surgical incision cannot be obtained without a high likelihood of motor block. The spread of the local injection after administration and, hence the area of anesthesia, differs with the formulation of the injection. Hyperbaric (diluted with dextrose and denser than CSF) and hypobaric (diluted with water and less dense than CSF) local anesthetic solutions are influenced by patient positioning and gravity, isobaric solutions are not. Hyperbaric solutions consistently produce upper thoracic dermatomal levels of anesthesia if a patient is placed in a supine position immediately after local anesthetic injection. Hyperbaric local anesthetics can be injected with the patient sitting to produce isolated lower lumbar and sacral anesthesia for perineal procedures. Hypobaric local anesthesia can be injected with the patient in Buie's (jackknife) position to produce isolated lower lumbar and sacral anesthesia for perineal procedures. When the same dose of bupivacaine was given in a hyperbaric, isobaric, or hypobaric solution to patients who were immediately turned supine, the hyperbaric solution yielded the greatest spread of anesthesia and the hypobaric technique yielded the least (Fig. 28.7). Local anesthetics for epidural injection (and plain spinal tetracaine) are nearly isobaric. Isobaric solutions have a greater delay of onset, longer duration, and less reliable anesthesia in thoracic dermatomes than hyperbaric solutions. The decline in local anesthetic concentrations in spinal fluid after injection results from uptake by vascular, neural, and adipose tissue. Vasoconstrictors (epinephrine 0.2–0.3mg, rarely phenylephrine 5–7mg) prolong hyperbaric tetracaine spinal anesthesia and maintain higher concentrations of tetracaine in spinal fluid in the first hour after local anesthetic injection compared with administration without epinephrine. Hyperbaric tetracaine and bupivacaine are minimally prolonged (at upper dermatomes)

Similar outcomes after general, spinal, or epidural anesthesia for peripheral vascular surgery				
Factor/outcome	General (*n*=138)	Spinal (*n*=136)	Epidural (*n*=149)	*p*
Age (years)	68 ± 12	68 ± 11	68 ± 11	0.95
History of myocardial infarction (%)	33	36	39	0.56
Perioperative myocardial infarction (%)	4	5	5	0.82
Perioperative death (%)	3	3	3	0.97

Figure 28.8 Similar outcomes after general, spinal, or epidural anesthesia for peripheral vascular surgery. There was no evidence for an outcome difference based on choice of anesthesia. (With permission from Bode et al., 1996.)

by vasoconstrictors. Isobaric spinal anesthesia is prolonged in a dose-dependent manner by epinephrine. Both subarachnoid and oral clonidine prolong spinal anesthesia, probably as a result of actions at α_2-adrenoceptors (Chapter 25).

The cardiovascular effects of spinal anesthesia increase with increasing dermatomal spread of anesthesia (and increased sympathetic block). Hypotension during spinal anesthesia is usually the result of the thoracolumbar sympathectomy induced by the local anesthetic and typically first appears when the sympathetic block includes the fourth thoracic dermatome. Spinal anesthesia has no direct actions on myocardial contractility but may have indirect effects from reduced systemic vascular resistance and venous pooling. The heart rate often declines during spinal anesthesia, particularly if pure α-adrenergic agonists (e.g. phenylephrine) are used to treat hypotension. Severe bradycardia can be the combined result of cardiac sympathectomy (block of T_2–T_4), diminished venous return, diminished right atrial distention, and possibly also of excessive sedation and respiratory depression. Hypotension rarely occurs during spinal anesthesia in small children. Because of the separation between sensory and sympathetic block, hypotension may occur in adults even when sensory anesthesia does not reach the upper thoracic dermatomes. Hypotension can be corrected by counteracting the drop in arterial resistance with α-adrenergic stimulation and the increased venous pooling with fluid administration, elevating the legs relative to the heart, or β-adrenoceptor stimulation. Treatment of hypotension with mixed adrenergic agonists rather than a pure agonist yields a higher cardiac output and a lower incidence of severe bradycardia.

Spinal anesthesia has minimal effects on organ blood flow or function in the absence of hypotension. Hepatic and renal blood flow and function are well preserved during spinal anesthesia when blood pressure is maintained. Mid-thoracic levels of spinal anesthesia (without phrenic nerve paralysis) produce minimal changes in tidal volume, respiratory rate, minute ventilation, and arterial blood gases. End-tidal CO_2 tension declines, and ventilatory responses to CO_2 and breath-to-breath variability of breathing both increase during spinal anesthesia. Phrenic nerve paralysis is uncommon even when sensory analgesia extends to cervical dermatomes. Apnea is a central feature of total spinal anesthesia and brain ischemia (from inadequately treated hypotension). The metabolic stress response to surgery [including increases in blood concentrations of adrenocorticotropic hormone (ACTH), cortisol, growth hormone, insulin, and glucose] is inhibited by spinal anesthesia, but only while the sensory block persists (Chapter 69).

Postdural-puncture headaches are a vexing problem after spinal anesthesia. They are relatively more common in younger, female, and (especially) pregnant patients. Headache is more common when needles larger than 25 gauge are used, and are more common with Quincke needles than with

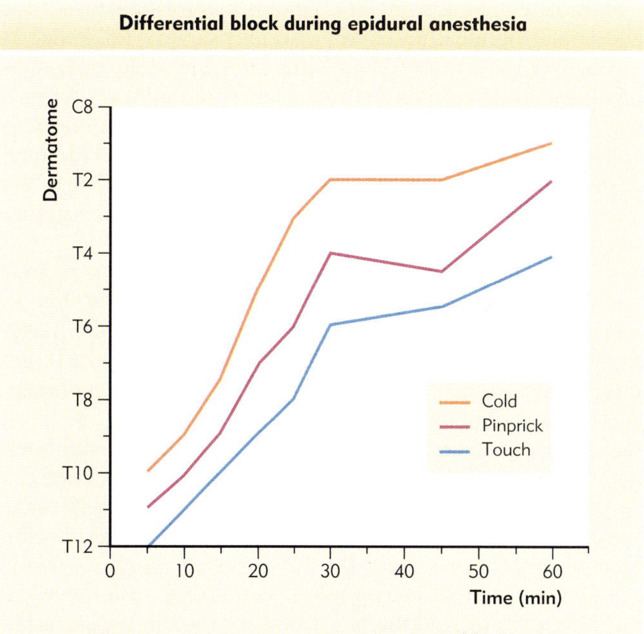

Figure 28.9 Differential block during epidural anesthesia. Patients received 2% lidocaine (lignocaine) with 5μg/mL epinephrine. The dermatomal levels of anesthesia were measured at 5-minute intervals. There was greater inhibition of cold compared with pinprick or light touch sensibility. (With permission from Brull and Greene, 1991.)

Whitacre, Sprotte, or Green needles (particularly with the 16–20 gauge needles used for continuous spinal techniques). The overall incidence is less than 10% in a general surgical population. Symptoms are positional (the headache is worse sitting or standing than supine), and include photophobia and nausea. An epidural blood patch is appropriate for persistent postdural-puncture headaches. Persistent neurologic deficits are distinctly rare after spinal anesthesia but are more common with this than with other regional techniques. Cardiac outcome is probably not altered by use of spinal (rather than epidural or general) anesthesia (Fig. 28.8).

Spinal anesthesia should never be performed if a patient refuses the technique or in patients with intracranial hypertension from mass lesions, CSF outflow obstruction (e.g. massive brain edema after anoxia), or infection (at the site of lumbar puncture or generalized septicemia). Most clinicians prefer not to perform spinal punctures in patients taking full anticoagulation therapy (heparin or warfarin), because of concerns about bleeding, or in patients with undiagnosed, progressive neurologic deficits. Current data suggest that conduction anesthesia techniques may be performed safely in patients who will receive anticoagulation after lumbar puncture therapy, or who have received aspirin. Because blood pressure will almost always decrease in the absence of treatment, the technique should be used only with caution in excessively afterload-sensitive patients (e.g. those with aortic stenosis or hypertrophic cardiomyopathy) or in excessively preload-sensitive or preload-'challenged' patients (e.g. after the Fontan procedure, massive hemorrhage, or excessive gastrointestinal fluid loss).

Epidural anesthesia

Epidural techniques are in common use for anesthesia for abdominal, perineal, and lower extremity surgery; for analgesia during labor (Chapter 65) and after thoracic, abdominal, perineal, and lower extremity surgery; and for treatment of a variety of pain syndromes. A continuous (catheter) technique is appropriate whenever duration of surgery or the need for analgesia cannot be predicted. This technique does not carry the increased risk of headache relative to single-shot techniques that occurs with spinal anesthesia.

Differences between spinal and epidural anesthesia include the shallower depth of needle placement, the use of 'loss of resistance' or 'hanging drop' to define correct needle placement, the larger size and contour of the needle, and the larger dose of local anesthetic required for the epidural technique. Advantages of epidural over spinal anesthesia include a low incidence of headache with continuous (catheter) techniques, and the ease with which continuing postoperative analgesia can be provided. Disadvantages of epidural relative to spinal anesthesia include the longer delay of onset, the decreased reliability of surgical anesthesia, the less consistent motor block, the possibility of systemic toxic side effects (from the larger local anesthetic dose), and the relatively large needles required to permit passage of catheters.

The mechanism by which local anesthetics produce epidural anesthesia remains uncertain but clearly does not require complete interruption of nervous transmission through the spinal cord. The initial onset of epidural anesthesia may reflect local anesthetic binding to Na^+ channels in nerve roots. Later on, epidural anesthesia may involve local anesthetic binding to multiple targets including sites within the cord, where the wide variety of ion channels and synapses makes strict definition of a molecular mechanism almost impossible. A zone of differential blockade is present with epidural as with spinal anesthesia. Cold sensibility is consistently inhibited over more dermatomal segments than pinprick (Fig. 28.9), which, in turn, is more extensively inhibited than light touch. There is greater dermatomal separation between sensory and motor block in epidural anesthesia compared with spinal anesthesia.

Lumbar epidural anesthesia has effects on the circulation that differ from those of spinal anesthesia. Specifically, absorption of the epidural local anesthetic solution may influence the hemodynamic state, especially with hypovolemia. Nevertheless, epidural anesthesia, like spinal anesthesia, induces arterial vasodilatation and pooling of venous blood. As a result, similar treatment for intraoperative hypotension is indicated. Epinephrine-containing local anesthetic solutions yield increased cardiac output and ability to withstand hemorrhage, and lower blood pressure, compared with plain local anesthetic solutions during lumbar epidural anesthesia. The probability of hypotension increases with increasing body weight and increasing dermatomal spread of anesthesia. Bradycardia is more common during epidural anesthesia in men than in women. Both hypertension and bradycardia are less common when a lower extremity tourniquet is used. There are also marked differences between thoracic and lumbar epidural anesthesia. Left ventricular contractility may be reduced when high thoracic epidural anesthesia (but not lumbar epidural anesthesia) is added to general anesthesia. A bolus of phenylephrine given to a patient receiving general anesthesia with isolated upper thoracic epidural anesthesia may lead to depressed left ventricular function. Thoracic epidural anesthesia increases upper extremity blood flow by 50% and produces a lesser increase in lower extremity blood flow. Lumbar epidural anesthesia decreases upper extremity blood flow by 35% but markedly increases lower extremity blood flow (by 500%).

Hepatic blood flow, primarily regulated by mean arterial pressure, is reduced (by about 20%) by epidural anesthesia. Lumbar epidural anesthesia prevents the endocrine stress response normally occurring during abdominal surgery; however, as the epidural block recedes, hormone concentrations rise towards the levels seen in the absence of epidural anesthesia.

Phrenic nerve inhibition is rarely caused by lumbar, thoracic, or cervical epidural anesthesia. The rare instances of respiratory arrest during epidural anesthesia usually result from sympathectomy, hypovolemia, inadequately treated hypotension, and reduced oxygen delivery to the brain. Epidural anesthesia does not change resting ventilation, arterial blood gases, the ventilatory response to hypoxia, or vital capacity and does not impair the ability to cough. Lumbar epidural anesthesia, like spinal anesthesia, increases the ventilatory response to hypercapnia. Studies have shown reduced lower-extremity deep venous thrombosis and reduced operative blood loss with lumbar epidural anesthesia compared with general anesthesia.

Some controversial studies in vascular surgery suggested that the addition of epidural anesthesia improved overall outcome and reduced vascular graft failure compared with general anesthesia alone. A more recent study of patients undergoing peripheral vascular surgery showed no difference in morbidity, cardiovascular outcomes, or vascular graft patency among patients receiving general, spinal, and epidural anesthesia (see Fig. 28.8). Similarly, long-term cognitive dysfunction and adverse cardiovascular outcomes were no less likely when epidural anesthesia was used rather than general anesthesia for total joint arthroplasty. Permanent neurologic deficits after epidural anesthesia are rare and significantly less common than with spinal anesthesia; transient neuropathy occurs in 0.02% of patients. Contraindications to epidural anesthesia are virtually the same as those for spinal anesthesia.

Entry of the needle into the epidural space is normally confirmed by 'loss of resistance' to injection of air or saline or by spontaneous aspiration into the hub of the needle of a 'hanging drop'. An experienced operator will usually also feel a 'grit' or 'crunch' as the needle passes through ligaments, and 'give' as it passes through the ligamentum flavum. Ideally, the site of epidural puncture should be chosen on the basis of the dermatomal location of surgery and should be located at the mid point of the dermatomal segments to be anesthetized. The caudal approach is used for lower abdominal, for anorectal, and lower extremity surgery, and for postoperative pain control in small children. Lumbar epidural anesthesia is used for lower abdominal and lower extremity surgery. Thoracic epidural anesthesia is used for surgery of the upper abdomen and thorax. Cervical epidural anesthesia can be used to provide surgical anesthesia but is a more common technique for managing upper extremity pain syndromes. In all cases, local anesthetic should always be administered incrementally to avoid the risks of CNS or cardiovascular toxicity from intravenous placement of the epidural needle or catheter. In adults, the dermatomal spread of epidural anesthesia increases with age, weight, body mass index, and local anesthetic dose. It also decreases with height and with higher site of injection.

Nerve blocks

Brachial plexus block

Brachial plexus block is suitable for nearly all surgery on the arms and hands. The three most common techniques – axillary, supraclavicular, and interscalene – produce predictable distributions of blocked and unblocked nerves. The anesthesiologist can tailor the technique to operative needs and by choice of local anesthetic can provide anesthesia of nearly any duration. Brachial plexus anesthesia appears to be the direct result of local anesthetic binding to Na^+ channels in the roots, trunks, divisions, cords, and branches of the brachial plexus.

Brachial plexus blocks can be performed using an electrical nerve stimulator to 'find' nerves near the tip of the needle, using techniques that seek paresthesias in the nerves to be anesthetized, or using techniques that rely on other physical parameters (the feel of the needle passing through the axillary sheath or aspiration of blood from the axillary artery).

The axillary approach

The axillary approach to the brachial plexus block is an easy and effective technique for providing anesthesia for hand and distal forearm surgery. Some clinicians advocate a single (large) injection technique; others prefer a more conservative approach in which at least two injections are made to reduce the possibility of an incomplete block. Accidental intravascular injection of local anesthetic is always possible during axillary block. Other complications (axillary hematoma, neuritis) other than unblocked nerves are uncommon. The nerves that most commonly remain unanesthetized after axillary block include the medial brachial cutaneous nerve, the intercostobrachial nerve, the lateral cutaneous nerve of the forearm (the sensory continuation of the musculocutaneous nerve), and the radial nerve. The first two of these may be blocked by infiltration of local anesthetic into the skin overlying the axillary artery pulse. This supplemental procedure must be performed if a tourniquet will be placed on the upper arm. The musculocutaneous nerve may be blocked in the axilla, or its sensory branch can be anesthetized selectively in the antecubital fossa. The radial nerve may be blocked in the antecubital fossa or the wrist. The total local anesthetic volume required for axillary block is usually about 0.6mL/kg, although with selective injection the volume can be reduced.

The supraclavicular approach

The supraclavicular approach to the brachial plexus has several important advantages, and one disadvantage, over the axillary and interscalene approaches. Of the three techniques, the supraclavicular approach has the fastest onset of anesthesia and is the least likely to produce incomplete anesthesia from unblocked nerves. However, it carries a risk of pneumothorax of at least 1%, and a higher risk of hemidiaphragmatic paralysis. The supraclavicular approach is appropriate for surgery of the upper arm, forearm, or hand and is superior to axillary block for operations on the elbow or proximal to it. Supraclavicular block carries a low risk of accidental intravascular injection; nevertheless, the initial test injection should be preceded by aspiration and followed by close observation. Following the initial injection, the patient often complains of an 'aching,' 'pressure' sensation. Between 0.3 and 0.5mL/kg is required to produce complete anesthesia.

The interscalene approach

The interscalene approach is preferable to other brachial techniques for providing regional anesthesia of the upper arm and shoulder. It is the brachial plexus technique least likely to provide complete anesthesia for hand surgery. Misdirected needles during attempted interscalene block can pierce carotid or vertebral arteries, or the epidural or subarachnoid spaces. Successful anesthesia will always be accompanied by ipsilateral Horner's syndrome and nearly always by ipsilateral phrenic nerve block. The total volume of local anesthetic necessary to achieve full anesthesia in an adult is usually about 0.6mL/kg, as for axillary block. The most commonly unblocked regions following interscalene block are served by C8 and T1. If C8 and T1 remain unblocked and anesthesia in the ulnar distribution is required for hand surgery, supplementation is easily accomplished by ulnar nerve block at the elbow or wrist. If surgery is on the forearm, anesthesia of the medial antebrachial cutaneous nerve, also a product of C8 and T1 nerve roots, must be obtained by supplementation in the antecubital fossa.

Lower extremity nerve blocks

Blocks of the sciatic and femoral nerves provide satisfactory anesthesia for surgery sited below the knee. Surgery at or proximal to the knee joint requires additional local anesthesia of the obturator and lateral femoral cutaneous nerves. If a tourniquet is applied to the thigh, block of the obturator (which innervates a small area of skin on the medial side of the knee and lower thigh and provides motor innervation of the hip adductor muscles) and lateral femoral cutaneous nerves is necessary, regardless of the site of the surgery. Generally, 50–60mL local anesthetic is required to anesthetize the femoral, sciatic, obturator, and lateral femoral cutaneous nerves.

Intravenous regional anesthesia

Intravenous regional anesthesia (or Bier's block) reliably produces distal anesthesia of the upper or (less commonly) lower extremity for surgery of less than 1 hour's duration. Whether anesthesia results from local anesthetic action on free nerve endings or action on nerve trunks remains unclear. To perform intravenous regional anesthesia, local anesthetic is injected through an intravenous catheter in the primarily exsanguinated operative extremity. A pneumatic tourniquet is inflated after exsanguination to contain the local anesthetic solution. Since the doses of local anesthetic (40–50mL of either 0.5% prilocaine or 0.5% lidocaine) are sufficient to cause severe CNS side effects (if given as an intravenous bolus), the pneumatic tourniquets must be fully inflated before the local anesthetic is injected.

Ankle block

Surgery of the toes and distal foot is well-suited to 'ankle block' anesthesia. A complete ankle block requires anesthesia of five peripheral nerves: superficial and deep peroneal, tibial, sural, and saphenous. Usually, block of all five nerves is not required. Ankle block anesthesia will not provide anesthesia for inflation of a thigh tourniquet; however, most patients tolerate an Esmarch bandage wrapped around the lower leg for the brief duration required for toe surgery. A total of 20–30mL of local anesthetic (typically, lidocaine 1%, mepivacaine 1%, or bupivacaine 0.25%) is required to anesthetize all five nerves.

Intercostal nerve blocks

Intercostal (or rib) blocks are useful for providing postoperative analgesia after upper abdominal and thoracic surgical procedures and to provide cutaneous anesthesia in the relevant dermatomes. Absorption of the injected local anesthetic after intercostal blocks is rapid, especially when epinephrine-free local anesthetic solutions are used. Intercostal blocks carry a finite but small risk of pneumothorax. Each intercostal nerve should be injected with 3mL local anesthetic (often bupivacaine 0.25%) containing epinephrine.

Cervical plexus block

Blocks of the cervical plexus are useful for providing regional anesthesia for operations on the neck. Superficial cervical plexus blocks can be used for carotid thromboendarterectomy, with the understanding that local infiltration by the surgeon may be required when dissection reaches the carotid sheath. Roughly 20–30mL of local anesthetic (often bupivacaine 0.25% or ropivacaine 0.5%) will be required. Deep cervical plexus blocks are used for more extensive or invasive neck surgery, such as thyroidectomy, and require an additional 20mL of local anesthetic.

Key References

Bode RH Jr, Lewis KP, Zarich SW, et al. Cardiac outcome after peripheral vascular surgery. Comparison of general and regional anesthesia. Anesthesiology. 1996;84:3–13.

Bromage PR. Epidural analgesia. Philadelphia, PA: Saunders; 1978.

Brull SJ, Greene NM. Zones of differential sensory block during extradural anesthesia. Br J Anaesth. 1991;66:651–5.

Butterworth JF IV, Strichartz GR. Molecular mechanisms of local anesthesia: a review. Anesthesiology. 1990;72:711–34.

Butterworth J, Ririe DG, Thompson RB, Walker FO, Jackson D, James RL. Differential offset ofmedian nerve block: randomized, double-blind comparison of mepivacaine with bupivaciane in healthy volunteers. Br J Anaesth. 1998;81(4):515–21.

Caterall WA. Structure and function of voltage-gated ion channels. Annu Rev Biochem. 1995;64:493–531.

Greene NM, ed. Physiology of spinal anesthesia. Baltimore, MD: Williams & Wilkins; 1969.

Hanck DA, Makielski JC, Sheets MF. Kinetic effects of quaternary lidocaine block of cardiac sodium channels: a gating current study. J Gen Physiol. 1994;103:19–43.

Lambert LA, Lambert DH, Strichartz GR. Irreversible conduction block in isolated nerve by high concentrations of local anesthetics. Anesthesiology. 1994;80:1082–93.

Strichartz GR, ed. Local anesthetics. Berlin: Springer-Verlag; 1987.

Strichartz GR, Sanchez V, Arthur GR, Chafete R, Martin D. Fundamental properties of local anesthetics. II. Measuring octanol:buffer partition coefficients and pK_a values of clinically used drugs. Anesth Analges. 1995;71:158–70.

van Gessel EF, Forster A, Schweizer A, Gaumlin Z. Comparison of hypobaric, hyperbaric, and isobaric solutions of bupivacaine during continuous spinal anesthesia. Anesth Analg. 1991;72:779–84.

Winnie AP. Plexus anesthesia. Philadelphia, PA: Saunders; 1983.

Further Reading

Auroy Y, Narchi P, Messiah A, et al. Serious complications related to regional anesthesia: results of a prospective survey in France. Anesthesiology. 1997;87:479–86.

Butterworth IV JF, Walker FO, Lysak SZ. Pregnancy increases median nerve susceptibility to lidocaine. Anesthesiology. 1990;72:962–5.

Caplan RA, Ward RJ, Posner K, Cheney FW. Unexpected cardiac arrest during spinal anesthesia: a closed claims analysis of predisposing factors. Anesthesiology. 1988;68:5–11.

Gage JG, Eisenach JC. New intra-axial agents and their safety issues. Anesth Clinic North Am. 1997;1:65–102.

Kane RE. Neurological deficits following epidural or spinal anesthesia. Anesth Analg. 1981;60:150–61.

Makielski JC, Limberis JT, Chang SY, Fan Z, Kyle JW. Coexpression of beta 1 with cardiac sodium channel alpha subunits in oocytes decreases lidocaine block. Mol Pharmacol. 1996;49:30–9.

Pierce ET, Pomposelli FB Jr, Stanley GD, et al. Anesthesia type does not influence early graft patency or limb salvage rates of lower extremity arterial bypass. J Vasc Surg. 1997;25:226–33.

Rauk RL. The anticoagulated patient. Reg Anesth. 1996;21:51–6.

Rowlingson JC. Toxicity of local anesthetic additives. Reg Anesth. 1993;18:453–60.

Wildsmith JAW, Rocco AG. Current concepts in spinal anesthesia. Reg Anesth. 1985;10:119–24.

Williams-Russo P, Sharrock NE, Mattis S, Szatrowski TP, Charlson ME. Cognitive effects after epidural vs general anesthesia in older adults. J Am Med Assoc. 1995;274:44–50.

Yeager MP, Glass DD, Neff RK, Brinck-Johnsen T. Epidural anesthesia and analgesia in high-risk surgical patients. Anesthesiology. 1987;66:729–36.

Chapter 29 Autonomic nervous system

Thomas J Ebert

Topics covered in this chapter

The autonomic nervous system (ANS) is a network of neural connections that maintains body homeostasis by integrating signals from a variety of somatic and visceral sensors to modulate tissue and organ function. The efferent components of the ANS are the sympathetic and parasympathetic nervous systems (SNS and PNS). Their tonic activity maintains visceral organs and vascular smooth muscle in a state of intermediate function (Fig. 29.1) from which rapid increases or decreases in autonomic outflow can adjust blood flow and organ function in response to the environment. There is generally no voluntary control of the ANS although conscious modulation can transiently occur (biofeedback or mental stress). The SNS has been called the 'fight or flight' division. Its activation under stress (e.g. blood loss, temperature change, or exercise) increases sympathetic neural activity to the heart and other viscera, peripheral vasculature, sweat glands, ocular muscles, and piloerector muscles. This leads to increases in cardiac output, blood glucose, pupillary dilation, and body temperature. In contrast, the PNS is responsible for 'rest and digest'. Activation of the PNS slows heart rate, respiration, digestion, and metabolism (Fig. 29.1).

Anesthesiologists should have a good understanding of the ANS and its function for several reasons. First, because the administration of either intravenous or inhaled anesthetics is severely limited by hypotension when autonomic control systems are dysfunctional. Autonomic reflexes oppose the relaxation of vascular smooth muscle and the depression of cardiac function that result from the direct effects of anesthetics. Second, most anesthetics alter the ANS and autonomic reflexes. Third, most vasoactive drugs mimic or modulate the ANS. Finally, the general goals of anesthesia can be considered to be unconciousness, amnesia, analgesia, immobility, and blockade of autonomic responses to noxious stimuli. In fact, most anesthetics are titrated based upon autonomic responses (heart rate and blood pressure).

CENTRAL ORGANIZATION

The basal 'tone' of the ANS is determined by input to various regions of the lower brainstem. The primary relay or integration region is called the medullary vasomotor center, which integrates neural information from the central autonomic network (CAN) and peripheral sensors. The CAN consists of four primary areas: the cerebral cortex, amygdala, hypothalamus, and medulla. The CAN receives input from peripheral visceral and somatic receptors. In addition, humoral substances modulate the CAN via regions of the circumventricular organs where the blood–brain barrier is absent. Circulating substances, including angiotensin, arginine-vasopressin, and various cytokines, appear to cross into the central nervous system (CNS) at the subfornical organ, in the lamina terminalis of the anterior wall of the third ventricle and at the area postrema in the fourth ventricle. These circulating substances modify various 'visceral' reflexes initiated from peripheral receptors in blood vessels and tissues.

There is increasing evidence that the CAN is not completely automatic or autonomous; rather, it can be transiently influenced by both environmental and somatic sensors. Consider biofeedback, whereby conscious relaxation methods reduce blood pressure and heart rate, or exercise, where the simple act of thinking about beginning exercise increases heart rate and where metabolic waste products from muscular activity trigger ascending neural signals that modify the ANS.

The medullary vasomotor center serves as the first relay station for afferent input from peripheral sensors including the baro- and chemoreceptors and gastrointestinal receptors. Ascending signals synapse in the nucleus tractus solitarius (NTS). The NTS relays information to higher centers of the CAN and also has connections with the ventrolateral medulla (VLM). The origin of efferent sympathetic outflow (i.e. preganglionic) is in the VLM. Preganglionic nerves from the VLM result in both sympathetic and respiratory (vagal) activity.

The SNS consists of preganglionic fibers that arise from the intermediolateral column and exit the spinal cord between the first thoracic (T1) and the third lumbar (L3) level (Figs. 29.1 and 29.2). Most of these fibers make synaptic connections in the 22 pairs of ganglia termed the bilateral sympathetic chain. The preganglionic fibers are so named because they have not yet synapsed with a ganglion cell. Likewise, postganglionic fibers are the terminal fibers of a ganglion cell and synapse with the appropriate end organ. However, some preganglionic fibers feed directly to peripheral ganglia before synapsing, and some make direct connections with the adrenal medulla. Because the adrenal medulla originates from neural tissue, it can be considered to be the postganglionic nerve. There is considerable dispersion in the SNS. For example, for every one preganglionic fiber there are 20–30 postganglionic fibers. Moreover, the sympathetic terminal in a

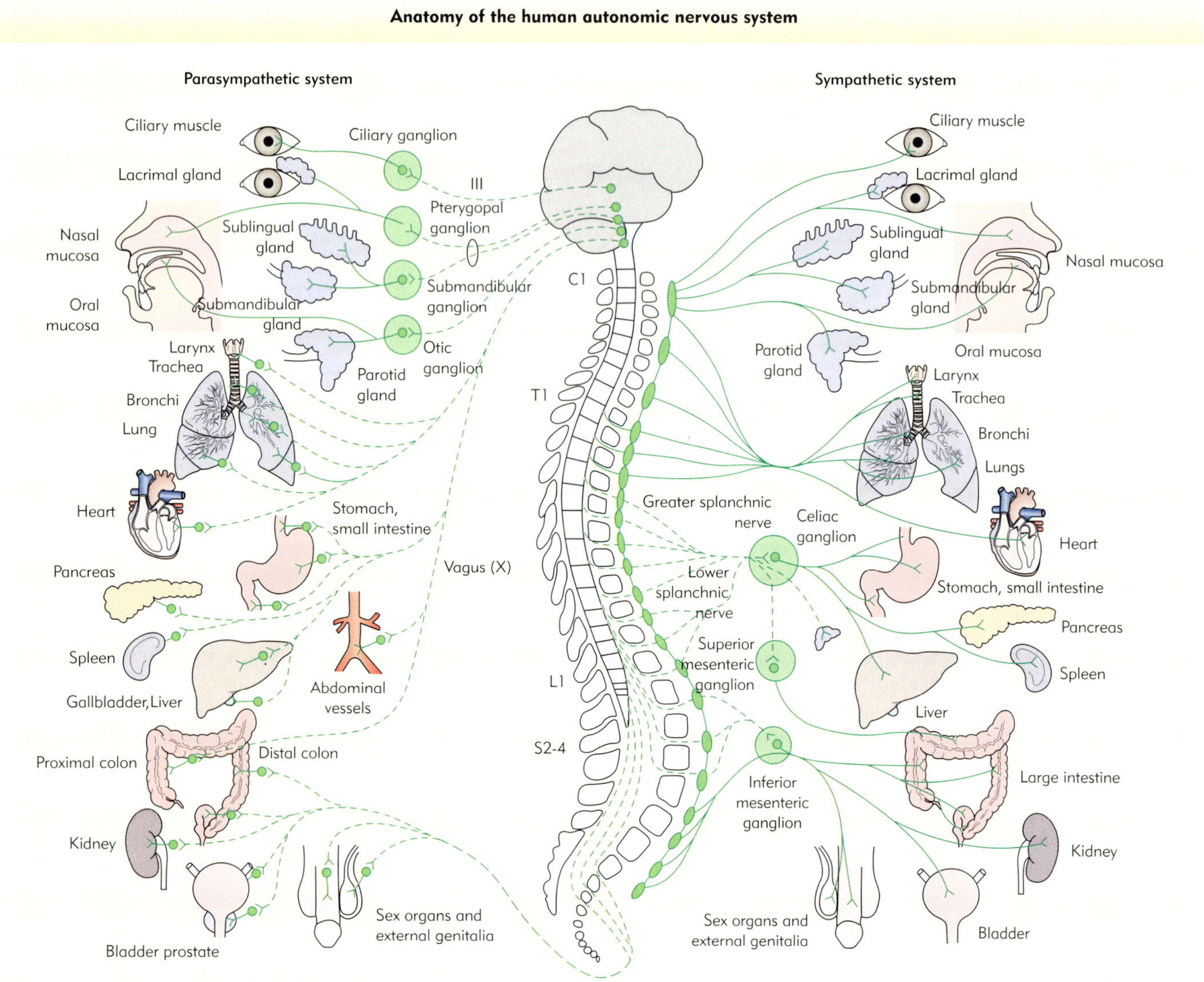

Figure 29.1 Anatomy of the human autonomic nervous system. Preganglionic and postganglionic fibers are indicated by broken and solid lines, respectively.

visceral organ or tissue is not a single terminal, rather it is a multiple, branched series of endings called a *terminal plexus*. A single postganglionic nerve can innervate up to 25,000 effector cells via the terminal plexus. Finally, when there is a great deal of sympathetic activity, the release of norepinephrine (noradrenaline), the postganglionic neurotransmitter, may exceed the capacity of the local uptake system and enzymatic breakdown that function to terminate its action. The excess norepinephrine (or spillover) can be dispersed by the circulatory system and can cause widespread humoral effects.

Historically, activation of the SNS has been considered a 'mass reflex' or response. Current understanding is that there is selectivity of sympathetic response although the site of differentiation or regulation of the selectivity is not known. A clear example of the selectivity of the SNS can be observed in the neural activity recorded from the skin and muscle sympathetic nerves in humans. The efferent sympathetic nerves to blood vessels, sweat glands, and piloerector muscles in the skin are generally silent during quiet resting conditions and during blood pressure perturbations but are activated when a sudden noise is imposed or an embarrassing question is asked. In contrast, the efferent sympathetic nerves that supply skeletal muscle blood vessels show significant tonic activity that is inversely modified by changes in blood pressure via the baroreflex. This sympathetic activity is not altered by startle maneuvers.

In the PNS, preganglionic fibers originate in two sites, the brainstem and the sacral spinal cord (see Fig. 29.1). Preganglionic neurons from the dorsal motor nucleus of the vagus and the nucleus ambiguus send efferent signals to the head, heart, and abdominal viscera via cranial nerves III (oculomotor), VII (facial), IX (glossopharyngeal), and X (vagus). The vagus nerve controls most visceral function within the thorax and abdomen and accounts for as much as 75% of the parasympathetic nerve activity. The sacral parasympathetic nucleus originates in the intermediolateral cell column at sacral segments 2–4 and controls bladder, bowel, and penile erector function. Unlike the SNS, preganglionic fibers pass

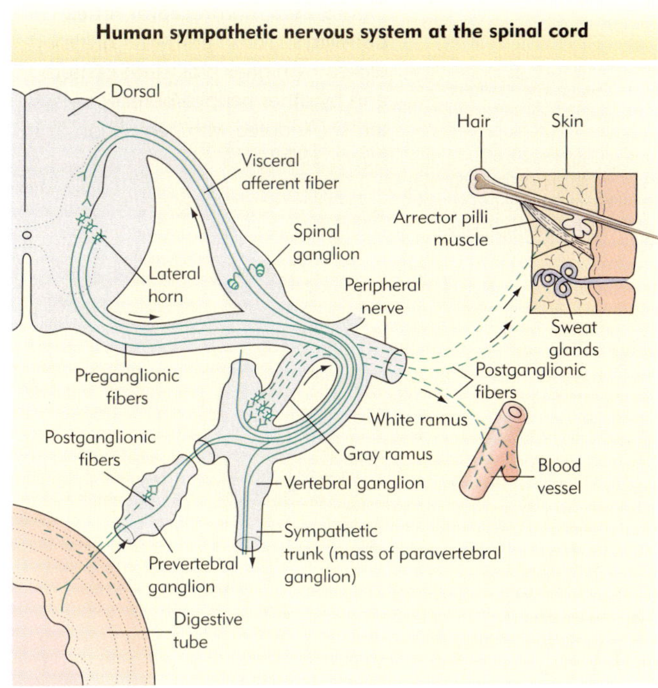

Figure 29.2 Anatomy of the human sympathetic nervous system at the spinal cord level. (Adapted with permission from Carpenter and Sutin, 1983.)

directly to ganglia that are close to, or within, specific organs. Very short cholinergic postganglionic fibers extend into the organ tissue. There are no interconnections between the components of the cranial and sacral outflows. In contrast to the SNS, there is very little dispersion of parasympathetic outflow. The ratio of pre- to postganglionic fibers is 1:1 to 1:3. This provides a fair degree of selectivity for the PNS. For example, vagal-mediated bradycardia can occur without increasing salivation or miosis.

ANATOMY OF THE PERIPHERAL SYMPATHETIC NERVOUS SYSTEM

Although autonomic outflow is segmental and somewhat parallels the somatic outflow to skeletal muscle, it differs from the somatic system in that it is disynaptic. Preganglionic autonomic cholinergic neurons synapse in peripheral ganglia and activate postganglionic neural fibers. In contrast, the somatic motor neurons have monosynaptic efferent pathways to skeletal muscle. A useful principle to facilitate understanding of the pertinent neuroanatomy is that the SNS 'disseminates' and 'amplifies' information related to maintenance of body homeostasis. The preganglionic sympathetic cell bodies lie in the intermediolateral cell columns of the spinal cord gray matter, extending from spinal levels T1 to L3. The preganglionic, or B, fibers are myelinated, small, having diameters less than 3μm, and conduct at a speed of 2–14m/s. Axons of these neurons leave the spinal cord in the ventral spinal roots, along with somatic, α and γ neurons, then branch off in the white rami communicantes and enter the paravertebral ganglia comprising the 'sympathetic chain'. The fine myelination of these fibers is responsible for their white appearance. The paravertebral ganglia are arranged as a bilateral vertical chain of ganglia running the length of the spinal column located anterolateral to the vertebral body. The preganglionic fiber has several potential destinations once it enters a paravertebral ganglion (see Fig. 29.2): it could synapse with one or more sympathetic neurons in the ganglion it has entered; it could ascend or descend in the paravertebral chain and synapse with neurons at other levels; it could synapse in the ganglion with a postganglionic fiber that leaves the paravertebral chain via gray rami communicantes to join a somatic nerve and travel to an effector site (e.g. blood vessels); or it could exit the sympathetic chain and synapse with an intermediate ganglion cell or with a prevertebral ganglion cell.

In addition to the 22 pairs of paravertebral ganglia referred to as the sympathetic chain, there are prevertebral, intermediate, and terminal ganglia. The intermediate ganglia are small structures, occasionally microscopic, that are located near the paravertebral chain. Their significance for the anesthesiologist is unclear. The prevertebral ganglia are composed of a network of pre- and postganglionic sympathetic fibers, parasympathetic fibers, and the ganglion cell bodies. The prevertebral ganglia that have the most importance to an anesthesiologist are the celiac ganglia and, possibly, the superior hypogastric (mesenteric) ganglia (see Fig. 29.1). Other prevertebral ganglia include the superior and middle cervical ganglia, the stellate ganglion (which is a fusion of the inferior cervical and the first thoracic ganglia), the aorticorenal ganglion, and the inferior mesenteric ganglion. The terminal ganglia lie in close proximity to their end organs (e.g. the urinary bladder and rectum).

The postganglionic noradrenergic sympathetic fibers, or C fibers, are largely unmyelinated and have diameters ranging from 0.3 to 1.3μm and conduction velocities of less than 2m/s. Like preganglionic fibers, one postganglionic fiber can synapse with a number of effector cells; however, a postganglionic fiber will synapse with only one type of end organ. In other words, one postganglionic fiber might synapse with several vascular smooth muscle cells but would not simultaneously synapse with a blood vessel, a sweat gland, and a piloerector muscle. The important end organs innervated by the SNS include the eye, secretory organs (including the sweat glands), the heart, blood vessels, the adrenal medulla, the abdominal and pelvic viscera, and the piloerector muscles.

Although the ANS has numerous functions, among the most important are temperature regulation and maintenance of blood pressure through baroreceptor-mediated reflex regulation of cardiac output and peripheral resistance. The autonomic reflexes are proving to play a more important role in anesthesiology than previously considered. For example, the degree of impairment of the basal function of autonomic reflexes correlates with the extent of hemodynamic instability after induction of anesthesia. Moreover, reduced autonomic function may be predictive of postoperative cardiac dysfunction; it has also been associated with an increased risk of adverse cardiac events (especially malignant arrhythmias) after myocardial infarction, and after anesthesia and surgery, and has been implicated in prolonging episodes of myocardial ischemia in patients with angina. Because of these important emerging relationships, the physiology of the baroreflex will be briefly reviewed.

THE BAROREFLEX AND OTHER NEURAL REFLEXES

Cardiopulmonary baroreceptors

Tonic activity of the ANS is regulated by strategically located pressure sensors in the blood vessels (Fig. 29.3). Low-pressure, cardiopulmonary baroreceptors are located primarily at the

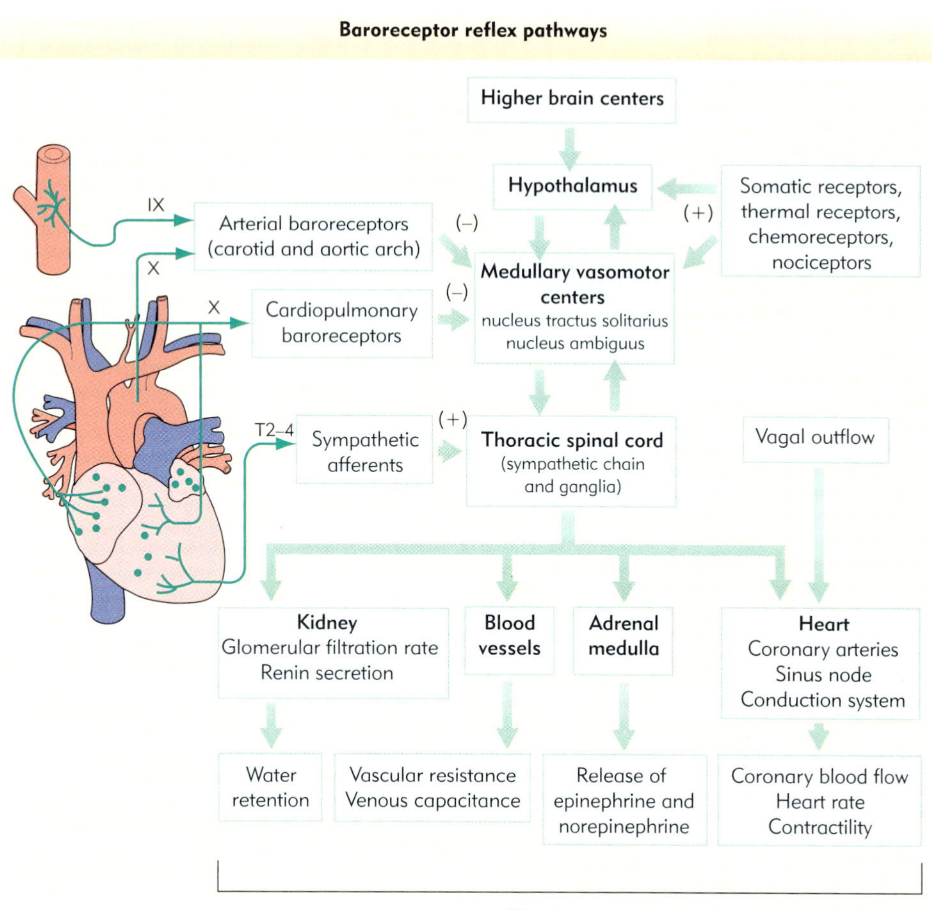

Figure 29.3 Baroreceptor reflex pathways. These pathways are modulated by higher brainstem centers and by other peripheral receptor systems. (Adapted with permission from Ebert, 1993.).

junction of the vena cavae and the right atrium, within the right atrium, and in pulmonary blood vessels. These appear to sense slight alterations in central blood volume and initiate reflex adjustments of peripheral sympathetic outflow. For example, when central venous pressure is reduced by 1 or 2mmHg, cardiac output decreases but blood pressure is well maintained because of a reflex increase in sympathetic activity. Thus, this reflex is the first line of defense against hypotension caused by dehydration or mild surgical blood loss. Halothane markedly attenuates this reflex in humans. In contrast, opioid–benzodiazepine anesthesia appears to preserve the low-pressure baroreceptor reflexes. Thus, the use of halothane for surgical procedures in which there is a potential for significant or rapid blood loss may be disadvantageous compared with an opioid–benzodiazepine technique.

Arterial baroreceptors

Arterial, or 'high pressure', baroreceptor reflexes are mediated by pressure sensors located in the arch of the aorta and in the carotid sinus (Fig. 29.3). The efferent component of this reflex regulates heart rate primarily through the vagal nerve and peripheral vascular tone through sympathetic outflow. Previous research investigating the cardiac limb of the baroreceptor reflex has found that both halothane and enflurane have a more pronounced effect on attenuating this reflex than does isoflurane, sevoflurane, or desflurane. Opioids may attenuate the cardiac baroreflex to a lesser degree than occurs with the volatile agents. For example, when fentanyl is employed in combination with a benzodiazepine, reflex heart rate slowing in response to phenylephrine-induced hypertension is well maintained.

ANESTHETICS AND THE SYMPATHETIC NERVOUS SYSTEM

Because of the difficulty in quantifying efferent SNS activity in humans, there is a relative paucity of information relating to the effects of intravenous anesthetics on both basal levels of sympathetic vasoconstrictor traffic and the reflex regulation of the SNS. The technique of sympathetic microneurography permits the recording of vasoconstrictor impulses directed to blood vessels within the skeletal muscle. This technique has been applied in several studies evaluating the effects of nitrous oxide in humans. An oxygen/nitrous oxide mixture (60%/40%) breathed by healthy volunteers provides a marked increase in sympathetic nerve traffic. Moreover, the reflex regulation of sympathetic outflow was well preserved during nitrous oxide breathing. Consequently, nitrous oxide may enhance sympathetic function when added to an anesthetic regimen. Both thiopental (thiopentone) and propofol result in near neural silence for a period of several minutes following their administration. Part of this sympathetic silence may be related to the concomitant loss of consciousness. However, when etomidate is infused, sympathetic outflow is well maintained despite loss of consciousness. This maintained sympathetic activity with

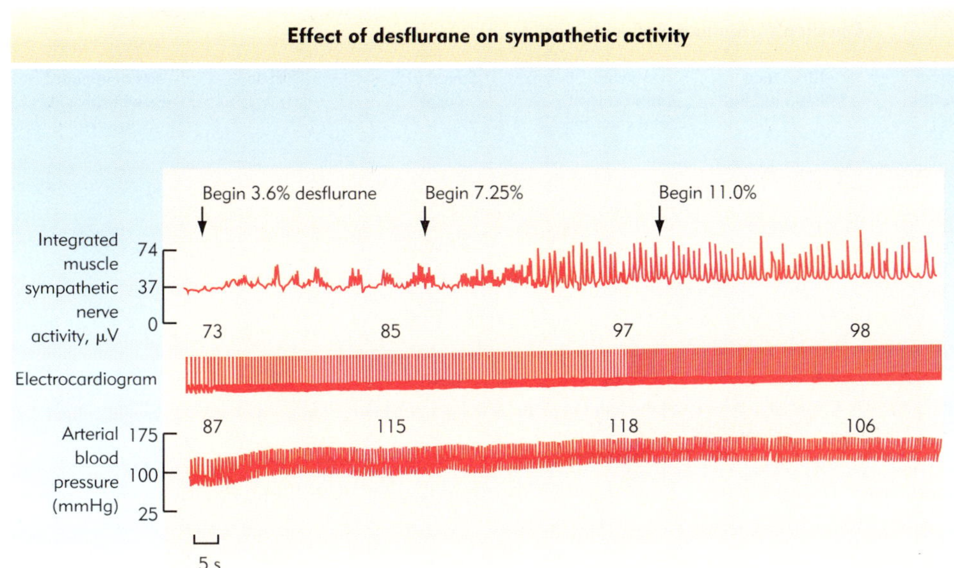

Figure 29.4 The effect of desflurane on sympathetic nerve activity, heart rate, and arterial pressure in a human volunteer following anesthetic induction with sodium thiopental (thiopentone). Sympathoexcitation occurred (top tracing) along with increases in heart rate and blood pressure. Heart rate and mean arterial blood pressure values are indicated over the electrocardiogram and blood pressure traces, respectively. (Adapted with permission from Ebert and Muzi, 1993.).

etomidate results in a very stable blood pressure. Thiopental and propofol appear also to abolish the normal reflex sympathetic discharge associated with hypotension. In contrast, etomidate preserves this reflex. Therefore, in the hypovolemic patient undergoing anesthesia, thiopental and propofol reduce tonic levels of sympathetic outflow and inhibit the normal reflex sympathetic compensation. This combination can lead to precipitous declines in blood pressure after bolus administration of either agent. Despite the profound influence of thiopental and propofol on sympathetic vasoconstrictor outflow, these agents do not appear to attenuate the sympathetic discharge associated with laryngoscopy and intubation. The marked sympathetic discharge recorded during tracheal intubation is followed immediately by hypertension and tachycardia. This suggests that the sympathetic neuroeffector response is preserved during the administration of these intravenous agents.

The volatile anesthetic desflurane has been associated with large increases in sympathetic activity and a generalized stress response (Fig. 29.4). The trigger for these responses is currently unknown, but two possibilities exist: it may irritate airway receptors, thereby triggering a sympathetic response leading to increases in blood pressure and heart rate and/or it may act centrally to disinhibit sympathetic outflow. This action might occur with many volatile anesthetics but may only be apparent when desflurane is used because of its rapid uptake into central neural sites and the need to deliver high concentrations of desflurane owing to its relative lack of potency.

AUTONOMIC PHARMACOLOGY

Parasympathetic nervous system

Acetylcholine (ACh) is a quaternary ammonium ester that is synthesized by acetylation of choline with acetyl coenzyme A. It is stored in mass quantities within synaptic vesicles at the nerve terminal, released by exocytosis during nerve depolarization, and its action is terminated by acetylcholinesterase at neuroeffector junctions. ACh may coexist with peptide cotransmitters (e.g. vasoactive intestinal peptide in the salivary gland). ACh has actions on two distinct receptor types: nicotinic and muscarinic (Chapter 19). Nicotinic receptor stimulation by ACh results in depolarization via increased channel permeability to sodium ions. Nicotinic receptors are located in four general areas: in skeletal muscle; on postganglionic neurons in the autonomic ganglia; on the adrenal medulla; and within the CNS. Muscarinic receptors are coupled to a family of G proteins that alter adenylyl cyclase activity (see Fig. 3.8). Five muscarinic receptors with distinct chemical and anatomic properties have been defined pharmacologically: m_{1-5}. The m_1 receptors are located in autonomic ganglia, the CNS, and secretory glands. The m_2 receptors exist in the sinoatrial and atrioventricular nodes of the heart and modulate both the rate and conduction of cardiac electrical activity. They also are found in atrial and ventricular myocardium and may modulate contractility of cardiac muscle. The m_3 receptors reside on select smooth muscle cells, where their stimulation results in contraction and secretion at localized glands. In addition to PNS postganglionic junctions, muscarinic receptors exist on the presynaptic membrane of sympathetic nerve terminals in the myocardium, coronary vessels, and peripheral vasculature. When these receptors are stimulated, the release of norepinephrine (noradrenaline) is inhibited, as occurs with α_2-adrenoceptor stimulation. Muscarinic blockade removes the inhibition of noradrenaline release, which augments SNS activity. In this manner, atropine blockade of muscarinic receptors elicits sympathomimetic activity as well as vagal blockade. Neuromuscular blocking drugs may elicit tachycardia via a similar mechanism.

Parasympathetic agonists

Cholinergic drugs can act at nicotinic receptors, muscarinic receptors, or both. The nicotinic receptor agonists consist primarily of the depolarizing neuromuscular-blocking drugs [e.g. succinylcholine (suxamethonium), hexamethonium], and some of these simultaneously stimulate autonomic ganglia (Chapter 32). Trimethaphan is an example of a drug that blocks specific autonomic ganglia by occupying receptors normally responsive to ACh. Muscarinic receptor agonists are divided into three groups: the choline esters [ACh, methacholine (amechol), carbachol (carbamylcholine), bethanechol] and the alkaloids [pilocarpine, muscarine, arecoline (arecholine)] that act directly, and

Dose (mg/kg)	Elimination half-time (min)		Volume of distribution (L/kg)		Clearance (ml/min per kg)		Renal contribution to total clearance (%)	Speed of onset	Duration (min)	Recommended dose of atropine[a] (μg/kg)
	normal	anephric	normal	anephric	normal	anephric				
Edrophonium (0.5)	110	206	1.1	0.7	9.6	2.7	66	rapid	60	7
Neostigmine (0.043)	80	183	0.7	0.8	9.0	3.4	54	intermediate	60	15
Pyridostigmine (0.35)	112	379	1.1	1.0	8.6	2.1	76	slow	90	15

[a] Dose to be co-administered with anticholinesterase during reversal of neuromuscular blockade.

Figure 29.5 Commonly used anticholinesterases. (Adapted from Stoelting RK. Pharmacology in Anesthetic Practice. Philadelphia: Lippincott; 1987.)

the anticholinesterases [physostigmine, neostigmine, pyridostigmine, edrophonium, echothiophate (ecothiophate)] that act indirectly. The direct-acting agonists have few clinical applications, with the exception of their topical use to produce miosis. In contrast, anticholinesterase drugs are frequently employed to reverse the action of nondepolarizing neuromuscular drugs and to improve neuromuscular function in myasthenia gravis.

The diffuse action and rapid hydrolysis by cholinesterase of ACh make it virtually useless as a therapeutic agent. However, ACh is used topically as a miotic agent during cataract extraction surgery when a rapid miosis is desired. Longer activity can be achieved with the synthetic drug methacholine, which contains a methyl group on the β position of choline; this modification prevents any nicotinic receptor effects. Carbachol is a long-acting synthetic parasympathetic agonist that has both nicotinic and muscarinic receptor activity, although its use is limited to that of a miotic agent. It has a carbamic-linked ester moiety that makes it resistant to hydrolysis by cholinesterase. Pilocarpine is derived from the South American shrub pilocarpa; it is a tertiary amine alkaloid with actions similar to methacholine. It is the only direct-acting cholinomimetic alkaloid that is used therapeutically. Its sole clinical use is as a standard treatment for glaucoma, where it is employed as a topical miotic drug to reduce intraocular pressure. Pilocarpine has minimal nicotinic effects unless given systemically, in which case hypertension and tachycardia may result. Bethanechol has both a methyl group on the β position of choline and a carbamic-linked ester, resulting in a long half-life. This structure makes it predominately specific for muscarinic receptors; it can be used parenterally since it has only minimal cardiac chronotropic or inotropic effects. The rare therapeutic systemic applications of bethanechol include treatment for abdominal or bladder distention and esophageal reflux.

The *anticholinesterase*, or indirect cholinomimetic, drugs are ionized, water-soluble agents that inhibit acetylcholinesterase at the synaptic cleft, thereby increasing local concentrations of ACh. The therapeutic use of anticholinesterases is to reverse nondepolarizing neuromuscular blockade at the nicotinic ACh receptor and to improve neuromuscular function in patients with myasthenia gravis. Because anticholinesterase drugs also activate muscarinic receptors, the administration of a muscarinic receptor antagonist such as atropine or glycopyrrolate (glycopyrronium) can reduce the side effects of bradycardia, bronchospasm, or intestinal spasm (Fig. 29.5). The speed of onset of action for the commonly employed cholinesterase inhibitors is edrophonium > neostigmine > pyridostigmine.

The anticholinesterase physostigmine is a tertiary amine that has the ability to cross the blood–brain barrier and is sometimes employed to reverse the CNS effects of cholinergic receptor antagonists, e.g. atropine or scopolamine (hyoscine). Edrophonium, neostigmine, and pyridostigmine are quaternary amines that do not cross the blood–brain barrier. The common therapeutic application of neostigmine is for reversal of neuromuscular blockade because it is the most potent anticholinesterase. It also has been used to treat paralytic ileus, atonic distended urinary bladder, and myasthenia gravis. The slow onset of action of pyridostigmine limits its application for reversal of neuromuscular blockade. Edrophonium has a rapid onset of action (peak effect in 1–2 minutes versus the 7–11 minute activation for neostigmine), short duration (1 to 2 hours), and fewer cholinergic side effects compared with neostigmine. It also is used in the diagnosis of myasthenia gravis and to differentiate cholinergic crisis (excessive ACh) from inadequate therapy (insufficient ACh) in myasthenic patients.

Irreversible anticholinesterases are mostly organophosphate compounds. They form a phosphorylated enzyme that is resistant to attack by water. They readily pass into the CNS and are rapidly absorbed through the skin, hence their use as pesticides and in chemical warfare. The only therapeutic agent in this group is echothiophate, a long-acting, irreversible anticholinesterase that is instilled into the eye to lower intraocular pressure by decreasing the resistance to aqueous humor outflow. Echothiophate is absorbed into the circulation and, therefore, can prolong the duration of action of succinylcholine because of a reduction in plasma cholinesterase levels. The action of ester-based, local anesthetics also might be lengthened in patients receiving echothiophate through slower metabolism of the local anesthetic. Enzyme activity may not return to normal for 4–6 weeks after discontinuation of chronic therapy.

Parasympathetic antagonists

Anticholinergic drugs (atropine, scopolamine, glycopyrrolate) competitively inhibit the action of ACh by reversibly binding at muscarinic cholinergic postganglionic receptors. They are considered selective for muscarinic ACh receptors because

Comparison of antimuscarinic and anticholinergic drugs

Drug	Sedation	Heart rate	Gastro-intestinal tone	Airway secretions	Mydriasis and cycloplegia	Duration IM	Duration IV
Atropine	+	+++	−−	−	+	15–30min	2–4h
Scopolamine	+++	−/+	−	−−−	+++	30–60min	4–6h
Glycopyrrolate	0	++	−−−	−−−	0	2–4h	6–8h

−−− markedly depressed −− moderately depressed − mildly depressed 0 no effect
+ mildly increased ++ moderately increased +++ markedly increased
IM, intramuscular; IV, intravenous

Figure 29.6 Comparison of antimuscarinic and anticholinergic drugs.

nicotinic ACh receptors are not affected by the doses usually employed in the clinical setting. However, selectivity is not predictable during oral administration and, therefore, the common routes of administration are intravenous or intramuscular. Sympathomimetic actions also have been demonstrated during muscarinic blockade, presumably through interruption of the normal presynaptic cholinergic inhibition of endogenous norepinephrine release from synaptic terminals.

Anticholinergic drugs can be used to inhibit salivary, bronchial, pancreatic, and gastrointestinal secretions. They relax bronchial smooth muscle and reduce airway resistance, increase heart rate, and act as gastrointestinal relaxants (Fig. 29.6). Atropine and scopolamine possess antiemetic action; scopolamine skin patches are used to control motion sickness. Atropinic drugs also produce mydriasis and cycloplegia. When bronchodilation without systemic side effects is desired, inhalation is the most effective route of administration. Ipratropium, a derivative of methylatropine, is an anticholinergic drug with bronchodilator capabilities as effective as the β-agonist isoproterenol (isoprenaline) when inhaled. Recent studies have shown that low doses of ipratropium decrease airway size via initial, preferential blockade of neuronal m_2 muscarinic receptors. However, following large ipratropium doses, bronchodilation results from blockade of m_3 muscarinic receptors on airway smooth muscle. The use of anticholinergic drugs as preanesthetic medication is sometimes avoided in patients where ventilation–perfusion matching might be impaired from inspissation of airway secretions. These drugs also are contraindicated in patients with narrow-angle glaucoma, in whom they may increase intraocular pressure.

The naturally occurring anticholinergic drugs atropine and scopolamine are derived from the belladonna plant. As tertiary amine alkaloids they are able to cross the blood–brain barrier. Their anticholinergic function is primarily via the levorotatory stereoisomer, although the drugs contain equal parts of both levorotatory and dextrorotatory isomers. Low doses of atropine and scopolamine (up to 2μg/kg) exert their effects within the CNS, augmenting vagal outflow, which may result in bradycardia. At normal clinical doses (15–70μg/kg), atropine acts at peripheral muscarinic receptors to block the action of ACh, thereby increasing heart rate and pupil size while reducing secretory gland activity, which results in both an antisialagogue effect and anhydrosis.

Scopolamine displays stronger antisialagogue and ocular activity but is less likely than glycopyrrolate or atropine to increase heart rate (see Fig. 29.6). Scopolamine crosses the blood–brain barrier more effectively than atropine and is commonly associated with amnesia, drowsiness, fatigue, and non-REM sleep. It is often used in conjunction with sedatives and opioids for preanesthetic medication. One limitation imposed by the central actions of scopolamine (and atropine) is an infrequent side effect termed the *central anticholinergic syndrome*. This consists of agitation, disorientation, delirium, hallucinations, and restlessness, but it may manifest as somnolence and needs to be considered in the differential diagnosis of delayed awakening from anesthesia. Physostigmine can be administered in intravenous doses of 15–60μg/kg for the treatment of central anticholinergic syndrome.

Glycopyrrolate is a quaternary amine and is, therefore, unable to cross the blood–brain barrier and exert CNS effects. It is more potent and longer acting at peripheral muscarinic receptors than atropine. It is used clinically as an antisialagogue and to inhibit cardiac muscarinic receptor side effects when anticholinesterase agents are employed to reverse the effects of muscle relaxants.

Sympathetic nervous system

The transmitters of the SNS are norepinephrine and epinephrine (adrenaline). Norepinephrine is released primarily from postganglionic neurons and epinephrine is discharged from the adrenal glands, which also release norepinephrine. A number of cotransmitters may be released simultaneously with norepinephrine including ATP and neuropeptide Y. In most vascular tissues, ATP causes synergistic vasoconstriction with norepinephrine (α_1-adrenoceptors) via P_{2X} purine receptors, but in the coronary circulation ATP produces dilation via P_{2Y} receptors. These catecholamines are synthesized from dopamine; their actions are terminated by local metabolism, by reuptake into nerve terminals, and by clearance in the pulmonary circulation. Most clinically employed catecholamines stimulate both α- and β-adrenoceptors, the exceptions being phenylephrine and methoxamine (pure α-agonists) and isoproterenol (pure β-agonist) (Fig. 29.7). The α-adrenoceptors respond to catecholamines with an order of potency: norepinephrine ≥ epinephrine > isoproterenol. Their order of potency on β-adrenoceptors is isoproterenol > epinephrine ≥ norepinephrine.

An understanding of the potency of each drug on arteriolar and venous smooth muscle is important when selecting a drug for clinical use. Each catecholamine has distinct qualitative and quantitative effects on arterial and venous smooth muscle. Knowledge of their net effect in different vascular beds permits a better understanding of their mechanism of secondary effect on cardiac output: in addition to the direct effect

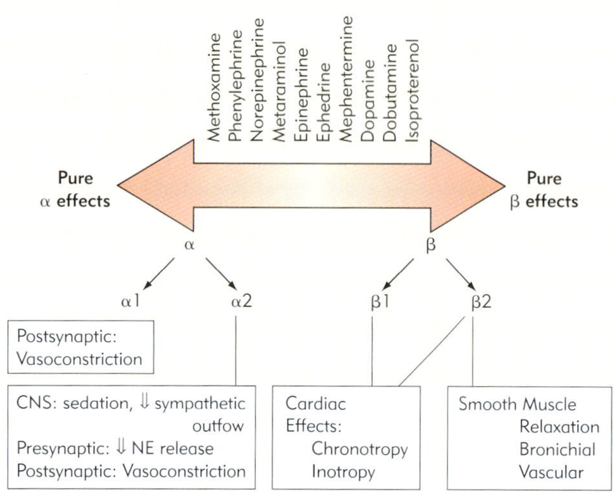

Figure 29.7 The effects of various catecholamines on adrenoceptor subtypes. Effects range from pure α-agonist to pure β-agonist. (Adapted with permission from Lawson and Wallfisch, 1986.)

Relative potencies of sympathomimetic amines

Resistance vessels		Capacitance vessels	
Drug	**Relative potency**	**Drug**	**Relative potency**
Norepinephrine	1.000	Norepinephrine	1.00
Metaraminol	0.0874	Phenylephrine	0.0570
Phenylephrine	0.0684	Metaraminol	0.0419
Tyramine	0.0148	Methoxamine	0.0068
Mephentermine	0.0049	Ephedrine	0.0025
Ephedrine	0.0020	Tyramine	0.0023
Methoxamine	0.0018	Mephentermine	0.0023

From Schmid PG, Eckstein JW, Abboud FM: Comparison of the effects of several sympathomimetic amines on resistance and capacitance vessels in the forearm of man. Circulation 1996;34(3):209.

Figure 29.8 Relative potencies of sympathomimetic amines in humans as constrictors of resistance and capacitance vessels. (Adapted with permission from Schmid, Eckstein and Abboud, 1993.)

of the catecholamine on inotropy, cardiac output also is influenced by the ability of the drugs to modify cardiac preload and afterload (Fig. 29.8).

The α-adrenoceptors

The α-adrenoceptors are widespread throughout the human body. They exist at both presynaptic and postsynaptic neuroeffector junction sites and are involved in cardiovascular regulation, metabolism, consciousness, and nociception. Seven subtypes of α-adrenoceptor have been identified, but for practical purposes this chapter will focus on the two 'primary' subtypes: α_1 and α_2. The α_1-adrenoceptors are characterized by their stimulation by phenylephrine and methoxamine and inhibition by low concentrations of prazosin, whereas α_2-adrenoceptors are selectively activated by clonidine and dexmedetomidine and are blocked by yohimbine. Both α-adrenoceptor subtypes respond with an order of potency of norepinephrine > epinephrine > isoproterenol, but the distinction is made on the greater strength of potency of norepinephrine for the α_1- versus the α_2-adrenoceptor. The α-adrenoceptors also can be differentiated based upon regulation of intracellular calcium ion and cAMP levels through specific G protein-coupled receptors. The α_1-adrenoceptors activate G_q and increase calcium ion levels via phospholipase Cβ. Stimulation of α_2-adrenoceptors activates G_i and, ultimately, results in a decrease in cAMP levels. Stimulation by α_1-adrenoceptors results in hydrolysis of membrane phospholipids, increases cytoplasmic calcium ion concentration, and results in smooth muscle contraction. Activation of α_2-adrenoceptors in the peripheral vasculature leads to vasoconstriction via inhibition of adenylyl cyclase. Physiologic effects of α_2-adrenoceptor stimulation include contraction of vascular smooth muscle via postsynaptic receptors and inhibition of norepinephrine release into the synaptic cleft via a presynaptic effect. In addition, central effects consist of sedation, anxiolysis, analgesia, and modulation of sympathetic and parasympathetic outflow from the CNS.

The β-adrenoceptors

The β-adrenoceptors are pharmacologically differentiated based upon their sensitivity to the β-agonists isoproterenol, epinephrine, and norepinephrine. The order of β_1-adrenoceptor sensitivity is isoproterenol > epinephrine ≥ norepinephrine, whereas that for β_2-adrenoceptors is isoproterenol > epinephrine >> norepinephrine (i.e. the potency of norepinephrine at the β_2-adrenoceptor is significantly less than that of epinephrine). Both β-adrenoceptors activate G_s and increase cAMP levels through activation of adenylyl cyclase. The β_1-adrenoceptors are located primarily in the sinoventricular node, myocardium, ventricular conduction system, and adipose tissue. The β_2-adrenoceptors are more widespread and are found in vascular smooth muscle beds (skin, muscle, mesentery, bronchi) and mediate vasodilatation and bronchial relaxation. Albuterol (salbutamol) is a selective agonist for β_2-adrenoceptors; there is no selective agonist for β_1-adrenoceptors. Pindolol is a specific antagonist of β_2-adrenoceptors and metoprolol is a selective β_1-antagonist.

Endogenous catecholamines

The basic catecholamine structure is a phenylethylamine with three hydroxy groups (Fig. 29.9). The naturally occurring catecholamines act on both α- and β-adrenoceptors. More pronounced α activity is observed when minimal α-carbon amino group catecholamine substitutions occur, whereas increased β activity results as catecholamine amino group substitutions increase.

Dopamine

Dopamine is the immediate precursor to norepinephrine and is located in the CNS, SNS postganglionic nerve terminals, and adrenal glands. Dopamine has dose-dependent actions as both a direct neurotransmitter via D_1 receptor activation and as an indirect agent through inhibition of norepinephrine release via a D_2 receptor (see Fig. 29.9). At low doses (1–2μg/min per kg body weight), renal and mesenteric vasodilatation occur and renal blood flow, glomerular filtration, and sodium ion excretion increase via D_{1A} receptor agonism (Fig. 29.10). At doses of 2–10μg/min per kg, β_1-adrenoceptor stimulation has positive inotropic and chronotropic effects. As dopamine doses

Adrenoreceptor activity of catecholamines

Drug, IV infusion dose (μg/min per kg)	Structure	Receptor site of activity $\alpha_1$art	$\alpha_1$ven	β_1	β_2	DA
Epinephrine, 0.015	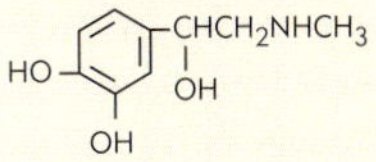 HO, OH; $-CHCH_2NHCH_3$, OH	0	0	++++	++++	0
0.03–0.15		++	++	++++	++++	
0.15–0.30		++++	++++			
Norepinephrine, 0.1	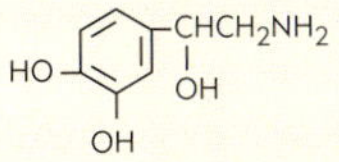 HO, OH; $-CHCH_2NH_2$, OH	+++++	+++++	++++	?+	0
Dopamine, 0.5–2	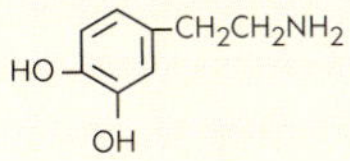	0	++++			+++++
2–10	HO, OH; $-CH_2CH_2NH_2$	0	+++	+++	+++++	
≥10		++++	+++	+++++		

$\alpha_1$art = α, receptor, arerial; $\alpha_1$ven = $\alpha_1$receptor, venous; DA = dopamine receptors
0 = no effect; += slight effect; +++++ = potent effect

Figure 29.9 Adrenoceptor activity of catecholamines.

Cardiovascular and renal actions of catecholamines

Drug, IV infusion dose (μg/min per kg)	Cardiovascular effects CO	Inotropy	HR	Preload	TPR	RBF
Epinephrine, 0.015	⇧–	⇧⇧	⇧⇧	⇧	⇧⇧	–⇩
0.03–0.15	⇧	⇧⇧	⇧⇧	⇧	⇧⇧⇧	⇩
0.15–0.30	⇧⇧	⇧⇧	⇧	⇧	⇧	⇧
Norepinephrine, 0.1	–⇩	–	Reflex⇩	⇧⇧⇧	⇧⇧	–⇩
Dopamine, 0.5–2	⇧	– – –	– – –	⇧	–⇩	⇧
2–10	⇧⇧	⇧	–⇧	⇧	–⇧	⇧
>10	⇧–⇩	⇧⇧	⇧⇧	⇧	⇧⇧	–⇩

CO = cardiac output, HR = heart rate, TPR = total peripheral resistance, RBF = renal blood flow
– = No change; ⇩ = decreased effect; ⇧ = increased effect.

Figure 29.10 Cardiovascular and renal actions of catecholamines.

reach 10μg/min per kg, α_1-adrenoceptor activation causes peripheral vasoconstriction and can reduce renal blood flow.

Norepinephrine

Norepinephrine is the endogenous mediator of SNS activity. Exogenous administration results in dose-dependent hemodynamic effects on α- and β-adrenoceptors (see Fig. 29.9). At low doses, β_1 actions predominate and cardiac output and blood pressure increase. Larger doses of norepinephrine cause further increases in blood pressure via arterial and venous smooth muscle contraction from α_1-adrenoceptor stimulation (see Fig. 29.10). Norepinephrine also causes feedback inhibition of further norepinephrine release from synaptic terminals via α_2-adrenoceptors.

Intravenous administration of norepinephrine causes marked arterial and venous vasoconstriction in most vascular beds; it is most often used therapeutically for the treatment of severe vasodilation and cardiogenic shock (see Fig. 29.10). Caution must be used in patients already exhibiting marked vasoconstriction, as norepinephrine administration may further increase vascular resistance such that organ blood flow is compromised and ischemia occurs.

Epinephrine

Epinephrine is an endogenous catecholamine that is synthesized, stored, and released from the chromaffin cells of the adrenal medulla. Epinephrine actions at α- and β-adrenoceptors are dose dependent (see Fig. 29.9). At low doses (0.015μg/min per kg), β_1- and β_2-adrenoceptor actions predominate. Specifically, β_1-adrenoceptor stimulation produces predictable cardiac effects, including increased heart rate, cardiac output, contractility, and conduction. Stimulation of β_2-adrenoceptors causes relaxation of bronchial smooth muscle, an increase in liver glycogenolysis, and vasodilatation in most regional vascular tissue. This last effect results in a decrease in diastolic blood pressure and redistribution of blood flow to low-resistance circulations. At higher doses of epinephrine (0.15–0.30μg/min per kg), α-adrenoceptors are activated, leading to vasoconstriction of the skin, mucosa, and renal vascular beds. These actions result in substantial blood flow redistribution away from these circula-

Adrenoreceptor activity of catecholamines

Drug, IV infusion dose	Structure	Receptor site of activity				
		$\alpha_1$art	$\alpha_1$ven	β_1	β_2	DA
Synthetic catecholamines						
Isoproterenol, 0.015 μg/min per kg	HO, OH, CHCH$_2$NHCH(CH$_3$)$_2$, OH	0	0	+++++	+++++	
Dobutamine, 5 μg/min per kg	HO, OH, CH$_2$CH$_2$NHCH(CH$_3$)CH$_2$CH$_2$, OH	+	?	++++	++	0
Synthetic noncatecholamines						
Indirect acting						
Ephedrine, 5–10 mg IV push	CH(OH) CH(CH$_3$)NHCH$_3$	++	+++	+++	++	0
Metaraminol, 0.5 μg/min per kg	OH, CH(OH)CH(CH$_3$)NH$_2$	+++++	++++	+++	0	0
Direct acting						
Phenylephrine, 0.15 μg/min per kg	OH, CH(OH)CH$_2$NHCH$_3$	++++	+++++	0	0	0
Methoxamine, 5–10 mg IV push	H$_3$CO, OCH$_3$, CH(OH)CH(CH$_3$)NH$_2$	++++	0 -+?	0	0	0

$\alpha_1$art = $\alpha_1$receptor, arterial; $\alpha_1$ven = $\alpha_1$receptor, venous; DA = dopamine receptors
0 = no effect; += slight effect; +++++ = potent effect.

Figure 29.11 Adrenoceptor activity of synthetic α- and β-agonists.

Cardiovascular and renal actions of synthetic α and β agonists

Drug, IV infusion dose	Cardiovascular effects					
	CO	Inotropy	HR	Preload	TPR	RBF
Synthetic catecholamines						
Isoproterenol, 0.015 μg/min per kg	↑–	↑↑↑	↑↑↑	↓	↓↓	–↑
Dobutamine, 5 μg/min per kg	↑↑	↑↑	–↑	?	–	–↑
Synthetic noncatecholamines						
Indirect acting						
Ephedrine, 5–10mg IV push	↑	↑	↑	↑↑	↑	↑–↓
Metaraminol, 0.5 μg/min per kg	–↓	↑	Reflex↓	↑	↑↑↑	↓↓↓
Direct acting						
Phenylephrine, 0.15 μg/min per kg	–↓	–	Reflex↓	↑↑↑	↑↑	–↓
Methoxamine, 5–10mg IV push	–↓	–	Reflex↓	–	↑↑	↓↓

CO = cardiac output, HR = heart rate, TPR = total peripheral resistance, RBF = renal blood flow
– = no change; ↓= decreased effect; ↑= increased effect.

Figure 29.12 Cardiovascular and renal actions of synthetic α- and β-agonists.

tions (Fig. 29.10). Stimulation of α-adrenoceptors eventually decreases skeletal muscle blood flow, inhibits insulin secretion, and contracts mesenteric vascular smooth muscle.

In addition to the use of epinephrine for improving myocardial function, exogenous administration of epinephrine is commonly employed in conjunction with local anesthetics to prolong their duration of action. Epinephrine also is employed as treatment for anaphylactic shock, localized bleeding, and bronchospasm.

Synthetic β-agonists

Isoproterenol

Isoproterenol shows almost pure β-adrenoceptor activity as a consequence of the increased size of the alkyl substituent on the ethylamine amino group (Fig. 29.11). Isoproterenol produces positive inotropic effects via β_1-adrenoceptor stimulation, and bronchodilatation and vasodilatation in vascular smooth muscle through β_2-activation (Fig. 29.12). Isoproterenol can produce arrhythmias and increase myocardial oxygen demand while reducing oxygen delivery via an increased heart rate and decreased perfusion pressure.

Dobutamine

Dobutamine is a direct-acting synthetic catecholamine that is derived from dopamine but does not have dopamine receptor effects. Dobutamine is predominately selective for β_1-adrenoceptors, resulting in positive inotropic effects but with surprisingly smaller increases in heart rate than seen with isoproterenol (see Fig. 29.12). Dobutamine is employed clinically as a 'cardioselective' inotrope. It improves cardiac output without major adverse effects on the myocardial oxygen supply/demand relationship because heart rate is relatively stable and afterload is maintained through reduced β_2-adrenoceptor-mediated effects and through some α-adrenoceptor activity.

Ephedrine

Ephedrine is a commonly used sympathomimetic noncatecholamine (see Fig. 29.11). The action of ephedrine is considered indirect because it competes with norepinephrine for local reuptake, thus resulting in elevated concentrations of norepinephrine at receptor sites. Generally, the cardiovascular effects

Beta adrenoreceptor antagonists								
Drug	β_1 potency ratio[a]	Relative β_1 selectivity	Intrinsic sympathomimetic activity	Membrane stabilizing activity	Lipid solubility	Elimination half-life (h)	Total body clearance (L/min)	Metabolism
Atenolol	1.0	++	0	0	low	6–9	0.13	renal
Esmolol	0.02	++	0	0	low	9 min	27	esterases[b]
Labetalol	0.3	0	+?	0	low	3–4	2.7	hepatic
Metoprolol	1.0	++	0	0	moderate	3–4	1.1	hepatic
Nadolol	1.0	0	0	0	low	14–24	0.2	renal
Pindolol	6.0	0	++	+	moderate	3–4	0.4	renal/hepatic
Propranolol	1.0	0	0	++	high	3–4	1.0	hepatic
Timolol	6.0	0	0	0	low	4–5	0.66	renal/hepatic

[a] β_1 Potency ratio is determined relative to propranolol (equal to 1).
[b] Red blood cell and nonspecific esterases.
0 = No selectivity or activity; ++ = significant selectivity or activity.
Adapted from Frishman WH. Clinical Pharmacology of the β-Adrenoceptor Blocking Drugs, 2nd edn, Norwalk, CT: Appleton-Century-Crofts, 1989.

Figure 29.13 Antagonists of β-adrenoceptors.

produced by ephedrine are similar to those of epinephrine (see Fig. 29.12). It is less potent but longer acting than a single intravenous dose of epinephrine. The primary mechanism for the increased myocardial performance associated with ephedrine is stimulation of β_1-adrenoceptors, although α-adrenoceptor-mediated venoconstriction has an important contribution through increasing preload and cardiac output. Intravenous ephedrine administration leads to increases in heart rate, systolic and diastolic blood pressure, cardiac output, and coronary artery blood flow.

In addition, ephedrine decreases renal and splanchnic blood flow, stimulates the CNS (e.g. increases MAC), and is associated with tachyphylaxis after extended use. Ephedrine can improve bronchial asthma. It is administered as a vasopressor during obstetrics because it has been shown to have no effect on uterine blood flow. During anesthesia, ephedrine is the most commonly employed noncatecholamine sympathomimetic drug. It is used in the treatment of hypotension during general or regional anesthesia when accompanied by relative bradycardia.

Amphetamines, mephentermine, and metaraminol are synthetic vasopressors with predominately indirect actions on α- and β-adrenoceptors. In particular, metaraminol produces a marked increase in both systolic and diastolic pressure through α-adrenoceptor-mediated vasoconstriction (see Figs 29.11 and 29.12).

Beta$_2$-agonists

The β_2-adrenoceptor agonists selectively relax bronchial and uterine smooth muscle. Metaproterenol (orciprenaline), albuterol, and isoetharine (isoetarine) are inhaled, relatively selective β_2-agonists that decrease airway resistance and are indicated in the treatment of acute bronchial asthma and chronic obstructive pulmonary disease. Side effects may result from higher doses of these agents and include tachycardia, pulmonary edema, hypokalemia, and hyperglycemia. The frequency of tachycardia is relatively low since these drugs are 10-fold less potent than isoproterenol at activating β_1-adrenoceptors.

Terbutaline and ritodrine are tocolytic drugs that are frequently used to manage premature labor contractions because they stimulate β_2-adrenoceptors in the myometrium, resulting in relaxation (Chapter 65). These tocolytic drugs stimulate both β_1- and β_2-adrenoceptors. They can be given via subcutaneous, intramuscular, or intravenous injection. Side effects include hyperglycemia, hypokalemia, cardiac arrhythmias, tachycardia, and pulmonary edema.

Beta antagonists (blockers)

Structurally, β blockers are derivatives of isoproterenol with various benzene ring substituents. These blockers bind selectively to β-adrenoceptors and competitively inhibit the effects of endogenous and exogenous β-agonists. This antagonism is reflected by a rightward shift of the dose–response curve for β-agonists. Beta blockers produce negative chronotropic and inotropic effects and, consequently, are used widely for the treatment of cardiovascular disease. Certain β blockers show a *relative selectivity* but not *specificity* for β_1-adrenoceptor subtypes, such that β_2-adrenoceptor antagonism may occur in all tissues as blood levels increase (Fig. 29.13).

The β-antagonists can be further subdivided as either partial or pure blockers based on the presence or absence of intrinsic sympathomimetic activity (ISA), respectively (see Fig. 29.13). Partial antagonists produce less myocardial depression and bradycardia than drugs without ISA but are unable to preserve ventricular function. Clinically, both partial and pure antagonists are used in the treatment of hypertension, dysrhythmias, and effort angina, but drugs with ISA have been employed particularly in patients with bronchial asthma, compromised left ventricular function, and peripheral vascular disease. The myocardial depression from inhaled and injected anesthetics is additive to that of β blockers yet is not excessive enough to limit the perioperative use of β blockers. Although the clinical significance remains uncertain, certain β blockers exhibit a membrane-stabilizing activity via the (+)-stereoisomer, which produces a local anesthetic-like effect on myocellular membranes.

Withdrawal symptoms can occur from discontinuing chronic β blocker therapy and is characterized by hyperadrenergic symptoms such as palpitations, tremors, and sweating. The principal contraindications to the use of β blockers are pre-existing obstructive airway disease, atrioventricular heart block, and/or cardiac failure.

Propranolol

Propranolol, a nonselective, pure β-adrenoceptor antagonist with limited ISA activity, is the prototypical β blocker (see Fig. 29.13). It causes a decrease in heart rate and cardiac output that is most pronounced during periods of SNS stimulation. Antagonism of β_2-adrenoceptors by propranolol can concomitantly increase peripheral and coronary vascular resistance, although this effect diminishes with chronic administration. Propranolol reduces myocardial oxygen consumption and reduces blood flow to major organs, except the brain.

Therapeutically, propranolol is useful because it is lipid-soluble and is readily absorbed from the small intestine; however, larger oral doses are required to achieve equivalent clinical effects to intravenous doses. Prolonged use of propranolol may cause depression, nightmares, fatigue, and/or sexual dysfunction. Marked bradydysrhythmias may result when propranolol is used in conjunction with halothane or opioids.

Esmolol

Esmolol is a selective β_1-adrenoceptor antagonist with a low potency but a rapid onset and short duration of action. Its structure, a phenoxypropanolamine, allows for rapid esterase degradation; the half-life of esmolol is only 10–20 minutes (see Fig. 29.13). These properties make esmolol particularly useful to reduce the transient β-adrenergic stimulation that occurs in the perioperative period. Indeed, 50–100mg intravenous esmolol administered only a few minutes prior to laryngoscopy and tracheal intubation can reduce or abolish the commonly observed tachycardia. As a consequence of its cardioselectivity and lack of β_2-adrenoceptor antagonism, minimal bronchial or vascular tone changes are observed. Esmolol is employed to manage short-duration tachycardia accompanied by hypertension and in the management of supraventricular tachycardia.

Labetalol

Labetalol is considered a mixed antagonist because of its actions at both α- and β-adrenoceptors (see Fig. 29.13). Intravenous labetalol administration has an α/β antagonistic potency ratio of 1:7 compared with 1:3 after oral administration. A lowered heart rate in the presence of lowered systemic blood pressure during labetalol therapy has certain advantages when employed in patients with coronary artery disease because the myocardial oxygen supply/demand ratio is improved. In addition, cardiac output is maintained since the decreased afterload compensates for reduced cardiac function. The duration of action of labetalol has been estimated to be 4–6 hours after a single intravenous dose.

Alpha$_1$-agonists

Agonists of α_1-adrenoceptors exert vasopressor actions on arterial and venous vessels, thereby increasing pressure and flow in certain beds. In healthy individuals, cardiac output is well maintained. In fact, cardiac output may improve because of increased preload. The concomitant increase in afterload can improve myocardial oxygen delivery via improved diastolic coronary blood flow. However, there is a potential for decreased organ blood flow through regional vasoconstriction.

Phenylephrine

Phenylephrine is a pure α-agonist that is longer acting but considerably less potent than norepinephrine. Phenylephrine increases both venous and arterial resistance and often enhances preload (see Figs 29.11 and 29.12). It is frequently employed in the perioperative period as treatment for hypotension accompanied by increased heart rate. It causes reflex slowing of the heart rate as blood pressure is increased by vasoconstriction. This vasopressor can be useful in reversing 'tet spells' (right-to-left shunt) in patients with tetralogy of Fallot.

Methoxamine

Methoxamine is a selective α_1-agonist similar to phenylephrine but without significant venoconstriction (see Figs 29.8, 29.11, and 29.12). Its clinical uses are limited, except for treatment of paroxysmal atrial tachycardia, where a single dose of intravenous methoxamine can counteract the tachycardia via baroreceptor reflex-mediated slowing of the heart.

Alpha$_2$-agonists

Agonists of α_2-adrenoceptors include the imidazolines, phenylethylamines, and oxaloazepines. They are utilized as antihypertensive agents because of their ability to decrease sympathetic outflow from the CNS and their ability to reduce local norepinephrine release at nerve terminals. Other actions of α_2-agonists include vasoconstriction via postsynaptic α_2-adrenoceptors, cardiac antiarrhythmic effects, decreased cerebral blood flow, and inhibition of insulin and growth hormone secretion. An attribute of α_2-agonists in the perioperative period is that they can sedate but do not significantly impair respiration. Side effects of α_2-agonists include bradycardia, sedation, and dry mouth. Their bradycardic actions seem to occur through a centrally mediated enhancement of vagal outflow.

The α_2-agonists lower the requirements for anesthetics and analgesics in the perioperative period because of their sedative, analgesic, and anxiolytic properties. Preoperative administration helps to diminish perioperative blood pressure variations, intraoperative plasma catecholamine levels, and the hemodynamic response to endotracheal intubation and surgical stimulation. The ability of α_2-agonists to attenuate the sympathoadrenal stress response has been demonstrated during both general and regional anesthesia.

Clonidine

Clonidine is a selective α_2-agonist that has potent antihypertensive effects. Decreased blood pressure results from inhibition of preganglionic sympathetic fiber activity following α_2-adrenoceptor stimulation in the CNS. Small oral doses of clonidine (2μg/kg) may have a beneficial role in reducing adverse myocardial events in patients with coronary artery disease having noncardiac surgery. Another clinical application of clonidine has been in the treatment of opioid withdrawal.

Dexmedetomidine

Dexmedetomidine, the (+)-stereoisomer of the imidazolidine compound medetomidine, is highly selective for the α_2-adrenoceptors. It is seven times more potent for the α_2-adrenoceptor and is considered a full agonist. Dexmedetomidine is being investigated for clinical utility as a strong analgesic with sedative and anxiolytic actions. When used in conjunction with volatile anesthetics, dexmedetomidine reduces the minimal alveolar concentration, reduces chest wall rigidity caused by opioids, and lessens postanesthetic shivering.

Alpha antagonists

Alpha antagonists include the β-haloethylamines, imidazoline analogs, piperanzinyl quinazolines, and indole derivatives (Fig. 29.14). These agents exhibit either competitive or noncompetitive inhibition. Important clinical actions of α-antagonists include reductions in blood pressure; however, reflex tachycardia, nasal stuffiness, diarrhea, and suppression of ejaculation can be troublesome.

Alpha-adrenoreceptor agonists and antagonists

Drug	Type of antagonism	Receptor selectivity
Agonists		
Phenylephrine		$\alpha_1 >> \alpha_2$
Methoxamine		α_1
Norepinephrine		$\alpha_1 = \alpha_2$
Epinephrine		$\alpha_1 = \alpha_2$
Clonidine		$\alpha_2 > \alpha_1$
Dexmedetomidine		$\alpha_2 >> \alpha_1$
Antagonists		
Prazosin	Competitive	$\alpha_1 >> \alpha_2$
Phenoxybenzamine	Noncompetitive	$\alpha_1 > \alpha_2$
Phentolamine	Competitive	$\alpha_1 = \alpha_2$
Tolazoline	Competitive	$\alpha_1 = \alpha_2$
Yohimbine	Competitive	$\alpha_2 >> \alpha_1$

Figure 29.14 Alpha-adrenoceptor agonists and antagonists.

Key References

Berkowitz DE, Schwinn DA. Basic pharmacology of α- and β-adrenoceptors. In: Bowdle TA, Hovita A, Kharasch ED, eds. The Pharmacological Basis of Anesthesiology. New York: Churchill Livingstone; 1994:581–606.

Carpenter MB, Sutin J. The autonomic nervous system. In: Carpenter MB, Sutin J, eds. Human Neuroanatomy, 8th edn. Baltimore, MD: Williams & Wilkins; 1983:220.

Ebert TJ. Preoperative evaluation of the autonomic nervous system. Adv Anesth. 1993;10:49–68.

Ebert TJ, Muzi M. Sympathetic hyperactivity during desflurane anesthesia in healthy volunteers: a comparison with isoflurane. Anesthesiology. 1993;79:444–53.

Wood M. Cholinergic and parasympathomimetic drugs. Cholinesterases and anticholinesterases. In: Wood M, Wood AJJ, eds. Drugs and Anesthesia. Pharmacology for Anesthesiologists. Baltimore, MD: Williams & Wilkins; 1982:111.

Wood M. Drugs and the sympathetic nervous system. In: Wood M, Wood AJJ, eds. Drugs and Anesthesia. Pharmacology for Anesthesiologists. Baltimore, MD: Williams & Wilkins; 1982:407.

Further Reading

Ahlquist RP. A study of the adrenotropic receptors. Am J Physiol. 1948;153:586–94.

Burnstock G. Integration of factors controlling vascular tone. Anesthesiology. 1993;79:1368–80.

Ebert TJ, Harkin CP, Muzi M. Cardiovascular responses to sevoflurane: a review. Anesth Analg. 1995;81:S11–22.

Ebert TJ, Muzi M. Propofol and autonomic reflex function in humans. Anesth Analg. 1994;78:369–75.

Flacke WE, Flacke JW. Cholinergic and anticholinergic agents. In: Smith NT, Corbascia AN, eds. Drug Interactions in Anesthesia. Philadelphia, PA: Lea & Febiger; 1986:160.

Lawson NW, Wallfisch HK. Cardiovascular pharmacology: a new look at the 'pressors'. In: Stoelting RK, Barash PG, Gallagher TJ, eds. Advances in Anesthesia. Chicago, IL: Year Book Medical Publishers; 1986:195.

Smiley RM, Kwatra MM, Schwinn DA. New developments in cardiovascular adrenergic receptor pharmacology: molecular mechanisms and clinical relevance. J Cardiothorac Vascular Anesth. 1998;12:80–95.

Ziegler MG. Antihypertensives. In: Chernow B, Lake CR, eds. The Pharmacologic Approach to the Critically Ill Patient. Baltimore, MD: Williams & Wilkins; 1983:303.

Chapter 30 Voluntary motor systems – skeletal muscle, reflexes, and control of movement

Philip M Hopkins

Topics covered in this chapter

Types of muscle
Control of muscle contraction
The basal ganglia
The cerebellum
Motor areas of the cerebral cortex
Drug treatment of movement disorders

TYPES OF MUSCLE

Muscles are the contractile tissues of the body. Morphologically, muscles can be described as striated or smooth, depending on the degree of organization of the contractile filaments. Physiologically and pharmacologically, smooth muscles are a markedly heterogenous group of tissues (Chapter 33). Striated muscles include cardiac and skeletal muscles. The skeletal muscles themselves are far from uniform. Examination of muscles from lower mammals reveals that some muscles are pale in color while others are more red. Examples are the extensor digitorum longus (pale) and soleus (red) of the rat. The redness of the muscles reflects the amount of myoglobin in the muscle fiber. *Myoglobin* is the specialized heme-containing oxygen-storage protein of striated muscle. A high myoglobin content endows the fiber with a high capacity for aerobic metabolism. The fibers with the highest myoglobin content have a relatively slow rate of shortening; these slow-twitch fibers are categorized as type I fibers. Most fast-twitch fibers have a low myoglobin content and are dependent on anaerobic metabolism (type IIb), while some have moderate myoglobin levels and aerobic capacity (type IIa).

All skeletal muscles in the human body contain a mixture of type I and type II fibers. However, be it through variation in the proportion of fiber type or other factors, different human muscles show subtle differences in their physiologic characteristics. Different degrees of response to some drugs can be demonstrated in isolated muscle strips taken by biopsy from various regions of the body. The diaphragm is an especially interesting example in that it shares some characteristics of cardiac muscle. This is presumably an adaptation to allow its continuous cycle of contraction and relaxation, as with the heart.

Structure of skeletal muscle

The skeletal muscles are the effector organs of voluntary movement. The muscle fibers are specialized, elongated excitable cells that range in diameter from 10 to 100μm and in length from 0.5 to 12cm. Most muscle fibers do not span the whole length of the intact muscle. At one end of the muscle, the fibers extend from the tendon and end in long tapering points that interdigitate with other fibers. The fibers are tightly bound together by intrafascicular connective tissue, the endomysium (Fig. 30.1). Several lengths of bound muscle fibers are often required before the final fibers reach the tendon at the other end of the muscle. Functionally, however, muscles behave as if they are groups of fibers extending from tendon to tendon.

The integrity of individual skeletal muscles is maintained by a framework of connective tissue: that enclosing the whole muscle is termed the epimysium. Smaller and smaller bundles of muscle fibers are enclosed by sleeves of connective tissue, the perimysium, that are protrusions of the epimysium into the body of the muscle. The smallest bundles visible to the naked eye are termed muscle fascicles; these are made up of 12 or more fibers enclosed by their perimysium. In addition to holding the individual fibers together, the endomysium also provides the architecture to hold capillaries and nerves in place.

Movement of the skeleton is achieved by shortening, or contraction, of muscles. Each muscle fiber contains thousands of contractile units, myofibrils, made up of *sarcomeres* arranged in series in the long axis of the fiber. The myofibrils contain filaments of two types, thin and thick, which are arranged to form the lines and bands that are visible microsopically. The thin myofilaments consist of three major types of protein: *actin*, *tropomyosin,* and *troponin*. Actin, an α-helical protein, is an important structural protein in most cell types but its organization in striated muscle enables a specialized role. Tropomyosin is a filamentous protein that lies in the groove of the actin helix. Troponin consists of three subunits, troponin I ('inhibitory'), troponin T (tropomyosin-binding) and troponin C (Ca^{2+} binding). Troponin is found at every seventh actin subunit.

The thick myofilaments are formed from bundles of *myosin*, which consists of helical chains and a double globular head formed by the folding of the *N*-terminal regions of the chains. The tertiary structure of the head is maintained by myosin elastic light chain. Phosphorylation of another light chain protein, the LC_{20} or regulatory light chain, alters the angle between the helical rod and the globular head. There are several isoforms of myosin, which determine the twitch speed of the fiber.

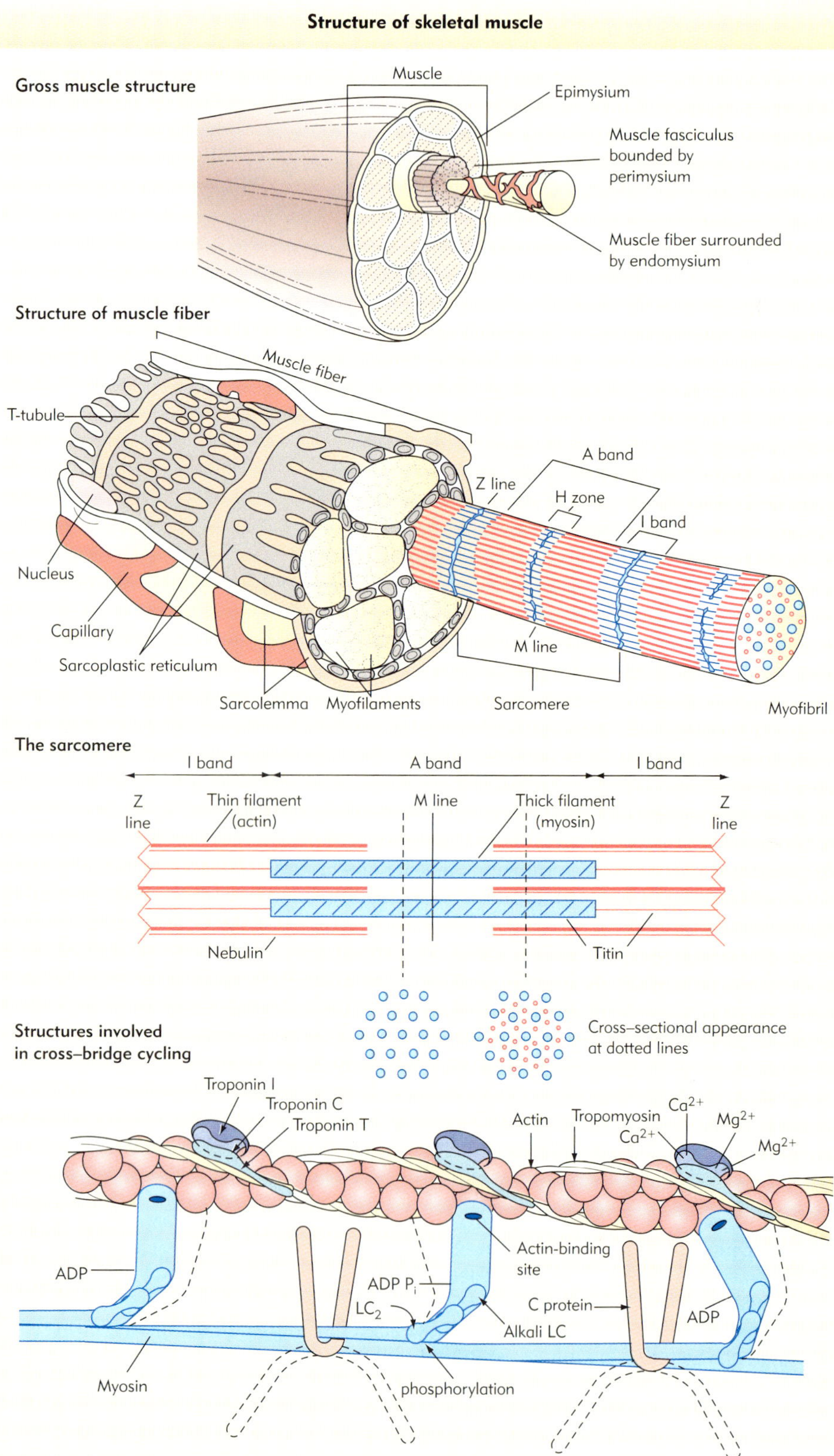

Figure 30.1 The structure of skeletal muscle. Note that within the muscle fiber the sarcoplasmic reticulum is arranged in parallel with the myofilaments whereas the T-tubules are perpendicular. The organization of the major proteins constituting the thick and thin filaments within the sarcomere is maintained by several structural proteins including nebulin and titin. The proteins forming the Z-line and M-line structures are closely related to actin. Each thick filament is surrounded by six thin filaments. The structural elements involved in cross-bridge cycling are shown. C protein is believed to be an additional regulator of actin–myosin interaction: its position is not known and hence it is illustrated in two potential configurations. (With permission from Moffett et al., 1993)

Muscle contraction

Shortening of the sarcomere is achieved by the drawing together of opposing thin filaments by a ratchet-like effect of the thick filaments (Fig. 30.2). Pure actin and myosin will readily interact with each other. The actin filament has a series of myosin-binding sites that sequentially bind with increasing affinity to the head processes of the myosin molecule. In resting muscle, the myosin-binding sites of actin are covered by the tropomyosin filaments; as a result the actin–myosin interaction is weak or prevented completely. Tropomyosin is lifted clear from the myosin-binding sites on the

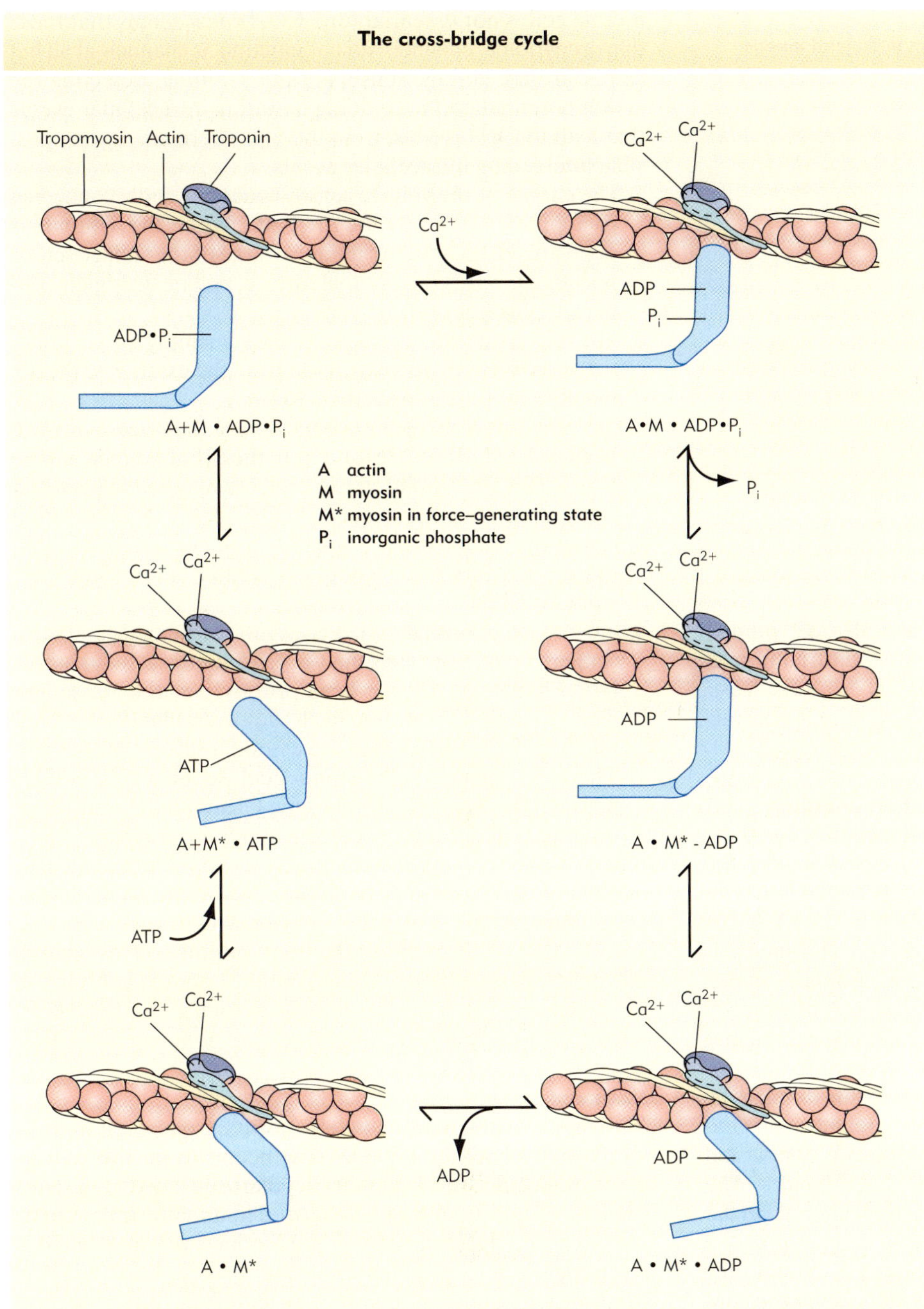

Figure 30.2 The biochemistry of the cross-bridge cycle. Activation starts with the addition of Ca^{2+} to the resting state (top left) and proceeds through various stages (in a clockwise direction here), returning to the resting state after hydrolysis of ATP.

actin molecule in response to a conformational change in troponin that is brought about by Ca^{2+} binding to troponin C. Binding of increasing intensity of myosin, which at this stage is complexed with ADP and inorganic phosphate, to actin leads to dissociation of the inorganic phosphate from the myosin head. This stage is associated with a strongly bound cross-bridge between actin and myosin. This strong chemical bonding is a dynamic process as it causes a conformational change in the myosin chain leading to a swivelling of the myosin head in relation to the actin-binding sites, moving the myosin filaments against the actin. This is the basis of the contractile process. Once the conformational myosin change has occurred, ADP dissociates from the myosin head and the actin–myosin bond is subject to ATP-dependent hydrolysis, enabling a further interaction with a myosin-binding site further down the actin filament.

The contractile process is dependent on the presence of Ca^{2+}. Indeed, regulation of muscle contraction is through control of the myoplasmic Ca^{2+} concentration. In contrast to heart muscle, skeletal muscle contraction is well maintained in the absence of extracellular Ca^{2+}, indicating that the source of Ca^{2+} for contraction in skeletal muscle is intracellular. The major internal store of Ca^{2+} in skeletal muscle is the sarcoplasmic reticulum (SR). In the SR, most Ca^{2+} is bound to a matrix formed by the low-affinity Ca^{2+}-binding protein calsequestrin, which is in equilibrium with the free, releasable Ca^{2+}. When muscle is stimulated, Ca^{2+} is released from the terminal cisternae of the SR through specialized Ca^{2+}-release channels (CRCs).

Following release of Ca^{2+} from the SR, myoplasmic Ca^{2+} concentration remains high only while further Ca^{2+} release is taking place, as Ca^{2+} is continually sequestered from the

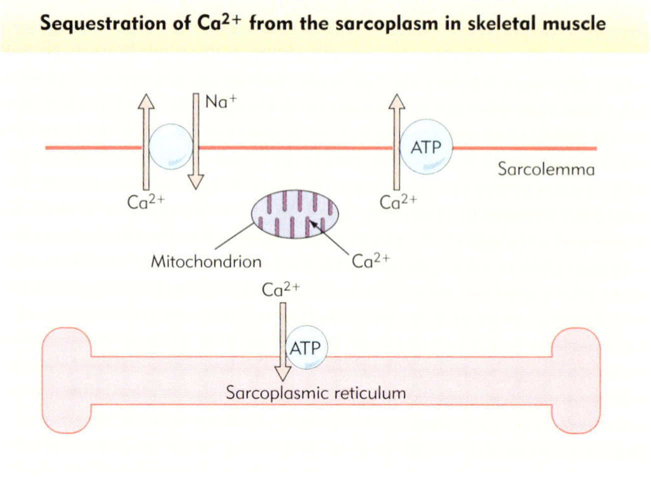

Sequestration of Ca^{2+} from the sarcoplasm in skeletal muscle

Figure 30.3 Mechanisms of sequestration of Ca^{2+} from the sarcoplasm of skeletal muscle.

myoplasm via the action of sarcolemmal and SR Ca^{2+} pumps, sarcolemmal Na^+/Ca^{2+} exchange, and mitochondrial uptake (Fig. 30.3). Therefore, when Ca^{2+} sequestration exceeds release, the muscle will relax. ATP is essential for both muscle contraction and relaxation as the immediate source of energy.

The motor unit and excitation–contraction coupling

The functional unit involved in skeletal muscle contraction is the motor unit. The motor unit comprises an α-motor neuron, the muscle fibers that it innervates, and the neuromuscular junctions that form the chemical synapse between the neuron and the muscle fiber. Each α-motor neuron branches at its terminus; as a result, it supplies from three to hundreds of muscle fibers. Stimulation of a muscle fiber follows the transduction of an action potential arriving at the terminal swelling of a motor neuron into an action potential at the postjunctional region of the neuromuscular junction (the motor end plate). This occurs through the action of acetylcholine (Chapter 31). An action potential generated at the motor end plate spreads across the sarcolemma and down the invaginations of this membrane, the *T-tubules*. The transduction of the electrical signal of the action potential in the T-tubule to produce physical interaction between the contractile proteins, or excitation–contraction coupling (ECC), is not fully understood. There is now overwhelming evidence that the contraction process is initiated by a rise in the myoplasmic Ca^{2+} concentration from a resting level of about 0.01μmol/L to 5μmol/L and that this rise is effected by the release of Ca^{2+} from the terminal cisternae of the SR. Here, the SR and T-tubule are separated by a gap of only 12–14nm, which is spanned at intervals by structures seen on electron microscopy as 'feet' (Fig. 30.4). These feet processes are large proteins that have affinity for the plant toxin ryanodine and are, therefore, known as *ryanodine receptors*. Purified ryanodine receptors incorporated into planar lipid bilayers behave as Ca^{2+} channels with identical properties to those of the CRC of isolated 'heavy' SR vesicles, indicating that the ryanodine receptor is the CRC of SR. High-power electron microscopy has revealed that this protein comprises four transmembrane subunits (M1–M4) (see Fig. 30.4).

The T-tubular membrane also contains Ca^{2+} channels and has the greatest density of dihydropyridine-binding sites in the body. However, the passage of extracellular Ca^{2+} into the muscle cell is not essential for ECC. It now seems that these dihydropyridine 'channels' do not function as channels at all but rather are the voltage sensors of the T-tubule, detecting the action potential and in so doing initiating intracellular events that lead to Ca^{2+} release from the SR. There are several possible intervening intracellular events.

1. The charge of the voltage sensor could be rigidly connected to a 'plug' that blocks the SR CRC. When the T-tubule is depolarized, the intramembrane charge of the voltage sensor is shifted towards the external surface, pulling the rigidly connected plug out of the channel lumen.
2. The dihydropyridine receptor may act simply as a conductor of the wave of depolarization from the exterior to the SR membrane, which opens the CRC.
3. Calcium ions have been shown to cause the release of Ca^{2+} from isolated SR vesicles and from the SR of skinned muscle fibers. This Ca^{2+}-induced Ca^{2+} release may be the basis of a second messenger system in which T-tubule depolarization causes the release of Ca^{2+} bound to its inner surface and this, in turn, triggers release of much greater amounts of Ca^{2+} from the SR.
4. Inositol trisphosphate (IP_3) is an intracellular second messenger capable of releasing Ca^{2+} from intracellular stores (see Chapter 3). IP_3 has been proposed as the messenger involved in ECC; it is more likely, however, that IP_3 is a modulator of ECC rather than the essential second messenger. There is considerable amino acid sequence homology between the M1–M4 region of the CRC and the transmembranous regions of IP_3 receptors in other cell types.

Recent evidence suggests there are two populations of CRC, one where the cytoplasmic part is apposed to the T-tubule voltage sensors and the other where it is not. This has led to the suggestion that activation of the first population by charge movement in the voltage sensor (option 1 above) leads to the local release of Ca^{2+}, which is the trigger for Ca^{2+}-induced Ca^{2+} release (option 3 above) from the second population of CRC.

Malignant hyperthermia

Malignant hyperthermia (MH) results from a pathologic increase in skeletal muscle Ca^{2+} concentrations that is triggered by volatile anesthetics and depolarizing muscle relaxants. The susceptibility to MH is inherited in an autosomal dominant pattern. Molecular genetic studies have revealed that it is a genetically heterogenous condition; that is, the same clinical disorder can be caused by abnormalities in one of several genes. Prime candidates for causative genes are those for the SR CRC and the T-tubule voltage sensor. There is evidence that mutations in genes coding for either of these structures are associated with some instances of MH. The clinical features of MH are secondary to increased myoplasmic Ca^{2+}, which causes muscle rigidity (increased myofilament interaction), hypermetabolism (secondary to increased demand for ATP and Ca^{2+}-calmodulin activation of glycolytic enzymes), and loss of integrity of the sarcolemma (lack of ATP and Ca^{2+} activation of membrane phospholipases).

Treatment of MH is dependent on early recognition of the developing reaction, withdrawal of trigger drugs, symptomatic treatment of the fever and metabolic disturbances, and the intravenous administration of dantrolene sodium, a drug that prevents release of Ca^{2+} into the muscle cells. The site of action of dantrolene is disputed but it either directly blocks the release of Ca^{2+} from the SR or reduces the stimulus to SR Ca^{2+} release

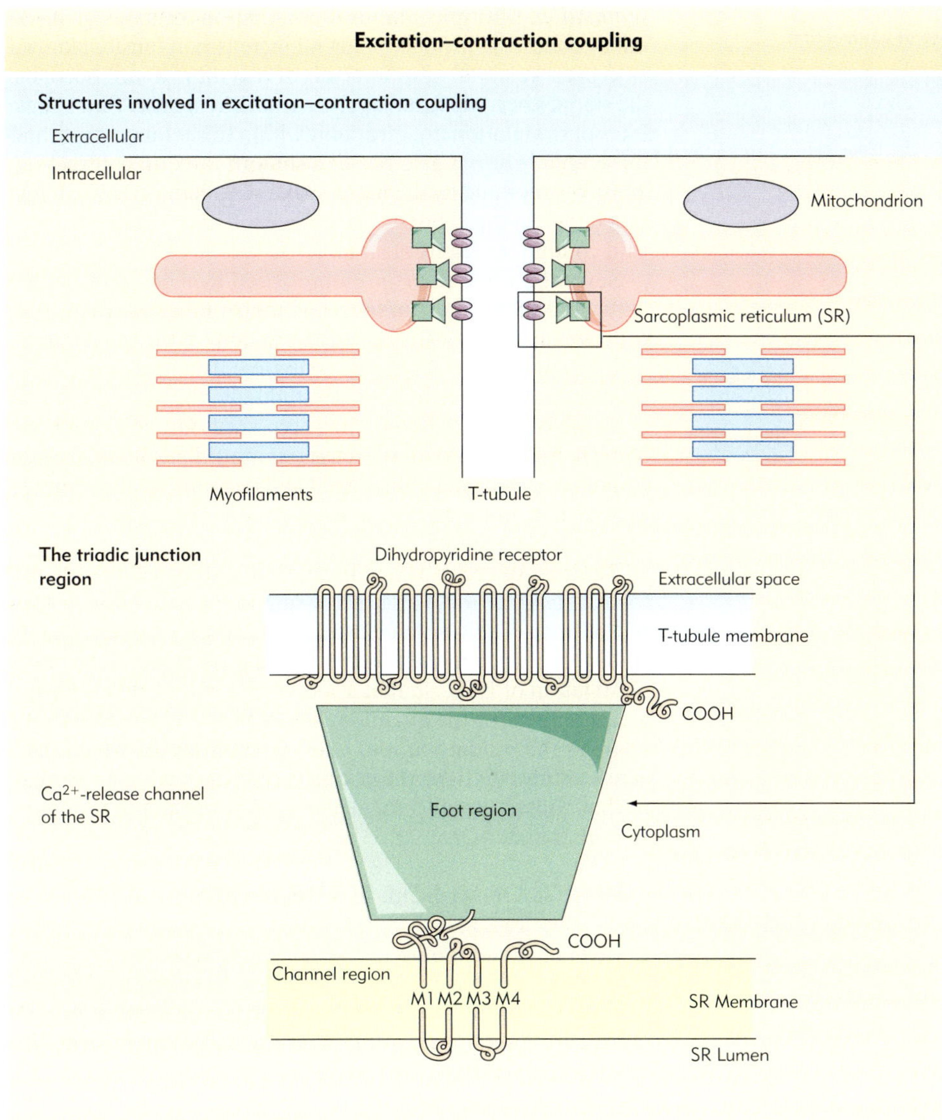

Figure 30.4 Excitation–contraction coupling. The structures involved in the coupling are shown (top) plus expansion of the triadic junction region to show the relationship of the dihydropyridine voltage sensor and the SR Ca^{2+}-release channel (CRC). The foot process of the CRC is presumed to be the regulatory region.

following arrival of the action potential at the voltage sensors of the T-tubules. Dantrolene is poorly soluble in water and is, therefore, presented for intravenous use as a lyophilized powder containing a mixture of 20mg dantrolene sodium, 3g mannitol, and sodium hydroxide (to produce a pH of 9.5 when reconstituted with 60mL sterile water). Dantrolene should be administered in intravenous doses of 1mg/kg, repeated until a maintained response is seen. Up to 10mg/kg has been required, but the usual total dose is 2–3mg/kg. Side effects of dantrolene in the treatment of MH are usually unnoticed because of the severity of the MH reaction, although severe reactions, such as acute hepatic dysfunction, can occur.

MH can be avoided by using drugs that are known not to trigger the condition (intravenous anesthetics, opioids, nondepolarizing muscle relaxants, local anesthetics). Some authorities have proposed the use of dantrolene as 'prophylaxis' against MH in known susceptible individuals requiring surgery. Its short-term use provokes nausea, vomiting, and muscle weakness in a high proportion of recipients as well as unpleasant CNS effects including euphoria and disorientation. The use of prophylactic dantrolene is, therefore, not warranted as part of a 'belt and braces' approach. The relatively weak effects of dantrolene on cardiac and diaphragmatic muscle may also become significant in those patients with pre-existing cardiac or respiratory disease, respectively.

Regulation of the force of muscle contraction

When stimulated by a single action potential, the force developed by a muscle fiber depends on the sum of the myosin–actin interactions. The Ca^{2+} release is probably sufficient to fully saturate all the Ca^{2+}-binding sites of tropinin C but the Ca^{2+} concentration is not maintained sufficiently to achieve a steady-state (maximal) activation of all potential actin and myosin bonds. The number of myosin heads that are aligned with potential binding sites on the actin filaments, which is determined by the degree of stretch applied to the muscle fiber, is also important. This concept is best understood by considering the basic contractile units, the sarcomeres, and more specifically the consequences of changing sarcomere length (distance between adjacent Z -lines) (Fig. 30.5). Essentially, there is a relatively narrow range of length of muscle at which stimulation will lead to a maximal response. For maximum efficiency, therefore,

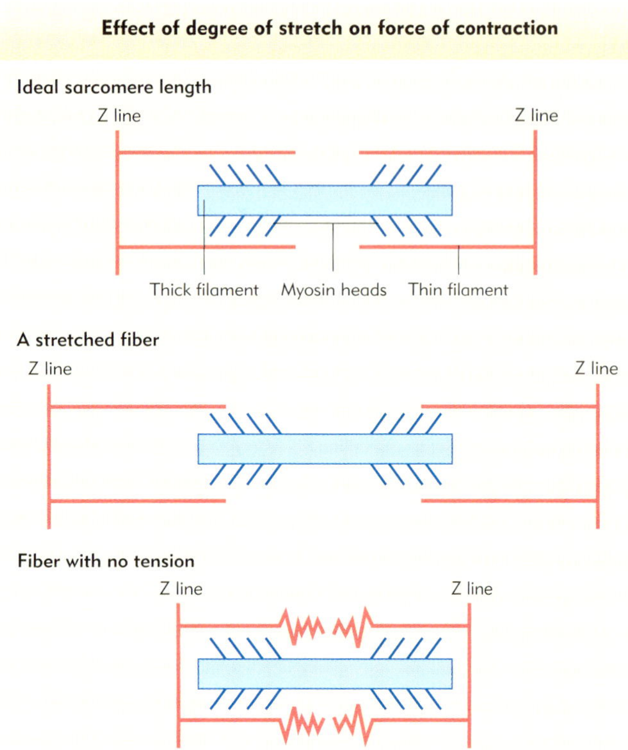

Figure 30.5 The effect of degree of stretch on the force of contraction. In the ideal situation, the sarcomere length is such that the thin and thick filaments overlap and align all the myosin heads adjacent to potential actin-binding sites; maximal force can then be generated if the fiber is stimulated. If the fiber is stretched so that the sarcomere length is increased, a point is reached where the ends of the thin filaments furthest from the Z lines are pulled beyond the most centrally situated myosin heads. In this situation, if the fiber is stimulated, there is redundancy of these myosin heads and the contractile response is submaximal. At the other extreme, if no tension is applied to the fiber, its elastic nature minimizes sarcomere length, causing overlap of thin filaments attached to adjacent Z lines. The response to stimulation would again be limited as the most distal myosin heads would 'run-out' of actin-binding sites as the thick filaments abutted onto the Z-line structures.

muscle shortening should be limited. This is achievable, while still enabling a large range of joint movement, because most muscle insertions are relatively close to the joint. The negative feature of this arrangement is that there is a six- to eightfold reduction in the maximum tension generated that can be applied to a distal load.

The previous discussion concerned a single stimulus applied to a single muscle fiber. Consider now what happens if a second stimulus is applied a short interval after the first (Fig. 30.6). If the second stimulus is within 8 milliseconds of the first, the plasmalemma will be electrically refractory and no second response will be seen. However, following the first stimulus, myoplasmic Ca^{2+} remains elevated for approximately 50 milliseconds and tension does not return to the prestimulation level for a further 30 milliseconds. Therefore, a second stimulus applied 8–80 milliseconds after the first will have an additive effect, known as *summation*. Multiple stimuli at stimulation intervals of 40–80 milliseconds will produce stepwise increases in tension, known as *steppe*. At stimulation intervals of less than 40 milliseconds, the steppes become fused to give a *tetanic* response. Physiologic rates of stimulation are invariably within this tetanic range, and these tetanic bursts give rise to a smooth forceful contraction. Tension generated by the muscle fiber will increase as the intervals between these bursts are decreased and will be maximal with continuous trains of stimuli.

Several muscle fibers are innervated by a common motor nerve and these fibers of the same motor unit will, therefore, contract simultaneously. Not all motor units in the same muscle will, however, contract at the same time. If a muscle at rest is required to increase its tension gradually, the smallest motor units will be activated first, with successively larger motor units being recruited as greater force is required. Thus *summation* of responses at the single fiber level and *recruitment* at the motor unit level combine to enable a continuum of tension development over a wide range.

The rate of cross-bridge formation, and consequently the force of contraction, varies according to the activation history of the fiber. The Ca^{2+} released as the result of one stimulus leads to a change in the position of the myosin heads, by phosphorylation of LC_{20}, so that a succeeding stimulus may have a greater effect for the quantal release of Ca^{2+}. The mechanism involves the binding of four Ca^{2+} to calmodulin, which then activates myosin light chain kinase (MLCK), which is similar to that contributing to the development of the latch state in smooth muscle (Chapter 33).

CONTROL OF MUSCLE CONTRACTION

Control of skeletal muscle contraction is achieved at several levels, ranging from involuntary simple reflex responses to consciously initiated complex patterns involving many different muscle groups. In order to carry out a particular maneuver, the effectors (agonists) of the response need to be activated and, in addition, the muscles having the opposite effect (antagonists) need to be inhibited. In many movements, compensatory responses are required: for example, to maintain posture and/or balance. As with any control system, feedback information is required if useful output is to be achieved. In the context of control of muscle contraction and movement of the skeleton, this feedback or sensory information is known as *kinesthesia*. Body position sense is a function of the proprioceptive receptors located in the joints, but there are also mechanisms for sensing the tension, length, and rate of shortening of the skeletal muscles. The receptors for detecting muscle tension are located in the tendons and are called the Golgi tendon organs. Afferent signals from the Golgi tendon organs are relayed up the spinal cord to higher centers but also synapse at the spinal cord level to inhibit the efferent supply to the muscle via its α-motor neurons. The receptors for muscle length and change in length are found in the muscle spindle complexes.

The muscle spindle and the stretch reflex

Muscle spindles are encapsulated adapted muscle fibers orientated so that the enclosed intrafusal fibers are arranged parallel to the force-generating, or extrafusal, fibers. Muscle spindles are located throughout the body of muscles, being more numerous in muscles with higher proportions of small motor units. The structure of the muscle spindle and its innervation is

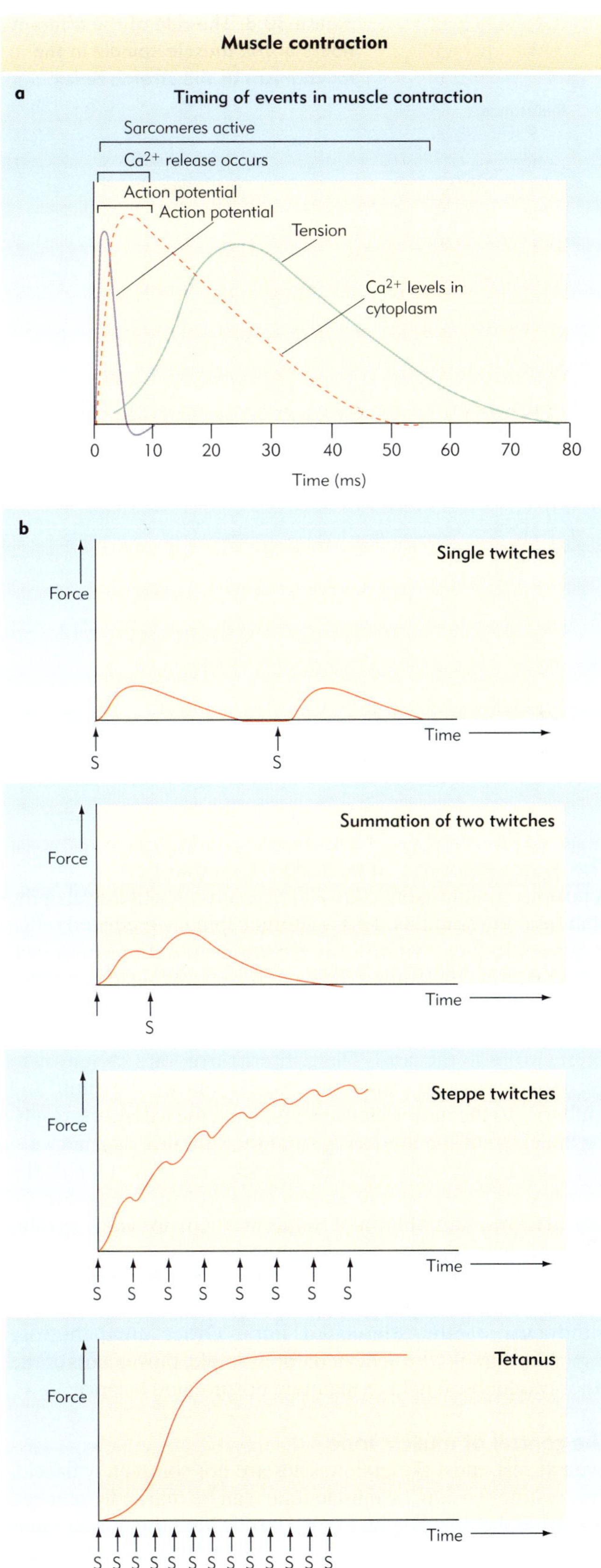

Figure 30.6 Muscle contraction. (a) The timing of events in muscle contraction. (b) The efffect of stimulus interval on the force of contraction: single twitches; summation of two twitches; steppe twitches; and tetanus.

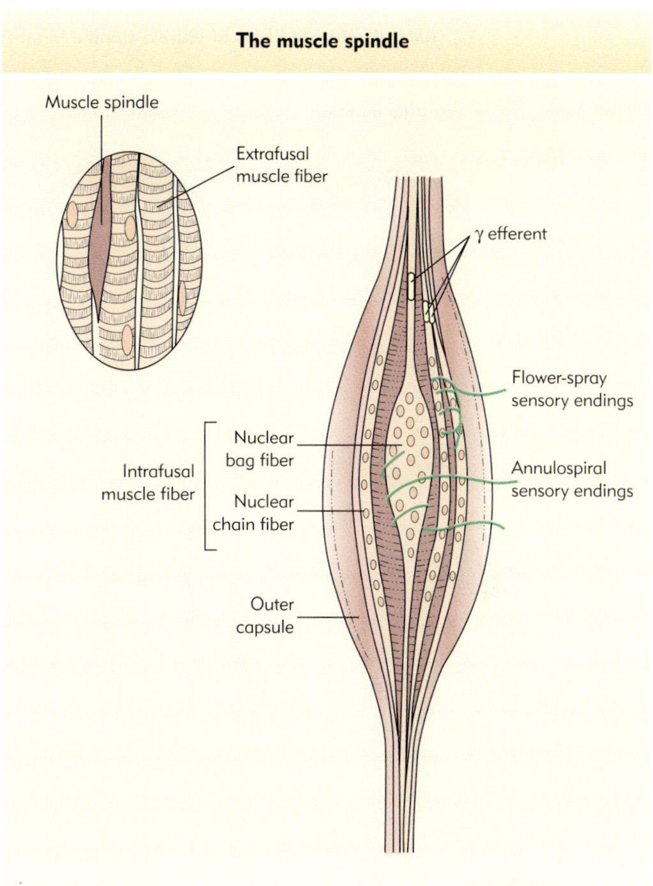

Figure 30.7 The muscle spindle. The intrafusal fibers have a central elastic portion with no myofibrils, making the nuclei prominent features. There are two types of intrafusal fiber: nuclear bag fibers, with a dilated central portion having annulospiral sensory endings; and nuclear chain fibers, with a more uniform diameter and flower-spray sensory endings at the central portion. Nuclear chain fibers detect muscle length, while nuclear bag fibers detect changing length or stretch. The neurons from both types of sensory ending are large myelinated fibers (Aα), which have high conduction velocities. (With permission from Moffett et al., 1993)

illustrated in Figure 30.7. The spindle afferent fibers enter the spinal cord through the dorsal root and branch to make connections at their segmental level of innervation and to pass up the dorsal columns to higher centers. Amongst the segmental connections in the spinal cord are direct single synaptic connections with the α-motor neurons supplying the same muscle and its synergists. These are excitatory synapses, and it is this pathway that is responsible for the stretch reflex typified by the knee-jerk response to tapping the patellar tendon (Fig. 30.8). The function of the stretch reflex is to maintain muscle length.

Efferent supply to the muscle spindles and control of muscle length

The muscle spindles are attached through the endomysium to the extrafusal fibers and are arranged so that intrafusal fibers are parallel to the extrafusal fibers. Contraction, relaxation, or passive stretching of the extrafusal fibers affects tension of the intrafusal fibers, and the resulting afferent impulses

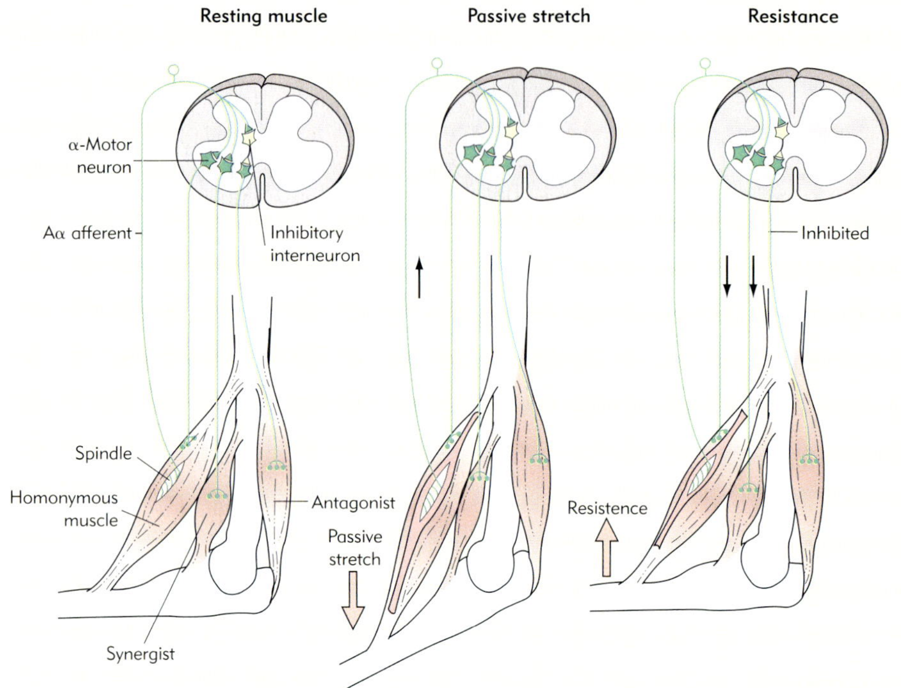

Figure 30.8 The role of the afferent fibers of the muscle spindle in the mechanism of the stretch reflex.

from the sensory fibers of the muscle spindle are relayed in order to return the muscle to the required length. However, the required length is not fixed but can be constantly changed depending on the desired movement or function. To enable appropriate sensory impulses from the muscle spindles, the degree of stretch of the central (sensory) regions of the intrafusal fibers can be controlled independently from the length of the extrafusal fibers by the action of γ-efferent neurons, which synapse on the peripheral regions of the intrafusal fibers. These regions contain contractile myofilaments; impulses from the γ-efferent neurons cause their contraction, resulting in stretching of the central regions of the intrafusal fibers and increased sensory feedback.

During voluntary muscle contraction, the γ-efferent neurons are activated simultaneously with the α-motor neurons supplying the extrafusal fibers of the muscle. Therefore, if the desired response is a shortening of the muscle, and this occurs, the muscle spindle sensory feedback will not change because the reduction in stimulus, owing to shortening of the intrafusal fibers secondary to shortening of the extrafusal fibers, is balanced by the tendency to increase the stimulus by contraction of the end regions of the intrafusal fibers with subsequent stretching of the central regions. If, however, an excessive load prevents the desired shortening of the muscle, muscle spindle sensory feedback will increase because the stretching of the central regions of the intrafusal fibers caused by γ-efferent discharge will be unopposed. The increased sensory feedback results in greater excitatory stimulus to the α-motor neurons in the spinal cord, increasing the contractile effort to try to overcome the load in order to achieve the desired muscle length.

The motor response to nociceptive stimulation

A noxious stimulus applied to a limb results in withdrawal of the limb from the stimulus. This is another spinally mediated reflex response. In fact, two reflexes are implicated: the withdrawal reflex affecting the injured limb and the crossed-extensor reflex affecting the contralateral limb. Nociceptive cutaneous afferents enter the dorsal horns of the spinal cord and send projections to interneurons in the cord. These interneurons are excitatory to the motor neurons supplying the flexors of the limb and inhibitory to the motor neurons supplying the extensors, resulting in flexion of the limb away from the stimulus. The nociceptive sensory afferents also have projections that cross to the contralateral side of the spinal cord before synapsing on interneurons. Stimulation of these interneurons leads to inhibition of the limb flexors and excitation of the extensors. The result of this crossed-extensor response is that the contralateral limb is made more rigid so that posture can be maintained during withdrawal of the stimulated limb. Other compensatory responses may also be activated: for example, movements of the other two limbs to help to maintain posture and balance.

The control of muscle tone

Even at rest, most skeletal muscles are not completely flaccid. This resting tension, or muscle tone, can be markedly reduced by cutting the dorsal spinal roots, implicating the muscle spindle afferents as important determinants of muscle tone. Inputs to α-motor neurons from higher CNS centers can have facilitatory or inhibitory effects on the basal excitation from the muscle spindle afferents.

The reticular formation and brainstem nuclei provide facilitatory inputs to spinal motor neurons. The vestibular nuclei are

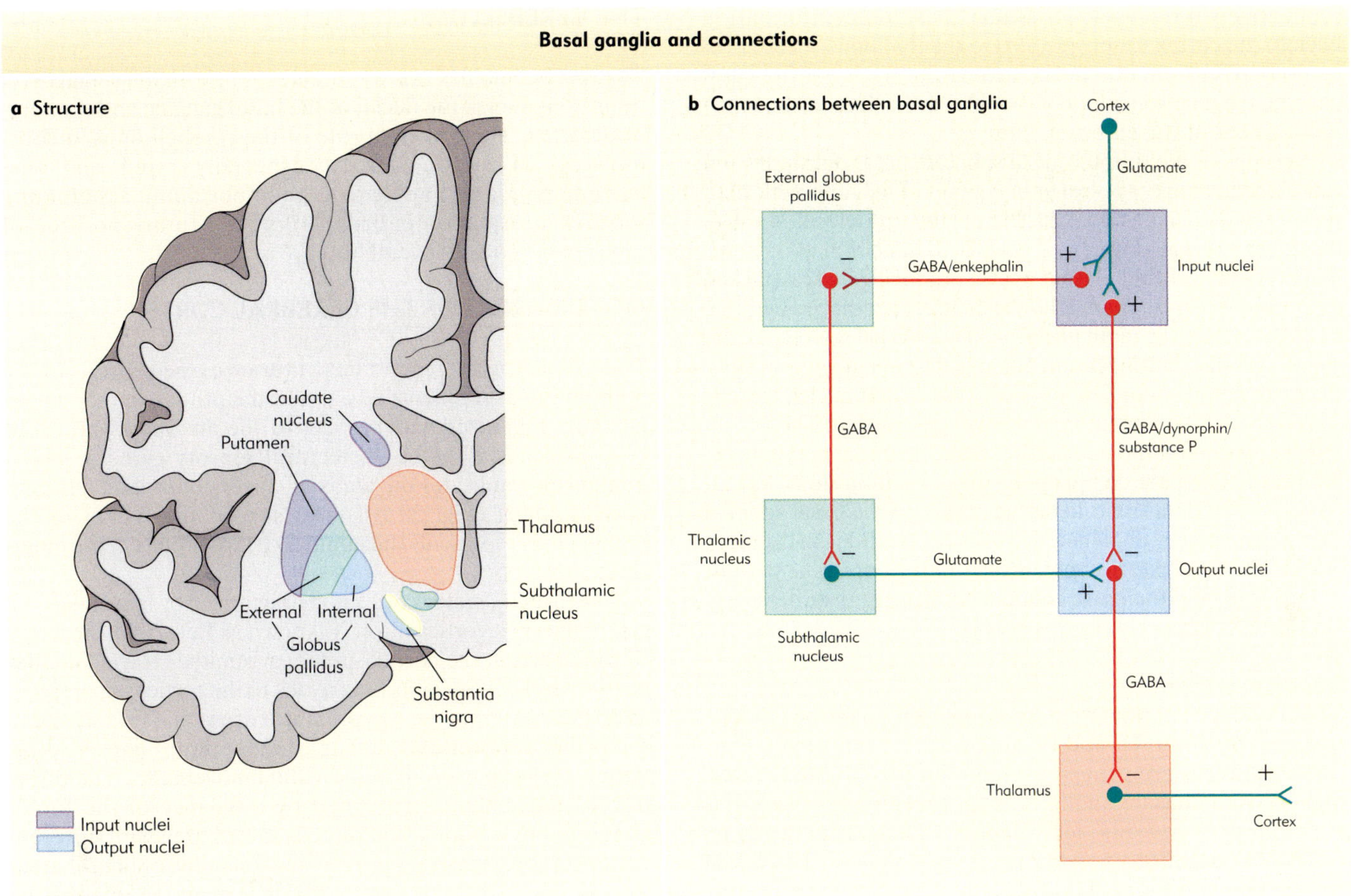

Figure 30.9 The basal ganglia and their connections.

specifically implicated in enhancing the tone of the postural muscles and are thought to coordinate actions to maintain posture against the influence of gravity. One example is the righting reflex, which is an ipsilateral extensor response to sudden tilting of the body to one side. A total spinal lesion, involving section of the spinal cord below the level of the vestibular nuclei, results in a flaccid paralysis. There is also a temporary loss of spinal reflexes below the level of section that recovers, possibly through development of a denervation sensitivity of the spinal motor neurons, enabling response to activation of muscle spindle afferents.

In contrast, section above the brainstem reticular formation (decerebration) in experimental animals dramatically increases muscle tone, especially in the postural and proximal limb muscles. Inhibition of the brainstem reticular formation is via the cerebellum and the basal ganglia, and it is through these centers that information from the cerebral cortex is relayed to the brainstem in order to make any reductions in postural muscle tone that are necessary for voluntary movements. Signals from the cortex to the peripheral muscle groups are carried in upper motor neurons that bypass the brainstem, running in the pyramidal tract (decussating in the medullary pyramids) and several extrapyramidal tracts.

Motor programs for the generation of stereotyped patterns of movement

Although the skeletal muscles are under voluntary control, most muscle activity is carried out at a subconscious level. In other words, we do not have to think about each movement necessary to carry out a task, let alone the individual muscles that we need to contract and relax in order to generate each movement. Rather, the cortical function is to activate motor programs that have been learned and from previous experience will result in the desired outcome. A motor program is defined as a set of commands that is generated in one area of the CNS before the onset of the relevant movement and that causes activation or inhibition of motor units in an appropriately timed sequence.

There is evidence from lower mammals that motor programs can be generated at all levels of the CNS. For example, section of the spinal cord above and below the segmental innervation of the leg results in walking movements, an example of a spinal motor program. In humans, the basal ganglia are recognized to be important regions for motor program generation; this is evidenced by dyskinesias, which result from diseases affecting the basal ganglia or their connections. Dyskinesias are repeated inappropriate movements of whole muscle groups that appear to be caused by spontaneous activity of the diseased basal ganglia.

THE BASAL GANGLIA

The basal ganglia consist of five subcortical nuclei (Fig. 30.9) that form one of the two major subcortical loops of the motor system: the other loop involves the cerebellum. The basal ganglia receive inputs from the entire cortex, which enter one of the two input nuclei, the caudate nucleus and putamen (collectively termed the striatum); these relay information back to the cortex via projections to the thalamus. These projections arise from one of the two output nuclei of the basal ganglia, the pars reticulata of the substantia nigra or the internal segment of the globus pallidus.

Neurons of the output nuclei spontaneously discharge and cause a reduction of the excitatory output of thalamocortic neurons. Excitation of the input nuclei from the cortex leads, through the direct pathway of the basal ganglia, to inhibition of the tonic inhibitory fibers of the output nuclei, producing increased excitation of the cortex. There is also an indirect neural circuit of the basal ganglia via the input nuclei and the external segment of the globus pallidus, causing disinhibition of the subthalamic nucleus. Excitatory fibers from here project to the output nuclei, thereby causing increased inhibition of the thalamic output. The overall effect depends on the balance between the direct and indirect pathways. The pars compacta of the substantia nigra has an important modulatory role on the output of the basal ganglia. This is mediated by dopaminergic neurons synapsing in the input nuclei. The basal ganglia contain 80% of the dopamine present in the brain, and the more common movement disorders (e.g. Parkinson's disease) affect this system.

Dopamine receptors

Seven subtypes of dopamine receptor have so far been identified in the brain; D_1 and D_2 are by far the most abundant. These subtypes are principally found in the striatum (input nuclei) of the basal ganglia. The D_1 receptor is linked to a stimulatory G protein (see Chapter 3); activation leads to increased formation of cAMP by adenylyl cyclase. The resultant increased protein phosphorylation causes increased conductance of several types of ion channel. Whether D_1 activation has an overall excitatory or inhibitory effect depends on the different ion channel populations of that particular cell. In the input nuclei of the basal ganglia, activation of D_1 receptors may lead to neuronal excitation or inhibition, depending on the subtype of the medium-sized spiny striatal neuron. Activation of D_2 receptors causes several cellular effects, including inhibition of cAMP formation via linkage to an inhibitory G protein and increased production of the second messengers IP_3 and diacylglycerol. However, perhaps the most important mechanism whereby stimulation of D_2 receptors produces reduced neuronal excitability is through increasing the conductance of K^+ channels, which leads to hyperpolarization of the cell.

In the input nuclei of the basal ganglia, dopamine activates the direct pathway via D_1 receptors and inhibits the indirect pathway via D_2 receptors. Both actions of dopamine lead to an increase in excitatory impulse transmission to the cortex. In Parkinson's disease, there is a striatal dopamine deficiency resulting from destruction of 70–90% of the dopaminergic neurons projecting from the pars compacta of the substantia nigra. This results in reduced cortical excitation, leading to rigidity through reduction of the inhibitory cortical effect on the brainstem nuclei and to bradykinesia through reduced corticospinal tract outflow.

The input nuclei of the basal ganglia also contain large cholinergic interneurons, stimulation of which opposes the effects of dopamine. The output of the basal ganglia tends to be phasic; damping of this variable output depends on the balance between dopaminergic and cholinergic activity. A resting tremor is another characteristic feature of Parkinson's disease.

THE CEREBELLUM

The cerebellum has two-way connections with the spinal cord, brainstem nuclei, the nuclei of the basal ganglia, and the cerebral cortex. The principal role of the cerebellum is in coordination of motor activity, especially rapid and fine movements. It also appears to be important in assimilating sensory information in order to predict future position of limbs in dextrous movements.

MOTOR AREAS OF THE CEREBRAL CORTEX

The primary motor cortex lies anterior to the central sulcus. Stimulation experiments reveal that the primary motor cortex is highly organized with respect to the anatomic pattern of responses. As with the postcentral sensory gyrus, a motor homunculus indicates the areas of cortex controlling different muscle goups (Fig. 30.10). The size of the region in the homunculus represents the number of motor units in the innervated muscles.

The primary motor cortex is characterized by large neuronal cell bodies in a cortical layer V, known as Betz cells, the axons of which run in the corticospinal (pyramidal) tracts. Smaller cells of layer V also contribute axons to the corticospinal tracts, as do neurons from the two premotor areas that lie anterior to the primary motor cortex. The primary motor cortex determines the force exerted in individual movements. The direction of movement is governed by a balance of the forces generated by a population of cells in this area with different vectors of force generation. The function of the premotor areas is to prepare the motor systems for movement. The medial and superior part of the premotor area, termed the supplementary motor area, programs motor sequences and coordinates bilateral movement. The lateral part of the premotor area, the premotor cortex, controls the proximal movements that project the arms to targets.

DRUG TREATMENT OF MOVEMENT DISORDERS

Parkinson's disease

Parkinson's disease, as described above, results from dopamine deficiency in the basal ganglia. Therapeutic approaches include the use of drugs to increase availability of dopamine, the use of dopaminergic receptor agonists, and the use of muscarinic cholinergic antagonists.

Levodopa (L-dihydroxyphenylalanine) is the amino acid precursor of dopamine but unlike dopamine, it is absorbed in the intestine and crosses the blood–brain barrier. It is taken up into cells by an amino acid transporter coupled to Na^+ transport. In the basal ganglia, it is converted into dopamine by DOPA decarboxylase. Decarboxylases are also found in many peripheral tissues; consequently, very little levadopa reaches the brain and the systemic dopamine production causes vomiting and hypotension. To increase availability of the drug to the brain, levadopa is administered in combination with *carbidopa,* a decarboxylase inhibitor that does not readily cross the blood–brain barrier. Side effects of levodopa/carbidopa combinations include nausea, vomiting, anorexia, postural hypotension, involuntary movements, and psychiatric disturbances.

Amantadine increases dopamine release from nerve terminals. Its principal use is in early disease before neuronal destruction is too advanced.

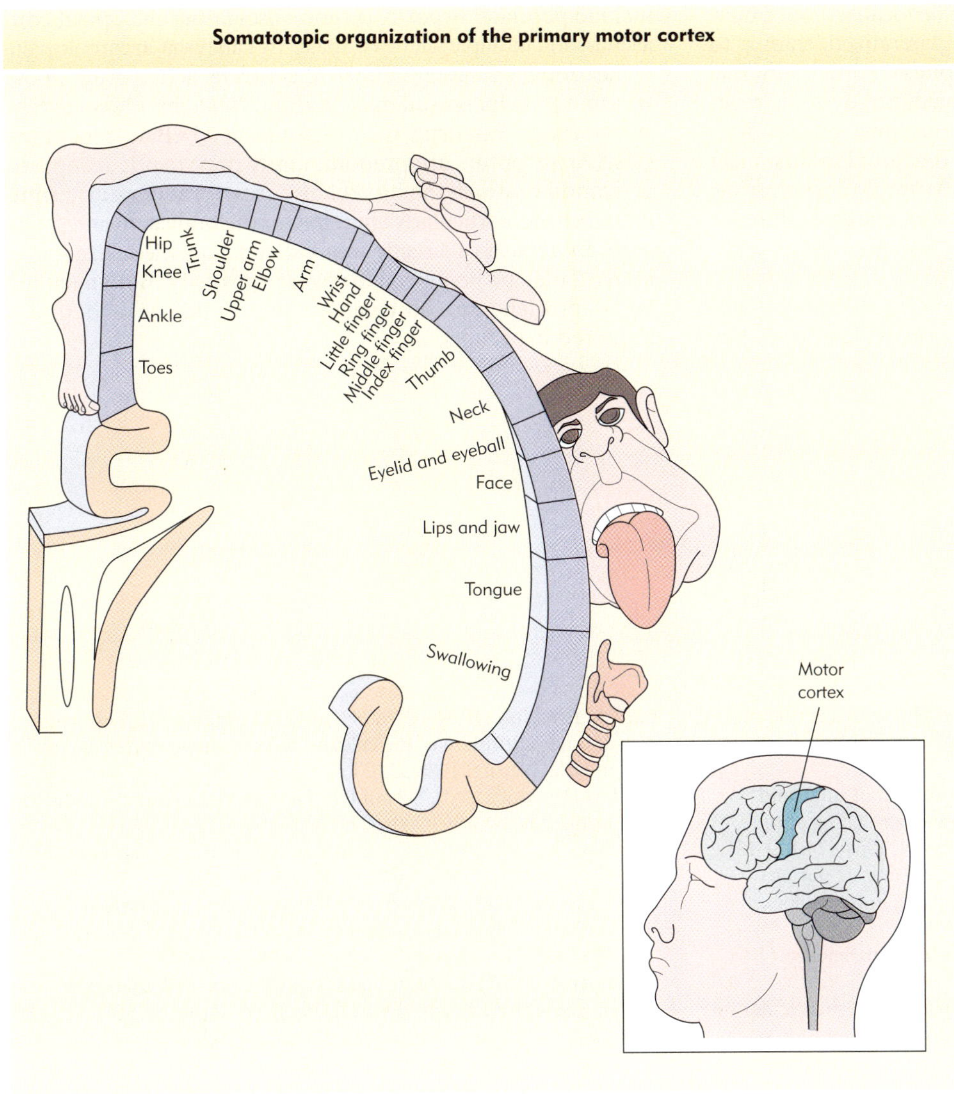

Figure 30.10 Somatotopic organization (motor homunculus) of the primary motor cortex. (With permission from Moffett et al., 1993)

Selegiline is a selective inhibitor of monoamine oxidase B (MAO-B) . It is effective in the treatment of Parkinson's disease In humans, MAO-B is primarily responsible for the degradation of dopamine in the basal ganglia, while MAO-A predominates in the periphery. Inhibition of MAO-A in the gut leads to sympathomimetic effects from tyramine-containing foods, but the use of selegiline is associated with few side effects. There does not appear to be a dangerous interaction with opioids as there is with nonselective MAO inhibitors.

Bromocriptine and *pergolide* are dopamine agonists that act at D_1 and D_2 receptors, although they are more potent at the D_2 subtype. This profile of dopaminergic effects provides the optimal therapeutic response in Parkinson's disease. Peripheral dopaminergic effects can cause nausea and vomiting, which can be treated with domperidone. Other side effects include hypotension, especially postural, and psychiatric disturbance. Bromocriptine is one of the known causes of retroperitoneal fibrosis. Bromocriptine has also been advocated in the treatment of neuroleptic malignant syndrome, a rare reaction to major tranquilizers which is characterized by severe rigidity, hyperpyrexia, and rhabdomyolysis. *Apomorphine* is a potent dopamine agonist that has been used in refractory parkinsonism. Administration must be preceded by domperidone to limit the severe emetic response.

Cholinergic antagonists were the first group of drugs used with benefit in Parkinson's disease, although they have largely been superseded by levodopa/carbidopa. They are most effective in early disease where tremor is the predominant feature. Peripheral anticholinergic side effects include dry mouth, blurred vision owing to mydriasis, urinary retention, and constipation; confusion and agitation are central side effects. The two most commonly used drugs of this class are benzatropine (benztropine) and trihexyphenidyl (benzhexol), which have the additional beneficial action of blocking dopamine reuptake into nerve terminals.

Parkinsonian and other extrapyramidal reactions

Similar symptoms to the more common idiopathic Parkinson's disease can be caused by drugs with antidopaminergic effects, such as the major tranquilizers (phenothiazines, butyrophenones) and metoclopramide. Such drugs are commonly used in the prophylaxis and treatment of postoperative nausea and vomiting, where parenteral administration can lead to acute dystonic reactions in which there is simultaneous activation of opposing muscle groups. Dystonias can be localized, for example to produce an oculogyric crisis, or generalized, leading to painful, abnormal postures (opisthotonus). Anticholinergic drugs are the drugs of choice for drug-induced dystonic reactions and can be given parenterally (benzatropine, procyclidine, diphenhydramine) when the reaction is acute. Parkinsonism may also be secondary to encephalitis or arteriosclerosis. Treatment here is the same as for the idiopathic condition.

Spasticity

Spasticity is caused by chronic dissociation of lower motor neurons from upper motor neuron influences. Common causes include perinatal hypoxia, cerebrovascular insults, spinal cord lesions, and multiple sclerosis. Spasticity can result in chronic pain.

Benzodiazepines are effective centrally acting drugs in the treatment of increased muscle tone. *Baclofen* is also extensively used; this drug is an agonist at $GABA_B$ receptors. $GABA_B$ receptors are predominantly presynaptic receptors, activation of which inhibits release of several neurotransmitters: they are particularly abundant in the brainstem and spinal cord. *Dantrolene*, a directly acting skeletal muscle relaxant (see above), may be beneficial in severe spasticity. Both baclofen and dantrolene can cause nausea, muscle fatigue, and, rarely, impaired liver function.

Key References

Carlsson A. The occurrence, distribution and physiological role of catecholamines in the nervous system. Pharmacol Rev. 1959;11:490–3.

Crowe A, Matthews PBC. The effects of stimulation of static and dynamic fusimotor fibers on the response to stretching of the primary endings of muscle spindles. J Physiol. 1964;174:109–131.

Huxley AF, Niedergerke R. Structural changes in muscle during contraction. Interference microscopy of living muscle fibers. Nature. 1954;173:971–3.

Huxley HE. The mechanism of muscular contraction. Science. 1969;164:1356–66.

Huxley H, Hanson J. Changes in the cross-striations of muscle during contraction and stretch and their structural interpretation. Nature. 1954;173:973–6.

Lai FA, Erickson HP, Rousseau E, Lui QY, Meissner G. Purification and reconstitution of the calcium release channel from skeletal muscle. Nature. 1988;331:315–19.

Moffett DF, Moffett SB, Schauf CL. Human Physiology, 2nd edn. St. Louis: Mosby; 1993:290–323.

Renshaw B. Central effects of centripetal impulses in axons of spinal ventral roots. J Neurophysiol. 1941;9:191–204.

Rios E, Brum G. Involvement of dihydropyridine receptors in excitation–contraction coupling in skeletal muscle. Nature. 1987;325:717–20.

Sherrington CS. Decerebrate rigidity, and reflex coordination of movement. J Physiol. 1898;22:319–32.

Somlyo AP. The messenger across the gap. Nature. 1985;316:298–9.

Further Reading

Freund H-J. Motor unit and muscle activity in voluntary motor control. Physiol Rev. 1983;63:387–436.

Grillner S, Wallen P. Central pattern generators for locomotion, with special reference to vertebrates. Annu Rev Neurosci. 1985;8:233–61.

Hopkins PM, Ellis FR. Inherited disease affecting anaesthesia. In: Healy TEJ, Cohen PJ, eds. A practice of anaesthesia, 6th edn. London: Edward Arnold; 1995:938–52.

Huxley AF. Review lecture: muscular contraction. J Physiol. 1974;243:1–43.

Kandel ER, Schwartz JH, Jessel TM. Principles of neural science, 3rd edn. New York: Elsevier; 1991:Chs 35–42.

Marsden CD, Rothwell JC, Day BL. The use of peripheral feedback in the control of movement. Trend Neurosci. 1984;7:253–7.

Moss RL, Diffee GM, Greaser ML. Contractile properties of skeletal muscle fibers in relation to myofibrillar protein isoforms. Rev Physiol Biochem Pharmacol. 1995;126:1–63.

Chapter 31 Neuromuscular junction physiology

Chris Prior and Ian G Marshall

Topics covered in this chapter

The neuromuscular junction
Acetylcholine metabolism
Acetylcholine release
Motor end-plate excitation
Regulation of transmission

The neuromuscular junction is an intercellular relay structure designed for the efficient communication between the motor axon and skeletal muscle fiber. It is the most studied and best understood mammalian synapse. The neuromuscular junction is a chemical synapse and, as such, behaves as a pair of transducers, the motor nerve terminal and the muscle motor end plate, arranged in series (Fig. 31.1). As with any transducer, each has an input and an output signal. In the case of the motor nerve terminal, the input signal is a depolarizing wave produced by an action potential in the terminal part of the incoming axon and the output signal is the synchronous release of the chemical neurotransmitter acetylcholine into the junctional cleft of the neuromuscular junction. For the muscle motor end-plate, the input signal is acetylcholine in the junctional cleft and the output signal is an action potential in the muscle fiber membrane. The entire functioning of the neuromuscular junction revolves around the efficient execution of these two transducer tasks. This complex signal transduction mechanism between the motor nerve and muscle cell allows for signal amplification and modulation. There is insufficient energy in the action potential to excite the muscle fiber membrane directly, so some form of energy-dependent signal amplification is necessary. By altering the amount of acetylcholine released in response to motor nerve terminal depolarization, or by altering the sensitivity of the postjunctional muscle membrane to acetylcholine, the neuromuscular junction can be fine-tuned for optimum performance. This chapter describes the cellular structures and processes required for efficient communication between the motor nerve and skeletal muscle fiber. First, the cellular and subcellular anatomy of the neuromuscular junction is described, followed by a discussion of the physiologic processes involved in the functioning of both the pre- and postjunctional elements of the system.

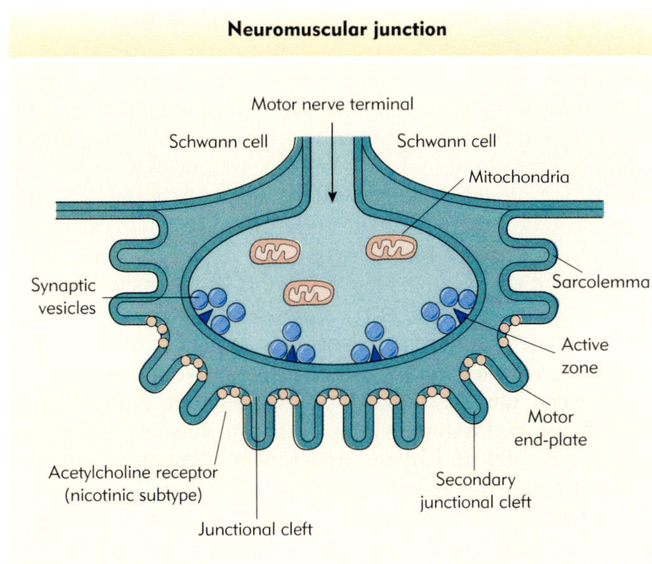

Figure 31.1 The neuromuscular junction showing key structural features.

THE NEUROMUSCULAR JUNCTION

Prejunctional morphology

As the motor nerve fiber (containing numerous axons) approaches a skeletal muscle, it branches extensively, sending terminal axons to many separate muscle fibers. A single motor neuron and the group of muscle fibers it innervates are collectively termed a motor unit. The muscle fibers within any single motor unit are not grouped together but are scattered throughout the muscle. All muscle fibers within a single motor unit contract simultaneously when excited. In mammalian skeletal muscle, as the terminal axon approaches the single muscle fiber it innervates it loses its Schwann cell myelin sheath (Chapter 18) and branches into a number of bouton-like structures that lie in close apposition to the muscle fiber membrane. This structure is referred to as the *motor nerve terminal*. The boutons are compact structures that contain all the essential elements for the synthesis, storage, and release of acetylcholine. The bulk of the motor nerve terminal cytoplasm is filled with numerous synaptic vesicles: spherical bilayer membrane structures of approximately 60–100nm in diameter that store acetylcholine. Synaptic vesicles are distributed throughout the motor nerve terminal but are particularly concentrated around electron-dense structures on the nerve terminal membrane, referred to as active zones. Active zones are thought to be the sites at which vesicular exocytosis of acetylcholine occurs; they are believed to comprise the molecular components required for synaptic vesicle docking and fusion with the nerve terminal cell membrane. Freeze-fracture electron microscopy reveals that active zones are not diffuse, disorganized structures but consist of an ordered arrangement of a number of large intramembranous particles, called active zone particles. Each active zone is composed of four parallel lines of such particles. Within the active zone, the lines are arranged in two pairs. Given their dimension, the active zone particles are thought to be large, multisubunited, membrane-spanning proteins. One obvious candidate for this protein is the nerve terminal membrane voltage-gated Ca^{2+} channel, which is instrumental in the evoked release of acetylcholine (Chapter 19 and below). Electron microscopy shows that synaptic vesicles close to the active zone are also arranged in a highly ordered fashion in a pair of parallel rows in line with the active zone particles (Fig. 31.2), which further implicates the latter in synaptic vesicle docking and fusion with the nerve terminal membrane.

Aside from synaptic vesicles, the only other major subcellular organelles present in the motor nerve terminal are mitochondria, which are necessary for the high levels of metabolism required for the synthesis, storage, and release of acetylcholine (see below). The motor nerve terminal has no protein synthesis or Golgi processing apparatus; these processes take place within the cell body of the motor neuron in the spinal cord. The motor axon possesses a highly developed bidirectional axonal transport system that allows the facilitated movement of cellular components between the nerve cell body and the axon terminals. Synaptic vesicles do not move around freely within the terminal cytoplasm; throughout the nerve terminal there is an extensive network of intracellular filaments, composed mostly of actin. Microtubules, although present as a component of the axonal transport systems, do not extend to the nerve terminal membrane. The nerve terminal actin filaments are thought to be important in the anchoring of synaptic vesicles within the nerve terminal and in the ordered movement of synaptic vesicles towards and away from the active-zone release sites. Although initially created in the cell body, there is clear evidence that mature synaptic vesicles within the motor nerve terminal can undergo repeated cycles of filling and exocytosis.

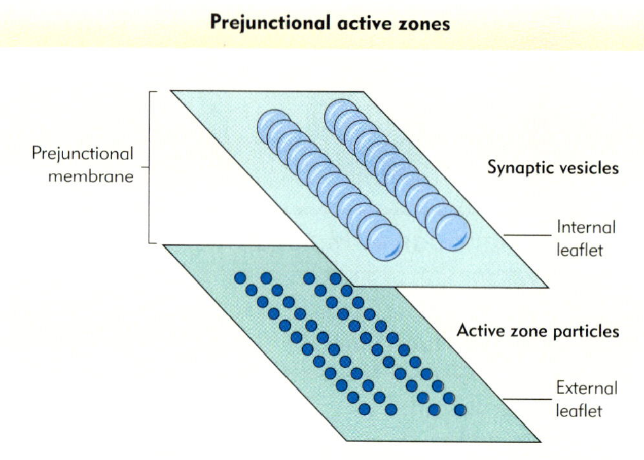

Figure 31.2 Structural organization of prejunctional active zones. Expanded view of the motor nerve terminal membrane showing the organization of synaptic vesicles and large intramembranous active zone particles, as revealed by electron microscopy.

Postjunctional morphology

The motor end-plate is the specialized region of the skeletal muscle fiber membrane that is chemically receptive to acetylcholine released from motor nerve terminals. In mammalian skeletal muscle, there is a deep recess in the muscle fiber membrane, the junctional cleft, at the contact of the terminal part of the motor nerve with the muscle fiber. The nerve terminal is essentially surrounded by the muscle fiber membrane and the terminal Schwann cell, which extends down to the muscle fiber membrane (Fig. 31.1). The muscle fiber membrane in apposition to the nerve terminal is folded into deep clefts, called secondary junctional clefts. The junctional gap is narrowest (~60nm) at the peaks of the postjunctional folds, between the secondary clefts. These crests are opposite the release sites on the prejunctional membrane and are the locations of postjunctional acetylcholine receptors (AChRs). These receptors are highly concentrated ($>10{,}000/\mu m^2$) in the shoulder regions between the secondary clefts. This is a consequence of their being fixed both to each other and also to an underlying cytoskeletal matrix. During development, AChRs aggregate and anchor to appropriate sites; the mechanisms by which this occurs are poorly understood. The receptors are also found on muscle membranes outside the region of the motor end-plate, but these receptors are sparsely distributed and have a much shorter half-life (20 hours) than the receptors at the motor end-plate (several weeks). The AChR at the motor end-plate is of the nicotinic subtype (nAChR) in that nicotine can mimic the effects of acetylcholine on this receptor.

The space between the muscle and nerve terminal membranes, the junctional cleft, is filled with a basement membrane material rich in collagen-like mucopolysaccharides. The basement membrane probably functions as a structural support, but it must also allow the free and rapid diffusion of acetylcholine through the junctional space. A second role of the basement membrane is to act as a trap for acetylcholinesterase, which has a strong affinity for the collagen-like components of the matrix (see below).

The acetylcholine receptor

The nAChR on the postjunctional membrane of the neuromuscular junction is the best characterized member of a 'superfamily' of closely related ligand-gated ion channels (see Chapters 3 and 19). This receptor superfamily includes excitatory receptors such as all central and ganglionic nAChRs, the 5-hydroxytryptamine $5HT_3$ receptor, the AMPA-type (α-amino-3-hydroxy-5-methyl-4-isoxazole) glutamate receptor and inhibitory receptors such as the $GABA_A$ (γ-aminobutyric acid type A) receptor and the glycine receptor. The general structure of channels in the family is believed to be similar, although there are some important differences. The nAChRs are acetylcholine-activated nonselective cation channels. Each macromolecular complex contains two binding sites for acetylcholine that, when occupied, trigger a conformational change to open the channel pore through which Na^+, K^+, and, to a lesser extent, Ca^{2+} can flow.

The nAChR at the neuromuscular junction is pentameric: it is composed of five individual protein subunits each with the same basic structure (Fig. 31.3a). The complex has a molecular weight of approximately 270,000. Each subunit is a single protein chain of 440–500 amino acid residues with both the N- and C-terminal ends on the extracellular side of the cell membrane.

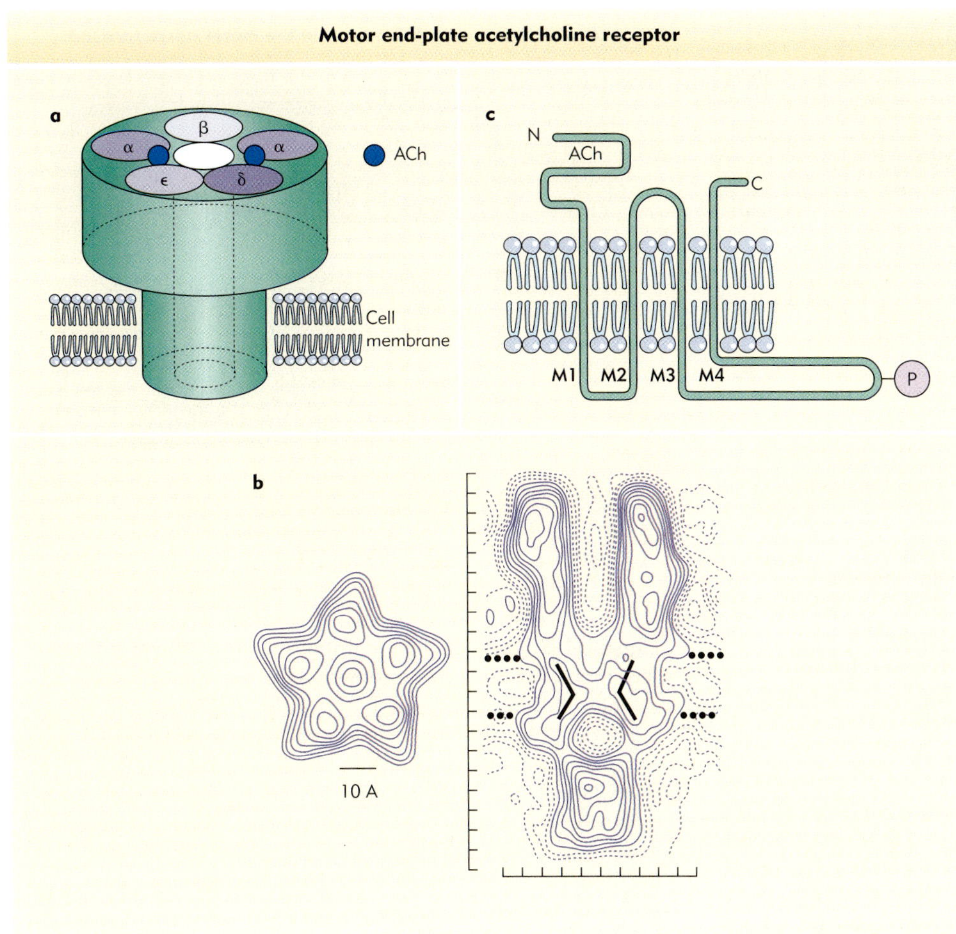

Figure 31.3 Motor end-plate acetylcholine receptor. (a) Structure of the nicotinic acetylcholine receptor (nAChR). The five protein subunits are arranged around the central ion channel pore. Two acetylcholine-binding sites (ACh) are shown at the interfaces of the α- and ϵ-subunits and the α- and δ-subunits. Note that the bulk of the receptor protein resides on the extracellular side of the cell membrane. (b) Electron-density maps of the *Torpedo* nAChR. High-resolution electron microscopy of the extracellular face (left) showing fivefold symmetry and a cross-sectional view (right) showing the extracellular portion and the likely gate (bent lines). Graduations are 1nm. (With permission from Unwin, 1993, 1995.) (c) An individual subunit of the nAChR. A Phosphorylation site (P) on the β- and δ-subunits.

The protein strand traverses the cell membrane four times; the hydrophobic transmembrane segments are designated M1, M2, M3, and M4. These membrane-spanning regions were originally believed to be α-helices, but there is now some evidence to suggest that they may be β-pleated sheets. There is a large (about 200 amino acid residues) extracellular segment at the N-terminus; in the appropriate subunits, this region contains the acetylcholine-binding site. There is an intracellular loop of around 80 to 100 amino acid residues between M3 and M4 that contains several phosphorylation sites thought to be involved in receptor desensitization.

Four different subunits are found in each nAChR complex at the adult motor end-plate. Two identical α-subunits are combined with one each of the β-, ϵ-, and δ-subunits ($\alpha_2\beta\epsilon\delta$). The α-subunits contain the bulk of the acetylcholine recognition site. They are characterized by two disulfide-coupled cysteine residues at sites 192 and 193, which are thought to be involved in acetylcholine binding. In fetal muscle, denervated adult muscle, and in the electric organ of *Torpedo* there is a γ-subunit rather than an ϵ-subunit ($\alpha_2\beta\gamma\delta$). In each nAChR complex, the five subunits are arranged in a structure that resembles a goblet spanning the cell membrane: the cup being made from the N-terminal regions of each subunit (Fig. 31.3b,c). The stem of the goblet spans the cell membrane and forms the transmembrane cation channel. The ordering for the subunits around the pore is α–β–α–ϵ–δ and the two acetylcholine-binding sites are thought to be located on the α-subunits at the interfaces with the ϵ- and δ-subunits.

Site-directed mutagenesis has been used to show that the ion specificity of the nAChR is determined by the amino acid sequence of the M2; this region of each subunit lines the ion channel pore. In the inactive state of the channel, M2 regions of each of the five subunits are close together and the channel is closed. When two acetylcholine molecules bind to their binding sites, the receptor undergoes a conformational change that leads to the movement of the membrane-spanning regions relative to each other and the opening of the channel.

Acetylcholinesterase

Acetylcholinesterase (AChE) catalyzes the hydrolysis of acetylcholine to choline and acetate. The enzymic activity of AChE resides in a globular catalytic subunit. Hydrolysis of acetylcholine by the catalytic subunit involves the formation of an acyl enzyme, which, given the high catalytic efficiency of the enzyme, must be short lived. Attack by water restores enzymic activity, liberating acetate. There is considerable diversity in the macromolecular assembly of AChE. At the neuromuscular junction, the principal form of AChE is the asymmetric or A_{12} species (Fig. 31.4). In this species of AChE, three groups of four catalytic subunits each are anchored by disulfide bonds to filamentous, collagen-containing structural subunits. The collagen-containing tail of the macromolecular complex associates with the basal lamina of the postjunctional membrane, rather than the postjunctional membrane itself. The macromolecular complex has the appearance of a bunch of flowers sprouting from the postjunctional motor end plate.

Structure of the motor end-plate acetylcholinesterase

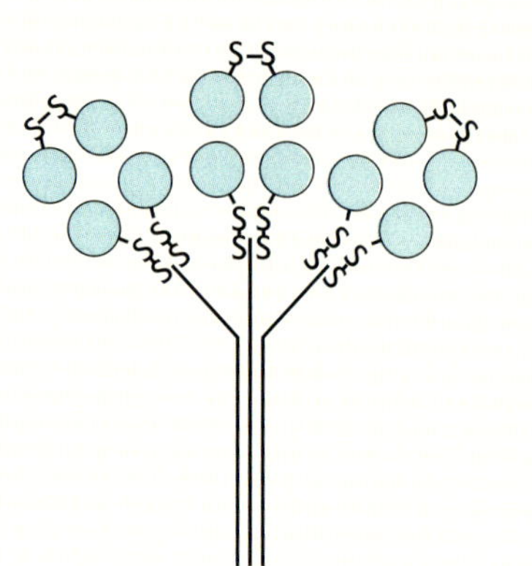

Figure 31.4 The structure of the motor end-plate acetylcholinesterase. At this site, 12 globular catalytic acetylcholinesterase subunits are organized into an asymmetric (A_{12}) macromolecular structure. The tail element of the macromolecular complex is largely composed of trihelical collagen and has a high affinity for the basal lamina within the junctional cleft of the neuromuscular junction.

Acetylcholine metabolism within the motor nerve terminal

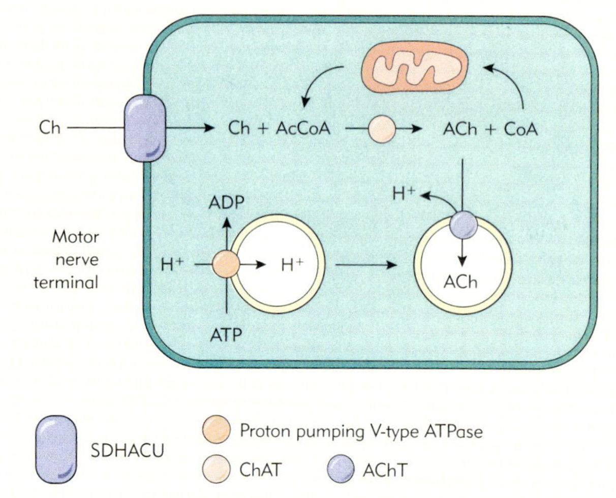

Figure 31.5 Acetylcholine metabolism within the motor nerve terminal. Choline is concentrated in the nerve terminal cytoplasm through the action of the plasma membrane sodium-dependent high-affinity choline uptake system (SDHACU). Cytoplasmic choline is acetylated by choline acetyl-O-methyltransferase, utilizing mitochondrially derived acetyl CoA as a substrate. Finally, a two-stage process loads acetylcholine into synaptic vesicles. The interior of the synaptic vesicle becomes acidic as a result of H^+ entry through a proton-pumping ATPase. The acetylcholine transporter exchanges vesicular protons for cytoplasmic acetylcholine. Ch, choline; AcCoA, acetyl coenzyme A; AChT, acetylcholine transporter; ChAT, choline acetyl-O-methyltransferase.

The catalytic sites have good access to acetylcholine in the junctional cleft while being firmly anchored to the motor end-plate region. A second class of cholinersterase enzyme (butyrylcholinesterase or pseudocholinesterase) exists that is encoded by separate genes and has different substrate specificity and tissue distribution. Butyrylcholinesterase is not present in the synaptic cleft of the neuromuscular junction but is present in plasma.

ACETYLCHOLINE METABOLISM

In order for the motor nerve terminal to release acetylcholine in response to activation, systems must exist for the accumulation of choline and the synthesis and storage of acetylcholine (Fig. 31.5).

Nerve terminal choline transport

The main precursor of acetylcholine is the quaternary amine, choline. Nerve cells of higher animals are unable to manufacture choline and so rely on external sources such as the diet or manufacture in the liver. Quaternary amines contain a nitrogen atom with a fixed positive charge. As such, these molecules are unable to cross lipophilic cell membranes by passive diffusion and require a carrier mechanism to allow the molecule access to the nerve terminal. Two separate choline transport mechanisms have been described in nervous tissue. One system has a relatively low affinity for choline (K_m = 50–200μmol/L), is widely distributed throughout all nervous tissue, and does not show marked energy dependence. The distribution of this low-affinity system does not correlate with the distribution of acetylcholine synthesis and is probably not related to cholinergic neurotransmission. More likely it is concerned with the supply of intracellular choline for phosphatidylcholine and sphingomyelin metabolism. The second membrane choline transport system is far more selective in its distribution and far more specific in its functional role. The sodium-dependent high-affinity choline uptake (SDHACU) is found only in cholinergic nerve terminals and, consequently, has a distribution in brain tissue that closely matches acetylcholine synthesis. Further, the normal functioning of the SDHACU system is a prerequisite for the efficient synthesis of acetylcholine by cholinergic nerve terminals. Under normal conditions, about half of the choline produced in the junctional cleft from the destruction of neurally released acetylcholine is returned to the nerve terminal through the action of SDHACU.

SDHACU has a relatively high affinity for choline (K_m = 1–5μmol/L) and a strict dependence on the presence of extracellular Na^+. SDHACU can transport choline against its concentration gradient, going from approximately 10μmol/L in the junctional cleft to around 30mmol/L in the nerve terminal cytoplasm. As such, it can be classified as an active carrier-mediated transport system. In addition to having a relatively high affinity for choline, SDHACU will transport all the *N*-ethyl derivatives of choline but is unable to translocate the transmitter molecule acetylcholine itself. The exact mechanism underlying choline transport by SDHACU is unclear. Given the existence of a large transmembrane Na^+ gradient, it is possible that choline uptake involves co-transport with Na^+ across the nerve terminal membrane.

Acetylcholine synthesis

Acetylcholine is synthesized in the nerve terminal cytoplasm by the addition of an acetyl group to choline in a reaction catalyzed by the enzyme choline acetyl-*O*-methyltransferase. This enzyme is synthesized in the cell body of motor nerve cells and transported to the nerve terminal by axoplasmic transport involving neurofilaments. The localization of choline acetyltransferase to cholinergic nerve endings is highly specific and, consequently, this enzyme has been used as a specific marker for cholinergic neurotransmission in the CNS. The acetyl moiety required for the synthesis of acetylcholine from choline is derived from acetyl CoA that is synthesized by the decarboxylation of pyruvate within the matrix of the nerve terminal mitochondria. Choline acetyltransferase exists in the nerve terminal in unbound (soluble) and membrane-bound isoforms. There is evidence that these two isoforms of the enzyme may not be identical, but the exact role of each in the normal synthesis of acetylcholine by motor nerve terminals is unknown. Acetylcholine synthesis appears to be intimately linked to choline uptake by SDHACU. This could be as a result of a physical coupling between choline acetyltransferase and SDHACU. Alternatively, it could reflect a rate-limiting kinetic interaction. The bulk of choline that is translocated by SDHACU is converted to acetylcholine; if SDHACU had a considerably lower rate than choline acetyltransferase (i.e. it was rate-limiting), then any change in the activity of SDHACU would result in altered acetylcholine synthesis.

Vesicular storage of acetylcholine

Once synthesized in the nerve terminal cytoplasm, acetylcholine is packaged into synaptic vesicles from which it can be released by exocytosis. Acetylcholine transport into synaptic vesicles is a distinct process from choline uptake mediated by SDHACU. The synaptic vesicle acetylcholine transporter is an exchange pump. The driving force for bringing acetylcholine into the interior of synaptic vesicles is a transvesicular membrane proton gradient. The interior pH of cholinergic synaptic vesicles have been estimated to be 5.2–5.5. This is considerably lower than the cytoplasmic pH of around 7.0 and represents an ample energy gradient to drive acetylcholine accumulation (acetylcholine/proton antiport). The acidic interior of the synaptic vesicle is produced by a Mg^{2+}-dependent vesicular membrane proton pumping (V-type) ATPase. Thus, the uptake of acetylcholine by synaptic vesicles is a two-stage process utilizing ATP as its energy source. There is evidence suggesting that synaptic vesicle filling is a dynamic process. There is considerable passive leakage of acetylcholine from synaptic vesicles and, under certain conditions, the total acetylcholine content of cholinergic synaptic vesicles appears to be dependent on the level of free acetylcholine within the nerve terminal cytoplasm.

In addition to high concentrations of acetylcholine, cholinergic synaptic vesicles contain high concentrations of ATP and Ca^{2+}. The reason for the presence of the former is uncertain, although it has been suggested that ATP may act as a co-transmitter released along with acetylcholine. In this respect, ATP would have a very different role to its role at the sympathetic neuroeffector junction. At the neuromuscular junction, ATP has no direct postjunctional excitatory or inhibitory effects. However, it is possible either ATP or enzymatically derived adenosine could have modulatory roles on nerve terminal function, either to increase or to decrease transmitter release. The presence of a high concentration of Ca^{2+} in cholinergic synaptic vesicles suggests that synaptic vesicles may act as a Ca^{2+} buffering system that removes Ca^{2+} from the nerve terminal cytoplasm via a vesicle membrane Ca^{2+} ATPase for extrusion to the extracellular space upon exocytosis.

ACETYLCHOLINE RELEASE

The release of acetylcholine from motor nerve terminals is quantal. At a typical mammalian neuromuscular junction, each time the motor nerve terminal is activated there is the Ca^{2+}-dependent synchronous release of 50–100 discrete packets (quanta) of acetylcholine, each comprising around 10,000 molecules. Each unit of released acetylcholine has been termed a quantum of transmitter and this unit has been correlated with the exocytotic discharge of the entire contents of a single synaptic vesicle. There are four identifiable phases involved in the synaptic vesicle exocytotic process. First, in order for the content of a synaptic vesicle to be released, the vesicle must be translocated to the release sites on the nerve terminal membrane (mobilization) and attached to these sites so that the exocytotic release process can be initiated (docking). Once mobilized and docked, the contents of the synaptic vesicle can be released. The physical process of exocytosis is initiated by a trigger and subsequent to this a host of specialized proteins on the synaptic vesicle and nerve terminal membrane participate in the formation of an exocytotic pore (fusion pore formation). Fusion pore formation leads to exocytosis and acetylcholine release. However, whether it inevitably leads to the total coalescence of the nerve terminal and synaptic vesicle membranes is uncertain. Following the depletion of the synaptic vesicle content, retrieval and recycling of the spent synaptic vesicles occurs (Chapter 19).

The release of acetylcholine from motor nerve terminals following depolarization is highly dependent on the presence of extracellular Ca^{2+}. The concentration of Ca^{2+} in the motor nerve terminal cytoplasm at rest is strictly regulated and very low (~0.1μmol/L, compared with approximately 1000μmol/L in the extracellular space). A rise in intracellular Ca^{2+} concentration is the trigger for exocytosis. In the absence of depolarization, increasing nerve terminal membrane permeabililty to Ca^{2+}, either by physical disruption or by use of a Ca^{2+} ionophore such as A23187, leads to the massive asynchronous release of quanta of acetylcholine. The link between nerve terminal membrane depolarization and a rise in the intracellular concentration of Ca^{2+} is the nerve terminal membrane voltage-gated Ca^{2+} channel. These channels are found in close apposition to the vesicular release sites, are opened in response to membrane depolarization, and allow Ca^{2+} access to the Ca^{2+}-dependent trigger mechanisms for exocytosis. The molecular mechanisms involved in synaptic vesicular exocytosis are complex and highly regulated processes (Chapter 19).

MOTOR END-PLATE EXCITATION

When acetylcholine interacts with its binding sites on the nAChR it produces a conformational change in the receptor that opens a nonselective cation channel (Fig. 31.6). Activitation of this channel leads to the generation of an action potential in the muscle sarcolemma. In its resting state, the motor end plate is at the same potential as the rest of the muscle fiber membrane (near –80mV in mammalian species). Opening of a nonselective cation channel allows Na^+ and K^+ to move across the sarcolemma down their

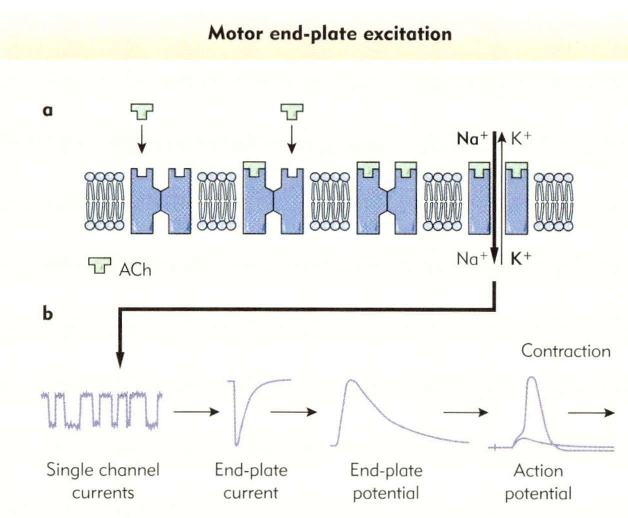

Figure 31.6 Motor end-plate excitation. (a) Agonist binding results in current flow. In its resting state, the nicotinic acetylcholine receptor is closed and impermeable to ions. Following acetylcholine (ACh) binding to its recognition sites, the protein undergoes a conformation change that leads to the formation of a pore through the cell membrane through which cations can freely pass, driven by their transmembrane electrochemical gradients. (b) Single channel current leads to muscle contraction. Cations flowing through many thousands of individual receptor proteins lead to considerable electrical current flowing across the motor end plate. This inward current (depicted as a downward curve) depolarizes the end plate, which triggers a depolarizing action potential in the muscle fiber membrane (depicted as an upward curve). This propagating signal, in turn, leads to the activation of the muscle contractile machinery.

respective electrochemical gradients. Their electrochemical gradients are determined by the membrane potential and the distribution of the ions on either side of the membrane. Because the resting membrane potential is much closer to the K^+ equilibrium potential (about –90mV) than to the Na^+ equilibrium potential (about +40mV), the predominant movement of ions through the open channel is Na^+ into the muscle cell. However, as the membrane becomes progressively depolarized through Na^+ influx, K^+ will flow outwards.

The sequence of electrical events leading from single channel currents to the generation of muscle contraction is illustrated in Figure 31.6b. The ion flow at individual channels can be measured by patch-clamp techniques as single channel currents. Single channel currents are brief, square-wave pulses, the duration of which represents channel open times and the amplitude of which represents current flow (Chapter 5). The closing of an open ion channel is a probabilistic event and, therefore, open times are exponentially distributed, such that there are many short openings and fewer longer openings. At the neuromuscular junction there are thousands of receptors available for interaction with released acetylcholine. The release of acetylcholine from an individual synaptic vesicle results in the near simultaneous opening of hundreds to thousands of ion channels. The result is a miniature end-plate current (MEPC), which represents the sum of all the single channel currents involved. Because of the exponential open-time distribution of single channel currents, the MEPC amplitude decays exponentially with time. The time course of this exponential decay is the same as the mean of the single channel open times. Each channel opening is an all-or-nothing event: the amplitude of the single channel current is independent of the acetylcholine concentration. However, the MEPC is a graded response, depending on the number of channel openings contributing to its occurrence. During normal evoked release there are tens of quanta of acetylcholine released simultaneously. This results in the evoked end-plate current (EPC), which, like the MEPC, can be measured under voltage-clamp conditions. As for MEPC, the EPC amplitudes are directly related to the amount of acetylcholine interacting with receptors (i.e. how many channels are open). Although much valuable mechanistic information has been gained from patch-clamp and voltage-clamp recording techniques, normal neuromuscular transmission does not operate under such conditions. The current changes described above result in changes in membrane potential, the miniature end-plate potential (MEPP) and end-plate potential (EPP), respectively. Like the EPC, the EPP is also graded according to the amount of acetylcholine released, although the relationship is not direct.

The single channel current, the EPC, and the EPP are all produced by acetylcholine action at the specialized, chemically receptive area of the muscle membrane at the neuromuscular junction. The remainder of the muscle membrane does not normally express acetylcholine receptors, but it is electrically excitable. The trigger for this excitation is the EPP. The EPP represents depolarization of the chemically excitable part of the muscle membrane (muscle end plate) relative to the adjacent electrically excitable membrane. Whenever two adjacent areas of unequal potential exist, local circuit currents flow in an attempt to equalize the potentials, which depolarizes the area just surrounding the neuromuscular junction. If this is great enough (reaches the threshold potential for Na^+ channel activation), Na^+ channels open in the electrically excitable membrane, which initiates a self-propagating muscle action potential that activates the contractile mechanism by inducing Ca^{2+} release from the sarcoplasmic reticulum (Chapter 30). The margin of safety for neuromuscular transmission is determined by the size of the EPP compared with the action potential threshold. The muscle action potential is an all-or-nothing response, as is the contraction response in an individual muscle fiber. However, the gross muscle contraction is made up of the sum of the contractions of individual fibers; it can, therefore, be graded according to how many fibers are contracting in an all-or-nothing fashion. Therefore, the whole process, from single channel current to contraction, represents a series of either graded or all-or-nothing responses occurring in populations of structures. This is an important consideration when interpreting data from tension studies such as those used when monitoring neuromuscular transmission and neuromuscular block in humans.

REGULATION OF TRANSMISSION

Prejunctional regulation

Neuromuscular transmission, like other forms of neurotransmission, is a highly regulated phenomenon. One of the main ways in which the performance of the system can be either enhanced or depressed is through the modulation of the amount of acetylcholine released by the motor nerve terminal in response to activation. There is abundant evidence that the motor nerve terminal membrane contains receptors that can alter the evoked release of acetylcholine. Perhaps the best characterized are those for acetylcholine itself (autoreceptors) and for adenosine. Others postulated to exist on motor nerve terminals include α_1- and β_1-adrenoceptors and receptors for ATP and CGRP (calcitonin-gene-related peptide).

Both muscarinic and nicotinic acetylcholine autoreceptors have been proposed to exist on motor nerve terminals. However, no clear picture has yet emerged as to the presence or role of these receptors. With respect to prejunctional nicotinic acetylcholine autoreceptors, some researchers claim a predominantly inhibitory role for these receptors, reducing acetylcholine release in response to activation while others postulate the existence of excitatory feedback mechanisms whereby acetylcholine can boost its own release during times of nerve terminal stress. Indeed, it is even possible that multiple subclasses of prejunctional nicotinic autoreceptors may exist on the motor nerve terminal and that both facilitatory and inhibitory control systems mediated by nicotinic acetylcholine receptors are present. Similarly, both facilitatory and inhibitory roles have been claimed for prejunctional muscarinic autoreceptors. It is clear that acetylcholine can influence its own release through actions on at least one, if not many, classes of prejunctional acetylcholine autoreceptor.

Both excitatory and inhibitory prejunctional receptors have also been proposed for adenosine. The role of these receptors is generally less confusing than that of the acetylcholine receptors. Inhibitory adenosine A_1 receptors on the motor nerve terminals are activated by adenosine produced by the enzymic destruction of vesicular ATP released from the nerve terminals. There is considerable, but less conclusive, evidence that there are also excitatory adenosine A_{2A} receptors on motor nerve terminals.

The process of vesicle mobilization increases the availability of synaptic vesicles for release. Mobilization is particularly important during times of high quantal output since in the absence of an enhanced supply of synaptic vesicles to the release sites the per impulse release of acetylcholine quanta cannot be sustained. Relatively little is known of the molecular mechanisms underlying mobilization at the neuromuscular junction; however, several candidate systems have been implicated. One of these involves the synapsins, a family of phosphorylated synaptic vesicle-associated proteins. Synapsin 1 interacts with synaptic vesicle associated Ca^{2+}/calmodulin-dependent protein kinase II and the actin cytoskeletal matrix (Fig. 31.7). Thus, synapsin 1 appears to be vesicle anchor protein that regulates the availability for exocytotic release. Binding of vesicles to the actin cytoskeleton would be expected to inhibit their availability of synaptic vesicles for exocytotic release. Activation of Ca^{2+}/calmodulin-dependent protein kinase II by Ca^{2+}-bound calmodulin leads to phosphorylation of synapsin 1, which causes it to dissociate from synaptic vesicles (Chapter 19).

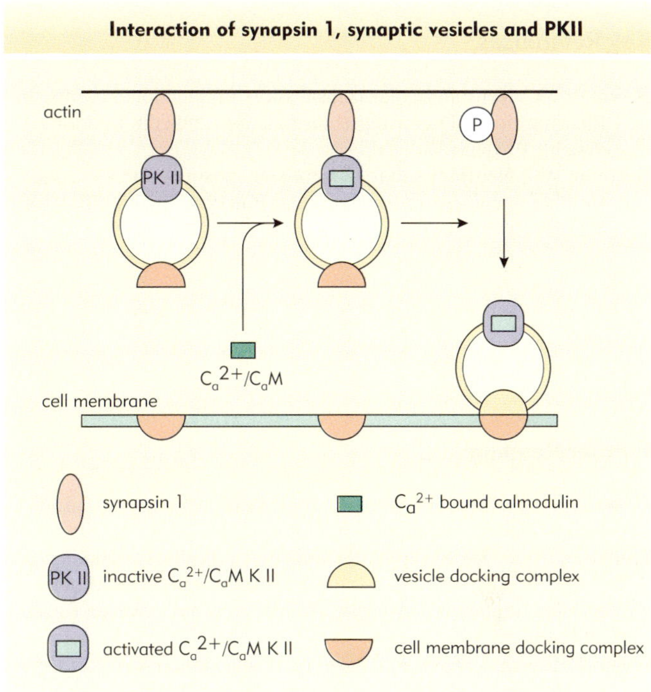

Figure 31.7 Interaction of synapsin 1, synaptic vesicles and PKII.

Postjunctional regulation

In addition to the prejunctional modulation of acetylcholine release, the efficiency of neuromuscular transmission is also influenced by the postjunctional modulation of nAChR function. The nAChR contains a number of potential phosphorylation sites, particularly on the M3–M4 intracellular loop of each of the five subunits. Various agents, including ATP and CGRP, can interact with their receptors on the muscle membrane at or near the motor end plate to influence the phosphorylation of the nAChR and modulate postjunctional sensitivity. Modulation by receptor desensitization often results from receptor phosphorylation activated by various intracellular signaling pathways. The fact that both pre- and postjunctional modulatory roles have been intimated for ATP is of considerable interest. It has been postulated that ATP has a genuine co-transmitter role at the neuromuscular junction but that, unlike sympathetic neuroeffector junctions, the ATP is modulatory rather than excitatory.

Key References

Bowman WC. Neuromuscular transmission: prejunctional events. In: Pharmacology of neuromuscular function, 2nd edn. London: Wright; 1990:65–84.

Bowman WC. Neuromuscular transmission: postjunctional events. In: Pharmacology of neuromuscular function, 2nd edn. London: Wright; 1990:100–26.

van der Kloot W, Molgo J. Quantal acetylcholine release at the vertebrate neuromuscular junction. Physiol Rev. 1995;74:899–991.

Zimmermann H. Exocytosis and endocytosis. In: Synaptic transmission: cellular and molecular basis. Oxford: Thieme; 1993:54–67.

Further Reading

Calakos N, Scheller RH. Synaptic vesicle biogenesis, docking, and fusion: a molecular description. Physiol Rev. 1996;76:1–29.

Holz RW, Fisher SK. Synaptic transmission and cellular signaling: an overview. In: Siegel GJ, ed. Basic neurochemistry: molecular, cellular, and medical aspects, 6th edn. New York: Raven Press; 1999:191–212.

Galzi JL, Revah F, Bessis A, Changeuz JP. Functional architecture of the nicotinic acetylcholine receptor – from electric organ to brain. Annu Rev Pharmacol. 1991;31:37–72.

Kuhar MJ, Murrin LC. Sodium-dependent, high affinity choline uptake. J Neurochem. 1978;30:15–21.

Lindstrom J, Schoepfer R, Conroy WG, Whiting P. Structural and functional heterogeneity of nicotinic receptors. In: Marsh J, Bock G, eds. The biology of nicotine dependence. New York: Wiley; 1990:23–52.

Parsons SM, Prior C, Marshall IG. Acetylcholine transport, storage and release. Int Rev Neurobiol. 1993;35:279–390.

Taylor P, Brown JH. Acetylcholine. In: Siegel GJ, ed. Basic neurochemistry: molecular, cellular, and medical aspects, 6th edn. New York: Raven Press; 1999:213–42.

Usdin TB, Eiden LE, Bonner TI, Erickson JD. Molecular biology of the vesicular ACh transporter. Trends Neurosci. 1995;18:218–24.

Chapter 32 Neuromuscular junction pharmacology

Cynthia A Lien and John J Savarese

Topics covered in this chapter

Depolarizing neuromuscular blockers
Nondepolarizing neuromuscular blockers
Onset of neuromuscular blockade
Recovery of neuromuscular function
Monitoring neuromuscular function
Neuromuscular block under altered physiologic conditions

DEPOLARIZING NEUROMUSCULAR BLOCKERS

Neuromuscular blocking agents are quaternary ammonium compounds that interact with acetylcholine-binding sites on the α-subunits of postjunctional nicotinic acetylcholine receptors (nAChRs). By interacting with these binding sites, they block neuromuscular function either by a depolarizing or a nondepolarizing mechanism of action.

Succinylcholine (suxamethonium) (Fig. 32.1) is the most commonly used depolarizing neuromuscular blocking agent. It causes rapid muscle relaxation or paralysis (onset 60–90 seconds) by a desynchronized depolarization of the muscle membrane (sarcolemma), resulting in disorganized muscle contractions called fasciculations; these are followed by a refractory period (relaxation). Succinylcholine binds to and activates the acetylcholine receptor (Chapter 31) but is not broken down by acetylcholinesterase; therefore, it has a longer duration of action than acetylcholine. Succinylcholine is metabolized by plasma cholinesterase, which is not found in the synaptic cleft. Therefore it must diffuse out of the synaptic cleft into the plasma to be hydrolyzed. Until this occurs, it is available to bind repeatedly with the acetylcholine receptor.

Succinylcholine has a number of adverse effects. Its cardiovascular side effects are quite varied because it stimulates autonomic cholinergic receptors (Fig. 32.2). Patients with muscular dystrophy and other neuromuscular diseases, extensive burns (sustained 1 day to 18 months prior to administration), trauma (sustained up to 60 days prior to administration), prolonged immobilization or intra-abdominal infections are at risk of hyperkalemia in response to succinylcholine that can result in cardiac arrest. In normal individuals, succinylcholine may result in small increases (1.0mEg/L) in serum K^+ concentration. Succinylcholine is also a potent trigger for malignant hyperthermia (Chapter 30).

The increase in intraoccular pressure seen following succinylcholine typically begins 1 minute following administration, peaks at 2–4 minutes, and subsides within 6 minutes. As a result, succinylcholine is relatively contraindicated in patients with an open anterior chamber. The increase in intraoccular pressure may be attenuated by sublingual nifedipine, 'precurarization' with a small dose of nondepolarizing muscle relaxant, or deepening anesthesia with a volatile agent.

Succinylcholine increases intracranial pressure. The mechanism of this phenomenon is not known but may involve increased cerebral blood flow secondary to proprioceptive cortical neuron activation by muscle spindle afferents (Chapter 30). It can be attenuated by precurarization with a nondepolarizing relaxant, thiopental (thiopentone) or lidocaine (lignocaine).

With prolonged infusion or administration of large doses of succinylcholine, a phase II block may develop. The characteristics of phase II blockade seen with monitoring of the neuromuscular blockade are similar to those seen with nondepolarizing muscle relaxants. Fade occurs in response to tetanic stimulation and train-of-four stimulation (see below), and post-tetanic facilitation is present. Recovery, which otherwise proceeds quite rapidly (5–10 minutes), becomes more prolonged. Antagonism of succinylcholine-induced phase II block is controversial, although administration of an anticholinesterase may hasten recovery.

Because of the number of adverse effects of succinylcholine, it is no longer recommended for the maintenance of neuromuscular block or for routine endotracheal intubation in pediatric patients. Research is ongoing to develop a nondepolarizing muscle relaxant with the favorable pharmacokinetic characteristics of succinylcholine in order to eliminate the need for depolarizing muscle relaxants and their attendant risks (massive K^+ efflux and malignant hyperthermia).

NONDEPOLARIZING NEUROMUSCULAR BLOCKERS

Nondepolarizing neuromuscular blocking agents act primarily by competitive inhibition of acetylcholine binding to the postjunctional nAChR. They block channels for periods of about 1 millisecond, which is longer than the normal lifetime of released acetylcholine. When either one or both of the two α-subunits of the pentameric nAChR bind a nondepolarizing neuromuscular blocker at the acetylcholine-binding site, the ion channel of the receptor cannot open and the sarcolemma remains at its resting membrane potential. Acetylcholine competes in a concentration-dependent manner with nondepolarizing relaxants for its receptor sites. Relaxant concentration must decrease below a critical level (determined by its affinity for the receptor) before acetylcholine can bind and activate the receptor.

Nondepolarizing relaxants can also have presynaptic effects by interacting with presynaptic muscarinic and nicotinic cholinergic

Chemical structures of muscle relaxants

Depolarizing

Succinylcholine (diacetylcholine)

Acetylcholine

Acetylcholine

Short-acting neuromuscular blocking agents

Mivacurium

Rapacuronium

GW280430A

Intermediate-acting benzylisoquinoliniums

Atracurium

Cisatracurium

(continued...)

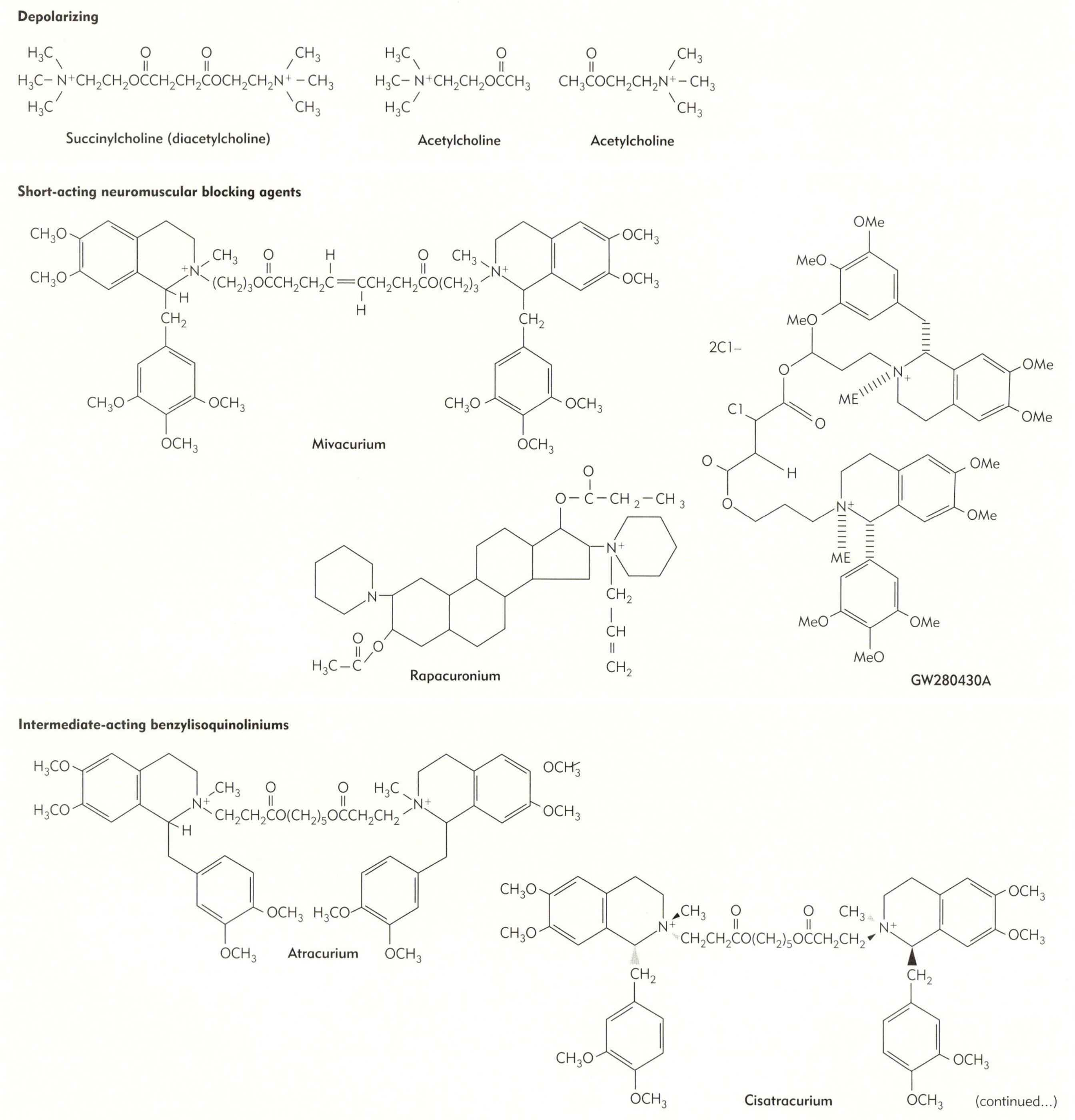

Figure 32.1 Chemical structures of muscle relaxants. Two molecules of acetylcholine are shown for comparison with succinylcholine. Cisatracurium is one of ten stereoisomers resulting from the four isomeric centers that occur in atracurium (the *1R-cis,1′R-cis*-configuration).

receptors. There they may decrease the release of acetylcholine from the nerve terminal, thereby enhancing their competitive postjunctional neuromuscular blocking potency. The specific presynaptic actions of nondepolarizing relaxants vary between agents.

Nondepolarizing neuromuscular blockers have a number of cardiovascular side effects resulting from their ability to cause histamine release, ganglionic blockade, or vagolysis. These are summarized in Figures 32.3 & 32.4. Nondepolarizing neuro-

Chemical structures of muscle relaxants (cont.)

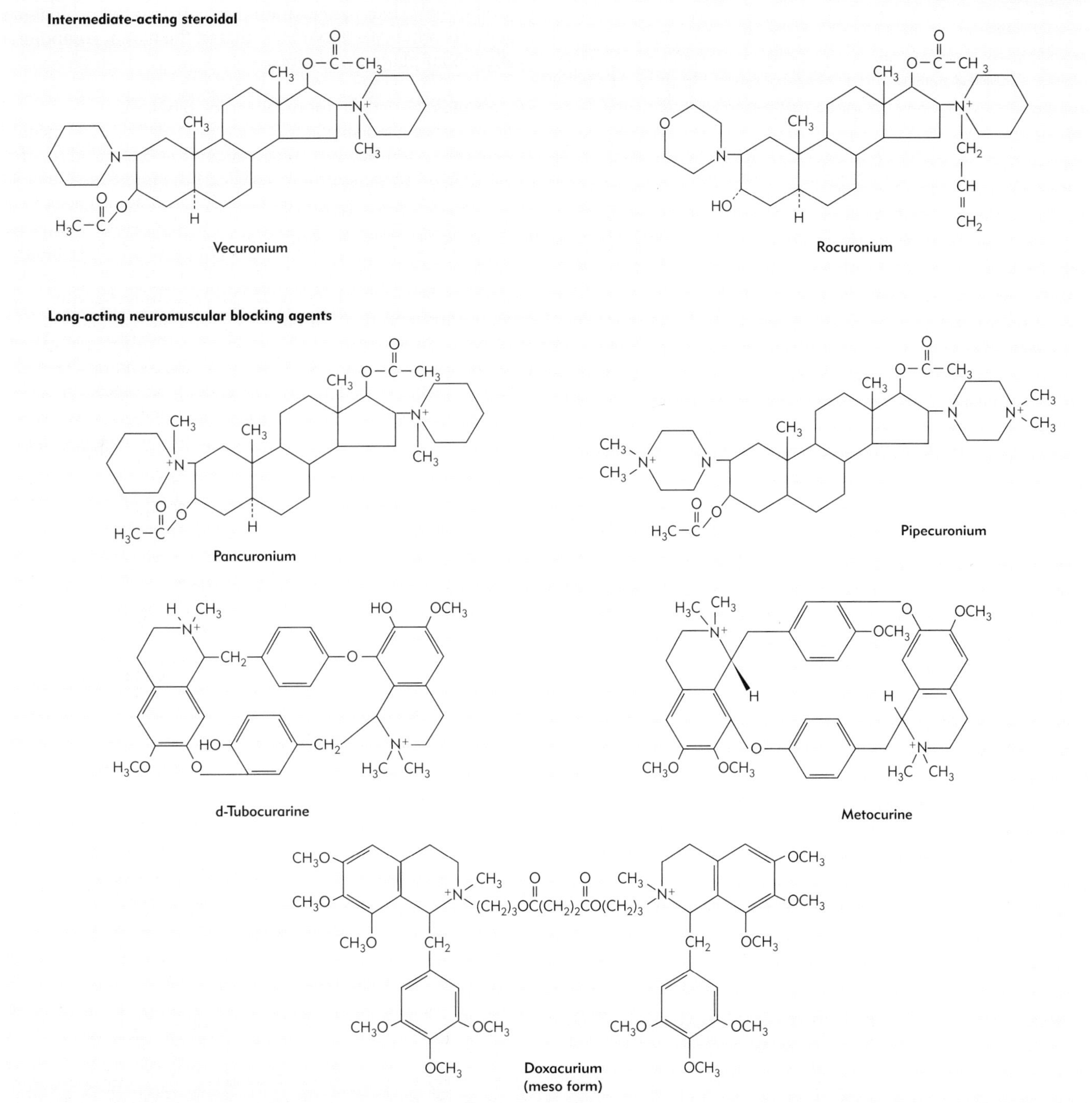

Intermediate-acting steroidal

Vecuronium

Rocuronium

Long-acting neuromuscular blocking agents

Pancuronium

Pipecuronium

d-Tubocurarine

Metocurine

Doxacurium (meso form)

muscular blocking agents can be categorized based on a number of characteristics, including duration of action, means of elimination, side effects, and underlying chemical structure.

Long-acting neuromuscular blockers

Long-acting muscle relaxants have a duration of action of 60 to 150 minutes. Included in this category are tubocurarine (d-tubocurarine), metocurine, doxacurium, gallamine, alcuronium, pancuronium, and pipecuronium (see Fig. 32.1). Following the administration of an intubating dose of muscle relaxant (typically two times the ED_{95}), at least 60 minutes are required for patients to recover to 25% of their baseline twitch strength. The ED_{95} is the dose that causes, on average, 95% neuromuscular blockade. The long duration of action of these neuromuscular blocking agents results from their low clearance (1.5–3mL/min per kg body weight). They are all eliminated primarily through the kidney and undergo little or no metabolism (see Fig. 32.3).

Of the long-acting neuromuscular blockers, only pancuronium undergoes significant metabolism. Most is eliminated unchanged primarily by renal mechanisms and secondarily by

Adverse effects of succinylcholine

- Cardiovascular effects
  - Arrhythmias
  - Sinus bradycardia
  - Junctional rhythms
  - Ventricular arrhythmias: unifocal premature ventricular contractions, ventricular fibrillation
  - Negative inotropic effect
- Hyperkalemia secondary to burns, trauma, neuromuscular disease, closed head injury, intra-abdominal infections
- Increased intraoccular pressure
- Increased intragastric pressure
- Myalgias
- Increased intracranial pressure
- Masseter spasm
- Malignant hyperthermia
- Phase II neuromuscular block
- Anaphylaxis: relatively high incidence of anaphylactoid reactions

Figure 32.2 Adverse effects of succinylcholine (suxamethonium).

hepatic mechanisms, but up to 20% is deacetylated at the 3-position in the liver. This metabolite is eliminated primarily by the kidney and to a lesser extent by the liver. The 3-hydroxy metabolite is, like pancuronium, a neuromuscular blocking agent. Its potency is about 50% that of the parent compound, with similar pharmacokinetics.

Intermediate-acting neuromuscular blockers

The intermediate-acting muscle relaxants (see Fig. 32.4) include atracurium, cisatracurium, vecuronium (Fig. 32.5), and rocuronium. These compounds have a clinical durations of action of 30 to 45 minutes, and spontaneous recovery occurs more quickly than for the long-acting relaxants. Their shorter durations of action are the consequence of their faster clearance rates (4–7mL/min per kg). These compounds are eliminated by a variety of means: primarily by hepatic and secondarily by renal mechanisms (e.g. vecuronium and rocuronium), by Hofmann elimination and hydrolysis by esterases [e.g. atracurium (Fig. 32.6)], or by Hofmann elimination alone (e.g. cisatracurium). Rocuronium is the only member of this class that does not undergo significant metabolism. Vecuronium, the other steroidal intermediate-acting relaxant, is the 2-desmethyl analog of pancuronium but is more

Long-acting neuromuscular blocking agents

Compound	ED_{95} (mg/kg)[a]	Dose for intubation[b]	Clinical duration of action (min)	Routes of elimination	Cardiovascular side effects	Chemical structure
d-Tubocurarine	0.5	1.0–1.2	60–100	Kidney, liver	Histamine release, ganglionic blockade	Benzylisoquinoline
Metocurine	0.3	1.0–1.3	60–120	Kidney	Mild histamine release	Benzylisoquinoline
Doxacurium	0.025	2–3	90–150	Kidney, liver	None	Benzylisoquinoline
Gallamine	3	1.3–2.0	90–120	Kidney	Strong vagolysis	Gallic acid derivative
Alcuronium	0.2	1.0–1.5	60–120	Kidney, liver	Ganglionic blockade, mild vagolysis	Toxiferine derivative
Pancuronium	0.06–0.07	1–2	60–120	Kidney, liver	Moderate vagolysis, sympathomimetic	Steroid
Pipecuronium	0.04–0.05	2–3	60–120	Kidney, liver	None	Steroid

[a]Effective dose for 95% of maximal blockade.
[b]Amount the ED_{95} (dose that, on average, causes 95% blockade) should be multiplied by.

Figure 32.3 Long-acting neuromuscular blocking agents.

Intermediate and short-acting neuromuscular blocking agents

Compound	ED_{95}(mg/kg)[a]	Dose for intubation[b]	Clinical duration of action (min)	Routes of elimination	Cardiovascular side effects	Chemical structure
Atracurium	0.25	2	30–45	Kidney: Hofmann elimination, ester hydrolysis	Mild histamine release	Benzylisoquinolinium
Cisatracurium	0.05	2–4	40–75	Liver: Hofmann elimination	None	Benzylisoquinolinium
Vecuronium	0.05	2	45–90	Liver, kidney	None	Steroid
Rocuronium	0.3–0.4	2–4	45–75	Liver, kidney	Mild vagolysis	Steroid
Mivacurium	0.07–0.08	3	15–20	Hydrolysis by plasma cholinesterase	Mild histamine release	Benzylisoquinolinium
Rapacuronium	0.75–1.0	2	8	Liver, kidney	Mild hypotension, vagolysis	Steroid
GW280430A	0.19	2–3	7	Chemical degradation	None	Chlorofumarate

[a]Effective dose for 95% of maximal blockade.
[b]Amount the ED_{95} (dose that, on average, causes 95% blockade) should be multiplied by.

Figure 32.4 Intermediate and short-acting neuromuscular blocking agents.

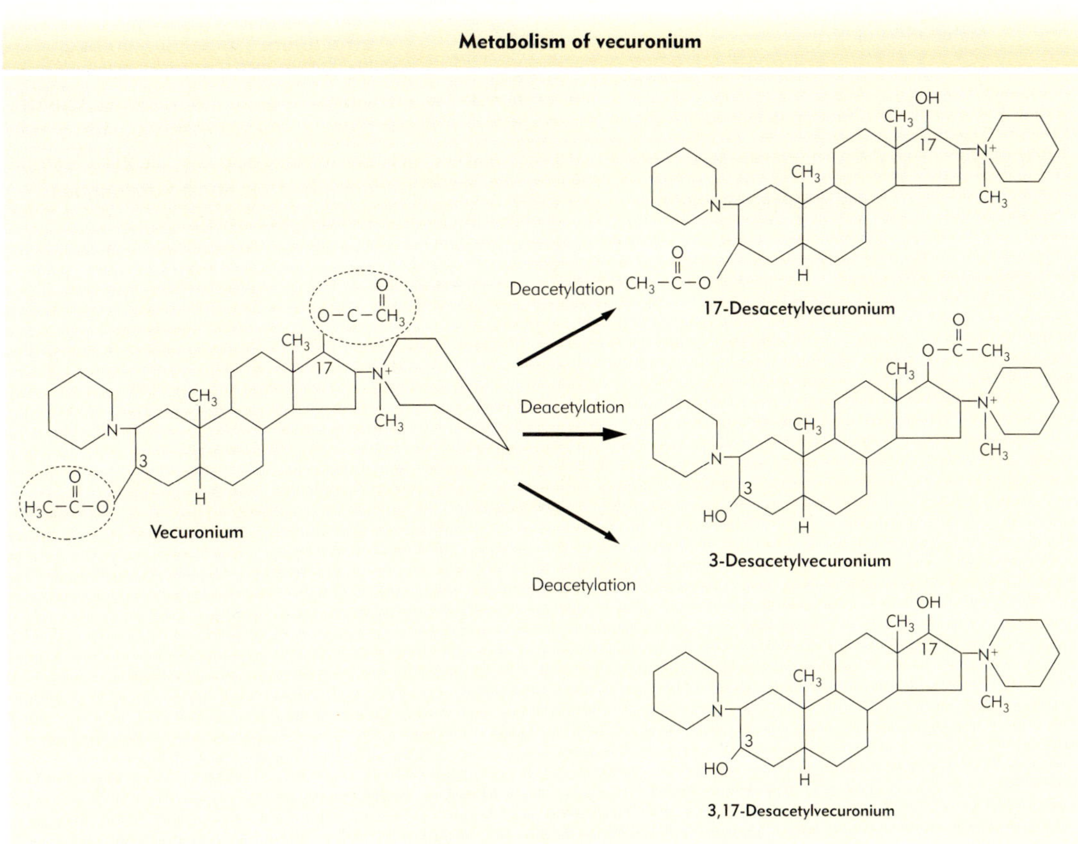

Figure 32.5 Metabolism of vecuronium. Vecuronium is deacetylated at the 3- and/or 17-positions to yield 17-desacetyl, 3-desacetyl-, or 3,17-desacetylvecuronium. Most deacetylation occurs at the 3-position.

extensively metabolized. Like pancuronium, it can be deacetylated at the 3-position, to yield 3-desacetylvecuronium (30 to 40%), which is 70% as potent as vecuronium (see Fig. 32.5). It can also be deacetylated at the 17-position, to yield 17-desacetyl- or 3,17-desacetylvecuronium. In contrast to vecuronium, 3-desacetylvecuronium has a long duration of action. Its accumulation may account for the prolonged action of vecuronium in patients in the intensive-care unit who have renal failure.

Both cisatracurium and atracurium depend on extensive degradation, rather than end-organ elimination, for their clearance from plasma. Cisatracurium is one of 10 atracurium isomers, but unlike atracurium does not significantly release histamine. Both compounds undergo Hofmann elimination (see Fig. 32.6), a chemical reaction in which a quaternary nitrogen atom is converted to a tertiary amine. This nonenzymatic reaction is base catalyzed and temperature dependent. Hofmann elimination of atracurium or cisatracurium yields laudanosine; this tertiary amine is excreted in the urine and bile and crosses the blood–brain barrier, where it is a potential CNS stimulant. Evidence of CNS excitement has been demonstrated in animals following administration of extremely large doses of atracurium, but this has not been reported in patients receiving the relaxant as an infusion in the intensive-care unit. Even in patients with renal failure receiving an infusion of atracurium, plasma laudanosine concentrations reach a plateau that is substantially lower than those anticipated to cause CNS stimulation. In part because of its greater potency, administration of cisatracurium results in less laudanosine formation than atracurium.

In addition to Hofmann elimination, atracurium undergoes ester hydrolysis to yield a quaternary alcohol and a quaternary acid (see Fig. 32.6). The esterase system that catalyzes this reaction is unrelated to plasma cholinesterase, which metabolizes succinylcholine and mivacurium. Less than 20% of atracurium or cisatracurium is eliminated unchanged through the kidney.

Short-acting neuromuscular blockers

The short-acting muscle relaxant mivacurium (see Fig. 32.4) exhibits rapid spontaneous recovery. Following administration of double the ED_{95}, patients spontaneously recover to 95% of baseline muscle strength within 30 minutes. Rapid recovery results from its extensive metabolism by plasma cholinesterase, the same enzyme that metabolizes succinylcholine. Mivacurium is metabolized at about 80% the rate of succinylcholine, with a comparable K_m value; its plasma clearance is 60–100mL/min per kg. Mivacurium metabolites are excreted in the urine and bile and do not appear to have pharmacologic activity (Fig. 32.7).

Rapacuronium

Rapacuronium (ORG 9487), an analogue of vecuronium, is a new steroidal neuromuscular blocking drug. Its onset of effect is rapid and intubating conditions following administration of 1.5 to 2.0 mg/kg approximate or are equivalent to those of succinylcholine. Maximal block occurs within 60 seconds at the laryngeal adductors following administration of 0.75 mg/kg and in about 90 seconds at the adductor pollicis following administration of 1.5 to 2.0 mg/kg. In addition to having a fast onset of effect, rapacuronium is a short-acting nondepolarizing neuromuscular blocking agent. In the larynx spontaneous recovery to a twitch height of 75% of baseline occurs in approximately

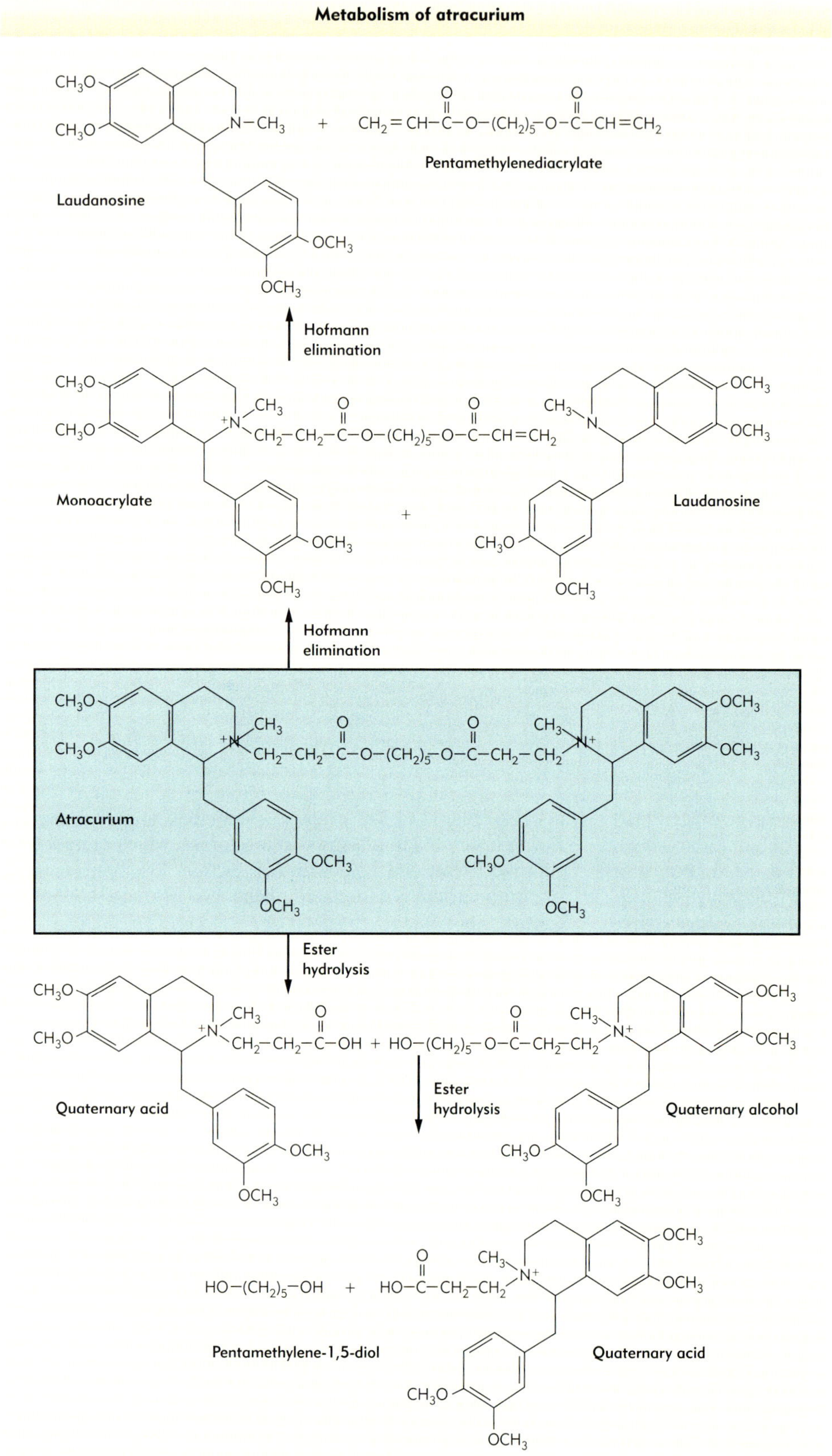

Metabolism of atracurium

Figure 32.6 Metabolism of atracurium. Atracurium undergoes Hofmann elimination to yield laudanosine and a monoacrylate as well as ester hydrolysis to yield a quaternary acid and alcohol. A small amount is eliminated unchanged through the kidney.

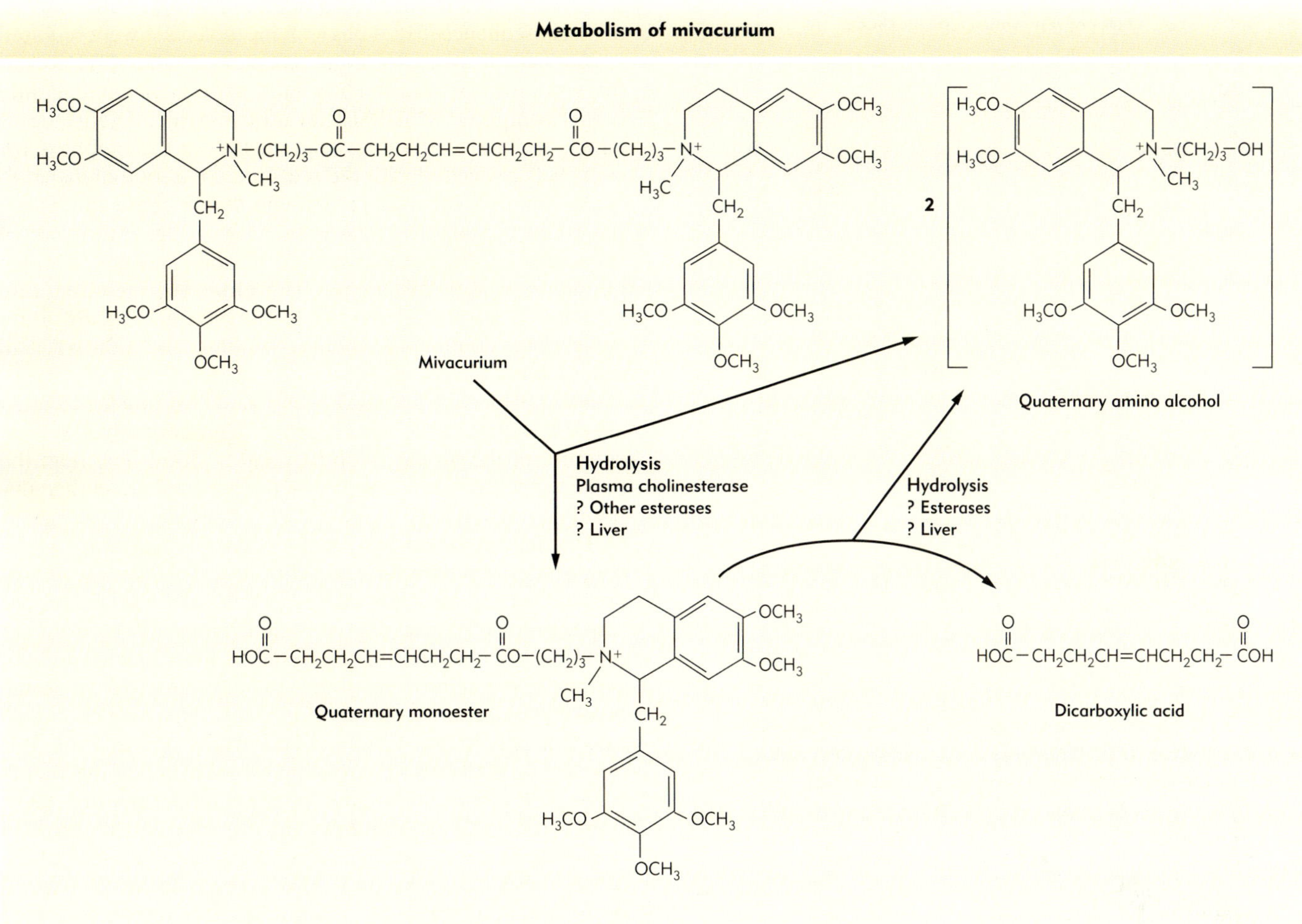

Figure 32.7 Metabolism of mivacurium. Mivacurium undergoes hydrolysis by plasma cholinesterase to yield a quaternary amino alcohol and a quaternary monoester.

5 minutes following a dose of 0.75 mg/kg, 6 minutes following 1.5 mg/kg and 17 minutes following 2.0 mg/kg.

Following administration of either an infusion or multiple doses of the compound, recovery occurs over an increasingly longer time similar to an intermediate-acting nondepolarizing relaxant. Rapacuronium has a clearance of 7 ml/min/kg. It is metabolized in the liver to ORG 9488, its 3-desacetyl metabolite. This compound is a long-acting neuromuscular blocking agent that is primarily excreted unchanged in the urine. Its clearance is 1 ml/min/kg. Formation of this metabolite accounts for the increasingly prolonged duration of action of subsequent or larger doses of action of rapacuronium. Recovery of neuromuscular function following administration of rapacuronium can be shortened, consistent with its nondepolarizing mechanism of neuromuscular block, by the administration of neostigmine.

Like most other nondepolarizing relaxants, rapacuronium has side effects. Across studies, following administration of intubating doses of 1.5 mg/kg or greater, it causes bronchospasm in 10% of patients. It also causes transient increases in heart rate, which are likely due to vagolysis, and decreases in mean arterial pressure, which may be due to calcium channel blockade.

GW280430A (see Fig. 32.1), a new nondepolarizing neuromuscular agent, is an asymmetrical mixed-onium chlorofumarate. Its ED_{95} is 0.19mg/kg and it has an ultra-short duration of action. A dose of 2.8 times the ED_{95} (0.54mg/kg) results in 100% neuromuscular block in 0.9 minutes in the laryngeal adductors and 1.5 minutes at the adductor pollicis. The onset times are similar to those observed following administration of succinylcholine (1mg/kg). Complete spontaneous recovery following 0.54mg/kg GW280430A is rapid. Recovery to a train-of-four ratio of 90% requires 15 minutes at both the larngeal adductors and the adductor pollicis. The times required for recovery from 5–95% of muscle strength and from 25% recovery of twitch height to a train-of-four ratio of 90% remain constant at 7 and 5 minutes, respectively, regardless of the ammount of relaxant administered. This short duration of action and lack of cumulation is likely due to its degradation by chemical mechanisms. Recovery from GW280430A-induced neuromuscular block can be further shortened by the administration of edrophonium.

ONSET OF NEUROMUSCULAR BLOCKADE

Onset of neuromuscular blockade is influenced by a number of factors, including neuromuscular blocking potency, bioavailability, clearance, and muscle blood flow. Perhaps the most important of these factors is neuromuscular blocking potency and blood flow to the affected muscles.

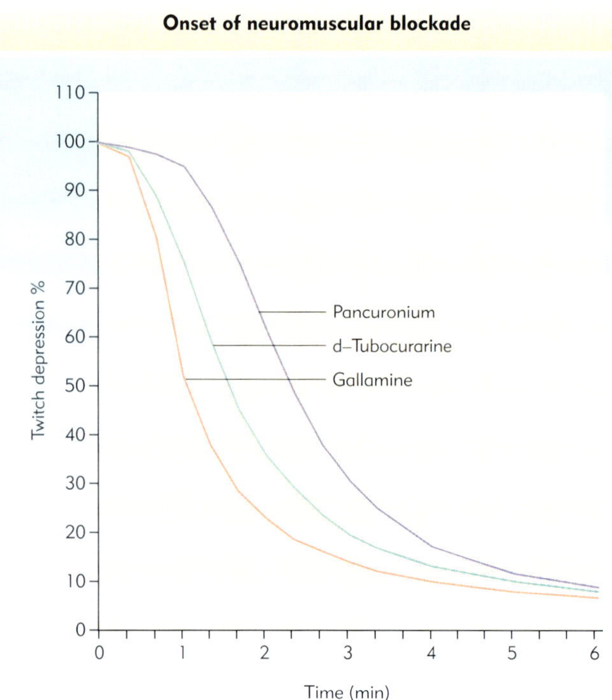

Figure 32.8 Onset of neuromuscular block with gallamine, pancuronium, or d-tubocurarine. Gallamine, which is the least potent of the relaxants tested, had the fastest onset. Pancuronium, the most potent of the three relaxants tested, had the slowest onset.

The onset time of neuromuscular blockade is a function of molar potency. The least potent relaxants have the fastest onset both experimentally and clinically (Fig. 32.8). These observations led to the development of rocuronium, a structural modification of vecuronium made with the intention of lowering its neuromuscular blocking potency. The potency is reduced eightfold by modification of the acetoxy substitution at position 3 to a hydroxyl group, the position 2 substitution of piperidino by morpholino, and the position 16 substitution of piperidino with methyl quaternization by pyrrolidino with allyl quaternization. The reduced potency results in a significantly faster onset compared with vecuronium or other available nondepolarizing neuromuscular blocking agents.

Why do relaxants with the lowest potency have the most rapid onset? The concept of 'buffered diffusion' is useful in explaining the biophase kinetics. According to the model of Armstrong and Lester, receptor affinity for nondepolarizing neuromuscular blockers is such that at 50% occupancy by tubocurarine, one drug molecule in 300 is free in the biophase (binding ratio 300:1). This binding ratio is higher for relaxants such as doxacurium that have greater potency than tubocurarine. Assuming that only one molecule of tubocurarine binds to each receptor, at 50% receptor occupancy a sample of 1800 receptors binds 900 molecules of drug with three molecules free in the biophase. The free biophase concentration (at equilibrium) is identical to the unbound plasma concentration. If an equipotent dose of a hypothetical relaxant that is one-tenth as potent as tubocurarine is used, plasma concentrations will be 10-fold higher and the diffusion gradient from capillary to the junctional cleft will also be 10 times as great. This would be of no consequence if 10 times as many molecules were required to produce the same degree of receptor occupancy. However, this is not the case. For the hypothetical drug, the binding ratio is 30:1 compared with 300:1 for tubocurarine. At 50% occupancy, there are 30 unbound molecules in the biophase for every 900 associated with the receptor, for a total of 930 molecules per 1800 receptors. Although the biophase concentration of the hypothetical relaxant is 10 times higher than that of tubocurarine, the actual number of molecules per receptor population is only 3% higher. Therefore, the increased rate of delivery resulting from the higher plasma concentration becomes the dominant element controlling onset time when all other factors are equal.

Onset of block is also affected by blood flow, and hence delivery of relaxant, to the muscle group. Consequently, the musculature of the airway, with its greater blood flow than the adductor pollicis, has a faster onset of maximal effect than this peripheral muscle.

The diaphragm and larynx are relatively resistant to neuromuscular blockers. In general their dose–response curves are shifted to the right and larger doses of relaxants are required for the same degree of neuromuscular blockade as required in a peripheral muscle such as the adductor pollicis. In spite of this relative resistance to neuromuscular blockade, block develops more quickly (Fig. 32.9). This may be important clinically for the timing of endotracheal intubation; it is not necessary to wait for complete loss of twitch of the adductor pollicis prior to laryngoscopy for good 'intubating conditions' (relaxed jaw, abducted vocal cords, and absence of diaphragmatic movement). In general, maximal blockade of airway musculature occurs 30 to 60 seconds earlier than in the periphery, at a point where the adductor pollicis response to ulnar stimulation is decreased to 70% of baseline. The onset of neuromuscular blockade in the orbicularis occuli coincides closely with onset in the larynx. Therefore, monitoring of onset in this muscle group more closely reflects effects on the larynx.

RECOVERY OF NEUROMUSCULAR FUNCTION

Spontaneous recovery of neuromuscular function following administration of a nondepolarizing neuromuscular blocking agent involves diffusion of the relaxant away from the nAChR and the motor end plate as well as its elimination from the body. Recovery is facilitated in the presence of anticholinesterases, which increase acetylcholine concentration at the motor end plate. Recovery is also influenced by depth of neuromuscular block at the time of antagonism, the clearance and half-life of the relaxant used, and any factors that affect neuromuscular blockade (Fig. 32.10). Factors that affect the opening and closing times of the nAChR, alter resting membrane potential, or influence the release of acetylcholine from the presynaptic terminal may affect neuromuscular block.

Anticholinesterases

Anticholinesterases (acetylcholinesterase inhibitors) effectively increase the concentration of available acetylcholine by inhibiting the action of acetylcholinesterase, the neuromuscular junction enzyme responsible for acetylcholine breakdown (Chapter 31). The increased concentration of acetylcholine at the neuromuscular junction increases the likelihood that an agonist rather than an antagonist will bind the nAChR.

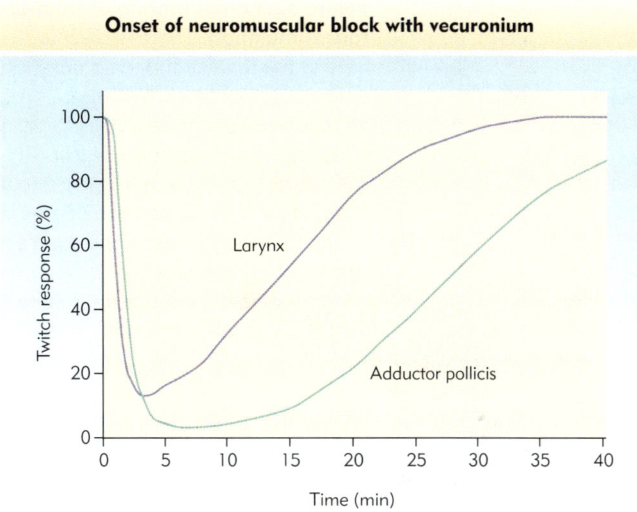

Figure 32.9 Onset of neuromuscular block with vercuronium in the larynx and in the adductor pollicis. While onset of block (using 0.07mg/kg vecuronium) occurs more quickly in the larynx, it is relatively resistant to neuromuscular block. Recovery also occurs more quickly in the larynx.

Factors potentiating neuromuscular blockade

Drugs

- Volatile anesthetics
- Antibiotics: aminoglycosides, polymyxin B, lincomycin, clindamycin, neomycin, tetracycline
- Dantrolene
- Verapamil
- Furosemide (frusemide)
- Lidocaine (lignocaine)

Electrolyte and acid–base disorders

- Hypermagnesemia
- Hypocalcemia
- Hypokalemia
- Respiratory acidosis

Hypothermia

Figure 32.10 Factors potentiating neuromuscular blockade.

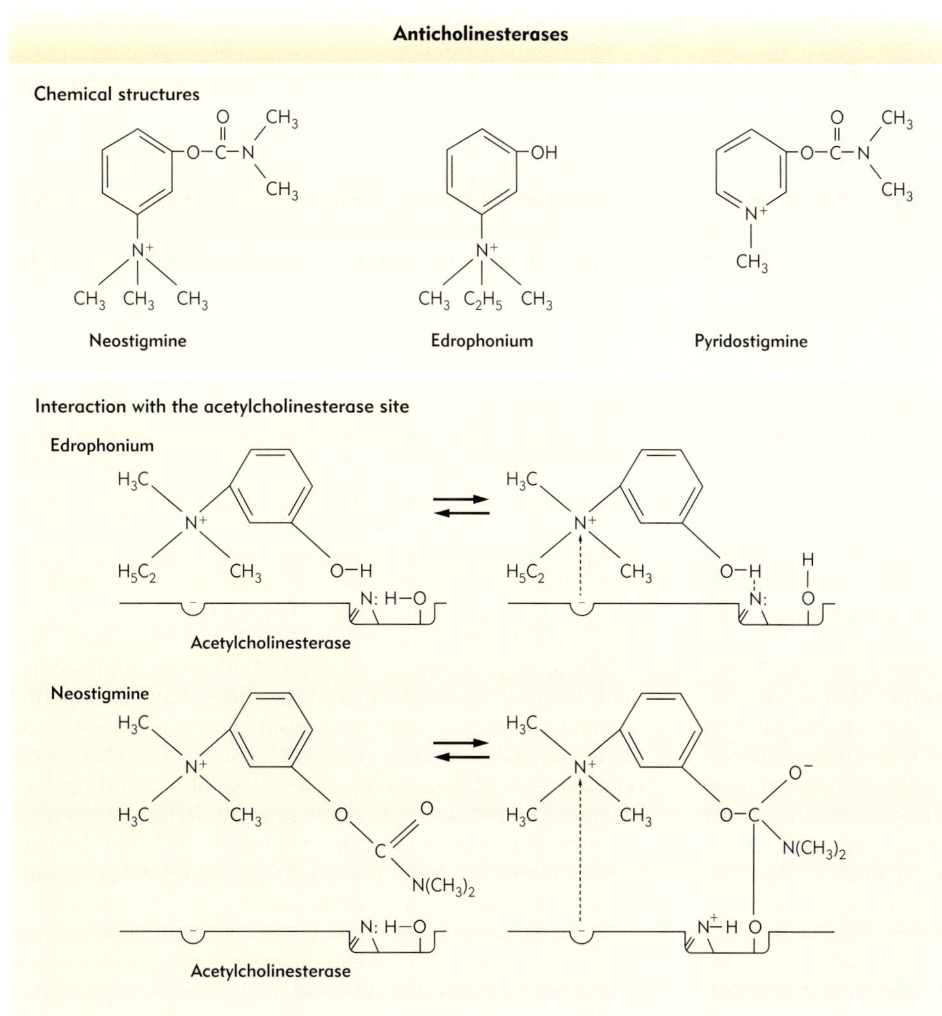

Figure 32.11 Anticholinesterases. The chemical structures of neostigmine, edrophonium, and pyridostigmine and the interaction of edrophonium and neostigmine with the acetylcholinesterase active site.

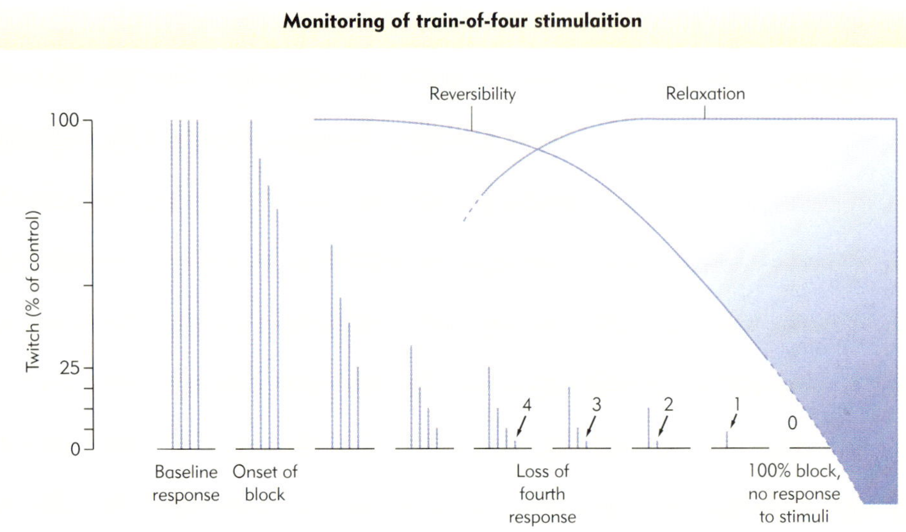

Figure 32.12 Monitoring of train-of-four stimulation. There is a 25% fade in the train-of-four with onset of neuromuscular block. With increasing depth of neuromuscular block, the fourth response is lost. At 100% block, there is no response to stimulation. The greater the degree of spontaneous recovery, the quicker and more complete is the pharmacologic antagonism. (See text for details of this method.)

Three anticholinesterases are used clinically to antagonize the effects of nondepolarizing neuromuscular blocking agents: edrophonium, neostigmine, and pyridostigmine (Fig. 32.11). The mechanism by which neostigmine and pyridostigmine inhibit acetylcholine is identical (see Fig. 32.11). The positively charged nitrogen atom in the anticholinesterase is attracted to the negatively charged anionic site at the acetylcholinesterase active site. Once bound to the enzyme, the anticholinesterase is slowly hydrolyzed and in the process its carbamate moiety binds covalently to (carbamylates) the catalytic site and inactivates the enzyme. The covalent bond can be cleaved by water (hydrolyzed) over the course of minutes, rendering the inhibition reversible. Edrophonium binds to acetylcholinesterase by electrostatic attraction; its presence in the active site denies acetylcholine access. Typical doses of neostigmine are up to 70μg/kg and doses of edrophonium are up to 1mg/kg, depending on the clearance of the relaxant and the depth of block to be antagonized.

When antagonizing moderate depths of neuromuscular block (three responses to train-of-four stimulation), the speed of action of the anticholinesterases is edrophonium > neostigmine > pyridostigmine. This ranking may be irrelevant at deep levels of neuromuscular block, where the faster action of edrophonium is lost. In fact, when comparing large doses of edrophonium (1mg/kg) with neostigmine (50μg/kg), the latter more rapidly and more completely antagonizes profound levels of neuromuscular block than the former.

Acetylcholine and acetylcholinesterase both function at muscarinic as well as nicotinic sites. Administration of an anticholinesterase increases acetylcholine concentrations at these sites as well as at the neuromuscular junction, causing undesirable muscarinic side effects (e.g. bradycardia). In order to minimize muscarinic side effects, anticholinesterases are usually administered concomitantly with an antimuscarinic agent such as glycopyrrolate (glycopyrronium) (10μg/kg) or atropine (20μg/kg).

There is a limit to the depth of neuromuscular blockade that can be antagonized by anticholinesterases. They cannot, for example, antagonize 100% twitch inhibition. This is readily understood if one remembers that antagonism of neuromuscular block involves increasing acetylcholine concentrations at the neuromuscular junction to compete with neuromuscular blockers for sites on available receptors. Recovery occurs more quickly if the anticholinesterases are administered once a significant amount of spontaneous recovery has occurred and more receptors are available.

The speed of antagonism of residual block is related to the depth of block present at the time of administration of the anticholinesterase (Fig. 32.12). Deeper levels of neuromuscular block require a longer time for the return of twitch strength to baseline values. The speed of antagonism of block by either tubocurarine or pancuronium depends on the dose of neostigmine administered; larger doses of anticholinesterase are required for more complete and faster recovery of neuromuscular function.

Volatile anesthetics potentiate neuromuscular blockade and impede antagonism of residual neuromuscular blockade. For example, during neostigmine antagonism of residual vecuronium-induced block, the train-of-four ratio reached a mean of 0.85 within 15 minutes when isoflurane was discontinued at the time of neostigmine administration. If 1.25% end-tidal isoflurane was continued during the antagonism, the train-of-four ratio was only 0.7 within 15 minutes of neostigmine administration. Volatile anesthetics can influence the depth of neuromuscular block and recovery of neuromuscular function by several possible mechanisms. These include alterations in local blood flow and interactions with Na^+ and Ca^{2+} channels.

Following neostigmine antagonism of profound pancuronium-induced neuromuscular block, there is an initial period of rapid but incomplete antagonism, which peaks within 10 minutes. Further recovery of neuromuscular function occurs relatively slowly; this second, slower stage of recovery appears to depend on the clearance of the relaxant. In the case of long-acting relaxants, with clearance values of 1.5–3.0mL/min per kg and elimination half-lives of 1.5–2 hours, little drug is eliminated during the first 10 minutes following neostigmine administration, since this 10-minute period represents only about one-tenth of one half-life. Consequently, during antagonism of long-acting relaxants the return of neuromuscular function to normal depends nearly entirely on the antagonistic effect of the anticholinesterase. For relaxants with shorter half-lives (2–20 minutes), a larger fraction of the relaxant is eliminated during the 10-minute period following administration of the anticholinesterase. Therefore, antagonism of residual blockade in the latter represents a combination of the pharmacodynamic effect of the anticholinesterase and the pharmacokinetic effect of clearance of the relaxant. The net result is that antagonism of residual effect is more rapid and more complete with shorter-acting relaxants than it is with long-acting relaxants. This results in a higher incidence of residual weakness in the recovery room following administration of long-acting nondepolarizing neuromuscular blockers compared with intermediate-acting drugs.

Cholinesterases

Plasma cholinesterase is a blood glycoprotein produced in the liver; its physiologic role is not known. Blood transfusions and a purified form of the human enzyme may be given to patients homozygous for atypical plasma cholinesterase in order to shorten recovery times from succinylcholine or mivacurium. This speeds recovery of neuromuscular function by providing a means of metabolizing succinylcholine or mivacurium where none exists. The risk of transfusion-acquired infection usually makes this an undesirable alternative compared with conservative management. Human plasma cholinesterase has also been evaluated for the routine antagonism of mivacurium-induced block in patients with normal plasma cholinesterase activity. By increasing the enzymatic breakdown of the relaxant, recovery times can be shortened without exposing patients to the adverse effects of anticholinesterases, and antagonism of more profound levels of block may be possible.

Plasma cholinesterase deficiency

Approximately 5 to 10% of patients have decreased plasma cholinesterase activity. They may be heterozygous for an atypical plasma cholinesterase gene, a clear example of genetic control of drug metabolism (see Chapter 7), or they may have decreased plasma cholinesterase activity because of chronic disease, as in chronic renal or hepatic failure, where less enzyme is synthesized. Reduced activity can also be seen in the elderly and in pregnancy. Rare individuals may also have up to threefold higher than average cholinesterase activity.

Recovery from neuromuscular blockade induced with agents that are metabolized by plasma cholinesterase (succinylcholine, mivacurium) is slowed because of decreased clearance in patients with reduced plasma cholinesterase activity. When succinylcholine is administered to facilitate intubation, its effect may be prolonged by 7 to 10 minutes, which may pass unnoticed. However, if mivacurium is used to maintain muscle relaxation, the 5–95% recovery interval (defined by the recovery from 5 to 95% of baseline muscle strength), is increased from 10–13 minutes (normal) to 20–25 minutes. In about 5% of patients, relatively slow recovery from mivacurium occurs; these patients can be identified by their response to an initial dose. In patients with normal plasma cholinesterase, the interval between the return of the first and the third twitch in response to train-of-four stimulation is about 3 minutes. If prolonged recovery following the initial dose is observed, exogenous anticholinesterase-facilitated recovery can be used.

Rarely, patients are homozygous for an atypical gene (incidence about 1 in 3000 in Caucasians). The duration of action of succinylcholine and mivacurium in these patients is markedly prolonged because the primary means of elimination is absent as a result of the absence or the reduced affinity (high K_m) of the enzyme for these substances. Elimination occurs through what would be secondary routes in genotypically normal individuals, such as the kidney and liver. In these rare individuals, mivacurium is the most potent, long-acting nondepolarizing muscle relaxant available. In patients homozygous for atypical plasma cholinesterase, a dose of 0.03mg/kg, which is less than 50% of the ED_{95}, causes 100% neuromuscular block within 5 minutes, and the time for recovery to 25% of baseline muscle strength is 1–2 hours. Following a typical intubating dose of 0.2 to 0.25mg/kg mivacurium, the duration of full paralysis is 2–4 hours, with complete spontaneous recovery in 48 hours. Once spontaneous recovery in these patients is demonstrable, the now long-acting neuromuscular blockade can be antagonized with neostigmine. In spite of pharmacologic antagonism, recovery from mivacurium block occurs more slowly than in patients with a normal genotype and is similar to that following antagonism of a long-acting nondepolarizing blocker such as pancuronium. While pharmacologic antagonism of mivacurium-induced block in such patients is recommended at the appropriate time, antagonism of succinylcholine block in these patients is not. Management of patients homozygous for the atypical gene who have received succinylcholine is conservative. These patients are sedated and mechanically ventilated until full spontaneous recovery to head lift has taken place.

MONITORING NEUROMUSCULAR FUNCTION

Activation or blockade of the nAChR depends upon the relative biophase concentrations of agonist and antagonist. Because the interaction of nondepolarizing relaxants with the acetylcholine-binding sites on the α-subunit is competitive, blockade can be overcome by increasing the concentration of acetylcholine (or intensified by reducing it). This fundamental concept is important in clinical monitoring and reversal of neuromuscular blockade. A second fundamental concept is the economy of acetylcholine synthesis, storage, and release in the motor nerve terminal. The quantity of acetylcholine released per motor nerve action potential is inversely proportional to the number of action potentials reaching the nerve terminal per unit time: the stimulus frequency. For this reason, low concentrations of nondepolarizing relaxants block responses to high-frequency peripheral nerve stimulation; however, relatively high concentrations of relaxant are required to abolish responses elicited to low-frequency stimulation. The depth of blockade of evoked neuromuscular responses in the presence of nondepolarizing relaxants is directly proportional to the stimulus frequency. Consequently, stimuli of increasing frequency are able to detect increasingly subtle degrees of neuromuscular blockade. This provides a distinct advantage for evaluating the depth of nondepolarizing blockade.

Peripheral nerve stimulation is employed at sites where motor nerve stimulation results in easily observed muscular contraction. The ulnar nerve/adductor pollicis response remains the most commonly observed and easily recorded response, and this is used in clinical studies of neuromuscular blockade or its antagonism. With single twitch stimulation at frequencies of 0.1 or 0.15Hz, the evoked response is still present but markedly reduced during conditions of deep paralysis (95% blockade of the twitch). The problem with the use of this stimulus frequency in monitoring depth of block is that the responses are so infrequent that one cannot judge with any certainty the effect of the muscle relaxant. Train-of-four stimulation is a more useful method of peripheral nerve stimulation (see Fig. 32.12). Four single stimuli are delivered at a frequency of 2Hz for 2 seconds to elicit four twitch responses at 0.5-second intervals. This pattern may be repeated every 12 to 20 seconds. The train-of-four ratio is used to determine the degree of muscle relaxation; it is calculated by dividing the height or strength of the fourth response by that of the first response. The train-of-four ratio cannot be calculated clinically without instrumentation but can be determined with precision by mechanomyography or electromyography. Clinically, evaluation of the number of responses present on train-of-four stimulation can be used to determine the depth of neuromuscular blockade. The presence of only one visible twitch in response to train-of-four stimulation correlates well with about 95% suppression of the single twitch response; the presence of two responses correlates with 80–85% suppression of twitch response; the presence of three twitches correlates with 75–80% neuromuscular blockade; and the presence of four responses with easily appreciable decrement in strength indicates recovery of the first twitch of the train-of-four response to at least 25% of control.

When the train-of-four ratio has no apparent decrement in response, some subtle degrees of paralysis may still be present. It is not until the train-of-four ratio is greater than 0.7 that respiratory mechanical parameters such as inspiratory force and vital capacity have returned to 95% of baseline values. The clinical utility of train-of-four monitoring is considerable. A control or baseline response is not needed and the stimulus pattern is not painful to the patient. It provides a good qualitative estimate of onset, depth, and recovery of block by simply counting the number of responses visible in the train and noting the presence or absence of fade in the response.

Double burst stimulation (DBS) is another, perhaps better, method of stimulation to detect residual neuromuscular block during recovery of neuromuscular function. This pattern of stimulation applies two short tetanic bursts at an interval of 0.75 seconds. The most common pattern of DBS ($DBS_{3,3}$) applies stimulation at 50Hz for three 60-millisecond impulses twice, separated by a 0.75-second interval, to produce two brief tetanic responses. If the second response is not as strong as the first, there is *fade*, which indicates a substantial degree of residual neuromuscular block. When the intensity of the second response is at least 60% of the first, fade is no longer detectable by either observation or palpation. This is important since a DBS ratio of 0.6 or more is usually compatible with clinically acceptable neuromuscular function such as ability to lift the head for 5 seconds. In this way, DBS is more useful clinically than the train-of-four pattern of stimulation because when no fade is clinically detectable in the train-of-four response, the patient may in fact have a train-of-four ratio of only 0.4, a level of block that is usually not compatible with substantial head lift.

Maximum voluntary muscular tension development occurs at 30 to 50 motor nerve action potentials per second. Since motor nerve activation at rates higher than 50Hz cannot be achieved voluntarily, external stimulation at 50Hz is the highest rate of artificial stimulation consistent with normal physiology. Tetanic stimulation is usually applied at 50Hz for 5 seconds during recovery from nondepolarizing block. The absence of easily visible or palpable loss of strength during tetanic contraction is an indicator of recovery of normal function. The most important aspect in monitoring of tetanic responses is the detection of fade in the response. Considerable fade can occur within the first fraction of a second of a 5-second tetanic stimulus, following which the response is sustained at a substantially weaker level. This pattern may easily be misinterpreted as full recovery of function when considerable weakness may exist. For this reason, tetanic stimulation is seldom used.

Tetanic stimulation at 50Hz for 5 seconds followed, 3 seconds later, by a period of single twitch stimulation at a fequency of 1Hz is used to assess post-tetanic stimulation. When twitch is elicited at 1.0Hz following tetanus during very deep levels of neuromuscular blockade, the number of twitch responses following the tetanus stimulation can be counted. This is the post-tetanic count (PTC), and is a means of determining the depth of block when no response can be elicited with single twitch or train-of-four monitoring. Once the PTC is 2 to 3, the train-of-four response will begin to reappear within 20 or 30 minutes during pancuronium-induced block and within 7 to 8 minutes during vecuronium- or atracurium-induced block. The PTC is useful following the administration of the large doses of muscle relaxant given to facilitate endotracheal intubation. PTC can be used to predict when neuromuscular function has recovered to a point where either redosing is necessary or pharmacologic antagonism with anticholinesterase is possible.

Given the possibility of inadequate recovery of neuromuscular function, it is important to monitor depth of neuromuscular blockade carefully whenever muscle relaxants are administered. Since monitors of neuromuscular blockade do not reliably detect subtle degrees of block, tests of function should also be employed. Sustained tetanic responses are indicated by strongly maintained antigravity muscular movements (e.g. the 5-second head lift). For patients who are too young to respond to verbal commands, leg lifting yields similar information regarding return of neuromuscular function. Recovery to a train-of-four ratio of 0.7 may not be adequate for hospital discharge: volunteers feel much better and less weak once the train-of-four ratio returns to 0.9. The only clinical test that indicates this degree of recovery of neuromuscular function is the ability to appose the teeth, which is assessed by asking the subject to hold a tongue blade between their teeth.

NEUROMUSCULAR BLOCK UNDER ALTERED PHYSIOLOGIC CONDITIONS

Patients with upregulated nAChR, which can occur in a number of pathologic conditions (e.g. disuse, burns, trauma, atrophy, myopathy, and upper motor neuron lesions) are subject to an exaggerated hyperkalemic response and cardiac arrest following administration of depolarizing neuromuscular blockers. The increased number of extrajunctional receptors provides more channels for K^+ efflux. Rhabdomyolysis can also occur if myopathy is present (e.g. as a result of high-dose chronic steroid therapy).

Burns

Patients with thermal injuries show a relative resistance to nondepolarizing neuromuscular blockers. The degree of resistance depends on the size of the burn; resistance to neuromuscular blockers may be seen if the burn covers 30% or more of body surface area. Resistance to neuromuscular blockers results partially from an increase in α_1-acid glycoprotein, to which muscle relaxants normally bind. Resistance may also be caused by a proliferation of extrajunctional nAChR as a result of the burn injury. Reduced duration of action may be observed because of increased hepatic and renal clearance of nondepolarizing blockers.

Disuse

Patients who undergo prolonged immobilization become resistant to nondepolarizing neuromuscular blocking agents whether or not they receive neuromuscular blocking agents for the period of immobilization, as a result of nAChR upregulation. Receptor upregulation is potentiated by pharmacologic denervation through the use of muscle relaxants, as can occur in patients in intensive care.

Key References

Ali HH, Savarese JJ. Monitoring of neuromuscular function. Anesthesiology. 1976;45:216–49.

Bevan DR, Donati F, Kopman AF. Reversal of neuromuscular blockade. Anesthesiology. 1992;77:785–805.

Donati F, Plaud B, Meistleman D. Vecuronium neuromuscular blockade at the adductor muscles of the larynx and at the adductor pollicis. Anesthesiology. 1991;74:833–7.

Donati F. Onset of action of relaxants. Can J Anaesth. 1988;35:S52-8.

Kopman AF, Yee PS, Neuman GG. Relationship of train-of-four fade to clinical signs and symptoms of residual paralysis in awake volunteers. Anesthesiology. 1997;86:765–71.

Schiere S, Proost JH, Schuringa M, Wierda JMKH. Pharmacokinetics and pharmacokinetic-dynamic relationship between rapacuronium (ORG 9487) and its 3-desacetyl metabolite (ORG 9488). Anesth Analg. 1999;88:640–647

Further Reading

Ali HH, Utting JE, Gray TC. Quantitative assessment of residual antidepolarizing block (parts I and II). Br J Anaesth. 1971;43:473–85.

Bevan DR, Bevan JC, Donati F. Muscle relaxants in clinical anesthesia, , Chicago, IL: Year Book Medical Publishers; 1988.

Boros EE, Bigham EC, Boswell GE, et al. Bis-and mixed-tetrahydroisoquinolinium chlorofumarates: New ultra-short-acting nondepolarizing neuromuscular blockers.J Med Chem. 1999;42:206–9

Donati F, Antzaka C, Bevan DR. Potency of pancuronium at the diaphragm and adductor pollicis muscles in humans. Anesthesiology. 1986;65:1–5.

Engbaek J, Östergaard D, Viby-Mogensen J. Double burst stimulation (DBS). A new pattern of nerve stimulation to identify residual curarization. Br J Anaesth. 1989;62:274–8.

Kisor D, Schmith V, Wargin W, et al. Importance of the organ-independent elimination of cisatracurium. Anesth Analg. 1996;83:1065–71.

Östergaard D, Jensen E, Jensen FS, Viby-Mogensen J. The duration of action of mivacurium-induced neuromuscular block in patients homozygous for the atypical plasma cholinesterase gene. Anesthesiology. 1991;75:A774.

Viby-Mogensen J, Howardy-Hansen P, Chraemmer-Jorgensen B. Post-tetanic count (PTC): a new method of evaluating an intense nondepolarizing neuromuscular blockade. Anesthesiology. 1981;55:458–61.

Martyn JAJ, White DA, Gronert GA, Jaffe RS, Ward JM. Up-and-down regulation of skeletal muscle acetylcholine receptors: effects of neuromuscular blockers. Anesthesiology. 1992;76:822–43.

Yanez P, Martyn JAJ. Prolonged d-tubocurarine infusion and/or immobilization cause upregulation of acetycholine receptors and hyperkalemia to succinycholine in rats. Anesthesiology. 1996;84:384–91.

Chapter 33 Smooth muscle

Hugh A O'Beirne and Philip M Hopkins

Topics covered in this chapter

Smooth muscle structure
Smooth muscle contraction
Regulation of contraction
Vascular endothelium

SMOOTH MUSCLE STRUCTURE

Smooth muscle is composed of small fibers measuring 2–5μm in diameter and 20–500μm in length. Smooth muscle is generally divided into two broad categories, multiunit and single unit (unitary). Multiunit smooth muscle is composed of discrete fibers, each operating independently and usually innervated by a single nerve ending, similar to skeletal muscle. Multiunit fibers may contract independently. This type of smooth muscle usually lacks spontaneous contractions. Examples of multiunit smooth muscle include the ciliary and iris muscles in the eye. Single unit smooth muscle acts as a large mass of fibers, which contract as a single unit – hence the name. The cells form large sheets or bundles and are connected via gap junctions. Multiunit smooth muscle is not discussed further in this chapter.

Smooth muscle differs from striated muscle in that the organization of the filaments appears to be less well defined – smooth muscle lacks the visible cross-striations found in skeletal and cardiac muscle. The major contractile proteins in smooth muscle are actin and myosin. The myosin molecules are bundled together, to form thick filaments. Thin filaments comprise actin, tropomyosin, and other proteins attached via membrane plaques to the cell membrane (vinculin, metavinculin, α-actinin, and talin). The precise structure of the smooth muscle cytoskeleton remains uncertain. Within the cytoplasm thin filaments insert into fusiform dense bodies, which contain α-actinin and are analogous to the Z-lines in striated muscle. Other structural proteins include desmin and vinmentin, which have been proposed as intermediate filaments that create a three-dimensional network holding the dense bodies together. Filamin crosslinks actin filaments. The organization of thick, thin, and intermediate filaments imparts the characteristic shape to the myocyte.

Myosin is composed of a dimer of two heavy chains (200kDa) and two sets of light chains, 20kDa (LC_{20}) and 17kDa (LC_{17}). The carboxyl terminal region of the heavy chain forms the α-helical tail structure of the myosin molecule. The tails are involved in the assembly of myosin molecules into filaments, while the heads contain the actin-activated Mg^{2+} adenosine triphosphatase (ATPase) site.

Smooth muscle myocytes are coupled via low-resistance pathways termed gap junctions (connexons). These junctions are membrane structures that contain nonselective channels, and thus link the cytoplasm of adjacent cells together. Each channel is formed by two hemichannels and a hexameric subunit array of 43kDa connexins. This structure allows equilibration of ions and small molecules between cells, and thereby electronic coupling. In vascular smooth muscle, at least, these gap junctions are responsible for coordinating the contraction of blood vessels.

The neuromuscular junction of smooth muscle consists of autonomic nerve fibers branching diffusely over the muscle sheet. These diffuse junctions consist of terminal axons with multiple varicosities that contain acetylcholine or norepinephrine (noradrenaline).

Calmodulin is a ubiquitous Ca^{2+} binding protein (16.7kDa) that binds up to four Ca^{2+} ions. The three-dimensional structure consists of a dumbbell-shaped molecule with two globular domains, each possessing two Ca^{2+} binding sites, connected by a long central helix. Binding of Ca^{2+} induces a conformational change that allows interaction with and regulation of a number of proteins.

Calponin (34kDa) is an actin-binding protein involved in smooth muscle cell regulation; it binds to actin and tropomyosin and inhibits actomyosin ATPase activity. This is reversed by Ca^{2+} and calmodulin, and by phosphorylation of calponin by protein kinase C or Ca^{2+}/calmodulin-dependent protein kinase II. Calponin may be involved in the modulation of Ca^{2+} sensitivity of smooth muscle contraction.

Caldesmon, which is a weak Ca^{2+}/calmodulin-binding protein, also binds to actin, but its precise function is unknown. Experimentally, caldesmon enhances binding of myosin subfragments to actin. Phosphorylated caldesmon, acting through actin and tropomyosin, slows crossbridge detachment, possibly by altering actinomyosin binding or ATPase kinetics.

Vascular smooth muscle contains the sarcoplasmic reticulum (SR) protein phospholamban. When phosphorylated, phospholamban possesses Ca^{2+} channel activity and is involved in cyclic adenosine monophosphate (cAMP) mediated Ca^{2+} uptake by the SR. β-adrenergic agonists increase cAMP, which leads to activation of cAMP-dependent protein kinase and phosphorylation of phospholamban, thus increasing Ca^{2+} uptake into the SR.

SMOOTH MUSCLE CONTRACTION

Energy

Smooth muscle has a skeletal role in the maintenance of organ dimensions. Continuous partial activation, which may vary to produce oscillations in force, is characteristic of smooth muscle. Organs such as the intestines and bladder must maintain tonic contraction. In smooth muscle cells there is no physiologic need for speed or a high-power output, compared with that of skeletal muscle. In this setting, in which power requirements are comparatively low, the efficiency of chemomechanical transduction becomes secondary to the energy cost of force maintenance (e.g. continued vascular smooth muscle tone) which may be measured as economy of action (force × time /ATP consumption). If vascular smooth muscle behaved as skeletal muscle in terms of energy requirements, maintenance of blood pressure would result in a doubling of the basal metabolic rate. Smooth muscle cells can generate a force per cell cross-sectional area similar to that of skeletal muscle cells, but utilize only 25% of the myosin content and several hundred-fold less ATP consumption in the process. This implies not only that smooth muscle regulates crossbridge cycling rates, but also regulates the power output, efficiency, and economy of contraction.

Role of calcium

Smooth muscle contraction occurs when $[Ca^{2+}]_i$ (intracellular Ca^{2+} concentration) increases. The rise in $[Ca^{2+}]_i$ may result from nerve stimulation, stretch, or hormonal stimulation (Fig. 33.1). Some smooth muscle is self-excitatory, exhibiting slow-wave activity that initiates action potentials; these slow waves are termed pacemaker waves. The controlling mechanism for this slow-wave activity is unknown, but pumping of Na^+ out of the cell has been postulated as a mechanism. Ca^{2+} binds calmodulin, and the resultant Ca^{2+}/calmodulin complex activates myosin light chain kinase (MLCK).

Myosin light chain kinase and phosphorylation

Contractile activity of smooth muscle is regulated by reversible protein phosphorylation (Fig. 33.1). Protein phosphorylation–dephosphorylation is an important mechanism in the regulation of a wide variety of cellular processes (Chapter 3). Phosphorylation of proteins results in a conformational change that alters the activity and function of that protein. The state of phosphorylation of the protein depends on the relative activity of the protein kinases (phosphorylation) and protein phosphatases (dephosphorylation).

Not only does MLCK phosphorylate the myosin light chain (LC_{20}), but it also activates actomyosin ATPase. The energy for crossbridge formation (one ATP molecule per crossbridge formed) and actin–myosin interaction is provided by ATPase. The resultant tension developed occurs because of a change of axis between actin and myosin heads, from 90° to 45° with respect to the long axis of the myosin chain. The effect of load on shortening velocity and power output is qualitatively (but not quantitatively) the same in striated and smooth muscle. This similarity of force–velocity relationship in both muscle types supports the hypothesis that a sliding filament–crossbridge mechanism occurs in smooth muscle analogous to that described for skeletal muscle (Chapter 30).

The rate-limiting step in the actomyosin ATPase cycle (i.e. the release of inorganic phosphate) is increased 1000-fold by the phosphorylation of LC_{20}. The resultant conformational change in the myosin molecule facilitates crossbridge formation. Phosphorylation of LC_{20} correlates closely with the velocity of smooth muscle shortening. It is possible to measure this mechanical parameter using the slack test, which is the time required to redevelop tension after abrupt shortening of a contracted

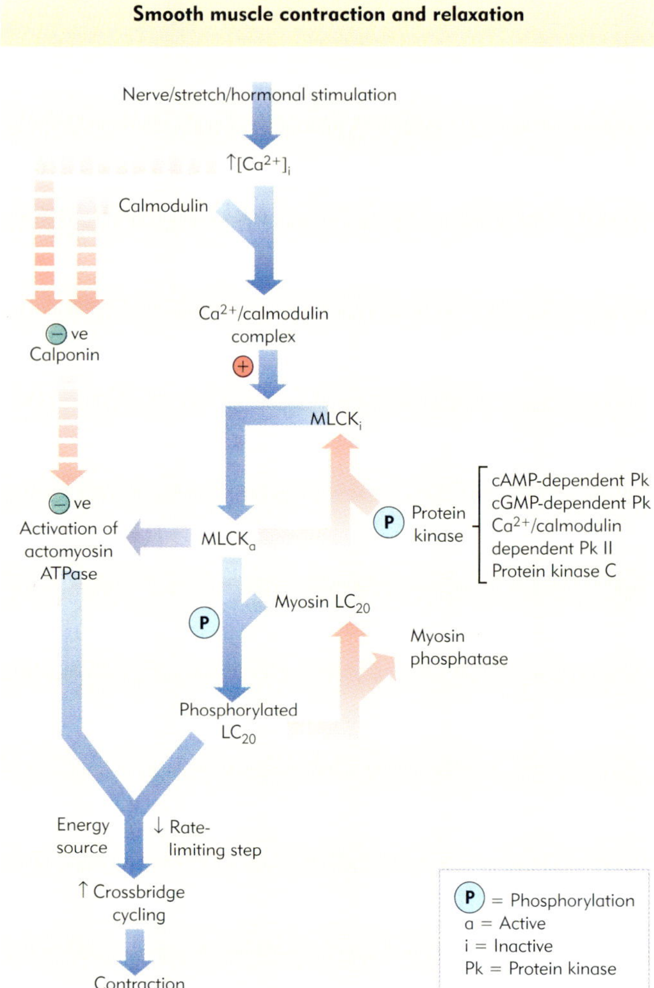

Figure 33.1 Smooth muscle contraction and relaxation. MLCK, myosin light chain kinase.

muscle. This is an estimate of the rate of actomyosin crossbridge cycling. Serine-19 residue on LC_{20} is phosphorylated by MLCK following activation by the Ca^{2+}/calmodulin complex. The MLCK enzyme is inactivated by phosphorylation. Protein kinases that phosphorylate MLCK include cAMP dependent protein kinase, cyclic guanosine monophosphate (cGMP)-dependent protein kinase, Ca^{2+}/calmodulin-dependent protein kinase II, and protein kinase C. This phosphorylation may play a role in enzyme regulation within the cell.

Dephosphorylation of LC_{20} by myosin phosphatase results in relaxation of smooth muscle, as demonstrated experimentally in skinned fiber preparations. Application of okadaic acid prevents relaxation of smooth muscle by inhibiting myosin phosphatase.

Latch state

Using Fura-2, a fluorescent dye, it is possible to measure changes in $[Ca^{2+}]_i$. LC_{20} phosphorylation changes parallel the change in $[Ca^{2+}]_i$. Tension development increases slowly in smooth muscle cells, reaching a peak level that is maintained despite a decrease in $[Ca^{2+}]_i$ and LC_{20} phosphorylation. This mechanical state of tension maintenance with slowly cycling crossbridges is the 'latch state', which is energy efficient because tension is maintained at the level of a slow-cycling actomyosin, with a resultant lower ATP consumption. The mechanism responsible for the latch state is unknown, but may involve dephosphorylation of LC_{20} while it is in a high-affinity binding conformation. A four-state crossbridge hypothesis has been proposed – free, attached, phosphorylated, and dephosphorylated myosin, each state having its own rate constant. Slowing of crossbridge detachment prolongs high-affinity binding and thus tension. This model varies from the classic Huxley model. In the Huxley two-state model, the distribution of active crossbridges, under steady-state isometric conditions, is determined by the relative rates of crossbridge attachment and detachment. During relaxation, crossbridges are at equilibrium between a dissociated state and a weak binding state in which crossbridge binding to actin is rapidly reversible and noncooperative. During contraction, crossbridges cycle through a strong-binding state, in which myosin cooperatively binds to actin with much greater affinity. Muscle shortening and force develops because of the transition from the weak-binding to the strong-binding state. The latch state differs from the rigor state of striated muscle in that the latch state is dynamic, requiring low but continuous LC_{20} phosphorylation and elevated Ca^{2+}.

REGULATION OF CONTRACTION

Excitation–contraction coupling

A resting membrane potential (RMP) of –40 to –55mV exists in smooth muscle cells. Mechanical factors such as stretch can depolarize the cell, which may involve a stretch-activated cation channel similar to that found in endothelial cells. Spike potentials similar to those in skeletal muscle occur in smooth muscle, and last about 10–50ms. In smooth muscle, action potentials are distinctive in that they have a long plateau phase, because Ca^{2+} is the major ion involved in action potential generation. Not only do Ca^{2+} channels open much more slowly than Na^+ channels but also they remain open for longer. Unlike skeletal muscle, Na^+ channels play little part in the generation of the action potential in smooth muscle.

The absence of either a refractory period or fatigue of smooth muscle is essential to its function. As discussed above, the latch state provides an energy-efficient mechanism for maintenance of force. To trigger smooth muscle contraction, Ca^{2+} is important. At rest $[Ca^{2+}]_i$ is about 0.1μmol/L, and rises to 10μmol/L during maximum activation. The rise in Ca^{2+} is mainly from influx through the sarcolemma, but also occurs because of release from intracellular stores (Fig. 33.2). Influx of Ca^{2+} is through voltage-dependent calcium channels (VDCCs), receptor-operated channels (ROCs), and nonselective cation channels (NSCCs), and by the Na^+/Ca^{2+} exchange pump. These cell membrane ion channels, cell membrane transporters, and a number of secondary messenger systems determine calcium homeostasis within the cell. The VDCCs are subdivided into long-lasting (L-type), transient (T-type), and resting (R-type) channels. Release of $Ca^{2+}$from the SR is via the ryanodine receptor channels (Ca^{2+}-induced Ca^{2+} release), which are caffeine sensitive, and through inositol-1,4,5-trisphosphate (IP_3) channels (heparin sensitive).

A fall in $[Ca^{2+}]_i$ is associated with relaxation of smooth muscle. At least three mechanisms are known to reduce intracellular calcium (Fig. 33.3):

- calcium–magnesium ATPase;
- sodium–calcium exchange; and
- uptake of Ca^{2+} into intracellular organelles, such as SR and mitochondria.

The Ca^{2+}–Mg^{2+} ATPase (calcium efflux pump) is found in the plasma membrane, and extrudes one calcium ion in exchange for two hydrogen ions. The enzyme is dependent on Mg^{2+} and ATP, and is stimulated by the Ca^{2+}/ calmodulin complex. This may act as a feedback mechanism to limit the rise in $[Ca^{2+}]_i$.

The Na^+/Ca^{2+}exchanger transports one Ca^{2+} in exchange for three Na^+ ions. The Na^+ gradient across the cell acts as the driving force, and Na^+,K^+-ATPase maintains this gradient. The distribution of Na^+/Ca^{2+}exchangers among different subtypes of smooth muscle cells is unclear, but some evidence suggests that this pump is present in some types of smooth muscle, namely tracheal smooth muscle.

Intracellular Ca^{2+} removal is by uptake into SR and mitochondria. Uptake of Ca^{2+} by the SR is via a Ca^{2+}-ATPase-dependent pump. Uptake into the SR is cAMP- and cGMP-dependent through activation of cAMP-dependent and cGMP-dependent protein kinases, respectively. Affinity for Ca^{2+} by this pump is enhanced by cGMP. Activated protein kinase C increases the activity of the pump, and thereby reduces $[Ca^{2+}]_i$ (Fig. 33.3).

The mitochondria take up Ca^{2+}, store it in a nonionic form (calcium phosphate complex), and release it into the cytosol via a Ca^{2+} efflux pathway. This may have a protective role in states of Ca^{2+} overload (e.g. anoxia, ischemia).

Potassium channels

A key role is played by K^+ channels in the regulation of cell excitability and smooth muscle contractility. These K^+ channels include Ca^{2+}-activated channels (BK_{Ca}), delayed rectifier K^+ channels (K_V), and ATP-sensitive K^+ channels (K_{ATP}). Also, K^+ is important in maintaining the RMP and in the repolarization after action potentials. In smooth muscle cells the RMP is –40 to –55 mV. Since $[K^+]_i$ is about 150mmol/L and $[K^+]_o$ is around 3–5mmol/L, the activation of K^+ channels results in an outward current of K^+ ions, down their electrochemical gradient, which leads to hyperpolarization of the cell. The membrane hyperpolarizes from –55mV toward the equilibrium potential of K^+ (E_{K+} = –80mV). Smooth muscle excitability is reduced at this hyperpolarized potential, and other important channels remain closed.

In particular, voltage-gated Ca^{2+} channels remain closed because the voltage threshold required for them to open is around –40mV. Hyperpolarization also activates the Na^+, K^+-ATPase pump, which reduces intracellular Na^+ and, as a consequence, drives the reversible Na^+/Ca^{2+} pump with increased extrusion of Ca^{2+} and influx of Na^+. Mobilization of Ca^{2+} from intracellular stores is reduced because of inhibition of the agonist-stimulated accumulation of IP_3 and there is a decrease in Ca^{2+} sensitivity of the contractile proteins. K^+_{ATP} channels open when ATP levels are reduced, and in response to K^+ channel activators (cromakalim, nicorandil, pinacidil). The effect of K^+ channel opening is relaxation of the smooth muscle cell. Sulfonylureas (glibenclamide, tolbutamide, chlorpropamide) block the K^+ channel.

Nitrovasodilators, nitric oxide (NO), and atrial natriuretic peptide lead to an increase in intracellular cGMP, which is broken down [by phosphodiesterase (PDE)] into 5′-GMP, and increases the open probability (P_o) of Ca^{2+}-activated K^+ channels. This results in hyperpolarization and vasorelaxation.

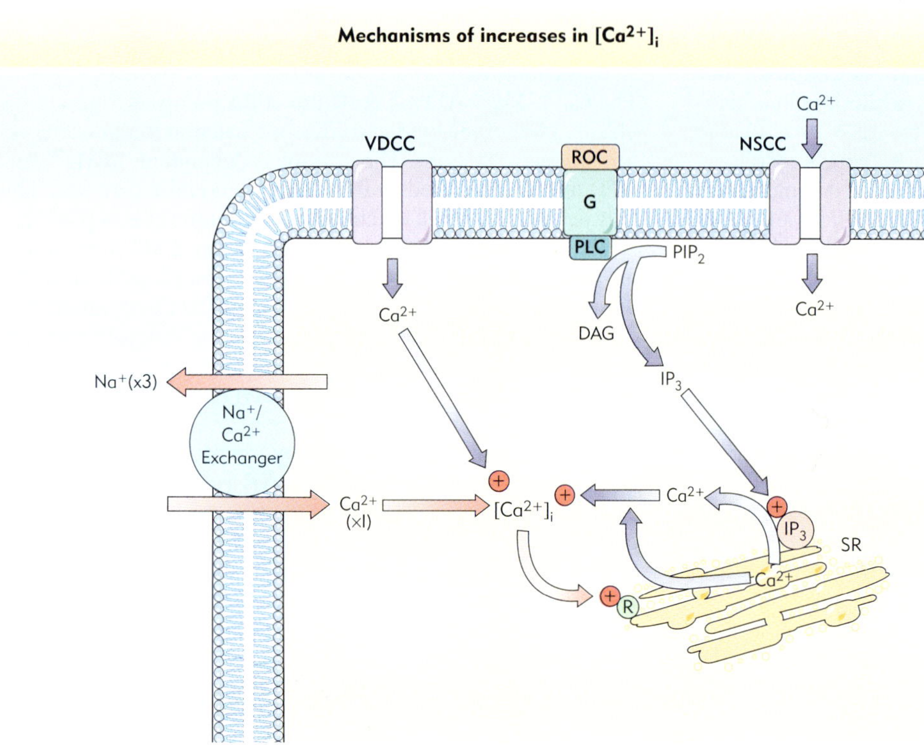

Figure 33.2 Mechanisms of increases in intracellular Ca^{2+} concentration. R, ryanodine receptor; SR, sarcoplasmic reticulum; VDCC, voltage-dependent calcium channel; ROC, receptor-operated channel; PLC, phospholipase C; G, G protein, PIP$_2$, phosphatidylinositol 4,5-bisphosphate; IP$_3$, inositol-1,4,5-trisphosphate; DAG, 1,2-diacylglycerol.

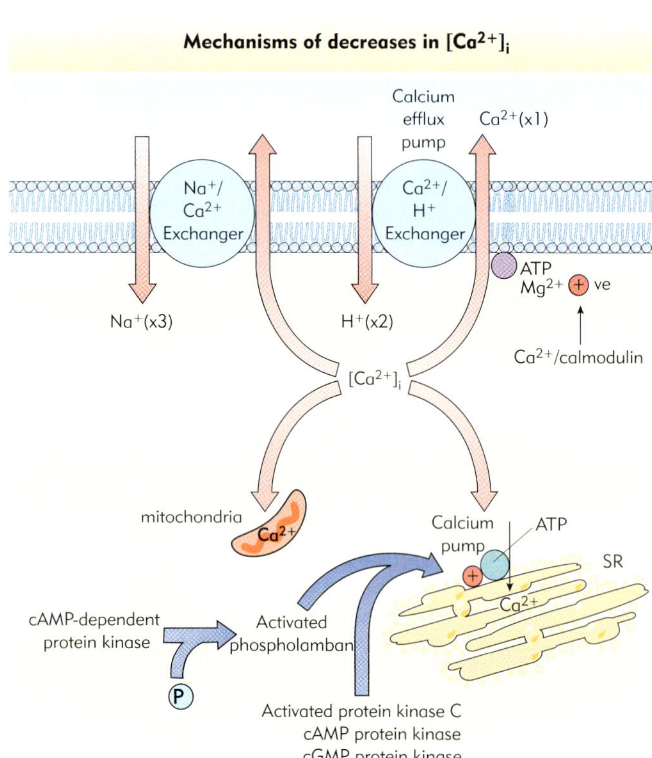

Figure 33.3 Mechanisms of decreases in intracellular Ca^{2+} concentration.

Receptor-operated channels

α_1-Adrenoceptors activate phospholipase and the resultant increase of IP$_3$ leads to release of Ca^{2+} from intracellular SR stores. The rise in $[Ca^{2+}]_i$ results in an opening of NSCCs, which leads to membrane depolarization. α_1-Receptor stimulation brings the cell membrane potential toward the equilibrium potential for Na^+ (E_{Na^+} = 50mV) which is more positive than the RMP of –55mV.

Norepinephrine (NE; noradrenaline) enhances the P_o of voltage-gated Ca^{2+} channels, and therefore increases $[Ca^{2+}]_i$ by release of Ca^{2+} from intracellular stores (namely SR), by IP$_3$, and stimulates extracellular Ca^{2+} influx through voltage-gated channels.

β_2-Adrenoceptors increase Ca^{2+} influx by G-protein coupled activation of Ca^{2+} channels and cell membrane depolarization. The population of α_1- and β_2-adrenoceptors varies between various vascular beds.

Second messengers within the smooth muscle cell: cyclic adenosine monophosphate and cyclic guanosine monophosphate

The cAMP pathway is an important relaxant signal transduction pathway in smooth muscle. The β_2-adrenoceptor is coupled through the stimulatory G protein (G_s) to adenylyl cyclase. The muscarinic receptor m$_2$ inhibits adenylyl cyclase through an inhibitory G protein (G_i). Activated cAMP-dependent protein kinase (protein kinase A) phosphorylates a number of different substrates, and thereby inhibits inositol phosphate hydrolysis to IP$_3$ and 1,2 diacylglycerol (DAG) and inactivates MLCK, increases uptake of Ca^{2+} into the SR, and activates ion channels including the Na^+,K^+-ATPase and K^+ channels (mainly the maxi-K^+ channel) (Fig. 33.4). Each of these pathways ultimately reduces $[Ca^{2+}]_i$ and causes relaxation. Agents that act through the cAMP mechanism include β_2-adrenoceptor agonists, vasoactive intestinal peptide (VIP), and various prostaglandins (e.g. PGE$_2$).

Elevation of cGMP within smooth muscle leads to relaxation. There are two types of guanylyl cyclase, a membrane-bound form and a cytosolic form. The membrane-bound form, also known as particulate guanylyl cyclase, is activated via membrane-bound receptors. This was discovered when the injection of guinea pig

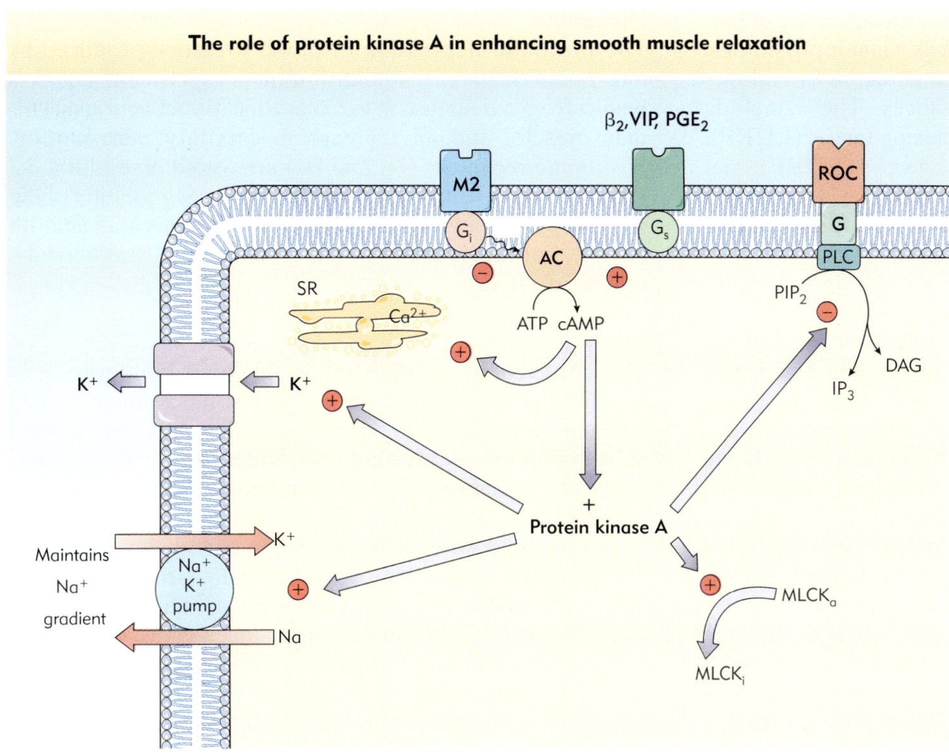

Figure 33.4 The role of protein kinase A in enhancing smooth muscle relaxation. G_s, G stimulatory; G_i, G inhibitory; AC, adenylyl cyclase; PLC, phospholipase C; PIP_2, phosphatidylinositol 4,5-bisphosphate; DAG, 1,2-diacylglycerol; IP_3, inositol -1,4,5-trisphosphate; G, G protein; MLCK, myosin light chain kinase; SR, sarcoplasmic reticulum; m_2, muscariunic tpe 2 receptor; β_2, β-adrenergic type 2 receptor; VIP, vasoactive intestinal polypeptide receptor; PGE_2, prostaglandin E_2 receptor; ROC, receptor operated channel.

atrial granules led to a diuresis; hence the term atrial natriuretic peptide (ANP). It was also noted that smooth muscle relaxation occurred. Since then, BNP (from porcine brain originally) and C-type natriuretic peptide (CNP) have been discovered. Soluble guanylyl cyclase is a heme protein heterodimer activated by NO. Since cGMP inhibits the hydrolysis of phosphatidylinositol 4,5-bisphosphate (PIP_2) to IP_3 and DAG, it reduces IP_3 production and thereby Ca^{2+} mobilization from the SR. Also cGMP increases Ca^{2+} uptake by the SR (via cGMP-dependent protein kinase), decreases the sensitivity of MLCK for Ca^{2+}, and interferes with receptor-operated Ca^{2+} channels.

Nitrates

Nitroglycerin and sodium nitroprusside relax smooth muscle by degrading to NO which stimulates soluble guanylyl cyclase and increase intracellular cGMP. *S*-Nitrosothiols consist of NO linked to a thiol group and are found endogenously. Endogenous NO is produced by epithelial cells and by the nonadrenergic noncholinergic nerves, which may be important for regulation of bronchomotor smooth muscle tone. Each of ANP, BNP, and CNP acts through cGMP production to cause smooth muscle relaxation.

The 3′-phosphoester bond on cAMP and cGMP is hydrolyzed and converted by PDE into the 5′-nucleotide metabolites 5′-AMP and 5′-GMP, respectively. At least seven classes of PDE (PDE I–VII) exist and each class has several isoforms. These PDE isoenzymes are present in differing distributions depending on the tissue. All of them may be inhibited, the physiologic consequences of which depend on the concentration of PDE within certain tissues and on the selectivity of the particular PDE inhibitor for that isoenzyme fraction. Airway smooth muscle, for example, contains a high concentration of PDE III and IV. The theophyllines and xanthine derivatives cause relaxation of airway smooth muscle *in vitro* and bronchodilatation *in vivo* through PDE inhibition, although other mechanisms may also be involved. Theophylline is a nonspecific inhibitor of PDE isoenzymes, and therefore has a narrow therapeutic window. Although inhibition of cyclic nucleotide PDE is often used to explain all the actions of theophylline, it is probably not the sole mechanism at therapeutic concentrations. The intracellular accumulation of cGMP may be partly responsible for mediating smooth muscle relaxation by theophyllines. However, methylxanthines act also as competitive antagonists of P1 purinergic receptors, which could explain some effects of theophylline on the central nervous and cardiac conduction systems, and may underlie the efficacy of theophylline in antagonizing bronchoconstriction. Newer, selective inhibitors (PDE III) include bipyridines (amrinone and milrinone) and imidazolones (piroximone and enoximone). The selective PDE inhibitors, which combine inotropic and vasodilator activity, act on the isoenzyme fraction present in cardiac and vascular smooth muscle.

Although PDE III isoenzymes exist in airway smooth muscle, bronchodilatation is not a predominant clinical feature of the current cardiotonic selective PDE III inhibitors. Some PDE inhibitors attenuate the release of inflammatory mediators, particularly those that affect PDE IV. It may be that PDE inhibitors that affect these isoenzyme systems and combine bronchodilatation, inhibition of platelet aggregation, and modification of airway inflammation could be developed for future treatment and prophylaxis of asthma. Sildenafil, an oral agent for erectile dysfunction, inhibits PDE V in the corpus cavernosum and, to a lesser extent, PDE VI in the retina, with little effect on PDE III. It acts by potentiating the response to NO released from nerve and endothelial cells, and potentiates the hypotensive effects of nitrates.

VASCULAR ENDOTHELIUM

The vascular endothelium constitutes a single layer of thin cells that lines the intimal surface of the circulatory system, and constitutes a very active tissue with a broad variety of biologic actions. Vascular endothelium plays a major physiologic role in the regulation of vascular tone mediated by endogenously synthesized vasoactive substances. These include prostacyclin, endothelium-derived relaxing factor (EDRF), endothelium-derived hyperpolarizing factor (EDHF), and endothelium-derived contracting factor (EDCF). Angiotensin I is converted into angiotensin II by the endothelial membrane-bound angiotensin-converting enzyme.

Endothelium-derived relaxing factor

The biologic half-life of EDRF is 6.3 seconds. The control of cellular superoxide anion levels by superoxide dismutase appears necessary for the action of EDRF and for the response of the nitrovasodilators on vascular smooth muscle. Smooth muscle relaxation caused by the endothelium-dependent vasodilators and nitrovasodilators (nitroglycerin and nitroprusside) known to release NO led to the hypothesis that EDRF and NO may be one and the same. Ignarro demonstrated that, indeed, EDRF is NO, which is synthesized by oxidation of L-arginine by constitutive NO synthase. This cytosolic enzyme is activated by interaction of Ca^{2+}/calmodulin and requires nicotinamide adenine dinucleotide phosphate and tetrahydrobiopterin as cofactors.

Since NO is a small non-polar molecule, it rapidly penetrates the smooth muscle cell membrane and binds to and activates the heme portion of soluble guanylyl cyclase. The increase of cGMP reduces intracellular Ca^{2+} levels and causes vasorelaxation (see above). Also, NO induces transient hyperpolarization of vascular smooth muscle by activating the Na^+, K^+-ATPase pump.

The production and release of NO is continuous. The continuous release may result from viscous shear stress and pulsatile arterial flow. The flow-induced shear stress, which acts on endothelial cells to produce EDRF (NO), is the most important stimulus for the endothelial-dependent control of vascular tone. This modulates systemic and pulmonary vascular resistance. Aside from this basal release, a variety of physiologic stimuli and vasoactive substances stimulate the endothelium to release EDRF. These include acetylcholine, adenosine diphosphate (ADP), ATP, bradykinin, calcitonin gene-related protein, cholecystokinin, histamine, norepinephrine, serotonin, substance P, thrombin, and VIP.

Increases in transmural pressure lead to a proportionate increase in EDRF with a resultant improvement in organ perfusion. Also, EDRF is released in response to hypoxia. When the partial pressure of oxygen falls to a critical level, however, endothelial cells cease to release EDRF and synthesize endothelium-dependent vasoconstricting factors (EDCF).

Purinoceptors

Purinoceptors are ATP and ADP receptors present on vascular endothelial and smooth muscle cells. Smooth muscle cells have two subclasses of purinoceptor population – stimulation of P_{2X} leads to vasoconstriction and of P_{2Y} leads to vasodilatation. The P_{2X} purinoceptor is an ATP-gated ion channel that mediates membrane depolarization and Ca^{2+} entry. The endothelial cell P_{2Y} purinoceptor produces vasodilatation via EDRF release, similar to acetylcholine stimulation. The ultimate smooth muscle cell response depends on the predominance of one subclass of receptor and the local production of EDRF. Release of purine transmitters is derived from aggregating platelets, specialized nonsympathetic purinergic neurons, and endothelial cells.

Histamine

The profound depression of blood pressure produced by intravenous histamine administration in experimental models results from a decrease in vascular tone, direct action on cardiac muscle, and an increase in capillary permeability. Histamine receptors (H_1 and H_2) are found on endothelial (H_1) and smooth muscle (H_1 and H_2) cells. Stimulation of the H_1 receptors causes vasoconstriction in vascular smooth muscle, but this is offset by endothelial H_1 receptor, which releases EDRF.

Bradykinin

The intravenous administration of bradykinin produces hypotension by decreasing peripheral resistance and increasing vascular permeability in the microcirculation. Under physiologic conditions, bradykinin contributes little to the maintenance of vascular tone because its plasma concentration is low. The cardiovascular actions of bradykinin are related to stimulation of a bradykinin receptor (B_2) on endothelial cells, stimulation of the production of prostaglandins from endothelial cells, and stimulation of bradykinin receptors on smooth muscle cells. The arterial vasodilatation produced via B_2 endothelial receptor stimulation is mediated by EDRF, prostacyclin PGI_2, and PGE_2 release. In veins, bradykinin preferentially liberates $PGF_{2\alpha}$ (vasoconstrictor) instead of PGE_2. The contractile effects of prostaglandins are mediated by thromboxane receptors at which PGE_2 is a weak agonist.

There are three PGE receptors – PG_1, PG_2, and PG_3. Each is coupled to a different cell signaling system. The relaxant effect of PGE_2 is mediated through stimulation of the EP_2 receptor, which is coupled to cAMP synthesis. Vasodilating prostaglandins probably play a determinant role in arterial vascular tone.

Another vasoactive compound released from aggregating platelets is thromboxane A_2. Thromboxane causes direct vasoconstriction but has no endothelial-mediated effects.

The release of platelet activating factor derived from platelets, neutrophils, mast cells, and endothelial cells produces endothelium-dependent vasodilatation only at higher concentrations. Platelet activating factor has a complex vasomotor effect because it is able to stimulate not only EDRF, but also effect thromboxane and leukotriene release. Also, ADP and ATP are released from platelets – their purinergic effects are discussed above.

The production of cGMP by ANP proceeds via particulate guanylyl cyclase. While ANP secretion increases in response to atrial stretching, released EDRF is able to influence the production and release of ANP by atrial myocytes, and thereby modulates in a negative fashion the release of ANP.

Prostacyclin

Prostacyclin (PGI_2) is a major vasodilatory prostaglandin produced by the endothelial cell. By activating platelet adenylyl cyclase, prostacyclin increases platelet cAMP levels and thereby inhibits platelet aggregation. Prostacyclin has a very short half-life of only one circulation time. Like EDRF, PGI_2 synthesis by endothelial cells is dependent on physical factors (pulsatile flow and shear stress) and endogenous mediators (bradykinin, thrombin, serotonin, platelet-derived growth factor, interleukin-1, and adenine nucleotides). Some drugs (calcium channel antagonists, captopril, dipyridamole, nitrates, diuretics, and streptokinase) can also stimulate its production.

Endothelium-derived hyperpolarizing factor

The release of EDHF follows acetylcholine stimulation; it causes transient changes in the membrane potential of smooth muscle cells. Acetylcholine causes endothelium-dependent relaxation and hyperpolarization in tissue contracted by norepinephrine. Acetylcholine activates m_1 muscarinic receptors to effect EDRF release, while m_2 muscarinic receptor stimulation leads to EDHF release.

Endothelium-derived contracting factor/endothelin

Endothelin/EDCF can be released from endothelium in response to changes of pressure, rapid stretching, anoxia, electrical stimulation, and large doses or repeated smaller doses of acetylcholine or arachidonic acid. In normal endothelium the basal release of EDCF has been reported. Endothelin exists as a family of isoforms, among the first of which to be identified was the peptide termed endothelin-1 (ET-1). It is a 21 amino acid, powerful vasoconstrictor peptide, originally isolated from porcine aortic endothelial cells. It is synthesized as a precursor protein called preproET-1 (203 amino acids), which is converted in two steps into ET-1. The ET peptides are not stored within synthesizing cells but are released in the extracellular medium at a steady rate. The only endothelin to be synthesized by the endothelial cells is ET-1. Unlike EDRF and EDHF, endothelin has a longer-lasting vasoconstrictor effect in most but not all vascular beds.

Endothelium-derived NO can interfere with endothelin production. Any agent that causes an increased level of cGMP inhibits endothelin synthesis. Activation of these endothelial receptors brings about increased production of EDRF and/or PGI_2. Endothelial cells can be stimulated by ET-1 to secrete different vasodilating substances depending on the origin of the vascular endothelial cells. The syntheses of NO and prostacyclin are also stimulated by ET-1.

The other isoforms of the endothelin family are endothelin-2 (ET-2), endothelin-3 (ET-3), and endothelin-b (ET-b). In many pathophysiologic states significant elevations in ET peptide concentrations have been observed. When administered intravenously (in animals), ET-1 and ET-3 are removed from the circulation with a half-life of <2 minutes. Binding sites for ET peptides are distributed throughout the body: ET receptors have been classified into two major subtypes, depending on the relative affinity for the receptor for the ET subtypes. At low concentrations, ET-1-induced vasoconstriction is dependent on extracellular Ca^{2+} and is effectively attenuated by dihydropyridine Ca^{2+} channel antagonists.

At higher concentrations, however, ET-1 causes vasoconstriction in Ca^{2+}-free solutions, which may involve an increase in cytosolic Ca^{2+} by IP_3 and activation of protein kinase C by DAG. These two second messengers are produced by receptor-mediated activation of phospholipase C, which catalyzes the hydrolysis of membrane phosphatidylinositol- 4, 5-bisphosphate. It has been shown that ET peptides stimulate this pathway of signal transduction in a number of cell types, including vascular smooth muscle cells. The ET-induced increases in cytosolic Ca^{2+} occur by IP_3-mediated mobilization from intracellular stores (initial transient increase) and by influx of extracellular Ca^{2+} via receptor-mediated or dihydropyridine-sensitive, voltage-gated Ca^{2+} channels (sustained increase).

Calcium channel antagonists

The VDCC antagonists include verapamil, diltiazem, nicardipine, nifedipine, and gallopamil. These agents inhibit the contractile response to depolarizing agents, and also inhibit the response to cholinergic agonists, histamine, and leukotriene D4. However, an in-vitro study in airway smooth muscle using these agents required high drug concentrations to elicit effects. A possible reason for this is that despite block by these agents of influx of Ca^{2+} through the Ca^{2+} channels (the main source of $[Ca^{2+}]_i$), increase in $[Ca^{2+}]_i$ may still be occurring because of release from intracellular stores, thus stimulating contraction.

Lithium

Lithium inhibits myoinositol phosphate synthesis, which results in a reduction in membrane phospholipid pools and causes relaxation of smooth muscle. In-vitro studies show a protective role of Li^+ against histamine-induced smooth muscle contraction in guinea pig airways.

Key References

Biebuyck JF, Watkins WD, Berkowitz DE, Gandhi CR. Endothelins: biochemistry and pathophysiologic actions. Anesthiology. 1994;80:892–8.

Knox AA, Tattersfield A. Airway smooth muscle relaxation. Thorax. 1995;50:894–9.

Large WA, Wang Q. Characteristics and physiological role of the Ca^{2+}-activated Cl^- conductance in smooth muscle. Am J Physiol. 1996:(2 Pt1);C435–50.

Murphy R. What is special about smooth muscle? The significance of covalent crossbridge regulation. FASEB J 1994;8:311–8.

Searle NR, Sahab P. Endothelial vasomotor regulation in health and disease. Can J Anesth. 1992;39:838–57.

Warner TD, Mitchell JA, Sheng H, Murad F. Effects of cyclic GMP on smooth muscle relaxation. Adv Pharmacol. 1994;26,171–94.

Further Reading

Bosnjak Z. Ion channels in vascular smooth muscle physiology and pharmacology. Anesthiology. 1993;79:1392–401.

Gerthoffer WT, Pohl J. Caldesmon and calponin phosphorylation in regulation of smooth muscle contraction. Can J Physiol Pharmacol. 1994;72:1410–4.

Guyton AC. Contraction and excitation of smooth muscle. In: Guyton AC, ed. Human physiology and mechanisms of disease, 6th edn. Philadelphia: WB Saunders; 1997; Chapter 8, 95.

Hathaway DR, March KL, Lash JA, Adam LP, Wilensky RL. Vascular smooth muscle, a review of the molecular basis of contractility. Circulation. 1991;83:382–90.

Johns R. Endothelium, anesthetics, and vascular control. Anesthiology. 1993;79:1381–91.

Su JY, Chang YI, Tang LJ. Mechanisms of action of enflurane on vascular smooth muscle: comparison of rabbit aorta and femoral artery. Anesthiology. 1994;81:700–9.

Chapter 34 Cardiac physiology

Daniel Nyhan and Thomas JJ Blanck

Topics covered in this chapter

Cardiac structure
Cardiac function
Anesthetic effects on cardiac function
Metabolism
Coronary blood flow
Regulation of coronary vasomotor tone

CARDIAC STRUCTURE

Cardiac muscle is a unique type of striated muscle; however, it resembles skeletal muscle in many of its basic features (Chapter 30). Myofibrils, which make up about half the volume of a cardiac myocyte, run parallel to the long axis of the cell. Myofibrils consist of ordered longitudinal arrays of interdigitating thick and thin filaments. The sarcomere is the repeating contractile unit found in each myocyte. The arrangement of the filaments gives rise to the lines and bands that can be seen by microscopy. Thick filaments are found in the center of the sarcomere and are made-up of intertwined myosin molecules with myosin heads extending out from the longitudinal axis in opposite directions (Fig 34.1). Thin filaments are made up of two chains of actin molecules intertwined to form a helical structure and are attached to the Z line in the sarcomere. The I band consists of thin filaments surrounding the Z line; the A band is made up of the area of overlap of the thick filaments with the thin filaments. Myocytes are joined together by specialized junctions known as intercalated disks. Actin filaments from adjacent cells insert into intercalated disks, as they do into Z lines (see Fig 34.1).

T-tubules, which are invaginations of the plasma membrane, are usually oriented transversely to the longitudinal axis of the myocyte; they allow closer access of the plasma membrane and extracellular fluid to the myocyte interior. The junctional sarcoplasmic reticulum (SR), which contains Ca^{2+}-release channels (CRC), is found in close apposition to the T-tubules. Voltage-dependent Ca^{2+} channels (VDCC) are found within the T-tubular membrane. Upon depolarization, they open and allow extracellular Ca^{2+} to enter. The Ca^{2+} interacts with the CRC resulting in Ca^{2+}-induced release of large amounts of Ca^{2+} from SR stores, which triggers contraction by a complex interaction with troponin and tropomyosin (Fig 34.2). The tropomyosin molecule, a linear regulatory protein of 70,000kDa, sits in the groove of the actin helix extended over seven actin monomers. The troponin complex is found bound to the thin filament at the end of each tropomyosin and serves to transmit the intracellular Ca^{2+} signal to actin and myosin. The troponin complex consists of three proteins: troponin C, which binds two molecules of Ca^{2+} during each heart beat, is complexed with troponin I, which inhibits the interaction of actin and myosin, and troponin T, which binds to tropomyosin. Binding of Ca^{2+} leads to a conformational change in troponin, resulting in a repositioning of tropomyosin and disinhibition of the actin–myosin interaction. The removal of tropomyosin from its inhibitory site allows the myosin head to bind to actin, resulting in the release of ADP, the binding and hydrolysis of ATP, and the utilization of ATP hydrolysis energy to allow the cycling of the myosin cross-bridge to another actin and, hence, shortening of the myocyte.

CARDIAC FUNCTION

The overall function of the cardiovascular system is to deliver oxygen and metabolic substrates to the tissues and to remove products of metabolism. This requires the normal and integrated function of the systemic arterial and venous circulations, right heart, pulmonary circulation, and left heart. Most abnormalities of cardiac function arise in the left ventricle (LV). However, normal and abnormal LV function is also critically influenced by interactions with both the systemic and pulmonary circulations and with the other cardiac chambers. Cardiac pump function (specifically LV function) will be discussed in the context of its main determinants: systolic function, diastolic function, and heart rate. Loading conditions (preload and afterload, the latter encompassing arterial compliance, impedance, and the Anrep effect) and contractility will be discussed under systolic function. Heart rate (including the treppe or Bowditch effect) will be discussed briefly in the context of its effect on systolic function (Chapter 35 covers mechanisms of conduction and dysrhythmias). It is now apparent that the concept of ascribing independent roles to preload, afterload, heart rate, and contractility in determining cardiac pump function is too simplistic. These determinants of pump function are all inter-related and have overlapping effects on the levels of Ca^{2+} to which the contractile elements are exposed and/or on the sensitivity of the contractile elements to Ca^{2+} (see below).

The cardiac cycle

Cardiac output is determined by heart rate and *stroke volume*. Normal stroke volume requires both normal systolic and normal diastolic LV function. Physiologists and cardiologists differ in

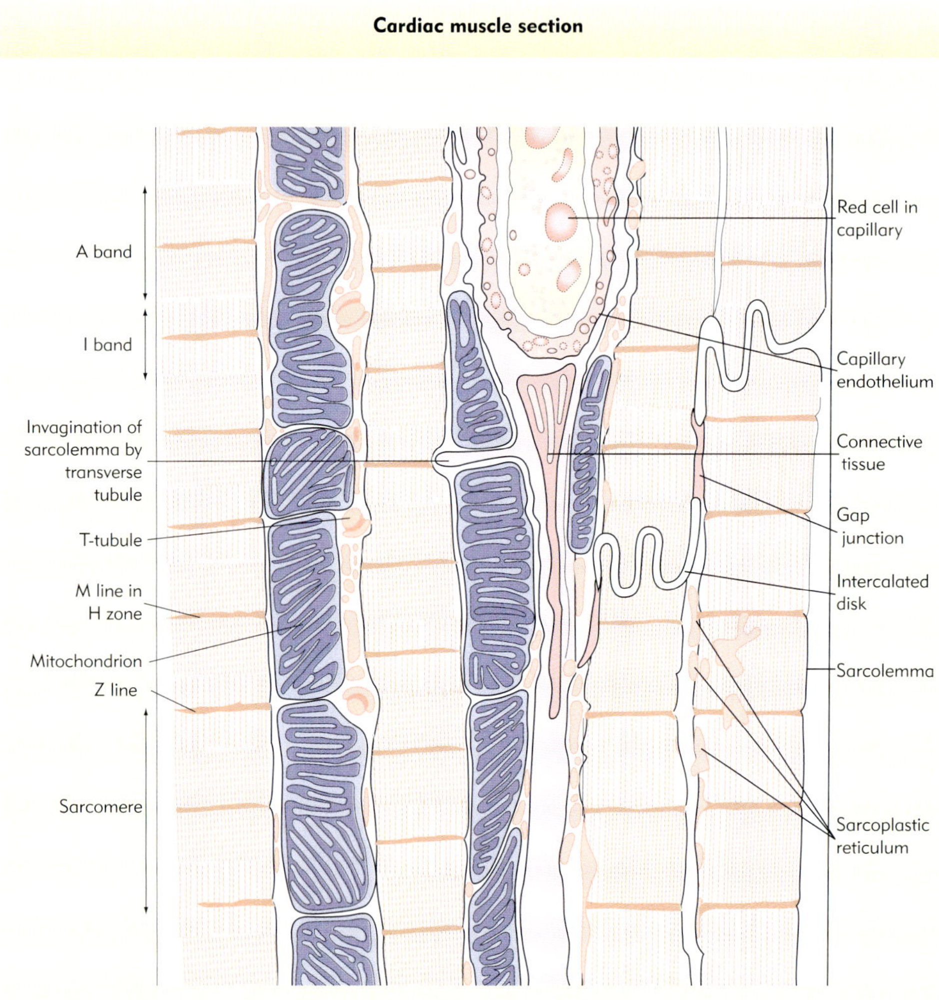

Figure 34.1 Cardiac muscle in longitudinal section. Cross-section showing components. Mitochondria bordering the myofibrils are dark elliptical structures (mit). The Z line demarcates the sarcomere, the repeating contractile unit. The dark structures in the cross-sectional view are myosin molecules, which form the thick filaments designated as the A band. The light I band on either side of the Z line consists of thin filaments composed of polymers. The T-tubule (T) is a membranous invagination of the sarcolemma. (Diagram from Berne and Levy, 1990.)

their definitions of systole and diastole. Physiologic systole begins at the start of isovolumic contraction when LV pressure exceeds atrial pressure (mitral valve closure occurs *after* this point) and extends to the peak of LV ejection. Physiologic diastole begins as LV pressure *starts* to fall. Aortic valve closure does not occur until LV pressure is less than or equal to aortic pressure. Cardiologists define systole as beginning with mitral valve closure and ending with aortic valve closure (both later in the cardiac cycle than the end points for physiologic systole). Depending on the circumstances, these are two operationally useful definitions of systole and diastole. However, the distinction is somewhat semantic when interpreted in the context of integrated pump function.

Both systole and diastole are active, energy-requiring processes. LV relaxation requires Ca^{2+} uptake by the SR and extrusion of Ca^{2+} across the sarcolemma. This results in reduced LV ejection, with LV pressure falling first below aortic pressure (with aortic valve closure) and then atrial pressure (with mitral valve opening and rapid ventricular filling). At the level of the sarcomere, LV relaxation, an important but not a unique determinant of LV filling, begins even as blood is being ejected into the aorta. Normal pump function depends on normal filling, which is critically determined by an active process (LV relaxation) that begins during LV emptying.

Multiple parameters are used to evaluate cardiac function. These range from those that evaluate overall cardiac function (e.g. family of Frank–Starling curves) to those that evaluate one specific feature of cardiac function [e.g. maximal velocity of contraction (V_{max}) and maximal pressure change with time (dP/dt)]. The LV pressure–volume relationship (Fig. 34.3) is conceptually useful in discussing both systolic and diastolic function. The assessment of cardiac function by any of these determinants depends on their proper interpretation.

Systolic function

Systolic function, defined as the ability of the LV to empty, is determined by the loading conditions of the heart (preload and afterload), contractility, and ventricular configuration.

Preload (the load on the heart at the end of diastole, preceding contraction) is determined by ventricular volume. Starling's original descriptions detailed the influence of LV volume on cardiac output. The frequently used surrogates for LV volume (LV end-diastolic pressure, pulmonary capillary wedge pressure) are, even under normal circumstances, imprecise because of the curvilinear relationship between LV end-diastolic volume and pressure. Measurement of pressure–volume loops is one of the best methods available to assess cardiac function. However, it is limited by difficulties

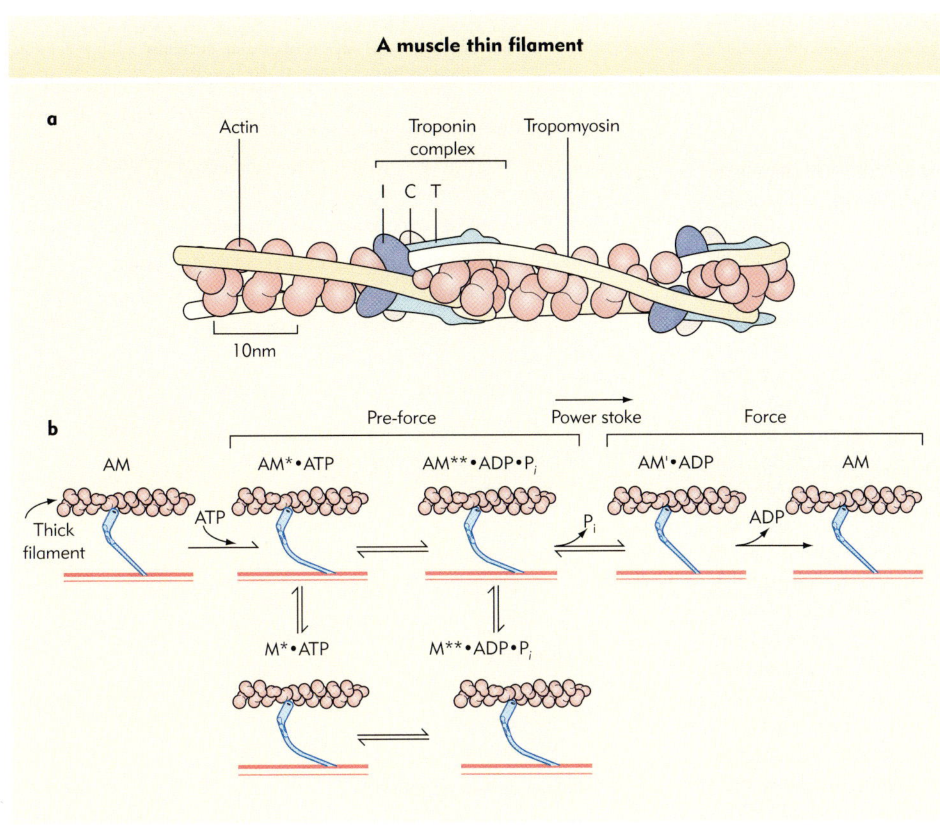

Figure 34.2 The actin filament and its interaction with the myosin head. (a) Tropomyosin and troponin fit along the actin polymer in a muscle thin filament. Binding of Ca^{2+} to troponin C relieves the tropomyosin blockade of the actin–myosin interaction, initiating contraction. (b) Schema modified from the Rayment five-step model for interaction between the myosin head and the actin filament. The cycle starts with the rigor state, in which the myosin head is still attached to actin at the end of the power stroke. ATP binds to the ATP-binding pocket to cause the head to assume the same molecular configuration as before the power stroke. Binding of the head of an adjacent actin monomer occurs first weakly and then strongly. Myosin ATPase activity splits the ATP into ADP and P_i (inorganic phosphate). As P_i is released, the power stroke occurs, and the actin filament is moved by 5 to 10nm. M, M*, M**, represent different conformations of the myosin molecule; A represents actin.

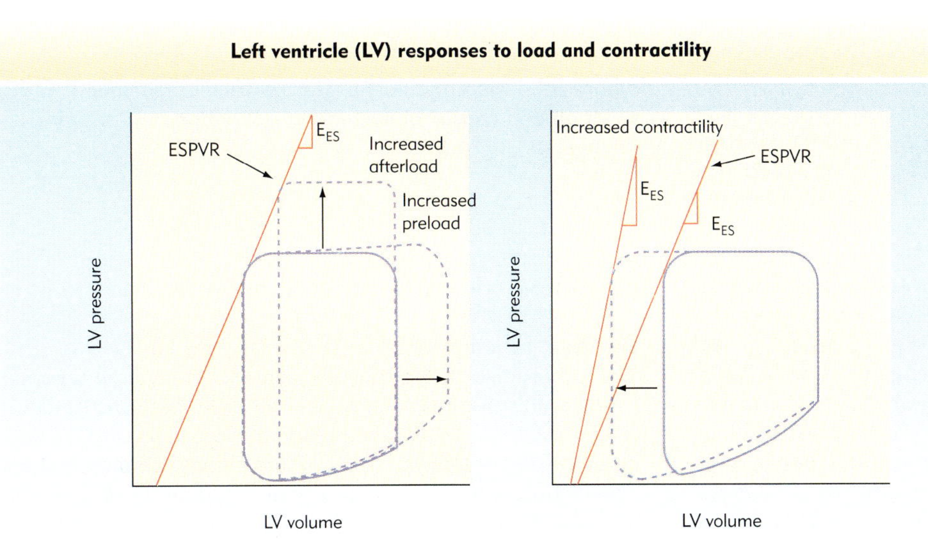

Figure 34.3 Left ventricle responses to load and contractility. The responses of the left ventricle to increased afterload, increased preload, and increased contractility are shown in the pressure-–volume diagram.

encountered with LV volume measurements throughout the cardiac cycle and by criticism of the assumption that the LV end-systolic pressure-volume relationship (ESPVR) is linear outside the empirically measured range. The effects of increasing preload on LV end-diastolic volume and, thus, on LV output, are readily discerned by inspection of the pressure–volume loop illustrated in Figure 34.3. At the level of the sarcomere, the phenomenon whereby increasing LV volume causes increased LV output (under conditions of constant contractility, afterload, and heart rate) has been ascribed to optimizing sarcomere length and overlap. However, extrapolation of this concept from skeletal to cardiac muscle is not justified. In cardiac muscle, little (~10%) force is developed even when the muscle is at <80% of maximum length. Consequently, cardiac muscle has to develop almost all its force over a relatively small range of shortening near its maximal length. This feature (length-activation) of cardiac muscle is attributable to increasing sensitivity of troponin C to cytosolic Ca^{2+} concentration as sarcomere length increases.

Afterload is defined as the load on the contracting myocardium (load after start of contraction). The LV systolic wall stress is directly proportional to LV radius and afterload as defined by the law of Laplace:

$$\text{wall stress} = \frac{(\text{pressure} \times \text{radius})}{(2 \times \text{wall thickness})}$$

Normally, afterload is determined mainly by blood pressure. Abnormal vascular compliance (e.g. hypertension, atherosclerosis) exerts a proportionally greater influence on afterload. Aortic impedance is a related but more specific term; it is defined as the quotient of instantaneous aortic pressure and flow. A decrease in afterload (decreased blood pressure and/or increased arterial compliance) results in a decrease in the LV systolic wall tension required for ejection (or increased ejection if LV wall tension is constant while afterload is decreased). Conversely, increasing afterload reduces LV ejection if LV systolic wall tension remains unchanged. Importantly, increases in afterload can decrease ejection *without* changes in contractility (one simply moves to a different point on the same LV ESPV relationship; see Fig. 34.3). However, sudden increases in afterload have a positive inotropic effect (Anrep effect), shifting to a different LV ESPV relationship. This is thought to result from activation of LV stretch receptors, which increase cytosolic Na^+; this in turn, causes an increase in cytosolic Ca^{2+} via the Na^+/Ca^{2+} exchanger.

Heart rate, within a wide range, directly influences cardiac output, as long as filling during diastole is not compromised. In addition, increases in heart rate result in a positive inotropic effect in isolated papillary muscle strips (treppe or Bowditch effect). This may result from a failure to remove cytosolic Ca^{2+} completely at rapid rates, resulting in an increase in the concentration of Ca^{2+} to which the contractile elements are exposed.

Contractility is one determinant of, but is not synonymous with, systolic function. Systolic function is also influenced by loading conditions and ventricular configuration. One can effectively augment ventricular emptying (systolic function) by decreasing afterload, or decrease ventricular emptying by increasing afterload at the same level of contractility (Fig. 34.3). The pressure–volume loop in Figure 34.3 also illustrates how changing contractility (seen in the pressure–volume loop as a change in the slope of the ESPVR) can change systolic function (ventricular emptying) under constant loading conditions. Increased contractility can be defined as a greater velocity of contraction that reaches a higher peak force when heart rate and loading conditions of the heart are kept constant. This definition is useful when analyzing *in vivo* or *in vitro* studies. However, its utility is limited at a subcellular level, where the mechanisms underlying the influences of preload, afterload, heart rate, and contractility overlap. The maximum velocity of contraction (V_{max}) of isolated, unloaded papillary muscle is a frequently used index of contractility since the preparation is unloaded and can be stimulated at a constant rate. However, V_{max} is not measured directly but extrapolated from the force–velocity relationship, which may not be linear. Studies utilizing sarcomeres indicate that V_{max} is not independent of length at shorter sarcomere lengths but is independent (and thus can be used as an index of contractility) at longer sarcomere lengths. As indicated above, cardiac muscle functions at the upper end of its length–tension relationship.

At the molecular level, it is not possible to separate the effects of heart rate, loading conditions, and contractility from each other. For example, inotropy is mediated by increased Ca^{2+} transients and/or increased sensitivity to Ca^{2+}; increasing heart rate results in increased cytosolic Ca^{2+} because of limited uptake of Ca^{2+} by the SR (treppe effect); increased preload causes length-activation mediated by increased sensitivity to Ca^{2+}; and increased afterload may increase cytosolic Ca^{2+} via stretch-sensitive channels.

Determinants of left ventricular diastolic function and causes of dysfunction

Myocardial relaxation and active elasticity
- Residual cross-bridge activation during part or all of diastole
- Slow relaxation (affects early diastolic filling)
- Incomplete relaxation (affects compliance throughout diastole)

Recoil of elastic components compressed during systole

Intrinsic ventricular chamber characteristics
- Passive ventricular elasticity (chamber stiffness)
- Ventricular wall thickness (mass)
- Ventricular wall compression (myocardial stiffness)
- Viscoelasticity

Factors extrinsic to the ventricle
- Pericardium
- Right ventricular loading and function
- Turgor of the coronary circulation
- Compression by mediastinal or pulmonary masses
- Pulmonary pathology or positive pressure ventilation

Left atrial structure and function
- Preload
- Wall thickness
- Inotropic state

Pulmonary venous return

Mitral valve competency

Heart rate and rhythm

Figure 34.4 Determinants of left ventricular diastolic function and causes of dysfunction. (With permission from Pagel et al., 1993.)

Diastolic function

The importance of diastolic function to overall pump function is now well recognized. Normal ventricular diastolic function can be defined as ventricular filling sufficient to produce an adequate cardiac output without elevated filling pressures. Systolic dysfunction is the most common cause of diastolic dysfunction in that systolic dysfunction results in elevated LV end-diastolic volume and filling pressures (Chapter 39). However, diastolic dysfunction can also occur in the absence of systolic dysfunction. There are many causes of 'primary' diastolic dysfunction (Fig. 34.4). They can be classified into those that result from abnormalities proximal to the LV (dysfunction of the mitral valve, left atrium, and pulmonary veins); those extrinsic to the LV; or those intrinsic to the LV. It is well recognized that structural abnormalities and dysfunction at the mitral valve, left atrium, or pulmonary veins can cause elevated pulmonary pressures and pulmonary congestion without systolic dysfunction. Similarly, any other cause of diastolic dysfunction (either extrinsic or intrinsic to the LV) can cause pulmonary congestion and symptoms of cardiac failure without systolic dysfunction. The effects of some causes of primary diastolic dysfunction on the pressure-volume loop are illustrated in Figure 34.5.

Diastole is divided into four phases: isovolumic relaxation (when aortic and mitral valves are both closed); rapid ventricular filling; slow ventricular filling (diastasis); and atrial systole. During isovolumic relaxation, LV pressure decreases because of LV relaxation. However, LV pressure continues to decrease following mitral valve opening as a result of continued LV relaxation, and also as a result of recoil of LV elastic and viscoelastic components. Relaxation requires removal of Ca^{2+} from troponin C-binding sites. This allows actin and myosin to dissociate. Removal of cytosolic Ca^{2+} involves reuptake by the SR and exchange of Ca^{2+} for Na^+ across the myocyte membrane (sarcolemma), both of which are active, ATP-dependent processes (the Na^+ gradient is maintained by the sarcolemmal Na^+, K^+ATPase). Under normal conditions, Ca^{2+} is effectively removed by the SR and sarcolemma. However, ineffective removal of Ca^{2+} can occur if there is insufficient time (excessive tachycardia), insufficient ATP (ischemia), or enhanced binding of Ca^{2+} to troponin C, each of which could result in impaired ventricular relaxation. Several invasive (isovolumic relaxation, early diastolic filling) and noninvasive (Doppler echocardiography) measurements are used to assess diastolic function, but their interpretation is difficult because diastolic function is influenced not only by several variables confined to diastole but also by variables that alter pump function during systole (loading conditions, heart rate, and contractility).

Systolic and diastolic function can be interpreted in the context of wall stress. An increase in diastolic wall stress occurs if LV end-diastolic pressure increases for any reason, and an increase in systolic wall stress occurs with increases in heart rate, afterload, or contractility. An increase in wall stress resulting from any cause leads to an increase in myocardial oxygen requirement. Coronary blood flow, including myocardial oxygen supply/demand, is discussed at the end of this chapter.

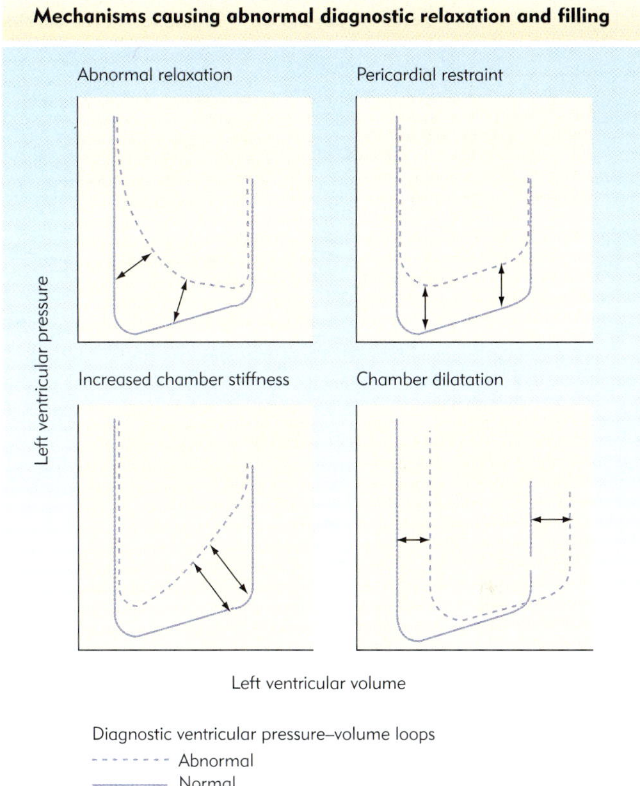

Figure 34.5 Mechanisms responsible for abnormal diastolic relaxation and filling.

Cellular and subcellular aspects of cardiac function

Cardiac myocytes, which make up the vast majority of cells in the heart, work in coordination to propel blood through the body. Each cardiac myocyte has the ability to contract and relax and to respond to positive and negative inotropic stimulation. An important feature of the heart that allows it to fulfill its pumping function is the integrated and coordinated action of billions of cardiac myocytes. The electrical impulse that initiates the heart beat originates in specialized cells in the sinoatrial node of the right atrium. The impulse is transmitted through a specialized conduction system to individual atrial and ventricular myocytes.

Cardiac myocytes are cylindrical in shape, approximately 120μm long, and 10–35μm in diameter (Fig. 34.6). The sarcolemma, or cell membrane of the myocyte, contains ion channels, ion pumps, substrate transporters, and receptors imbedded in its lipid bilayer, allowing communication with neighboring cells and the extracellular environment. Low-resistance contact between myocytes is provided by gap junctions, which allow instantaneous transmission of electrical impulses from one myocyte to the next.

Voltage-dependent Na^+ channels in the sarcolemma open in response to the electrical impulse and allow Na^+ entry, which depolarizes the cell and results in the opening of VDCC. These channels remain open for several milliseconds and result in the plateau phase of the action potential (Chapter 35). VDCC permit the entry of extracellular Ca^{2+} down a concentration gradient. The entry of Ca^{2+} to the myocytes (once thought to generate a common pool of Ca^{2+} that would activate the opening of multiple CRCs located in the junctional SR) is now believed to occur in small amounts in specific well-demarcated zones (adjacent to T-tubules), activating one or, at most a few CRCs in the SR, resulting in a Ca^{2+} 'spark'. The opening of multiple L-type (long-lasting) VDCC results in the activation of many 'zones' and leads to the generation of many 'sparks' and a global increase in myoplasmic Ca^{2+} concentration: from 0.1μmol/L (10^{-7}M) to 10μmol/L (10^{-5}M).

Excitation–contraction coupling offers many potential sites for regulation of contractile activity. Any site that Ca^{2+} passes through or binds to in the cardiac myocyte is a potential site at which contractility or relaxation (lusitropy) can be enhanced or depressed (Fig. 34.6). Negative or positive inotropy can result from decreased or increased Ca^{2+} entry through the VDCC, respectively. The Ca^{2+} channel antagonists, such as nifedipine, diltiazem, or verapamil, decrease Ca^{2+} influx (Ca^{2+} current: I_{Ca}) and, consequently, contractility. Communication between the VDCC and the CRC is another important site of regulation. The responsiveness of the CRC to a given amount of Ca^{2+} is decreased in myocytes isolated from hypertrophied hearts; in this situation, for a fixed I_{Ca} the CRC responds with less release of Ca^{2+} and hence less Ca^{2+} is available to activate troponin C. Another important site at which contractility can be regulated is through the Ca^{2+} load present in the SR. A decreased load might lead to a decreased number of 'sparks', resulting in decreased 'contractility' because of the decrease in the number of troponin C molecules binding Ca^{2+}.

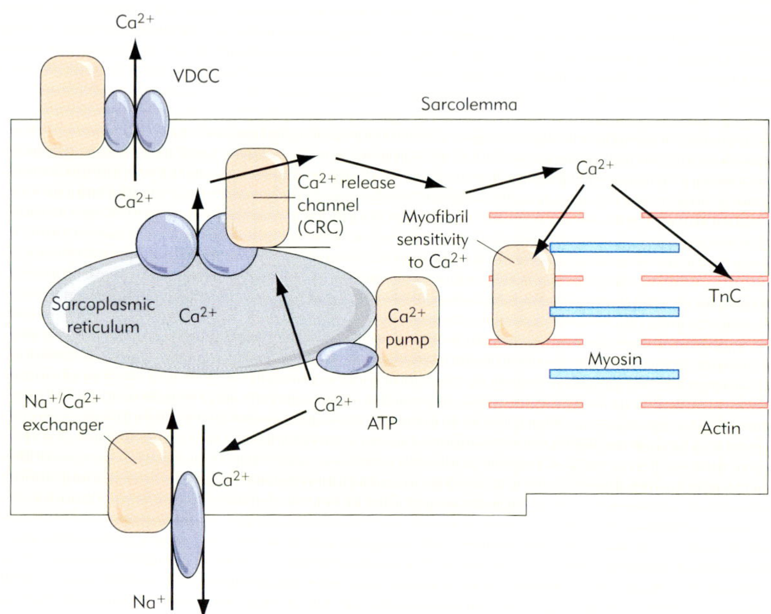

Figure 34.6 Schematic representation of a cardiac myocyte showing potential calcium regulatory sites in the cardiac myocyte. Myofibril sensitivity to Ca^{2+} can be either increased or decreased and the Ca^{2+} pump can sequester more or less Ca^{2+}, leading to changes in both systolic and diastolic function. The Na^+/Ca^{2+} exchanger is important for maintenance of Ca^{2+} homeostasis. VDCC, voltage-dependent Ca^{2+} channels; TnC, troponin C.

The regulation of Ca^{2+} (and, therefore, contraction) is linked to activation of β-adrenoceptors, which have multiple effects at various sites in the myocyte (Fig. 34.7). Phosphorylation of VDCC via adenylyl cyclase stimulation and cAMP-dependent protein kinase activation increases the open time of the L-type VDCC and enhances I_{Ca}, resulting in greater stimulation of the CRC and an increase in the availability of Ca^{2+} for contraction. Beta-adrenoceptor activation also leads to phosphorylation of phospholamban, a pentameric protein found in the SR membrane that is linked to Ca^{2+} ATPase function (Fig. 34.8). Phosphorylation of phospholamban leads to disinhibition of the SR Ca^{2+} pump, an enhancement in the rate of relaxation (lusitropic effect), and an increase in the amount of Ca^{2+} sequestered in the SR for subsequent contractions. Recent studies with a transgenic mouse model suggest that not all Ca^{2+} ATPase molecules in the heart are linked to phospholamban, and, therefore, modulation of Ca^{2+} pump activity is only partial. Finally, removal of inhibition by phospholamban of Ca^{2+} pump activity results in a greater sensitivity of the Ca^{2+} pump to Ca^{2+}.

ANESTHETIC EFFECTS ON CARDIAC FUNCTION

Contractile activity of the heart depends on extracellular Ca^{2+}. The negative inotropic activity of anesthetics appears to a large extent to be related to the interference with delivery to or response of myofibrils to Ca^{2+}. Figure 34.7 illustrates the major sites at which anesthetics could interfere with Ca^{2+} homeostasis and contractile activity. Current research suggests that the two sites most affected by volatile anesthetics are the L-type VDCC and the SR CRC, also known as the ryanodine receptor. Many studies have supported the notion of a reversible, inhibitory alteration of the L-type VDCC in cardiac myocytes, leading to a decrease in the entry of Ca^{2+} and, hence, a smaller stimulus for Ca^{2+}-induced Ca^{2+} release.

The other major site of importance, the CRC, responds to the entry of activator Ca^{2+} with the release of larger amounts of Ca^{2+}, which can go on to activate the myofibrils. The SR capacity for Ca^{2+} appears to be decreased by volatile anesthetics, especially halothane. This effect is apparently related to an increased open time of the CRC, allowing Ca^{2+} to leak more or less continuously at a low level (i.e. a level not leading to a measurable increase in diastolic pressure nor to increased inotropy). The final important site of potential negative inotropic activity is the myofibrils. It has been demonstrated that the rate of cycling of actin–myosin cross-bridges is unaffected by halothane, enflurane, and isoflurane, and that the force generated by each cross-bridge is the same in the presence or absence of anesthetic. However, the sensitivity of myofibrils and, in particular, troponin C, to Ca^{2+} appears to be decreased by volatile anesthetics, potentially contributing to their negative inotropic effect.

METABOLISM

The heart uses predominantly free fatty acids and glucose as its metabolic substrates. Throughout the day its use of these substrates varies; following a meal with a carbohydrate load, glucose will be the main substrate, while the fasting patient will have elevated free fatty acids, which will be the major substrate for aerobic metabolism. The exercising individual will produce lactate from skeletal muscle and this will then become the predominant energy substrate. The heart is an aerobic organ, as indicated by the large volume of the cell occupied by mitochondria (approximately 23% of total cell volume): 90% of cardiac metabolism is aerobic and 10% anaerobic. Contractile activity consumes 60% of the metabolic energy generated by the heart, while the SR Ca^{2+} ATPase consumes 15%. The Na^+ gradient is maintained by the Na^+/K^+ ATPase at the cell membrane; this process consumes 5% of available cellular energy. The 20% of energy remaining is used for basic cellular maintenance.

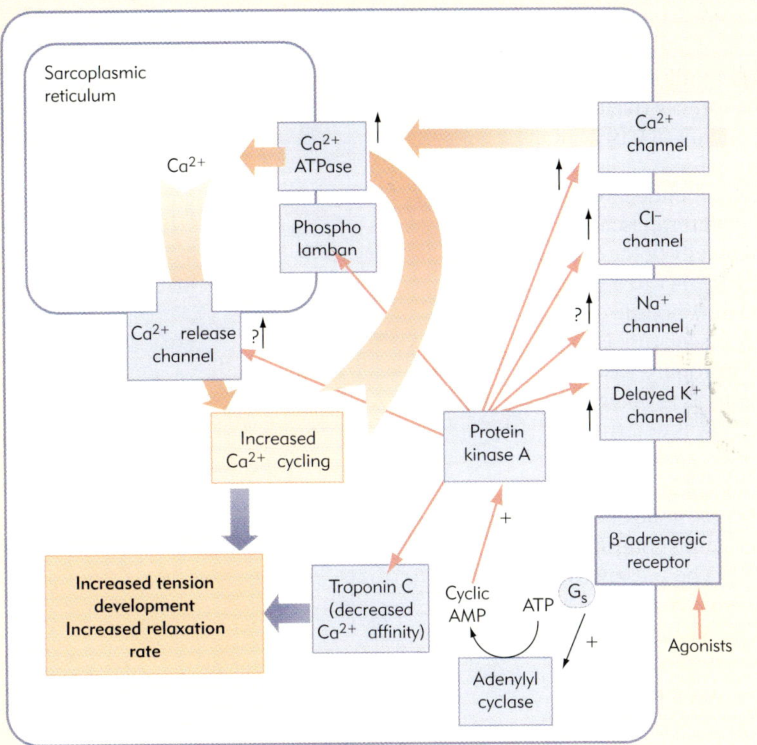

Figure 34.7 Signalling systems involved in positive inotropic and lusitropic (enhanced relaxation) effects of β-adrenergic stimulation. When β-adrenergic agonists interact with the β-adrenoceptor, the associated G protein (Gs), stimulates adenylyl cyclase, leading to a series of changes (activation of adenylyl cyclase by the stimulatory G protein Gs, increase in cAMP, and activation of protein kinase A) that stimulate metabolism and phosphorylate Ca^{2+} channels. The result is an enhanced opening probability of the Ca^{2+} channel, thereby increasing Ca^{2+} entry through the sarcolemma of the T-tubule. In turn, increased intracellular Ca^{2+} stimulates release of more Ca^{2+} from the sarcoplasmic reticulum and activates troponin C. Enhanced myosin ATPase activity explains the increased rate of contraction, with increased activation of troponin C causing increased peak force development. (With permission from Lynch, 1998.)

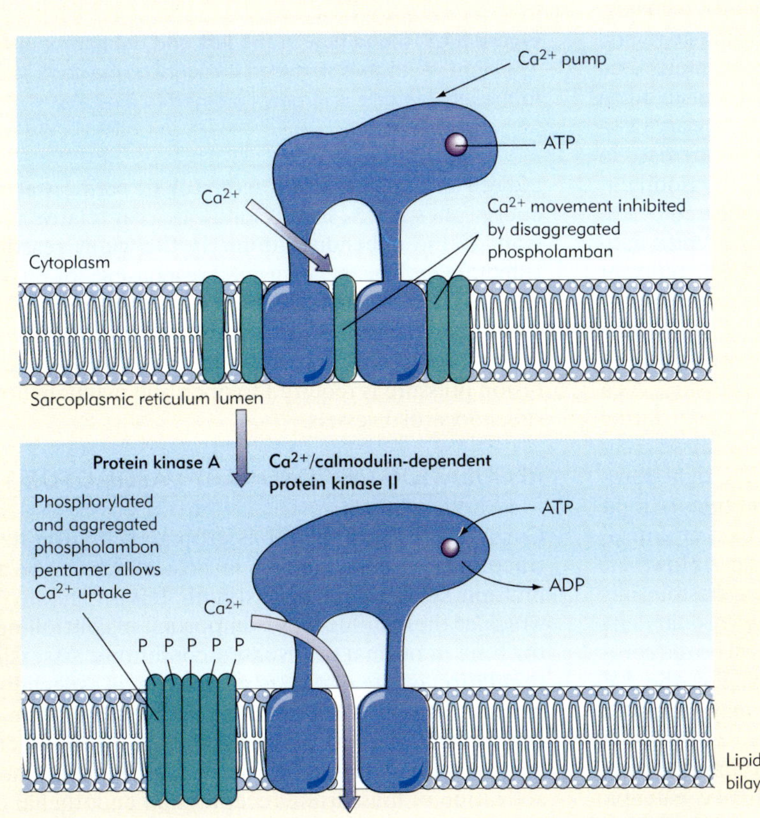

Figure 34.8 Uptake of calcium by the energy-requiring Ca^{2+} pump into the sarcoplasmic reticulum. Enhanced cytosolic Ca^{2+} or β-adrenergic stimulation results in phosphorylation of phospholamban at distinct sites. This removes the inhibition exerted by its unphosphorylated form. An increased rate of relaxation (lusitropy) follows because of the increased Ca^{2+} uptake.

CORONARY BLOOD FLOW

Coronary blood flow (CBF) is directly proportional to the pressure gradient and inversely proportional to the resistance of the vascular bed. Although extreme disturbances of coronary perfusion pressure can alter CBF, under normal conditions perfusion pressure is relatively stable and vascular resistance (including regional resistance) predominates as a determinant of CBF. The use of advanced techniques to study local or regional variations in CBF (small vessels including microvessels, subendocardium versus subepicardium, collateral versus noncollateral, ischemic versus nonischemic) demonstrates the heterogeneity of the coronary vasculature. Different vessels relax or contract to a given stimulus with varying intensity and may respond in opposite directions to the same stimulus. While the coronary vasculature is subject to systemic influences, local control of coronary vascular resistance (and, thus, CBF) predominates in this as in other vital organs. The resistance of coronary vessels to flow is determined by compressive forces generated by contracting cardiac muscle and by a profuse, complex interacting array of local and systemic factors. Even under normal physiologic conditions, none of these factors exert uniform influences across the heart; this contributes to the regional heterogeneity observed in CBF. The presence of coronary disease adds additional variables to the control of CBF.

The metabolic demands of the heart (i.e. a contractile pump with high energy and oxygen requirements) result in high basal oxygen extraction and low coronary sinus oxygen content. Therefore, increasing oxygen extraction is not an adequate mechanism for meeting increasing myocardial oxygen demand, which must be accommodated by increasing CBF. By extension, local mechanism(s) coupling oxygen supply to demand are pivotal in controlling local CBF. Clinically, the myocardial oxygen supply/demand ratio is optimized by manipulating global parameters (heart rate, afterload, contractility, preload), recognizing that the results of interventions may differ from one region of the myocardium to another. Results must also be interpreted in the context of both the direct and indirect effects of an intervention. For example, α_1-adrenoceptor-mediated coronary vasoconstriction may be superseded by a concomitant increase in contractility, with metabolically induced coronary vasodilatation and increases in CBF. This is further complicated by the recent recognition that endothelial cell α_2-adrenoceptor activation causes release of endothelium-derived relaxant factor/nitric oxide (EDRF/NO) with resultant relaxation of underlying vascular smooth muscle.

Under normal conditions, the upstream pressure for perfusion of the coronary arteries is aortic diastolic pressure. As a result of myocardial compression, CBF to the LV ceases during parts of systole, especially in the subendocardium where compressive forces are highest (Fig. 34.9). Flow in the right coronary artery may also be compromised under conditions of right ventricular hypertrophy. The effective downstream or critical closing pressure in the coronary circulation is unclear. However, since CBF to the LV occurs predominantly during diastole, it is unlikely that a 'vascular waterfall' occurs in the coronary circulation and the effective downstream pressure will be the coronary sinus pressure or a value close to this. For the LV subendocardium, the LV end-diastolic pressure may be a more accurate reflection of the downstream pressure.

It is well recognized that the LV subendocardium is vulnerable to ischemia. Studies of transmural (endocardial versus epicardial) myocardial blood flow (and thus oxygen supply) and of indices of oxygen utilization (glycolytic pathway activity, high-energy phosphates, lactate) indicate that relative underperfusion of the subendocardium is the main reason for this vulnerability. The mechanism(s) responsible for this may be the greater systolic compressive force in the subendocardium causing increased compression and stretching (and, thus, resistance) in these vessels. In the ensuing diastole, a relatively greater perfusion pressure is required to open and maintain flow in these subendocardial vessels.

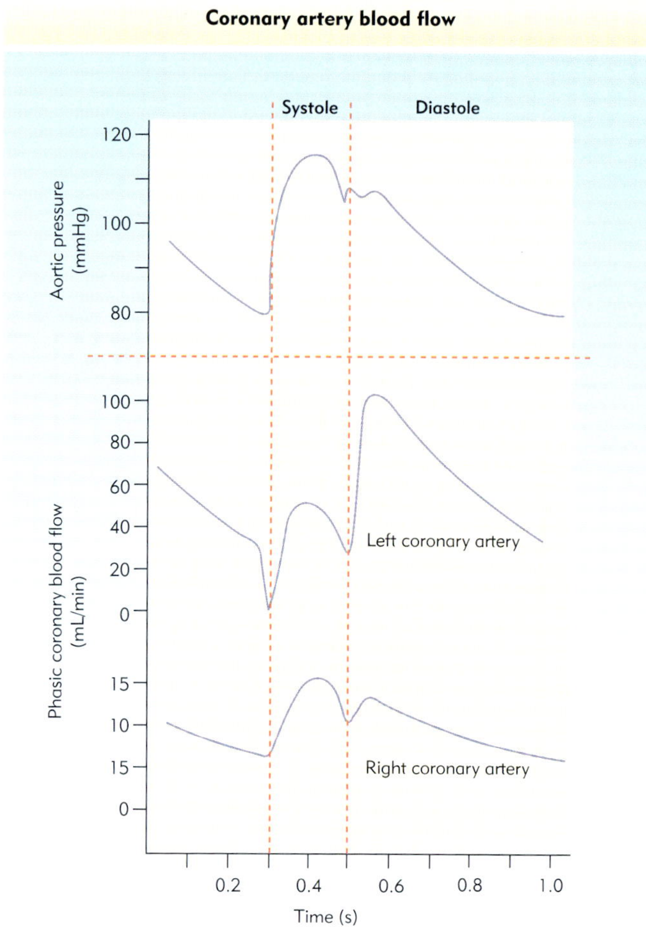

Figure 34.9 Blood flow in the left and right coronary arteries. The right ventricle is perfused throughout the cardiac cycle. Flow to the left ventricle is largely confined to diastole.

REGULATION OF CORONARY VASOMOTOR TONE

Coronary vasomotor tone is ultimately determined by contraction of vascular smooth muscle, which can be altered by multiple systemic and local stimuli. It is difficult to determine which of these influences is important in controlling vasomotor tone in normal or diseased conditions. Assessing neural regulation of the coronary circulation is especially difficult because of both direct and indirect effects. When indirect effects (metabolism) are controlled, parasympathetic activation consistently causes coronary vasodilatation mediated by activation of muscarinic receptors on endothelial cells (Fig. 34.10), although the parasympathetic nervous system is not an

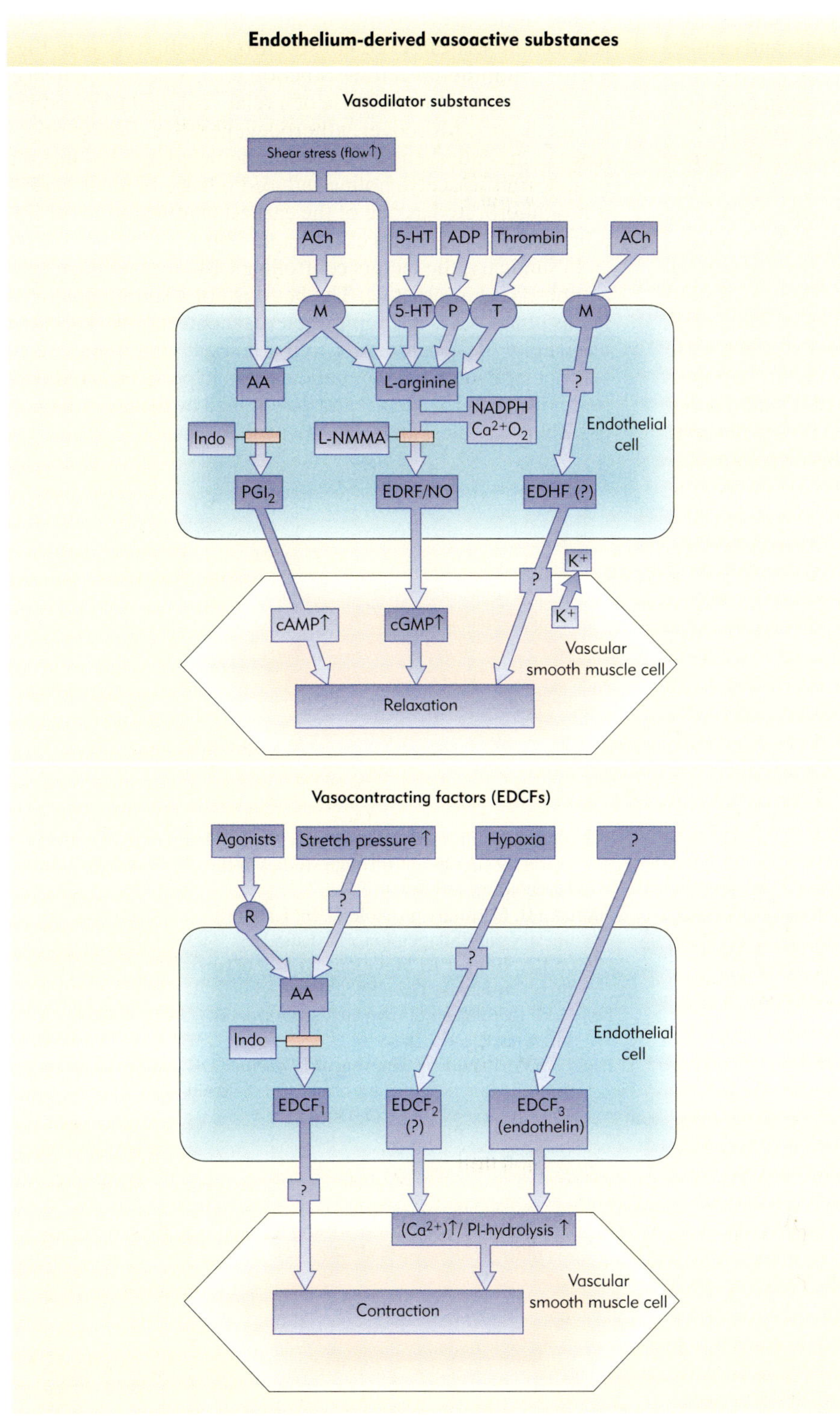

Figure 34.10 Endothelium-derived vasoactive substances. The endothelium produces both vasodilator and vasoconstrictive factors. Endothelium-derived vasodilator substances include prostacyclin. This is produced by the cyclooxygenase pathway, which can be blocked by indomethacin and aspirin. Endothelium-derived relaxing factor may be nitric oxide (NO) or a closely related compound. Its production can be blocked by arginine analogs, such as L-NMMA (Nγ-monomethyl-L-arginine). There are a number of endothelium-derived contracting factors (EDCFs). The release of $EDCF_1$ can be inhibited by cyclooxygenase inhibitors, such as indomethacin. $EDCF_2$ is released by hypoxia and is indomethacin insensitive. $EDCF_3$ is a potent vasoconstrictor peptide known as endothelin. 5-HT, serotonin; AA, arachidonic acid; PGI_2, prostacyclin; cGMP, cyclic GMP; cAMP, cyclic AMP; EDRF/NO, endothelium-derived relaxant factor/ nitric oxide; M, muscarinic receptor; P, purinergic receptor; T, thrombin receptor; Indo: indomethacin; ACh, acetylcholine; PI, phosphatidylinositol; R, receptor; EDHF, endothelium-derived hyperpolarizing factor that hyperpolarizes the smooth muscle membrane.

important regulator of coronary vasomotor tone. However, defects in muscarinic receptor activation may be a manifestation of endothelial cell dysfunction. Similarly, the role of direct effects of α- and β-adrenoceptor activation (vasoconstriction and vasodilatation, respectively) in coronary vasoregulation is likely to be modest. Alpha-adrenoceptor activation may play a role in diverting CBF to areas of relatively greater oxygen need (e.g. the subendocardium in exercise and to ischemic areas) as indicated by canine models. Studies in humans indicate that α-adrenoceptor activation can cause ischemia by constricting diseased vessels. Hormones (e.g. vasopressin, atrial natriuretic factor) or drugs that alter endogenously produced hormone levels (e.g. angiotensin-converting enzyme inhibitors) are not important regulators of coronary vasomotor tone. Potential mediators for metabolic regulation of coronary vasomotor effects [e.g. K^+, H^+, oxygen (or lack thereof), carbon dioxide, and osmolarity] may act either directly on vascular smooth muscle or indirectly via endothelial cells. A complex interaction of local factors (which differ from region to region) regulates vasomotor tone and couples oxygen delivery to oxygen demand.

Endothelial cells have a diverse array of biological functions, including modulation of underlying vascular smooth muscle and interaction with factors at the luminal surface (Chapters 33 and 38).

Temporary occlusion of coronary vessels causes an increase in CBF above baseline following reinstitution of flow, indicating the presence of coronary reserve and reactive hyperemia. The absence of reactive hyperemia indicates that basal CBF is maximal and that vasodilator capacity has been exhausted. Autoregulation describes the phenomenon whereby CBF returns towards baseline following a change in coronary perfusion pressure and CBF. The mechanisms underlying reactive hyperemia and autoregulation are likely to be multifactorial, involving one or more of the mechanisms described above.

The influence of endothelial cells on vasomotor tone reflects the net effect of constrictors and dilators (see Fig. 34.10). Endothelial cell dysfunction results in an imbalance favoring constrictors because of a relative deficit of vasodilator mediators. Moreover, atherodegenerative disease originates in the endothelium. Indeed, endothelial cell dysfunction (e.g. defects in acetylcholine-induced release of nitric oxide) is now interpreted as one of the earliest manifestations of the atherodegenerative process (Chapter 39).

In summary, the factors controlling CBF are multifactorial, complex, and interactive. The heart is not a simple homogeneous pump but is a complex heterogeneous organ. This heterogeneity is accentuated in pathologic conditions (e.g. ventricular hypertrophy in patients with hypertension). Blood flow is also heterogeneous and determined by the net influence of local mechanical and vasoactive influences.

Key References

Bassenge E, Busse R. Endothelial modulation of coronary tone. Prog Cardiovasc Dis. 1988;30:349–80.

Berne RM, Levy MN. Principles of physiology. Mosby; 1990:215.

Langer GA, ed. The myocardium. San Diego, CA: Academic Press; 1997.

Lynch C III. Myocardial excitation–contraction coupling. In: Yaksh et al., eds. Anesthesia: biologic foundations. Philadelphia, PA: Lippincott-Raven; 1997: 1041–79.

Lynch C III, Vogel S, Sperelakis N. Halothane depression of myocardial slow action potentials. Anesthesiology. 1988;55:360–8.

Marcus ML, Chilian WM, Kanatsuka H, et al. Understanding the coronary circulation through studies at the microvascular level. Circulation. 1990;81:1–7.

Nathan HJ. Coronary physiology. In: Kaplan JA, ed. Cardiac anesthesia. Philadelphia, PA: Saunders; 1993:235–60.

Olsson RA, Bunger R. Metabolic control of coronary blood flow. Prog Cardiovasc Dis. 1987;29:369–87.

Opie LH. Regulation of myocardial contractility. J Cardiovasc Pharmacol. 1995;26:S1–9.

Pagel PS, Grossman W, Haering JM, Warltier DC. Left ventricular diastolic function in the normal and diseased heart. Anesthesiology. 1993;79:836–54.

Further Reading

Flavahan NA. Atherosclerosis or lipoprotein-induced endothelial dysfunction. Circulation. 1992;85:1927–38.

Harrison DG, Bates JN. The nitrovasodilators: new ideas about old drugs. Circulation. 1993;87:1461–7.

Luscher TF, Tanner FC, Tschudi MR, Noll G. Endothelial dysfunction in coronary artery disease. Annu Rev Med. 1993;44:395–418.

Moncada S, Higgs EA, Vane JR. Human arterial and venous tissues generate prostacyclin (prostaglandin X), a potent inhibitor of platelet aggregation. Lancet. 1977;i:18–19.

Opie LH. Mechanisms of cardiac contraction and relaxation. In: Braunwald E, ed. Heart disease: a textbook of cardiovascular medicine. Philadelphia, PA: Saunders; 1997:361–93.

Shibata T, Blanck TJJ, Sagawa K. Hunter W. The effect of volatile anesthetics on dynamic stiffness of rabbit papillary muscle. Anesthesiology. 1988;70:496–502.

Chapter 35 Cardiac electrophysiology

Jeffrey R Balser and John L Atlee

Topics covered in this chapter

Cardiac arrhythmias, irregular patterns of contraction, are a major cause of death (estimated at 400,000 annually in the USA) and contribute to prolonged hospitalization if they occur in patients undergoing anesthesia and surgery. Fortunately, the application of basic molecular science to the problems of cardiac excitability has yielded significant advances in our understanding of cardiac arrhythmias. The pioneering work of Hodgkin and Huxley in the 1950s unambiguously defined voltage-gated ion channels as the molecular species that underlie membrane excitability. The development of 'patch-clamp' technology by Sakmann and Neher in the 1980s allowed measurement of ionic current through individual ion channels and exponentially increased our understanding of these proteins. At the same time, the use of molecular biological methods to clone and sequence ion channels has offered unparalleled insight into the basic structure of the cardiac ion channels and is also providing novel targets for antiarrhythmic drug therapy.

BASIC CARDIAC ELECTROPHYSIOLOGY

Ion channels and the action potential

The action potential represents the time-varying transmembrane potential of the cardiac cell during systole and diastole. Similarly, the surface electrocardiogram (ECG) represents the temperospatial average of the action potentials from all myocardial cells (Chapter 12). Figure 35.1 shows the approximate relationship between the action potential from a single ventricular myocyte and the ECG. The rate of upstroke of the action potential defines the time necessary for an individual cardiac cell to depolarize, while the duration of the QRS complex approximately represents the time necessary for the entire ventricle to depolarize. Similarly, the action potential duration defines the time required for a single cardiac cell to repolarize, while the Q–T interval represents the time required for complete ventricular repolarization.

The cardiac action potential can be divided into five phases that reflect time variation in the composition of ionic currents flowing during the cardiac cycle. These ionic currents arise mainly from passive movement of ions through ion channels: pore-forming transmembrane proteins in the cardiac cell membrane. In general, inward sodium (Na^+) and calcium (Ca^{2+}) currents depolarize the cell membrane, while outward potassium (K^+) currents repolarize the membrane. In atrial and ventricular muscle cells and Purkinje fibers, the initial depolarization period (phase 0) of the action potential results from inward flux of Na^+ current (I_{Na}) through Na^+ channels. In the atrioventricular (AV) and sinoatrial (SA) nodal cells, inward Ca^{2+} currents (I_{Ca}) through T- and L-type Ca^{2+} channels produce a slower depolarizing upstroke. This heterogeneity in tissue excitability has profound implications (discussed below) for both cardiac arrhythmogenesis and antiarrhythmic drug therapy.

The remaining phases of the action potential (see Fig. 35.1) involve repolarization. The earliest repolarization period (notch, phase 1) results from the transient outward K^+ current (I_{To}) and the inward Cl^- current (I_{Cl}). This is followed by a plateau (phase 2) during which repolarization is delayed, and depolarization is maintained primarily by inward I_{Ca}. The action potential is terminated (phase 3) by the rapid (I_{Kr}) and slow (I_{Ks}) components of delayed rectifier K^+ current (I_K). The actual duration of the action potential is determined by a delicate balance between these and many other smaller inward and outward currents from both ion channels and electrogenic pumps (Na^+/Ca^{2+} exchanger, Na^+,K^+-ATPase). $I_{Na/Ca}$ is the current carried by the Na^+/Ca^{2+} exchanger, and is the primary means of the Ca^{2+} efflux. Phase 4 is the period when the action potential is maximally repolarized. In atrial and ventricular muscle, the resting potential is maintained near the K^+ equilibrium potential of –90mV (E_K) by inward rectifier K^+ channels (I_{K1}) and the electrogenic Na^+,K^+-ATPase. In the absence of an applied stimulus (via conduction from a neighboring cell) or an injury that induces inward current (ischemia), these cells remain hyperpolarized and rarely fire action potentials spontaneously. Conversely, SA and AV nodal cells and Purkinje fibers possess inward pacemaker currents (I_f), backround Na^+ current ($I_{Na\text{-}B}$), and electrogenic pumps (I_{pump}) that shift the resting membrane potential to more positive values (–50 to –70mV), allowing spontaneous depolarization (pacemaking).

Structure and function of voltage-gated ion channels

Voltage-gated cation channels are the principal source of transmembrane ionic currents in the heart. The major pore-forming α-subunits of these channels are transmembrane proteins that possess striking sequence and structural homology and, in fact, are members of a common gene family (see Chapter 15).

Ionic currents during the cardiac action potential

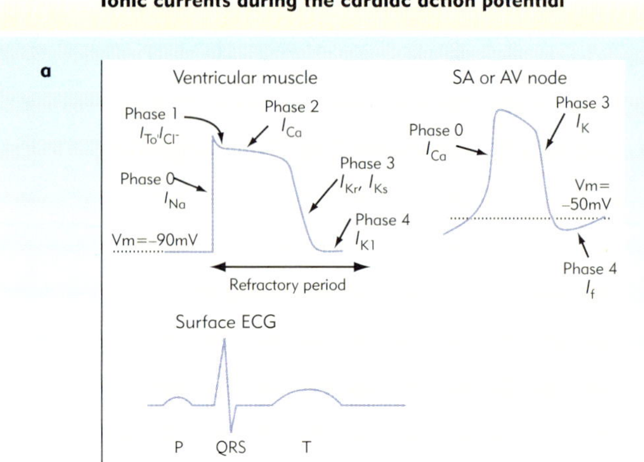

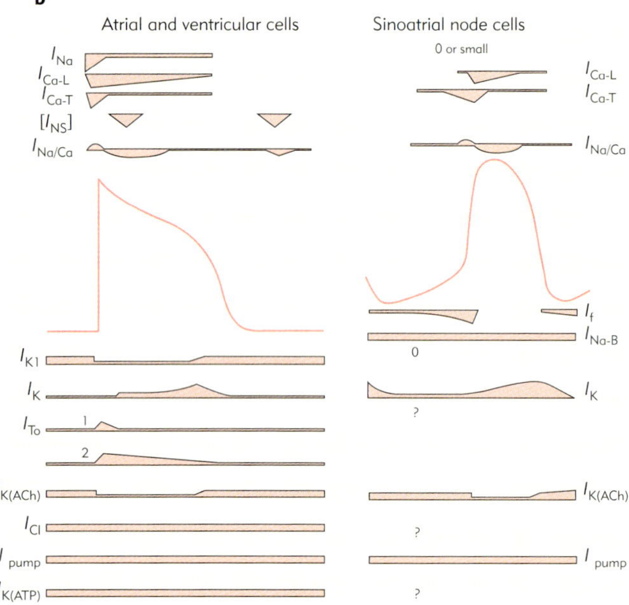

Figure 35.1 Ionic currents during the action potential. (a) The ventricular muscle action potential is shown in relation to the surface electrocardiogram (ECG). A sinoatrial (SA) or atrioventricular (AV) nodal action potential is also shown for comparison. The phases of the action potential (0–4) are shown along with the principal ionic currents (see text) flowing during each phase. Major tissue differences between phase 0 and phase 4 underlie the rationale for several antiarrhythmic therapeutic strategies. (b) The time course of a stylized action potential of atrial, ventricular, and sinoatrial node cells is shown with the various channels and pumps that contribute the currents underlying the electrical events. Where possible, the approximate time courses of the currents associated with the channels or pumps are shown symbolically without effort to represent their magnitudes relative to each other. The channels identified by brackets imply that they are active only under pathologic conditions. For the sinoatrial node cells I_{Na} and I_{K1} are small or absent. $I_{NS,}$ nonselective. (From the Task Force of the Working Group on Arrhythmias of the European Society of Cardiology, 1991.)

Figure 15.10 shows the α-subunits of the three classes of voltage-gated cation channel as they are thought to reside in the cardiac cell membrane. The Na^+ and Ca^{2+} channels contain four homologous domains (I–IV), each composed of six transmembrane repeats (S1–S6). Similarly, many voltage-gated K^+ channels (Shaker/Kv families) resemble a single domain of a Na^+ or Ca^{2+} channel and assemble as tetramers to form functional ion-conducting channels.

Figure 35.2 shows a structural model of the outer pore of the voltage-gated Na^+ channel. Each of the four homologous domains assemble together and individually contribute approximately 25% of the amino acids that form the outer pore. The structure of the pore is critical not only for conducting permeant ions (Na^+ in this case) but also for binding blocking ions, toxins, and drugs. Using *site-directed mutagenesis* (Fig. 35.2), single amino acid residues in the pore (or other sites) of the channel can be selectively replaced, and the permeation and binding characteristics after these manipulations re-evaluated using ‘patch-clamp’ single-channel recordings. Using these methods, the residues critical for ‘normal’ ion channel function may be determined. This hybrid approach, fusing single-channel electrophysiology with molecular biology, has greatly increased our knowledge of ion channel structure–function relationships.

Although voltage-gated ion channels conduct cations passively, they are nonetheless dynamic in nature, continuously opening and closing in response to changes in membrane potential. This capability, known as ‘gating’, was first described by Hodgkin and Huxley from recordings in squid giant axons. Generally speaking, the channels open only transiently in response to membrane depolarization; hence, the two gating processes critical to ion channel function are *activation* and *inactivation* (Fig. 35.3). Site-directed mutagenesis studies have defined specific regions of the channel critical to gating function; specific regions also appear to have consistent functional importance across the ion channel families. For example, in both Na^+ and K^+ channels, the S4 domain contains highly conserved positively charged arginine residues that appear to affect voltage-dependent channel activation during depolarization. By comparison, inactivation processes are more varied. For many K^+ channels, the N-terminal domain ‘swings’ into the pore like a ball on a tether, occluding the pore from the inside. In an analogous manner, the rapid inactivation process in Na^+ channels seems to involve movement of the domain III–IV linker over the cytoplasmic face of the channel (Fig. 35.3). Receptors for this ‘hinged-lid’ mechanism are disputed but may reside on the cytoplasmic ends of the S5 and S6 segments. In addition, slower inactivation mechanisms that involve direct approximation of external pore-lining segments are described for K^+ channels and may also exist in Na^+ channels. Further, activation and inactivation gating may be mechanistically coupled. For example, covalent modification of the *external* S4 arginine residue in the Na^+ channel ‘locks’ the S4 segment in the outward configuration. This has the paradoxical effect of speeding inactivation, presumably by facilitating binding of the *internal* inactivation gate to its receptor. These coupling interactions underscore the emerging view that ion channel gating processes are truly allosteric, involving the ensemble motion of multiple domains rather than individual amino acid residues.

Voltage-gated cation channels are subject to many forms of physiologic modulation. Subsidiary (β, γ) subunits are attached

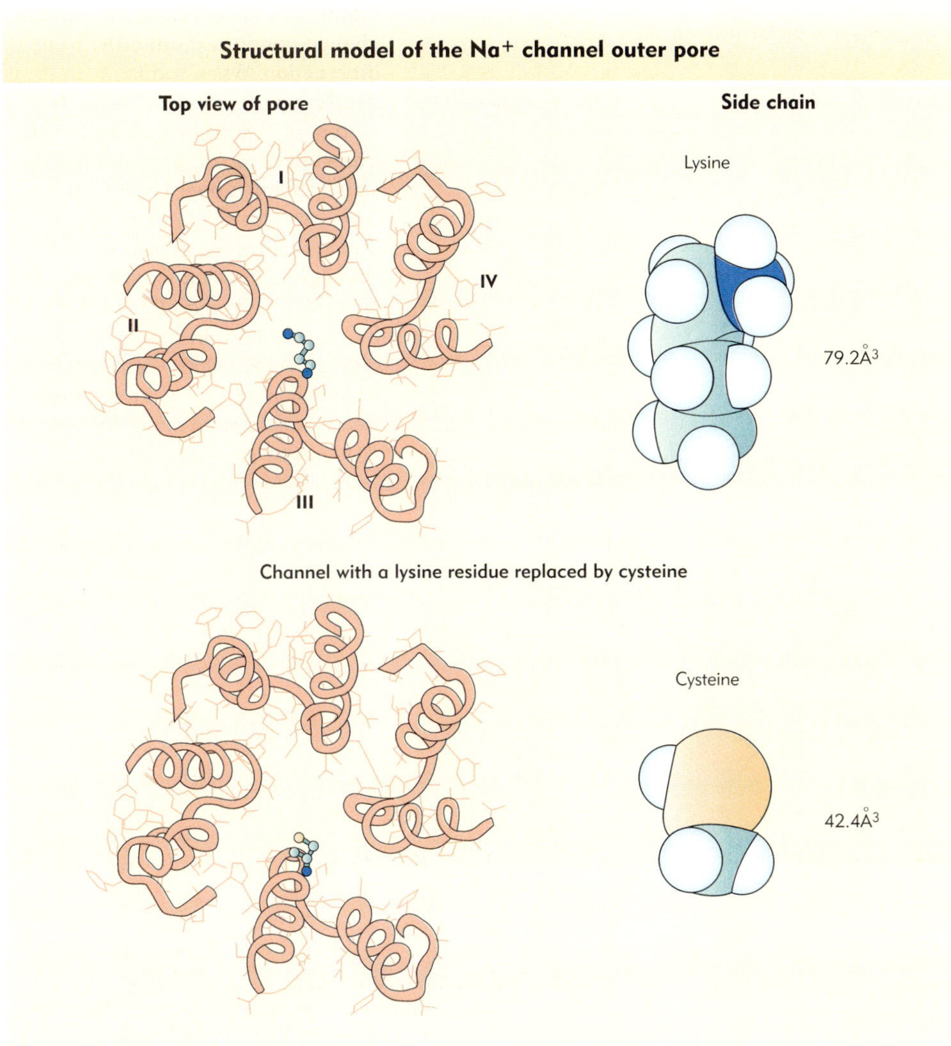

Figure 35.2 Structural model of the Na^+channel outer pore. The channel is shown as viewed from outside the cell, looking longitudinally down the pore. Selective replacement of a lysine residue by a cysteine residue using site-directed mutagenesis induces changes in both cation block and ion permeation. (With permission from Pérez-Garcia et al., 1997.)

to most of the major pore-forming α-subunits. The functional importance of many subsidiary subunits is unknown; however, it is clear that β-subunits critically modify the inactivation gating behavior of both Na^+ and K^+ channels. Further, β_1-subunit coexpression modifies the action of class I antiarrhythmic drugs on voltage-gated cardiac and skeletal muscle Na^+ channels, suggesting that subsidiary subunit interactions may serve as potential target sites for pharmacologic modulation of cardiac excitability. Many of the voltage-gated cation channels also contain consensus phosphorylation sites for a variety of protein kinases on both their principal and subsidiary subunits and are, thus, subject to regulation by G protein-coupled second messenger systems (Chapter 3). A prime example is Ca^{2+} channel modulation by the cAMP pathway. L-type Ca^{2+} channel currents increase in response to β_1-adrenergic stimulation, most likely through phosphorylation by cAMP-dependent protein kinase (Chapter 5). Single-channel experiments have shown that under cAMP stimulation, Ca^{2+} channels exhibit altered gating behavior and spend much more time in the open configuration. Additionally, recent studies have shown that catecholamines and other hormones alter the total number of functional Ca^{2+} channels in the cardiac cell membrane by regulating Ca^{2+} channel gene expression. Hence, the autonomic nervous system exerts exquisite control over cardiac excitability through voltage-gated ion channels, modulating not only the number of channels inserted into the sarcolemma but also their functional (gating) behavior. These regulatory mechanisms all provide potential sites for antiarrhythmic pharmacologic modulation.

ANTIARRHYTHMIC DRUGS

Classification

In addition to indirect autonomic regulation, voltage-gated cation channels are principal targets for the direct action of many antiarrhythmic compounds. The manner in which drugs and hormones modify the cardiac action potential may be predicted from their effects on ion channel classes (Fig. 35.4). Antiarrhythmic agents possess overlapping affinities for different molecular targets because of the high degree of structural similarity among the ion channel classes. Hence, some antiarrhythmic agents that block Na^+ channels may also block Ca^{2+} and K^+ channels at low doses. The most popular and well-known antiarrhythmic drug classification system was developed as a means of grouping antiarrhythmic agents by their electrophysiologic actions. However, our evolving understanding of molecular pharmacology suggests a more useful classification based on molecular targets. A 'hybrid' classification generally similar to the original grouping but linked to the principal mol-

Site-directed mutations change gating and antiarrhythmic drug action

Changes from sudden depolarization

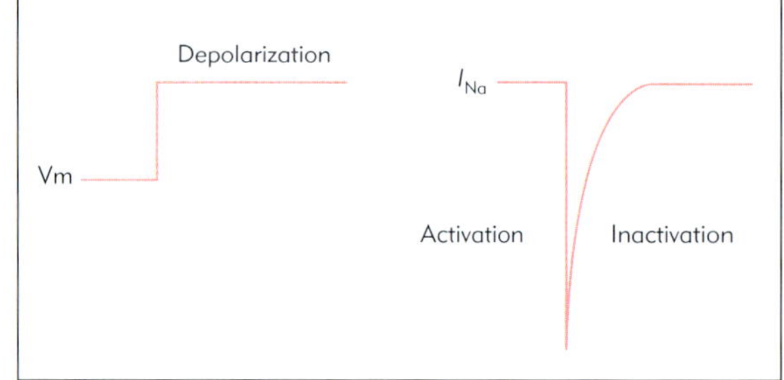

Effect of mutations on Na^+ channel structure and fuction

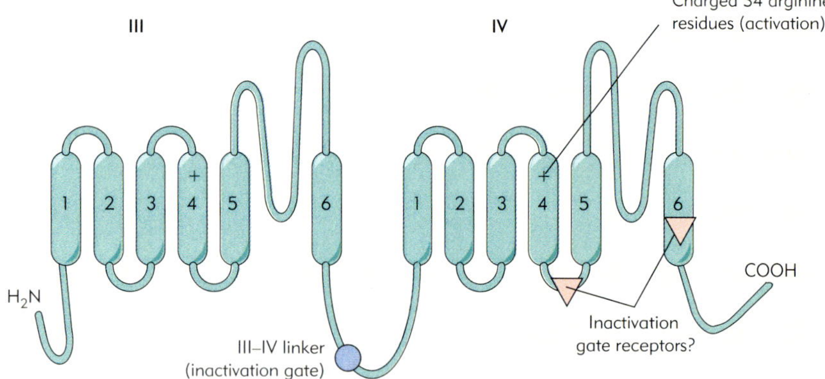

Figure 35.3 Site-directed mutations change gating and antiarrhythmic drug action. When suddenly depolarized, a transient inward Na^+ current (I_{Na}) flows into cardiac cells. This current rapidly activates (as single channels open) and then inactivates (as single channels close) during maintained depolarization (throughout the action potential plateau, phases 2 and 3 in Fig. 35.1). Mutations in specific locations alter gating functions (activation, inactivation) of Na^+ channels and may also attenuate antiarrhythmic drug action.

Antiarrhythmic drug classification

Class[a]	Molecular target	Antiarrhythmic agents
IA	Na^+ and K^+ channels	Procainamide, quinidine, amiodarone[b]
IB	Na^+ channels	Lidocaine (lignocaine), phenytoin
II	β-Adrenoceptors	Esmolol, propranolol, amiodarone
III	K^+ channels	Bretylium, ibutilide, amiodarone[b]
IV	Ca^{2+} channels	Verapamil, diltiazem, amiodarone

[a]Class IC agents (propafenone, flecainide) are potent Na^+ channel antagonists but are approved in the USA for oral administration only.

[b]Amiodarone i.v. does not induce Q–T prolongation acutely but these effects do develop with prolonged administration (hours to days).

Figure 35.4 Antiarrhythmic drug classification. These antiarrhythmic agents are available in intravenous form and used in anesthesiology and critical care. Agents are listed according to their preferred molecular target but generally follow the original classification described by Vaughan Williams.

ecular target of the agent (ion channels, adrenergic receptors) is proposed for didactic purposes (Fig. 35.4). This emphasizes antiarrhythmic agents available in intravenous form and, therefore, of use in anesthesiology and critical care. Because of receptor nonspecificity, some agents (amiodarone) are listed in multiple categories.

Molecular pharmacology

The earliest observations of local anesthetic/antiarrhythmic drug action on Na^+ currents revealed that the blocking action was markedly enhanced by rapid, repetitive depolarization, so-called 'use dependence'. The earliest robust models (modulated receptor models) of antiarrhythmic drug action viewed drug binding to Na^+ channels in cardiac and neuronal tissues similarly; that is, binding affinity is a function of the gated conformational state. Most antiarrhythmic drugs were viewed as potent blockers of inactivated and open channels, since these conformational states are induced by depolarization. This preference for binding to depolarized channel conformations may partly underlie antiarrhythmic drug efficacy, since ischemic cardiac tissues are depolarized relative to healthy tissues.

The evolution in our understanding of the structural basis of ion channel gating processes figures critically in the modern view of antiarrhythmic drug action. Site-directed mutagenesis studies have shown that mutations that modify or eliminate specific gating processes also alter the use-dependent action of antiarrhythmic agents. In Na^+ channels, mutations disabling the fast-inactivation gating apparatus (see Fig. 35.3) markedly attenuate use-dependent lidocaine (lignocaine) action. In particular, S6 residues seem to play a critical role in the blockade of multiple channel classes by clinically useful agents. In addition to effects on Na^+ channels, similar S6 residues appear to modulate block of Ca^{2+} channels by both dihydropyridines and phenylalkylamines and block of delayed K^+ channels by quinidine. Nonetheless, it remains uncertain whether these S6 mutations modify antiarrhythmic drug action through altering gating

Arrhythmia	Mechanism	Adenosine response
AV nodal re-entry	Re-entry within the AV node	Termination
AV reciprocating tachycardias	Re-entry involves AV node and accessory pathway (WPW)	Termination
Unifocal, multifocal atrial tachycardias	Re-entry in the atrium	Transiently slows QRS rate
Atrial flutter/fibrillation	Re-entry in the atrium	Transiently slows QRS rate
Other atrial tachycardias	Abnormal automaticity or cAMP-mediated triggered activity	Transient suppression or termination
Junctional rhythms	Variable	Variable

Responses of supraventricular arrhythmias to adenosine

AV, atrioventricular; WPW, Wolff–Parkinson–White syndrome.

Figure 35.5 Supraventricular tachyarrhythmias and their typical responses to bolus adenosine administration.

processes (such as inactivation) or by eliminating the drug-binding site altogether. Recent studies on mutant Na^+ channels with inactivation only *partly* disrupted confirm that lidocaine not only binds preferentially to inactivated channels but also *enhances* the native inactivation gating process. Similarly, quaternary ammonium blockers produce use-dependent block of K^+ channels through promoting an intrinsic inactivation mechanism, known as 'C-type' inactivation. Therefore, while defining the channel residues that underlie drug binding is essential, future drug development efforts will also require a more detailed understanding of how antiarrhythmic agents function as allosteric effectors to modify ion channel gating processes.

Tissue diversity and antiarrhythmic drug action

Diversity in the molecular basis for phase 0 among cardiac tissues figures critically in the physiology and pharmacology of cardiac arrhythmias (see Fig. 35.1). The rate of the upstroke of the action potential is a determinant of conduction velocity through excitable tissue. Therefore, since I_{Ca} develops much more slowly than I_{Na}, impulses conduct through atrial and ventricular muscle far more rapidly than in the AV node. This tissue diversity protects the ventricle from fibrillation during very rapid atrial arrhythmias. Further, because β-blockers and Ca^{2+} channel blockers (Fig. 35.4) reduce Ca^{2+} current (through G protein-mediated pathways and direct channel blockade, respectively), these agents slow conduction in the SA and AV node but not in ventricular myocardium. Hence, these agents slow the rate of ventricular stimulation during rapid atrial arrhythmias (a principal indication for their use) and may also terminate supraventricular rhythms that involve the SA or AV node primarily in a re-entrant pathway. Conversely, agents that selectively block Na^+ channels (local anesthetics, class IB; Fig. 35.4) are not useful in these settings, but may be useful in terminating arrhythmias that arise in ventricular muscle where I_{Na} predominates. Although β-blockers are effective in *chronic* management of ventricular arrhythmias, the molecular mechanisms are ill-defined and may ultimately involve voltage-gated ion channels indirectly through second messenger systems. The acute effect of most agents that reduce I_{Ca} (β-blockers indirectly via G protein-coupled pathways and Ca^{2+} channel blockers directly) in ventricular muscle is attenuation of the action potential plateau. This reduces intracellular Ca^{2+} and may induce negative inotropic effects (see Chapter 34).

Phase 4, like phase 0, is another period where major differences exist between atrial and ventricular muscle and SA and AV nodal tissue (see Fig. 35.1). Adenosine A_1 receptors exist in both atrial and nodal tissues and cause activation of the K^+ current $I_{K(ACh,Ado)}$, which hyperpolarizes the cell membrane potential (transiently) to more negative potentials. This has less effect in atrial tissue (already at –90mV) but drives pacemaker cells in the AV and SA nodes farther from the action potential firing threshold, slowing their rate. Adenosine also antagonizes adenylyl cyclase and thereby slows AV nodal conduction by a second mechanism: inhibition of I_{Ca}. Hence, adenosine has effects on supraventricular tachycardias that relate specifically to the tissue responsible for their generation.

It is mechanistically useful to group supraventricular arrhythmias by their responses to adenosine (Fig. 35.5). Supraventricular arrhythmias arising from re-entry in the atrium exhibit transient slowing of the ventricular rate in response to adenosine; however, the rate of atrial discharges (P waves) does not change significantly. Moreover, slowing the rate of QRS complexes in this manner may unmask P waves on the surface ECG and facilitate diagnosis. Atrial tachycardias resulting from abnormal phase 4 depolarization may transiently slow, or even stop, with adenosine if they are caused by cAMP-mediated triggered activity. Arrhythmias that involve AV nodal tissue in the re-entry pathway are terminated by adenosine. AV junctional rhythms (common during general anesthesia) have an inconsistent response to adenosine based on their variable etiology (re-entrant, automatic). Ventricular arrhythmias usually originate in tissues distal to the conduction system and, therefore, exhibit no response to adenosine administration. Conversely, adenosine administration should induce some change (termination, ventricular rate reduction) in the R–R interval of wide complex supraventricular rhythms. Diagnostic use of adenosine in this setting may prevent inappropriate therapy of ventricular tachycardia with Ca^{2+} channel blockers, which have longer elimination kinetics.

CELLULAR MECHANISMS AND ANTIARRHYTHMIC THERAPY

Cell-to-cell coupling

An intrinsic feature of cardiac excitability is conduction of electrical impulses from cell to cell. Cardiac cells are electrically 'coupled'; as a result, the electrical behavior of one cell heavily influences that of its neighbors. Coupling effects may even supercede the intrinsic electrical behavior of the cell with the result that it behaves differently from its behavior in isolation.

Quantitative models suggest that coupling is a critical factor in arrhythmogenesis. Spatial inhomogeneities in cardiac conduction are not essential for induction or maintainence of arrhythmias; nonetheless, they make it easier to generate re-entrant arrhythmias. Such spatial inhomogeneities may result from either naturally occurring barriers to conduction (heart valves, tissue bundles) or from pathologic remodeling after myocardial infarction.

The molecular site of cell-to-cell coupling is the gap junction, a structure that interconnects cells with small channels and allows for the passage of ions. The distribution of gap junctions partly dictates the rate of conduction through tissue. For example, fast-conducting tissue (atrial and ventricular muscle, Purkinje fibers) has more extensive cell-to-cell coupling than slow-conducting tissue (SA and AV nodes). Each individual gap junction channel (known as connexons) comprises six connexin molecules, which coassemble to form pores. It remains unclear whether primary abnormalities in the genes coding for these molecules form the basis of congenital disorders in conduction. The molecular substrates of cell-to-cell coupling may prove to be viable targets for pharmacologic or gene-therapeutic arrhythmia interventions.

Re-entry and arrhythmogenesis

Re-entry, which underlies most supraventricular and ventricular arrhythmias, involves continuous movement of an impulse around a re-entrant loop (Fig. 35.6). The loop must be long enough to allow recovery of Na^+ and Ca^{2+} channels from inactivation (the refractory period) between passes. The 'excitable gap' refers to the time between recovery of tissue in the re-entrant loop and the arrival of the next impulse and is related to the size and speed of conduction in the re-entrant loop. Anatomic sites for re-entry that can be affected by disease include the AV node (AV nodal re-entrant tachycardia), accessory pathways (Wolff–Parkinson–White syndrome, AV reciprocating tachycardia), and ventricular myocardium (ventricular scar after myocardial infarction: monomorphic ventricular tachycardias). These re-entrant pathways are thought to possess long excitable gaps. In contrast, a more *functional* form of re-entry occurs when an impulse propagates around a refractory core. During myocardial ischemia, re-entry may result from disparities in repolarization rates across tissues, both between normal and ischemic epicardium and between epicardial and endocardial layers. The electrical impulse finds the shortest circuit that allows tissue beyond the leading edge of excitability to recover, producing a short excitable gap. More sophisticated models of re-entry include the leading circle model, the figure-of-eight model, the anisotropic model, and the spiral wave model. Fibrillation in either the atrium or ventricle may involve numerous coexistent functional re-entry circuits (micro re-entry).

Our ability to relate mechanisms of re-entry to pharmacologic intervention is primitive; nonetheless, it is possible that re-entrant arrhythmias exhibit differential sensitivity to antiarrhythmic agents based on the length of their excitable gap. Drugs with class I activity (Na^+ channel blockers; see Fig. 35.4) should suppress currents responsible for the action potential upstroke in atrium and ventricle, while drugs with class II or IV activity should do the same in the SA or AV node. Hence, these drugs should provide antiarrhythmic action by slowing or blocking conduction. Re-entrant circuits with long excitable gaps may be most susceptible to this mechanism, since long excitable gaps may be insensitive to small changes in the refractory period.

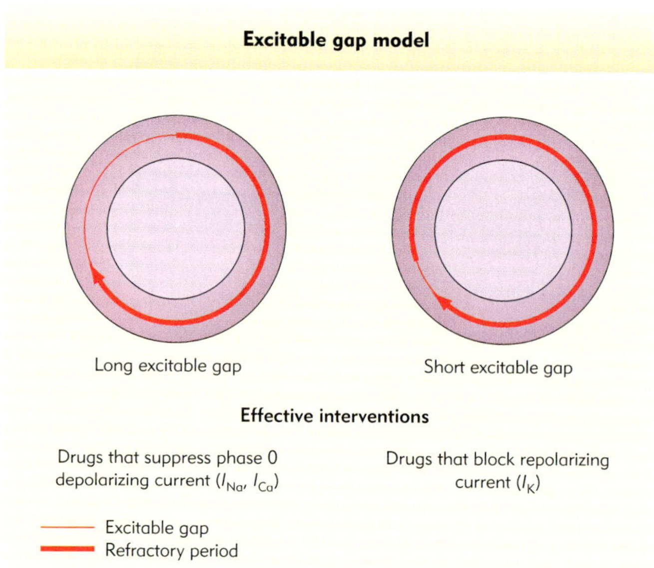

Figure 35.6 Excitable gap models for re-entry and pharmacologic intervention. Long-gap re-entry implies that the conduction loop is very long relative to the tissue refractory period, so a long period exists between complete recovery of tissue excitability and the next impulse. Short excitable gap re-entry implies the opposite: there is little time for the tissue to recover between impulses. While fixed anatomic pathways for re-entry may have long excitable gaps (scar, accessory bundles), functional re-entry circuits are thought to possess short excitable gaps (fibrillating myocardium).

Alternatively, drugs that prolong repolarization (class IA or III agents, see Fig. 35.4) prolong the refractory period and might, therefore, extinguish the leading edge of impulse propagation in a re-entrant circuit with a short excitable gap. In support of this concept, agents that prolong the refractory period have been most successful in suppressing fibrillation of both the atrium and the ventricle.

Automaticity and arrhythmia suppression

Normally, atrial and ventricular tissues do not spontaneously undergo phase 4 depolarization (see Fig. 35.1). *Abnormal automaticity* or *depolarization-induced automaticity* refers to spontaneous depolarization caused by a pathophysiologic process, such as ischemia. Such automaticity may underlie unifocal and multifocal atrial tachycardias and ventricular tachycardias in the initial days following acute myocardial infarction. Maneuvers to hyperpolarize the atrial cell during phase 4 (adenosine) may be clinically effective. *Triggered automaticity* includes arrhythmias that arise from after depolarizations during or following complete repolarization. 'Early afterdepolarizations' (EADs) arise during phase 2 or 3, while 'delayed afterdepolarizations' (DADs) begin after completion of phase 3 and result from mechanisms distinct from EADs. The ion channels that underlie the depolarizing currents responsible for EADs and DADs are debated.

The major factor predisposing to EAD formation is action potential prolongation in the ventricle. Low serum K^+ concentrations, slow heart rates, and repolarization-prolonging (class IA or III) antiarrhythmic drugs provoke EADs *in vitro,* and identical factors induce QT interval prolongation and torsades de pointes in patients. Ironically, these conditions are not pathologic in the atrium, and repolarization-prolonging drugs are the most common pharmacologic means of converting atrial fibrillation (see below). Specific ion channel mutations induce congenital forms of the long QT syndrome, which genetically predispose patients to torsades de pointes. One subtype (LQT2) results from a defect in a distinct component of repolarizing current (I_{Kr}; see Fig. 35.1). The relative importance of this current in ventricular repolarization is enhanced by slow heart rates. Further, low K^+ concentrations reduce the magnitude of I_{Kr}. Notably, I_{Kr} is a molecular target for most of the available antiarrhythmic agents that prolong repolarization. Therefore, the QT-prolonging effects of antiarrhythmic drug therapy appear to be analogous to the mechanisms involved in the congenital arrhythmias.

The major factor underlying DADs is an increase in intracellular Ca^{2+}. Although many conditions produce Ca^{2+} overload, digitalis toxicity and unopposed catecholamines are common causes. Catecholamines may underlie triggered activity during exercise, acute myocardial infarction, or perioperative stress. As such, DADs may underlie either supraventricular or ventricular tachycardias in perioperative patients who have no structural heart disease. Digitalis toxicity produces Ca^{2+} overload indirectly by inhibition of the Na^+,K^+ pump. Consequent high intracellular Na^+ limits the normal Ca^{2+} extrusion from the cell by the Na^+/Ca^{2+} exchanger. Catecholamines induce Ca^{2+} overload indirectly by increasing I_{Ca} through G protein-mediated pathways. DAD-induced arrhythmias may respond to maneuvers aimed at lowering intracellular Ca^{2+}, including Ca^{2+} channel blockade.

Perioperative atrial fibrillation

Atrial fibrillation is the most common perioperative tachyarrhythmia requiring pharmacologic intervention and it provides an opportunity to examine the relationship between arrhythmia mechanisms and drug selection. The agents most often used intraoperatively to control ventricular rate are the Ca^{2+} channel blockers because of their effects on AV nodal conduction. These agents do not influence conduction in normal atrial tissue and, therefore, have little or no potential for converting atrial fibrillation. Nonetheless, in patients with accessory pathways, these agents may paradoxically (either directly or indirectly) facilitate conduction through the accessory pathway and thereby induce malignant ventricular arrhythmias. Procainamide and amiodarone, agents with blocking activities in both Na^+ channel and K^+ channels, are most commonly used to attempt intravenous pharmacologic conversion of atrial fibrillation. Procainamide prolongs repolarization through both its own action and the action of its principal metabolite, *N*-acetylprocainamide. The efficacy of intravenous procainamide for conversion of atrial fibrillation is not well established. Largely owing to its repolarization-prolonging action, intravenous amiodarone has been used to treat atrial fibrillation in patients where procainamide or other agents fail. The risk--benefit ratio for using intravenous amiodarone in this setting has not been established, and valid concerns exist regarding potential pulmonary toxicity with perioperative use. As with procainamide, studies have not shown that intravenous amiodarone provides conversion to sinus rhythm at a rate exceeding placebo. Ibutilide is a potent, rapid-acting class III antiarrhythmic compound with 'pure' cardiac action potential-prolonging activity and few noncardiac side effects. Conversion rates for atrial fibrillation among nonsurgical patients have been remarkably high (~30% within 30 minutes), suggesting that selective K^+ channel blockade is an effective mechanistic strategy for converting atrial fibrillation. Unfortunately, the pure repolarization-prolonging action of ibutilide manifests as well in the ventricle, and significant numbers of patients (>5%) receiving this agent experience torsades de pointes. It has been advised that this drug be used cautiously in patients in uncontrolled settings or in patients with underlying heart disease, and the risk–benefit ratio for its use in perioperative patients is not yet clear. Because of this potential for inciting torsades de pointes, current strategies for therapeutic intervention in atrial fibrillation include the development of more selective K^+ channel blockers that may inhibit K^+ channel activity in the atrium but not the ventricle.

Some AV nodal blocking agents may also effect conversion to sinus rhythm. Trials have recently shown that intravenous Mg^{2+} effects conversion of atrial fibrillation at a rate exceeding that with either verapamil or amiodarone. In surgical and nonsurgical patients with recent onset atrial fibrillation, ventricular rate control with β-blockers produces a more rapid rate of conversion to sinus rhythm than rate control with Ca^{2+} channel blockers. Serum catecholamine levels are elevated following major surgery, and the arrhythmogenic potential of catecholamines in the human atrium is well established. Hence, unopposed β-adrenergic stimulation may be a factor contributing to atrial fibrillation in both perioperative and other settings. Because Mg^{2+} influences numerous voltage-gated ion channels and second messenger systems in cardiac cells, the mechanism by which it accelerates conversion of atrial fibrillation is unclear. It may partly mimic β -blockade through downregulation of catecholamine release from both peripheral and adrenal sources.

Ventricular arrhythmias

Coordinated ventricular contractions are essential for effective cardiac output from the ventricles. Ventricular arrhythmias are grouped according to their ECG morphology (Fig. 35.7). Because direct correlation between morphology and molecular mechanism is incomplete, the therapeutic principles are also somewhat empiric. Nonsustained ventricular tachycardias, including premature ventricular beats or runs of ventricular tachycardia lasting 30 seconds or less, often require no therapy. In fact, clinical studies in which patients were treated with class I antiarrhythmic drugs for nonsustained ventricular arrhythmias found death rates from proarrhythmic effects that exceeded placebo.

Sustained ventricular tachycardias may have either a monomorphic or a polymorphic morphology. In monomorphic ventricular tachycardia, the amplitude of each QRS complex mimics its predecessor; the converse is true in polymorphic ventricular tachycardia, in which the QRS complex amplitude and axis changes continuously in a sinusoidal or irregular pattern. Monomorphic ventricular tachycardia is thought to result from re-entry associated with scar tissue from a healed myocardial infarction. Although lidocaine is the traditional primary therapy for this arrhythmia, a small trial recently showed procainamide may be more effective. Our understanding of antiarrhythmic mechanisms and vulnerable parameters does not adequately explain why the addition of repolarization-prolonging activity with procainamide should markedly increase antiarrhythmic efficacy against monomorphic ventricular arrhythmias that presumably have a long excitable gap. If in

Classification of ventricular arrhythmias by ECG morphology

Arrhythmia	Usual substrate	Usual therapy
Nonsustained ventricular tachycardia (VT)	Normal ventricle	None
Sustained VT		
Monomorphic VT[a]	Prior myocardial infarction (scar)	Lidocaine (lignocaine), then procainamide, bretylium or amiodarone
Polymorphic VT with normal Q–T interval	Acute ischemia, infarction, idiopathic cardiomyopathy	Defibrillation, same as for monomorphic VT
Ventricular fibrillation	Acute ischemia, infarction, idiopathic cardiomyopathy	Defibrillation, same as for monomorphic VT
Polymorphic VT with long Q–T interval (torsades de pointes)	Congenital, prior therapy with drugs prolonging repolarization	Mg^{2+}, pacing, lidocaine, or phenytoin; consider amiodarone[b]

[a]Hemodynamically stable patients may respond better to procainamide than to lidocaine.
[b]Amiodarone induces polymorphic VT but is less proarrhythmic in this regard than other antiarrhythmics (class IA, IC, and III) and may be useful when other measures fail.

Figure 35.7 Classification of ventricular arrhythmias by electrocardiographic morphology.

addition to the anatomic substrate, the re-entry loop involves tissue with inhomogenous refractory periods (epicardial versus endocardial), and procainamide has differential effects on refractory period in these tissues, the agent may suspend re-entry by making repolarization more uniform.

When ventricular tachycardia is polymorphic, the mechanism of the arrhythmia profoundly influences the selection of antiarrhythmic therapy. Polymorphic ventricular tachycardia in the presence of corrected QT interval (QT_c) prolongation, whether acquired (e.g. from class IA or III antiarrhythmics or other drugs that prolong repolarization) or congenital, is torsades de pointes. Interventions for torsades de pointes are aimed at reducing the likelihood of EAD and, therefore, include measures to increase heart rate and normalize QT_c (pacing, catecholamines, electrolytes). Conversely, polymorphic ventricular tachycardia without QT_c prolongation, common in settings of ischemia or structural heart disease, is managed with therapy similar to that of monomorphic ventricular tachycardia or ventricular fibrillation (Fig. 35.7).

PACING AND CARDIAC ELECTROVERSION

This section will examine how molecular and cellular electropharmacology influence therapy with electronic assist devices.

Pacing and capture

Pacing has assumed a prominent place among the therapies for pathologic bradycardias and some tachycardias. Drug therapies are often limited in their ability to restore a hemodynamically effective cardiac rhythm in the face of sinus node dysfunction or severe conduction block. Temporary or permanent pacing can reduce the requirement for drug therapies, which often carry unwanted side effects. Pacemakers stimulate the heart by delivering a constant voltage (2.5–5.0 volts) to the endocardial or epicardial surface of the atrium, the ventricle, or both. The amount of current that enters the myocardium depends on the impedance of the lead/tissue interface and the pulse characteristics (duration, strength). The minimum amount of current needed to stimulate and capture the myocardium (pacing threshold) is determined by both tissue and pacemaker variables.

'Failure to capture' is a common difficulty with temporary pacing in the operating room, as well as with permanent pacemakers, and requires consideration of both the pacemaker technology and the cellular events that underlie cardiac impulse propagation. Pacemakers stimulate the cardiac cell through cathodal stimulation; that is, the stimulating electrode injects current into the underlying cardiac tissue, causing direct depolarization of cells in its vicinity. This results in activation and opening of Na^+ channels, producing further intrinsic depolarization of these cells. Once an action potential is generated, the impulse spreads throughout the heart via cell-to-cell coupling through gap junctions. Inability to capture is caused by failure either to deliver stimulation or to depolarize sufficient myocardium for action potential propagation. Ongoing studies attempt to define novel mechanisms by which electrical stimulation may excite the heart (anodal and cathodal break stimulation, virtual cathode effects) and these may dramatically alter our approach to pacing.

Pacing failure usually results from mechanical factors (battery depletion, lead fracture or dislodgement, etc.), while depolarization and action potential propagation failure results from inflammation and fibrosis at the electrode–tissue interface. The latter process, termed 'lead maturation', is less problematic with the use of steroid-eluting electrodes. Loss of capture months to years postimplantation, known as exit block, frequently results from failure of myocardial cells to propagate action potentials and may be caused by a variety of conditions. Pathophysiologic states that cause cardiac tissue to depolarize, such as hyperkalemia, acidosis, and ischemia, induce Na^+ channel inactivation and prevent action potential generation (and propagation). Virtually all antiarrhythmic agents, especially those with class I activity, raise pacing thresholds. Similarly, drugs that impair conduction through other mechanisms (β-blockers) raise pacing thresholds. Inhalational anesthetics do not significantly affect pacing thresholds or impulse propagation. Drugs that enhance conduction, such as sympathomimetic agents, lower the pacing threshold, as do physiologic conditions that raise sympathetic tone such as exercise and stress. Recognition of these important physiologic and pharmacologic variables is helpful in perioperative situations where pacing thresholds may change.

Defibrillators

Electroversion, through either external defibrillators or implanted (internal) cardioverter-defibrillators (ICD), involves application of high-energy capacitor discharges to depolarize a large mass of myocardium simultaneously with the goal of abruptly terminating an abnormal rhythm. *Cardioversion* is utilized specifically for re-entrant tachycardias (either atrial or ventricular) and refers to the application of discharges that are synchronized with the QRS complex. Cardioversion terminates re-entrant arrhythmias by simultaneously depolarizing the entire re-entrant pathway, thus removing the arrhythmia substrate. Antiarrhythmic agents have limited efficacy for converting re-entrant arrhythmias and have undesirable side effects. Nonetheless, cardioversion may fail primarily or secondarily. Successfully cardioverted tachyarrhythmias may recur if the conditions inducing the re-entrant pathway are not corrected; hence, antiarrhythmic drug therapy may be a necessary supplement to cardioversion. Arrhythmias resulting from automatic or triggered automaticity may be resistant to cardioversion (ectopic atrial tachycardia, torsades de pointes).

Defibrillation refers to the asynchronous discharge of current to the myocardium and is indicated for pulseless ventricular arrhythmias including ventricular fibrillation. The higher energy requirements for converting ventricular fibrillation reflect the involvement of the entire ventricle in multiple, functional re-entry circuits (micro re-entry). With external defibrillation, the major factor determining success is transthoracic resistance, which is a function of not only tissue variables but also ventilatory phase and electrode size. Consequently, internal defibrillation, either via internal devices (internal cardioverter-defibrillators) or open-thoracotomy, dramatically lowers the energy requirement. Most antiarrhythmic drugs raise the defibrillation threshold (bretylium and lidocaine are possible exceptions). Additionally, physiologic factors including hypothermia, acidosis, or hypoxemia may lower the success of defibrillatory shocks. As with cardioversion, antiarrhythmic drugs are useful as adjuncts to defibrillation in patients where ventricular fibrillation is recurrent and prompt elimination of the arrhythmia substrate is not feasible.

Key References

Atlee JL. Periooperative cardiac dysrhythmias: diagnosis and management. Anesthesiology. 1997;86:1397–424.

Catterall WA. Structure and function of voltage-sensitive ion channels. Science. 1988;242:50–61.

Engelstein ED, Lippman N, Stein KM, Lerman BB. Mechanism-specific effects of adenosine on atrial tachcycardia. Circulation. 1994;89:2645–54.

Hondeghem LM, Katzung BG. Time- and voltage-dependent interactions of the antiarrhythmic drugs with cardiac sodium channels. Biochim Biophys Acta. 1977;472:373–98.

Pérez-Garcia MT, Chiamvimonvat N, Ranjan R, et al. Mechanisms of sodium/calcium selectivity in sodium channels probed by cysteine mutagenesis and sulfhydryl modification. Biophys J. 1997;72:989–96.

Ragsdale DS, McPhee JC, Scheuer T, Catterall WA. Common molecular determinants of local anesthetic, antiarrhythmic, and anticonvulsant block of voltage-gated Na^+ channels. Proc Natl Acad Sci USA. 1996;93:9270–5.

Stühmer W, Conti F, Suzuke H, et al. Structural parts involved in activation and inactivation of the sodium channel. Nature. 1989;339:597–603.

Task Force of the Working Group on Arrhythmias of the European Society of Cardiology. The Sicilian Gambit: a new approach to the classification of antiarrhythmic drugs based on their actions on arrhythmogenic mechanisms. Circulation. 1991;84:1831–51.

Trautwein W, Hescheler J. Regulation of cardiac L-type calcium current by phosphorylation and G proteins. Annu Rev Physiol. 1990;52:257–74.

Further Reading

Lukas A, Antzelevitch C. Differences in the electrophysiological response of canine ventricular epicardium and endocardium to ischemia: role of the transient outward current. Circulation. 1993;88:2903–15.

Peterson BZ, Tanada TN, Caterall WA. Molecular determinants of high affinity dihydropyridine binding in L-type calcium channels. J Biol Chem. 1996;271:5293–6.

Platia EV, Michelson EL, Porterfield JK, Das G. Esmolol versus verapamil in the acute treatment of atrial fibrillation or atrial flutter. Am J Cardiol. 1989;63:925–9.

Roden DM. Ibutilide and the treatment of atrial arrhythmias. Circulation. 1996;94:1499–502.

Roden DM, Hoffman BF. Action potential prolongation and induction of abnormal automaticity by low quinidine concentrations in canine Purkinje fibers. Relationship to potassium and cycle length. Circ Res. 1985;56:857–67.

Sauguinetti MC, Jiang C, Curran ME, Keating MT. A mechanistic link between an inherited and an acquired cardiac arrhythmia: HERG encodes the I_{Kr} potassium channel. Cell. 1995;81:299–307.

Spach MS, Heidlage JF. The stochastic nature of cardiac propagation at a microscopic level. Electrical description of myocardial architecture and its application to conduction. Circ Res. 1995;76:366–80.

Yeola SW, Rich TC, Uebele VN, Tamkun MM, Snyders DJ. Molecular analysis of a binding site for quinidine in a human cardiac delayed rectifier K^+ channel: role of S6 in antiarrhythmic drug binding. Circ Res. 1996;78:1105–14.

Chapter 36 Regulation and assessment of cardiac function

Paul M Heerdt

Topics covered in this chapter

Anatomy and physiology
Dynamic determinants of ventricular function
Ventricular–vascular interaction
Clinical assessment of ventricular function

In the course of a normal life span, the human heart beats between 2 and 3 billion times. Each heart beat represents multiple electrical, biochemical, and mechanical events that occur over milliseconds, and translocate a volume of oxygenated blood into the peripheral circulation that is sufficient to meet metabolic needs of the body. Regulation of contraction and relaxation of the heart and its performance as a pump involves acute and prolonged events that are both intrinsic and extrinsic to the heart proper. In this chapter a brief review is given of the anatomy and physiology of the heart, both as a muscle and a pump, and the clinical assessment of its performance is discussed. In Chapter 37, a more detailed discussion of cardiac mechanics is provided and a systematic approach for interpreting hemodynamic monitoring is presented.

ANATOMY AND PHYSIOLOGY

Multiple structures form individually and eventually fuse to form 'the heart' during organogenesis. Although the heart is regarded as a single organ, it actually represents two interdependent pumps (the right and left hearts) which are connected in series and contained in a common sac (the pericardium). Unlike the right ventricle (RV) inflow tract and the entire left ventricle (LV), which arise from the ventricular portion of the primitive cardiac tube, the RV outflow tract is derived from the bulbus cordis. In some phylogenetically lower animals this portion of the heart takes on specific functions; in sharks, for example, the bulbus is retained as a separate chamber involved with providing flow across the gills, and in turtles the RV outflow tract regulates the distribution of blood flow between the systemic and pulmonary circulations as it is ejected from an essentially common ventricle.

The atria are grossly similar in size and dimension while the ventricles are quite different; the RV is crescent-shaped and largely wrapped around the interventricular septum, which represents the medial wall of the elliptic LV. Functionally, the pattern of contraction varies between the LV and RV. The LV contracts in a relatively homogeneous fashion, with both the short and long axes shortening simultaneously. In contrast, the RV contracts sequentially from the inflow tract to the outflow tract. The mechanical significance of this sequential pattern of contraction is unclear, but the process is altered by sympathetic stimulation, positive inotropic drugs, total autonomic blockade, and volatile anesthetics. At the cellular level, the myocardium of both ventricles comprises individual myofibrils, which are linked by specialized gap junctions to form a functional syncytium that allows rapid conduction of electrical charge. Fundamentally, all myocytes display five basic characteristics – excitability (bathmotropy), conductivity (dromotropy), rhythmicity (chronotropy), contractility (inotropy), and relaxation (lusitropy).

At the center of cardiac mechanical function is the process of excitation–contraction coupling (Chapter 34). Myocyte depolarization leads to influx of extracellular Ca^{2+} via voltage-dependent Ca^{2+} channels and, to a lesser extent, electrogenic Na^+–Ca^{2+} exchange. This relatively small amount of Ca^{2+} functions primarily as 'activator Ca^{2+}' which stimulates the sarcoplasmic reticulum (SR) to release a larger amount of Ca^{2+} in a process known as Ca^{2+}-induced Ca^{2+} release. Storage and release of Ca^{2+} by the SR are relatively complex processes modulated by the high capacity Ca^{2+}-binding protein calsequestrin and the ryanodine-sensitive Ca^{2+} release channel, respectively. Once myoplasmic Ca^{2+} concentration exceeds about 1μmol/L, Ca^{2+} binds to troponin C to produce a conformational change in tropomysin that allows interaction between actin and myosin myofilaments and mechanical shortening. As soon as the stimulus to release Ca^{2+} is terminated, reuptake of Ca^{2+} by SR leads to a rapid decline in intracellular Ca^{2+} concentration, which facilitates dissociation of Ca^{2+} from troponin C and relaxation. Reuptake of Ca^{2+} into the SR is energy-dependent and involves Ca^{2+}-adenosine triphosphatase (ATPase) and its regulatory protein phospholamban. Most factors that influence contractility of the heart – from pharmacologic manipulation to idiopathic failure – alter intracellular Ca^{2+} cycling.

Multiple factors intrinsic to the heart influence excitation–contraction coupling, the process of relaxation, and ultimately performance of the heart. In general, intrinsic processes influence initial sarcomere length, the number of active crossbridges between actin and myosin, the rate of crossbridge cycling, and the time course of activation and inactivation. Extensive research has characterized the impact of these factors upon myocardial contraction at the cellular and subcellular level. However, *in vivo* the interaction between intrinsic and extrinsic regulators of myocyte function dictate performance of the heart as a pump.

Chamber geometry

While each myocyte is capable of contracting (changing length and developing tension), it is the association of millions of myocytes in a three-dimensional configuration that allows the heart to develop pressure and function as a pump. Consideration of the LV as a thin-walled sphere allows relatively simple characterization of the relationship between intraventricular pressure (distending force at right angles to the wall) and wall stress (tension per unit area reflecting a shear force applied circumferentially) within the context of the law of Laplace (Equation 36.1), in which P is ventricular pressure, r is internal radius, σ is stress, and h is uniform wall thickness. Equation 36.1 can be simplified to give Equation 36.2, since $r >> h$ (Chapter 37).

■ Equation 36.1

$$Pr = \sigma h\left(2 + \frac{h}{r}\right)$$

■ Equation 36.2

$$\sigma = \frac{Pr}{2h}$$

Application of the law of Laplace to a spherical model of the LV requires three assumptions:

- wall thickness and internal radius remain constant;
- the wall itself is thin relative to the internal radius – thus stress is constant throughout the wall; and
- the chamber is at rest.

In reality, the LV is more of an elongated ellipse than a sphere, and stress is not uniform across the LV wall. Nonetheless, the law of Laplace provides useful information in the qualitative assessment of pathophysiologic alterations in wall stress. For example, although both aortic stenosis and regurgitation increase LV wall stress, the concentric hypertrophy associated with stenosis can lead to a substantial increase in wall thickness, which tends to reduce stress by offsetting increases in pressure and radius (Chapter 40). This has clinical importance because of a direct relationship between wall stress and oxygen consumption.

In contrast with the LV, the complex geometry (essentially a crescent) and contraction pattern of the RV defies simple application of spherical models. Although the general relationships between pressure and wall stress remain, it is impossible to incorporate global terms such as internal radius; distribution of wall stress throughout the walls of the RV is probably even more heterogeneous than that in the LV. Conceptually, although RV systolic pressure is about 20% that of the LV, RV volume tends to be higher and the free wall thinner. Thus, RV wall stress during systole is probably not as different from that of the LV as may be anticipated from their differences in pressure. However, in the setting of a modest increase in afterload, RV wall stress increases more than that of the LV because of a more prominent relative rise in both its pressure and volume.

DYNAMIC DETERMINANTS OF VENTRICULAR FUNCTION

The fundamental determinants of ventricular pump function are generally regarded as rate and rhythm, preload, afterload, and contractility. The concepts of preload, afterload, and contractility are largely derived from studies of isolated muscle and as such are difficult to apply precisely to the intact heart. Nonetheless, with increased understanding of the complexities of cardiac physiology, improved techniques for determining intracavitary volume, and the widespread access to real-time images of the heart, these determinants – and their limitations – have assumed an expanded meaning to clinicians. Appreciation of how these determinants interact to influence performance of the heart as a pump can be enhanced by considering cardiac pressure–volume relationships.

Although often regarded as a relatively novel approach to the assessment of cardiac function, ventricular pressure–volume loops were first constructed for frog hearts by Frank in the late 1800s. Figure 36.1 depicts an LV pressure–volume diagram in which specific phases of the cardiac cycle are easily recognized. Two particular areas of the loop are especially important. The 'upper left corner' designates the end of ejection and is widely used in assessing LV contractility based upon the load-variable end-systolic pressure–volume relationship (ESPVR). The 'lower right corner' denotes the end-diastolic point and is used to assess diastolic function based upon the load-variable end-diastolic pressure–volume relationship (EDPVR), and contractility based upon the relationship between end-diastolic volume (EDV) and stroke work. End of ejection is not always clearly defined, which can complicate use of the upper left corner for ESPVR analysis. This is evident in representative LV and RV pressure–volume loops (Fig. 36.2a). The RV loop is more triangular, with an ill-defined end-ejection point and a minimal period of isovolumic relaxation. To study regional myocardial function in conjunction with, or as an alternative to, global function, segmental dimension measurements can be obtained to create pressure–segment length loops. As shown in Figure 36.2b, these loops are morphologically similar to pressure–volume loops, and the same principles as those for ESPVR and EDPVR analysis can be used.

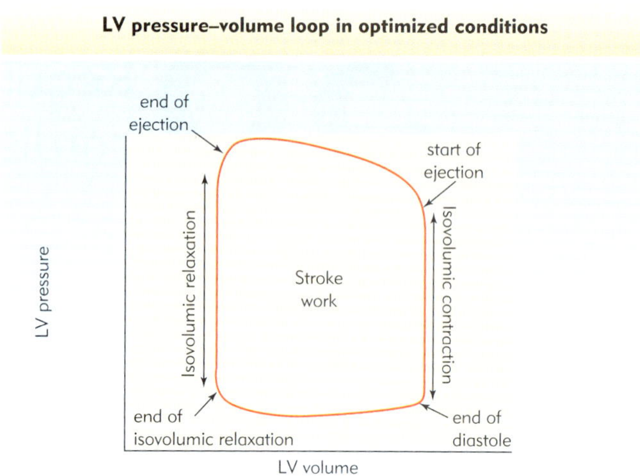

Figure 36.1 A left ventricular pressure–volume loop obtained under optimized conditions in an experimental animal. In general, the loop is rectangular with relatively well-defined phases that correspond to the beginning and end of ejection, and the beginning and end of filling.

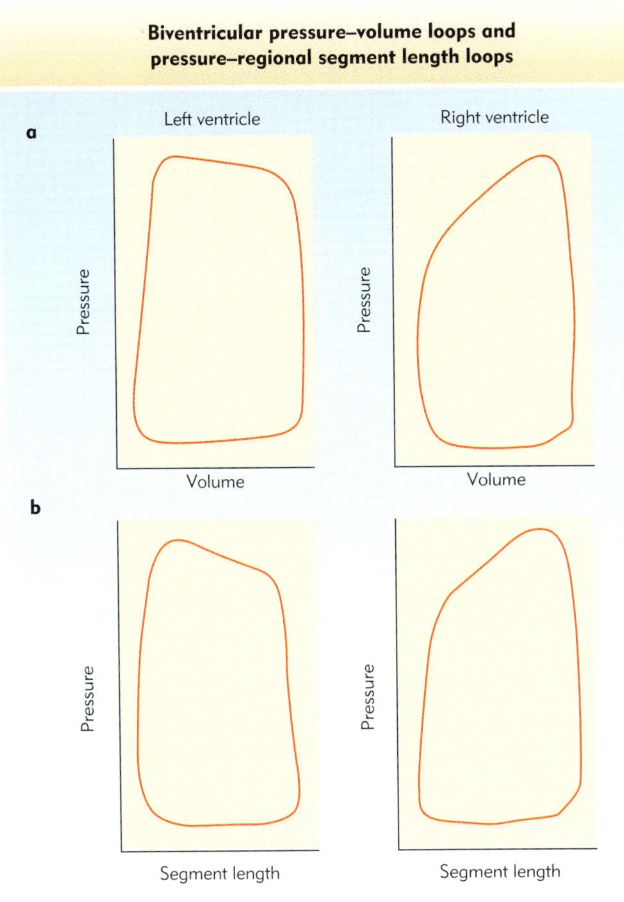

Figure 36.2 Comparison of left and right (a) ventricular pressure–volume loops and (b) pressure–regional segment length loops recorded simultaneously from the same heart. Under normal conditions, right ventricular loops tend to be more triangular with a poorly defined 'upper left corner'.

Rate and rhythm

Although it is intuitive that changes in heart rate and rhythm influence cardiac pump performance, subtle complexities exist. For example, when the contraction rate of a normal heart increases, so initially does the force of contraction (positive force–frequency relationship). In the setting of heart failure, however, an increase in heart rate can produce a decrease in contractile force (negative force–frequency relationship). Similarly, while the impact of arrhythmias on ventricular filling and ejection are easily visualized, subtle factors that alter the synchrony (but not necessarily electrical activity) of regional ventricular contraction can influence cardiac pump performance. Under normal circumstances, a substantial amount of work performed by the RV is actually performed by the LV and septum with up to 60% of RV pressure and 80% of RV ejection produced by LV contraction and septal movement in the absence of RV free wall contraction (ventricular interaction). This magnitude of RV dependency upon LV function has become clinically evident in situations in which mechanical assistance and unloading of a failing LV contributes to failure of an adequately functioning RV.

Factors that influence ventricular compliance and filling

Extrinsic

a intrathoracic pressure
b pericardial inflammation or effusion
c intrapericardial mass

Intrinsic

a concentric hypertrophy (chronic hypertension or valvular stenosis)
b chronic cardiomyopathy
c acute ischemia
d infarction

Figure 36.3 Factors that influence ventricular compliance and filling.

Preload

Preload represents the volume (and to a lesser extent pressure) that produces 'stretch' of myofibrils and determines sarcomere length prior to contraction; it is directly related to end-diastolic wall stress. Limitations to measuring intracardiac volumes have led to reliance upon intracardiac pressures as an indirect indicator of preload. Recent advances in techniques to measure intraventricular volume have greatly enhanced the clinical appreciation of diastolic pressure–volume relationships and thus diastolic function. Pressure and EDV are determined by many processes that extrinsically affect venous return to the heart, and intrinsically influence relaxation and the ability of the heart to fill (Fig. 36.3). The ventricle normally has four phases of diastole – isovolumic relaxation, early rapid filling, diastasis, and atrial systole. Of these phases, only isovolumic relaxation is an active process that requires expenditure of energy by ventricular myocytes. Characterized as ventricular lusitropy, this active relaxation process can be quantified by the minimum value of the first derivative of ventricular pressure versus time ($-\partial P/\partial t$), or more precisely as a time constant of isovolumic pressure decline (τ). Both methods require measurement of ventricular pressure with high fidelity, and the utility of $-\partial P/\partial t$ is limited by a dependence upon developed pressure and that the maximal rate of pressure decline is determined from a single point. Calculation of τ is based upon the monoexponential decline of pressure during the isovolumic phase of the cycle: that is, from end-ejection (commonly defined as the point of peak $-\partial P/\partial t$) to opening of the mitral valve. This gives Equation 36.3, in which P is ventricular pressure, A is ventricular pressure at $-\partial P/\partial t$, t is the time after $-\partial P/\partial t$, and τ is the relaxation time constant.

■ Equation 36.3

$$P = A^{-t/\tau}$$

As a consequence of the relative lack of an isovolumic phase in the RV, calculation of τ is problematic. In the LV, two facets of τ calculation and interpretation are controversial:

- precisely which portion of the LV pressure curve should be used and whether or not a 0 pressure asymptote should be assumed; and
- the afterload dependence of the measurement.

Nonetheless, relaxation is delayed, and τ increased, in chronic processes such as hypertrophy or cardiomyopathy, or in acute processes such as ischemia or with negative inotropic drugs. In contrast, relaxation is enhanced, and τ is reduced, by increases in heart rate or administration of positive inotropic drugs.

Rapid ventricular filling follows isovolumic relaxation and begins when ventricular pressure falls below atrial pressure. During this period, elastic recoil of the myocardium in combination with continued relaxation create an atrial–ventricular pressure gradient (sometimes characterized as suction), which greatly facilitates ventricular filling. As the atrial–ventricular pressure gradient diminishes, the phase of diastasis (slow ventricular filling) begins, and continues until atrial systole. Early rapid filling normally accounts for 75–80% of ventricular EDV; diastasis and atrial systole provide about 3–5% and 15–25%, respectively. Multiple processes can alter diastolic filling dynamics, most notably ectopy arising from the atrioventricular node and ventricular pacing (no atrial systole), and reductions in ventricular compliance (e.g. concentric hypertrophy). Alterations in diastolic compliance can significantly impact early diastolic filling. The characteristics of ventricular compliance in pathologic states can be quantified by measurements of chamber stiffness (the monoexponential relationship between chamber pressure and volume changes) and myocardial stiffness (a material property of the myocardium that reflects its resistance to stretching). Increased understanding of the relationship between ventricular relaxation, chamber stiffness, diastolic filling, and sarcomere length reveals that heart failure, manifest as low cardiac output and pulmonary vascular congestion, can result not only from impaired systolic function but also from impaired diastolic function (diastolic dysfunction).

Afterload

Despite the intuitive nature of the concept of afterload, it is actually somewhat difficult to apply to the intact heart in that ejection is opposed by the variable hydraulic load imposed by the outflow circulation. Perhaps the closest parallel to afterload as defined in isolated muscle is instantaneous wall tension, but this parameter is difficult to quantify, particularly in the clinical setting. Accordingly, ventricular afterload is commonly summarized as the relationship between *mean* pressure and *mean* flow, expressed as systemic (SVR) or pulmonary (PVR) vascular resistance. Vascular resistance alone, however, is an incomplete expression of ventricular afterload, since the pressure and flow generated by the heart are not steady and continuous, but intermittent and pulsatile. Thus, in addition to steady-state resistive forces, ejection is opposed by elastic (large vessels are distended with each beat) and reflective (pressure waves reflected backward) forces.

To incorporate both pulsatile and nonpulsatile components into a single index of afterload, the concept of effective arterial elastance [the total change in aortic or pulmonary artery (PA) pressure divided by the volume change that occurs during a beat] has been proposed. While this approach enables the quantification of total load, it does not dissociate pulsatile from nonpulsatile components. To achieve this, proximal aortic or PA pressure and flow characteristics can be resolved into individual frequency components (since each waveform actually represents the summation of forward and backward waves of multiple frequencies) and used to calculate input impedance (Z_{IN}). This 'frequency domain' analysis of pressure and flow throughout the entire cardiac cycle allows the creation of an impedance spectrum in which the pressure–flow amplitude and phase ratios at each frequency are plotted over a range of frequencies (Fig. 36.4). Specific components of the input impedance spectrum can then be used to represent different components of ventricular afterload when:

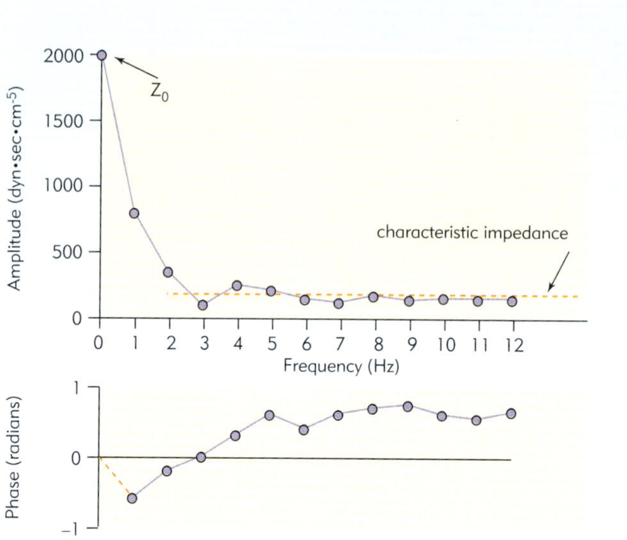

Figure 36.4 Aortic input impedance spectrum generated from pressure and flow recorded in the aortic root. Amplitude designates the ratio of pressure and flow at each frequency; Z_0 designates the ratio at zero frequency, which is essentially equal to systemic vascular resistance and reflects the contribution of small resistance vessels to afterload. Characteristic impedance designates the average of values between 3 and 12Hz and reflects the contribution to afterload of large elastic vessels. Phase designates the phasic relationship between the pressure and flow wave at each frequency; when its value is negative, flow precedes pressure. This information is useful in determining the characteristics of wave reflection.

- analyzed to determine the location and magnitude of wave reflection; and
- fit to a three-element model of the circulation, which emulates an electrical circuit.

Such a 'lumped parameter' model contains:

- a direct current (DC) component (frequency-independent), which represents nonpulsatile load and is characterized by Z_0 at zero frequency;
- an alternating current (AC) component (frequency-dependent), which represents pulsatile load and is described by the 'characteristic' Z (Z_C) defined as the average of values at 3Hz and higher; and
- a capacitor (energy storage element), which is characterized by the compliance of the proximal aorta or PA which through elastic recoil transmits energy downstream during diastole.

This 'Windkessel' model is based upon similarities with early firehose systems that allowed water to be pumped by hand (pulsatile work or AC component) into a distensible chamber (energy-storage element), which dampened the pulsations and discharged the water as a continuous stream (steady-state or DC component).

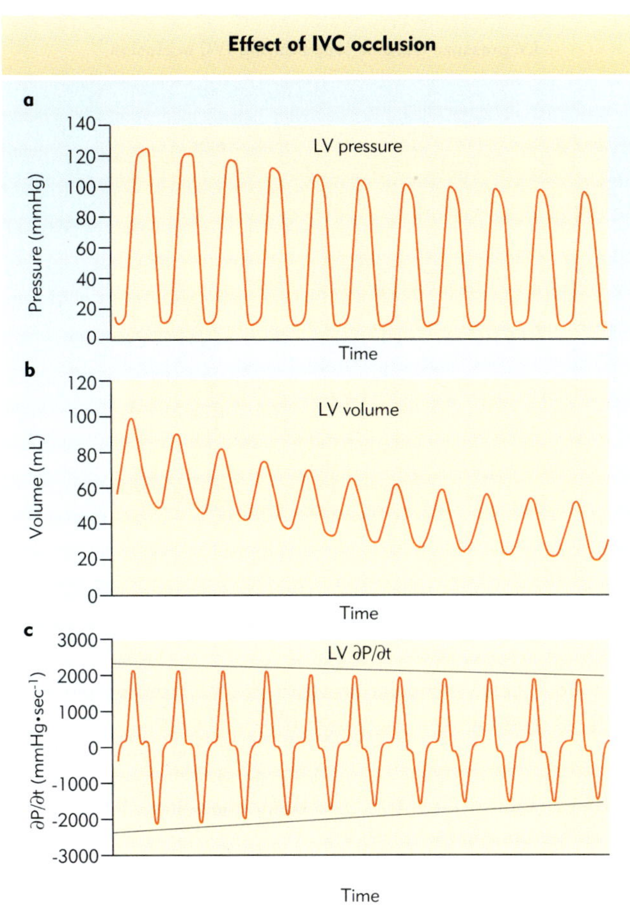

Figure 36.5 Effect of an acute reduction in preload [inferior vena cava (IVC) occlusion]. (a) Left ventricular pressure, (b) volume, and (c) ∂P/∂t. Despite no intrinsic change in contractility, ∂P/∂t falls with the decline in volume, which demonstrates the preload dependence of this index.

Contractility

Contractility reflects the ability of the myocyte to generate tension given a specific load; when the relationship is shifted such that tension is developed more rapidly and/or to a greater degree for the load, contractility is increased. While relatively easy to quantify in isolated muscle systems or intact hearts beating isovolumically, for which loading conditions can be strictly controlled, quantification of contractility in the ejecting heart is much more complex. Load-independent methods to assess contractility in the intact heart have proved extremely valuable in experimental preparations, but clinical applications have not been uniformly successful. In general, indices of contractility can be derived from the phase of isovolumic contraction, the phase of ventricular ejection, the ESPVR, or the relationship between stroke work and EDV.

Indices derived from isovolumic contraction

One of the most common and useful indices of contractility is the first derivative of developed pressure, or $\partial P/\partial t$MAX, which is sensitive enough to detect acute alterations in contractility, easy to interpret, and relatively independent of afterload. Disadvantages include the need for high-fidelity measurements of pressure, distortion by wall properties and valve dysfunction, and a substantial influence by preload (Fig. 36.5). To compensate for preload dependence, the ratio of $\partial P/\partial t$ to developed pressure has been used, as has $\partial P/\partial t$ from a fixed pressure [e.g. 40mmHg (5.3kPa)], and the relationship between $\partial P/\partial t$MAX and EDV.

Ejection phase indices

The most frequently used clinical index of global contractile function is ejection fraction (EF). Calculated as stroke volume (SV) divided by EDV, the normal LV EF is 60–70%, and the normal RV EF is 45–50%. Both invasive and noninvasive techniques have been used to determine EF from image-based volume measurements (echocardiography, angiography, magnetic resonance imaging, positron emission tomography scanning) or indicator dilution techniques. While EF provides useful information about systolic pump performance, it is heavily influenced by afterload, which reduces its value as a specific index of contractility. Such load dependence is common to virtually all indices of contractility based upon ejection-phase parameters, with the possible exception of the maximal rate of power generation (the product of pressure and flow per unit time) during ejection. In this, the relationship between pressure and flow is largely determined by afterload (i.e. at low afterload more flow and less pressure is generated), and the maximal rate of power generation is less sensitive to alterations in afterload within the physiologic range.

Indices derived from pressure–volume relationships

In the late 1970s Suga and Sagawa began to describe the use of ESPVR to characterize ventricular contractility in a load-independent manner based upon the concept of volume elastance (E), defined as $\Delta P/\Delta V$, or the inverse of compliance. If the empty heart is considered to behave like an elastic sac or balloon, as filling begins an initial increase in volume occurs without significant pressure change. Eventually a volume is reached (V_0) at which the contents go from being unstressed (no pressure) to stressed (under pressure), and pressure begins to rise as volume increases. If the subsequent pressure–volume relationship is linear, the slope of this line at any volume (V) and corresponding pressure (P) is $P/(V–V_0)$, which represents E. However, unlike a balloon, the heart actively increases wall tension during contraction. As the wall stiffens, the relationship between pressure and volume, and therefore E, changes. The pressure–volume ratio increases over the course of contraction to reach a maximum approximately at the end of systole (Fig. 36.6). In the intact heart, end-systolic elastance (Ees) can be determined by varying loading conditions to provide a range of pressures and volumes, and regressing the point of end systole for each beat; the slope of this regression is Ees, and the x (or volume) intercept is V_0 (Fig. 36.7). This method assumes that V_0 stays relatively constant and that the $P/(V–V_0)$ slope remains linear, which is valid under most physiologic conditions. However, acute alterations in contractility (e.g. the negative inotropic effect of volatile anesthetics) can alter both the slope and volume intercept of ESPVR (Fig. 36.7). Furthermore, nonlinear (monoexponential and quadratic) ESPVR relationships have been described. Also, Ees can be influenced by how end-systole is defined. The assumption is often made that end-ejection and the point of maximal P/V ratio (EMAX) occur at essentially the same time, but under some circumstances this is not so. Thus, many investigators use only the point of maximal P/V ratio to calculate EMAX instead of Ees.

An alternative to Ees is preload recruitable stroke work (PRSW), which essentially represents a linearization of the

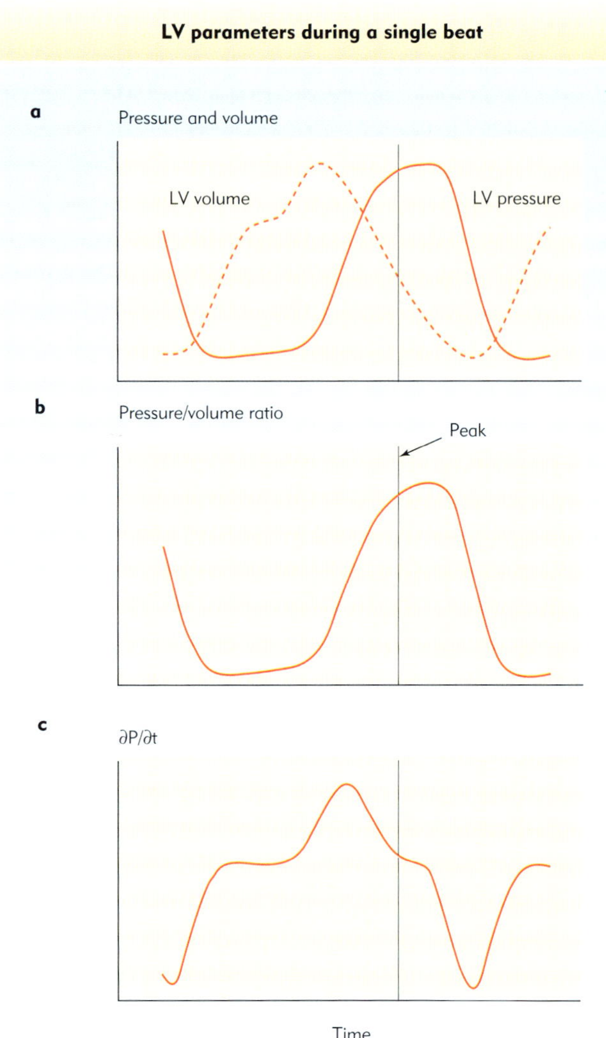

Figure 36.6 Left ventricular parameters during a single beat. (a) Pressure and volume, (b) pressure–volume ratio, and (c) ∂*P*/∂*t* for a single beat. Timing of the maximal pressure–volume ratio relative to peak pressure and minimum volume (which occurs at the upper left corner of the pressure–volume loop and represents end systole) is evident.

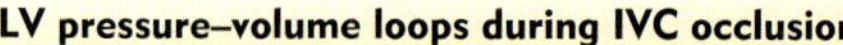

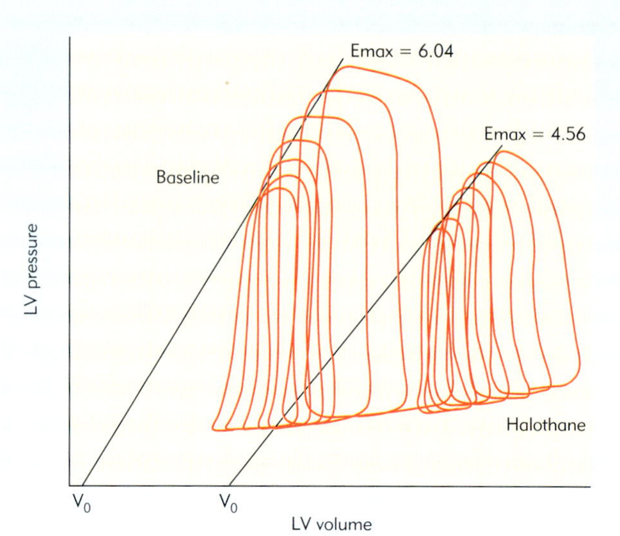

Figure 36.7 Left ventricular pressure–volume loops obtained during an acute preload reduction (IVC occlusion). Measurements were taken before and during the administration of halothane 1%. Changes in both the slope of the end-systolic pressure–volume relationship (*E*MAX) and the volume intercept (V_0) were produced by halothane.

Frank–Starling relationship. To measure PRSW, venous return to the intact heart is acutely decreased and the area of each *P*/*V* loop, which represents the external work performed during the beat, is plotted as a function of the EDV (Fig. 36.8). The slope of this relationship determines how much work the heart is capable of at any given preload. When contractility increases or decreases, the slope rises or falls as the heart performs more or less work for a given preload. In the assessment of acute alterations in contractility, this technique appears to have less variation in the volume intercept and more shift in slope than does *E*MAX.

Multiple physiologic and pharmacologic factors can directly alter contractility (Fig. 36.9), while others (e.g. nitroprusside with its systemic vasodilation) produce indirect effects by stimulating regulatory autonomic responses. Since the fundamental basis of contraction is Ca^{2+} binding to troponin C, the final common pathway of most processes is either intracellular Ca^{2+} availability or a change in sensitivity of troponin C to Ca^{2+}. Alteration in contractility can be either acute or chronic, and a shift in dose–response to most drugs occurs over time as a consequence of changes either in membrane receptor binding affinity or number, or disruption of postreceptor events.

VENTRICULAR–VASCULAR INTERACTION

With each beat, the heart expends a certain amount of energy toward tension development to produce pressure and myocyte shortening to produce flow. The balance between tension and shortening dictates performance and efficiency of the chamber as a pump and is influenced by both afterload and contractility. Understanding the interaction between contractility and afterload can be very important clinically in the treatment of patients with compromised ventricular performance.

A number of methods have been described to characterize 'ventricular–vascular interaction'. By far the most common is EF (see above), which provides general information about how well the heart can pump, but not about how efficiently the heart is working. A relatively simple approach to this question is to examine the hydraulic work performed by the ventricle (the product of pressure and flow) over a range of vascular resistances. At low resistances, hydraulic work is low because the pressure term is very small; at high resistances hydraulic work is low because the flow term is small. In between, if contractility is kept constant there is a point at which the pressure–flow product reaches a maximum and the afterload is said to be 'optimally matched' with contractility. As noted above, afterload is determined not only by steady-state resistance but also by pulsatile factors presented

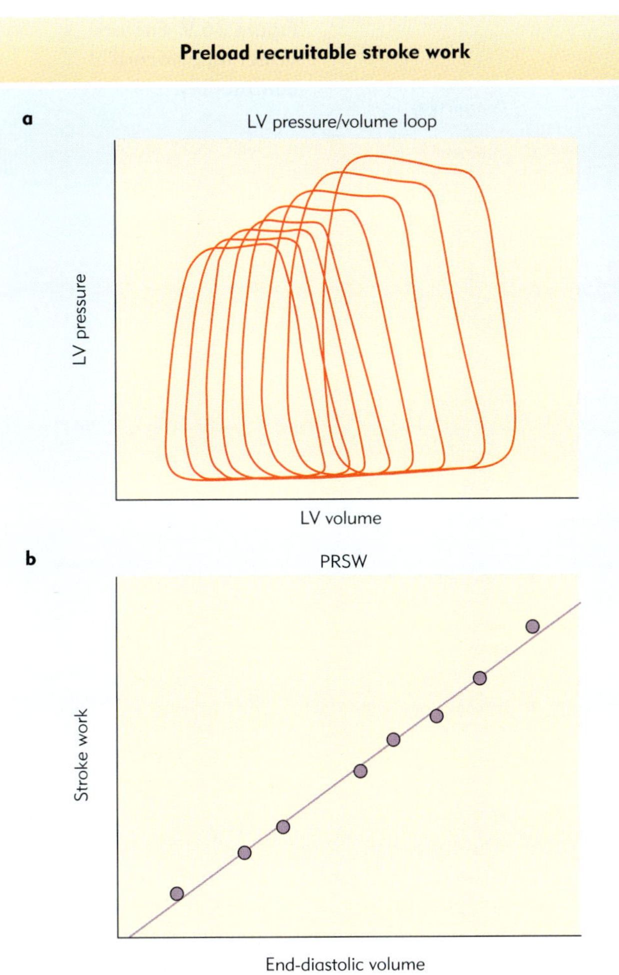

Figure 36.8 Preload recruitable stroke work (PRSW). (a) Left ventricular pressure–volume loops obtained during an acute preload reduction in an experimental animal. (b) The area of each loop (which represents stroke work) is plotted as a function of the end-diastolic volume to derive PRSW as an index of contractility.

by the large elastic vessels. An extension of ventricular–vascular matching concepts based upon the product of pressure and flow considers pump performance in both nonpulsatile and pulsatile (oscillatory) terms. This enables characterization of how much work done (or power generated) by the system helps move blood forward, and how much is lost to pulsatility (i.e. helps distend the system). Power output (W), which represents work performed per unit time, is calculated by multiplying instantaneous pressure and flow, with the area under the waveform for each cardiac cycle representing the total power (W_T) for the duration of that beat. These values are averaged over a series of beats. If the mean pressure and flow over the same sequence of beats are multiplied, steady-state power (W_{SS}) is derived. Since W_T represents the sum of W_{SS} and oscillatory power (W_{OS}), the W_{OS} value can be calculated by subtraction. Examining the amount of work required to move a milliliter of blood through the system per unit time and the distribution of W_T between steady-state and oscillatory components provides a convenient means to quickly assess the nature of energy transfer from the ventricle to the circulation

Perhaps the most complete approach to assessing ventricular–vascular interaction is based upon the expression of both contractility and afterload in the common term of elastance. As noted above, end-systolic ventricular elastance summarizes contractility, and vascular elastance summarizes total afterload. When the end-systolic vascular–ventricular elastance ratio is 0.5 (afterload low relative to contractility), the heart achieves maximal efficiency in terms of the amount of work performed for oxygen consumed. Alternatively, when the vascular–ventricular elastance ratio is 1.0, the heart is performing maximal stroke work. Since end-systolic elastance measurements represent pressure–volume relationships, it is possible to calculate EF as (ventricular elastance)/(vascular elastance + ventricular elastance). When this relationship is considered in the context of optimal matching for stroke work that occurs when the vascular–ventricular elastance ratio is 1.0, it is evident that optimal matching is associated with an EF of 50%.

CLINICAL ASSESSMENT OF VENTRICULAR FUNCTION

Of the multiple techniques used to evaluate cardiac function, some are exclusively diagnostic while others are applicable to continuous monitoring at the bedside. A variety of methods to characterize ventricular pump function based upon estimates of volume have been described. Chamber imaging techniques (angiography, echocardiography, magnetic resonance) are the most common. In general, accuracy of the imaging techniques is far better for the LV than the RV because of the complex geometry of the RV. Alternative techniques that avoid the problems associated with complex geometry are radionuclide time–activity relationships (e.g. wash-out curves). These methods allow not only determination of EF, but also of the indices of filling rates and ejection time, and thus have been widely used for pre- and postoperative evaluation of ventricular function.

Two main approaches to continuous perioperative evaluation of ventricular function are currently available – placement of a pulmonary arterial (PA) catheter and echocardiography. An additional technique that uses changes in thoracic bioimpedance to estimate SV and cardiac output is also available, but general experience with this method has not been favorable.

Pulmonary artery catheterization

Since the introduction of the Swan–Ganz PA catheter to clinical use in the early 1970s, this device has become the mainstay for assessment of cardiac function in critical care and intraoperative settings. The PA catheter allows direct measurement of right atrial, RV, and PA pressure, indirect measurement of left atrial pressure, and indicator dilution-based calculation of cardiac output. Recent refinements include the addition of fast-response thermistors, high-fidelity pressure transducers, fiberoptics to determine mixed venous oxygen saturation, and miniaturized electronics located on the catheter to measure PA flow. A wide variety of variables can be derived from PA catheter data to characterize facets of biventricular function.

Pulmonary artery blood flow

A central feature of PA catheterization is the measurement of cardiac output by the indicator (cold fluid) dilution technique (Chapter 14). Since PA and aortic flows are essentially matched at steady state, PA flow represents cardiac output. Since heart rate can greatly influence cardiac output, the calculation of SV is often a more valuable clinical index than that

Factors affecting myocardial contractility

	Primary effect	Secondary effect	Contractility
cardiac glycosides	inhibition of Na^+ K^+ -ATPase	increase intracellular Ca^{2+}	increase
β-adrenergic agonists, glucagon, histamine (H_2) agonists, phosphodiesterase III inhibitors	increase cAMP, protein kinase A activation	increase SR Ca^{2+} release, increase troponin C Ca^{2+} affinity	increase
α-adrenergic agonists, angiotensin II, endothelin	phospholipase C activation → increase IP_3 and DAG, protein kinase C activation	increase myofilament Ca^{2+} sensitivity, possibly increase SR Ca^{2+} release and reuptake	increase
myofilament sensitizers	increase sensitivity to Ca^{2+}	+/− inhibit phosphodiesterase III	increase
Ca^{2+} channel agonists	increase Ca^{2+} transient with depolarization	enhance SR Ca^{2+} loading	increase
thyroid hormone	mitochondrial stimulation, increase Na^+ transient, increase intracellular Ca^{2+} pool	alteration in myosin isoenzymes, increase expression of β-adrenergic receptors	increase
hypoxia	decrease ATP	impair Ca^{2+} uptake into SR, increase resting level in myoplasm	reduce; increase resting tension
acidosis	decrease intracellular Ca^{2+} transient; decrease myofilament Ca^{2+} sensitivity	increase Na^+ entry secondary to enhanced H^+/Na^+ exchange	reduce

Figure 36.9 Factors affecting myocardial contractility.

of cardiac output alone. The thermodilution method of flow measurement utilizes a modification of the Stewart–Hamilton equation, which considers specific gravity, specific heat, and temperature of both cold injectate and blood, as well as injectate volume and a correction factor for warming of the injectate along the catheter. In the denominator of the equation is the area under the curve for dilution of cold injectate back to baseline temperature. Since other variables in the equation stay relatively constant, blood flow is inversely proportional to the area under the dilution curve. Accuracy and reproducibility of the thermodilution technique is dependent upon characteristics of cold indicator injection (speed, proper volume, timing of respiratory cycle), complete and rapid mixing of the indicator in the RV, and proper calibration of the measuring system. When measurement conditions are strictly controlled, thermodilution measurements are remarkably accurate. However, variation in measurement technique, inappropriate injectate volume, and physiologic abnormalities such as tricuspid regurgitation can combine to produce significant error.

The ability to measure beat-to-beat changes in blood temperature with fast-response thermistors allows the estimation of RV EF from the difference between successive diastolic temperature plateaus. This measurement is used along with SV to calculate end-systolic volume (ESV) and EDV based upon the relationships EDV = SV/EF and ESV = EDV – SV. However, in that the technique is an indicator dilution method, clinical thermodilution measurements of RV EF are subject to error associated with catheter position, right heart dilation, and tricuspid regurgitation. Data have also been reported from beat-to-beat flow measurements obtained with a modified PA catheter for continuous assessment of RV contractile function. This device, which was once commercially available but failed in the marketplace, contains two Doppler transducers and two ultrasonic transit time transducers 12–13cm from the tip. When positioned in the root of the PA, these transducers continuously measure blood velocity, catheter angulation, and internal diameter of the vessel. The angulation-corrected diameter measurement is subsequently used to determine cross-sectional area of the PA, which is multiplied by the angulation-corrected velocity signal to yield instantaneous flow.

Preload

Although preload is more a function of volume than pressure, RV preload can be indexed with measurements of mean right atrial and RV end-diastolic pressures. Right atrial pressures should be carefully interpreted in the context of pressure wave morphology. For example, a dampened waveform may not accurately reflect RV end-diastolic pressure, and rhythm disturbances such as ectopy arising from the atrioventricular node may produce waveform distortion (cannon A-waves) and a mean right atrial pressure that is substantially higher than the true RV end-diastolic pressure. Commonly, LV preload is assessed by the measurement of pulmonary capillary wedge pressure (PCWP). Determined by measuring pressure distal to an occluding balloon in a branch of the PA, PCWP reflects left atrial pressure that has been transmitted back through the pulmonary venous, capillary, and distal arterial circulation. Thus, PCWP provides an index, but not a direct measure of, mean left atrial pressure, which is an index, but not a direct measure of, LV end-diastolic pressure, which is an index, but not a direct measure of, LV EDV. Given the indirect nature of PCWP as a monitor of preload, factors that affect the pulmonary circulation (e.g. lung injury, mechanical ventilation) can influence the utility of the absolute number. However, when measurement conditions are kept relatively consistent, changes in PCWP over time can provide useful information.

Afterload

As noted above, LV and RV afterloads are commonly expressed as SVR and PVR, respectively. While these variables are incomplete in terms of expressing total afterload, they nonetheless remain useful clinical indices when considered in the context of their limitations. The value for SVR is calculated as (mean arterial pressure – right atrial pressure)/cardiac output; PVR is calculated as (mean PA pressure – PCWP)/cardiac output. In that right atrial pressure is usually quite small relative to mean arterial pressure, abnormalities in the waveform or absolute pressure frequently have little impact upon SVR. In contrast, PCWP is usually much higher relative to mean PA pressure and can significantly influence the calculation of PVR. Additionally, PVR measurements are much more heavily influenced by flow than those for SVR, such that even in the absence of significant direct effects on the pulmonary circulation, a fall in cardiac output can produce a substantial increase in PVR. Refinements in PA catheter design now allow the characterization of RV afterload in terms of characteristic impedance and compliance calculated from internal measurements of PA diameter and flow. However, the clinical use of these devices is not widespread.

Contractility

Despite the utility of PA catheters, they provide little direct information regarding LV contractility. In contrast, because of the direct access afforded to the right heart and pulmonary circulation, techniques have been described to assess RV contractility. Two reported approaches to assess RV contractility include the use of:

- Doppler flow and PA pressure measurements to index RV power generation; and
- thermodilution-derived measurements of RV end-systolic and EDVs to calculate PRSW.

Echocardiography

Both imaging and Doppler echocardiography are useful in perioperative monitoring of ventricular function. Transesophageal echocardiography (TEE) in particular is easily used in the operating room, and with standard transverse views provides reasonably clear images of biventricular morphology, structures, and both global and regional ventricular function (Chapter 16). When carefully and skillfully performed, a TEE examination can provide much of the same information as can a PA catheter. Recent refinements such as automated border detection and 3D imaging have further increased the yield of information from TEE.

Blood flow

Multiple techniques have been described to calculate cardiac output from Doppler measurements of blood velocity and ultrasonic transit-time measurement of vessel (or valve) cross-sectional area (flow = velocity × area). Since TEE is able to quantify blood velocity in the PA, across the mitral valve, through the LV outflow tract, and within the aortic root, cardiac output determinations from each of these areas have been described. However, as a result of anatomic variation and technical problems with optimal imaging, failure rates of up to 24% have been reported from PA and mitral measurements. Perhaps the best location is the LV outflow tract, which may provide the most reliable source of adequate Doppler velocity signals and allows the application of different models to calculate aortic valve area.

Preload

The ability to observe the cross-sectional area of the LV continuously with TEE has enhanced our appreciation that preload is a manifestation of EDV, not just pressure. Indeed, TEE assessment of LV dimensions under variant intraoperative conditions has clearly demonstrated that changes in end-diastolic dimension are not necessarily closely linked to alterations in PCWP. This observation underscores the importance of considering LV compliance in the assessment of diastolic function. In addition to direct imaging of the LV chamber, Doppler assessment of systolic pulmonary venous flow (both systolic and diastolic components) into the left atrium and visual inspection of interatrial septal motion can provide information about LV filling pressures, which may be particularly valuable when interpretation of direct LV dimension data is complicated by significant regional wall motion abnormalities. In general, when the systolic component of pulmonary venous flow is <55%, or the interatrial septum does not exhibit paradoxic motion during the initial phase of exhalation following a positive pressure breath, left atrial pressure is at least 15mmHg (2kPa).

Also, TEE allows the evaluation of diastolic filling characteristics based primarily upon transmitral flow patterns. Under normal circumstances, the majority of LV filling occurs during the early, rapid filling phase of diastole with the remaining fraction provided by atrial systole. Accordingly, transmitral flow patterns exhibit two velocity peaks, reflecting these filling intervals, designated as the 'E' (early) and 'A' (atrial systole) waves. The ratio of these two waves provides a convenient means to evaluate LV filling dynamics; in the normal, compliant LV the E/A ratio is well over 1. In contrast, when compliance is reduced, atrial systole becomes much more important for filling and the ratio is less than 1.

Afterload

As noted above, vascular resistance is an incomplete index of afterload because it assumes the ventrical is a steady-state pressure/flow generator. Since TEE allows the derivation of end-systolic wall stress from ventricular dimension, thickness, and pressure it potentially provides a more complete index of afterload.

Contractility

While continuous visual images of the contracting heart give the observer a general feel of contractility, real-time quantification with TEE is not reliable. Multiple techniques for off-line assessment have been described, including the relationship between end-systolic wall stress and dimension or rate-corrected fiber shortening. Unfortunately, these indices are load-sensitive. Application of pressure–dimension or pressure–volume analysis techniques to echocardiographic images has been enhanced by the introduction of automated border detection software that allows the generation of a continuous LV dimension (and by calculation, volume) waveform. With these data, pressure–volume loops somewhat similar to those generated by more invasive techniques have been generated and used to index contractility in a load-independent manner. To obviate the need for LV pressure, some investigators described the use of a peripheral arterial pressure and TEE-derived volume to construct loops that resemble the systolic portion of a true LV pressure–volume loop. While these techniques have been shown to predict trends in contractility correctly, the use of absolute values for subject-to-subject comparison is potentially problematic.

Ventricular–vascular interaction

Since EF reflects the forces of both contractility and afterload, it provides a quantifiable means to assess the mechanical interaction between the heart and circulation. The reported accuracy of EF predicted by TEE has ranged from excellent to fair, but probably is not as good as that determined by transthoracic echo, because of limited imaging of the LV apex. More refined imaging techniques now provide better apical views and may enhance TEE accuracy. An alternative TEE technique, LV fractional area change, measured at the midpapillary level in the short-axis (cross-sectional) view, is a reasonable approximation of EF and is now widely used. Another technique measures the distance between the point of mitral leaflet coaptation and the interventricular septum at end-systole. While somewhat complex, this method provides data (expressed in millimeters) that have a high predictive value for LV dysfunction.

Key References

Kass DA, Kelly RP. Ventriculo-arterial coupling: concepts, assumptions, and applications. Ann Biomed Eng. 1992;20:41–62.

Sagawa K, Maughan L, Suga H, Sunagawa K. Cardiac contraction and the pressure volume relationship. New York: Oxford University Press; 1988:110–52.

Tuman KJ, Carroll GC, Ivankovich AD. Pitfalls in interpretation of pulmonary artery catheter data. J Cardiothorac Vasc Anesth. 1989;3:625–41.

Further Reading

Benson MJA, Cahalan MK, Seeberger MD, Sutton DC, Rouine-Rapp K. The echocardiographic assessment of left ventricular function. In: Warltier DC, ed. Ventricular function. Baltimore: Williams and Wilkins; 1995:253–77.

Damiano RJ, La Follette P, Cox JL, et al. Significant left ventricular contribution to right ventricular systolic function. Am J Physiol. 1991;261:H1514–24.

Heerdt PM Dickstein ML. Assessment of right ventricular function. Sem Cardiothorac Vasc Anesth. 1997;1:215–24.

Heerdt PM, Pond CG, Blessios GA, Rosenbloom M. Comparison of cardiac output measured by intrapulmonary artery Doppler, thermodilution, and electromagnetometry. Ann Thorac Surg. 1992;54:959–66.

Kadota LT. Theory and application of thermodilution cardiac output measurement: A review. Heart Lung. 1985;14:605–11.

Lang RM, Borow KM, Neumann A, Janzen D. Systemic vascular resistance: an unreliable index of left ventricular afterload. Circulation. 1986;74:1114–23.

O'Rourke MF. Steady and pulsatile power energy losses in the systemic circulation under normal conditions and in simulated arterial disease. Cardiovasc Res. 1967;1:313–26.

Perrino AC, Harris SN, Luther MA. Intraoperative determination of cardiac output using multiplane transesophageal echocardiography. Anesthesiology. 1998;89:350–7.

Spiess BD, McCarthy RJ, Tuman KJ, Ivankovick AD. Bioimpedance hemodynamics compared to pulmonary artery catheter monitoring during orthotopic liver transplantation. J Surg Res. 1993;54:52–6.

Chapter 37 Integrative view of cardiovascular function

Richard Teplick

Topics covered in this chapter

Flow through a tube
Venous return
Mean systemic and mean pulmonic pressures
Venous coupling with the ventricles
Mechanical properties of the ventricles
The starling curve
Integrating the cardiovascular system
Summary

Basic physiologic principles provide a systematic method by which hemodynamic data and the integration of the cardiovascular system can be understood.

FLOW THROUGH A TUBE

Flow through a rigid tube is governed by the pressure difference across the tube and the resistance.

■ **Equation 37.1**

$$Q = (P_u - P_d)/R$$

where Q is flow, and P_u and P_d are upstream and downstream pressures, respectively. For laminar flow, resistance is inversely proportional to the fourth power of the tube radius (r^4). If a sample of blood is forced in one end of the rigid tube, an equal volume must exit the other end because blood is nearly incompressible. An abrupt increase in P_u results in an almost instantaneous increase in flow out of the tube. By comparison, flow from the downstream end of a tube that can distend, does not immediately increase as the tube is distended by a portion of the fluid entering it. It's ability to distend is characterized by its compliance (C). Compliance is defined as the change in volume (V) for a given pressure change ($C = \Delta V/\Delta P$, or more accurately $C = dV/dP$). The increase in volume of the tube also raises the pressure exerted by its walls by an amount equal to $\Delta V/C$. Eventually, the diameter of the tube increases such that the pressure exerted by its walls equals that exerted by the fluid within. Subsequently, the flow of fluid out of the tube equals that entering it.

For most physiologic purposes, flow through a compliant tube can be simplified by modeling it as a cylindrical reservoir with a rigid tube affixed to its base (Fig. 37.1). If flow into the reservoir is increased, the height of the fluid gradually rises. The rate of rise is governed by the resistance of the rigid tube and the area of the reservoir. The higher the resistance or the smaller the area, the more rapid the rise. The compliance of a distensible tube is approximated by the area of the reservoir. The rise in P_u with an increase in flow into the reservoir increases flow through the affixed tube. The height of fluid in the reservoir continues to increase until flow out of the tube equals flow into the reservoir. The time required to reach this new equilibrium depends upon the time constant of the system, which is proportional to the product of the reservoir area, the force of gravity, and the pipe resistance. It takes approximately five time constants before flow through the pipe equals the new flow rate into the reservoir. The time constant can be quite large if the pipe has a high resistance or if the reservoir represents a large compliance (i.e. has a large area). Intuitively, this occurs because if the resistance is high the increase in flow will be small for a given increase in P_u. Conversely, if the reservoir has a large area, the rate at which pressure (height) rises is small for a given increase in flow into the reservoir. In either case it will take longer for the outflow to increase to equal the inflow. A more complete model can be derived by regarding the circulation as many small reservoir-pipes in series, but the single reservoir-pipe model is adequate to explain the basic properties of the circulation.

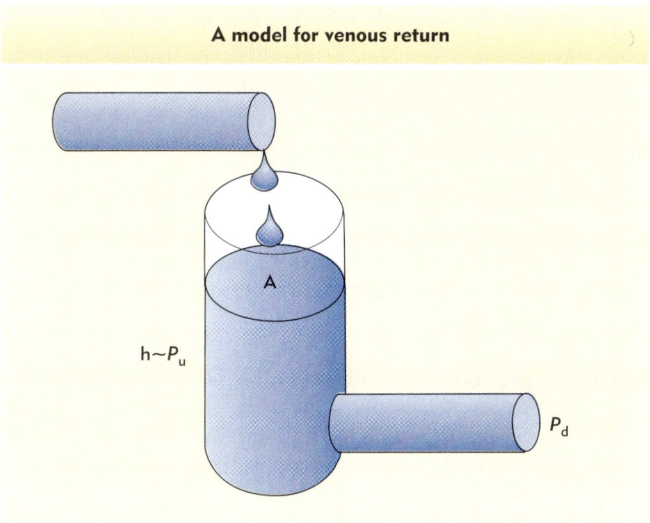

Figure 37.1 A model for venous return. Flow through a distensible tube can be approximated by a reservoir affixed to the end of a rigid pipe with fluid flowing freely into the reservoir. The upstream pressure (P_u) is determined by the height of the fluid in the reservoir (h) multiplied by the fluid density.

VENOUS RETURN

Implicit in the calculation of systemic vascular resistance is the premise that the circulation is modeled as a single vessel that includes both the arterial and venous system. For this model, cardiac output is determined by the difference between the mean arterial (P_a) and right atrial (P_{ra}) pressures divided by the systemic vascular resistance (R). To understand the factors that determine venous return (Q_v), Guyton and colleagues recognized the advantages of dividing this single vessel circulation into two distinct (arterial and venous) vascular beds (Fig. 37.2). The pressure difference driving blood through the arterial portion of the circulation is the difference between P_a and a hypothetical pressure at the end of the arterial bed termed the mean systemic pressure (P_{ms}). P_{ms} should not be confused with mean arterial pressure. Therefore, cardiac output through the arterial bed (Q) is given by Equation 37.2.

■ Equation 37.2

$$Q = (P_a - P_{ms})/R_a$$

where R_a is the resistance of the arterial vessels. Because the flows through the arterial and venous beds are usually the same, cardiac output is also given by Equation 37.3.

■ Equation 37.3

$$Q = (P_{ms} - P_{ra})/R_v$$

where R_v is the resistance of the venous bed. Therefore, $P_{ms} - P_{ra}$ is the driving pressure for Q_v. If P_{ms} and R_v remain constant, a decrease in P_{ra} will increase Q_v by increasing the driving pressure across the venous bed.

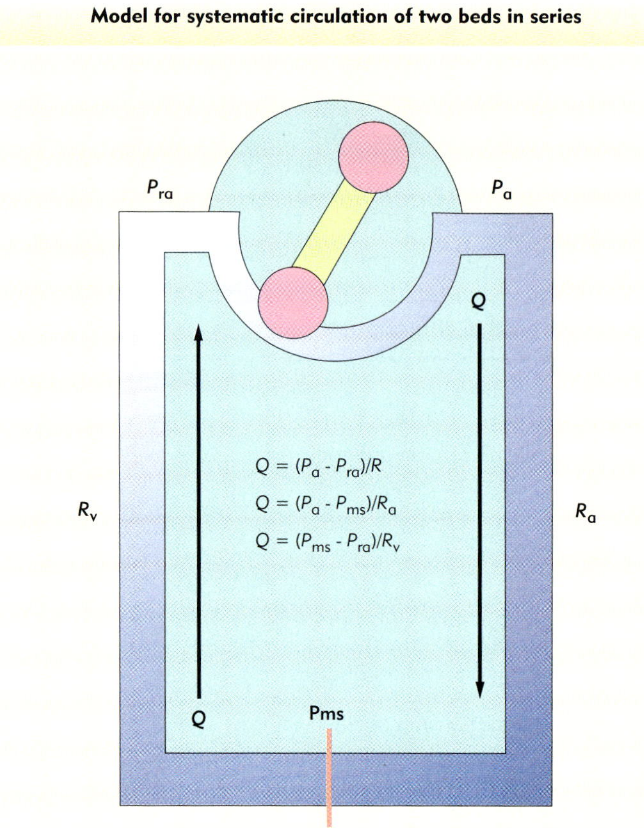

Figure 37.2 Model of the systemic circulation divided into two vascular beds in series, arterial and venous. Flow through the arterial bed [$(P_a - P_{ms})/R_a$] must equal flow through the venous bed [$(P_{ms} - P_{ra})/R_v$].

MEAN SYSTEMIC AND MEAN PULMONIC PRESSURES

Guyton and colleagues used a right-heart bypass preparation to determine R_v and P_{ms} in dogs. Blood from the venae cavae was diverted from the right atrium (RA) into a reservoir and outflow from the reservoir was pumped into a cannula inserted into the main pulmonary artery (PA), thus bypassing the RA and right ventricle (RV). The height of the blood in the reservoir relative to the heart determined P_{ra} and pump flow replaced RV output. It is interesting to note that when pump flow was increased, the left ventricle (LV) output had to increase to match the output of the pump. This occured because of increased LV end-diastolic volume (EDV), which causes LV end-diastolic pressure (EDP) and, thus, the PA pressure to rise. Under these conditions, the only way that the LV can affect cardiac output is by increasing its EDP, causing a passive increase in PA pressure to the point where the pump can no longer maintain its output. This would decrease the output of the pump by what might be termed its *afterload*.

Using this experimental preparation, the transient effects on Q_v resulting from changes in P_{ra} caused by adjusting the reservoir height can be measured. For example, elevating the reservoir increases P_{ra} thereby causing a transient decrease in Q_v because $P_{ms} - P_{ra}$ decreases (assuming that P_{ms} does not change). Because pump flow would remain constant while Q_v decreased, blood would be translocated from the reservoir into the systemic blood vessels. After about five time constants (approximately 10 minutes), Q_v would reach a new equilibrium that would depend on the area of the reservoir, the amount of blood it initially contained, and its height. If the initial change in Q_v is determined for different reservoir heights, the relation between Q_v and reservoir height (i.e. P_{ra}) should be linear (Fig. 37.3), assuming P_{ms} and R_v are constant. As shown by rewriting Equation 37.3, Q_v can be calculated as follows.

■ Equation 37.4

$$Q_v = \frac{P_{ra}}{R_v} + \frac{P_{ms}}{R_v}$$

This equation describes a straight line with a slope of ($-1/R_v$). This line is termed the venous return line. Below approximately 1.5mmHg, Q_v is independent of P_{ra} because P_{ra} is less than intrathoracic pressure, creating a waterfall so that the downstream pressure for Q_v is essentially intrathoracic pressure, not P_{ra}. By determining Q_v for a wide range of values for P_{ra} and finding the straight line that relates these two parameters, venous resistance and P_{ms} may be determined. The value of P_{ra} at which Q_v is zero is P_{ms} (i.e. $P_{ms} = P_{ra}$ when $Q_v = 0$). These same principles apply to the pulmonary circulation and the LV and left atrium (LA), except the relevant pressures are mean pulmonic and LA pressure.

Although this experiment allows P_{ms} and R_v to be determined, it provides no insight into the mechanical factors that determine P_{ms}. Since $P_{ra} = P_{ms}$ when $Q_v = 0$, P_{ms} could be determined by

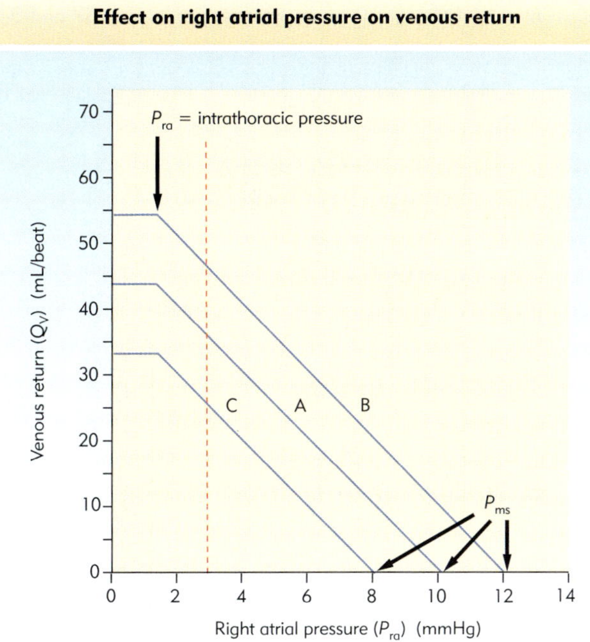

Figure 37.3 Relationship between venous return (Q_v) and right atrial pressure (P_{ra}). The slope of curve A ($-1/R_v$, from Equation 37.4) is –5.3mL/mmHg per beat. If the heart rate were 100 beats/min and venous return is expressed in L/min, then R_v is 1.9mmHg/L per min. If volume were infused or the venous compliance decreased, P_{ms} increases, shifting the curve to the right (B). Conversly, volume loss or increase in venous compliance decrease P_{ms} (C). If P_{ra} is kept constant at 3mmHg (vertical dashed line) and at a heart rate of 100beats/min, venous return at P_{ms} values of 8 (C), 10 (A), and 12mmHg (B) would be 2.6, 3.7, and 4.7L/min, respectively (26, 37, and 47mL/beat, respectively).

causing all blood flow to stop (e.g. fibrillating both ventricles and clamping the aortic and pulmonary arterial roots to isolate the respective circulations). Pressure does not drop to zero because blood within the pulmonary and systemic circulations distends the vessels, which exert a counterbalancing force because of their compliance. The pressure at zero flow depends upon both the volume of blood and the vascular compliance in the respective circulatory beds. Although the pressures at zero flow must be equal everywhere within each circulatory bed (neglecting the effects of venous valves), the zero-flow pressure in the pulmonary and systemic beds need not be equal because they are isolated from each other. The zero-flow pressure within the systemic bed is P_{ms}, and the zero-flow pressure within the pulmonary bed is P_{mp}. Thus, the blood volume and vascular compliance in each circulation determine the upstream venous pressure for that circulatory bed. Intuitively, changes in venous blood volume should affect venous resistance because a change in diameter of the veins should alter their resistance. Experimentally this does not seem to occur, presumably because most of the volume change occurs in relatively large vessels, which contribute little to resistance.

The concept of P_{ms} can be further simplified because the systemic arterial compliance is approximately 5% that of the veins and at least 75% of the blood volume resides in the veins. Consequently, P_{ms} is predominately determined by the volume of blood in the veins and their compliance. When a patient receives a volume infusion, initially most of the fluid resides in the systemic venous bed. This results in an increase in P_{ms} that causes a parallel shift to the right of the venous return line (see Fig. 37.3). Consequently, if P_{ra} remained the same, Q_v would increase. However, as discussed below, P_{ra} also increases by an amount that depends on RV contractility, PA pressure, and RV and RA compliances. The relative increases in P_{ms} and P_{ra} determine the overall change in Q_v that ultimately results from changes in systemic volume.

VENOUS COUPLING WITH THE VENTRICLES

Changes in volume status

The coupling of Q_v with the ventricles can be visualized using Starling curves. These curves take many forms, for example mean atrial or ventricular EDP versus stroke work, cardiac output, or stroke volume (SV); however, the relation between EDP and SV lends itself well to characterization of ventricular–venous coupling. Starling curves shift upward or downward with changes in contractility, arterial pressure, and compliance (Fig. 37.4) and tend to become flat as atrial pressure increases, which reflects the steepness of the compliance curve at high EDP.

In a steady state, SV must equal Q_v/beat. This corresponds to the intersection of the plot of Q_v with the Starling curve. The effects of changing P_{ms} are shown in Figure 37.5a for the systemic veins and the RV. At point A, curve 1 for Q_v, corresponding to a P_{ms} of 12mmHg, intersects the Starling curve at a SV of 48mL/beat. As a result of an abrupt decrease in P_{ms} from 12 to 8mmHg (e.g. caused by acute bleeding), the line for Q_v shifts downward and to the left (curve 2), and a new equilibrium point is reached at point C. In the first instant following the decrease in P_{ms}, P_{ra} would not change. Consequently, Q_v would decrease along the rightmost vertical dashed line in Figure 37.5a from point A to A′, which would cause Q_v to decrease from 48 to 27mL/beat. Because the RV would still be ejecting 48mL/beat, RV volume would begin to decrease. The associated decrease in RV EDP would cause RV SV to move leftward on the Starling curve toward point B. The decrease in RV EDP would also decrease P_{ra}, causing Q_v to increase toward point B′. However, RV SV would still exceed Q_v (in Fig. 37.5a being approximately 41 and 32mL/beat, respectively). Therefore, RV would continue to eject more than it received from the systemic veins and its EDV would continue to fall, resulting in a continuous decrease in RV EDP along the Starling curve. The resultant fall in P_{ra} would cause Q_v to continue to increase along curve 2. This process would continue until RV, SV and Q_v equalize (point C, 35mL/beat), the end result being a decrease in both P_{ra} and SV.

A volume infusion produces a rise in SV by the same mechanisms that occur in acute hypovolemia, which decreases it (Fig. 37.5b). If enough volume were infused to raise P_{ms} from 4 to 9mmHg (Fig 37.5b, line 2), SV would increase from 27 to 54mL/beat. If additional volume were infused, increasing P_{ms} by the same increment to 14mmHg (line 1), the SV increases by only 10mL/beat to 64mL/beat. The larger rise in SV that occurs if the patient is hypovolemic is a consequence of the steepness of the Starling curve at lower P_{ra}.

Because identical changes in P_{ms} can result both from changes in venous compliance and blood volume, it seems reasonable to refer to the functional volume status of a patient rather than trying to separate compliance from actual blood

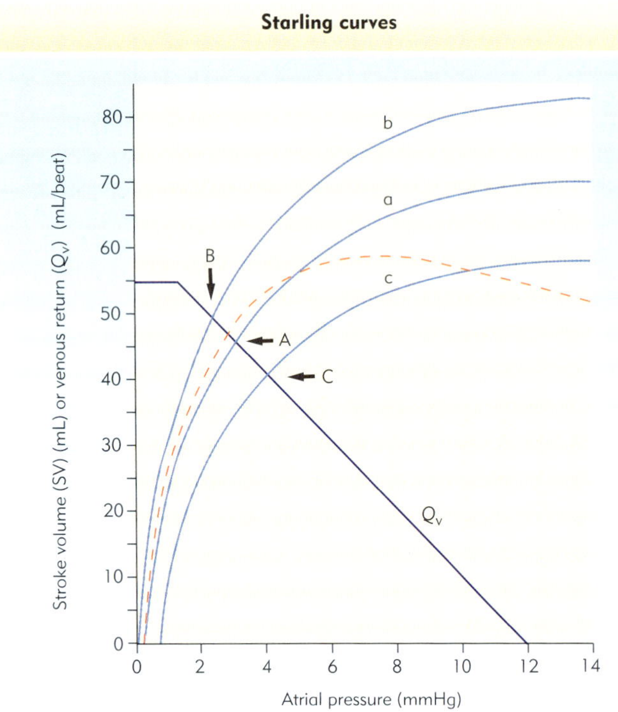

Figure 37.4 A family of Starling curves relating stroke volume (SV) to atrial pressure. An increase in arterial pressure or decrease in contractility shifts the curve downward abd to the right (curves a–c). A decrease in ventricular compliance will have the same effect but it will also alter the shape of the curve. The dashed curve shows a decrease in SV as atrial pressure increases above 8mmHg. This descending limb does not actually exist but may appear to occur if an increase in atrial pressure shifts the Starling curve downward, for example by causing ischemia or atrioventricular valvular regurgitation. The equilibrium SV is determined by the points of intersection of a venous return line with the Starling curves (A, B, and C). As expected, increasing pressure, decreasing contractility, or decreasing compliance all cause a decrease in SV and an increase in atrial pressure.

volume. For example, assuming normal values for P_{ra} and P_{ms} (5 and 12mmHg, respectively), the pressure gradient causing Q_v is 7mmHg. A patient with a P_{ra} of 15mmHg and a SV of 70mL (assuming normal SV of 60mL) would be functionally hypervolemic because to have a supranormal Q_v with a P_{ra} of 15mmHg, P_{ms} would still have to be 7mmHg greater (22mmHg) than P_{ra}. The requisite increase in P_{ms} to 22mmHg could only be achieved by hypervolemia or by a decrease in venous compliance, which could only be inferred from knowledge of the disease state and previous therapy, not by measurement. Consequently, it seems reasonable to refer to such a patient as functionally hypervolemic and to a patient's functional volume status as being determined by actual blood volume and venous compliance. This implies that measurement of absolute blood volume might be less useful than expected because a patient could still be 'functionally' euvolemic owing to changes in venous compliance despite abnormal absolute blood volume.

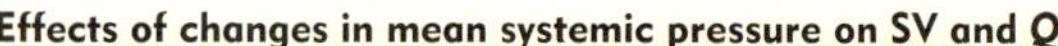

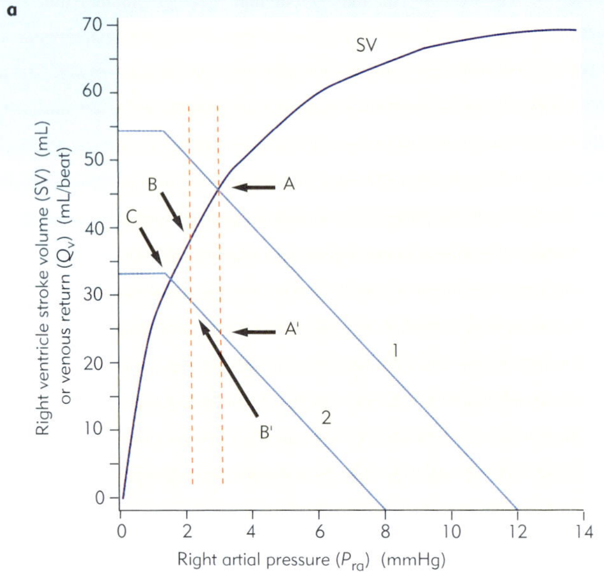

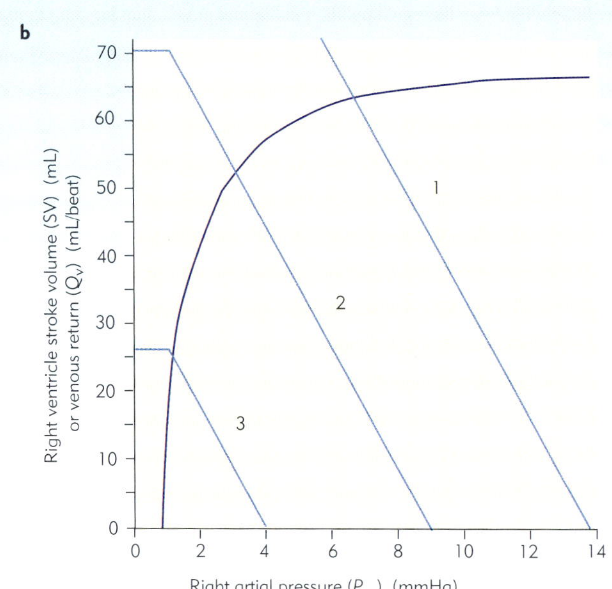

Figure 37.5 Effects of changes in mean systemic pressure on stroke volume (SV) and venous return. (a) Changes in the equilibrium point between venous return and right ventricular SV following an abrupt decrease in mean systemic pressure (P_{ms}), from 12–18mmHg. The end result is move from point A to a new equilibrium point at C (see text). (b) Changes in SV with volume status. Volume infusion increases SV and acute hypovolemia (curve 3) decreases it. Volume infusions at normovolemia are less effective in increasing SV (2 to 1) than at hypovolemia (3 to 2) because the Starling curve is relatively flat above the normal operating point.

Changes in the Starling curve

Changes in the Starling curve affect EDP and SV. In contrast to acute hypovolemia, a downward shift in the Starling curve leads to an increase in P_{ra} despite the decrease in SV. This can be explained through the steps outlined in Figure 37.6. At the initial equilibrium (point A), SV and Q_v equal 48mL/beat. In the instant following the shift in the Starling curve from curve a to b, SV falls to 33mL/beat (point A′) because of the decrease in ejection fraction. However, atrial pressure, and therefore Q_v, do not change, which causes ventricular volume to begin to increase. The resultant increase in EDP causes Q_v to decrease along line 1 from point A toward point B. Because Q_v would still exceed SV, EDV and, thus, EDP increase toward point B′, resulting in an increase in SV. However, Q_v still exceeds SV (approximately 43 and 37mL, respectively). Therefore, the ventricle would continue to eject less than it received from the Q_v. This process continues until the SV equals Q_v (point C, SV 37mL/beat). The end result would be a decrease in SV and an increase in P_{ra}.

The Starling curve does not provide a unique measure of intrinsic ventricular function because arterial pressures and ventricular compliance also affect its appearance. Therefore, before developing an integrated model of the circulation by coupling both ventricles and the arterial circulation, a more basic approach to cardiac mechanics will be discussed.

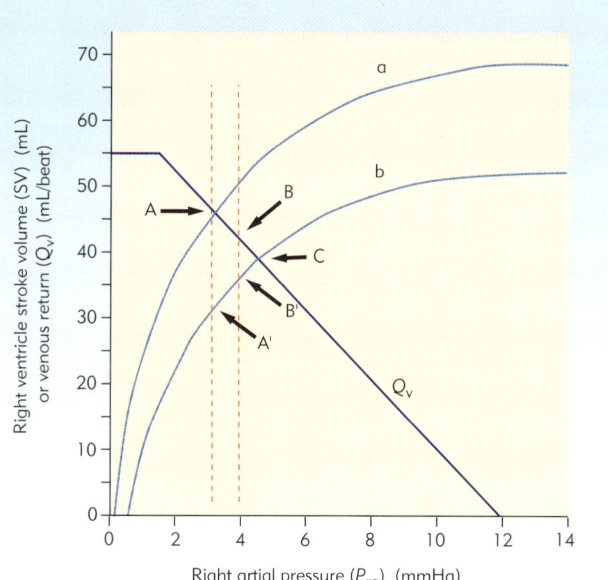

Figure 37.6 The effect of a downward shift in the Starling curve on the equilibrium point between venous return (Q_v) and right ventricular (RV) stroke volume (SV). An abrupt downward shift in the Starling curve (a to b) might occur with global ischemia or hypertension. A downward shift in the Starling curve (from the initial equilibrium point, A) leads to a fall in ejection from the RV until SV equals Q_v (point C). The end result would be a decrease in SV and an increase in right atrial pressure (see text).

MECHANICAL PROPERTIES OF THE VENTRICLES

Stroke volume versus cardiac output

In describing cardiac function, cardiac output is usually the central focus. However, this can be misleading. Consider a patient about to undergo major vascular surgery who has a history of episodic pulmonary edema and mild, stable angina. An exercise history cannot be elicited because of claudication. A PA catheter is placed before induction of anesthesia; the data obtained are shown in Figure 37.7. Although the pressures appear relatively normal, the cardiac output of 3.5L/min seems quite low. However, as the heart rate is only 50 beats/min, the SV is 70mL (3500/50), which is normal. Although SV does tend to decrease somewhat with age, indexing for body surface area or weight does not decrease individual variation. Normal values for younger individuals are 60–70mL/beat, falling to 60mL/beat or less for elderly patients.

Following induction of anesthesia and tracheal intubation, the patient's central pressures rise substantially and new ST segment depression is noted in the lateral precordial lead. Are the elevations in central pressures secondary to ischemic dysfunction? The cardiac output has increased from 3.5 to 5.6L/min accompanied by an increase in heart rate from 50 to 70 beats/min. Therefore, the SV has increased from 70 to 80mL. Using the arguments developed above, it is evident that the increase in central pressures could not have occurred solely because of LV dysfunction. Were this the case, without an increase in P_{ms} and P_{mp} the elevated atrial pressures would have caused a decrease in Q_v and, thus, SV. Consequently, regardless of the effects ischemia might have had on the ventricles, it could not account for an increase in SV without a concomitant increase in P_{ms} and P_{mp}. Viewed somewhat differently, acute LV dysfunction would shift the LV Starling curve downward, causing an increase in P_{LA} and a decrease in SV (see Fig. 37.6). This would cause a passive increase in PA pressures, which would impair RV ejection. The resultant downward shift in the RV Starling curve would increase P_{ra} and decrease systemic Q_v. The net effect would be an increase in central pressures and a decrease in SV.

From these considerations, the data in Figure 37.7 are not consistent with primary ventricular dysfunction but, in fact, are more consistent with acute hypervolemia. Increased myocardial oxygen consumption and decreased perfusion secondary to the increases in ventricular volumes and filling pressures could have caused the ischemia. It is possible that if the ischemia were not present, the SV would have increased above 80mL, but this cannot be determined from these data. Because the patient did not receive a rapid volume infusion, it seems likely that he had an acute decrease in the compliance of the systemic venous bed. This, in effect, would reduce the volume of the container for blood in the systemic circulation (e.g. the veins), resulting in functional hypervolemia (i.e. an increase in P_{ms}). Consequently, the changes in pressures observed likely resulted from inadequate anesthesia leading to sympathetic nervous activation and causing, among other things, a decrease in the compliance of the venous bed and functional hypervolemia. This interpretation suggests that therapy should be directed toward deepening anesthesia and thereby blunting the sympathetic response rather than toward treating the ischemia.

In contrast, consider the same data shown in Figure 37.7 but with a heart rate of 100 beats/min following intubation. In this case, the SV would have decreased from 70 to 56mL. These data, using the arguments presented above, are consistent with ischemic dysfunction. An important point is that if central pressures are acutely increased from ventricular dysfunction, the SV (but not necessarily the cardiac output) must decrease. This example illustrates that the interpretation of data obtained from a PA catheter is critically dependent upon the heart rate as this is the only number that differs in the two

Hemodynamic data for patients about to undergo major vascular surgery

Hemodynamic data for a patient with a history of episodic pulmonary edema and angina

Pressures (mmHg)	Initial	Following intubation
Systemic	120/70 (90)	150/90 (115)
Pulmonary artery	28/12 (17)	40/25 (32)
Pulmonary capillary wedge	12	22
Central venous	6	15
Cardiac output (L/min)	3.5	5.6
Heart rate (beats/min)	50	70

Initial hemodynamic data for a patient about to undergo infrarenal aortic cross-clamping

Pressures (mmHg)	Initial
Systemic	130/70 (100)
Pulmonary artery	25/12 (16)
Pulmonary capillary wedge	12
Central venous	4
Cardiac output (L/min)	4.8
Heart rate (beats/min)	80

Initial hemodynamic data for a patient with biventricular dysfunction

Pressures (mmHg)	Initial
Systemic	90/60 (70)
Pulmonary artery	50/30 (37)
Pulmonary capillary wedge	30
Central venous	12
Cardiac output (L/min)	3.0
Heart rate (beats/min)	100

Figure 37.7 Hemodynamic data for patients about to undergo major vascular surgery. Numbers in parentheses are mean pressures.

different conditions just discussed. There are two other important points illustrated by this example. First, an increase in cardiac output does not necessarily indicate an improvement in ventricular function. Second, changes in filling pressures cannot be interpreted without measuring the associated changes in cardiac output and calculating SV.

Determinants of stroke volume

The terms preload, afterload, and contractility are often used in describing ventricular performance. Preload and afterload have precise definitions in papillary muscle experiments. However, because the geometry and dynamics of a functioning ventricle differ so radically from those of a papillary muscle, these terms are not directly applicable to an intact ventricle. Although a definition analogous to preload is possible in an intact ventricle, functionally it is more useful to define ventricular preload as the EDV. Because the force generated by a ventricle changes constantly during ejection, the term afterload, which is the constant force during shortening in papillary muscle experiments, cannot be applied directly to ejecting ventricles. Rather than struggling to find an analogous definition, it seems more important to define the factors that have a major influence upon SV. Because SV is, by definition, the difference between the EDV and the end-systolic volume (ESV), the problem becomes delineating the determinants of these two volumes.

End-diastolic volume

Although the pressure–volume relationship at end diasole (EDPVR), which relates EDV to EDP under different conditions, is usually referred to as the compliance curve, it is actually an elastance curve that is defined as the change in pressure per unit change in volume (dP/dV). Therefore, end-diastolic elastance is the slope of the EDPVR at any point. In contrast, compliance is the change in volume with pressure (dV/dP). The EDPVR is relatively flat over the normal operating range of ventricles (100–150mL) so that changes in EDV cause relatively small changes in EDP. However, as the EDV increases above normal, the EDPVR becomes steep and a small rise in EDV causes a large increase in EDP (Fig. 37.8a). If the shape of the EDPVR were known, the EDV could be determined from the EDP. However, the shape of the EDPVR is not precisely known even in normal individuals, let alone for patients with heart disease. Consequently, accurate determination of the EDV from the EDP is not generally possible. Therefore, although the EDV increases with a rise in EDP, the magnitude of this increase is unpredictable. For this reason, the effects of changes in EDP on SV are more useful than the exact value of the EDP.

End-systolic volume

The isovolumic peak pressure–volume relation

If the outflow of the LV or RV were occluded to prevent ejection, it would develop the maximum peak pressure possible for that EDV and contractile state. This type of beat is termed isovolumic because there is no volume change during systole (i.e. EDV = ESV). These beats may be characterized by plotting ventricular pressure against volume (Fig. 37.8b). When beats at different EDV are plotted in this way, keeping contractile state constant, the relation between peak pressure and volume is nearly linear and is termed the end-systolic pressure–volume relation (ESPVR). For a given ESPVR, the peak pressure of an isovolumic beat could be determined from the EDV and vice versa. This is analogous to the relation between pressure and volume at end-diastole except that the EDPVR is highly nonlinear. The ESPVR intersects the volume axis at V_0, which is the volume at which the ventricle does not develop any pressure. If the contractile state increases (e.g. by an inotrope), peak isovolumic pressure at any volume also increases. However, the increase would be proportionally greater at larger volumes, causing a counterclockwise rotation of the ESPVR around V_0. Therefore, for isovolumic beats, the slope of the ESPVR becomes steeper with an increase in contractility, and flatter with a decrease in contractility and its slope provides a volume-independent measure of contractility for isovolumic beats.

The end-systolic pressure–volume relation for ejection

The ESPVR model can be extended to describe end-systole for ejecting beats, providing a load-independent definition of contractility that relates ESV and end-systolic pressure (ESP) in a simple manner. The period of systole preceding ejection is isovolumic because both valves are closed, and it appears on a pressure–volume diagram as a vertical line positioned at the EDV (Fig. 37.9a). When the pressure within the ventricle exceeds that in the aorta or PA, the aortic or pulmonic valve opens and ejection begins. The onset of ejection is marked by an abrupt change

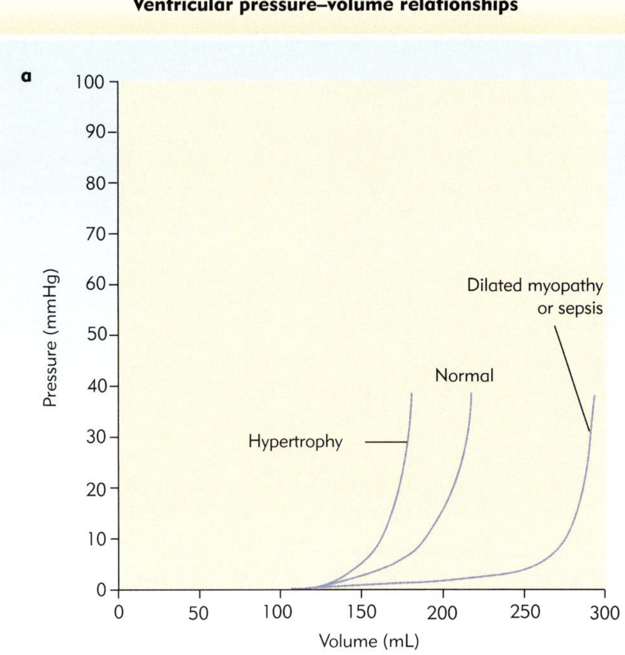

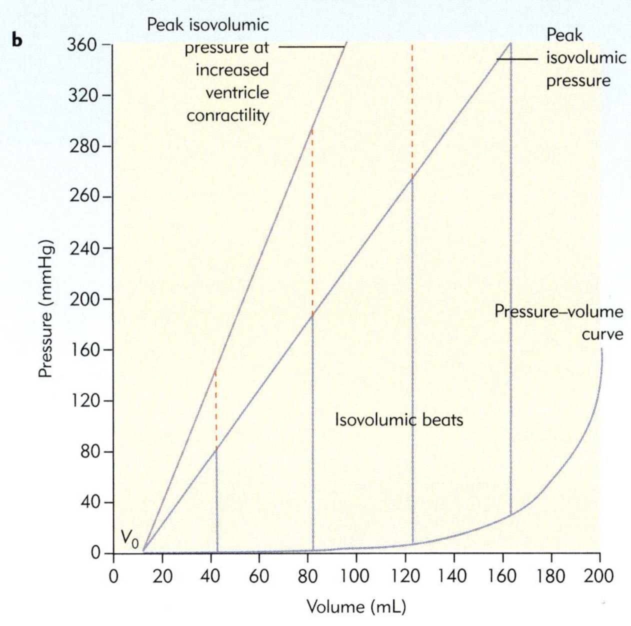

Figure 37.8 Ventricular pressure–volume relationships. (a) End-diastolic pressure–volume relationship (EDPVR) varies among individuals and disease processes. (b) End-systolic pressure–volume relationship (ESPVR) determined from isovolumic contractions. The solid vertical lines represent isovolumic beats at different end-diastolic volumes. An increase in the contractile state of the ventricle causes the peak pressure of each isovolumic contraction to increase in direct proportion to its volume, $-V_0$, which is reflected in the increased height of each vertical line (dotted portions). The relations between peak pressures and volumes at any contractile state are nearly linear.

from a vertical line to a curve with decreasing volume and increasing pressure. The rise in pressure depends upon complex interactions between the arterial tree and ventricle. If ejection were interrupted by clamping the aorta or PA, the respective ventricle would continue to develop pressure until the pressure equaled the maximum possible for an isovolumic beat at the clamped volume (dashed line 1 in Fig 37.9a). That is, the pressure would rise until it touched the ESPVR. This maximum decreases later in ejection because of the decreasing volume (dashed line 2). At end-ejection, the pressure falls on the ESPVR. That is, the ESP is determined by the volume at this point (ESV) and the contractile state of the ventricle defined as the slope of the ESPVR. The aortic or pulmonic valve then closes and isovolumic relaxation begins. When ventricular pressure decreases below atrial pressure, the mitral or tricuspid valve opens and the ventricle again fills until atrial ejection ends returning the ventricle to its EDV, and the cycle repeats itself.

If ejections are repeated with different vascular properties (Fig. 37.9b) or starting from different EDV (Fig. 37.9c), the end of ejection still always falls approximately on the ESPVR. This property allows SV to be described by two pressures and two elastances. Specifically, EDV is determined by EDP and EDPVR, and ESV by ESP and ESPVR (Fig. 37.9d). That is, end-diastolic and end-systolic elastances define the relationships between pressures and volumes at end-diastole and end-systole, respectively. Consequently, if these elastances are known, the pressures at end-diastole and end-systole will determine the respective volumes.

The time-varying elastance model

During an ejection, the pressure at any instant falls on the same line (Fig. 37.10). The slope of this time-varying elastance line increases with time during a beat until end-systole is reached. That is, it becomes progressively steeper until it reaches a maximum value, which corresponds to the time at which ESP is developed. The same time-varying elastance lines define the instantaneous relation between pressure and volume for both isovolumic beats and ejections if contractility is constant. For this reason, this description is called the time-varying elastance model of cardiac contraction. Unfortunately, relaxation cannot be defined accurately using a time-varying elastance model. This model has important implications in predicting myocardial oxygen consumption.

Limitations of end-systolic parameters

Although the ESPVR provides a very useful approach to understanding ventricular performance, it has limitations. First, end-ejection does not always occur precisely at the ESPVR, especially for large or rapid LV ejections or in the RV. As SV increases with increasing EDV, ESP begins to fall below that predicted by the ESPVR (shortening deactivation). This has been attributed to an internal resistance in the contracting ventricle. Second, the ESPVR appears to be nonlinear, especially if measured over a wide range of EDV and at different contractile states. As contractility increases, the ESPVR tends to become convex away from the volume axis. Conversely, the ESPVR for depressed ventricular activity tends to be concave away from the volume axis. Third, elastance at end-systole is not always the same as maximum elastance, probably because of resistive and inertial forces affecting end-ejection. The slope of the maximum elastance may be steeper than that for the end-systolic elastance. While maximum elastance is conceptually more appealing and more useful for modeling of cardiac mechanics, end-systole elastance is clinically a more useful

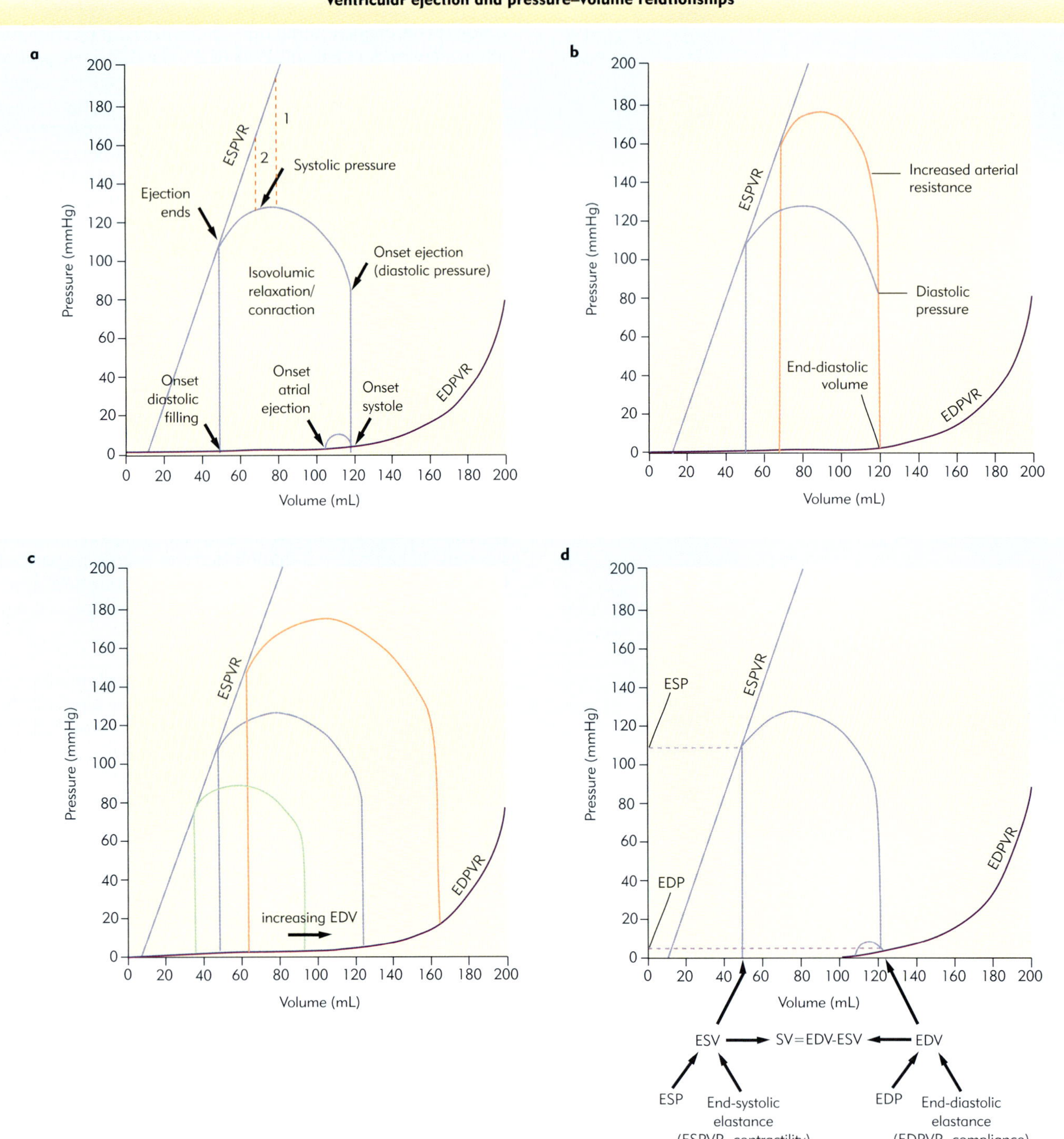

Figure 37.9 Ventricular ejection and pressure–volume relationships (PVR). (a) Normal stages in an ejection cycle. Ejection occurs in a counterclockwise direction. Vertical dashed lines 1 and 2 indicate pressures that would developed if further ejection were prevented at the respective volumes. (b) Effects of changes in vascular properties on ventricular ejection. At unchanged end-diastolic volume (EDV) and pressure at ejection (diastolic pressure), an increase in arterial resistance would develop higher ejection pressures and a smaller stroke volume (SV). (c) Effects of changes in left ventricular EDV with constant vascular properties on ejection. Arterial pressures and SV change, although end-systole still occurs when the ejection intersects the ESPVR. (d) The SV is determined by two elastance curves, the ESPVR and EDPVR, and two pressures, end-systolic (ESP) and end-diastolic (EDP).

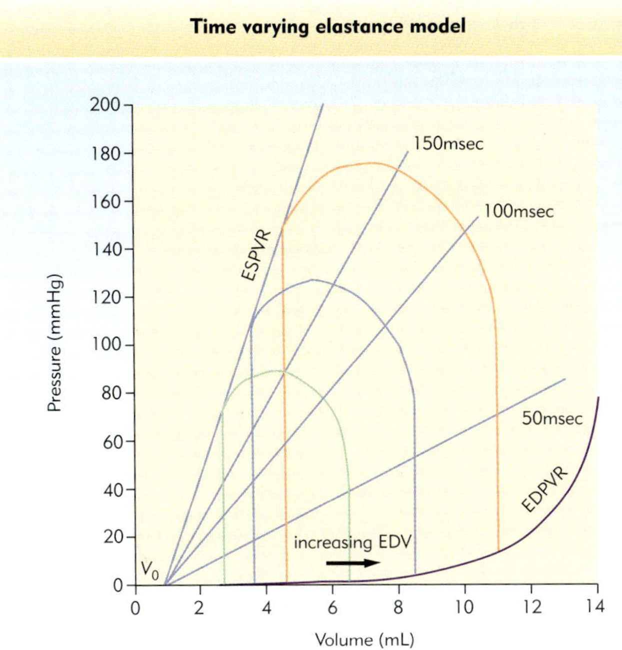

Figure 37.10 Time-varying elastance model. During ejection, the ventricular pressure at a given time after the onset of systole is related linearly to ventricular volume. As systole progresses, the line defining this relationship rotates counterclockwise around V_0. That is, it becomes progressively steeper until it reaches a maximum value, the end-systolic pressure–volume relation, a change that can be viewed as progressive stiffening of the ventricle.

measure of contractility. The ESPVR will refer to this unless otherwise stated.

Afterload

Despite these limitations, the ESPVR provides a clinically useful framework for assessing ventricular performance and predicting how changes in blood pressure will affect cardiac performance. In contrast, making such assessments using the term afterload is difficult if not impossible. As discussed, the definition of afterload as defined for papillary muscles is difficult to apply to the intact ventricle. Systemic vascular resistance (SVR) is often used as a surrogate for afterload in the intact ventricle. However, this definition can be misleading. First, it is evident from the discussion of the ESPVR that SVR can only affect ejection by changing the ESP. Second, because ESP can also be affected by vascular compliance, even with a constant resistance, and because both compliance and resistance are greatly simplified vascular concepts, SVR is not a reasonable definition of afterload. Third, even if vascular compliance is constant, ESV is generally impossible to calculate from SVR alone, so that changes in SVR cannot be directly related to changes in ventricular performance. Consequently, vascular properties such as resistance and compliance are not measures of ventricular afterload but only modifiers of load as measured by pressure. Therefore, rather than attempting to apply the papillary muscle definition of afterload to the intact ventricle, it seems more sensible to relate the simpler concepts based on the ESPVR and EDPVR to performance. Moreover, because the time-varying elastance model shows that ventricular volume at any instant during systole depends mostly upon the pressure at that instant, instantaneous pressure and, more importantly, ESP provide more information about ventricular ejection than do vascular properties.

THE STARLING CURVE

The Starling curve is useful for understanding the coupling of the heart and the vasculature. However, it is affected not only by the contractile state of the heart but also by the ESP and EDPVR. Some insight into the interaction of these factors on the Starling curve may be gained by considering the factors that can cause a decrease in SV for a given EDP. By definition, a decrease in SV can result from a decrease in EDV or an increase in ESV. For a fixed EDP, the EDV can decrease only if the EDPVR is shifted upward, that is, if the ventricle becomes stiffer. Such a change leads to a decrease in SV for any EDP simply because the corresponding EDV is smaller. This emphasizes the importance of the EDPVR in determining the shape of the Starling curve. In fact, as shown below, the shape of the Starling curve is largely a reflection of the EDPVR.

Probably the most common mechanism for an upward shift in the compliance curve is ventricular interaction. Because the ventricles share a common septum and are enclosed by the pericardium, an increase in size of one chamber changes the pressure–volume relation in the other chambers so that a higher pressure is required to achieve the same volume. Although it is often stated that a decrease in ventricular compliance occurs with ischemia, this is probably unusual and never occurs without systolic dysfunction. In contrast, ischemia-induced systolic dysfunction probably occurs commonly without stiffening of the ventricle and actually may be accompanied by an increase in ventricular compliance. As discussed above, ESV is determined predominantly by two factors: the ESPVR (the contractile state) and the ESP. Therefore, an increase in ESV can occur if either ESP increases or the slope of the ESPVR decreases, the latter reflecting a decrease in contractility. Either change would shift the Starling curve downward because, for a given EDP and EDV, the ESV would increase, thereby decreasing SV. Thus, the Starling curve can be shifted downward by a decrease in diastolic compliance, a decrease in contractility, or an increase in ESP. This greatly simplifies analysis of changes in SV. For example, if LV SV decreases without a change in systemic arterial pressures but with an increase in LV EDP, either contractility has decreased or the ventricle has become stiffer. The latter would be unusual without marked increases in the RV EDV causing RV interaction.

Derivation of Starling curves

Although the Starling curve is often described as being shifted downward by increases in load or decreases in contractility, the definitions of load and contractility are usually vague and quantitation of their interactions is lacking. Deriving Starling curves from pressure–volume diagrams can overcome these limitations by defining contractility as the slope of the ESPVR and load as ESP (Fig. 37.11). The shape of the Starling curve is essentially a reflection of the portion of the EDPVR for a volume greater than the ESV.

The effects of load on the Starling curve can be derived using the same process with different ESP and, therefore, ESV. Curve 2 in Figure 37.11b was generated as described above except the ESP was decreased to 50mmHg (ESV = 20mL). The origin of this Starling curve is shifted slightly to the left

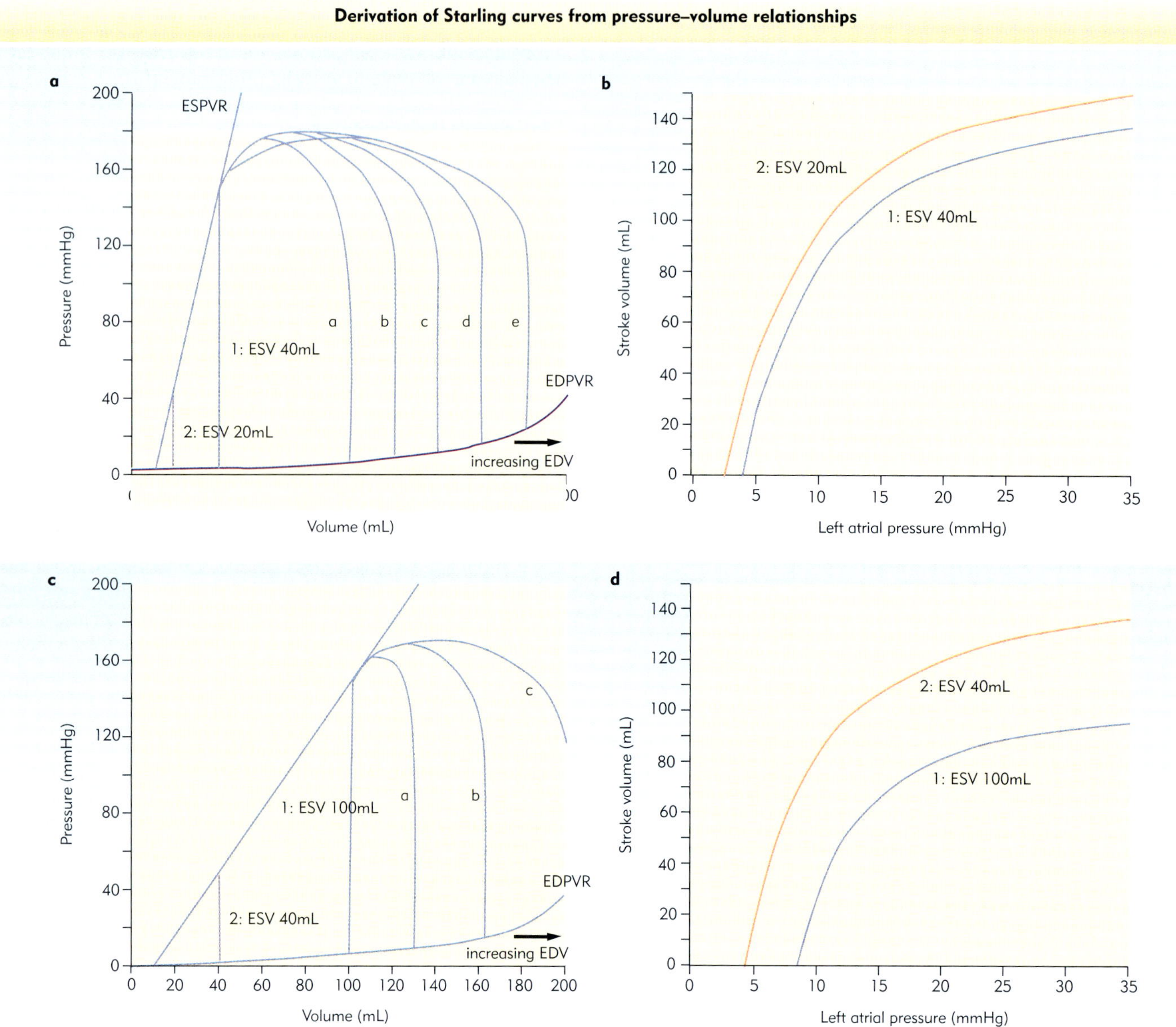

Figure 37.11 Derivation of Starling curves from pressure–volume relationships. (a) Ejections with the same end-systolic volume (ESV, 40mL) but progressively increasing end-diastolic volumes (EDV, a through e). Contractility is defined as the slope of the end-systolic pressure–volume relation (ESPVR); here it is 5mmHg/mL. (b) The effect of load (ESP) on the Starling curve. Data for the end-diastolic pressure (EDP) derived from panel a are plotted against stroke volume (SV). Lowering the ESV by decreasing ESP to 50mmHg results in a larger SV for the EDV a–e. This shifts the Starling curve slightly upward and to the left. (c) Starling curves at depressed contractility (slope of the ESPVR 1.7mmHg/mL). (d) The effect of load at depressed contractility. Curve 1 was generated at an ESP of 150mmHg as in (a). Curve 2 was derived by fixing the ESV at 40mL [identical to curve 1 in (b)]. However, the ESP is only 50mmHg compared with 150mmHg in (a) because the ESPVR is much flatter. For any EDP the SV is much smaller than in (a) because ESP is increased.

because an isovolumic contraction at an ESV of 20mL has a lower ESP than one at 40mL. Moreover, the entire curve is shifted upward because for any EDV, SV is larger than that for curve 1 because of the smaller ESV while the EDP is unchanged. However, because of the high contractile state (i.e. the steep ESPVR, 5mmHg/mL), the change in ESV with changes in ESP is small, and the resultant shift in the Starling curve also is small.

The interaction of contractility and load on the shift of Starling curves can also be derived. Curve 2 in Figure 37.11d was generated with the same ESV as in Figure 37.11b, whereas curve 1 corresponds to the same ESP. Because the ESPVR is relatively flat, the ESV of 40mL reflects an ESP of only 50mmHg (line 2 in Figure 37.11c). The corresponding Starling curve is identical to curve 1 in Fig. 37.11b because the ESV at an ESP of 50mmHg is the same as that for the ventricle in Figure 37.11a with an ESP of 150mmHg. However, the Starling curve for the ESP of 150mmHg in the depressed ventricle (curve 1 in Figure 37.11d) is shifted markedly downward and to the right, because for an ESP of 150mmHg, the ESV must increase to 100mL. This shift is much greater for a depressed than for a normal ventricle because of the greater change in ESV for a given change in ESP. This is consistent with the observation that an increase in 'load' (ESP) has a much greater effect on the EDP and SV of a ventricle with depressed activity than of a normal ventricle. The Starling curves resulting from a decrease in contractility or an increase in load are indistinguishable if the ratio of the ESP to the slope of the ESPVR is constant. Consequently, the Starling curve cannot be used to assess contractility.

If the ventricle is both depressed and very compliant (e.g. dilated myopathy), the corresponding Starling curve appears almost normal for low loads. However, it would still shift markedly downward and to the right with an increase in blood pressure because of the large increase in ESV and, therefore, EDV and EDP. This illustrates why a patient with a dilated myopathy may have a normal EDP and SV if the blood pressure is well controlled but have a decrease in SV and large increases in filling pressures with hypertension.

INTEGRATING THE CARDIOVASCULAR SYSTEM

At equilibrium not only must Q_v equal SV for each ventricle, but also SV of both ventricles must also be equal (they may not be exactly equal because of coronary and bronchial circulations or cardiac lesions producing intracardiac shunts). One way to analyze the effects of changes in any component of the circulation upon other components is to plot ventricular pressure–volume curves, Starling curves, and curves for Q_v for each ventricle adjacent to each other. The interactions of the critical elements of these idealized hemodynamic analyses can then be visualized. Three important basic principles in such analyses are:

- EDV and ESV are controlled by two pressures, the EDP and ESP, and two elastances, the EDPVR and the ESPVR;
- The value of Q_v is determined by the difference between P_{ms} or P_{mp} and their respective atrial pressures divided by their respective venous resistances;
- P_{mp} and P_{ms} are largely determined by the volumes of blood and the compliances in the respective venous beds (normal values for both P_{ms} and P_{mp} are 10–15mmHg).

These principles are used below to establish some basic behaviors of the circulation. The following discussion shows intuitively that transient changes in SV resulting from alterations in LV performance cannot be sustained unless there is a secondary effect on P_{ra}. Changes in P_{ra} are usually mediated by alterations in RV performance or by ventricular interactions.

Increasing LV contractility in a normal ventricle

Consider the effects of a hypothetical drug that can increase LV contractility and therefore its ejection fraction (EF), without directly affecting the RV or any vascular bed. Suppose that initially both ventricles have an EDV of 100mL and EF of 60%, and that this drug increased the EF of the LV to 80%. Assume also that this drug was applied in such a way that the increase in LV EF occurred just before the onset of systole. The effects, which are derived from simulations in which the slope of the LV ESPVR was increased from 3mmHg/mL to 5mmHg/mL, are summarized in Figure 37.14. On the beat 1 after the drug was applied, the LV would eject 80mL while the RV still ejected 60mL. This, in effect, would translocate 20mL of blood from the pulmonary circulation into the systemic circulation, which is equivalent to infusing 20mL of blood directly into the systemic venous circulation, Clinically, such an infusion would not increase systemic venous return appreciably because P_{ms} would not change significantly, for several reasons. First, the compliance of the systemic venous bed is very large so that such a change in volume would produce relatively little change in the size of the veins and thus their distending pressure, P_{ms}. Second, regardless of venous compliance, because 20mL is less than 0.5% of systemic venous blood volume it is too small a volume to increase P_{ms} appreciably. However, the situation in the pulmonary circulation is much different. Because the pulmonary circulation contains only 200mL to 300mL of blood, a 20mL volume loss is 7–10% of the total pulmonary blood volume. Consequently, P_{mp} would decrease, thereby reducing venous return to the LV. Moreover, assuming that systemic pressure did not change much, the increase in contractility would cause a decrease in the LV ESV from 40mL to 20mL. Consequently, it would take an additional 20mL to fill to the original EDV of 100mL. Extracting this additional 20mL from the pulmonary circulation would also decrease P_{mp}. The LV would then fill to an EDV of only 88mL instead of 100mL. Therefore, for beat 2, the LV will eject only 70mL (0.8 × 88mL) instead of 80mL. Moreover, because the EDV of the LV has decreased from 100mL to 88mL, the LV EDP will also decrease slightly resulting in a slight drop in pulmonary artery pressures. Therefore, the RV ESP will also decrease slightly causing an ejection to a slightly lower RV ESV. Consequently, on beat 2 the RV EF will increase from 60% to 61% so that the RV will eject 62mL (101 × 0.61) instead of 60mL. Thus, on the second beat, an additional 9mL (70.4–61.6mL, to be exact) will be translocated from the pulmonary to the systemic circulation, bringing the total translocated to 29mL. For the reasons stated above, this still will not appreciably increase systemic venous return. However, the total loss from the pulmonary circulation is now 29mL, which is 10–15% of the initial total pulmonary blood volume. Accordingly, LV filling will decrease further so that in beat 3 the LV would fill to only 81mL. As this process continues, the pulmonary circulation will become hypovolemic enough, i.e. P_{mp} will decrease enough to reduce the LV EDV substantially with very little increase in systemic venous return. Because of this, and only a small change in RV EDP due to LV interaction from the slight decrease in LV EDP, the SV of the RV will not change appreciably. Thus, when a new equilibrium is finally reached, the SV will still be close to 60mL/beat (actually 62mL/beat) and the LV EDV will be reduced to approximately 77mL. That is, the increase in LV EF will have resulted in a decrease in LV size without an appreciable increase in SV.

It is noteworthy that in this example, a pulmonary artery catheter (PAC) would show a decrease in pulmonary capillary wedge pressure (PCWP) and pulmonary artery pressures (PAP), but essentially no change in P_{ra} or SV. Clearly, the patient's blood volume has not changed. This illustrates why the PCWP cannot be used to assess volume status. The decrease in PCWP without a change in SV indicates that the pulmonary circulation has become functionally hypovolemic. That is, P_{mp} must have decreased otherwise the pressure gradient for pulmonary venous return, P_{mp} – left atrial pressure (P_{la}), would have increased, thereby increasing venous return to the left atrium. The unchanged SV and P_{ra} indicate that the functional volume of the systemic circulation, P_{ms}, did not change. Therefore the CVP,

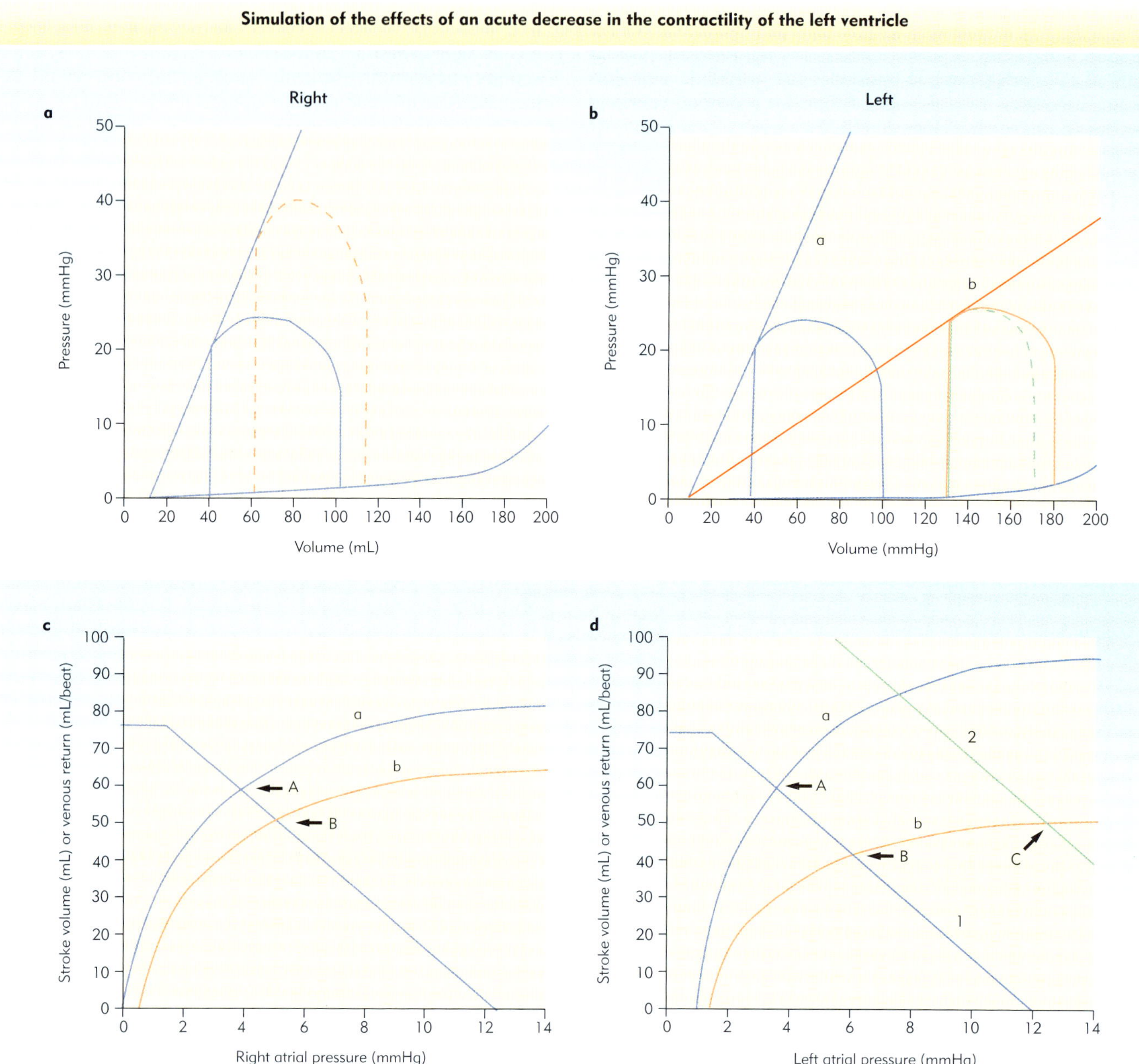

Figure 37.12 Simulation of the effects of an acute decrease in the contractility of the left ventricle (LV) on hemodynamics with initially normal ventricles and vascular volumes. The decrease in contractility is depicted by the shift in the end-systolic pressure–volume relationship (ESPVR) from curve a to the flatter curve b in (b), giving the downward shift in the Starling curve from curve a to curve b in (d). If blood were not translocated into the pulmonary circulation, venous return (Q_v) would still have to lie on line 1 in (d). The Starling curve would intersect this line at point B, corresponding to the dashed ejection curve in (b). However, because the LV stroke volume (SV) would then be only 40mL compared with the right ventricle (RV) SV of 60mL, blood would be translocated from the systemic into the pulmonary circulation until the SV of the two ventricles was again equal. This movement has little effect in the large systemic blood volume [change in mean systemic pressure is too small to show in (c)], but a relatively large effect in the smaller pulmonary blood volume [mean pulmonary pressure increases markedly in (d) from line 1 to line 2]. When the new equilibrium is reached, SV is decreased because the increase in LV end-diastolic pressure (EDP) [point C in (d)] increased pulmonary artery pressure [dashed ejection in (a)], impairing RV ejection. As a result, the RV Starling curve shifts downward from a to b in (c). The new RV equilibrium occurs on essentially the same Q_v line [point B in (c)] at a higher RV EDP. A lower RV contractile state would cause a greater depression in the RV Starling curve. In this case, the equilibrium SV and pulmonary capillary wedge pressure would be lower and right atrial pressure would be higher.

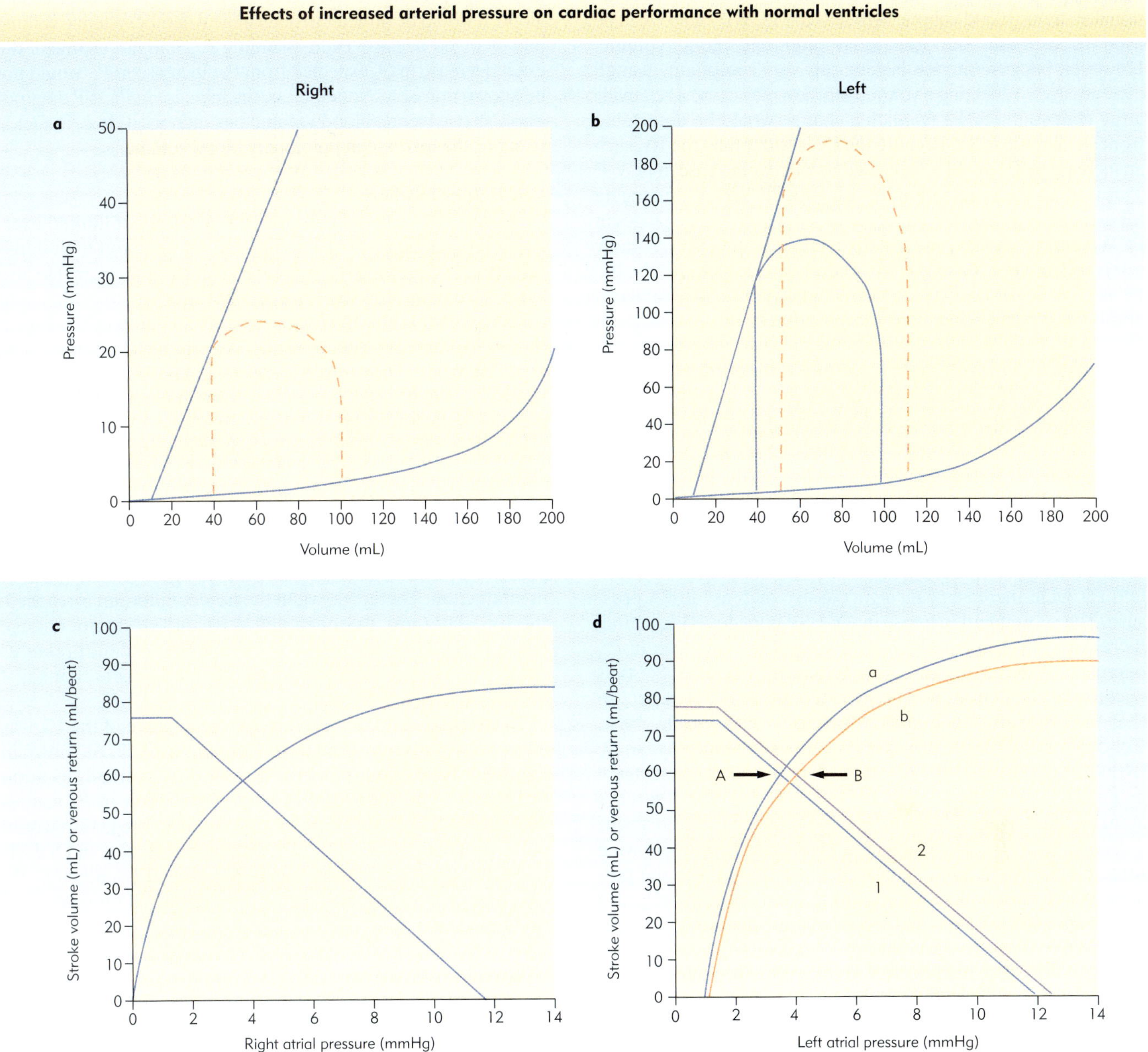

Figure 37.13 Effects of increased arterial pressure on cardiac performance with normal ventricles. Because of the steepness of the LV end-systolic pressure–volume relationship (ESPVR), the end-systolic volume (ESV) is normal (40mL) at an end-systolic pressure (ESP) of 130mmHg. To achieve a 60mL stroke volume (SV), the end-diastolic volumes (EDV) must be 100mL. If the LV ESP were increased abruptly to 180mmHg by, for example, aortic cross-clamping, and there were no reflex changes in contractility, LV ESV would increase by only 15mL because the ESPVR is steep [dashed ejection in (b)]. This would cause a slight downward shift in the LV Starling curve [curve b in (d)]. The LV SV would decrease by 15mL on the first beat, translocating this volume from the systemic into the pulmonary circulation. This would have virtually no effect on mean systemic pressure or on systemic venous return (Q_v) (c) but would increase the blood volume of the pulmonary circulation by approximately 10% and P_{mp} slightly [line 2 in (d)]. Consequently, Q_v to the LV would increase slightly but the increase in LV EDP would be negligible; both the LV Starling curve and Q_v curve would shift slightly and the intersection would occur at a slightly higher LV EDP [B in (d)]. Pulmonary artery pressure would not change. The RV would not detect the alteration in the LV; right atrial pressure would not change and, thus, Q_v and the SV of the RV would remain 60mL. At the new equilibrium, the central pressures and SV would not have changed measurably. But the LV EDV would have increased by 15ml.

which approximates P_{ra}, and SV can be used to estimate the functional systemic blood volume, whereas the PCWP and SV can be used to estimate the functional pulmonic blood volume. However, because the RV is generally very compliant, a small increase in P_{ra} reflecting a volume infusion may cause a relatively large change in RV EDV. Such a change would be detectable from an increase in SV. Because the LV is stiffer than the RV, such an increase in SV might be reflected by a larger increase in PCWP. This is often the justification for using the PCWP as a surrogate for evaluating systemic volume status. However, such changes in PCWP may be variable and systemic volume status (SVS) is easily inferred from the SV and CVP. Therefore, physiologically, the PCWP can be, at most, a very indirect indicator of SVS but it can also be misleading when used for this purpose.

Decreasing contractility in a normal left ventricle

The methods described above can also be used to analyze the effects of an acute decrease in LV ejection fraction, for example from 60 to 30%, as might occur with severe global ischemia (Fig. 37.12). For simplicity, assume that systemic pressures and RV contractility do not change. Because the decrease in LV contractility causes the LV initially to eject less than the RV, blood is translocated from the systemic to the pulmonary circulation, increasing P_{mp} and, thus, Q_v to the LV. Consequently, LV EDV and LV EDP increase, causing a passive increase in PA pressure. The subsequent increase in RV ESP impedes RV ejection, increasing RV EDV and EDP. The resultant increase in P_{ra} decreases systemic Q_v. As this process continues, RV SV falls because of the continuing passive increase in PA pressure, so that translocated volumes decrease with each beat. Concomitantly, LV SV increases because of the increase in Q_v to the LA. Eventually, the SV of the two ventricles would again be equal but less than the initial 60mL and greater than the 30mL ejected by the LV immediately following its depression.

These hemodynamic changes are governed by the following three mechanisms. First, translocation of blood into the pulmonary circulation increases P_{mp} and Q_v to the LV thereby also increasing LV EDV and the LV SV. Second, increased LV EDV causes LV EDP to rise and passively elevates PA pressure, RV ESP, and RV ESV, thus decreasing RV SV. This increases P_{ra} because systemic Q_v initially exceeds that required to fill the RV to its initial EDV from the now increased ESV. The resultant increase in P_{ra} without a change in P_{ms} causes systemic Q_v to decrease. Third, the increase in LV EDV effectively decreases compliance of the RV and RA by shifting the septum rightward - further increasing P_{ra} and decreasing systemic Q_v. The equilibrium SV depends upon both RV contractility and compliance. A normal RV will not increase its ESV much with the increase in PA pressure. Therefore, the equilibrium SV will be closer to the initial 60mL than the initial depressed LV SV of 30mL, and P_{ra} will not change much. In contrast, if the RV was initially depressed, the rise in PA pressure increases RV ESV more than for a normal RV, ultimately leading to a greater increase in P_{ra} and a lower equilibrium SV.

This simulation illustrates that the LV can affect cardiovascular function mainly only by altering (in this case increasing) P_{ra}. The increase in P_{ra} without a significant change in P_{ms} causes systemic Q_v to decrease, which can occur both from ventricular interaction and from passive increases in PA pressure. As will be seen below, this concept allows for a much simpler analysis of circulatory dynamics. As in the preceding example, the patient's volume status did not change appreciably, yet both the pulmonary capillary wedge pressure (PCWP) and P_{ra} increased. From these data alone, it would be difficult to determine whether systemic volume had changed because even assuming P_{ms} had not changed, the exact decrease in Q_v expected from the increase in P_{ra} would not be known precisely. Nonetheless, the increase in PCWP does not imply that systemic blood volume has increased. It is, in fact, a result of the increase in pulmonary blood volume.

Ventricular loading

Consider a 67-year-old man who has a history of limited exercise tolerance because of claudication who is about to undergo resection and grafting of an infrarenal aortic aneurysm. He also suffers from chronic stable angina but there is no evidence of cardiac dysfunction. Because of the uncertainty of the extent of his coronary artery disease, a PA catheter is inserted. The initial data are shown in Figure 37.7. These data, although showing a slightly elevated PCWP, show a normal SV and are, therefore, consistent with ventricles that function relatively normally. The effects of increased arterial pressure with aortic cross-clamping are shown in Fig. 37.13. For simplicity, assume that the systolic pressure corresponds to ESP, although the actual ESP is always lower than systolic pressure. The LV EDV has to rise by 15mL to match the SV of the RV, which does not produce a physiologically significant change in the LV EDP, or in interaction. Therefore, when the new equilibrium is reached, the LV EDP (and, therefore, PCWP) and SV do not change measurably. This illustrates why changes in systemic pressures usually do not produce measurable hemodynamic changes if both ventricles are normal.

In contrast, suppose that the contractile state of the LV was lower than suspected from the data in Figure 37.7. As shown in Figure 37.14, at equilibrium there would be a marked elevation in LV EDP and thus PCWP, a small elevation in P_{ra}, and a decrease in SV. These changes are similar to those that would occur with depression of the LV without an increase in LV ESP. If the RV contractile state was depressed, at equilibrium P_{ra} would be greater whereas the SV and left atrial pressure (P_{la}) would be lower.

Ventricular unloading

It is sometimes stated that an arterial vasodilator increases blood pressure if a patient has a dysfunctional LV because the resultant increase in cardiac output is greater than the decrease in arterial resistance. However, analysis using the ESPVR indicates that this is not possible unless the contractile state also increases. Consider a patient who has a LV myopathy of unknown etiology who presents with an acute decrease in contractility of his already compromised LV. The patient, who is is complaining of increased dyspnea, an inability to lie flat, and severe fatigue, is found to have pulmonary edema and is transferred to an intensive-care unit where a PA catheter is placed (see Fig 37.7 for typical data). Pressure–volume diagrams, Starling curves, and Q_v plots for this patient are depicted in Fig. 37.15. Because the P_{ra} is as high as the normal P_{ms} of 12mmHg, P_{ms} must have increased substantially. That is, the patient must be functionally hypervolemic in the systemic circulation to maintain a sufficient venous pressure between P_{ms} and P_{ra} to provide systemic Q_v even to match the low SV. Furthermore, the SV cannot be readily increased with additional volume because any further increment in LV EDV would markedly increase the LV EDP because of the steepness of the EDPVR in this region. This would further limit RV performance and exacerbate the

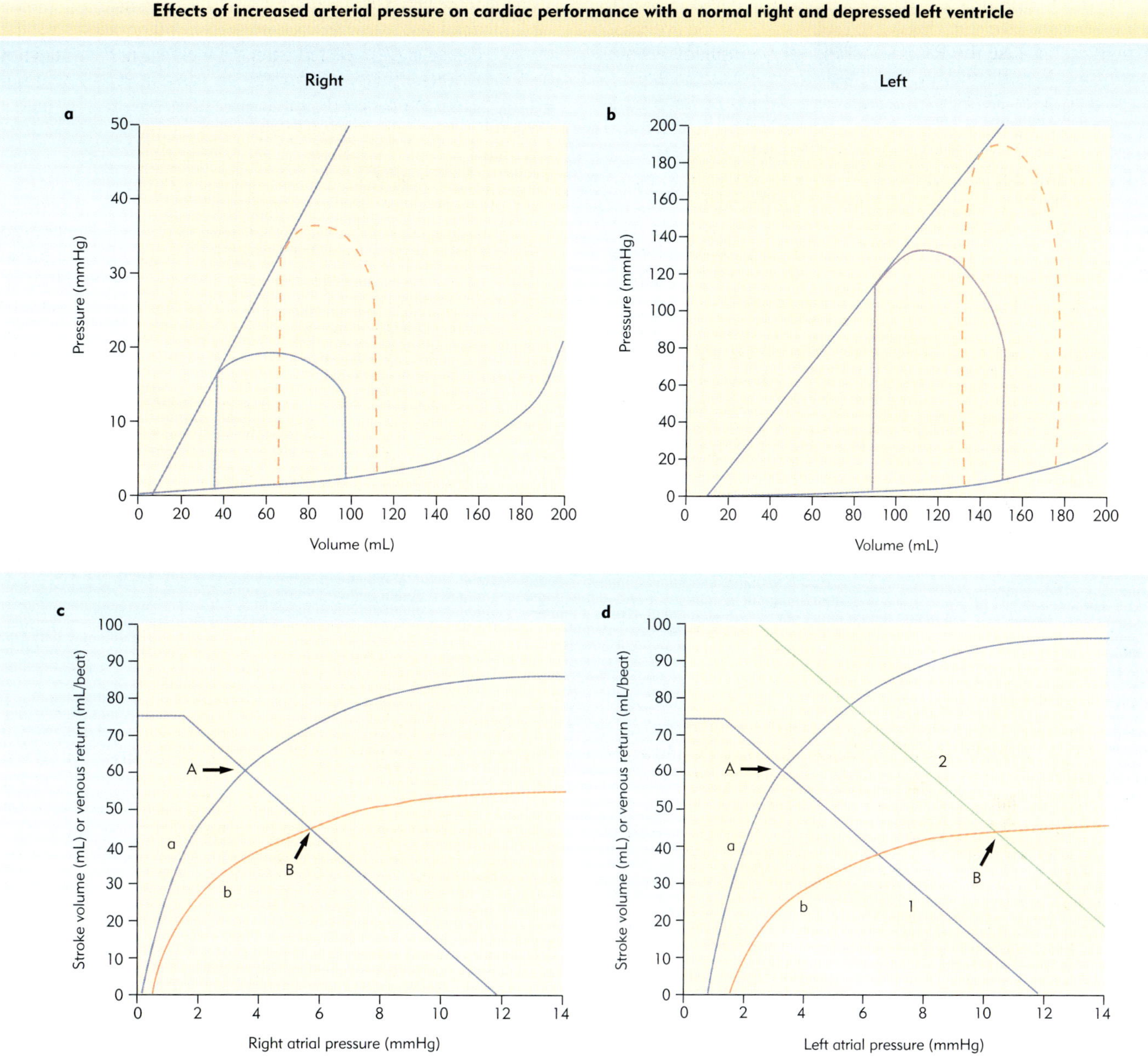

Figure 37.14 Effects of increased arterial pressure on cardiac performance with a normal right and depressed left ventricle (LV). The slope of the LV end-systolic pressure–volume relationship (ESPVR) is flatter than in Fig. 37.13, consequently the LV end-diastolic volume (EDV) corresponding to an LV end-systolic pressure (ESP) of 130mmHg is 90mL rather than 40mL. For a 60mL stroke volume (SV) LV EDV must then be 150mL. End-diastolic pressure–volume relationship (EDPVR) is slightly more compliant than in Fig. 37.13 so that LV end-diastolic pressure (EDP) is still 12mmHg despite the larger LV EDV. Because the LV is depressed, an increase in LV ESP to 180mmHg (e.g. by aortic cross-clamping) causes LV end-systolic volume (ESV) to increase by 40mL to 130mL instead of by only 15mL. Consequently, the Starling curve is shifted downward more [curve b in (d)] by aortic cross-clamping than in Fig. 37.13. Moreover, a much larger volume of blood is translocated into the pulmonary circulation, causing a greater increase in mean pulmonary pressure [line 2 in (d)] and, therefore, in LV EDV. The new equilibrium would occur at point B in (d). Mean systemic pressure and, therefore, the systemic venous return (Q_v) line would not change appreciably (c). However, as LV EDV increases, LV EDP also begins to rise substantially because the LV EDPVR is relatively flat at higher volumes. The rise in LV EDP causes a passive rise in pulmonary artery pressure, thereby increasing RV ESP and ESV. Consequently, RV EDV increases [dashed ejection in (a)] because systemic Q_v initially exceeds that required to fill the RV to its original 100mL EDV. However, with the increase in RV EDV and, therefore, RV EDP, the RV Starling curve shifts downward [curve b in (c)]. Right atrial pressure (P_{ra}) would increase, causing systemic Q_v to fall [point B in (c)]. At equilibrium, there is a marked elevation in LV EDP and thus pulmonary capillary wedge pressure, a small elevation in P_{ra}, and a decrease in SV. The effects of ventricular interaction are not shown but would stiffen the RV and RA, further increasing P_{ra} and decreasing the equilibrium SV.

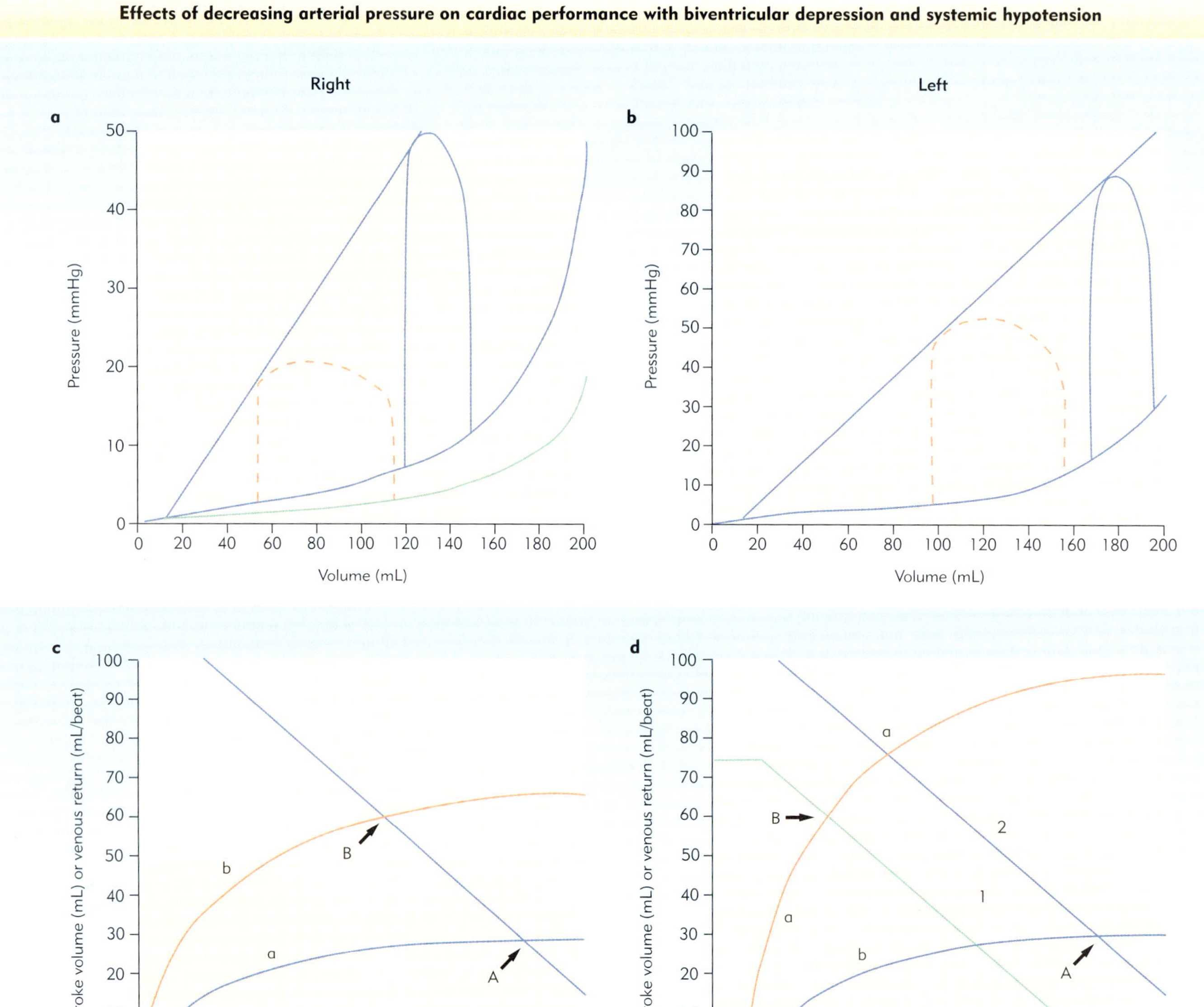

Figure 37.15 Effects of decreasing arterial pressure (unloading) on cardiac performance with biventricular depression and systemic hypotension. The slope of the left ventricular (LV) end-systolic pressure–volume relationship (ESPVR) is very flat, giving an LV end-systolic volume (ESV) of 165mL and pressure (ESP) of only 90mmHg. The stroke volume (SV) is only 30mL because with a LV end-diastolic volume (EDV) of 195mL, the LV end-diastolic pressure (EDP) is 30mmHg, resulting in elevated pulmonary artery pressure. The resultant elevation in right ventricular (RV) ESP causes RV ESV to increase to 115mL. Compared with the RV in Fig. 37.12, the RV ESPVR is somewhat flattened, indicating some RV depression. In addition, because of ventricular interaction resulting from the acute increase in LV size and rightward septal displacement, the RV EDPVR is considerably stiffer than in Fig. 37.12. Therefore, even though the RV EDV is only 145mL, the RV ESV and EDP also are increased. The high RV EDP (and, thus, right atrial pressure) impedes venous return. Arterial dilation would decrease LV ESP, causing a reduction in both LV EDV and EDP [dashed ejection, (b)]. This would cause a passive reduction in pulmonary artery pressure and, thus, RV ESP, which would cause a decrease in RV EDV and EDP [dashed ejection, (a)]. These changes cause a shift in the equilibrium point from A to B in (c) and (d).

pulmonary edema. Very large increases in RV EDP would be required to produce even small increases in RV EDV.

If this patient were given a pure arterial dilator, the resultant decrease in the LV ESP would increase LV SV, causing blood to be translocated from the pulmonary to the systemic circulation (Fig. 37.15). Even if Q_v to the LV did not change, the LV EDV would decrease because of the reduction in the LV ESV. However, the actual LV EDV after application of the dilator would depend upon two factors. First, the decrease in P_{mp} resulting from the translocation of blood into the systemic circulation would reduce LV filling. Second, because the LV EDP (actually P_{la}) is the downstream pressure for pulmonary Q_v, the decrease in the LV EDP resulting from the decrease in the LV EDV would tend to increase LV filling. Regardless of which factor dominates, the LV EDV would decrease somewhat, resulting in a decrease in LV EDP and, thus, PA pressure and RV ESP. This, in turn, would reduce RV ESV thereby improving RV ejection, reducing RV EDV and, therefore, P_{ra}. The final result would be an increase in Q_v and a new equilibrium at which SV increases and both right- and left-sided EDP decrease. Importantly, this effect could not be achieved without the decrease in systemic blood pressure, which caused the initial decrease in LV ESV. This is consistent with published data on unloading. These results suggest that the only way that blood pressure could increase with 'unloading' would be if the contractile state of the LV improved (e.g. by resolution of global ischemia). This analysis leads to the conclusion that if systemic blood pressure increases with the use of an arterial or venous dilator, the LV most likely was ischemic.

The principle point in these examples is that changes in LV SV cannot be sustained unless systemic Q_v is also affected. Because of the relatively large blood volume of the systemic circulation and the high venous compliance, the systemic vasculature is essentially unaffected by (uncoupled from) changes in forward flow of the LV. That is, the LV can only change Q_v by altering P_{ra} because it cannot move sufficient blood out of the pulmonary vasculature to affect P_{ms}. Conversely, changes in RV or LV performance can move enough blood from the systemic to the pulmonary circulation to increase P_{mp} and, therefore, Q_v to the LV. However, this still cannot be sustained unless P_{ra} also changes enough to cause systemic Q_v to match this change. The LV can cause the requisite changes in P_{ra} either directly by changing the effective compliance of the RV and RA by ventricular interaction or indirectly by affecting RV ejection via changes in the PA pressure. If the RV is normal, the former mechanism seems to be more important.

CONCLUSIONS

An understanding of basic physiologic principles simplifies analysis of data obtained with invasive cardiovascular monitoring. Moreover, it allows prediction of the effects of interventions on mechanical performance. Because the volumes of the ventricles are usually unknown, often one can only guess at the contractile state of the ventricles. However, as illustrated in the examples, perturbation of the system (e.g. by a drug or volume infusion) yields considerable information about the state of the ventricles. In this way, a hypothesis can be tested; if it proves to be wrong and things are not changing in a salutary direction, it may be revised and another therapy tried. By repeated perturbations, the principles described can usually be used to estimate the relative contractile state of both ventricles, the functional central and peripheral blood volumes, and the likely effect of various interventions upon ventricular mechanics.

Key References

Guyton AC, Jones CE, Coleman TG. Circulatory physiology: cardiac output and its regulation, 2nd edn. Philadelphia PA: Saunders; 1973.

Kass DA, Maughan WL. From Emax to pressure-volume relations: a broader view. Circulation. 1988;77:1203–12.

Janicki JS, Reeves RC, Hefner LL. Factors influencing left ventricular shortening in isolated canine heart. Am J Physiol. 1976;230:419–26.

Further Reading

Bunnell E, Parrillo JE. Cardiac dysfunction during septic shock. Clin Chest Med. 1996;17:237–48.

Burkhoff D, Sugiura S, Yue DT, Sagawa K. Contractility-dependent curvilinearity of end-systolic pressure–volume relations. Am J Physiol. 1987;252:H1218–27.

Guyton AC, Lindsey AW, Abernathy JB, Richardson T. Venous return at various right atrial pressures and the normal venous return curve. Am J Physiol. 1957;189:609.

Little WC, Freeman GL. Description of LV pressure–volume relations by time-varying elastance and source resistance. Am J Physiol. 1987;253:H83–90.

Kass DA, Beyar R, Lankford E, et al. Influence of contractile state on curvilinearity of in situ end-systolic pressure–volume relations. Circulation. 1989;79:167–78.

Maughan WL, Kass DA, Heard M, Sagawa K. Erroneous estimation of the end-systolic pressure–volume relationship from time-varying elastance in patients. Circulation. 1987;76:IV-545.

Shroff SG, Janicki JS, Weber KT. Evidence and quantitation of left ventricular systolic resistance. Am J Physiol. 1985;249:H358–70.

Suga H, Sagawa K, Demer L. Determinants of instantaneous pressure in canine left ventricles. Circ Res. 1980;46:256–63.

Suga H, Yamakoshi K. Effects of stroke volume and velocity of ejection on end-systolic pressure of canine left ventricle. End-systolic volume clamping. Circ Res. 1977;40:445–50.

van der Velde ET, Burkhoff D, Steendijk P, et al. Nonlinearity and load sensitivity of end-systolic pressure–volume relation of canine left ventricle in vivo. Circulation. 1991;83:315–27.

Chapter 38 The peripheral circulation

Simon Howell and Pierre Foëx

Topics covered in this chapter

The primary role of the peripheral circulation is to deliver nutrients to and remove waste products from the tissues. However, it is not a passive conduit. It is structurally adapted to meet the differing needs of various tissues and is subject to complex regulatory mechanisms to control local and global blood flow.

VESSELS OF THE PERIPHERAL SYSTEM

Apart from capillaries, all blood vessels have the same basic three-layered structure (Fig. 38.1). The outermost layer, the adventitia, is a fibrous connective tissue sheath that holds the vessel loosely in place. The adventitia of the larger vessels, such as the aorta, pulmonary arteries, and iliac vessels, contain a plexus of small vessels, the vasa vasorum. These provide nourishment for the media of large vessels. In the largest arteries, they penetrate into the outer two-thirds of the media.

The media is bounded by the inner and outer elastic laminae and consists of smooth muscle cells embedded in a matrix of collagen and elastic fibers. It provides the vessels with mechanical strength and compliance.

The innermost layer is the intima; it is the main barrier to the passage of plasma proteins but is mechanically weak. It consists of a flat layer of endothelial cells lying on a thin layer of connective tissue. The intima synthesizes and secretes a number of vasoactive substances and has an important role in the local regulation of the circulation.

The pulmonary arteries, the aorta, and major branches such as the iliac vessels have a tunica media rich in elastin and are classified as elastic arteries. They expand during systole to receive the blood ejected by the heart and then recoil during diastole, so smoothing the pulsatile ejection of blood by the heart into a more continuous flow. The medium and small arteries, such as the popliteal and radial arteries, act as low-resistance conduits. They have a tunica media that is thick relative to the vessel diameter and that is rich in smooth muscle. These vessels have a rich sympathetic innervation and can con-

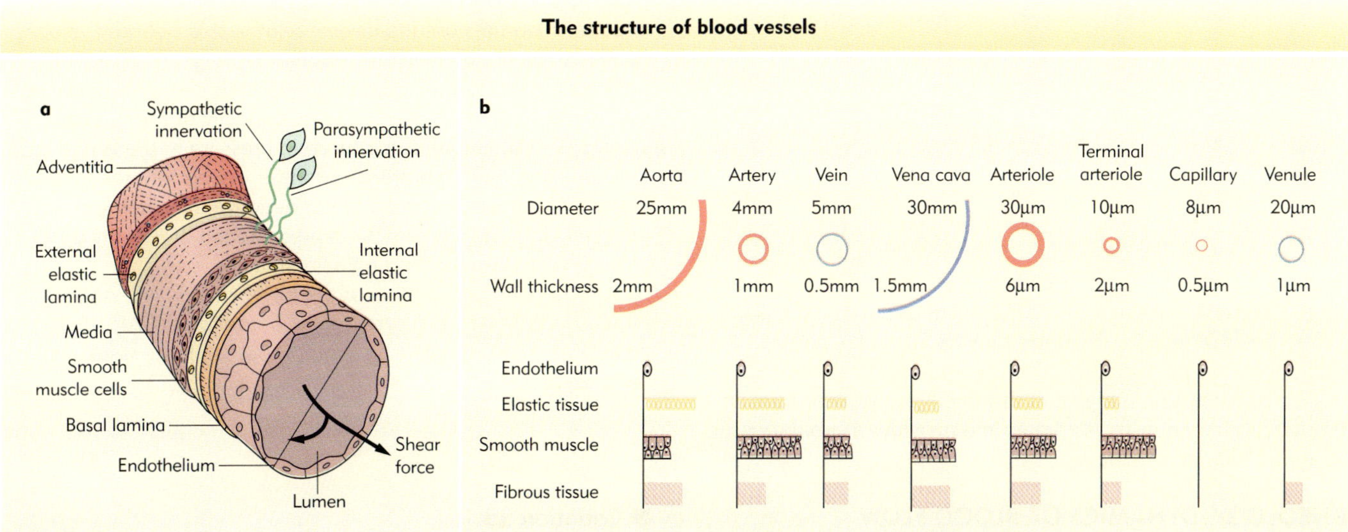

Figure 38.1 The structure of blood vessels. All blood vessels have the same general structure (a). Different vessels have varying internal diameters, wall thickness, and relative amounts of the principal components of the vessel walls (b). Cross-sections of the vessels are not drawn to scale because of the huge range from aorta and vena cavae to capillary. (Redrawn from Burton, 1954).

tract. Their resistance is low, however, and they are not important in the regulation of blood flow. Their thick walls help to prevent collapse at sharp bends such as the knee, and their ability to produce a profound contraction may prevent exsanguination from a severed vessel in the event of trauma.

The wall of veins and venules (diameter 50–200μm) follow the same three-layered structure seen in the arterial system. In the limbs, the intima is formed into semilunar valves, which act to prevent back flow. Valves are absent from the large central veins and the veins of the head and neck. The venous media is thin and the vessels are easily collapsed and distended. Venules and veins outnumber arteries and arterioles, and the overall cross-sectional area of the venous system is greater than that of the arterial system; consequently, resistance to flow in the venous system is low. The venous system functions as a reservoir of variable capacity. It is capable of holding up to two-thirds of the circulating volume. Much of this capacity is located in small veins and venules; sympathetically mediated vasoconstriction of these vessels can actively displace blood into the arterial circulation.

The microcirculation consists of the fine plexus of vessels that ramifies through the tissues and comprises arterioles, capillaries, and venules. The smallest arteries branch into first-, second-, and third-order arterioles, and finally into terminal arterioles. Arterioles are the main resistance vessels of the systemic circulation; the pressure drop across arterioles is greater than that in any other vessels in the systemic circulation (Fig. 38.2). They have the thickest walls of all arteries relative to the diameter of the vessel lumen because of their large complement of medial smooth muscle cells. First-order arterioles are innervated and controlled by sympathetic nerves, while in terminal arterioles control is dominated by local metabolites. Arteriolar constriction and dilatation controls local blood flow. Each terminal arteriole gives rise to a cluster or module of capillaries. The smooth muscle tone of the terminal arteriole determines the extent to which the capillary module is perfused. In a few tissues, notably the mesentery, there is a ring of smooth muscle at the capillary entrance, the precapillary sphincter. Capillaries are devoid of smooth muscle and are effectively long thin tubes of endothelium 5 to 8μm in diameter. Despite their small diameter, capillaries offer only a moderate resistance to flow. This is partly because of bolus flow (see below) and partly because the total cross-sectional area of the capillary bed is very large (see Fig. 38.2). The distal ends of capillaries unite to form postcapillary (pericytic) venules; their walls contain pericytes but no smooth muscle. Smooth muscle reappears in the walls of venules when diameters reach 30–50μm.

Blood flow waxes and wanes every 15 seconds or so in many capillary modules. It may stop entirely for brief periods because of the spontaneous rhythmic contractions in the terminal arterioles (vasomotion). In well-perfused capillaries, the transit time is typically 0.5 to 2 seconds. This may fall to 0.25 seconds during exercise.

In skeletal muscle, capillary density provides an area for exchange of approximately $100 cm^2/g$ muscle. In tissues where oxygen consumption is high and sustained (e.g. myocardium and brain), capillary density is greater and provides a capillary area of about $500 cm^2/g$ tissue.

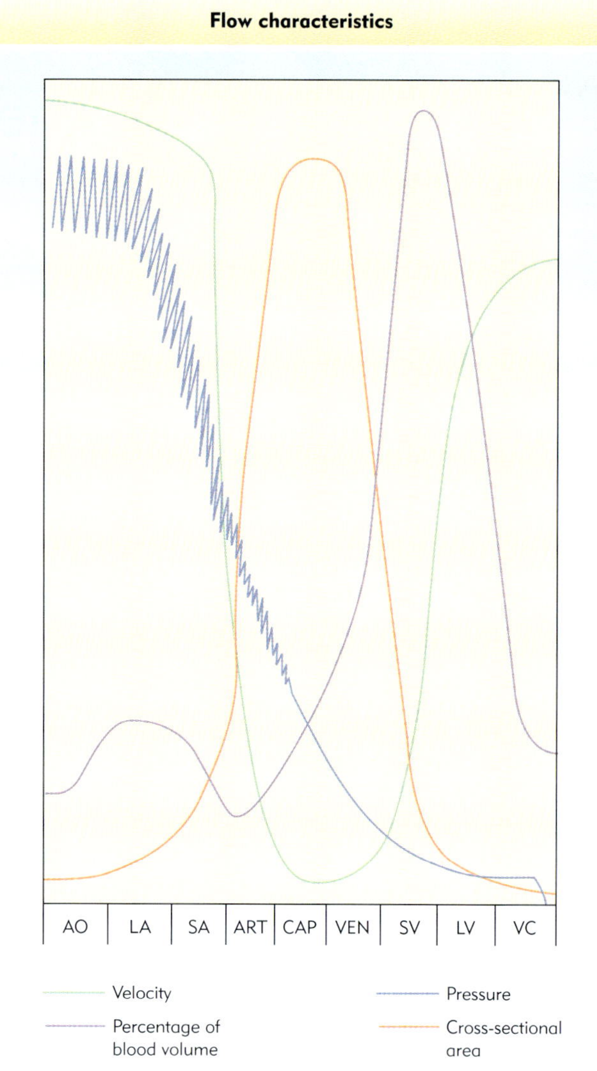

Figure 38.2 Flow characteristics in systemic vessels. The important features are the inverse relationship between velocity and cross-sectional area, the major pressure drop across the arterioles, the maximal cross-sectional area and minimal flow rate in the capillaries, and the large capacity of the venous system. The small but abrupt drop in pressure in the venae cava indicates the point of entrance of these vessels into the thoracic cavity and reflects the effect of the negative intrathoracic pressure. To permit schematic representation of velocity and cross-sectional area on a single linear scale, only approximations are possible at the lower values. AO, aorta; LA, large arteries; SA, small arteries; ART, arterioles; CAP, capillaries; VEN, venules; SV, small veins; LV, large veins; VC, vena cava.

RHEOLOGY: DYNAMICS OF BLOOD FLOW

The flow of fluid through tubes is governed by Darcy's law of flow. This states that flow in a steady state (Q) is linearly related to the pressure difference between two points ($P_1 - P_2$):

■ Equation 38.1

$$Q = K(P_1 - P_2) = \frac{(P_1 - P_2)}{R}$$

where K is the hydraulic conductance and R is the hydraulic resistance. For the circulation, cardiac output (CO) equals the difference between mean arterial and the central venous pressure (P_a – CVP) divided by total peripheral resistance (TPR). Central venous pressure is close to zero compared with atmospheric pressure and the expression may be simplified by omitting this term:

■ Equation 38.2

$$CO = \frac{(P_a - CVP)}{TPR} \approx \frac{P_a}{TPR}$$

Darcy's law applies to laminar flow, in which fluid flows in smooth streamlines and the velocity of flow increases from the perimeter to the center of the tube. It takes several tube diameters from the tube entrance to establish laminar flow. In the entrance region, a broad core of fluid flows at a uniform velocity (Fig. 38.3). Therefore, in the ascending aorta, the near uniform velocity allows estimation of aortic flow by the Doppler method. With a particulate suspension such as blood, shearing forces of lamina against lamina tend to orientate red cells parallel to the direction of flow. Also cells tend to be displaced towards the central axis (axial flow), leaving a thin, cell-deficient layer of plasma at the margins. This marginal layer is only 2–4μm thick, but it is important in arterioles, where it improves flow.

As the pressure difference across a tube is progressively raised, a point is reached where laminar flow is lost and flow becomes turbulent. At this point, Darcy's law breaks down and flow no longer increases linearly with pressure but changes with the square root of pressure. Turbulent flow is encouraged by a high mean fluid velocity (v), large tube diameter (D), and high fluid density (ρ). Turbulence is discouraged by a high viscosity (η). These factors can be combined to give a dimensionless ratio called the Reynolds' number (Re):

■ Equation 38.3

$$Re = \frac{vD\rho}{\eta}$$

For steady flow down a straight rigid uniform tube, turbulent flow begins at a Reynolds' number of about 2000. Despite the fact that blood flow is pulsatile and the vessels are neither straight nor uniform, flow is laminar in most vessels. Turbulence occurs in the ventricles where it helps to mix the blood and produce a uniform blood gas content. It also occurs in the aorta during peak flow, where the Reynolds' number reaches approximately 4600. Turbulence can also develop in arteries roughened by atheromatous plaques.

Resistance to laminar flow arises from the shearing between adjacent laminae. Because the lamina in contact with the tube is stationary, it is not affected by friction between the tube and the fluid. Resistance is affected by tube geometry because the radius of the tube alters the rate of shear of the laminae. The determinants of resistance for laminar flow of a Newtonian fluid along a straight cylindrical tube are given by Poiseuille's equation. For a fluid of viscosity (η) traveling along a tube of length (l) and radius (r), resistance (R) is given by:

■ Equation 38.4

$$R = \frac{8\eta l}{\pi r^4}$$

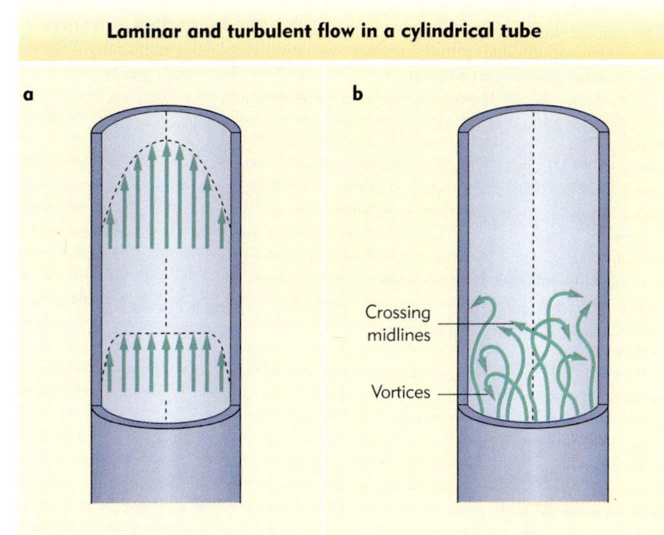

Figure 38.3 Laminar and turbulent flow in a cylindrical tube. The arrows indicate the velocity of flow, which increases from the edge to the center of the tube. Note that laminar flow takes some distance to become established and at the mouth of the tube a plug of fluid flows at uniform velocity. In laminar flow (a) all elements of the fluid move in streamlines (laminae) that are parallel to the axis of the tube; movement does not occur in a radial or circumferential direction. The layer of fluid in contact with the wall is motionless; the fluid that moves along the axis of the tube has the maximal velocity. In turbulent flow (b) the elements of the fluid move irregularly in axial, radial, and circumferential directions. Vortices frequently develop.

Resistance is inversely proportional to the fourth power of the radius. The increase in resistance from the human aorta of about 1cm in radius to an arteriole of radius 0.01cm is 10^8. Further, vasoconstriction producing a 16% reduction in arteriolar radius doubles resistance. This is why arterioles are the main site of resistance. It may seem at first sight that capillaries (radius 3μm) should offer an even greater resistance to flow. However, there are a huge number of capillaries arranged in parallel, and blood in capillaries tends to move by bolus flow. The diameter of capillaries (5–6μm) is less than the width of the human red cell (8μm). Red cells, therefore, deform to enter capillaries and travel through the capillary circulation in single file. Classical laminar flow is impossible and the bolus of plasma trapped between each red cell is forced to travel along at uniform velocity. This is described as *bolus* or *plug flow*. Bolus flow eliminates some of the friction associated with laminar flow. The efficiency of bolus flow depends on the deformability of the red cell. This is reduced when the red cells have a sickle shape, as in sickle cell anemia. In hypoxic conditions, the red cell adopts a rigid sickle shape that impairs capillary flow and causes tissue damage (sickle cell crisis).

The viscosity of blood is affected by the diameter of the tube through which it is flowing; that is to say it is a non-Newtonian fluid. In tubes of diameter greater than 1mm, blood viscosity is independent of bore. This is known as the Fahraeus–Lindquist effect. In capillaries, bolus flow reduces viscosity. In arterioles, viscosity is reduced by the peripheral plasma stream produced by axial flow. Shear rates are highest peripherally and a reduction in friction at the margin has a marked effect. The effect

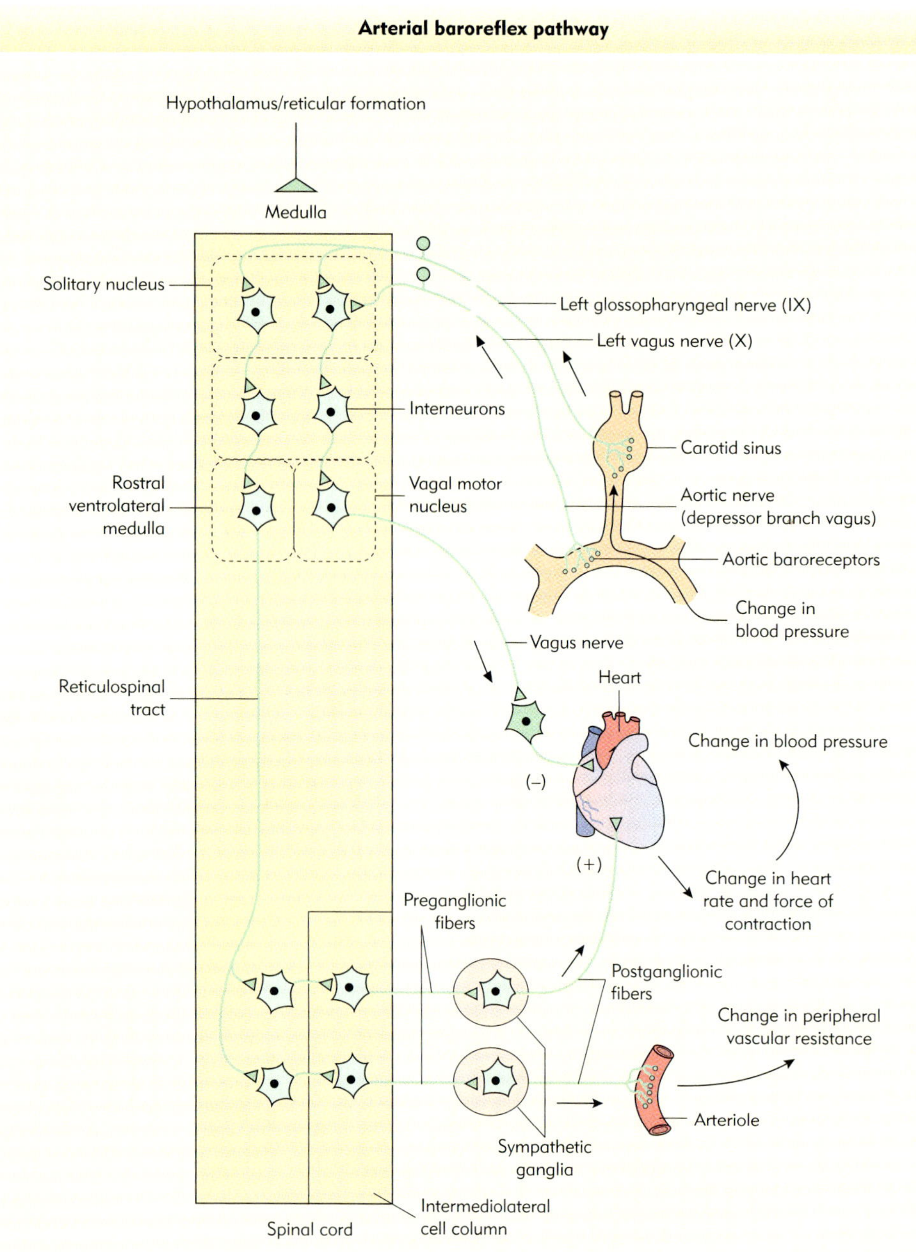

Figure 38.4 Schematic of the arterial baroreflex pathway. The afferent fibers travel in the glossopharyngeal (IX) and vagus (X) nerves, while the efferent fibers travel in the sympathetic nerves and vagus nerve.

declines in wider tubes because the thickness of the marginal layer becomes insignificant relative to the tube diameter. Viscosity also increases drastically as the hematocrit increases, and increases to a lesser degree with increasing plasma proteins. Thus, blood flow is impeded by increases in hematocrit (polycythemia) and facilitated by decreases (anemia, hemodilution).

CARDIOVASCULAR REGULATORY MECHANISMS

Long-term control of the circulation involves a number of mechanisms that control the circulating volume. These mechanisms respond to persistent elevation of arterial pressure by increasing salt and water output from the kidneys, which reduces extracellular fluid volume, blood volume, and cardiac filling pressures (Chapter 54). The reduction in cardiac filling leads to a fall in cardiac output and blood pressure. Over the following weeks, cardiac output returns to baseline but a persistent reduction in systemic vascular resistance develops so that lower arterial pressure is maintained.

Baroreflex control

In contrast to renal mechanisms that control circulating blood volume, cardiovascular reflexes are mediated by the autonomic nervous system and are rapid acting (Chapter 29). They control heart rate and vascular tone over a period of seconds rather than days. Arterial baroreflexes effect rapid control of arterial pressure (Fig. 38.4). The sensors for this baroreflex are arterial baroreceptors, which are stretch receptors in the walls of the aortic arch and the carotid sinus of the internal carotid arteries. Fibers from the carotid sinus baroreceptors travel in the carotid sinus nerves, which join the glossopharyngeal nerves. Those from the aortic baroreceptors travel in the aortic nerves, which join the vagus

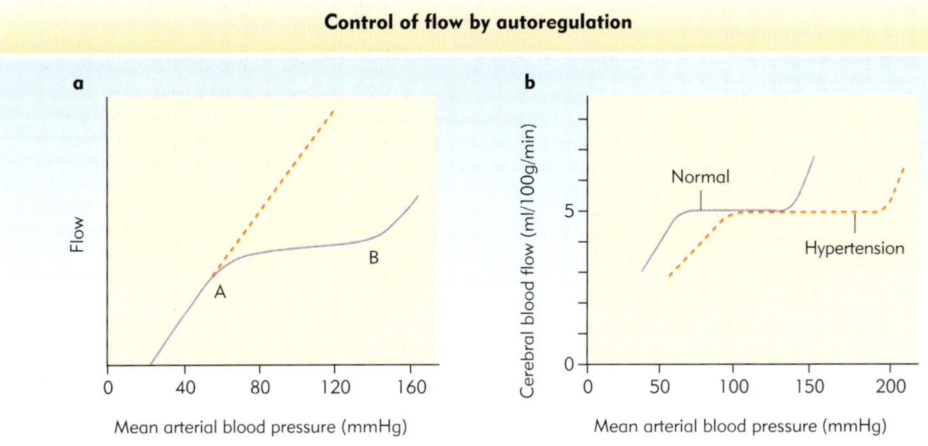

Figure 38.5 Control of flow by autoregulation. Pressure–flow curve showing autoregulation (left). Between A and B there is little change in flow with changes in perfusion pressure. Outside of this range, flow increases approximately linearly with pressure. The dotted line shows the pressure–flow relationship during absence of the autoregulatory response. Adaptation within the microcirculation is capable of shifting the autoregulated range to higher or lower pressures, as illustrated for the effect of chronic hypertension on cerebral blood flow (right).

nerves. The fibers travel to a sensory area in the nucleus tractus solitarius (solitary nucleus) in the medulla, from which they project to the pressor and depressor areas in the medulla. The former lies in the anterolateral portion of the upper medulla and the latter more medially in the lower medulla. There is a background tonic discharge from the baroreceptor afferents at normal arterial pressure. The discharge rate of the baroreceptor afferents increases in proportion to the stretching of the vessel wall by increasing arterial pressure: the greater the arterial pressure, the greater the rate of discharge. This, in turn, increases activity in the medullary depressor area and decreases activity in the pressor area. This results in an increase in vagal tone, which decreases heart rate and the sympathetic outflow to the heart and peripheral vasculature; in turn, this produces a decrease in myocardial contractility and a reduction in vascular tone and thus a fall in systemic vascular resistance. The baroreflex also affects the splanchnic arterioles and venules. Vasodilatation of the latter reduces venous return. The opposite effects are seen in response to a fall in blood pressure, when a pressor response is elicited, resulting in increases in heart rate, myocardial contractility, and vascular tone. The primary effect of the arterial baroreflex is on heart rate and contractility. The effect on systemic vascular resistance is of secondary importance.

The arterial baroreflex does not have a role in the long-term regulation of blood pressure. Rather the baroreflex resets (adapts) in the face of long-term increases or decreases in blood pressure. Decreased baroreflex responses are seen in hypertensive patients and with advancing age. Diseases such as diabetes and Parkinson's disease, which cause autonomic dysfunction, may attenuate or abolish the arterial baroreflex, as may drugs that interfere with autonomic function. The baroreflex response is also depressed by most anesthetic agents, most notably propofol. The arterial baroreflex response is most effective in the pressure range 80–150mmHg and responds more vigorously to decreases in pressure than increases. It is important for the rapid regulation of blood pressure: for example, in maintaining blood pressure when rising from supine.

Flow is locally controlled in certain vascular beds by *autoregulation*, or the ability of an organ to maintain relatively constant blood flow in the face of variations in perfusion pressure. At lower perfusion pressures, there is vasodilatation while higher perfusion pressures produce vasoconstriction. The result is a characteristic autoregulatory curve, as shown in Fig. 38.5. Within the limits of autoregulation, flow is constant despite variations in pressure. Outside the limits of autoregulation, flow is directly dependent on driving pressure. Autoregulation is seen in the kidneys, brain, and heart. In the skin and lungs, there is minimal autoregulation.

Autoregulation is an intrinsic property that is present even in denervated tissues. Two principal hypotheses attempt to explain the mechanism of autoregulation. According to the *myogenic hypothesis,* elevations in perfusion pressure stretch smooth muscle cells in the vessel wall and cause contraction and vasoconstriction. A reduction in pressure and stretch leads to relaxation. The *metabolic hypothesis* suggests that reduced perfusion pressure reduces blood flow and consequently causes a reduction in tissue oxygen partial pressure and an increase in tissue carbon dioxide partial pressure and other metabolites (lactic acid, adenosine, and potassium and hydrogen ions). The accumulating metabolites and reduced oxygen content then directly cause vasodilatation. Conversely, high perfusion pressures increase blood flow, providing ample tissue oxygen and washing out metabolites. This causes vasoconstriction and a reduction in blood flow.

REGIONAL BLOOD FLOW

Heart

Myocardial capillary density is very high (3000–5000 capillaries per mm^2), which provides extensive endothelial surface area for exchange and reduces the maximum diffusion distance to approximately 9μm. Myocardial oxygen consumption is also very high, of the order of 8mL/min per 100g tissue, or 20 times greater than skeletal muscle. With exercise, cardiac work can increase five-fold and oxygen delivery must increase accordingly.

The myocardium extracts 65–75% of the oxygen from coronary blood, compared with whole body extraction of approximately 25% at rest. Consequently, the extra oxygen required for high work rates must be provided by increased blood flow. During light to moderate work, coronary blood flow increases almost linearly with myocardial oxygen consumption. At high work rates, blood flow lags behind somewhat and myocardial oxygen extraction increases. During exercise, coronary oxygen extraction can rise to 90%. This increase in blood flow is an example of metabolic hyperemia. Myocardial arteries and arterioles are well innervated by sympathetic vasoconstrictor fibers and their tonic discharge contributes to arteriolar tone. This effect is overcome by metabolic vasodilatation with increasing myocardial work, although the predominant vasodilator substance remains unclear. Autoregulation is well developed in the coronary circulation and is reset by metabolic vasodilatation to operate at a higher flow.

The branches of the coronary arteries within the myocardium are compressed during systole. This effect is most marked in the left ventricle during isovolumic contraction, when pressure in the ventricular wall may reach 240mmHg and coronary blood pressure is at its nadir, approximately 80mmHg (Chapter 34). Consequently in the left ventricle, coronary blood flow ceases briefly and may even reverse during systole. Flow is only fully restored in diastole, and at basal heart rates 80% of coronary blood flow occurs during diastole.

Lungs

The whole output of the right ventricle flows through the alveolar capillary bed (Chapter 44). Therefore, perfusion greatly exceeds pulmonary needs, and metabolic factors do not influence flow. There is an independent systemic bronchial circulation that meets the needs of the bronchi. Pulmonary vascular resistance is about one-eighth of the systemic vascular resistance; as a result, pulmonary arterial pressure is low (20–25mmHg in systole and 6–12mmHg in diastole). Pulmonary arteries and arterioles are shorter and thinner than systemic vessels. There is low basal tone in the pulmonary circulation and no autoregulation. Sympathetic motor nerves exist but have a poorly defined role. Resistance is shared between the arteries, microvasculature, and veins. Consequently, pulmonary capillary pressure is approximately midway between mean pulmonary arterial pressure and left atrial pressure (8–11mmHg). Elevation of left atrial pressure to 20–25mmHg raises capillary pressure sufficiently to cause pulmonary edema. Vascular conductance increases with perfusion pressure (Fig. 38.6), probably through vascular distension and the recruitment of vessels that were initially closed by airway pressure.

Pulmonary vessels also differ from systemic vessels in their response to hypoxia. If ventilation to a local region falls, alveolar oxygen content falls and carbon dioxide content increases. The small pulmonary arteries that pass close to the surface of small airways respond to this change by vasoconstriction, while bronchial smooth muscle responds to airway hypercapnia by relaxation. These changes tend to maintain an optimal ventilation/perfusion ratio (Chapter 44).

The pulmonary circulation can act as a blood reservoir. Pulmonary blood volume is about 600mL in a supine man. If intrathoracic airway pressure is raised by a Valsalva maneuver, the external pressure on the blood vessels can expel up to half the blood content. On forced inspiration, which lowers intrathoracic pressure, pulmonary blood volume can increase to about 1L. The pulmonary capacitance vessels act as a transient source of blood for the left ventricle when output begins to increase at the start of exercise.

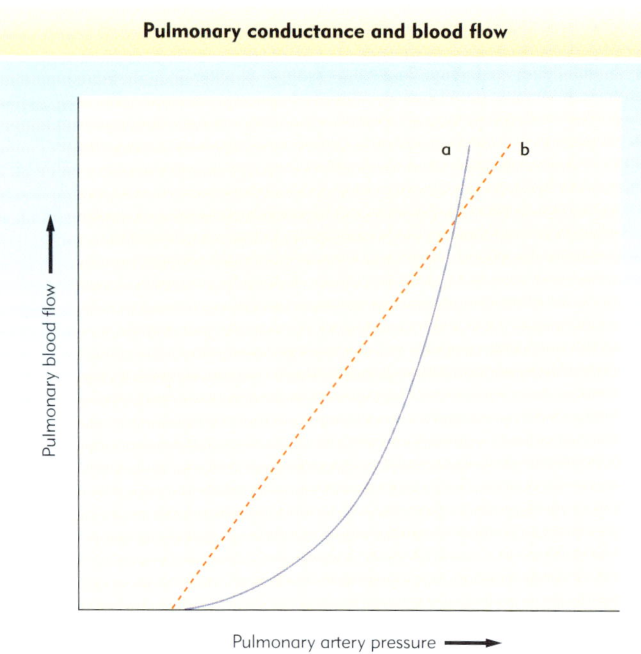

Figure 38.6 Pulmonary conductance and blood flow. A non-linear relationship is observed between perfusion pressure and flow (a). A linear relationship would be expected with constant pulmonary vascular resistance (b).

Splanchnic circulation

The splanchnic circulation comprises the gastric, small intestinal, colonic, pancreatic, hepatic, and splenic circulations. They are arranged in parallel and are fed by the celiac artery and the superior and inferior mesenteric arteries. Resistance arterioles are the primary determinants of vascular resistance in the splanchnic circulation. Neuronal control of the mesenteric circulation is almost entirely sympathetic; parasympathetic fibers from the vagus nerves have little effect on blood flow. Mechanoreceptor reflexes, particularly the low-pressure cardiopulmonary systems, are closely involved in splanchnic arterial and venous vascular tone. Overall, splanchnic blood flow receives about 25% of cardiac output. The splanchnic venous capacitance reservoir contains about one-third of the total blood volume. Sympathetic postganglionic fibers cause arteriolar vasoconstriction and decrease splanchnic perfusion. Sympathetic stimulation also contracts the smooth muscle of the capacitance veins in the splanchnic circulation and may expel a large volume of pooled blood from the splanchnic into the systemic circulation. Autoregulation in the splanchnic circulation is less marked than in the cerebral, cardiac, or renal circulations. The response is present, however, and serves to restore blood flow to hypoperfused areas. The splanchnic circulation also responds to reduced perfusion pressure by the redistribution of blood flow within individual organs. For example, in hypovolemic shock perfusion usually favors the mucosa of the gut at the expense of the mucosa muscularis.

The liver is unique in that it has both an arterial and venous afferent blood supply. In the resting adult, the liver receives approximately 0.5L/min blood via the hepatic artery and a further 1.3L/min from the portal circulation (see Chapter 61).

Kidneys

The kidneys constitute less than 0.5% of body weight, yet they receive about 20% of the cardiac output, and this percentage can be increased further. Renal blood flow is regulated to maintain optimum delivery of filtrate to the nephrons and adequate reabsorption of fluid back into the vascular system (Chapter 54).

Flow is well beyond that required to supply the metabolic needs of the kidneys.

The renal vasculature has a sympathetic innervation. Both norepinephrine (noradrenaline) and epinephrine (adrenaline) released from the adrenal medulla activate α_1-adrenoeptors and cause renal vasoconstriction, which decreases renal blood flow and glomerular filtration. The renal innervation also includes dopaminergic nerves. Activation of dopamine D_1receptors in the kidneys causes significant increases in both cortical and medullary blood flow. The kidneys display autoregulation of blood flow over a range of mean perfusion pressure from 75 to 180mmHg. Outside this range, flow is pressure-dependent. Autoregulation is demonstrable in isolated kidneys and is, therefore, assumed to be mediated by factors intrinsic to the kidney.

The renin–angiotensin system is described in Chapter 56. Angiotensin II is a potent vasoconstrictor. Although it does have an effect on afferent arterioles, its primary effect appears to be constriction of efferent arterioles. It acts to maintain renal glomerular filtration even when renal plasma flow is reduced. Prostaglandins E_2 and I_2 are produced within the kidney during hemorrhagic hypovolemia. They cause dilatation of the efferent and afferent arterioles and so help to prevent severe vasoconstriction and ischemia in the face of hypovolemia.

Muscle

The blood supply to skeletal muscle must supply metabolic needs that vary greatly between rest and vigorous exercise. Skeletal muscle constitutes 40% of adult body mass. The resistance of this large vascular bed has a substantial effect on blood pressure. Skeletal muscle arterioles are innervated by sympathetic vasoconstrictor fibers and their tonic discharge maintains a high vascular tone. This is essential if marked vasodilation is to be possible during exercise. Further vasoconstriction is also possible. During strenuous exercise, muscle blood flow accounts for 80–90% of cardiac output. Muscle hyperemia results almost entirely from a fall in vascular resistance through metabolic-mediated vasodilatation rather than from changes in arterial blood pressure. Blood flow increases almost linearly with local metabolic rate. The nature of the vasodilator agents is controversial. Initial vasodilation appears to be caused by local increases in interstitial K^+ concentration and osmolality. Perfusion during exercise is also increased to some extent by the effect of the skeletal muscle pump, whereby the rhythmic massaging of the calf muscles on the deep veins assists limb perfusion. Resting skeletal muscle extracts only 25–30% of oxygen from the blood. In severe exercise extraction can reach 80–90%. Despite this, intracellular oxygen tension may fall so low in severe exercise that anaerobic metabolism predominates, leading to the production of lactic acid and an oxygen debt.

Skin

Skin blood flow is controlled primarily by sympathetic vasomotor fibers; the activity of these fibers is linked to temperature regulation. Certain skin areas possess abundant direct connections between dermal arterioles and venules called arteriovenous anastomoses (AVAs) (Fig. 38.7). They occur at exposed sites with a high surface area to volume ratio (e.g. fingers, toes, palm, sole, lips, nose, and ears) and are coiled muscular walled vessels of 35μm average diameter. They are controlled almost exclusively by sympathetic vasoconstrictor fibers, the activity of which is controlled by a temperature-regulating center in the

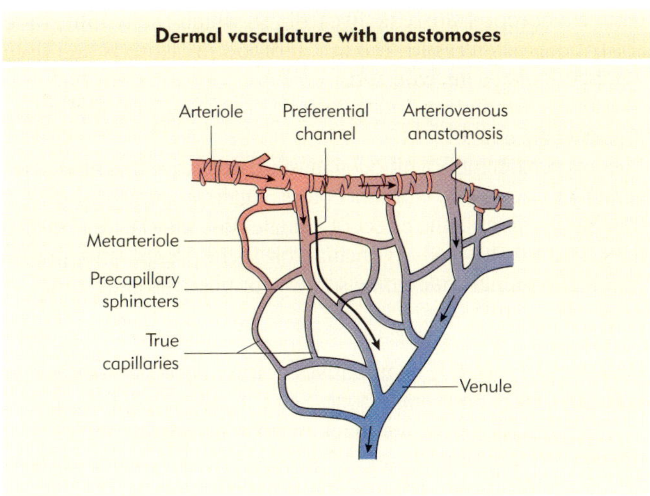

Figure 38.7 The dermal vasculature, showing arteriovenous anastomoses.

hypothalamus (Chapter 64). When core temperature is high, vasomotor drive is reduced and the AVAs dilate. They offer a low-resistance shunt pathway that increases cutaneous blood flow and heat delivery to the skin. Heat readily crosses the walls of the dermal venous plexus fed by the AVAs so skin temperature rises and heat loss increases. Conversely, AVAs are constricted to conserve heat under cold conditions.

The cutaneous circulation participates in many cardiovascular reflexes. Hypotension reflexly elicits constriction of the cutaneous veins and arterioles, producing the pale cold skin characteristic of shock. The rise in cutaneous vascular resistance helps to support blood pressure while the venoconstriction displaces blood centrally and helps to support central venous pressure.

Areas of skin may be subject to high pressures for long periods during sitting, standing, and lying and this may compromise local blood flow. Ischemic damage is prevented by the high tolerance of skin for hypoxia, reactive hyperemia on removal of the stress, and the onset of restlessness as metabolites accumulate and stimulate skin nociceptors. The last mechanism fails in patients such as paraplegics, the frail elderly, and, of course, patients under anesthesia and in the intensive-care unit. If appropriate precautions are not taken, such patients may suffer pressure necrosis (bed sores).

PHARMACOLOGIC CONTROL OF BLOOD PRESSURE

Perioperative hypertension may put undue strain on the heart and lead to myocardial ischemia. Perioperative hypotension may compromise the perfusion of the heart, the brain, and other organs. Conversely, a degree of hypotension may be useful in some types of surgery. A number of vasoconstrictors and vasodilators are available for the manipulation of blood pressure. Vasodilators and vasopressors affecting the sympathetic and parasympathetic nervous system are also discussed in Chapter 29.

Vasodilators

Phentolamine

Phentolamine binds reversibly to postsynaptic α_1-adrenoceptors and presynaptic α_2-adrenoceptors. Postsynaptic blockade causes marked arterial vasodilatation and a fall in blood pressure. This causes a compensatory tachycardia to which the α_2-blockade contributes; as a result, the fall in blood pressure is less than would otherwise be expected.

Phenoxybenzamine

Phenoxybenzamine is a nitrogen mustard derivative that binds irreversibly to α_1- and α_2-adrenoceptors. Again it causes vasodilatation but in this case the effect of a single dose may last for several days. The drug has had a particular role in the preoperative preparation of patients undergoing surgery for pheochromocytoma.

Prazosin

Prazosin is a selective competitive α_1-adrenoceptor blocker that reduces arterial and venous tone. Since α_2-adrenoceptors are not blocked, the negative feedback of norepinephrine on its own release is not inhibited and tachycardia does not occur. It has a greater affinity for α_1-adrenoceptors in veins than in arteries and for this reason its effects resemble those of nitroglycerin (glyceryl trinitrate) more than those of phentolamine or hydralazine.

Labetalol

Labetalol combines α_1-adrenoceptor-blocking and nonselective β-receptor-blocking activity. It produces a decrease in systemic arterial pressure because of simultaneous reductions in systemic vascular resistance and cardiac output. When given intravenously, the β-blocking effect is seven-fold more potent than the α_1-blocking effect.

Sodium nitroprusside

Sodium nitroprusside (SNP) consists of a ferrous iron atom bound with five cyanide molecules and one nitric group. Contact with blood decomposes the molecule, releasing nitric oxide. The nitric oxide binds to the ferrous ion moiety of guanylyl cyclase, with subsequent production of cGMP. Increased levels of intracellular cGMP reduce cytosolic calcium ion levels and cause dephosphorylation of the myosin light chains, leading to smooth muscle relaxation (Chapter 33). SNP acts within 1 to 2 minutes and its effect dissipates within a few minutes of discontinuation of the infusion. The ferrous iron reacts with sulfhydryl groups in red blood cells and releases cyanide. This cyanide is reduced to thiocyanate in the liver and is excreted in the urine. However, the half-life of thiocyanate is 4 days and this is considerably increased in renal failure. The potential for thiocyanate toxicity (treated with thiosulfate and nitrite) limits the dose and duration of use of SNP.

Organic nitrates

Organic nitrates such as nitroglycerin and isosorbide mononitrate and dinitrate also act by the release of nitric oxide. Unlike SNP, their dose and duration of use is not limited by thiocyanate accumulation.

Calcium channel blockers

Calcium channel blockers act by blocking membrane Ca^{2+} channels (Chapter 33). They inhibit transmembrane Ca^{2+} influx to reduce smooth muscle tone and cause vasodilatation.

Hydralazine

Hydralazine is a potent vasodilator of arterioles; it has little or no effect on venous smooth muscle. Its precise mode of action is unclear. Its action is endothelium-dependent, suggesting a role for nitric oxide. It also interferes with the mobilization of calcium ions in vascular smooth muscle. Its use is associated with a baroreflex-mediated increase in sympathetic activity, causing increased heart rate and contractility and an increase in plasma renin activity. The drug has a slow onset (15–30 minutes). The elimination half-life is about 4 hours, but the effective half-life is approximately 100 hours because of its avid binding to smooth muscle. Because of these unfavorable properties, it is giving way to newer drugs for the short-term control of blood pressure.

Fenoldopam

Fenoldopam is a new rapid-acting vasodilator with a unique mechanism of action. It is a dopamine D_1 receptor agonist that causes smooth muscle relaxation and vasodilatation in a variety of vascular beds, including renal and coronary. Fenoldopam induces rapid and reversible reductions in blood pressure that are comparable to those seen with SNP but without the problems with stability and cyanide toxicity.

Phosphodiesterase inhibitors

Phosphodiesterase inhibitors prevent cyclic nucleotide breakdown and cause vasodilatation and reduced peripheral vascular resistance in addition to their inotropic effect. Such 'inodilators' include the specific phosphodiesterase III inhibitors amrinone, milrinone, and enoximone.

Vasopressors

Vasopressors raise blood pressure, but their use is associated with a number of other cardiac and regional hemodynamic effects. Peripheral vasoconstriction produces a reflex bradycardia and reduction in cardiac output mediated via baroreflexes. Increased preload (owing to venoconstriction) and afterload (owing to arteriolar constriction) increases myocardial oxygen demand. Vasoconstriction may be most marked in the renal, hepatic, and splanchnic beds and carries the risk of severe hypoperfusion and organ failure. In anesthetic practice, vasopressors are used to counteract the hypotension produced by sympathetic blockade during regional anesthesia or by vasodilatation during general anesthesia. They are used to control perfusion pressure during cardiopulmonary bypass and to support the circulation during cardiopulmonary resuscitation and in the treatment of septic shock.

The sympathomimetic amines are the principal vasopressors currently in clinical use. Vasoconstriction caused by sympathomimetic amines is mediated by stimulation of α_1- and α_2-adrenoceptors. They may exert their effects directly on the receptors or indirectly by displacing endogenous norepinephrine from adrenergic nerve terminals. They should be used with considerable caution in patients taking monoamine oxidase (MAO) inhibitors because of the potential for unpredictable hypertensive responses.

Phenylephrine

Phenylephrine is a potent α_1-adrenoceptor agonist with no activity at β-adrenoceptors in clinical doses. Following a single dose, mean arterial pressure rises mainly through an increase in diastolic pressure. Systemic vascular resistance increases and a baroreflex-mediated reduction in heart rate and cardiac output is observed. These effects are seen within about 1 minute of injection and last for about 10 minutes. Doses of 50 to 100μg or an infusion of up to 3μg/min per kg body weight are generally used.

Methoxamine

Methoxamine is an α-adrenoceptor agonist with β-adrenoceptor-blocking actions. It increases systolic and diastolic pressure by increasing systemic vascular resistance. A response is seen within about 1 minute of injection and lasts for about 20 minutes. Heart rate decreases because of the β-adrenoceptor-blocking action and the baroceptor response to raised blood pressure.

Ephedrine

Ephedrine has direct β_1- and β_2-adrenoceptor agonist effects and indirectly releases norepinephrine from adrenergic nerve endings. It increases myocardial contractility and heart rate and, thus, increases cardiac output. Its vasoconstrictive effects tend to be counterbalanced by its tendency to cause β_2-mediated vasodilatation; consequently, there is usually little change in systemic vascular resistance. Diastolic and systolic pressure both increase. Doses of 3–6mg titrated to effect are usually given and its duration of action may be up to 20 minutes. Ephedrine reduces uterine contractility and tends to restore and maintain uterine blood flow. It is, therefore, widely used in obstetric anesthetic practice.

Metaraminol

Metaraminol acts both directly and indirectly to stimulate both α- and β-adrenoceptors. Like ephedrine, it tends to increase cardiac contractility and cardiac output. However, it also increases systemic vascular resistance and may produce a reflex bradycardia.

HYPERTENSION AND ANTIHYPERTENSIVE THERAPY

Hypertension is common and is associated with considerable cardiovascular morbidity. Individuals with persistently elevated blood pressure are at increased risk of stroke, coronary artery disease, left ventricular hypertrophy (LVH), and left ventricular failure. Systolic and diastolic blood pressures are continuous variables, and there are a number of definitions of what constitutes hypertension. With regard to drug treatment, the Joint National Committee of the National High Blood Pressure Education Program in the United States suggested that treatment is justified for a diastolic blood pressure above 94mmHg over a period of 3–6 months. The British Hypertension Society recommends treatment for a diastolic blood pressure over 100mmHg during the assessment period. In 'white coat hypertension', subjects who have a normal blood pressure on ambulatory monitoring or self-administered home blood pressure examination have raised blood pressure when examined by a doctor or nurse.

A specific cause for elevated blood pressure can be found in 6–8% of patients; this is secondary hypertension. The remainder of hypertension is described as primary or essential hypertension. The precise mechanisms of hypertension are not fully understood, and different mechanisms may operate in different patients. Hypertension is probably multifactorial and subject to both genetic and environmental influences. There is also increasing evidence for a relationship between intrauterine growth rate on blood pressure in later life.

A distinction is made between low-renin and high-renin hypertension. In the former, plasma renin activity is low, systemic vascular resistance is moderately elevated, and there is increased plasma volume and an elevated cardiac output. In high-renin hypertension, plasma renin activity is elevated and systemic vascular resistance is raised to a greater extent than in low-renin hypertension. Plasma volume and cardiac output are reduced and blood viscosity may be increased.

Hypertension produces structural changes in the cardiovascular system. Blood vessels exhibit endothelial dysfunction, smooth muscle replication or hypertrophy, intimal thickening, and migration of smooth muscles into the subintimal space. These changes are accompanied by alterations in collagen and elastin content. One result of these changes is an increased ratio of wall to inner radius. This, in turn, results in exaggerated changes in luminal diameter for any given change in vascular smooth muscle tone.

LVH is found in 50% of patients with stage I or II hypertension and is produced by changes in myocyte size, shape, and number. It is an ominous sign, as mortality from ischemic heart disease is increased three-fold in patients with LVH. It is not uncommon for LVH to progress to left ventricular failure. Stroke is a major cause of death in hypertensive patients. Indeed the most marked benefit from the treatment of hypertension is a reduction in the incidence of cerebrovascular accidents. Hypertension may be a cause and/or a consequence of renal impairment and adds considerably to the morbidity of renal disease.

Antihypertensive therapy has been shown to reduce the incidence of stroke, coronary events, congestive heart failure, and all-cause mortality. There is no absolute agreement as to the blood pressure at which treatment should be initiated. Many practitioners initiate drug therapy for stage I hypertension, while the British Hypertension Society recommends such patients undergo 3 to 6 months of nondrug therapy and observation before drug treatment is considered. There is also disagreement regarding the targets for treatment, but the view is emerging that treatment should be tailored to the patient and take into account age, sex, and other risk factors. Again there is disagreement about initial therapy. The Fifth National Committee on the Detection, Evaluation, and Treatment of High Blood Pressure recommended that diuretics or β-adrenoceptor agonists be the preferred first-line therapy. Many disagree with this and it has been suggested that treatment should be prescribed following a 24-hour urine collection for Na^+ measurement and an estimation of plasma renin activity. Patients with high plasma renin activity are candidates for β-adrenoceptor antagonists and angiotensin-converting enzyme (ACE) inhibitors, while those with low plasma renin activity should receive diuretics, α-adrenoceptor antagonists, or calcium channel blockers.

Antihypertensive therapy

Beta-adrenoceptor antagonists

Antagonism of β_1-adrenoceptors is valuable for the suppression of renin production. Characteristics of particular β-blockers are relevant with regard to pharmacokinetic profile, duration of action, side-effect profile, and so forth.

Angiotension-converting enzyme inhibitors

ACE inhibitors are useful for monotherapy or for combined therapy in the treatment of high-renin hypertension. Their acute hypotensive effect occurs through the reduction in circulating angiotensin II. Their longer-term effects seem to depend on other mechanisms, including tissue angiotensin inhibition, degradation of bradykinin, or an increase in endothelium-dependent relaxation. The combination of β_1-adrenoceptor antagonists and ACE inhibitors may be of particular value in preventing vascular damage in high-renin hypertension.

Diuretics

Diuretics are ineffective in high-renin hypertension but are the cornerstone of the treatment of low-renin hypertension. Low doses may provide satisfactory control of blood pressure without producing hypokalemia.

Calcium channel blockers

Calcium channel blockers are best used in low-renin hypertension. In these circumstances, Na^+ administration may paradoxically enhance the hypotensive effect.

Alpha-adrenoceptor antagonists

The α-adrenoceptor antagonists include prazosin and the longer-acting drugs terazosin and doxazosin. Again they are best used in low-renin hypertension.

Hypertension and anesthesia

It was established in the early 1970s that treated hypertensive patients, especially those treated with β-blockers, exhibited smaller hemodynamic responses to anesthesia and awakening than untreated hypertensive patients (Fig. 38.8). The β-blockers almost abolish the risk of myocardial ischemia and dysrhythmias. The greater blood pressure stability in adequately treated hypertension suggests that all hypertensive patients should have their hypertension properly controlled before elective surgery. Of course, such a policy would result in a large number of operations being canceled as, even now, a large proportion of hypertensive patients are untreated and among those who are treated, many have blood pressure that is still outside the normal range (i.e. not fully controlled). The issue is further complicated by the fact that several epidemiologic studies including those of Goldman *et al.* (1977) and Detsky *et al.* (1986) have failed to identify hypertension as a significant predictor of adverse outcome. As yet, no study, has shown conclusively that treatment of hypertension brings about a significant improvement in outcome.

Because of this uncertainty, an empirical approach to elective surgery has evolved. Patients with stage III hypertension (diastolic arterial pressure greater than 110mmHg) are referred for treatment; those with stage II hypertension (diastolic arterial pressure between 100 and 109mmHg) are considered for treatment especially if they have signs of coronary artery disease, cerebrovascular disease, or impaired renal function; those with mild hypertension do not usually have their operations canceled. This approach reduces the number of operations canceled but does not necessarily prevent complications because some patients with untreated mild or moderate hypertension can be extremely unstable.

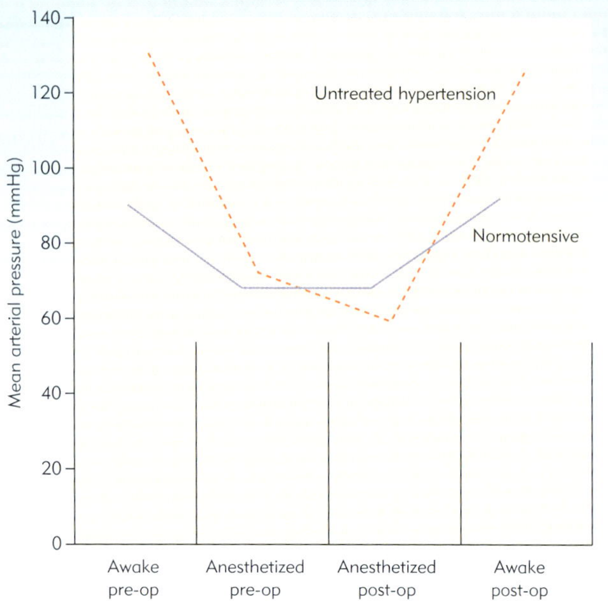

Figure 38.8 Changes in arterial blood pressure with induction of anesthesia. Normotensive patients (treated) and patients with uncontrolled hypertension (untreated) react differently to anasthesia. (Modified with permission from Prys-Roberts et al., 1971.)

Key References

Bristow DJ, Prys-Roberts-C, Fisher A, Pickering TG, Sleight P. Effects of anesthesia on baroreflex control of heart rate in man. Anesthesiology. 1969;31:422–8.

Burton AC. Physiol Rev. 1954;34:619.

Detsky AS, Abrams HB, McLaughlin JR, Drucker DJ, Sasson Z, Johnston N, Scott JG, Forbath N, Hilliard JR. Predicting cardiac complications in patients undergoing non-cardiac surgery. J Internal Med. 1986; 1:211–9.

Goldman L, Caldera DL, Nussbaum SR, et al. Multifactorial index of cardiac risk in noncardiac surgical procedures. N Engl J Med. 1977;297:845–50.

Marshall BE, Marshall C. Active regulation of the pulmonary circulation. In: Will J, Dawson CA, Weir EK, Buckner CK, eds. The pulmonary circulation in health and disease. Orlando, FL: Academic Press; 1987:252.

Prys-Roberts C, Meloche R, Foëx P. Studies of anesthesia in relation to hypertension I. Cardiovascular responses of treated and untreated patients. Br J Anaesth. 1971;43:122–37.

Further Reading

Priebe H-J, Skarvan K, eds. Cardiovascular physiology. London: BMJ Publishing; 1995.

Levick JR. An introduction to cardiovascular physiology. Oxford: Butterworth Heinemann; 1991.

Chapter 39 Ischemic heart disease and heart failure

Uday Jain

Topics covered in this chapter

Myocardial ischemia
Myocardial infarction
Heart failure
Toxic cardiomyopathy
Pericardial tamponade
Pulmonary embolism

Ischemic heart disease and heart failure are the most common forms of heart disease in the adult. Heart disease may lead to limitation of functional capacity, which has been classified by the New York Heart Association (NYHA):

class I: ordinary physical activity does not cause symptoms of fatigue, palpitation, dyspnea, or angina;
class II: ordinary physical activity causes symptoms that are not present at rest;
class III: less than ordinary physical activity causes symptoms that are not present at rest;
class IV: any physical activity causes symptoms, which may also be present at rest.

Patients with heart disease have greater perioperative morbidity [e.g. myocardial infarction (MI), congestive heart failure], and mortality, with greatest problems in those with more severe NYHA class disease (Fig. 39.1). Because of the high risk of cardiac complications, only emergency surgery should be performed in patients with unstable angina or decompensated heart failure (NYHA class IV).

Coronary artery disease (CAD) resulting from atherosclerosis is the usual cause of ischemic heart disease. Ischemia and infarction may result when there is increased myocardial oxygen demand through increases in contractility, volume or pressure load, and tachycardia and/or when supply is reduced because of lower coronary perfusion pressure, tachycardia, thrombi, emboli, vasospasm, and platelet plugging. Left coronary artery flow is predominantly diastolic, whereas right coronary artery flow to the right ventricle (RV), which is at a lower pressure, occurs in systole as well as in diastole (see Fig. 34.9). As the diastolic duration is substantially reduced at higher heart rates, coronary perfusion is impaired (Fig. 39.2). Myocardial perfusion depends primarily on aortic pressure, which is generated by the heart itself. The back pressure for flow in the left coronary artery is at least the higher of left ventricular (LV) end-diastolic pressure (EDP) and coronary sinus pressure. LV coronary perfusion pressure is the difference between aortic diastolic blood pressure and the back pressure. Coronary autoregulation maintains a constant coronary blood flow for perfusion pressures of 60–120mmHg by changes in coronary resistance, which is determined primarily by intramyocardial arterioles (Fig. 39.3). Adenosine, and to a lesser extent oxygen and carbon dioxide tensions, pH, and lactic acid and K^+ concentrations, affect coronary vascular resistance and may mediate the close link between coronary blood flow and metabolism. Increase in perfusion pressure

Clinical predictors of increased perioperative cardiovascular risk

Major

Unstable coronary syndromes
- Recent myocardial infarction[a] with evidence of important ischemic risk based on clinical symptoms or noninvasive study
- Unstable or severe[b] angina

Decompensated congestive heart failure

Significant arrhythmias

High-grade atrioventricular block
- Symptomatic ventricular arrhythmias in the presence of underlying heart disease
- Supraventricular arrhythmias with uncontrolled ventricular rate
- Severe valvular disease

Intermediate

Mild angina pectoris

Prior myocardial infarction based on history or electrocardiographic changes

Compensated or prior congestive heart failure

Diabetes mellitus

Minor

Advanced age

Abnormal electrocardiographic findings (left ventricular hypertrophy, left bundle branch block, ST–T abnormalities)

Rhythm other than sinus (for example, atrial fibrillation)

Low functional capacity (for example, unable to climb one flight of stairs while carrying bag of groceries)

History of stroke

Uncontrolled systemic hypertension

[a]The American College of Cardiology National Database Library defines recent myocardial infarction as greater than 7 days but less than or equal to 1 month (30 days).
[b]May include 'stable' angina in patients who are unusually sedentary.

Figure 39.1 Clinical predictors of increased perioperative cardiovascular risk (myocardial infarction, congestive heart failure, or death).

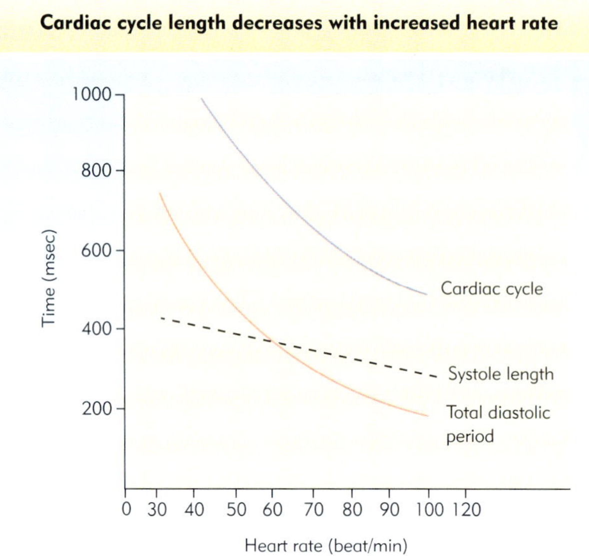

Figure 39.2 Increase in heart rate causes a decrease in the length of each cardiac cycle. The decrease in the length of systole with increase in heart rate is far less dramatic than the decrease in the length of diastole. Small changes in heart rate cause large decreases in the percentage of time spent in diastole.

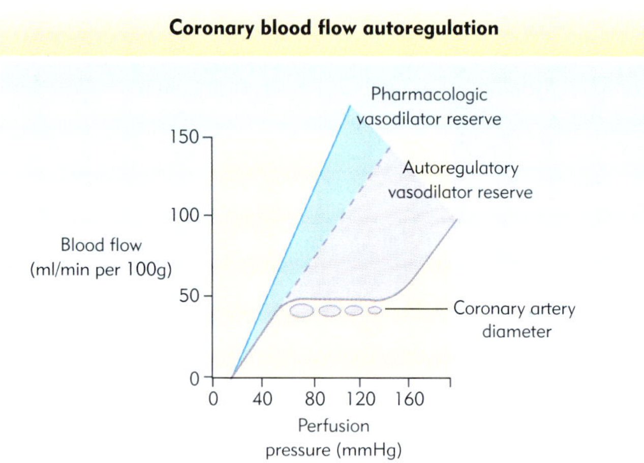

Figure 39.3 The variation of coronary blood flow with coronary perfusion pressure. Coronary blood flow is constant (autoregulated) over coronary perfusion pressures from 60 to 140mmHg. At 60mmHg, there is maximal autoregulatory vasodilatation to maintain coronary blood flow. Further decreases in coronary perfusion pressure result in decreases in coronary blood flow. At pressures above 60mmHg, vasodilatation provides autoregulatory vasodilator reserve (coronary reserve). This reserve provides the increased coronary blood flow necessary to meet increases in myocardial oxygen consumption such as those induced by exercise. Infusion of vasodilators at perfusion pressures below the autoregulation range may further increase coronary blood flow. The flat (autoregulatory) portion of the curve is shifted up to higher flow levels by increases in the metabolic state of the heart, myocardial oxygen consumption.

causes reflex coronary vasoconstriction (autoregulation). Acetylcholine, bradykinins, and prostaglandins release endothelium-derived relaxing factor (EDRF; nitric oxide), causing vasodilatation. Coronary vasodilatation is also caused by β_2-adrenoceptor stimulation, whereas vasoconstriction is caused by parasympathetic stimulation and α_1-adrenoceptor stimulation; these primarily affect large epicardial arteries. Interruption of coronary blood flow for as little as 1 second leads to a great transient increase in coronary flow, termed reactive hyperemia, through local myogenic responses.

Arrhythmias of many types are frequent complications of ischemia and infarction. Re-entry in the ischemic epicardium or ectopic foci in endocardial Purkinje fibers surviving in the infarct zone are frequent causes (see Chapter 35). Ischemia and infarction of the inferior-posterior LV is associated with first-degree block, Mobitz type I second-degree block, and transient atrioventricular third-degree blocks. Ischemia and infarction of the anterior LV is associated with Mobitz type II second-degree block, occasional permanent infranodal block, and intraventricular conduction defects.

A number of noninvasive tests are used for the detection of CAD and to evaluate patients with known CAD whose condition has worsened. During these tests, ischemia is provoked by increasing myocardial oxygen demand and possibly by reducing supply (e.g. via exercise or use of dobutamine). Alternatively, agents such as dipyridamole or adenosine are used to cause myocardial blood flow redistribution (steal) via collaterals from poorly perfused (flow restricted) to well-perfused areas, leading to ischemia. Ischemia or flow redistribution may be detected via electrocardiography (ECG), echocardiography, or scintigraphy.

Medical management should be optimized in patients with provocable ischemia. If coronary angiography and revascularization are indicated, they should be performed prior to elective noncardiac surgery. The diagnostic testing and medical management of a patient are generally the same whether or not surgery is to be performed. Even in patients with CAD, postoperative mortality is not primarily from cardiac causes.

MYOCARDIAL ISCHEMIA

Normal myocardial oxygen consumption ($M\dot{V}O_2$) is 6–8mL/min per 100g tissue. Of this, about 20% is for basal metabolism, 1% for electrical activation, 15% for volume work, and about 65% for pressure work. If heart rate, pressure work, or contractility increase by 50%, myocardial oxygen consumption also increases by 50%. An increase in wall stress (chamber pressure × chamber radius/wall thickness) by 50% causes about a 25% increase in myocardial oxygen consumption. An increase in volume work by 50% causes only about 5% increase in myocardial oxygen consumption.

Ischemia leads to contractile dysfunction. On re-establishment of adequate perfusion, reversible contractile dysfunction may persist for hours to days in the absence of necrosis; this is termed stunning. Patients with ischemic heart disease may have chronic contractile dysfunction that can be reversed by revascularization; this is termed hibernation.

With myocardial ischemia, anerobic glycolysis, which accounts for up to 50% of glycolytic flux, replaces oxidative phosphorylation as the primary source of ATP. Fatty acids that normally undergo β-oxidation are instead converted to triglycerides and deposited in the tissue. During ischemia, there is an increase in lactate, ADP, AMP, glucose 6-phosphate, and fructose 6-phosphate. There is a decrease in creatine phosphate, ATP, glycogen, and fructose 1,6-bisphosphate. The deterioration in ventricular function is measurable after 1 minute of ischemia and is substantial after 10 minutes even though ATP levels deteriorate more slowly.

Damage to the myocardium on reperfusion following prolonged ischemia is termed reperfusion injury. It results, in part, from rapid exchange of mitochondrial protons with cytoplasmic Ca^{2+} ions. Intracellular accumulation of free radicals leads to reduced high-energy phosphate production and ultrastructural damage.

In the preoperative period, an episode of reversible ischemia occurring in a resting patient with a history of chronic stable angina may be triggered by pain, discomfort, psychologic stress, or physiologic derangement. The occurrence of reversible ischemia indicates that the patient is under greater stress than can safely be withstood. Stressful conditions that lead to ischemia may also lead to MI. Hence, reversible ischemia should be treated and the precipitating causes removed.

Perioperative ischemia is frequently silent (i.e. not associated with symptoms such as angina). The modalities commonly used for perioperative ischemia detection include ECG and transesophageal echocardiography (TEE). The term ischemia usually refers to reversible ischemia; however, many changes observed perioperatively via ECG and TEE result from irreversible ischemia (i.e. infarct-in-evolution). During cardiac surgery, coronary vasospasm and thrombosis are frequent causes of ischemia that may progress to infarction. However, there are also many nonischemic causes of changes in ECG, TEE, and pulmonary artery pressures that are similar to those seen with ischemia.

Coronary steal

Intercoronary steal is a reduction in perfusion to collateral-dependent myocardium accompanied by an increase in perfusion to the area of the myocardium from which the collaterals originate. Vasodilatation of coronary vessels, caused by anesthetics or other agents, in previously nonischemic myocardium increases total flow and leads to a greater reduction in pressure across a stenosis. Lower pressure distal to the stenosis causes a reduction in flow to the ischemic myocardium as the vessels to that part of the myocardium are already fully dilated (Fig. 39.4). Anesthetics rarely cause ischemia via this mechanism, partly because they depress myocardial contractility, reducing oxygen demand. Transmural coronary steal involves increased subepicardial and decreased subendocardial perfusion. This can occur since subendocardial vessels are more dilated (have less vasodilator reserve) than subepicardial vessels in the resting state.

Electrocardiography in diagnosis and monitoring

Though ischemia may affect several features of the ECG, new ST segment deviation is used as a marker perioperatively because it is the only parameter with adequate sensitivity and specificity (see Chapter 12). The orthogonal leads III, V_2, and V_5 are suitable for recording ST segment depression and elevation in various regions of the heart during cardiac surgery. During noncardiac surgery, leads II and V_5 are adequate. RV and inferior ischemia and infarction, which are common during coronary artery bypass graft (CABG) surgery, may be detected using lead V_{4R}.

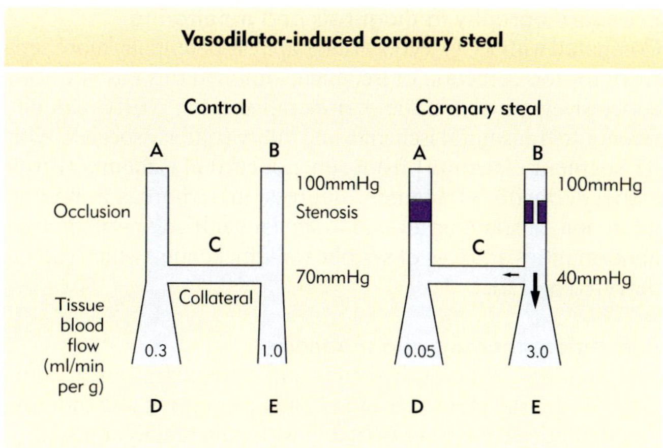

Figure 39.4 The mechanism of vasodilator-induced coronary steal in the coronary circulation. Collateral vessels (C) are maximally dilated in the control state and during coronary steal. During vasodilatation of E, perfusion pressure at the origin of the collateral vessels is reduced from 70 to 40mmHg, resulting in decreased perfusion of ischemic tissue (D). In contrast, vasodilatation to areas distal to the stenosis causes an increase in blood flow to tissue (E) supplied by the stenotic artery and coronary steal has occurred.

ST segment deviation may also have nonischemic causes. Fixed deviation may be caused by cardiac conduction changes and LV hypertrophy with strain. New deviations may be caused by changes in body position or acid–base and electrolyte status, and by hyperventilation, Valsalva maneuver, hyperglycemia, and pancreatitis. ST segment elevation observed on cooling at the beginning of cardiopulmonary bypass (CPB) and on electrical defibrillation after CPB is likely to be unrelated to ischemia. On termination of CPB, new ST segment deviation, in association with a widened QRS complex, may occur as a result of cardiac conduction abnormalities; it is usually of the opposite polarity to the terminal QRS complex. These cardiac conduction changes usually subside within a few hours after CPB but do indicate myocardial injury, even when transient. New postoperative ST segment elevation caused by pericarditis after cardiac surgery usually occurs in multiple leads and is associated with PR depression and J-point and concave-upward ST segment elevation, with an upright T wave.

A nonischemic etiology may be suggested for a new 1mm ST segment deviation if a temporal or other association is noted with the above causes. Perioperative ischemia often occurs in response to known stimuli. During noncardiac surgery, ischemia is most common during emergence from general anesthesia. This ischemia may result from a hyperdynamic circulation through pain, apprehension, or administration of muscarinic anticholinergic agents in combination with cholinesterase inhibitors for reversing muscle relaxation. Stimuli during CABG surgery include manipulation of old grafts during reoperation, administration of protamine, and an increase in myocardial oxygen consumption. Episodes of ST segment deviation are most common in the first 8 hours after release of aortic occlusion. Patients with perioperative ECG changes are more likely to have adverse cardiovascular outcomes after noncardiac or CABG surgery.

Echocardiography in diagnosis and monitoring

Compared with ECG, echocardiography is potentially more sensitive for the detection of ischemia, although this has not been conclusively proven in the perioperative setting. ECG can differentiate transmural ischemia and injury (often associated with ST segment elevation) from subendocardial ischemia (often associated with ST segment depression), whereas ischemia, infarction, or stunning all lead to similar ventricular wall motion abnormalities and loss of systolic wall thickening, which can be detected by TEE.

Prevention, therapy, and prognosis

Maintenance of hemodynamics and administration of anti-anginals are the mainstays of ischemia prevention and therapy. Sympathetic activation associated with pain and light anesthesia should be avoided. Patients with unstable angina prior to CABG surgery are placed on heparin infusion. Low-molecular-weight heparins also control ischemia but are associated with greater perioperative bleeding. If ischemia continues, nitroglycerin (glyceryl trinitrate) infusion is administered, though hypotension must be avoided to ensure adequate coronary perfusion pressure. Patients with continued ischemia qualify for intra-aortic balloon pump (IABP) or emergency CABG surgery. Prophylactic administration of nitroglycerin during surgery does not reduce the incidence of perioperative infarction.

MYOCARDIAL INFARCTION

Mechanism

In the presence of a vulnerable atherosclerotic plaque, onset of MI may be triggered when stressors produce hemodynamic, vasoconstrictive, and prothrombotic forces. These triggers, or acute risk factors, cause plaque disruption (Fig. 39.5). If the plaque disruption causes a major thrombogenic stimulus, an occlusive thrombus forms, leading to MI or sudden cardiac death. Circulation platelets rapidly adhere to damaged endothelium, a process mediated by the interactions between various membrane receptors and ligands present in the endothelium and sub-endothelium. Inhibitors of the platelet membrane receptor glycoprotein (GP) IIb/IIa interaction with fibrinogen, which mediates platelet aggregation, show considerable promise as antiplatelet agents for treating ischemia. If the plaque disruption causes a minor thrombogenic stimulus, platelet aggregates and thrombin generation may produce unstable angina or non-Q wave MI as the thrombus expands. Other triggers may then cause the artery to constrict, the thrombus to become occlusive, or the clot to grow, leading to complete occlusion and MI. The cellular mechanisms underlying atherosclerotic plaque formation are summarized in figure 39.6. Aggressive lipid-lowering therapy using inhibitors of 3-hydroxy-3-methylglutaryl coenzyme A reductase (e.g. lovastatin) to reduce plasma LDL concentration can reverse endothelial and vascular wall dysfunction and improve outcome in patients with CAD.

Diagnosis

Most perioperative MI involves subendocardial necrosis, though MI after cardiac surgery may consist of diffuse necrosis. Perioperatively, chest pain is masked by analgesics and other symptoms of MI lack specificity. The occurrence of arrhythmias, cardiac conduction changes, and new-onset pacemaker dependence has low sensitivity and specificity for the detection of MI. The commonly used tests for MI include ECG, serum levels of cardiac enzymes, and echocardiography. There is no generally accepted standardization of these tests for the detection of MI, and the results of different tests are often discordant. Most tests, including ECG and echocardiography, are more sensitive for detecting transmural MI than subendocardial MI. Some tests, such as elevation of serum cardiac enzyme levels, do not become positive for several hours after the onset of MI. Hence, they are not well suited for detecting the onset and trigger of MI. ECG and echocardiography are useful for continuous perioperative monitoring and may show changes at the onset of MI.

Identification of Q wave MI on the ECG is the most commonly used method for the detection of pre-existing and perioperative MI. For the identification of Q wave MI on the ECG, different criteria with differing sensitivities and specificities are available. The sensitive criteria used in nonsurgical patients suspected of having acute MI identify a large number of patients undergoing CABG as positive for Q wave MI. However, many of these patients do not have an adverse prognosis, suggesting that more conservative criteria should be used to identify Q wave MI in the setting of cardiac surgery.

CK-MB (MB isoenzyme of creatine kinase) is a commonly used enzymatic marker of MI that is detected in the serum 4–6 hours after the onset of MI. Immunoenzymatic measurement of CK-MB in mass units is the current standard, though in the past electrophoretic determination of activity was performed. Ventricular and atrial myocytes contain 20–30% CK-MB. Skeletal muscle trauma during surgery releases large amounts of CK, containing approximately 1% CK-MB. Serum CK-MB levels greater than 1–2% are associated with poor prognosis in surgical patients. In patients undergoing CABG , a peak level of CK-MB over 100ng/mL is commonly used for the detection of MI.

Serum cardiac troponin T and troponin I are used for the detection of MI because of their high sensitivity and specificity and their persistent elevation after MI. The assay for troponin I is virtually 100% specific for cardiac damage, and that for troponin T is about 99% specific. Troponin T becomes elevated within 3–5 hours of coronary occlusion and retains good diagnostic sensitivity until the fifth day. Troponin I becomes elevated 4–6 hours after coronary occlusion and retains good diagnostic sensitivity until the fourth day. After noncardiac surgery, patients with levels of serum troponin I exceeding 3.1ng/mL demonstrated new regional wall motion abnormalities on echocardiography. The threshold level of troponin T used for the detection of MI after cardiac surgery is 1–3.5ng/mL.

Echocardiography can be used for the detection of MI and can also provide clinically useful information about the structure and function of the heart. Currently, it is not routinely used because of the expense, difficulty in performing a transthoracic examination after cardiothoracic surgery, and difficulty in distinguishing MI from reversible ischemia and stunning.

Predictors

Intraoperative occurrence of ischemic ST segment deviation and major cardiac conduction changes, duration of post-CPB hypotension, and duration of CPB are independent predictors of MI after CABG surgery. These predictors suggest that the risk of MI depends primarily on the perioperative course rather than on the patient's preoperative status. The setting of noncardiac surgery is different. As the incidence of perioperative MI is low, the predictors of MI have not been adequately studied. Risk indices have been developed by

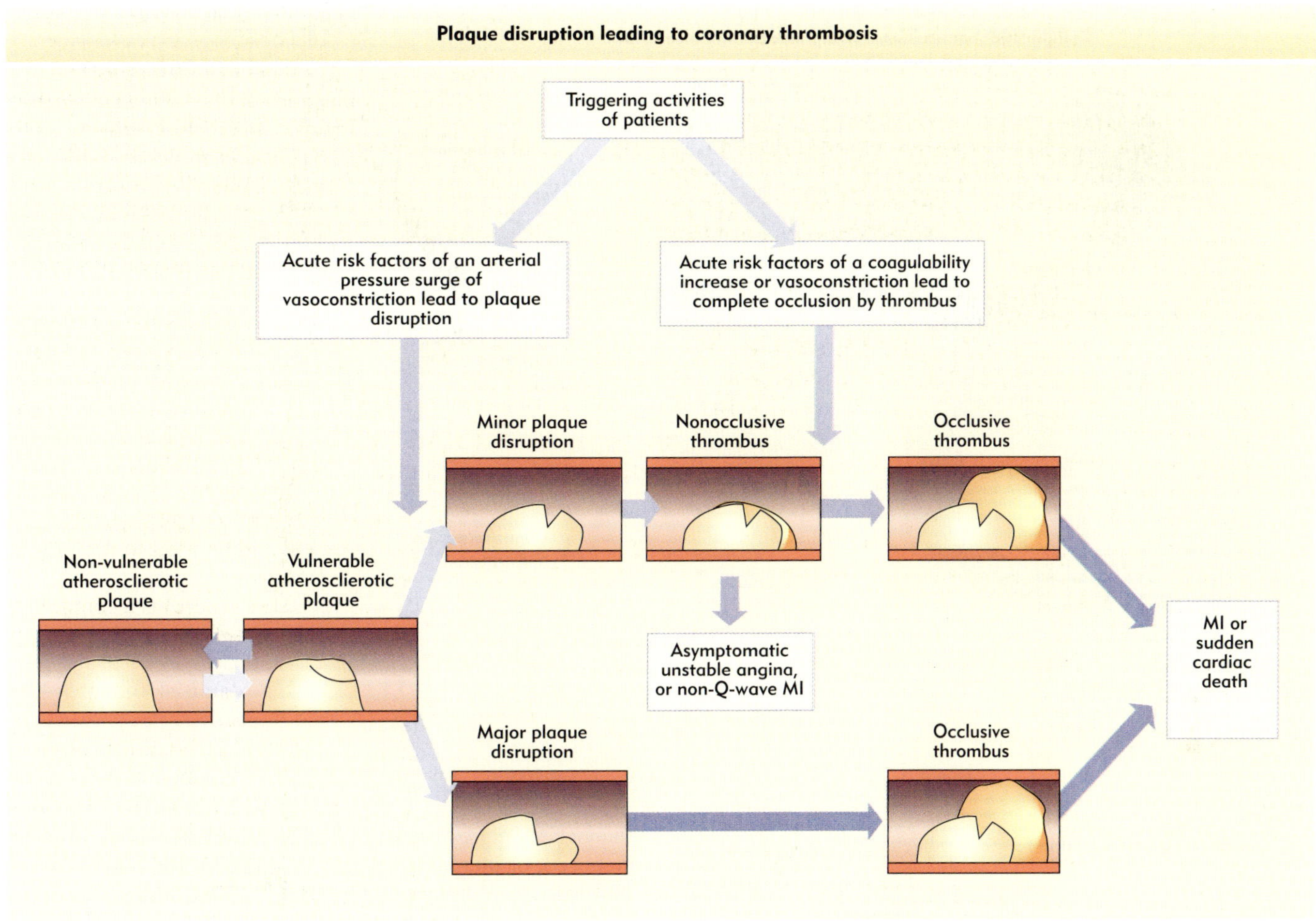

Figure 39.5 Hypothetical mechanisms by which hemodynamic changes leading to plaque rupture, increase in coagulability, and vasoconstriction trigger coronary thrombosis, unstable angina, myocardial infarction, and sudden cardiac death. (With permission from Muller et al., 1994.)

Goldman, Detsky, and others to predict the risk of cardiovascular mortality and morbidity, including MI. These indices indicate that the preoperative status of the patient (see Fig. 39.1) and the type of surgery (Fig. 39.7), rather than the perioperative course, are the primary determinants of MI after noncardiac surgery.

Prevention, therapy, and prognosis

Aspirin or heparin can prevent infarction by reducing coagulability, while β-adrenoceptor blockade may reduce hemodynamic stress, which can lead to plaque disruption. In the nonoperative setting, reflow in the infarct-related artery may be acutely achieved via thrombolysis or angioplasty. Thrombolysis is not applicable in the operative setting and the role of angioplasty may be limited by the involvement of smaller vessels. Medical therapy may be beneficial in the operative setting. In patients with CAD undergoing noncardiac surgery, the perioperative use of atenolol reduces mortality and other adverse outcomes on follow-up over 2 years. After CABG surgery, treatment with warfarin does not reduce graft occlusion rate, but the use of lovastatin and colestyramine (cholestyramine) to reduce cholesterol levels does. Treatment with antiplatelet drugs such as aspirin, dipyridamole, sulfinpyrazone (sulphinpyrazone), and triclopidine can also reduce occlusion rate.

The magnitude of the increase in adverse cardiac events and mortality after MI varies among different studies primarily because of differences in the methods used for detection and follow-up. Long-term follow-up of patients who have MI after noncardiac surgery indicates that they are more likely to have adverse cardiac events and mortality. The in-hospital mortality was 10% in patients with new Q wave MI and 1% in patients without new Q wave MI after CABG surgery. In another study, MI was an important predictor of late survival, surpassed only by LV function, age, and the number of associated illnesses.

Surgery in patients with myocardial infarction

Morbidity and mortality after MI varies between patients, especially during the first 6 months. In those who survive without morbidity for a long time after MI, the risk is low for subsequent surgery. Hence, elective surgery should be postponed for 6 months after MI if possible. If earlier surgery is necessary, cardiac risk stratification should be performed using tests such as exercise treadmill, dipyridamole–thallium scintigraphy, and coronary angiography.

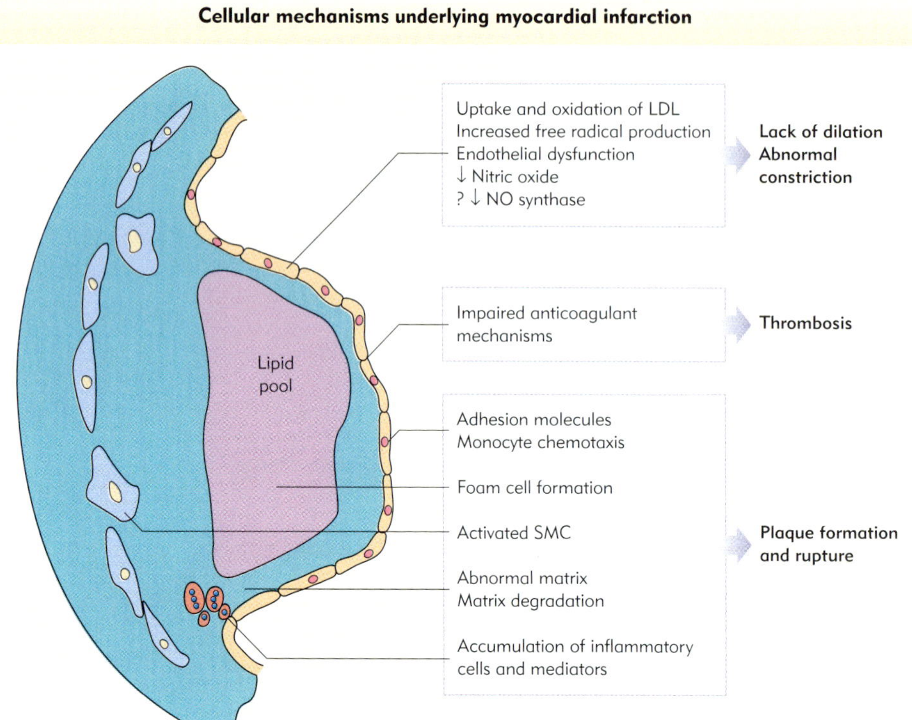

Figure 39.6 Cellular mechanisms underlying myocardial infarction. The changes in endothelium and other parts of the cell lead to plaque formation and rupture, lack of luminal dilation and abnormal contraction, and thrombosis.

Cardiac risk[a] stratification for noncardiac surgical procedures

High risk (reported cardiac risk often >5%)

- Emergent major operations, particularly in elder patients
- Aortic and other major vascular operation
- Peripheral vascular operation
- Anticipated prolonged surgical procedures associated with large fluid shifts or blood loss (or both)

Intermediate risk (reported cardiac risk generally <5%)

- Carotoid endarterectomy
- Head and neck operation
- Intraperitoneal and intrathoracic operation
- Orthopedic operation
- Prostate operation

Low risk (reported cardiac risk generally <1%)[b]

- Endoscopic procedures
- Superficial procedures
- Cataract operation
- Breast operation

[a]Combined incidence of cardiac death and nonfatal myocardial infarction.
[b]Further preoperative cardiac testing is generally unnecessary.

Figure 39.7 Cardiac risk stratification for noncardiac surgical procedures.

HEART FAILURE

Left ventricular failure

Acute and/or chronic LV and/or RV failure (i.e. impaired pump function) is prevalent perioperatively. Myocardial disease or damage, increased pressure load (e.g. hypertension and aortic stenosis), or increased volume load (e.g. aortic insufficiency) may lead to LV failure. High-output cardiac failure may occur in the presence of anemia, arteriovenous fistula, pregnancy, or thyrotoxicosis.

The pump function of the ventricle is commonly represented by the pressure–volume loop constrained between end-systolic and end-diastolic lines (Fig. 39.8 and see Chapter 36). The following changes occur as a result of heart failure. Decreased inotropy results in a shift of the end-systolic line downwards and the end-systolic pressure (ESP) is reduced. Stroke volume can be maintained by increasing LV end-diastolic pressure (EDP) and LV end-diastolic volume (EDV), shifting the pressure–volume loop to the right. With decreased lusitropy, the end-diastolic line moves upwards; the increased ventricular stiffness increases the pressure for a given volume. Lusitropy is a measure of relaxation, an energy-requiring process (Chapter 34). If stroke volume is to be maintained in the presence of a combination of low inotropy and lusitropy, the EDP must be increased whereas the systolic pressure is reduced. To maintain systolic pressure, compensatory vasoconstriction occurs, which shifts the loop to the right, leading to a reduction in stroke volume.

LV EDP, or its correlate pulmonary capillary wedge pressure (PCWP), is often used as a measure of preload. Depending on the above derangements, for a given PCWP, the LV EDV can vary widely. In patients who start with a low LV EDV, expansion of the intravascular volume increases stroke volume. Though PCWP is a poor measure of LV EDV, it is a good measure of propensity to develop pulmonary edema. If there is a disproportionately large change in PCWP after volume infusion, further volume loading will not substantially increase LV EDV but may cause pulmonary edema.

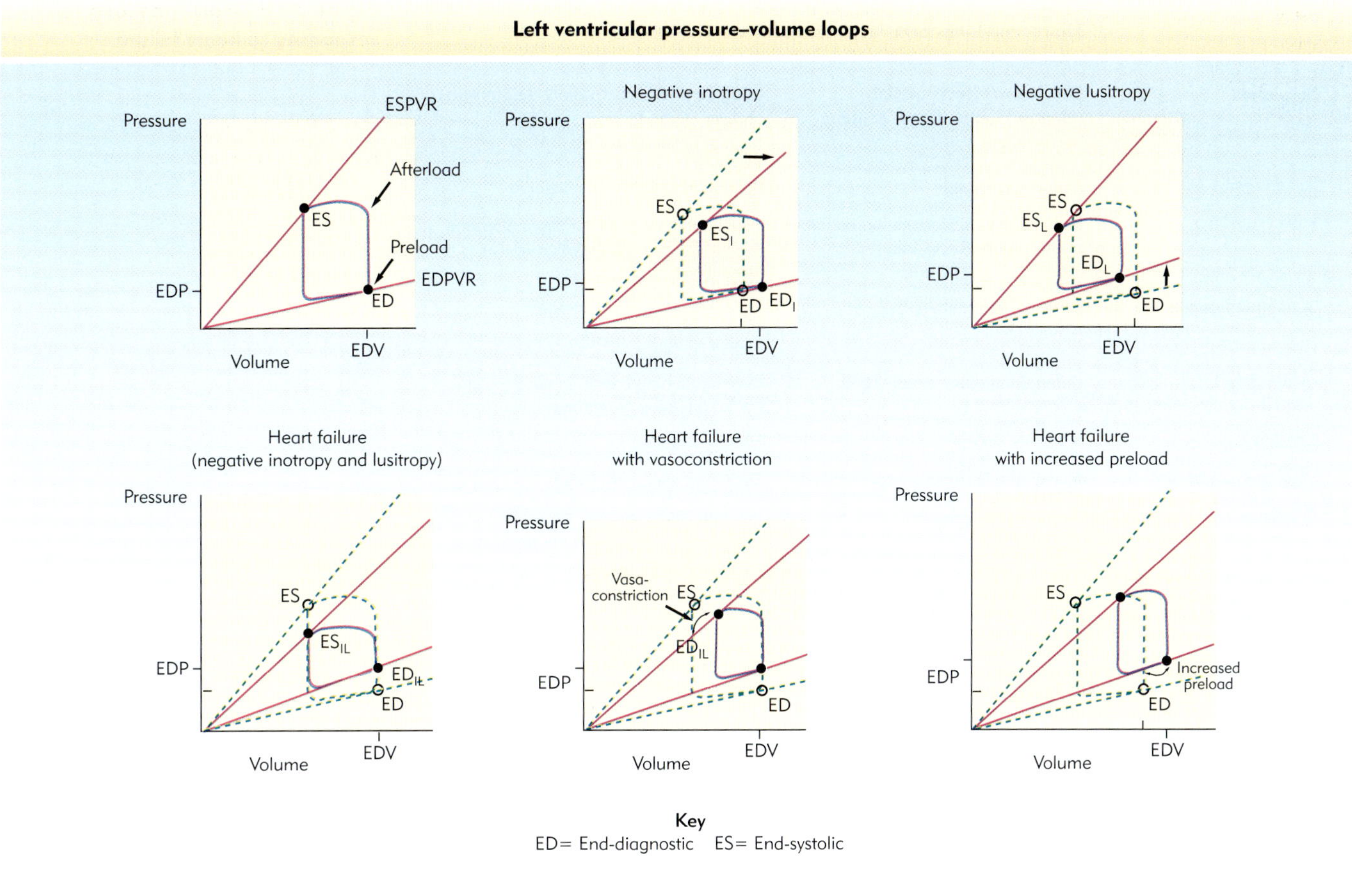

Figure 39.8 Schematic diagrams of left ventricular pressure–volume loops. The normal relationship between the end-diastolic (lower line) and end-systolic (upper line) pressure–volume relationships (EDPVR and ESPVR, respectively). Systole begins at the end-diastolic point (ED) and ends at the point (ES). The ventricle encounters its afterload when the aortic valve opens, at the end of isovolumic contraction. Filling begins at the end of isovolumic relaxation, but the ventricular preload is defined by the pressure and volume at end-diastole (EDP and EDV). This control pressure–volume loop is reproduced as the dashed line in the other graphs. A negative inotropic state shifts the ESPVR downward and to the right; if stroke volume remains constant, the pressure–volume loop shifts to the right, EDP increases, and developed pressure is reduced. A negative lusitropic state shifts the EDPVR upward and to the left; if stroke volume remains constant, the pressure–volume loop shifts to the left, EDP increases, and developed pressure is reduced. The combination of negative inotropic and lusitropic states, as commonly occurs in heart failure, 'compresses' the pressure–volume loop between the abnormal EDP– and ESP–volume relationships. In this illustration, where stroke volume is shown as remaining constant, EDP is increased, and developed pressure is reduced. The effect of vasoconstriction on the pressure–volume loop found in heart failure (curved arrow) shifts the ESP upward and to the right along the depressed ESPVR. This circulatory adjustment returns blood pressure toward normal but at the expense of a fall in stroke volume. Increased preload shifts the EDP upward and to the right along the abnormal EDPVR. Although this leads to a further increase in blood pressure through the operation of Starling's law of the heart, it does so at the expense of both a rise in filling pressure and an increased EDV. Both the negative inotropic and negative lusitropic effects of heart failure reduce the area of the pressure–volume loop, index of myocardial work. (With permission from Katz, 1991.)

The response to acute heart failure is to maintain circulation (Fig. 39.9). However, the chronic effects of heart failure are predominantly deleterious. The above adaptations increase myocardial oxygen requirements and contribute to symptoms such as edema. Myocardial hypertrophy and altered apoptosis of myocytes occur. The capillary supply is inadequate and mitochondrial density is reduced. Appearance of slow myosin decreases contractility and velocity of shortening. The prolongation of the action potential increases contractility and energy expenditure. Collagen is increased whereas the sarcoplasmic reticulum is reduced, both of which impair relaxation.

Perioperative management of heart failure focuses on optimizing hemodynamics. In patients with low cardiac output in spite of high central venous pressure (CVP), arterial vasodilators reduce LV afterload, which improves ejection and compliance and reduces $M\dot{V}O_2$. Vasodilator-induced reduction in ventricular stiffness reduces filling pressures and increases the LV EDV and stroke volume without causing pulmonary edema.

Ventricular interaction

Because of the constraining effect of the pericardium, failure of one ventricle affects the other. Compared with the LV,

Figure 39.9 Short- and long-term responses to heart failure.

Short- and long-term responses to heart failure

Response	Short-term effects (mainly adaptive) hemorrhage, acute heart failure	Long-term effects (mainly deleterious) chronic heart failure
Salt and water retention	Augments preload	Pulmonary congestion, anasarca
Vasoconstriction	Maintains blood pressure for perfusion of vital organs (brain, heart)	Exacerbates pump dysfunction (afterload mismatch), increases cardiac energy expenditure
Sympathetic stimulation	Increases heart rate and ejection	Increases energy expenditure
Desensitization	–	Energy sparing
Hypertrophy	Unloads individual muscle fibers	Deterioration and death of cardiac cells: cardiomyopathy of overload
Capillary deficit	–	Energy starvation
Mitochondrial density	Increase; helps meet energy demands	Decrease; energy starvation
Appearance of slow myosin	–	Increases force integral; decreases shortening velocity and contractility; energy-sparing
Prolonged action potential	–	Increases contractility and energy expenditure
Decreased density of sarcoplasmic reticulum Ca^{2+} pump sites	–	Slows relaxation, possibly energy sparing
Increased collagen	May reduce dilatation	Impairs relaxation

the RV is more susceptible to failure in the presence of increased afterload. RV dilatation leads to ischemia. The resulting leftward movement of the ventricular septum reduces LV EDV, compliance, and stroke volume, whereas LV EDP and $\dot{M}VO_2$ increase. The resulting LV failure may further accentuate RV failure.

The inferior-posterior wall of the LV and the RV free wall are common locations for perioperative MI after cardiac surgery. In the presence of cardiogenic shock associated with RV infarction, RV compliance is reduced, leading to a prominent *y* descent of the CVP waveform similar to that in constrictive pericarditis. Tricuspid regurgitation leads to volume overload of the right atrium and a large V wave in CVP.

In the treatment of RV failure, though a high preload may be required, the CVP should be kept below the PCWP to avoid leftward shift of the ventricular septum. Cardiac output may be substantially reduced if atrial contraction is lost. Adenosine, inhaled nitric oxide, prostaglandin E_1, isoproterenol (isoprenaline), or low-dose nitroglycerin may reduce elevated pulmonary artery pressure without substantially reducing systemic pressure. IABP increases coronary perfusion and improves RV dynamics.

Intrathoracic pressure

As peak end-expiratory pressure (PEEP) increases lung volume to the functional residual capacity, pulmonary vascular resistance decreases because of reduced compression of small vessels. Further increases in PEEP increase pulmonary vascular resistance, possibly leading to dilatation of the RV and a shift of the interventricular septum to the left, reducing LV compliance. The level of PEEP that is optimal for oxygenation may cause a reduction in stroke volume and hence cardiac output. Though PCWP may not change, LV EDV is reduced, which leads to a reduction in stroke volume. PEEP reduces ventricular diastolic compliance by shifting the pressure–volume curve up and to the left (see Fig. 39.8). Increased RV afterload from increases in PEEP causes paradoxical leftward shift of the ventricular septum. PEEP also causes an increase in lung volume, which raises juxtacardiac pressures, decreasing the transmural distending pressure.

Pulmonary vascular congestion caused by LV failure leads to reduced compliance. During spontaneous inspiration, venous return is augmented by the substantial negative intrathoracic pressure needed for lung inflation and by increased downward movement of the diaphragm, which increases intra-abdominal pressure. Reduced intrathoracic pressure increases LV afterload by increasing the transmural pressure across the aorta for a given systemic pressure. Accordingly, discontinuation of mechanical ventilation can precipitate myocardial ischemia and pulmonary edema. In the presence of isolated LV failure, mitral regurgitation, or ischemic dysfunction, high intrathoracic pressure (as occurs with mechanical ventilation) may improve cardiac performance.

Conversely, in the presence of RV failure, intrathoracic pressures should be minimized without compromising adequate gas exchange. PEEP should be minimized and tidal volume should be kept below 7mL/kg. High intrathoracic pressure increases right atrial pressure. This reduces venous return and hence cardiac output. As the intrathoracic pressure is increased, dilation of the RV reduces its coronary blood flow and contractility. Increased intrathoracic pressure and lung distension may slightly reduce contractility of the LV by stimulating vagal afferents and releasing prostaglandins.

TOXIC CARDIOMYOPATHY

Hypersensitivity or toxic reactions to a number of agents can lead to dilated (congestive) cardiomyopathy, which will affect perioperative management. These agents include alcohol, antiarrhythmic agents (e.g. digitalis), cancer chemotherapeutic agents (e.g. daunorubicin, doxorubicin, cyclophosphamide), antimony, antiretroviral agents [e.g. azidothymidine (zidovudine), dideoxyinosine (didanosine)], carbon monoxide, carbon tetrachloride, cobalt, cocaine, corticosteroids, emetine, hydralazine, interferon alfa, methysergide, phenothiazines, phenytoin, procainamide, thioridazine drugs, and tricyclic antidepressants (e.g. amitriptyline, imipramine). Dilated cardiomyopathy is associated with biventricular dilatation; reduced ejection fraction, stroke volume, and cardiac output; and increased LV EDP. Progressive worsening of heart failure and ventricular arrhythmias and systemic or pulmonary embolism (PE) may occur. Therapy includes diuretics, vasodilators, angiotensin-converting enzyme (ACE) inhibitors, digitalis, anticoagulants, immunosuppressives, antiarrhythmics, implantable cardioverter-defibrillator, and cardiac transplantation.

PERICARDIAL TAMPONADE

Blood or other fluid in the pericardial cavity reduces the transmural pressure across the atria, limiting their filling and reducing stroke volume. When less than about 200mL of fluid accumulates rapidly in a 70kg person, CVP is usually 10–12cmH_2O. Activation of the sympathoadrenal system leads to increased heart rate and constriction of capacitance vessels, causing augmentation of filling pressure, which maintains cardiac output. If pericardial fluid volume increases further, CVP and arterial blood pressure decrease, leading to shock followed by cardiac arrest. When pericardial fluid accumulates slowly, up to 400mL may accumulate before symptoms are observed. Trauma caused by catheters placed inside the heart and external trauma to the heart (e.g. rib fracture from blunt trauma or cardiopulmonary resuscitation) may cause tamponade. Localized tamponade may develop after cardiac surgery even though the pericardium is usually left open. After cardiac surgery, more than 80% of patients have pericardial effusion. Most effusions are asymptomatic and tamponade occurs in about 1% of the patients.

Signs and symptoms of tamponade include weakness, pulsus paradoxus (see below), and signs of right heart failure including dyspnea on exertion, orthopnea, hepatomegaly, ascites, peripheral edema, jugular venous distention, and prerenal azotemia. Beck's triad consists of distant heart sounds, hypotension, and elevated CVP, usually up to 15cmH_2O. Decreased urine output and Na^+ excretion occur as a result of reduced cardiac output, sympathetic activation, and a reduction in atrial natriuretic factor release subsequent to the lower atrial distending pressure.

ECG shows low-voltage, ST–T wave changes, and P and QRS alternans. Widening of the cardiac silhouette is observed on chest radiograph. Echocardiography is the most commonly used diagnostic technique. Transthoracic imaging is often adequate, though occasionally TEE is required. In the presence of a bloody effusion containing thrombi, identification of ventricular wall interface is difficult. Pericardial fluid may be observed as an echo-free crescent between the RV wall and the pericardium or the posterior LV wall and the pericardium. Two distinct echoes from the posterior wall may be caused by pericardial fluid.

With tamponade, the diastolic pressures in all cardiac chambers and the PCWP equal intrapericardial pressure. If reduced cardiac output and elevated CVP are observed, tamponade or biventricular failure may be present. If a large respiratory variation in blood pressure is also observed, tamponade is likely. In atrial waveforms, *x* descent during systole is accentuated whereas the *y* descent caused by opening of atrioventricular valves is depressed.

Pulsus paradoxus is a decrease of more than 10mmHg in systolic blood pressure during quiet inspiration, accompanied by a greater than normal decrease in pulse pressure and heart rate. There is greater than normal blood flow into the right atrium during inspiration, which increases intrapericardial pressure. As the ventricular septum is displaced leftward, LV volume and blood pressure are reduced. The flow of blood from the right to the left heart is slowed and may occur during expiration. The reduction of intrathoracic pressure during inspiration reduces blood pressure and inspiration directly decreases LV contraction.

Volume loading and inotropic agents (e.g. isoproterenol or dobutamine) are used to maintain cardiac output. Pericardiocentesis is often diagnostic, as well as therapeutic; it is falsely negative in about 20% of patients because of pericardial blood clots. If pericardiocentesis does not have the necessary therapeutic effect, surgical drainage can be performed. In patients with hemodynamic instability, drainage can be performed under local anesthesia through a small incision just below the xiphoid process. Cardiac performance often improves on pericardiotomy, though this is less likely in patients with constrictive pericarditis.

PULMONARY EMBOLISM

Pulmonary embolism is a common cause of perioperative heart failure and respiratory failure. Thrombi embolize most commonly from proximal deep veins of the lower extremities. Vascular damage, venous stasis, and hypercoagulability promote deep vein thrombosis (DVT). Risk factors for venous thromboembolism include previous venous thromboembolism, immobility, advanced age, malignancy, heart failure, use of oral contraceptives, obesity, and surgical procedures on the lower extremity, pelvis, and abdomen. Untreated proximal DVT is associated with a 50% risk of PE, resulting in death in approximately 1% of patients. Two-thirds of the deaths occur during the first hour after PE and the rest 4–6 hours later. Predictors of PE include perioperative MI, atrial fibrillation, blood type A, and CABG surgery. Massive PE is defined as greater than 50% obstruction of pulmonary outflow, which may lead to RV failure and death. Hypoxic pulmonary vasoconstriction occurring with PE further accentuates pulmonary hypertension.

Signs and symptoms of PE are nonspecific. Mild PE may cause dyspnea, tachypnea, tachycardia, hemoptysis, and chest pain. Severe PE may cause dyspnea and circulatory collapse. Arterial blood gases may show hypoxia, high alveolar to arterial oxygen gradient, acidosis, and respiratory alkalosis caused by hyperventilation. Hypercapnia may occur in the presence of a large embolus. Pressure measurements with a pulmonary artery catheter demonstrate elevated pulmonary artery pressure with normal PCWP and reduced cardiac output. ECG may show sinus tachycardia, supraventricular arrhythmia (especially atrial fibrillation), incomplete right bundle branch block, and nonspecific ST–T wave changes. Occasionally, a large S wave in lead I, and large Q and T waves in lead III (S_1 Q_3 T_3) may be observed. Right precordial leads may reveal downward sloping ST segment depression indicative of RV strain.

A ventilation–perfusion lung scan with xenon and technetium is the most common test for the diagnosis of PE. The negative predictive accuracy of this scan is high, while the positive predictive accuracy is lower. After thoracic or cardiac surgery, which alter both ventilation and perfusion, a ventilation–perfusion scan is likely to show intermediate probability of PE. TEE is increasingly popular for the diagnosis of PE. It can diagnose a saddle embolus, which may be missed by a ventilation–perfusion scan, and can identify sources of emboli in the right heart. Pulmonary angiography is the gold standard for the detection of PE. Impedance plethysmography and duplex ultrasound evaluation of the deep veins may identify the source of emboli.

For prophylaxis, intermittent compression of the lower extremities may be used perioperatively. Patients should walk and perform lower extremity exercises as early after surgery as possible. Subcutaneous heparin or low-molecular-weight heparin may be used for prophylaxis. Pulmonary vasodilators/inotropes such as prostaglandin E_1 or isoproterenol may be used to treat hemodynamic compromise. Ventilation may have to be supported. In patients with confirmed PE, fibrinolytic agents such as streptokinase, urokinase, or tissue plasminogen activator may lyse the emboli, as well as the underlying source. If anticoagulation is contraindicated, a filter (e.g. Greenfield filter) may be placed transvenously in the inferior vena cava to prevent further embolization. However, collaterals may develop over time and this will allow embolization.

Key References

Eagle KA, Brundage BH, Chaitman BR, et al. Guidelines for perioperative cardiovascular evaluation for noncardiac surgery. Report of the American College of Cardiology/American Heart Association Task Force on Practice Guidelines. Committee on Perioperative Cardiovascular Evaluation for Noncardiac Surgery. Circulation. 1996, 93:1278–317.

Jain U, Laflamme CJA, Aggarwal A , for the Multicenter Study of Perioperative Ischemia (McSPI) Research Group. Electrocardiographic and hemodynamic changes and their association with myocardial infarction during coronary artery bypass surgery. Anesthesiology. 1997;86:576–91.

Katz AM. Heart failure. In: Fozzard HA, Haber E, Jennings RB, Katz AM, Morgan HE, eds. The heart and cardiovascular system: scientific foundations, 2nd edn. New York: Raven Press; 1991:333–53.

Mangano DT, Layug EL, Wallace A Tateo I. Effect of atenolol on mortality and cardiovascular morbidity after noncardiac surgery. N Engl J Med. 1996;335:1713–20.

Muller JE, Abela GS, Nesto RW, Tofler GH. Triggers, acute risk factors and vulnerable plaques: the lexicon of a new frontier. J Am Coll Cardiol. 1994;23:809–13.

Palda VA, Detsky AS. Perioperative assessment and management of risk from coronary artery disease. Ann Intern Med. 1997;127:313–28.

Warltier D, ed. Ventricular function. Baltimore, MD: Williams & Wilkins, 1995.

Further Reading

Jain U. Myocardial ischemia after cardiopulmonary bypass. J Card Surg. 1995;10:520–6.

Kaplan J, ed. Cardiac anesthesia. 4th edn. Philadelphia, PA: Saunders, 1999.

Selwyn AP, Kinlay S, Creager M, Libby P, Ganz P. Cell dysfunction in atherosclerosis and the ischemic manifestations of coronary artery disease. Am J Cardiol. 1997;79:17–23.

Theroux P. Antiplatelet therapy: do the new platelet inhibitors add significantly to the clinical benefits of aspirin? Am Heart J. 1997;134:562–70.

Wallace A, Layug B, Tateo I, for the McSPI Research Group. Prophylactic atenolol reduces postoperative myocardial ischemia. Anesthesiology. 1998;88:7–17.

Chapter 40 Valvular heart disease

Susan Garwood and David L Lee

Topics covered in this chapter

Aortic insufficiency
Mitral regurgitation
Aortic stenosis
Mitral stenosis
Tricuspid stenosis
Pulmonic stenosis
Congenital valvular disease

AORTIC INSUFFICIENCY

The aortic valve consists of three cusps (left, right, and noncoronary) that lie in the aortic root separating the left ventricle from the ascending aorta. Historically, rheumatic fever and syphilitic aortitis have been the primary etiologies of aortic insufficiency (AI), but with advances in antibiotic therapy and treatment, AI secondary to these causes is far less frequent. Bacterial endocarditis, trauma, aortic dissection, and congenital abnormalities have recently emerged as the more common etiologies of AI.

The physical findings of both chronic and acute AI (Fig. 40.1) include a widened arterial pulse pressure with the hallmark 'water-hammer' pulse that represents a rapidly falling arterial pressure during late systole and diastole (Corrigan's pulse). The left ventricle is often hyperdynamic and produces a cyclic expansion/retraction of the apex corresponding to systole and diastole. A systolic thrill palpable in the jugular notch and radiating upward to the carotid arteries results from increased blood flow across the aortic valve and does not necessarily reflect any coexisting aortic stenosis (AS). The high-pitched, blowing diastolic murmur of AI is best heard in the left third intercostal space. As the severity of AI increases, the murmur may radiate down the lower sternal edge. A musical quality to this murmur suggests eversion and luffing of the aortic cusp in the regurgitant flow. An additional soft, low-pitched, mid-diastolic rumble, or Austin Flint murmur, is also frequently heard in patients with AI and results from displacement of the anterior mitral leaflet by the regurgitant jet. These murmurs are best heard in the apex and may be difficult to distinguish from the murmur of mitral stenosis (MS). An Austin Flint murmur with earlier onset in diastole and/or increased duration often correlates with the severity of AI. In acute AI, the sudden rise in left ventricular end-diastolic pressure (EDP) may lead to early closure of the mitral valve with a soft first heart sound and a soft short diastolic murmur. On electrocardiography (ECG), there may be evidence of left ventricular hypertrophy as the severity of AI increases. The effect of AI on the normal cardiac cycle is illustrated by the pressure–volume loop in Figure 40.2.

Pathophysiology

Chronic aortic insufficiency

The left ventricle responds to the increased volume load of AI with eccentric hypertrophy (Fig. 40.3), characterized by marked cardiomegaly with increased end-diastolic wall tension as the chamber radius increases. By dilating with respect to both left ventricle size and wall thickness, the compliance remains fairly normal and the ratio of ventricular wall thickness to chamber radius is maintained. In addition, peripheral vasodilatation aids in forward blood flow and, as such, myocardial oxygen consumption does not increase despite an increase in stroke volume and contractility. The heart continues to compensate for the increased regurgitant volume up to approximately 40% of the forward stroke volume. As the degree of AI exceeds this, irreversible myocardial tissue damage occurs. The earliest manifestation of this permanent change is a rise in left ventricular EDP, which is indicative of left ventricular dysfunction. This is accompanied by an increase in pulmonary artery pressure, with the development of dyspnea and congestive heart failure. Eventually, angina occurs as myocardial oxygen consumption increases in an effort to maintain adequate peripheral perfusion and maintain cardiac output, while myocardial oxygen supply decreases as coronary perfusion is compromised by a combination of increased wall tension from chronic hypertrophy and decreased diastolic perfusion pressure. The reflex sympathetic response to the failing heart leads to peripheral vasoconstriction that further compromises forward blood flow and worsens regurgitant flow.

Acute aortic insufficiency

With the development of acute AI, the normal ventricle experiences a major volume load that leads to a sudden increase in left ventricular EDP and end-systolic pressure (ESP). Severe ventricular distension as a result of limited distensibility can result in mitral annular dilation and regurgitation. Decreased diastolic perfusion pressure and elevated left ventricular EDP can lead to ischemia. In an effort to maintain adequate forward flow and cardiac output, sympathetic tone is increased, with accompanying tachycardia, vasoconstriction, and increased contractility. This is usually insufficient since vasoconstriction increases regurgitant flow, and emergent surgical intervention is warranted. The hemodynamic management of AI is summarized in Figure 40.4.

MITRAL REGURGITATION

The mitral valve consists of anterior and posterior leaflets; these lie in the mitral annulus separating the left atrium from the left

Physical and diagnostic findings of severe aortic insufficiency

Clinical findings	Acute presentation	Chronic presentation
Onset	Acute	Chronic and gradual dyspnea
Appearance	Severely ill	Normal or mildly dyspneic
Blood pressure	Normal or low	Wide pulse pressure
Tachycardia	Always	Variable
S1	Soft	Usually normal
S2	Soft	Usually normal (soft calcific valve)
S3	Common	Common with LV failure
Peripheral arterial signs	No	Obvious
Apical impulse	No	Displaced and forcible (very large heart)
Basal diastolic thrill	More common (perforation)	Rare
Basal systolic thrill	No	Common
Basal ejection systolic murmur	Common and soft	Common and harsh
Basal early diastolic murmur	Short and soft, or loud and musical (perforation)	Long, blowing, and decrescendo
Apical rumbling, diastolic murmur	No	Common
Electrocardiography		
Left ventricular (LV) hypertrophy	No	Almost always
Echocardiography		
LV size	Normal	Severely dilated
LV function (ejection fraction)	Hyperactive	Variable
Premature closure of mitral valve	Common	No
Diastolic mitral regurgitation	Common	No
Late mitral valve opening	Common	No
Chest X-ray		
Cardiomegaly	No	Severe
Lung fields	Pulmonary edema	Usually normal

Figure 40.1 Physical and diagnostic findings of severe aortic insufficiency. (With permission from Braunwald, 1997.)

ventricle. The tips of each leaflet are tethered by chordae tendinae to the anterior and posterior papillary muscles of the ventricular myocardium. The causes of mitral regurgitation (MR) vary tremendously depending upon whether the presentation is chronic or acute in nature (Fig. 40.5). The physical findings in both are depicted in Figure 40.6. These include a normal arterial pressure with a rapid upstroke of the arterial pulse, a prominent *a* wave in the jugular venous pulse, a prominent V wave in the pulmonary artery pulse, and pulmonary hypertension. A systolic thrill may be palpable at the cardiac apex, and apical contraction may be displaced laterally. If the left atrium is markedly enlarged, its expansion may be palpated on the lateral sternal border. On ECG, there may be evidence of left atrial enlargement and/or atrial fibrillation, right ventricular hypertrophy associated with pulmonary hypertension, and left ventricular hypertrophy associated with chronic severe MR. The effect of MR on the normal cardiac cycle is illustrated by the pressure–volume loop in Figure 40.2.

Pathophysiology

Chronic mitral regurgitation

In MR, the left ventricle initially propels a portion of its volume into the left atrium during the early part of the ejection phase (see Fig. 40.3). As a result, there is a reduction in ventricular size and wall tension, and an overall reduction in stroke volume, although a high normal ejection fraction is maintained through the reduced afterload. The initial compensatory response is to increase ventricular emptying by increasing contractility, which increases forward stroke volume and preserves cardiac output. In the early, asymptomatic stages of the disease process, the ventricle enlarges eccentrically with both hypertrophy and dilatation to accommodate the volume overload. However, unlike other forms of valvular heart disease, the ventricular compliance increases during the early phases of chronic MR, so there is often little change in the EDP despite the increase in ventricular size and end-diastolic volume. Likewise, the distensible nature of the left atrium allows for a large increase in atrial size with minimal change in the left atrial pressure, which helps to protect the pulmonary vascular beds. The V waves are often enhanced with MR, as the pulmonary veins experience increased filling from the left atrium as well as the regurgitant left ventricle. The degree of V wave enlargement is dependent on left atrial and pulmonary compliance and is more marked with acute MR.

As the severity of MR progresses, the ability of the heart to compensate for the reduction in forward blood flow by increasing size and contractility diminishes. The degree of ventricular dysfunction may be underestimated because of the optimal loading conditions (maximal preload and minimal afterload), which support ventricular ejection despite myocardial dysfunction.

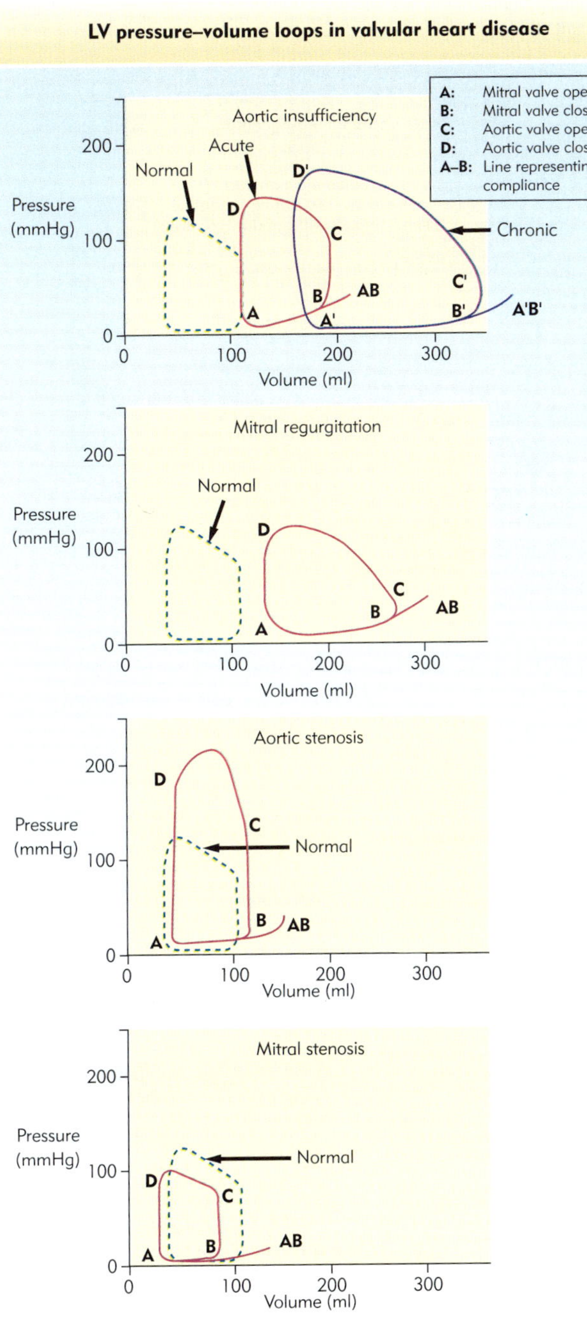

Figure 40.2 Left ventricular pressure–volume loops in valvular heart disease. Points A, B, C, and D correspond to opening and closing of the mitral and aortic valves, respectively. Line AB represents the diastolic pressure–volume relationship corresponding to compliance. In aortic insufficiency, there is a shift in the loop to the right that results in a low aortic diastolic pressure and early ejection of a large stroke volume. There is no period of isovolumic relaxation. In mitral insufficiency, there is no period of isovolumic contraction as blood is ejected directly into the left atrium with the onset of systole; the ejection volume is normal. In aortic stenosis, there is chronic pressure overload resulting from the reduced orifice, end-systole pressure is elevated, and there is reduced left ventricular compliance. Stroke volume is preserved. In mitral stenosis, left ventricular filling and stroke volume are reduced.

Symptoms result from the inability of the atrium to distend further. This leads to backflow of regurgitant blood into the low-pressure pulmonary system, which produces pulmonary vascular congestion and right-sided heart failure. Most patients eventually develop atrial fibrillation secondary to atrial enlargement. Whereas previously the distended atrium emptied itself rapidly into the left ventricle, the absence of an atrial kick may result in a reduced left ventricular end-diastolic volume and an associated decrease in forward systemic blood flow. The inability of the fibrillating left atrium to decompress itself adequately may further exacerbate pulmonary congestion.

Congestive heart failure typically develops once the regurgitant fraction (Fig. 40.7) exceeds 60%. The severity of MR is graded, based on the regurgitant fraction, with less than 30% considered mild, 30–60% moderate, and greater than 60% severe.

Acute mitral regurgitation

Unlike chronic MR, where left atrial compliance gradually increases to accommodate the regurgitant blood flow, the development of sudden MR leads to left atrial volume overload. This results from the inability of the left atrium to distend under acute demands and leaves the pulmonary vasculature unprotected; as a result; regurgitant blood flow produces pronounced congestion and edema. Most cases of acute MR are severe, based on the regurgitant fraction, with a consequent drop in systemic blood flow. The heart compensates by increases in contractility and heart rate. Increased sympathetic stimulation, however, may further exacerbate the MR by creating subendocardial ischemia subsequent to increased myocardial oxygen demand. Consequently, most patients with acute MR, especially those with ischemia-induced papillary muscle dysfunction, have 'giant' V waves. The hemodynamic management of MR is summarized in Figure 40.4.

AORTIC STENOSIS

The normal adult aortic valve orifice has an area of 2.6–3.5cm^2. In most adults, obstruction to flow does not become critical until the area is reduced to less than 0.8cm^2 (or 0.5cm^2/m^2 body surface). AS is most frequently diagnosed after the incidental finding of a murmur (Fig. 40.8), since symptoms appear late in the disease (see below).

Pathophysiology

Degenerative AS results in fibrosis and calcification of the valve. The cusps are rendered immobile by the deposition of calcium along their lines of flexion. Commissural fusion is rarely seen. Calcification of the aortic annulus is common and may be accompanied by calcification of the mitral annulus and MR. Congenitally, bicuspid or unicuspid aortic valves are more prone to degenerative calcification and endocarditis. In rheumatic AS the free borders of the cusps become stiff and retracted as a result of adhesions and fusion of the commissures; consequently, AS is often accompanied by AI as well as involvement of other valves, particularly the mitral valve.

Impedance to left ventricular outflow results in progressive concentric hypertrophy of the left ventricle characterized by increased wall thickness with no change in chamber size. Individual myocardial cells thicken markedly and multiply in parallel, producing an increase in the thickness of the free wall and the septum and a reduction in ventricular compliance. Late in the disease, as stenosis becomes severe, left ventricular dilatation may

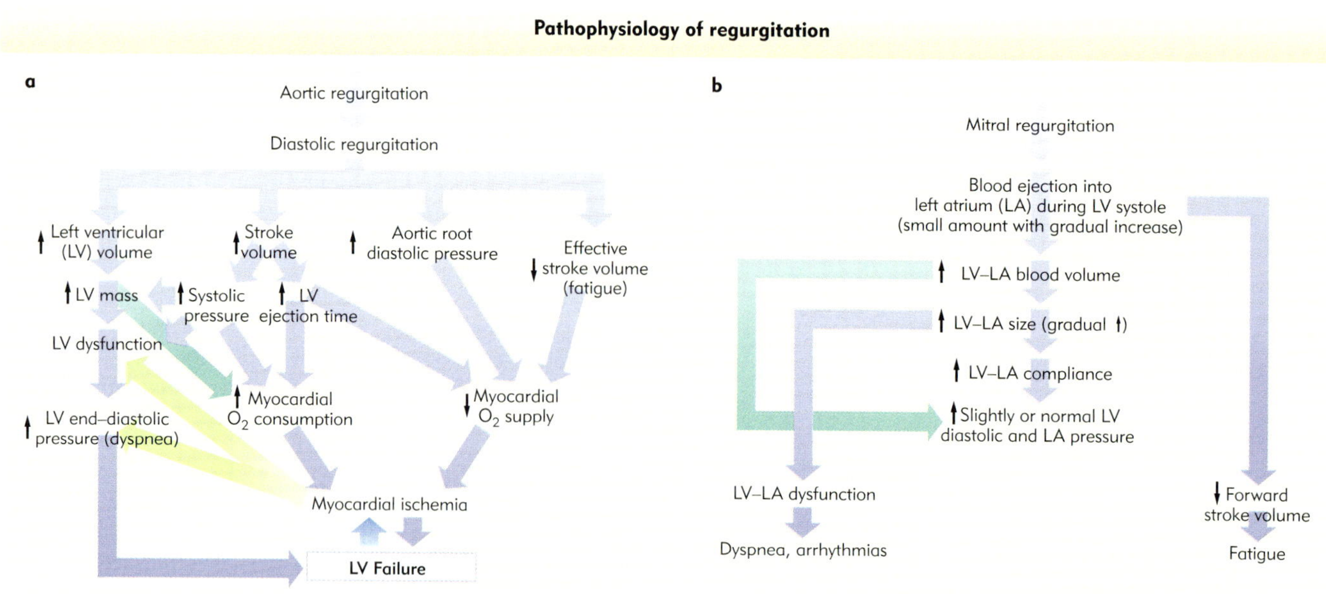

Figure 40.3 Pathophysiology of regurgitation. In aortic regurgitation (left), there are increases in left ventricular volume, mass, and ejection time, which eventually alter myocardial supply and demand and lead to ischemia and failure. In mitral regurgitation (right), increases in left atrial and ventricular volumes, sizes, and compliance eventually cause myocardial dysfunction and decreased forward cardiac output.

Hemodynamic management of specific valvular lesions

	Aortic insufficiency	Mitral regurgitation	Aortic stenosis	Mitral stenosis
Preload	Normal to slightly raised	Usually full; need to keep that way, although preload reduction may reduce regurgitant flow	Full; high ventricular filling pressure may be necessary to ensure adequate ventricular volume because of a noncompliant ventricle	Maintain to ensure adequate flow across stenotic valve
Afterload	Reduction by anesthetics or vasodilators beneficial to reduce regurgitant flow; increase augments regurgitant flow	Decreases are beneficial; increases augment regurgitant flow	Already elevated by lesion but relatively fixed; maintain blood pressure (BP) to ensure adequate coronary perfusion	Avoid raised right ventricular afterload (pulmonary vasoconstrictors); use inotropes for systemic hypotension if right ventricular dysfunction is present
Contractility	Usually adequate; depressed late	Unrecognized myocardial depression possible; titrate myocardial depressants carefully	Usually not a problem; inotropes may be helpful preinduction in patients with low BP	Left ventricle usually not clinically impaired; right ventricle may be impaired with long-standing pulmonary hypertension
Rate	Modest tachycardia reduces ventricular volume, raises aortic diastolic pressure	A faster rate decreases ventricular volume	Not too slow (reduces cardiac output); not too fast (ischemia)	Slow, to allow time for ventricular filling and reduce transmitral pressure gradient
Rhythm	Usually sinus; not a problem	Atrial fibrillation can be a problem	Maintain sinus rhythm! Cardioversion if unstable with supraventricular arrhythmia	Often atrial fibrillation; control ventricular response
Ischemia	At risk owing to low diastolic pressure	May be a problem if secondary to complication of coronary artery disease	Ischemia is an ever-present risk; increased heart rate and decreased BP must be avoided	Usually not a problem

Figure 40.4 Hemodynamic management of specific valvular lesions (With permission from Hemmings and Thomas, 1996.)

occur, causing MR. Women tend towards smaller, thicker-walled ventricles while men more frequently demonstrate eccentric hypertrophy and ventricular dilatation. Left atrial enlargement, pulmonary changes, and subsequent right-sided involvement, similar to those seen in MS (see below), can occur late in the course of the disease. The effect of AS on the normal cardiac cycle is illustrated by the pressure–volume loop in Figure 40.2. The increase in wall thickness serves to normalize wall stress in spite of the marked increase in intraventricular pressure (see Fig. 40.7: law of Laplace).

Etiologies of mitral regurgitation

Acute presentation

Mitral annulus disorders
- Infective endocarditis (abscess formation)
- Paravalvular leak owing to suture interruption (surgical technical problems or infective endocarditis)

Mitral leaflet disorders
- Infective endocarditis (perforation or interfering with valve closure by vegetation)
- Trauma (tear during percutaneous mitral balloon valvotomy or penetrating chest injury)
- Tumors (atrial myxoma)
- Myxomatous degeneration
- Systemic lupus erythematosus (Libman–Sacks lesion)

Rupture of chordae tendineae
- Idiopathic, e.g. spontaneous
- Myxomatous degeneration (mitral valve prolapse, Marfan syndrome, Ehlers–Danlos syndrome)
- Infective endocarditis
- Acute rheumatic fever
- Trauma (percutaneous balloon valvotomy, blunt chest trauma)

Papillary muscle disorders
- Coronary artery disease
- Acute global left ventricular dysfunction
- Infiltrative diseases (amyloidosis, sarcoidosis)
- Trauma

Primary mitral valve prosthetic disorders
- Porcine cusp perforation (endocarditis)
- Porcine cusp degeneration
- Mechanical failure (strut fracture)
- Immobilized disc or ball of the mechanical prosthesis

Chronic presentation

Inflammatory
- Rheumatic heart disease
- Systemic lupus erythematosus
- Scleroderma

Degenerative
- Myxomatous degeneration of mitral valve leaflets (Barlow's click–murmur syndrome, prolapsing leaflet, mitral valve prolapse)
- Marfan syndrome
- Ehlers–Danlos syndrome
- Pseudoxanthoma elasticum
- Calcification of mitral valve annulus

Infective
- Infective endocarditis affecting normal, abnormal, or prosthetic mitral valves

Structural
- Ruptured chordae tendineae (spontaneous or secondary to myocardial infarction, trauma, mitral valve prolapse, endocarditis)
- Dilatation of mitral valve annulus and left ventricular cavity (congestive cardiomyopathies, aneurysmal dilatation of the left ventricle)
- Hypertrophic cardiomyopathy
- Paravalvular prosthetic leak

Congenital
- Mitral valve clefts or fenestrations
- Parachute mitral valve abnormality in association with endocardial cushion defects, endocardial fibroelastosis, transposition of the great arteries, anomalous origin of the left coronary artery

Figure 40.5 Etiologies of mitral regurgitation. (Adapted with permission from Braunwald, 1997.)

The obstruction to left ventricular outflow in AS usually develops over a number of years, with an absence of symptoms until significant stenosis has developed. As the orifice diminishes in size, adaptive changes take place in order to maintain left ventricular output. The left ventricle hypertrophies and generates a pressure gradient across the valve, which varies inversely with the fourth power of the radius of the orifice (r^4) (see Fig. 40.7: Poisseuille–Hagen formula). Stroke volume becomes dependent on the length of the ejection phase of the cardiac cycle, and these patients typically have an increased period of systolic ejection. In spite of the chronic left ventricular pressure overload, wall stress remains within normal limits. The combination of hypertrophy, transvalvular gradient generation, and prolonged ejection time allows most patients to remain symptom free until late in the disease process. However, hydraulic considerations dictate that at any given orifice size, the transvalvular gradient is a

Physical and diagnostic findings of severe mitral regurgitation		
Clinical	**Acute presentation**	**Chronic presentation**
Onset	Acute	Chronic and gradual dyspnea
Appearance	Severely ill	Normal or mildly dyspneic
Blood pressure	Variable	Variable
Tachycardia	Almost always	Variable
S1	Usually normal or mildly increased	Normal or soft
S2	Usually normal	Wide splitting
S3	Common	Common
S4	Common	Rare
Apical impulse	Not displaced	Displaced and forcible (large heart)
Apical systolic thrill	No	Common
Apical mitral murmur	Soft or absent (early systolic) and decrescendo	Harsh (parasystolic)
Radiation of murmur	Axilla, spine, or base	Axilla
Basal ejection systolic murmur	With posterior chordal rupture	No
Apical rumbling diastolic murmur	Common and short	Infrequent
Electrocardiography		
Left ventricular (LV) hypertrophy	No	Almost always
Echocardiography		
LV size	Normal	Dilated
LV function	Hyperactive	Variable
LA (left atrium) size	Normal	Dilated
Chest X-ray		
Cardiomegaly	No cardiomegaly	Severe cardiomegaly
Lung fields	Pulmonary edema	Pulmonary venous congestion

Figure 40.6 Physical and diagnostic findings of severe mitral regurgitation. (Adapted with permission from Braunwald, 1997.)

function of the square of the transvalvular flow rate (see Fig. 40.7, Gorlin formula). As the severity of AS increases, patients become symptomatic during periods of augmented flow (exercise, tachycardia, fever, pregnancy).

In later stages, the hypertrophied left ventricle exhibits reduced compliance and diastolic relaxation, with increased EDP. High diastolic pressures are necessary to fill the hypertrophied left ventricle and are reflected in increased left atrial, pulmonary capillary, pulmonary arterial, and, eventually, right-sided pressures. Patients report dyspnea upon exertion, but later also at rest, and may experience episodes of pulmonary edema. The hypertrophied ventricle is exquisitely sensitive to ischemia. Increased ventricular wall stress increases myocardial oxygen demand. Elevated left ventricular EDP along with a shortened diastolic period of coronary artery perfusion can compromise oxygen supply to the point where infarction can occur in the absence of coronary artery disease (CAD). There is also evidence for reduced capillary density, abnormal arteriolar thickening, and impaired vasodilator reserve. Diastolic dysfunction as a result of hypertrophy and ischemia with intact or even increased systolic function progresses to a point at which the left ventricle begins to dilate and fail (Fig. 40.9). The hemodynamic management of AS is summarized in Figure 40.4.

MITRAL STENOSIS

The circumference of the mitral valve is 10cm in the adult, with the greatest diameter extending from the anterolateral to the posteromedial commissure. The commissures do not normally extend out to the ring, leaving an orifice of 4–6cm^2. The valve is bicuspid; the anterior leaflet is about twice the size of the posterior leaflet. Typical symptoms and signs of MS have a gradual onset (Fig. 40.8).

Pathophysiology

In rheumatic MS, the stenotic mitral valve results from fusion and thickening of the mitral apparatus. The leaflets fuse at their edges and the chordae shorten. Calcium deposits involve the leaflets and may spread to encompass the annulus. MR may be present secondary to the inability of the rigid leaflets to approximate, or because of shortening and fusion of the chordae with little involvement of the leaflets. Pure MS is seen in 25% of patients; 40% have combined MS and MR, and the remainder have coexisting lesions involving other valves. As the mitral valve orifice becomes smaller, the left atrium enlarges and undergoes fibrotic changes. Left atrial thrombi may be present. Structural pulmonary artery changes accompany long-standing MS, with dilatation of the major branches together with muscular hypertrophy, intimal proliferation, and fibrosis of the arterioles. Within the parenchyma, the basement membranes of the capillaries thicken and there is interstitial edema, fibrosis, and hemosiderin deposition. As the pulmonary arteriolar resistance rises secondary to these changes, right ventricular hypertrophy and right atrial and right ventricular dilatation develop, with progression to failure. The effect of MS on the normal cardiac cycle is illustrated by the pressure–volume loop shown in Figure 40.2. There is chronic

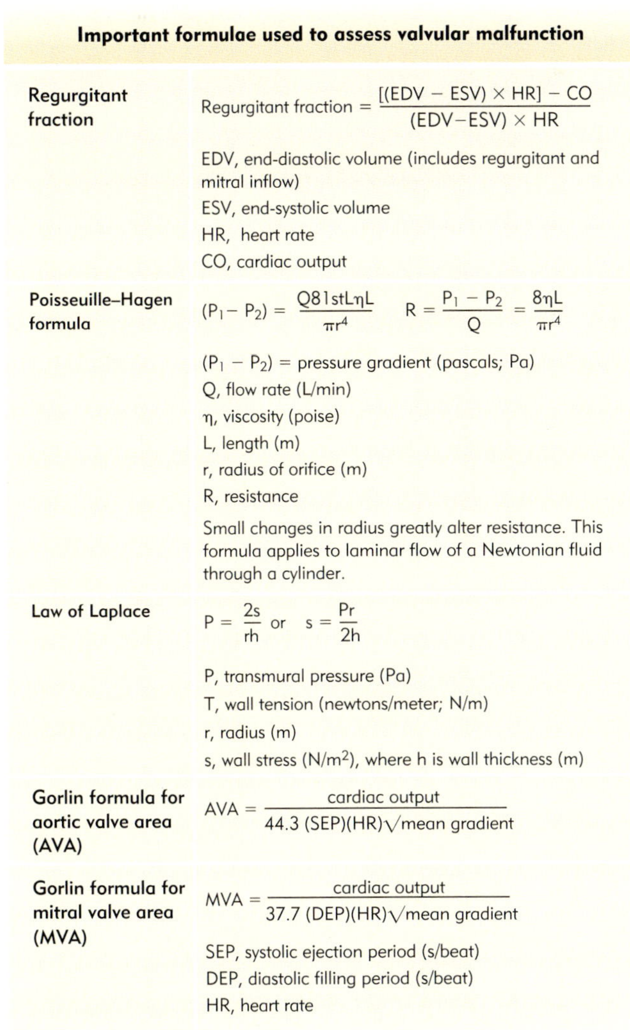

Important formulae used to assess valvular malfunction

Regurgitant fraction	$\text{Regurgitant fraction} = \frac{[(EDV - ESV) \times HR] - CO}{(EDV - ESV) \times HR}$ EDV, end-diastolic volume (includes regurgitant and mitral inflow) ESV, end-systolic volume HR, heart rate CO, cardiac output
Poisseuille–Hagen formula	$(P_1 - P_2) = \frac{Q81stL\eta L}{\pi r^4} \quad R = \frac{P_1 - P_2}{Q} = \frac{8\eta L}{\pi r^4}$ $(P_1 - P_2)$ = pressure gradient (pascals; Pa) Q, flow rate (L/min) η, viscosity (poise) L, length (m) r, radius of orifice (m) R, resistance Small changes in radius greatly alter resistance. This formula applies to laminar flow of a Newtonian fluid through a cylinder.
Law of Laplace	$P = \frac{2s}{rh}$ or $s = \frac{Pr}{2h}$ P, transmural pressure (Pa) T, wall tension (newtons/meter; N/m) r, radius (m) s, wall stress (N/m^2), where h is wall thickness (m)
Gorlin formula for aortic valve area (AVA)	$AVA = \frac{\text{cardiac output}}{44.3\ (SEP)(HR)\sqrt{\text{mean gradient}}}$
Gorlin formula for mitral valve area (MVA)	$MVA = \frac{\text{cardiac output}}{37.7\ (DEP)(HR)\sqrt{\text{mean gradient}}}$ SEP, systolic ejection period (s/beat) DEP, diastolic filling period (s/beat) HR, heart rate

Figure 40.7 Important formulae used in assessing the degree of valvular malfunction.

volume underload of the left ventricle with pressure and volume overload of the left atrium and proximal structures.

In mild MS (orifice 2–4cm^2), blood flow across the valve requires a small but nevertheless abnormal transvalvular pressure gradient to maintain cardiac output (Fig. 40.9). As can be seen from a rearrangement of the Gorlin formula (see Fig. 40.7), the pressure gradient increases as the square of the flow rate. Although the orifice is fixed at any one time, the transvalvular gradient may be dynamic, depending on the flows across it. To maintain cardiac output during tachycardia, even higher transvalvular gradients must be generated. Pulmonary venous pressures follow the transvalvular gradients and, therefore, these become markedly increased during times of augmented flow rate (tachycardia, exercise, fever, pregnancy, hypovolemia). This results in a reduced pulmonary compliance and increased work of breathing (dyspnea).

As the orifice continues to diminish in size, the gradient reaches 20–25mmHg across a 1cm^2 valve area at rest. The patient experiences dyspnea with minimal exertion and even nocturnal cough, paroxysmal nocturnal dyspnea, orthopnea, and hemoptysis. With relatively little exercise, pulmonary capillary pressures increase to 30–40mmHg. At this stage, capillary hydrostatic pressure greatly exceeds plasma oncotic pressure. A reversible vasoconstriction of the smaller branches of the pulmonary artery reduces preload to the left ventricle, thereby allowing left atrial and pulmonary capillary pressures to remain below the pulmonary edema level. However, the rising pulmonary artery pressure is now out of proportion to pulmonary capillary pressure and may approach systemic levels. Patients experience extreme fatigue associated with low cardiac output (secondary to the reduced left ventricular preload) and right-sided failure.

Early in the progression of MS, most patients remain in sinus rhythm. As the orifice diminishes and the left atrial pressure and size increase, atrial fibrillation may occur. The onset of clinical MS is frequently heralded by the development of atrial fibrillation, which reduces cardiac output through an increase in heart rate; the atrial kick contributes less to ventricular filling in MS than under normal conditions. Rapid atrial fibrillation is associated with a short diastolic filling time, increased flow rates across the stenotic valve, increased transvalvular gradients, and sudden elevations in left atrial and pulmonary capillary pressures, resulting in pulmonary edema.

It is commonly thought that the left ventricle is 'protected' in MS. Although symptoms of left ventricular failure are rare, laboratory findings demonstrate evidence of left ventricular impairment in 25% of patients. The pathophysiology of this dysfunction includes myocardial scarring from the rheumatic process (particularly in the posterobasal region and associated with regional wall abnormalities), continued subclinical rheumatic carditis, increased right ventricular volume with flattening or bulging of the septal wall, chronic effects of underloading on the left ventricle (likened to a disuse atrophy), and insufficient coronary artery blood flow secondary to reduced cardiac output and concurrent CAD. Patients over 50 years of age or with significant risk factors for CAD, should have coronary artery angiography prior to surgical correction. Similarly, those patents with chronic obstructive pulmonary disease should also have coronary artery angiography to clarify the clinical picture. The hemodynamic management of MS is summarized in Figure 40.4.

TRICUSPID STENOSIS

Tricuspid stenosis (TS) is an uncommon lesion that is virtually always rheumatic in origin. It is seen at autopsy in 15% of patients with a history of rheumatic fever, of which only a third will have been symptomatic. When presenting with MS, it occurs most commonly during the third decade in females. The diagnosis of TS may be confused with more rare forms of right atrial obstruction, including congenital tricuspid atresia, right atrial tumors, carcinoid syndrome, tricuspid vegetations, and endomyocardial fibrosis.

Pathophysiology

As in rheumatic MS, rheumatic TS results in thickening and fusion of the leaflets at their edges and shortening and fusion of the chordae tendinae. This shortening of the chordae can produce regurgitation and, therefore, TS is often a mixed stenotic and regurgitant lesion. Calcification of the leaflets or annulus is rare. As the orifice reduces in size, the right atrium enlarges and hypertrophies, with passive, peripheral venous congestion that is often severe.

As in MS, the pressure gradient across the stenotic valve increases with increased flow (e.g. exercise, fever, tachycardia). However, only a very small mean gradient (as low as 2mmHg) will cause symptoms. Consequently, venous congestion, with associated hepatosplenomegaly, ascites, peripheral edema, and even anasarca, is noted early. These symptoms are out of pro-

Physical findings in aortic and mitral stenosis

Findings	Aortic stenosis	Mitral stenosis
Onset	Latent period ≥10 years	Gradual
Appearance	Normal	Normal 'mitral fascies' (pink, purplish patches on cheeks)
Blood pressure	Reduced systolic and diastolic blood pressures in advanced stages	Normal or even low
Rhythm	Sinus; atrial fibrillation late	Sinus, atrial fibrillation, varying degrees of conduction defects
Peripheral arterial signs	Slow rising, small volume, sustained; anacrotic notch felt in carotids; lag between apex and carotid pulses	Normal or small in volume
Thrill	Systolic thrill at 2nd left intercostal space (leaning forward) in full expiration	Palpable tapping S1 apical thrill of diastolic murmur at apex (left lateral recumbent position); right ventricular (RV) lift at left parasternal border in pulmonary hypertension
Apical impulse	Presystolic distension of left ventricle (LV) visible and palpable	Rare
Heart sounds		
S1	Normal or soft	Accentuated
S2	May be single; paradoxical splitting suggests LV failure	Accentuated P2, as pulmonary hypertension rises, split S2 narrows then becomes single and accentuated
S3	Rare	Present in combined mitral stenosis (MS) and mitral regurgitation (MR)
S4	Prominent	Rare
Murmur	Ejection click in bicuspid aortic valve without significant stenosis at left sternal border radiating to apex; loud 'spindle shaped' late peaking systolic murmur across precordium radiating to apex and carotids; 'blowing' decrescendo diastolic murmur in aortic regurgitation	Opening snap at apex; low-pitched rumbling diastolic murmur; if soft limited to apex, louder radiates to axilla and/or lower left sternum; duration (not intensity) of murmur correlates with severity
Electrocardiography	LV hypertrophy (LVH); T wave inversion and ST depression of severe LVH. Left atrial enlargement (LAE)	Left and right atrial enlargement (LAE, RAE), RV hypertrophy (RVH); atrial fibrillation
Chest X-ray		
Cardiac	Normal cardiac silhouette; rounded LV border and apex; poststenotic aortic dilatation, calcified aortic valve	Enlarged atrial appendage LAE, RV enlargement (RVE), RAE, pulmonary artery enlargement if severe MS; calcified mitral valve
Lung fields	Pulmonary venous hypertension	Kerley B-lines, Kerley A-lines; hemosiderosis; evaluation of left main bronchus
Echocardiography	Can measure orifice, gradients and velocities across valve; LVH, LV function normal, supranormal, or depressed; LAE	Readily diagnosed by M-mode and two-dimensional mode; measure gradients and velocities across valve; LV size and function normal/reduced; LAE, RVE, RAE
Look for clues for underlying etiology	Degenerative: age, calcium deposits Rheumatic fever: previous history, other valvular involvement, pericarditis, conduction defects Other: Paget's disease, rheumatoid arthritis	Rheumatic fever: as for aortic stenosis Other: systemic lupus erythematosus, rheumatoid arthritis, amyloidosis

Figure 40.8 Physical findings in aortic and mitral stenosis.

portion to the fatigue and dyspnea, resulting from the low right-sided output state. The reduction in hepatic blood flow may be severe enough to cause liver dysfunction.

In patients with coexisting TS and MS, the typical symptoms of MS (shortness of breath, paroxysmal nocturnal dyspnea, hemoptysis, and pulmonary edema) may be attenuated by the low output from the right ventricle, which fails to rise during exercise. Therefore, even with a severely stenotic mitral valve, left atrial and pulmonary pressures may remain normal or only mildly elevated. Consequently, patients with MS who have minimal symptoms or lower left-sided pressures than expected should be evaluated for TS.

PULMONIC STENOSIS

Pulmonic stenosis (PS) as an acquired lesion is extremely rare. It may occur as a sequela of rheumatic fever but invariably is part of a multivalvular picture. Very rarely, the pulmonic valve may be associated with malignant carcinoid, which results in shortening and fusion of the valve leaflets. These shortened leaflets may produce an incompetent valve with ensuing regurgitation.

CONGENITAL VALVULAR DISEASE

Congenital valvular lesions may exist in isolation, or more commonly as part of a more complex cardiac anomaly. These lesions are typically obstructive and cause reduced outflow from, as well as pressure overload of, the corresponding chambers upstream from the obstruction. In the neonatal period, shunting will occur across patent shunt orifices. If the obstruction is severe or complete, an obligatory shunt must exist downstream to the obstruction to maintain circulation. The magnitude of the downstream shunt is variable and depends on the relative balance of pulmonary and systemic vascular resistance. Manipulation of either controls the amount of blood flow across the shunt, and determines the relative pulmonary and peripheral perfusion. Therefore, an under-

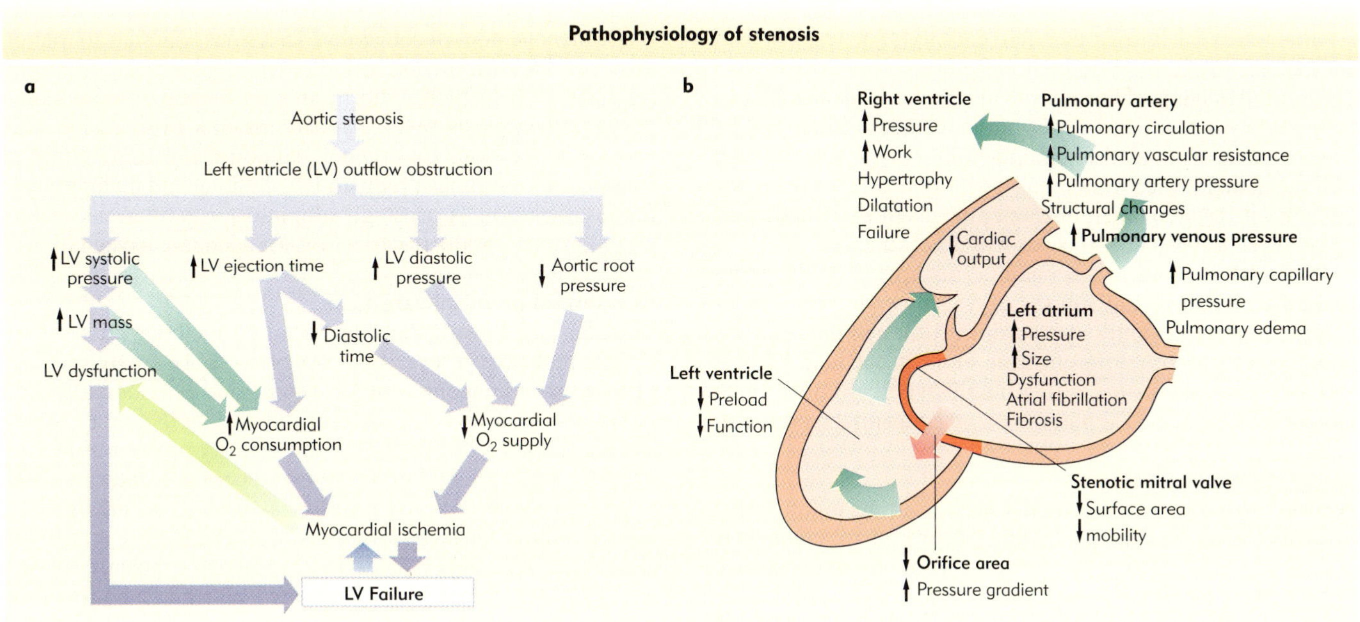

Figure 40.9 Pathophysiology of stenosis. In aortic stenosis (left), left ventricular outflow results in structural and function changes, leading eventually to left ventricular failure. In mitral stenosis (right), an increased transvalvular gradient is reflected in increased left atrial, pulmonary capillary, pulmonary artery, and right-sided pressure. Structural and function changes follow as depicted.

standing of the control of pulmonary vascular resistance is particularly important because abnormal pulmonary vasculature is often found in patients with congenital heart disease.

Congenital aortic stenosis

Valvular stenosis

Congenital valvular AS is one of the more common congenital cardiac defects. It occurs in approximately 5% of patients with congenital cardiovascular lesions, although this is probably an underestimate since congenital bicuspid AS is a frequent unsuspected autopsy finding. In 20% of congenital AS, other associated cardiac defects are present, the most common being coarctation of the aorta and patent ductus arteriosus.

The pathophysiology of congenital AS, as with the acquired form, centers around the gradient generated across the reduced orifice. In the infant or child, effective orifice sizes are expressed on a body surface area basis, with $2.0cm^2/m^2$ being normal. Below this, orifice sizes above $0.8cm^2/m^2$ are considered as mild, those $0.5–0.8cm^2/m^2$ as moderate, and those less than $0.5cm^2/m^2$ as severe. Cardiac output must be taken into account when considering the transvalvular gradient (see above), and a peak gradient of 75mmHg or more with a normal cardiac output is considered critical stenosis.

Symptoms differ in the newborn from the older child. In the neonate, AS can be a life-threatening lesion. Since the left ventricle is bypassed *in utero*, exposure to sudden severe obstruction at birth produces left ventricular failure, pulmonary venous congestion, and systemic hypoperfusion, with substantial left-to-right shunting at the atrial level accompanying right-sided failure. The severely affected infant is hypotensive with poorly palpable pulses, irritable, pale, cyanotic, tachypneic, and tachycardic. There is cardiomegaly and congestive heart failure. This picture is clinically indistinguishable from hypoplastic left heart syndrome or aortic arch syndrome and requires echocardiography or cardiac catheterization for rapid diagnosis and identification of other associated cardiac and noncardiac anomalies. Severely symptomatic neonates require emergency balloon aortic valvuloplasty.

In the older infant, congenital AS is compensated by the development of left ventricular hypertrophy, and symptoms may not arise until subendocardial oxygenation is compromised because of an inadequately developed network of collateral arteries. Ischemia, infarction, papillary muscle dysfunction, and fibroelastosis may occur, with resultant left ventricular failure and even functional MR.

Most children with congenital AS grow and develop normally. The resting cardiac output and stroke volume tends to fall within normal limits, with left ventricular hypertrophy maintaining supernormal ventricular function and lower than normal wall stress throughout systole. Nevertheless, high transvalvular gradients still exist with high end-diastolic filling pressures that result from pressure-overload hypertrophy. Studies suggest that the extent of early diastolic dysfunction is related to the degree of hypertrophy rather than to wall stress.

Early diagnosis is made by the incidental finding of a murmur. Interestingly, the aortic orifice itself does not tend to diminish progressively in size with congenital AS as it does in acquired AS. Rather the stenotic orifice becomes *relatively* smaller and transvalvular flows increase as cardiac output rises to meet the demands of growth. Children with moderate to severe AS should have their physical activity restricted until the defect is surgically corrected, as arrhythmias and sudden death can occur.

Subaortic and supravalvular stenosis

Subaortic and supravalvular stenotic lesions present as obstruction to left ventricular outflow; however, they are distinct entities that require brief mention. Subaortic stenosis accounts for approximately 10% of congenital AS and is clinically indistinguishable from valvular AS. However, the nature of the lesion (a subaortic fibrous ring or membrane) creates a high-velocity jet directed at the aortic valve that leads to tissue trauma, with subsequent thickening and immobilization of the leaflets. The differential diagnosis between valvular and subvalvular AS can be made by echocardiography or cardiac catheterization. Unlike congenital valvular AS, the pathophysiology of this lesion is such that the actual orifice will diminish with time and aortic regurgitation will develop. Therefore, once the diagnosis is made, surgical correction usually proceeds in a timely manner.

Supravalvular AS is a congenital narrowing of the aorta immediately above the sinuses of Valsalva which produces obstruction to left ventricular outflow. Although the hemodynamic effects are no different from those in valvular AS, this lesion is often associated with infantile hypercalcemia, which can itself be expressed as part of several congenital syndromes.

Congenital mitral stenosis

A varied spectrum of congenital lesions resulting in functional obstruction across the mitral valve occur and are commonly associated with other cardiac defects. Symptoms of congestive heart failure with pulmonary edema and a low-output state appear early; the underlying pathophysiology is similar to acquired MS (see above). The presence of other associated congenital cardiac defects changes the clinical and hemodynamic picture accordingly. The prognosis of congenital MS is extremely poor without early correction.

Congenital tricuspid stenosis

There are a number of anomalies of the tricuspid valve that produce stenosis or atresia, and in most patients form part of a complex of congenital anomalies. In the neonatal period, the degree of shunting and amount of pulmonary blood flow determine the clinical picture. There will always be a degree of cyanosis because of right-to-left shunting, but in patients where the pulmonary blood flow is greatly restricted, severe hypoxia results. This is in comparison with lesions where associated anomalies predispose to increased pulmonary blood flow and the clinical picture is similar to congestive heart failure. Medical, surgical, and anesthetic management of congenital TS lesions is similar to that of acquired TS, with the exception of tricuspid atresia. Tricuspid atresia is often diagnosed shortly after birth when these neonates persist with cyanosis, severe hypoxia, systemic hypotension, and venous congestion. Emergency balloon atrial septostomy is required to re-establish right-to-left shunting and maintain systemic circulation. A prostaglandin infusion is often needed to maintain a patent ductus arteriosis for adequate oxygenation.

Congenital pulmonic stenosis

Valvular and subvalvular congenital PS includes an array of lesions that vary in severity. It occurs in approximately 7% of patients with congenital heart disease and is associated with Noonan's syndrome. The clinical and hemodynamic consequences of PS will depend on the severity of the lesion and whether it is expressed in the neonatal period or later in life.

In the neonate, severe PS is associated with extreme right-to-left shunting at the atrial level (or ventricular if there is an associated ventricular septal defect) with profound hypoxia, cyanosis, and acidemia. Administration of prostaglandin E_1 maintains a patent ductus arteriosis and increases pulmonary blood flow with improvement of symptoms. Balloon valvuloplasty is the procedure of choice and may be life saving. In patients with hypoplasia of the right ventricle or pulmonic valve, corrective surgery is required that may involve a left-to-right shunt.

In the older child, PS is usually mild to moderate with little progression and is often noted as an incidental finding. However, in patients with more severe forms of the lesion, stenosis tends to be progressive and hemodynamically more significant as cardiac output increases with growth. Symptoms depend on the severity of stenosis; a peak transvalvular gradient of 75–100mmHg indicates moderate stenosis and values greater than 100mmHg indicate severe stenosis. There is an inability to increase pulmonary flow during exercise, and symptoms of fatigue, chest pain, and even syncope occur. Right ventricular failure occurs in more severe disease.

Key References

Chatterjee K, Cheitlin MD, Karliner J, et al., eds. Cardiology: an illustrated text reference, Section 9, Vol. 2. Philadelphia, PA: Lippincott; 1991:9/1–124.

Braunwald E, ed. Heart disease. A textbook of cardiovascular medicine, 5th edn, Ch. 32. Philadelphia, PA: Saunders; 1997:1007–76.

Fauci AS, Braunwald E, Isselbacher KJ, et al., eds. Harrison's principles of internal medicine, 14th edn, Ch. 237. New York: McGraw-Hill; 1998:1311–24.

Bell DB, Kain ZN, eds. The pediatric anesthesia handbook, 2nd edn, Ch 7. St Louis, MO: Mosby; 1997:133–73.

Carabello BA, Crawford Jr FA. Valvular heart disease. N Engl J Med. 1997;337:31–41.

Further Reading

Exadactylos N, Sugrue DD, Oakley CM. Prevalence of coronary artery disease in patients with isolated aortic valve stenosis. Br Heart J. 1984;51:121–4.

Gahol K, Sutton R, Pearson M, et al. Mitral regurgitation in coronary heart disease. Br Heart J. 1997;39:13–18.

Grossman W, Jones D, McLaurin LP. Wall stress and patterns of hypertrophy in the human left ventricle. J Clin Invest. 1975;56:56–64.

Hartman GS. Management of patients with valvular heart disease. Anesth Analg. 1994;78:141–51.

Hemmings HCJ, Thomas SJ. Management of patients with valvular disease. In: Prys-Roberts C, Brown BRJ, eds. International practice of anesthesia. Oxford, UK: Butterworth Heinemann; 1996:1/39/1–14.

Mattina CJ, Green SJ, Tortdani AJ, et al. Frequency of angiographically significant coronary artery narrowing in mitral stenosis. Am J Cardiol. 1986;57:802–5.

Meisner JS, Keven G, Pajaro OE, et al. Atrial contribution to ventricular filling in mtral stenosis. Circulation. 1991;84:1469–80

Ross J Jr. Afterload mismatch in aortic and mitral valve disease: implications for surgical therapy. J Am Coll Cardiol. 1985;5:811–26.

Chapter 41 Cardiac anesthesia

Lisa Warren and Stephen J Thomas

Topics covered in this chapter

Cardiovascular effects of anesthetics
Cardiopulmonary bypass
Pathophysiology of cardiopulmonary bypass
Pharmacokinetics during cardiopulmonary bypass

The practice of cardiac anesthesia requires a thorough understanding of normal and pathologic cardiac physiology and anatomy, the pharmacology of anesthetic and cardiovascular drugs, as well as the physiologic adaptations to cardiopulmonary bypass (CPB) and surgery. In this chapter a brief review of these topics is presented, bringing together concepts introduced in the preceding chapters to illustrate the mechanical and technical considerations in the clinical care of cardiac surgical patients.

CARDIOVASCULAR EFFECTS OF ANESTHETICS

Since anesthetic medications frequently induce changes in systemic vascular resistance, heart rate, contractility, and coronary blood flow, alterations in myocardial oxygen demand and supply may occur. Understanding the cardiovascular consequences of the drug combinations used and their effects on patients with coronary artery disease (CAD) and valvular heart disease (VHD) is imperative to safely induce and maintain anesthesia. The pharmacology of the various classes of anesthetic agents is discussed elsewhere (Chapters 22–28). The hemodynamic effects of inhalational and intravenous anesthetics, opioids, benzodiazepines, and muscle relaxants are summarized here (Fig. 41.1).

Hemodynamic effects of myocardial contractility drugs used in anesthesia

Agent	Parameters				
	HR	MAP	Myocardial Contractility	CO	Arrhythmia Potential
Inhalational					
Halothane	↓	↓	↓	↓	↑
Enflurane	↑	↓	↓	↓	
Isoflurane	↑	↓	↓	↓↑	
Desflurane	↑	↓	↓	↓	
Sevoflurane	–	↓	↓	↓	
Nitrous Oxide	–	↑	↓	↓	
Intravenous					
Thiopental	↑	↓	↓	↓	
Benzodiazepines	–	↓	–	–	
Etomidate	–	–	–	–	
Ketamine	↑	↑	↓	↑	
Propofol	–	↓	↓	↓	
Opioids					
Fentanyl	↓	–	–	–	
Morphine	↓	↓	–	–	
Meperidine	↑	↓	–	–	
Muscle Relaxants					
Pancuronium	↑	–	–	↑	
Vecuronium	–	–	–	–	
Atracurium	↑↓	↓	–	–	
Rocuronium	–↑	–	–	–	
Succinylcholine	↑↓	↑	–	–	↑

Abbreviations: HR, heart rate; MAP, mean arterial pressure; CO, cardiac output.

Figure 41.1 Hemodynamic effects of drugs used in anesthesia.

Inhalational anesthetics

All volatile anesthetics cause direct dose-dependent myocardial depression: halothane and enflurane cause the greatest degree, isoflurane, sevoflurane, and desflurane the least. The mechanism of myocardial depression is most likely related to effects on intracellular Ca^{2+} regulation (Chapter 34) and depression of sympathetic tone. Volatile agents reduce blood pressure: halothane predominantly by myocardial depression and a reduction in cardiac output; isoflurane, desflurane, and sevoflurane by a reduction in smooth muscle tone and vasodilation; and enflurane by a combination of both. The effect on heart rate varies among the agents. Halothane tends to reduce heart rate and slow conduction through the atrioventricular node and His–Purkinje system, which increases the chance of arrhythmia development. Halothane may also precipitate a junctional rhythm as a result of suppression of the sinus node. Enflurane, isoflurane, and desflurane increase heart rate, and sevoflurane causes little change in heart rate except at high inspired concentrations. Volatile agents attenuate the baroreceptor reflex to hypotension. Isoflurane has the least effect, such that the elevation of heart rate with isoflurane is compensatory in the setting of decreased systemic vascular resistance and cardiac output. Halothane sensitizes the myocardium to the arrhythmogenic effects of epinephrine (adrenaline), while the other inhalational agents do not. Nitrous oxide is also a myocardial depressant, but is less potent than the volatile anesthetics. Its direct depressant effects are countered by sympathetic activation.

Coronary effects

Halothane has a minor coronary vasodilating action but does not alter autoregulation. Enflurane also causes coronary vasodilation. Isoflurane is more potent than halothane and enflurane, and may lead to redistribution of blood flow in the presence of coronary stenosis (coronary steal phenomenon). Theoretically, the potential for ischemia exists with the use of high concentrations of isoflurane in the setting of steal-prone anatomy and hemodynamic alterations (tachycardia, hypotension). However, the clinical significance of isoflurane-induced coronary vasodilation remains unproved, since only a small proportion of patients with CAD demonstrate steal-prone anatomy, and isoflurane is generally used in combination with other anesthetic agents and rarely reaches concentrations high enough to cause coronary vasodilation. Desflurane and sevoflurane cause coronary vasodilation in animals, but are not associated with coronary flow redistribution. No evidence suggests an increased risk of ischemia or infarction when isoflurane is compared with sevoflurane in cardiac surgery patients. Nitrous oxide does not appear to affect coronary blood flow distribution.

Intravenous anesthetics

Thiopental reduces contractility and arterial blood pressure, and increases heart rate. A transient reduction of blood pressure is seen on induction because of peripheral vasodilation, which is partially offset by a baroreceptor-mediated increase in heart rate. Pooling of blood in capacitance vessels (venodilation) leads to a reduction in filling pressures and a potential decrease in cardiac output. Histamine release may also occur with rapid intravenous administration.

The benzodiazepines diazepam and midazolam cause a small decrease in arterial pressure with generally little effect on heart rate or contractility. When combined with other anesthetic drugs, such as fentanyl, a significant drop in blood pressure can be seen because of a reduction in systemic vascular resistance. Induction of anesthesia in patients with CAD or VHD using midazolam alone is associated with minimal changes in cardiac output, heart rate, or blood pressure.

Etomidate is noted for its hemodynamic stability. In patients with compensated CAD no significant changes are seen in heart rate, cardiac output, or systemic vascular resistance. Compared with other intravenous anesthetics, etomidate produces the least change in myocardial oxygen balance. Systemic blood pressure remains unchanged, except in patients with VHD or with concomitant opioids.

Ketamine stimulates the cardiovascular system by releasing catecholamines, which results in increased heart rate, cardiac output, systemic vascular resistance, and systemic and pulmonary arterial blood pressure. It is a useful agent in patients with hemodynamic compromise caused by hypovolemia or cardiac tamponade. However, negative inotropic effects, which can be demonstrated by direct application to cardiac tissue in vitro, may be seen in severely ill patients who have depleted catecholamines.

Propofol significantly decreases blood pressure, predominantly as a result of a reduction in systemic vascular resistance, with minimal change in heart rate. Blood pressure effects may be exaggerated in the setting of hypovolemia or poor left ventricular (LV) function. Propofol resets the baroreceptor reflex control of heart rate, eliminating the increase in heart rate normally induced by reduced blood pressure. Propofol decreases coronary blood flow (as a result of reduced blood pressure) and myocardial oxygen demand (MVO_2) proportionately.

Opioids

Opioids have negative inotropic effects, but at doses much higher than those used clinically. Morphine may cause a significant reduction in vascular resistance because of histamine release. The synthetic opioids fentanyl and sufentanil have little effect on vascular resistance when used alone, thus their popularity for hemodynamic stability. All opioids cause bradycardia as a result of central vagal stimulation except meperidine (pethidine), which is vagolytic. Sufentanil-induced bradycardia may be severe enough to reduce cardiac output significantly; this effect is attenuated by the concomitant use of vagolytic drugs and potentiated by negative chronotropic drugs (e.g. β-blockers and Ca^{2+} channel blockers).

Muscle relaxants

Pancuronium increases heart rate, blood pressure, and cardiac output. Heart rate increases because of vagal blockade with increased blood pressure and cardiac output may result from sympathetic stimulation and inhibition of catecholamine reuptake. Atracurium and mivacurium decrease mean arterial blood pressure when given in rapid bolus doses because of histamine release. Vecuronium is not associated with significant hemodynamic changes. Rocuronium is similar to vecuronium, although it occasionally has a mild vagolytic effect. The depolarizing muscle relaxant succinylcholine, when given in repeated doses, frequently causes sinus bradycardia as a result of muscarinic receptor stimulation at the sinus node. Succinylcholine may also precipitate arrhythmias during anesthesia because of generalized autonomic stimulation. Additionally, succinylcholine lowers the threshold of the ventricle to catecholamine-induced arrhythmias.

CARDIOPULMONARY BYPASS

To replace heart and lung function, the CPB technique must pump oxygenated blood through the patient and remove carbon dioxide. It is the standard method used whenever the operation requires a still heart. Where surgery of the aortic arch is planned, the technique of deep hypothermic circulatory arrest may be employed to achieve an adequate surgical field not obscured by bleeding while reducing the consequences of ischemia to the heart and brain. Minimally invasive techniques using endoscopic or endovascular methods which in some cases obviate the necessity for CPB and cardiac arrest.

Cardiopulmonary bypass circuit

The CPB machine (heart–lung machine), developed by Gibbon, was first employed successfully in 1953 for the repair of an interatrial septal defect. Prior to this, most intracardiac procedures were perforce performed on the beating heart and were hurried, incomplete, and usually unsuccessful, except for closed mitral commisurotomy. Elements of a simple CPB system include a venous reservoir, an 'artificial lung' or oxygenator to deliver oxygen and remove carbon dioxide, a heat exchanger for the extracorporeal blood, and an arterial pump (Fig. 41.2). Over the ensuing years, many investigators have contributed to advances in CPB technology, but the fundamental design remains the same. Two cannulae, venous and arterial, are placed either centrally in the right atrium and ascending aorta, respectively, or peripherally in the femoral vein and artery. Blood is drained via gravity to a venous reservoir, passed through an oxygenator in which gas exchange occurs, filtered to remove gas bubbles and particulate matter, heated or cooled as necessary, and pumped back to the patient through the arterial cannula. Parallel circuits

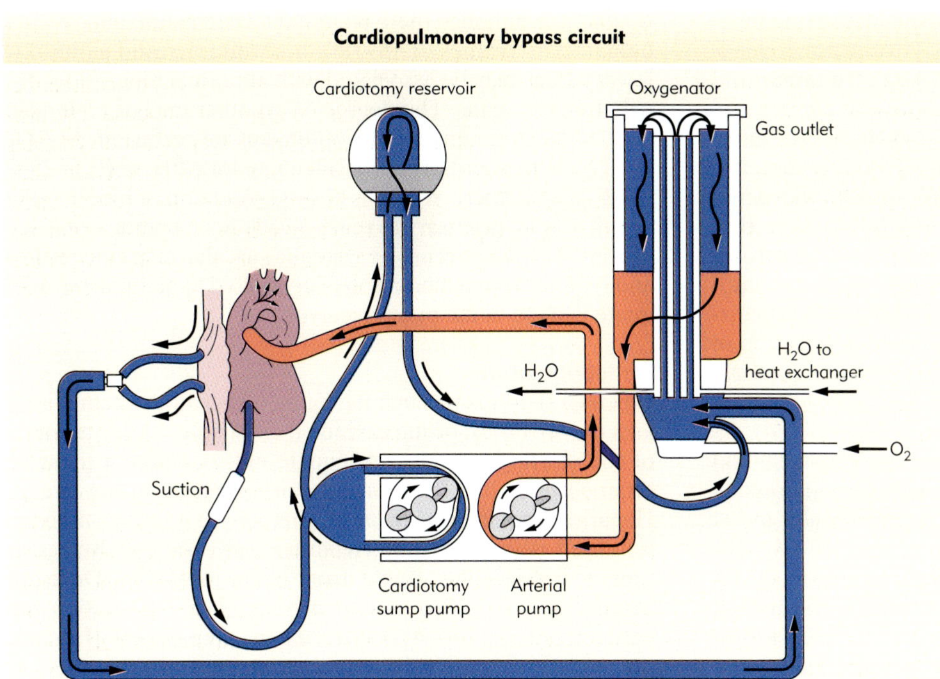

Figure 41.2 Cardiopulmonary bypass circuit.

with additional pumps can be added to this primary circuit, and may include cardiotomy suction (which removes shed blood and debris from the surgical field), an LV vent (which decompresses the heart), and a cardioplegia circuit (described below).

Cannulae

A single, large-bore, right atrial cannula, most frequently a dual-stage cannula, is placed through the right atrial appendage into the inferior vena cava. Venous blood is drained from the lumen in the inferior vena cava and from multiple right atrial fenestrations, which allows effective venous drainage from the upper and lower body and coronary sinus. Alternatively, for open cardiotomies two venous cannulae are often used to assure unobstructed venous return. These smaller cannulae are placed through the right atrium into each vena cava and secured with tourniquets. All venous blood, except coronary sinus return, is diverted from the right heart. Venous drainage is dependent upon gravity, and therefore the surgical table must be above the height of the venous reservoir. Inadequate venous drainage may result from kinking of the cannulae or tubing, or from the development of an air lock within the tubing. Jugular venous hypertension may also occur when the heart is rotated during surgery or from kinking of the superior vena cava cannula.

Oxygenated blood is returned to the patient through an arterial cannula placed either in the ascending aorta or the femoral artery. Aortic rupture, dissection, and misdirection of blood flow are potential complications. Usually a microfilter, 20–40μm in size, is placed in the arterial inflow line to prevent microemboli from entering the arterial circulation.

The cardioplegia cannula is a small-bore cannula placed in the aorta proximal to the arterial cannula. Cross clamping of the aorta just distal to this cannula, but proximal to the aortic cannula, allows the selective perfusion of cardioplegia to the coronary circulation. Cardioplegia solution is delivered to the heart from a parallel circuit on the bypass machine, either through the cannula or directly into the coronary ostia by hand-held cannulae if the proximal aorta is opened for aortic valve replacement or aortic repair. Alternatively, or additionally, cardioplegia may be injected in a retrograde fashion via a cannula placed in the coronary sinus. The ability to monitor cardioplegia line pressure is important to diagnose problems with cardioplegia delivery (e.g. dissection, aortic insufficiency).

Oxygenators

Bubble and membrane oxygenators are currently employed, although recently the membrane oxygenator has gained greater popularity. Bubble oxygenators are composed of an oxygenating column, a debubbling–defoaming chamber, and an arterial reservoir. Venous blood is passed through the oxygenating column, in which microbubbles form a large blood–gas interface for gas exchange. Oxygenation depends upon the size of the blood–gas interface, and carbon dioxide elimination is determined by the oxygen flow rate. The blood–gas mixture flows through a defoaming chamber in which the majority of microbubbles are removed, and finally oxygenated blood enters the arterial reservoir. Additional microbubbles rise out of the blood during transit in the reservoir, but microbubbles cannot be removed completely and gaseous emboli can be detected in the arterial inflow.

Membrane oxygenators separate blood and gas by a semi-permeable membrane across which gas exchange occurs. Membrane technology has advanced from the initial coil or parallel plate design to the modern hollow-fiber configuration. Oxygen from the membrane oxygenator diffuses along a concentration gradient through the membrane material to the blood flowing through it. Carbon dioxide from the venous blood diffuses along a concentration gradient through the membrane to the gas path of the device. Gas exchange depends on the total surface area of the membrane, the concentration gradients developed across the membrane, and the permeability of the membrane to the particular gases.

The direct blood–gas interface formed by the bubble oxygenator causes damage to cellular elements, platelets, and proteins, and results in a high level of gaseous microemboli. Hemolysis, leukocyte damage, and platelet and complement activation occur. Leukopenia and diminished leukocyte function may impair the host immune system. Postoperative bleeding may occur from the reduction in platelet number and function and result in increased postoperative blood loss and transfusion requirements. Although the blood–membrane interface of the membrane oxygenator can cause blood damage, it is believed that the membrane quickly becomes coated with denatured protein and results in a blood–protein interface that causes less damage. Theoretically, the membrane oxygenator is favored over the bubble oxygenator, although only a few studies have demonstrated its superiority as evidenced by less disturbance in platelet number and function and a reduction in microvascular retinal perfusion defects caused by microemboli.

Pumps and priming

A pump, either roller or centrifugal, returns oxygenated blood to the arterial circulation. Roller pumps work by compressing a segment of collapsible tubing against a semicircular metal plate. Centrifugal pumps contain rotor cones that are magnetically driven to spin rapidly and impart motion to the blood via centrifugal force. Roller pumps are not sensitive to the arterial vascular resistance and therefore obstruction to arterial return can result in the development of high line pressure with potential rupture of the tubing. In contrast, centrifugal pumps are sensitive to changes in arterial pressure and flow decreases as pressure increases. For this reason, electromagnetic flowmeters are required to measure flow rate from centrifugal pumps. Centrifugal pumps cause less damage to blood components than do roller pumps. Blood flow on CPB is nonpulsatile. No data indicate that pulsatile flow is of greater benefit to patients, except in the setting of preexisting renal insufficiency.

The bypass circuit is primed with 1.5–2L of crystalloid solution, which causes significant hemodilution and a reduction in the oxygen-carrying capacity. Hemodilution, however, has several beneficial effects. The risk of exposure to blood-borne viruses is reduced by avoiding the use of additional blood products for priming, improvement in oxygenation occurs by increasing the red blood cell and/or hemoglobin exposure to oxygen in the oxygenator, and viscosity is decreased (which improves blood flow, reduces peripheral resistance, and thereby increases tissue perfusion, especially during hypothermia). In small children, infants, and neonates the priming volume may exceed the blood volume and therefore blood prime is added to the circuit to achieve appropriate hemodilution.

Normal CPB flow is generally 50mL/kg per minute or 2L/m^2 per minute. Hypothermia is utilized during CPB to augment myocardial protection. A reduction in temperature increases peripheral resistance because of vasoconstriction and increases viscosity. Since viscosity is directly related to hematocrit, hemodilution improves blood rheology and ameliorates these effects.

The essential element of prime is crystalloid, which is similar to plasma in electrolyte content and osmolality. Additives to crystalloid prime may reduce some of the untoward effects of CPB. Colloid solution added to the crystalloid prime may prevent edema formation when the duration of extracorporeal circulation is prolonged. Other additives may include heparin (10–25U/mL) as a safety factor for inadequate systemic heparinization; $CaCl_2$ (200–1000mg), which balances Ca^{2+} chelation by citrate when blood products are used; mannitol (25–50g) to induce diuresis and perhaps renal protection; and corticosteroids to prevent or attenuate the immune response to CPB.

Blood is not usually needed in the priming solution since some hemodilution is desirable. The ideal hematocrit on CPB is unknown, although there is a trend toward maintaining higher hematocrits. Values of 15–18% are well tolerated generally; lower values may be associated with abnormal blood-flow distribution to organs. The degree of hypothermia has an impact on the hematocrit that allows optimal tissue perfusion. At 30°C (86°F) a hematocrit of 30% is adequate for CPB, while at 25°C (77°F) a hematocrit <25% is desired. Addition of blood to the circuit may be necessary to reach an adequate hematocrit if significant bleeding occurs or systemic vascular resistance is low and requires supplementation of crystalloid to maintain an adequate volume in the pump reservoir.

Anticoagulation

When CPB occurs through the pump oxygenator system it initiates the intrinsic clotting cascade (see Chapter 51 for a review of the clotting cascade). Adequate anticoagulation must be attained prior to CPB to avoid clot formation in the circuit. Heparin, derived from bovine lung or porcine intestinal mucosa, is utilized as anticoagulant. Heparin is a glycosaminoglycan that ranges in molecular weight from 3kDa to 40kDa. Doses of heparin are quantified as activity units, since the relationship between potency and mass varies among preparations. Heparin has a relatively small volume of distribution and a dose-dependent half-life; elimination occurs primarily from biotransformation in the liver and reticuloendothelial system, and from renal excretion. Heparin binds to and potentiates antithrombin III (Fig. 41.3), an inhibitor of thrombin and Factor Xa (Chapter 51). Thrombin increases the rate of fibrin clot formation via the common and intrinsic pathways by splitting fibrinogen into fibrin and activating cofactors V and XIII. Antithrombin III is an intrinsic limiting factor of clot formation; heparin increases the thrombin inhibitory potency of antithrombin III by a factor of 10^3.

A bolus heparin dose reduces arterial pressure and systemic vascular resistance (SVR) by 10–20% without affecting cardiac output or heart rate; this may be related to a reduction in the level of ionized Ca^{2+}. Heparin-bonded CPB circuits may reduce the intravenous dose of heparin necessary for anticoagulation.

Methods available to assess the level of anticoagulation for CPB fall into two categories – those that evaluate clotting time or those that measure heparin concentration. The activated clotting time (ACT), an activated whole blood coagulation test, is the standard method used because of its ease, rapidity, and reproducibility. The normal ACT ranges from 90–130 seconds; an ACT of 400–480 seconds is often accepted as adequate anticoagulation for CPB. The ACT is a measure of the intrinsic clotting cascade, which is affected by many factors including hypothermia, hemodilution, thrombocytopenia, platelet dysfunction and lysis, protamine, aprotinin, and surgical incision.

Heparin concentration can be measured utilizing protamine titration of heparinized whole blood. The protamine concentration that optimally neutralizes heparin (by fastest clot formation) can be identified and converted into blood heparin concentration if the neutralization ratio of protamine to heparin is known. Adequate anticoagulation generally occurs between heparin concentrations of 2–4U/mL. Since heparin concentration does not necessarily correlate with functional activity, clot formation may still occur despite attaining an 'adequate blood level'. Therefore, heparin concentration may be best used to identify residual heparin levels and estimate protamine requirements for post-CPB reversal of anticoagulation.

Thromboelastography (TEG) tests whole blood clot strength development over time and was originally used during liver trans-

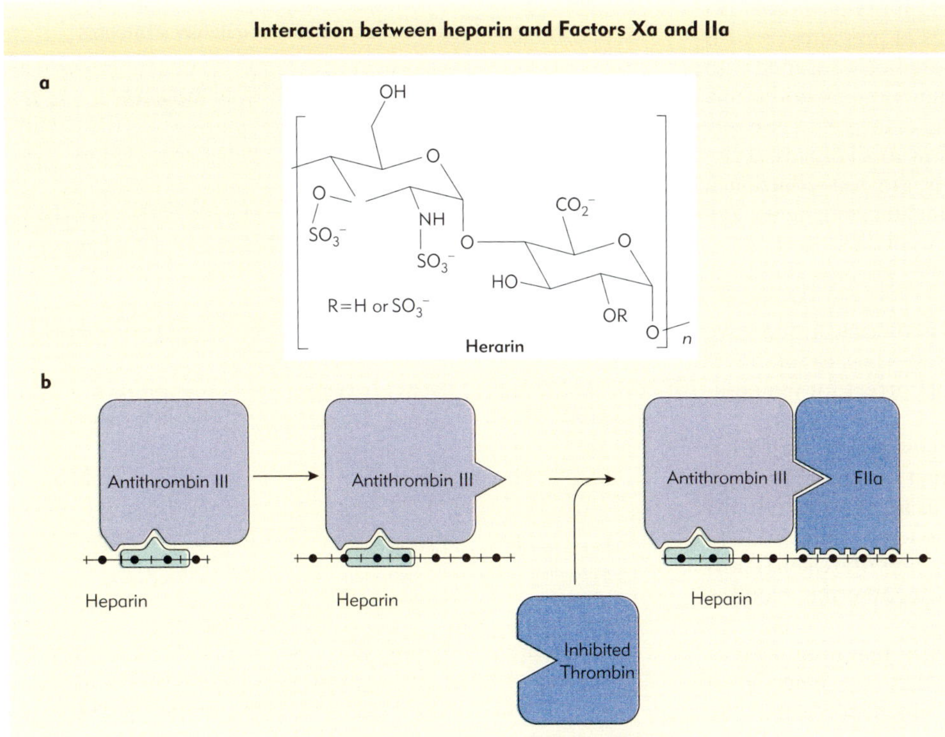

Figure 41.3 Heparin structure and function. Heparin is a sulfated polysaccharide (a) synthesized by most cells. Its high negative charge density contributed by sulfate and carboxylate groups facilitates strong interactions with several plasma clotting factors including IX, X and the α2 glycoprotein antithrombin III. A stoichiometric interaction between heparin and antithrombin III facilitates simultaneous binding and inhibition of activated serine proteases, including thrombin (b). In the absence of heparin, inhibition of thrombin by antithrombin III occurs at a slower rate

plantation to help guide therapy for coagulopathy (Chapter 51). This method involves measuring viscoelastic properties of blood clot formation (rate of clot formation and growth, clot strength, and lysis) and activity of the intrinsic cascade. Multiple parameters of TEG are analyzed and aid in identifying causes of coagulopathy. Although TEG is extremely sensitive to heparin, it is time consuming to perform and, as such, is infrequently used.

Heparin resistance, defined as the need for a higher than normal heparin dose to attain sufficient anticoagulation for CPB, is often encountered in cardiac patients. Multiple factors have been implicated in the development of heparin resistance, most notably antithrombin III deficiency (inherited or acquired), ongoing heparin therapy, and thrombocytosis. Increased doses of heparin generally overcome this effect, although the addition of antithrombin III in the form of fresh frozen plasma or concentrate may be necessary.

After successful separation from CPB, anticoagulation is reversed with protamine, a polycationic protein derived from salmon sperm. It binds ionically to heparin to produce a stable salt, preventing heparin interaction with antithrombin III. Protamine neutralizes heparin in a ratio of 1mg to 85U. The usual calculated reversal dose is 1mg protamine to 100U heparin; this excess amount prevents heparin rebound associated with releases from tissue stores and compensates for the shorter biologic activity of protamine. Protamine also exerts a mild anticoagulant effect independent of heparin, and therefore protamine doses should be guided by heparin concentration or anticoagulant studies.

Three types of adverse protamine reactions are described. First, transient systemic hypotension is related to the speed of administration and is caused by histamine release. Secondly, anaphylactic reactions result from the antibody-mediated release of vasoactive and bronchospastic substances. In anaphylactoid reactions these substances are released in the absence of antibody–antigen interaction. Patients predisposed to these types of reactions include those with a history of prior exposure to protamine, use of neutral protamine Hagedorn insulin (protamine complexed to insulin to prolong duration of insulin action), true fish allergy, and vasectomized males. Thirdly, catastrophic pulmonary vasoconstriction that causes elevated pulmonary artery pressure, right heart failure, low left atrial pressures, and systemic hypotension, appears to be related to heparin–protamine-induced thromboxane B_2 generation. The other reactions are not dependent upon the heparin–protamine complex. Protamine should be administered slowly via a peripheral vein with vigilant attention to development of these problems.

PATHOPHYSIOLOGY OF CARDIOPULMONARY BYPASS

Principles of organ protection

Systemic hypothermia reduces metabolism and oxygen consumption. The Q_{10} value is used to describe the dependence of the reaction rate of metabolic processes on temperature. Total body oxygen consumption has a Q_{10} of approximately 2, which means that a 10°C (28°F) increase in temperature doubles oxygen consumption. Conversely, a 10°C decrease in temperature halves oxygen consumption. Clinical use of mild-to-moderate hypothermia [>25°C] is mainly limited to cardiac surgery, vascular procedures, and intracranial surgery. Profound selective myocardial hypothermia is often used to protect the myocardium from ischemia induced by cross-clamp. Deep hypothermia [18–22°C] with circulatory arrest is used for protective effects when cessation of circulation is necessary, typically for cases that involve surgery of the aortic arch and great vessels or repair of complicated congenital lesions in pediatric patients. The safe duration of circulatory arrest depends upon the degree of systemic cooling.

In cardiac surgery, hypothermia combined with CBP allows for lower pump flows, less blood trauma, and better myocardial and organ protection. Lower flow rates improve visualization of the surgical field by reducing noncoronary collateral flow, which warms the heart and can jeopardize myocardial protection. Since

CNS infarcts are mainly embolic in nature, lower flow rates theoretically minimize injury. Low flow rates or pressures on CPB combined with moderate hypothermia are not associated with postoperative renal or neurologic dysfunction. Hypothermia adversely affects tissue perfusion because of increased viscosity vascular resistance and reduced blood flow to all organs; skeletal muscle and extremities demonstrate the greatest reduction in perfusion followed by the kidneys, splanchnic bed, heart, and brain. Hemodilution helps to offset this problem.

Acid–base management

Two methods of managing pH during hypothermic bypass have been described, 'α-stat ' and 'pH-stat' (Fig. 41.4). α-Stat refers to blood gas management that does not correct for temperature, while 'pH-stat' does correct for it.

The pH at electrochemical neutrality ($[H^+] = [OH^-]$) increases as temperature decreases. In other words, pH becomes more alkaline relative to normothermic values. In addition, the partial pressure of a gas is directly related to temperature. As temperature declines, the arterial partial pressures of oxygen ($Pa{O_2}$) and carbon dioxide ($Pa{CO_2}$) decrease; hypothermic blood is hypocarbic relative to normothermic values.

pH-Stat management aims to maintain temperature-corrected $Pa{CO_2}$ at 40mmHg (5.3kPa) and pH at 7.40. When blood gases are corrected for temperature during hypothermia, the reported values are alkalotic and hypocarbic relative to normothermia [37°C (98.6°F)]. Carbon dioxide is added to the gas inflow to achieve these values. Since the cerebral blood flow response to $Pa{CO_2}$ is maintained during hypothermia, pH-stat management results in cerebral vasodilation and increased cerebral blood flow.

α-Stat blood gas management does not correct for temperature and aims to maintain $Pa{CO_2}$ at 40mmHg (5.3kPa) and pH 7.40 regardless of temperature. Reported blood gas values [37°C] are hypercarbic and acidotic relative to hypothermic (actual *in vivo*) values. Increasing oxygen flow rates on the gas inlet to normalize this relative hypercarbia and acidemia increases the actual (*in vivo*) hypocarbia and alkalemia. Electrochemical neutrality is maintained with α-stat management, as reflected by the ionization state of histidine imidazole groups on proteins. Consequently, enzyme structure and function are better preserved. In theory, the disadvantages of this strategy include reduced cerebral blood flow and a leftward shift of the oxyhemoglobin dissociation curve with impaired oxygen delivery to the tissues.

Which hypothermic blood gas management strategy is appropriate? The pH management controversy focuses mainly on the brain, and which strategy may minimize neurologic complications that result from CPB. pH-Stat management results in cerebral vasodilation, increased cerebral blood flow, and loss of cerebral pressure autoregulation and flow–metabolism coupling. Cerebral blood flow in excess of metabolic need theoretically could increase embolic load. With α-stat, it appears that autoregulation and the coupling between cerebral metabolism and blood flow is preserved. Proponents of α-stat suggest that lower cerebral blood flow reduces embolic risk and neurologic complications. In patients who undergo moderately hypothermic CPB, postoperative neurologic and neuropsychiatric outcome is slightly but statistically better with α-stat management. In children who undergo deep hypothermic circulatory arrest (DHCA), pH-stat management provides an advantage by allowing faster and more even brain cooling, and reduced brain oxygen depletion.

Different hypothermic acid-base regulatory strategies

Strategy	pH-stat	Alpha-stat
Aim	Constant pH	Constant OH^-/H^+
Total CO_2 content	Increases	Constant
pH and PaCO maintenance	Normal corrected values	Normal uncorrected values
Intracellular State	Acidotic (excess H^+)	Neutral ($H^+ = OH^-$)
Alpha-Imidazole and buffering	Excess (+) charge, buffering decreased	Constant net charge, buffering constant
Enzyme structure and function	Altered and activity decreased	Normal and activity maximal
Cerebral blood flow and coupling	Flow close to normothermic, ?flow and metabolism uncoupled	Flow decreases (appropriate), ?flow and metabolism coupled

Modified from Hickey PR, Hansen DD. Temperature and blood gases: the clinical dilemma of acid-base management for hypothermic cardiopulmonary bypass. In: Tinker JH, ed. Cardiopulmonary bypass: current concepts and controversies. Philadelphia: WB Saunders, 1989; 16.

Figure 41.4 Different hypothermic acid–base regulatory strategies.

Myocardial protection

The major determinants of myocardial oxygen demand are LV wall tension and contractility; minor factors include heart rate, basal metabolism, ionic homeostasis, and oxidative energy for myocellular metabolism, (Chapter 34). The role of cardioplegia is to reduce myocardial oxygen demand and limit ischemic injury during intentional interruptions in regional or total coronary blood flow.

In the 1950s it was recognized that systemic hypothermia protected against ischemic injury induced by aortic cross-clamping. Further attempts to improve myocardial protection involved local myocardial hypothermia and chemical arrest of the heart, achieved in the late 1970s. Current principles of myocardial protection by cardioplegia include asystole, cardiac hypothermia, oxygen radical scavenging, buffering, edema prevention, amino acid enhancement, and oxygen delivery. Asystole reduces myocardial oxygen demands by 80–90% compared with those of the working heart and conserves myocardial energy reserves by avoiding depletion of high energy phosphates such as adenosine triphosphate (ATP). When ATP is generated by anaerobic metabolism it is channeled to support cellular metabolism rather than useless contractile activity. Hyperkalemia is the basic element for inducing electromechanical quiescence, by depolarizing the myocyte membrane and rendering the myocardium inexcitable. In general, the heart is stopped with a high concentration of KCl (140mmol/L) blood cardioplegia solution, followed by a multidose lower concentration of KCl (70mmol/L) solution during the rest of the surgery, since hypothermia potentiates electromechanical quiescence and further hyperkalemia is not necessary.

Myocardial hypothermia reduces metabolic rate and oxygen demands and increases the tolerance of the heart to ischemia (Fig. 41.5). The greatest drop in myocardial oxygen demand in the quiescent heart occurs between 37 and 25°C (98.6 and 77°F); more profound hypothermia may not be beneficial unless the period of ischemia is prolonged to 4–6 hours. The combination of intermittent hypothermic cardioplegia infusion with topical myocardial cooling using saline slush prevents rewarming of the myocardium from noncoronary collateral flow. The disadvantages of hypothermia include edema by inhibition of Na^+K^+-ATPase, impaired oxygen dissociation, and increased blood viscosity. Oxygen in crystalloid cardioplegia restores tissue oxygenation after an interval of myocardial ischemia, repays the oxygen debt developed during antecedent ischemia or between infusions, and replenishes high-energy phosphate supplies. Postischemic LV function is better preserved when cold cardioplegia contains blood saturated with oxygen than with unsaturated cardioplegia. Despite the hypothermia-induced shift in the oxyhemoglobin dissociation curve, ischemic myocardium is able to extract oxygen from cold blood. Blood provides a large extractable source of oxygen, endogenous free-radical scavengers, improved rheologic properties, and effective buffering capacity.

Several studies have shown the generation of oxygen free radicals during CPB and cardioplegic arrest. However, the clinical benefits of antioxidant therapy to reduce oxygen free radical injury are unclear. Anaerobic metabolism during periods of ischemia produces tissue acidosis and lactate, which inhibits catalyzed metabolic reactions and further reduces diminished energy production. Intermittent reinfusion of cardioplegia allows wash-out of metabolites and buffering (endogenous capabilities of blood or the addition of exogenous buffers) to counteract the accumulation of hydrogen ion in the myocardium. Edema is a consequence of ischemia–reperfusion injury and may be aggravated by the composition of cardioplegic solutions, hypothermia, and perfusion pressure. Edema increases microvascular resistance, impedes blood flow (no reflow phenomenon), and reduces myocardial compliance. Mannitol or glucose, which increase oncotic pressure, may counteract edema formation. Amino acid enhancement of cardioplegia (glutamate and aspartate replenish key Krebs cycle intermediates that are depleted during ischemia) may help maintain adequate levels of high-energy phosphates.

The cardioplegia solution components, temperature and mode of delivery may vary widely from surgeon to surgeon and from institution to institution. Hyperkalemic blood cardioplegia was introduced in 1978 and was shown to have an improved buffering capacity and oxygen transport over earlier crystalloid cardioplegia solutions. Blood cardioplegia also has the added benefit of limiting reperfusion injury (myocardial injury possibly caused by the generation of free radicals, activation of neutrophils and platelets, intracellular Ca^{2+} accumulation, and microvascular injury with impaired blood flow). The advantage of a cold solution is the generation of local myocardial hypothermia, which reduces myocardial metabolism and oxygen demands. Disadvantages of hypothermia include leftward shifting of the oxyhemoglobin dissociation curve, reduced membrane stability, increased blood viscosity, activation of platelets, leukocytes and complement, and coagulopathy.

Warm blood cardioplegia was subsequently developed to prevent problems associated with hypothermia. The patient and heart are maintained at 37°C and cardioplegia is delivered continuously when feasible. The advantages of this method include electromechanical quiescence, avoidance of reperfusion injury since the heart remains in a constant aerobic state, and avoidance of detrimental systemic effects of hypothermia (other organs, coagulation). However, warm cardioplegia has not been shown to be superior to the intermittent cold cardioplegic technique in protecting areas of jeopardized myocardium. Warm continuous cardioplegia must be intermittently interrupted to perform distal anastamoses, which can be dangerous to vulnerable regions, whereas intermittent cold cardioplegia offers a sustained period of protection. Warm cardioplegia delivered briefly before aortic unclamping reduces reperfusion injury as long as the formulation limits Ca^{2+} influx, buffers acidosis, and maintains cardiac arrest. Intermittent cold cardioplegia followed by a 'hot shot' of warm cardioplegia safely protects normal and ischemically damaged hearts for 2–4 hours of aortic cross-clamping, so it does not seem wise to favor the complete warm approach until further data are available.

Positive and negative physiologic effects of hypothermia on the myocardium

Positive	Negative
Decreases myocardial metabolism	Decreases rate of reparative processes
Decreases oxygen requirements	Increases myocellular swelling by altering Donnan equilibrium of Cl^- and inhibiting Na^+/K^+-ATPase
Decreases rate of degradative reactions	Increases inotropic state and MVO_2 per beat
Retards progression of ischemic injury	Induces fibrillation
Increases the tolerable period of ischemia	Impairs O_2 dissociation
Prolongs arrest	Impairs autoregulation
Does not alter transmural blood flow distribution	Promotes rouleau formation of erythrocytes
Inhibits intracellular Ca^{2+} gain	Decreases membrane fluidity
	Inhibits sarcoplasmic reticulum sequestration of Ca^{2+}

Figure 41.5 Positive and negative physiologic effects of hypothermia on the myocardium.

Cardioplegia benefits ischemic myocardium only if delivery is adequate to all regions. Anterograde delivery may be impeded by severe coronary artery obstructions, which may be overcome by retrograde infusion through the coronary sinus or by perfusing cardioplegia down vein grafts after distal anastomoses have been connected. Retrograde flow facilitates even distribution of cardioplegia, avoids direct coronary cannulation, and is useful in reoperative situations with patent internal mammary artery grafts and in aortic insufficiency that limits anterograde delivery. However, retrograde cardioplegia may not adequately protect the right heart because delivery may be compromised by anatomic variations. The use of alternating anterograde and retrograde flow provides the advantages of both techniques. Methods of simultaneous anterograde and retrograde flow exist since most drainage is through the thebesian vessels and therefore venous hypertension and myocardial edema are avoided. Wash-out of cardioplegia occurs over time because of noncoronary collateral flow, mainly from the bronchial circulation. Temperature and electrolyte changes caused by blood flow from the extracorporeal circuit promote electromechanical activity and therefore cardioplegia must be delivered intermittently or continuously to restore hypothermia, wash-out accumulated metabolites, and counteract acidosis and edema.

Ischemic preconditioning

Ischemic preconditioning refers to the reduced injury size when prolonged and severe myocardial ischemia is preceded by short episodes of ischemia followed by reperfusion. The mechanism of preconditioning involves activation of adenosine A_1 receptors, bradykinin receptors, and ATP-dependent K^+ channels (K^+_{ATP} channels). In animals, preconditioning and cardioplegia alone afford similar protection of postischemic contractile and vascular functions. Ischemic preconditioning may provide myocardial protection in cardiac operations that do not involve CPB or cardioplegia. In humans in small clinical trials, elevation of creatine kinase MB fraction and transmyocardial lactate gradient suggested no protective effect of ischemic preconditioning. The clinical utility of this technique remains to be seen.

Cerebral protection

Dysfunction of CNS after CPB ranges from catastrophic stroke to subtle injury detected only by detailed neuropsychiatric testing. The risk of severe injury is ≤ 5%, but the subtle variety can be found in 50% of patients. The mechanisms of CNS injury after CPB include embolism (micro- and macroemboli) and cerebral hypoperfusion caused by systemic hypotension, low pump flow, nonpulsatile pump flow, incorrect cannula placement, and acquired cerebrovascular disease. Factors that predispose to increased cerebrovascular risk include increasing age, open cardiac procedures, presence of LV thrombus, presence of ascending aortic atherosclerosis, preoperative symptomatic cerebrovascular disease, and duration of procedure. A variety of approaches are employed to reduce CNS injury, but no single method has been found ideal.

Bypass machine factors may be associated with neurologic injury. For example, bubble oxygenators are associated with greater retinal microvascular lesions compared with membrane oxygenators. Arterial inflow filters reduce microemboli counts and neuropsychiatric dysfunction.

The effect of pump flow on cerebral protection is unclear. Study results are controversial demonstrating either no change or a direct relationship between cerebral blood flow or oxygen consumption and perfusion flow rate. Conventional pump flows during hypothermia are 1.75–2.5L/min per m^2 (45–65cc/kg per minute), but lower flow rates of 1–1.75L/min per m^2 (25–45cc/kg per minute) are potentially beneficial as they reduce trauma to blood cells and platelets, and reduce noncoronary collateral flow. The incidence of neurologic injury has not been shown to be related to flow, but interpretation of the data is difficult since many studies do not distinguish between perfusion pressure and flow rate.

Cerebral blood pressure autoregulation of normotensive individuals occurs with mean arterial pressures between 50 and 150mmHg (6.6 and 20kPa; Chapter 20). When acid–base balance is managed by pH-stat, blood flow varies directly with perfusion pressure, whereas during α-stat management blood flow is independent of cerebral perfusion pressure (autoregulation is maintained). Although a lower threshold of 50mmHg (6.6kPa) for blood pressure during CPB is supported by a long history of safe practice, recent studies suggest that higher levels [70–80mmHg (9.3–10.6kPa)] for older patients with preexisting neurologic disease or severe aortic atheroma may reduce neurologic morbidity.

Since severe aortoatherosclerotic disease predisposes to stroke, identification of diseased aorta may allow modification of the surgical technique to avoid dislodgment and embolization of plaque from the aorta. Diseased aorta may be diagnosed from the chest radiograph, by the surgeon, or intraoperative ultrasonography. Altering the aortic cannulation site, the use of a single cross-clamping period, retrograde cardioplegia, or circulatory arrest may be necessary.

Moderate hypothermia induced for myocardial protection probably provides cerebral protection during nonpulsatile bypass by decreasing oxygen consumption. Deep hypothermia [20°C (68°F)] in the repair of complex congenital lesions or the thoracic aorta provides neuroprotection during circulatory arrest. Additional use of retrograde cerebral perfusion (cerebroplegia) via the jugular veins may augment neuroprotection during circulatory arrest.

Hyperglycemia has been shown in multiple studies to worsen ischemic brain injury (from trauma or cerebrovascular accident). During cardiac surgery, hyperglycemia occurs as a result of multiple mechanisms that involve insulin resistance and suppression of insulin secretion (Fig. 41.6). However, no evidence thus far suggests that tight glucose control during CPB improves neurologic outcome.

Barbiturates and Ca^{2+} channel blockers may reduce neurologic injury. Barbiturates reduce cerebral metabolic oxygen requirements when given in doses that produce an isoelectric electroencephalogram. During cardiac surgery barbiturates appear useful only in the setting of circulatory arrest. Those Ca^{2+} channel blockers that penetrate the blood–brain barrier are neuroprotective for acute cerebral ischemia, possibly by cerebral vasodilation and prevention of postischemic hypoperfusion or attenuation of ischemia-induced intracellular acidosis.

Renal protection

Renal failure occurs in 8% of patients after CPB, and the severity of renal insufficiency is related to mortality. Patients with preoperative renal insufficiency, advanced age, history of congestive heart failure, a longer duration of CPB and low CO peri-operatively are more likely to develop postoperative renal dysfunction. The etiology of renal failure after CPB is multifactorial. Renal blood flow, renal plasma flow, and urine output all diminish during CPB. Hypotension at the onset of CPB stimulates the renin–angiotensin–aldosterone system, which increases renal vascular resistance. Elevated levels of antidiuretic hormone may also contribute to renal vasoconstriction and reduced urine output and free water clearance. Hypothermia increases renal vascular resistance and depresses glomerular filtration, renal tubular function, and concentrating ability. Hemolysis with the production of hemoglobin casts, as well as microemboli of air and fat, may also contribute to renal dysfunction. Bubble oxygenators are associated with a rise in serum creatinine compared with membrane oxygenators. Finally, the immune response to CBP may play a role in the development of renal dysfunction.

Compared with other organs, the kidney shows the largest proportional decrease in blood flow during CPB. However, reduced perfusion pressure and flow on CPB have not been shown to deleteriously affect the normal kidney. A more likely predictor of post-CPB renal failure is a low perfusion state prior to and following sugery. Renal protection involves methods to improve perfusion of the kidney during and after CPB. Pulsatile flow preserves renal blood flow during CPB and, at rates of 80–100mL/kg per minute, decreases systemic vascular resistance and increases renal blood flow, but appears to be beneficial only in patients with pre-existing renal insufficiency. Furosemide (frusemide) improves renal blood flow and increases creatinine clearance in patients exposed to CPB for longer than 1 hour. Mannitol also increases renal blood flow and glomerular filtration and reduces renal tubular swelling and injury after ischemia. Dopamine improves renal blood flow because of renovascular vasodilation and improves glomerular filtration rate and Na^+ excretion. Pretreatment with furosemide and mannitol prior to ischemic insult may preserve renal function; the effects of dopamine remain inconclusive.

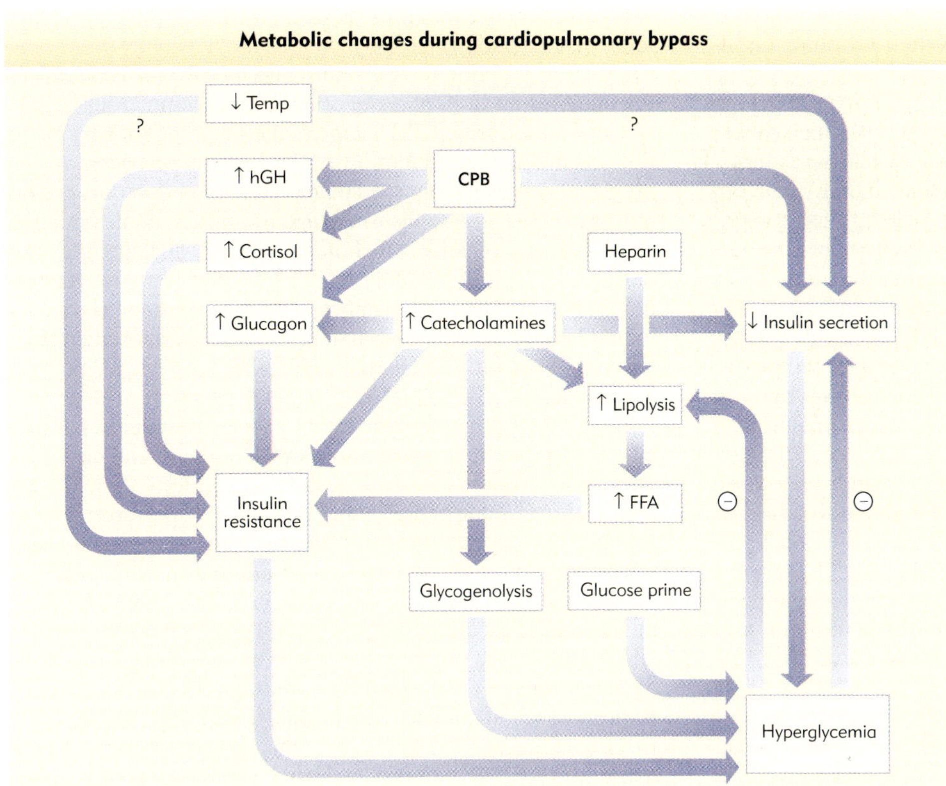

Figure 41.6 Metabolic changes during cardiopulmonary bypass. A complex system of factors contributes to the development of hyperglycemia early after initiation of CPB. Hyperglycemia, in turn, provokes hyperinsulinemia later in the course of CPB and also acts to restrain lipolysis. FFA, free fatty acid; hGH, human growth hormone.

Immune response

CBP is also associated with changes in cellular and humoral immunity and in reticuloendothelial function, which increase susceptibility to infection and contributes to organ dysfunction. Adverse effects on cellular immunity include a decrease in the number of leukocytes and lymphocytes, leukocyte activation and sequestration, diminished phagocytic activity, depressed chemotactic migration, decreased number and function of natural killer cells, reduced helper-T cells, reversal of the helper:supressor ratio of T cells, and depressed local graft versus host reaction. Adverse effects of CPB on humoral immunity include decreases in levels of complement, IgM, IgA, and IgG, and depressed opsonic capacity. The oxygenator may cause denaturation of serum proteins, making them antigenic and capable of activating complement. Reticulendothelial blockade occurs with CPB and results in depressed phagocytosis. Additionally, drugs (antibiotics and anesthetics), shock, and fever depress the immune system. Cardiac surgical patients are at higher risk for postoperative infection because of the aforementioned immune suppression and the nature of the surgery (long duration of procedure, sternal osteotomy, and use of prosthetic and intravascular foreign bodies). Prophylactic antibiotic therapy has been clearly demonstrated to lower the morbidity of cardiac surgery caused by infection.

Inflammatory response

Exposure of blood to a foreign surface, which initiates a systemic inflammatory response by activation of polymorphonuclear neutrophils and subsequent release of cytotoxic products and proteolytic enzymes (e.g. elastase) that trigger tissue and cell injury. The contact activation systems, Factor XII–kallikrein system, and complement and thrombin generation by the coagulation system are highly interactive and implicated in the damaging effects of CPB. Activation of Factor XII leads to elevated concentrations of kallikrein and bradykinin. Bradykinin is associated with increased capillary permeability and tissue edema. Contact with foreign surfaces initiates the complement cascade and leads to generation of fragments C3a and C5–9 particularly, and consequently the vasoactive, chemotactic, immunoregulatory, and cytolytic activities of complement. Early studies showed that an increased concentration of fragment C3a may be related to the incidence and degree of abnormalities of function of the heart, lung, and kidney. The lung is particularly susceptible since it receives the entire cardiac output and is therefore exposed to the full load of circulating mediators. Subsequent studies failed to show a relationship of C3a levels to pulmonary dysfunction, although the terminal complement component (C5b–C9) appears to have deleterious effects on myocardial performance after ischemia–reperfusion. Thrombin is able to initiate activation and release of humoral mediators involved in the inflammatory and hemostatic systems. Additionally, proinflammatory cytokines [interleukin-1 (IL-1), IL-6, IL-8, and tumor necrosis factor], activated neutrophils, and adhesion molecules have been implicated as mediators of tissue (myocardial) damage. Much attention is currently placed on improving biocompatability of the cardiopulmonary circuit and reducing the inflammatory response to CPB. Serine protease inhibitors inhibit surface activation and are known to reduce coagulopathy, but recent analysis reveals that they can also reduce the inflammatory response associated with CPB.

PHARMACOKINETICS DURING CARDIOPULMONARY BYPASS

The physiologic changes induced by CPB include hemodilution, hypothermia, and nonpulsatile blood flow that subsequently alter the disposition, metabolism, and elimination of many drugs. Sequestration within certain organs and acid–base status also affect drug concentrations. Understanding the pharmacokinetics of drugs during CPB enables their rational administration during this period.

At the initiation of CPB, the addition of pump prime to the blood volume results in significant hemodilution, which causes a decrease in hematocrit and an increase in plasma volume. Changes in both drug distribution and protein binding occur. An immediate reduction in total plasma drug concentration is counteracted by redistribution of the drug from tissues to plasma. For drugs with a large volume of distribution, after the initiation of CPB and equilibration, plasma drug concentrations are only slightly lower than those before hemodilution. Conversely, plasma concentrations of drugs with a small volume of distribution are significantly reduced with the onset of CPB. For drugs that are highly protein bound, the decreased concentration of binding proteins as a result of hemodilution leads to an increase in the fraction of free, active drug. The addition of heparin causes a rise in the level of free fatty acids, which can compete with drugs for protein binding. As a result drugs are displaced and plasma levels of unbound drugs rise. A rise in the level of α,-1 acid glycoprotein is seen post-CPB, and leads to an increase in the binding of basic drugs such as lidocaine (lignocaine), propranolol, and disopyramide and a resultant fall in free plasma levels of these drugs in the days after surgery.

Hypothermia and nonpulsatile flow result in alterations of regional blood flow with decreased perfusion of hepatic, renal, cerebral, and skeletal systems. Reduced renal perfusion affects the active secretion of drugs, whereas the degree of protein binding affects glomerular filtration. Hepatic metabolism of drugs is affected by blood flow to the organ, degree of protein binding, and enzymatic activity. Hypoperfusion and hypothermia decrease renal and hepatic function and drug elimination during CPB. With rewarming, drugs sequestered in previously low perfusion organs (muscle, skin) wash-out once perfusion improves. Hypothermia also increases the sensitivity of the neuromuscular junction to neuromuscular blockers which reduces the need for additional doses of muscle relaxant.

Generally, during CPB a large reduction in pulmonary blood flow occurs as the circulation to the lungs is restricted to the bronchial vessels. Diminished pulmonary blood flow during CPB may impair the metabolism of biogenic amines, contributing to an increase of plasma catecholamine levels during CPB. The plasma concentrations of basic drugs, such as fentanyl, propranolol, and lidocaine, with significant lung distribution fall with the initiation of CPB. When mechanical ventilation is resumed prior to separation from CPB, wash-out from the lung reservoir occurs and results in a rise of plasma drug concentrations. Adsorption to the CPB circuit and oxygenator occurs with opioids, particularly the lipophilic drugs fentanyl and sufentanil, and nitroglycerin. The amount of drug lost to the pump depends on temperature, timing of drug administration, composition of prime solution, and oxygenator type. Changes in acid–base status affect the fraction of unionized drug and binding to plasma proteins. Additionally, ion trapping may occur in certain tissue compartments in which acidic conditions prevail (skeletal muscle, brain).

How does this information relate to anesthetic drug management during CPB? Basically, if adequate plasma concentrations of opioid and benzodiazepine have been attained prior to CPB, supplemental doses are probably not necessary during hypothermic CPB. Additional dosing may be necessary during the rewarming and post-CPB periods. Since muscle relaxants are significantly diluted with the onset of CPB, an additional dose should be given at that time. Muscle relaxation is prolonged during hypothermia and even after rewarming and therefore further dosing should be guided by evidence of muscle activity (shivering or train-of-four monitoring).

Key References

Beckley PD, Holt DW, Tallman RD. Oxygenators for extracorporeal circulation. In: Mora CT, ed. Cardiopulmonary bypass: principles and techniques of extracorporeal circulation. New York: Springer-Verlag; 1995:199–228.

Buckberg GD. Update on current techniques of myocardial protection. Ann Thorac Surg. 1995;60:805–14.

Buckberg GD, Brazier JR, Nelson RL, Goldstein SM, McConnell DH, Cooper N. Studies of the effects of hypothermia on regional myocardial blood flow and metabolism during cardiopulmonary bypass I, II. J Thorac Card Surg. 1977;73:87–95.

Mills SA. Risk factors for cerebral injury and cardiac surgery. Ann Thorac Surg. 1995;59:1296–9.

Newman MF, Croughwell ND, Blumenthal JA, Lowry E, White WD, Reves JG. Cardiopulmonary bypass and the central nervous system: potential for cerebral protection. J Clin Anesth. 1996;8:53–60.

O'Dwyer C, Prough DS, Johnston WE. Determinants of cerebral perfusion during cardiopulmonary bypass. J Cardiothorac Vasc Anesth. 1996;10:54–65.

Royston D. The inflammatory response and extracorporeal circulation. J Cardiothorac Vasc Anesth. 1997;11(3):341–54.

Wegner JA. Oxygenator anatomy and function. J Cardiothorac Vasc Anesth. 1997;11:275–81.

Further Reading

Gravlee GP, Davis RF, Utley JR, eds. Cardiopulmonary bypass: principles and practice. Baltimore: Williams & Wilkins, 1993.

Hartman GS, Yao FS, Bruefach M, et al. Severity of aortic atheromatous disease diagnosed by transesophageal echocardiography predicts stroke and other outcomes associated with coronary artery surgery: a prospective study. Anesth Analg. 1996;83:701–8.

Hindman BJ. Choice of α-stat or pH-stat management and neurologic outcomes after cardiac surgery. Anesthesiology. 1998;89:5–7.

Kron IL, Joob AW, Van Meter C. Acute renal failure in the cardiovascular surgical patient. Ann Thorac Surg. 1985;39:590–8.

Palanzo DA. Perfusion safety: past, present, future. J Cardiothorac Vasc Anesth. 1997;11:383–90.

Slogoff S, Reul GJ, Keats AS, et al. Role of perfusion pressure and flow in major organ dysfunction after cardiopulmonary bypass. Ann Thorac Surg. 1990;50:911–8.

Stammers AH. Historical aspects of cardiopulmonary bypass: from antiquity to acceptance. J Cardiothorac Vasc Anesth. 1997;11:266–74.

Chapter 42 Respiratory mechanics

Andrew T Cohen and Alison J Pittard

Topics covered in this chapter

Anatomy
Forces
Time constants
Positive end-expiratory pressure
Non-elastic forces: resistance
Work of breathing

ANATOMY

The respiratory system consists of two mechanical components: the *lungs* and the surrounding *thoracic cavity*.

The lung comprises conducting airways, parenchyma, and pleura. The airways are a system of branching tubes starting at the mouth and nose and ending at the terminal bronchioles. No gas exchange occurs in these tubes. The terminal bronchioles divide into the respiratory bronchioles, which have occasional alveoli branching off their walls. Respiratory bronchioles lead to alveolar ducts, which are lined with alveoli and make up the bulk of the parenchyma. The number of alveoli is variable (2×10^8 to 6×10^8) and correlates with the height of the patient. The alveolar wall consists of two types of epithelial cell. Type I cells line the alveoli and form a thin sheet approximately 0.1μm thick. Type II cells do not function as gas-exchange membranes but are responsible for surfactant production. The pleura is in two parts: the parietal pleura, which coats the inner part of the thoracic cavity; and the visceral pleura, which surrounds the lung. In health, the two layers of pleura are closely applied and move as one. The pressure in the potential space between them, the intrapleural pressure, is usually subatmospheric because of the elastic properties of the lung. Commonly, this subatmospheric pressure is referred to as a negative pressure (that is, relative to atmospheric pressure). Intrapleural pressure varies in upright humans from the lung apex to the base; it is less negative (higher) at the base because of the weight of the lung.

The chest wall acts as a rigid expandable box that encases the lungs. The bony rib cage is reinforced by intercostal muscles. The diaphragm and abdominal contents function as a piston, forcibly aspirating gas into the lungs during inspiration and encouraging expiration by passive relaxation. Elastic forces tend to make the lung collapse to residual volume. This is prevented by the elasticity of the chest wall, which would otherwise expand (Fig. 42.1). The volume of chest and lung at the end of quiet expiration is a balance between these elastic forces.

Gases and liquids flow from high pressure to low pressure. Flow rate is determined by pressure difference and resistance. The relationship between pressure difference and flow depends on the nature of the flow. This may be laminar, turbulent, or transitional (see Fig. 42.1). Gas movement in an unbranched cylinder below its critical flow rate is streamlined, with a higher flow at the center than at the periphery. Laminar gas flow is inaudible. Under these circumstances, the flow rate is directly proportional to driving pressure when the resistance is constant. The Poiseuille equation describes the relationship between flow and the fourth power of the radius and explains the importance of airway narrowing. The nature of the airway and the gas velocity determine whether flow remains streamlined or becomes turbulent. Turbulence is characterized by irregular movement of gas, in contrast to the smooth velocity profile seen in laminar flow. Flow in the trachea has a high velocity and will normally be turbulent; as the airways divide and the flow rate reduces, it is more likely to become laminar. In parts of the bronchial tree where branching and reduction in tube diameter occur, eddies form and are carried for some distance down the airway: this is known as transitional flow. A substantial proportion of respiratory gas flow is transitional. These relationships are discussed in more detail in Chapter 10.

Ventilatory muscles

The muscles of ventilation are the intercostal, accessory, and abdominal muscles, and the diaphragm. The accessory muscles, including scalenus anterior and medius, sternocleidomastoid, and trapezius, are recruited during periods of respiratory difficulty, at which time the abdominal musculature will also contribute to respiratory effort. Contraction of the external and internal intercostal muscles and the transversus thoracic muscles results in the ribs being raised and drawn closer to their neighbors, causing an increase in the diameter of the thoracic cavity. The diaphragm has a central muscular and a peripheral tendinous component. Contraction of the central muscle causes flattening of the diaphragm and further increases thoracic volume.

The intercostal muscles receive their nerve supply from the intercostal nerves. The diaphragm is supplied by the phrenic nerve. Respiratory drive is affected by many factors; for example, it is increased in acidosis or depressed by anesthetic drugs (Chapter 46). Muscle function itself can be compromised under certain circumstances, such as failure to reverse muscle relaxant drugs adequately (Chapter 32). Muscle fatigue is a problem in the critically ill.

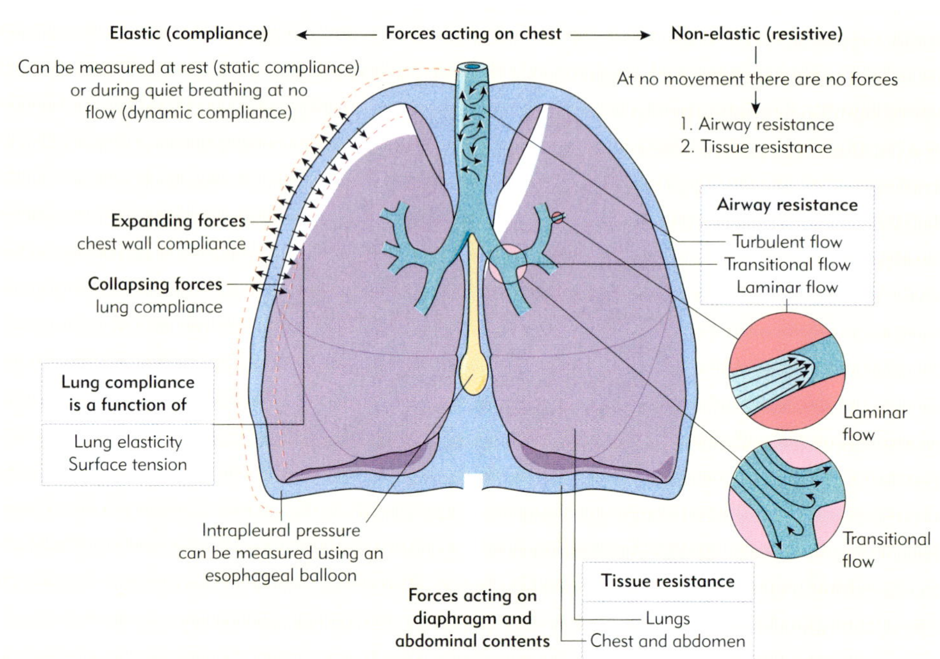

Figure 42.1 Forces acting on the lungs and chest wall during breathing. The elastic forces tending to cause chest wall expansion at rest balance the forces tending to cause pulmonary collapse. In both cases, the force results from elastic recoil. Elastic forces are measured as compliance, the slope of the pressure–volume curve when there is no gas flow or tissue movement. Large airways where gas flow is high have turbulent flow. Flow is laminar in smaller airways where gas flow has slowed, giving a parabolic velocity front. At junctions and branches eddy currents occur and flow is a mixture (or transitional).

FORCES

A clear idea of the forces moving gas in and out of the chest helps in understanding the effects of disease and artificial ventilation on pulmonary physiology. The physics of flow and factors involved in the transition from laminar to turbulent flow are covered in Chapter 10.

The SI unit of force, the newton, is defined as the force required to accelerate 1kg by $1 m/s^2$ or

Force = mass × acceleration

In *friction*, resistance is a measure of friction and

Force = velocity × resistance

In *elasticity*, stiffness is a measure of distensibility:

Force = displacement × stiffness

Considering gas movement, force can be substituted by pressure and displacement substituted by volume. When a force acts, work is done. Energy is the ability to do work. Kinetic energy is that energy related to the current state of motion of a body, whereas potential energy is the capacity to do work – for example, the energy held in a tensioned clock spring. A gas possesses potential energy by virtue of its pressures and kinetic energy by virtue of its movement or flow.

The *work* done by moving gases can be expressed as

Work = pressure × volume

At the end of expiration, the lungs are at rest. The intrapleural space is virtually obliterated and the lung and chest wall move as one. During inspiration, work is done by the muscles of respiration to overcome lung elastic forces, chest wall elastic forces, lung tissue resistive forces, chest wall resistive forces, and airway resistive forces.

Resistive forces can only be measured during movement as they have no value at rest. *Elastic forces* are present at all times but are measured in the absence of resistive forces when there is no tissue movement or gas flow. *Lung compliance* is the relationship of volume displaced and pressure change and can be measured by calculating the gradient of a pressure–volume line. Anesthetists will be familiar with the difference in tidal volume delivered by the application of the same airway pressure in an adult and a child. This is because compliance is higher in the larger lung of the adult. It is possible to compensate for the volume effect by measuring *specific compliance* (compliance divided by lung volume). There are two ways of assessing compliance. *Static compliance* is assessed by observing the relationship between lung volume and pressure at steady state. *Dynamic compliance* measurement is a way of assessing compliance during breathing. It is helpful to consider these forces individually.

Lung compliance: the lung elastic forces

The elastic property of lung results from the nature of its connective tissue as well as its architecture. Lung expansion results in increasing tissue tension because of stretching and distortion of interwoven elastin and collagen fibers. Surface tension effects are also important, comprising about 60% of the necessary force required to expand the lung. Surface tension effects would be even greater in the absence of surfactant.

Static compliance

Static lung compliance is measured in various ways. An isolated lung preparation can be inflated to known volumes and a static pressure–volume relationship plotted, which is linear throughout most of its range. At high lung volumes, at the limit of distensibility, compliance is reduced and the curve is flattened. The curve obtained during expiration does not overlap that of inspiration. Failure of stretched materials to return exactly to their relaxation length is seen in all elastic substances and can be termed *hysteresis*. Similar data can be obtained by placing an isolated lung in a jar and evacuating gas from around the lung. The curve now looks more physiologic as the distending pressure is negative, simulating intrapleural pressure.

In humans, it is not possible to measure intrapleural pressure directly, but it can be estimated from the pressure measured in a balloon placed at the lower end of the esophagus. It is not possible to validate absolute values measured but the changes in pressure are considered accurate. Static lung compliance can be estimated by instructing a subject to breathe in a predetermined volume and measuring the esophageal pressure. If the glottis is open, the force measured by an esophageal balloon is that required to stop the lung collapsing. This can be plotted against the change in lung volume to produce a compliance curve (Fig. 42.2). These measurements are performed in an upright subject breathing from functional residual capacity (FRC).

Surface tension

Molecules are closer together in a liquid than they are in a gas; consequently, at a gas–liquid interface, molecules are attracted to their neighbors in the liquid with a greater force than to molecules in the gas. This results in a tension tending to pull molecules at the gas–liquid interface into the liquid, causing it to adopt a minimum area. The surface tension (T) is measured as force per unit length (l) of surface. The relationship between pressure and radius of a sphere such as a bubble or alveolus is also important.

Surface tension can be demonstrated easily in the laboratory. An oblong wire frame is constructed with one side moveable. A soap film is placed on the frame. The force acting on the moveable side of frame of length l is lT. However, since the soap film has two surfaces (upper and lower), the force is actually $2lT$.

The surface tension of water is 70mN/m. This is reduced in biological fluids such as plasma to 50mN/m. A bubble in a liquid or a soap bubble in air takes a shape with the minimum surface area, which is a sphere. The relationship between the pressure in a bubble and the tension in the wall is described by the Laplace relationship:

$$P \propto T/r$$

This allows estimation of the pressure (P) above ambient required to prevent collapse of a hollow curved object if the tension in the wall is T and the radius of curvature is r. This relationship can be explored further if it is imagined that the sphere is cut down the middle. The force acting on one half is the product of pressure and cross-sectional area, which is balanced by the force acting on the other side, which is the product of surface tension and the length of circumference. In the case of a soap bubble, there are two surfaces so length is doubled

$$P\pi r^2 = T2(2\pi r)$$

or

$$P = 4T/r$$

Various factors affect the proportionality constant or numerator of this equation, such as the number of planes of curvature and the number of surfaces being considered. For an alveolus the equation reads

Lung compliance

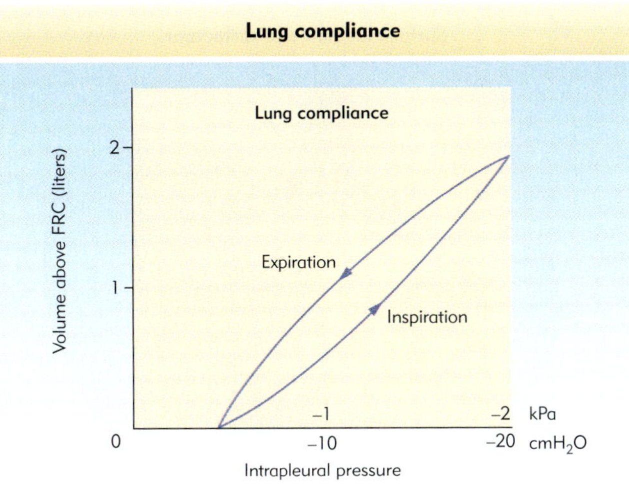

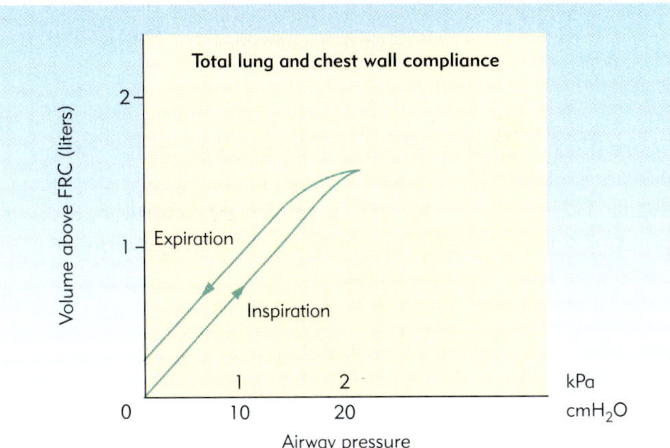

Figure 42.2 Static compliance curves. Lung compliance is the slope of the curve of static esophageal relaxation pressure versus the volume above the functional residual capacity (FRC) in a laboratory subject. The curve exhibits hysteresis: at a given pressure the volume during expiration is higher than inspiration. This phenomenon is caused by a number of factors such as alveolar recruitment, surfactant, and the nature of elastic tissue. Total lung and chest wall static compliance can be obtained experimentally in a ventilated relaxed patient. A curve is plotted of volume injected and airway pressure.

$$P = 2T/r$$

Therefore, as the radius of an alveolus becomes smaller, the pressure required to balance the tension in the wall and so prevent collapse must rise. It also explains why if two alveoli of different radii are connected together, theoretically the smaller one with the higher pressure should empty into the larger. Unique properties of pulmonary surfactant compensate for this phenomenon and also prevent the surface tension increasing as the lung reduces in volume (Fig. 42.3).

The importance of surface tension on static compliance can be demonstrated experimentally by plotting a compliance curve for an experimental lung inflated with saline. The absence of the air–fluid interface abolishes surface tension and results in a considerably more compliant lung.

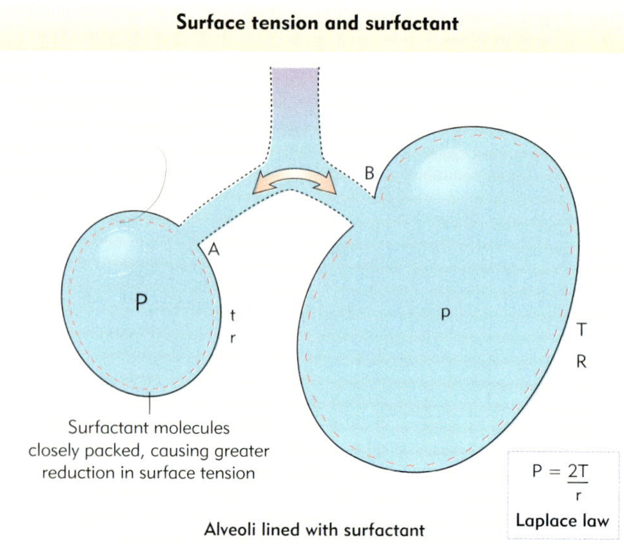

Figure 42.3 The effect of surface tension and surfactant on alveolar stability. The presence of surfactant helps to stabilize alveoli. T, large surface tension; t, small surface tension; R, large radius; r, small radius; P, large pressure; p, small pressure.

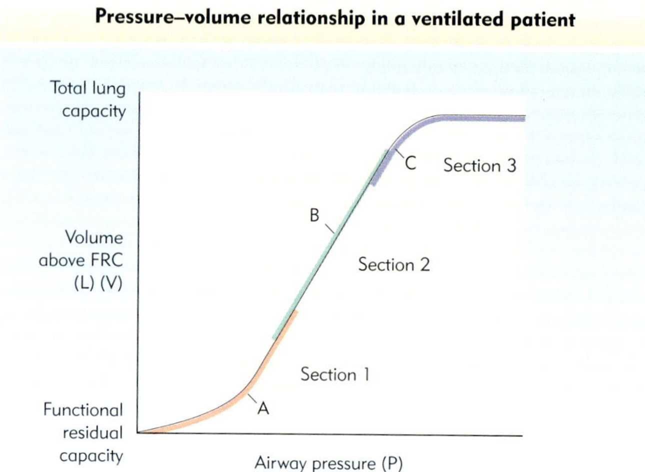

Figure 42.4 A pressure–volume curve in a ventilated patient. The slope at any point from the functional residual capacity (FRC) to the total lung capacity (TLC) indicates total compliance (lung and chest wall). The lag seen in section 1 is caused by the FRC being less than the closing capacity, allowing basal collapse to occur during expiration. At the upper section (3) the curve flattens as a result of alveolar overdistention from using a high tidal volume or excessive positive end-expiratory pressure (PEEP). Ideally the tidal volume in a ventilated patient will sit on section 2, which represents optimal compliance. Above this, it may be possible to increase compliance by reducing tidal volume or the level of PEEP. At section 1, it should be possible to increase compliance by applying increased PEEP. Point A represents the lower inflection point of the compliance curve, where the compliance suddenly increases. Ideally PEEP should be set to match the pressure at point A.

Surfactant

Surfactant is made up of phospholipids, which contain both hydrophobic and hydrophilic portions. The former project into the alveolus, the latter remain in the alveolar lining fluid. The most important constituent of surfactant is dipalmitoyl lecithin. Surfactants are detergents that lower the surface tension in proportion to their concentration at the interface. As alveoli expand during inspiration, surfactant becomes less concentrated and surface tension increases. During expiration, the concentration of surfactant increases again and reduces surface tension, splinting open alveoli and making them generally more stable (see Fig. 42.3). The surface tension in alveoli ranges between 5 and 30mN/m.

Lung compliance in disease

Lung compliance is affected in diseases in which there is reduction in production of surfactant or alteration in elastic tissue or bronchial mucous. In pulmonary fibrosis, elastic tissue is replaced by fibrous tissue, causing a reduction in compliance. Age or emphysema causes an increase in compliance from loss of elastic tissue. Pulmonary edema also causes a reduction in compliance. Surfactant is not normally produced until the late stages of gestation and can be inadequate in premature babies, causing respiratory distress syndrome. Absence or reduction in surfactant causes instability in alveoli, reduces compliance, and by increasing surface tension increases forces that can precipitate pulmonary edema.

Chest wall compliance

At end-expiration, elastic forces tending to cause the lung to collapse balance forces tending to make the chest wall expand. Static chest wall compliance can be measured using appropriate relaxation pressures but is often calculated (this is discussed below). Chest wall compliance can be reduced by obesity, by loss of skin elasticity (for example, caused by scarring from burns) or by skeletal problems such as fusion of costochondral joints.

Total compliance

The relaxation pressure for the whole respiratory system can be obtained by asking a subject to breathe in a quantity of air and then relax against an airway obstruction. This is a similar method to that described above where the positive pressure required to expand an isolated lung is used to measure lung compliance. The pressure measured at the mouth during relaxation is equal to the intra-alveolar pressure at that time. The gradient of volume of gas inhaled against the relaxation pressure represents total compliance. A problem with this method in an awake subject is the inability to completely relax the muscles of respiration. Total compliance (TC) is related to lung compliance (LC) and chest wall compliance (CWC):

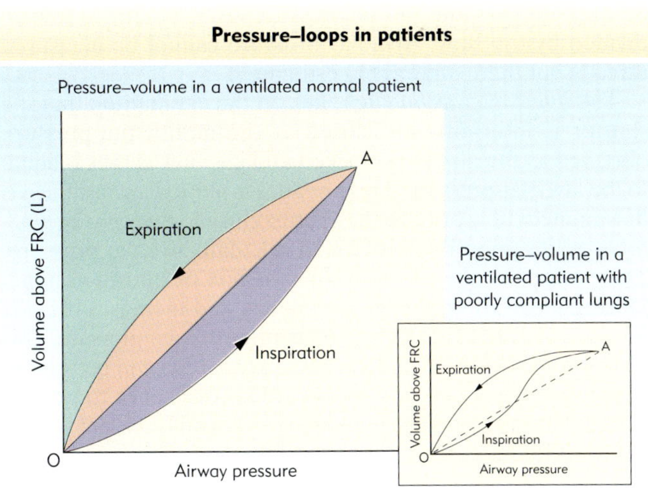

Figure 42.5 Dynamic pressure–volume loops obtained wiith a ventilated patient. The pressure–volume loop obtained from a ventilated normal patient (left) is a similar shape to that obtained from a subject breathing spontaneously. OA connects the beginning of inspiration to the end and represents the dynamic compliance as the flow is nominally zero at these points. Work done during inspiration against elastic forces is the sum of the areas shaded green and orange. Work done during inspiration against resistive forces is the area shaded purple. Total work done during inspiration is the sum of the areas shaded green, orange, and purple. Work done during expiration against resistive forces is the area shaded orange. An increase in resistive work seen in bronchospasm would be shown by larger purple (inspiration) and orange (expiration) areas.The pressure–volume loop in a patient with poorly compliant lungs (right) would be more sloped towards the x-axis. At higher pressures, there is no increase in lung volume. Dynamic compliance is represented by line OA. This loop represents a patient on section 3 of the curve in Figure 42.4.

$$\frac{1}{TC} = \frac{1}{LC} + \frac{1}{CWC}$$

Normal values (in L/kPa) are TC = 1; LC = 2; CWC = 2.

For practical reasons compliance is usually assessed clinically by measuring dynamic compliance, but there is a method for measuring static total compliance in patients on artificial ventilation in intensive care. An automated gas delivery system is used based on a large syringe that injects gas into the airway in steps, allowing time for stabilization. By monitoring the accompanying changes in pressure, compliance can be calculated (Fig. 42.4).

Dynamic compliance

The concept of dynamic compliance can be confusing as all compliance measurements are made in the absence of gas flow. Dynamic compliance is measured in a similar way to static compliance except that, instead of the measurement being made when the lung is at rest after having allowed time for settling, it is measured by analyzing the slope of the line joining the zero flow parts of a dynamic pressure–volume loop. Zero flow occurs as gas flow changes direction at the end of inspiration immediately prior to expiration and again at the start of inspiration. It is important to realize that the shape of the dynamic loop does not affect compliance measurements: only the line joining points is relevant (OA in Fig. 42.5). The width of the loop is a consequence of the greater pressure differentials needed to work against frictional forces at any point than required at rest. The area of the loop reflects tissue and airway resistance.

In the normal subject, dynamic compliance measurements should be similar to compliance measured statically, although they will never be identical. One reason for different values includes stress relaxation, which is seen in all elastic tissue through the tension of the stretched material reducing over time after stretching has occurred. Physiologic reasons include varying tone of pulmonary musculature, redistribution of blood, and the effects of alveolar time constants. These effects are more pronounced in lung disease.

Lung stability: interdependence

Stability of lung units is a balance between collapsing forces (e.g. surface tension) and stabilizing forces preventing collapse (e.g. airway pressure and surfactant). Stability is encouraged by the lung architecture as each alveolus is supported by surrounding alveoli, alveolar ducts, and other airways. It is unlikely that alveoli of greatly varying diameters could exist side by side because they share septal walls. This mutual support, known as interdependence, is helped by other structures such as blood vessels and fibrous tissue that penetrate from the lung surface and add to lung stability.

TIME CONSTANTS

The alveolar time constant is the time required for inflation if the initial gas flow were maintained throughout inspiration. It is the product of compliance and resistance. Compliance, resistance, and, therefore, the time constant are dependent on lung volume. A poorly compliant alveolus has reduced capacity compared with its normal neighbor. Its maximum volume is not affected by respiratory pattern and it will achieve it quickly: it has a fast time constant. A second alveolus has a high airway resistance but a normal compliance. This alveolus takes some time to fill but its capacity is not reduced as long as inspiration is long enough: it has a slow time constant. In disease, the lung comprises alveoli with a mixture of time constants. Those with fast time constants under certain circumstances may empty into those with shorter time constants. Differing time constants cause a reduction in dynamic compliance. This effect is exaggerated at high respiratory rates and the associated short inspiratory times.

POSITIVE END-EXPIRATORY PRESSURE

In lung disease, careful use of positive end-expiratory pressure (PEEP) can increase compliance and improve pulmonary function. The compliance curve in Figure 42.4 represents changes from FRC to total lung capacity: a volume of approximately 4L. This is significantly greater than a normal tidal volume, which lies on part of the curve. If the tidal volume is at low lung volumes, the compliance will be reduced but can be improved by increasing PEEP. Minor adjustments to PEEP can have a significant effect. Generally, it is possible to optimize the respiratory effects of PEEP by setting the level to match the lower inflection point of the pressure–volume loop. It is important to monitor the effect of PEEP on cardiovascular stability.

A tidal volume lying at the upper part of the curve in Figure 42.4 represents overdistension (seen expressed as a dynamic loop in the inset of Fig. 42.5). Higher airway pressure results in no increase in volume but increases the risk of barotrauma. Reducing PEEP will increase compliance.

NON-ELASTIC FORCES: RESISTANCE

An ideal lung would have elastic properties with no hysteresis and with no frictional or resistance effects. The relationship between intrapleural pressure and lung volume would be linear, inspiration overlapping expiration. In practice, such a graph plotted during breathing shows intrapleural pressure is always more negative than this during inspiration and more positive during expiration. This is because of the nonelastic forces. The area of the loop generated is a consequence of the work done against these forces. Generally, resistance relates the forces producing movement to the movement produced. In the case of gases, resistance is given by pressure difference/flow.

The total pulmonary resistance is the sum of the airway resistance and the tissue resistance. Energy is required to move the lung, chest wall, diaphragm, and abdominal contents during breathing to overcome tissue resistance even if there is no gas flow in the airway. Tissue resistance cannot be measured directly but has to be estimated by subtracting the measured airway resistance from the total pulmonary resistance. Quiet expiration is mainly powered by energy stored during stretching of elastic tissue during inspiration. If there is an increase in tissue resistance in disease, less energy will be available to overcome airway resistance and expiration will be prolonged. Tissue resistance is normally about 20% of resistive forces. It is increased by conditions causing pulmonary fibrosis, such as sarcoidosis and carcinomatosis. It can also be increased in musculoskeletal conditions limiting mechanical movement, such as kyphoscoliosis.

Resistance to flow in the airways (airway resistance) is affected by their radius and the flow characteristics of the gas. When flow is slow, it is likely to be laminar. If flow increases or there is a change in airway characteristic such as a constriction or branch, the parabolic profile flow is lost and it is said to be turbulent. In many parts of the bronchial tree the flow pattern is transitional, which is a mixture of these two extremes. In those parts of the respiratory tract where flow is laminar, flow is proportional to pressure drop. Small reductions in radius (r) have a marked effect on the resistance:

$$\text{Airway resistance} = \frac{8l\sigma}{\pi r^4}$$

where l is the length of the airway and σ is the gas viscosity.

In areas of turbulence, flow is no longer directly proportional to pressure drop but varies with its square root. As this relationship is no longer linear, the resistance is not constant but varies with the flow. Turbulent flow is not affected by gas viscosity but is inversely proportional to the square root of the gas density, which is why breathing gas at high pressures increases airway resistance (density increases with increasing pressure). Similarly, helium, which has a low density, reduces the work of breathing and can be used temporarily to help patients with upper airway obstruction (Chapter 49). Airway resistance can be measured as the fall in pressure from mouth to alveoli divided by the flow. Alveolar pressure cannot be measured directly but there are ways to estimate it.

The *interrupter technique* relies on the assumption that if a shutter is intermittently closed at the mouth the pressure obtained as the airway is blocked and gas flow ceases is equal to the alveolar pressure. This pressure is plotted against the gas flow immediately prior to the shutter closing. *Body plethysmography* relies upon Boyle's Law to calculate alveolar pressure. The patient is placed in an airtight box of known volume. During inspiration, the chest expands and increases the box pressure in association with a fall in intra-alveolar pressure. This allows calculation of alveolar pressure, which can be related to measured gas flow and allows airway resistance to be estimated. The normal range is about 0.05–1.5cmH_2O/L per second (0.005–0.15kPa/L per second) in adults.

Using measurements of the pressure in an esophageal balloon (see above) and the gas flow, total lung resistance can be obtained. Tissue resistance can be calculated as the difference between total lung resistance and measured airway resistance.

Factors affecting airway resistance include lung volume. As the lung expands, airways become wider and longer. The overall effect is a reduction in airway resistance. Airway resistance is increased if the bronchi become narrowed through bronchospasm, mucosal edema, mucous plugging, and epithelial desquamation. The parasympathetic system is of major importance in the control of bronchomotor tone. Afferents from the bronchial epithelium pass centrally to the vagus. Efferent preganglionic fibers also run in the vagus to ganglia located in the walls of small bronchi. Short postganglionic fibers lead to nerve endings that release acetylcholine to act on muscarinic receptors in the bronchial smooth muscle. Stimulation of any part of this reflex arc results in bronchoconstriction. Many drugs also affect the bronchial muscle tone.

All airways can be compressed by reversal of the normal transmural pressure gradient during forced expiration. The cartilaginous airways have considerable structural resistance. The smaller airways have no structural rigidity and rely on elastic recoil of the lung tissue surrounding them. This results in expiratory flow limitation.

During anesthesia, airway resistance can be increased by airway obstruction from a number of causes. The oropharyngeal airway can become obstructed as normal pharyngeal reflexes are lost during anesthesia, in a comatose patient, or during REM sleep, particularly in the elderly. The lumen of the pharynx and larynx may become obstructed with foreign material such as tumor, gastric contents, or blood. The larynx can also become obstructed by laryngeal spasm or subglottic edema. Airway obstruction can be detected by analyzing a flow–volume loop (Fig. 42.6).

WORK OF BREATHING

Work is done during inspiration against elastic and resistive forces. Work done combating the resistive forces is dissipated as heat. Energy used displacing elastic tissue can be compared with that used in stretching a spring; it is stored as potential energy that is available to power expiration. Expiration is passive in mechanically ventilated patients and at rest in health; expiratory work is not normally important.

The energy used by muscles of respiration can be calculated by measuring *oxygen cost*. This is small in a resting

Flow–volume loop in a patient

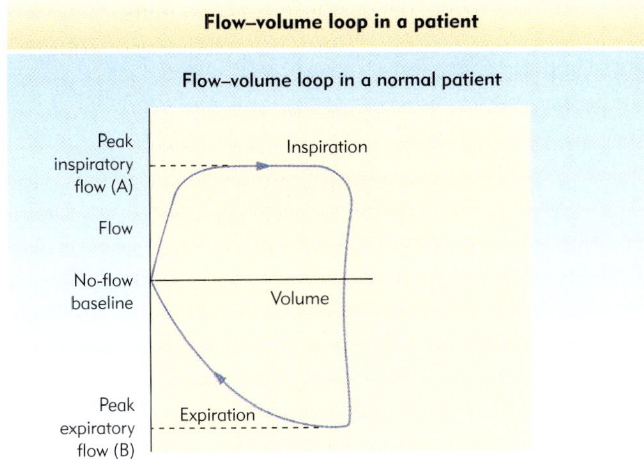

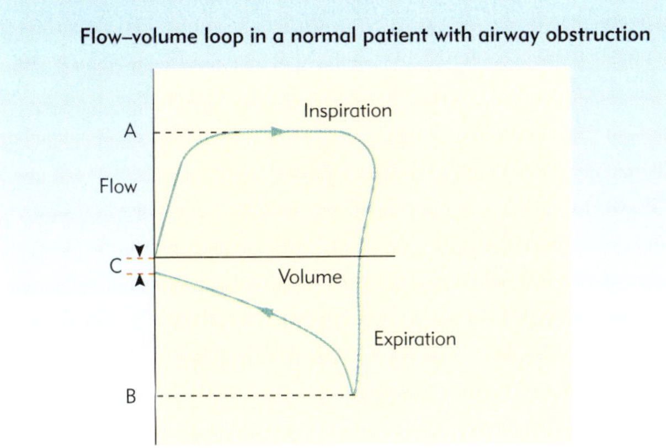

Figure 42.6 Flow–volume loops obtained during volume-controlled mechanical ventilation. Flow pattern is affected by the mode of ventilation. In pressure-controlled ventilation, the peak inspiratory flow is achieved early in inspiration and is followed by a decelerating pattern. Expiration is unchanged. In a patient with airway obstruction (bottom), there is a lower peak expiratory flow (B) that drops off suddenly and ultimately has a flatter shape than the normal curve (top). This indicates the expiratory flow limitation seen in bronchospasm. This loop is also incomplete: the expiratory curve does not reach the no-flow baseline (indicated by C). This may occur because of airtrapping, incomplete expiration, or gas leakage from the circuit.

healthy individual: less than 2% of total oxygen uptake. Respiratory efficiency is expressed as the percentage of the calculated energy that is actual work done. It is normally less than 10%; the majority of energy is lost as heat generated within muscles.

Work is performed when a force moves its point of application. In terms of the lungs, it is measured using pressure and volume changes. Pressure–volume loops monitored during mechanical and spontaneous ventilation supply information about many aspects of lung mechanics as well as the work of breathing. The work of breathing can be assessed from analyzing different areas of the loops (see Fig. 42.5) from which elastic and resistive work can be calculated. Further information can be obtained by observing the pattern of the flow–volume loop displayed on many modern intensive-care ventilators (see Fig. 42.6). Reduction in peak flow rates implies increased airway resistance.

Patients tend to optimize their respiratory pattern to match compliance and airway resistance. The work of breathing is increased if either compliance is reduced or airway resistance is increased. When compliance is reduced, increased work is done against elastic forces. It is possible to compensate by reducing the tidal volume and increasing the respiratory rate. Conversely, patients with high airway resistance reduce the resistive component of the work of breathing by reducing the respiratory rate and increasing the tidal volume.

Further Reading

Artigas A, Lemaire F, Suter P, Zapol W, eds. Adult respiratory distress syndrome. Edinburgh, UK: Churchill Livingstone; 1992.

Nunn JF. Applied respiratory physiology, 4th edn. Oxford, UK: Butterworths; 1993.

Scurr C, Feldman S, Soni N. Scientific foundations of anesthesia: the basis of intensive care, 4th edn. Oxford: Heinemann Medical; 1990.

West JB. Respiratory physiology – the essentials, 5th edn. Baltimore, MD: Williams & Wilkins; 1995.

Chapter 43 Lung function testing

Roger Hainsworth

Topics covered in this chapter

Although the principal role of the lungs is the exchange of respiratory gases between the blood and the atmosphere, lungs do have other functions, some which may impinge on their respiratory role. One of the most important secondary functions is that of a blood filter, trapping emboli returning from the systemic circulation and preventing them from blocking vital parts of the circulation. Clearly, pulmonary vessels blocked by microemboli can no longer function for gas exchange and excessive embolization results in pulmonary hypertension and impairment of respiratory function. The lungs are also a reservoir of blood that can change in volume: for example, to allow the cardiovascular system to adjust to the sequestration of blood in dependent veins when standing. In the supine position, the increased volume of blood in the pulmonary vessels and in the chambers of the heart reduces the volume of air that can be accommodated in the alveoli. The lung also has metabolic functions, perhaps the best known of which is the conversion of angiotensin I to angiotensin II. However, it is the respiratory function of the lung that is of main interest in this chapter.

Respiratory function refers to the uptake of oxygen and the elimination of carbon dioxide by the body; this should be adequate to maintain normal levels of blood gases both at rest and at all levels of exercise. The ideal lung is able to achieve this with a minimum expenditure of work both against elastic forces and against the resistance to gas flow in the airways. A minimum amount of ventilated air should be wasted in the conducting airways and in poorly perfused regions of the lung. Each breath should effectively exchange the pulmonary alveolar gases; this requires that the volume remaining in the lungs after each expiration [the functional residual capacity (FRC)] is not excessively large. Finally, the distribution of the pulmonary blood flow and the ventilation of the alveoli should be as even as possible and there should be a minimal barrier to the diffusion of gases.

The overall function of the lungs can really only be assessed by determining the effects of exercise on arterial blood gases and ventilation. This, however, is time consuming and requires medical supervision; therefore, it is applicable only to selected patients. Most lung function tests are carried out by technicians and examine various specific aspects of lung function. The simplest level of study is spirometry, which allows not only measurement of vital capacity and its subdivisions but also may permit expiratory and possibly inspiratory flow rates to be assessed. Laboratories specializing in lung function assessment also have facilities for the measurement of lung volumes by inert gas dilution or, possibly, the nitrogen washout method, and probably also possess a body plethysmograph. Pulmonary gas transfer can be assessed by the single-breath carbon monoxide method. Larger respiratory units are equipped for more specialized investigations including exercise tests, compliance studies, and studies of ventilatory control.

SPIROMETRY

Spirometer types

A spirometer is a device for measuring the volumes of air that can be breathed. If the volume signal is differentiated, either electronically or by manual measurements from the volume–time traces, spirometers can also be used to derive the gas flow rates. The most accurate type of spirometer is the *water-sealed bell spirometer*. This is an inverted bell, sealed under water and counterbalanced (Fig. 43.1). Assuming the bell is a perfect cylinder, the displacement of the counterweight and attached pen is directly related to the change in volume. If the recording kymograph is set to move rapidly, it is possible to determine the rate of change of volume and, hence, the expiratory and inspiratory flow rates.

Although this type of spirometer is inherently very simple, there are a number of precautions relating to its use. Generally, the bell will have a diameter to match the calibration on the recording device or the supplied paper. Nevertheless, a check should be made by injecting accurately known volumes of gas. The readout gives volumes at ambient pressure and temperature, although the volumes actually within the lung are at body temperature and atmospheric pressure saturated with water vapor (BTPS). This is usually about 10% greater than the measured volume and should be corrected accordingly by applying the gas laws or by the use of appropriate tables.

For accurate measurements of high flow rates, the spirometer bell and counterweight should have minimum inertia, and bells constructed of lightweight plastic materials are preferred. Another problem may be leaks in the system; these can easily be checked by occluding the connecting tubing and applying a weight on the top of the bell. The bell should not continue to move.

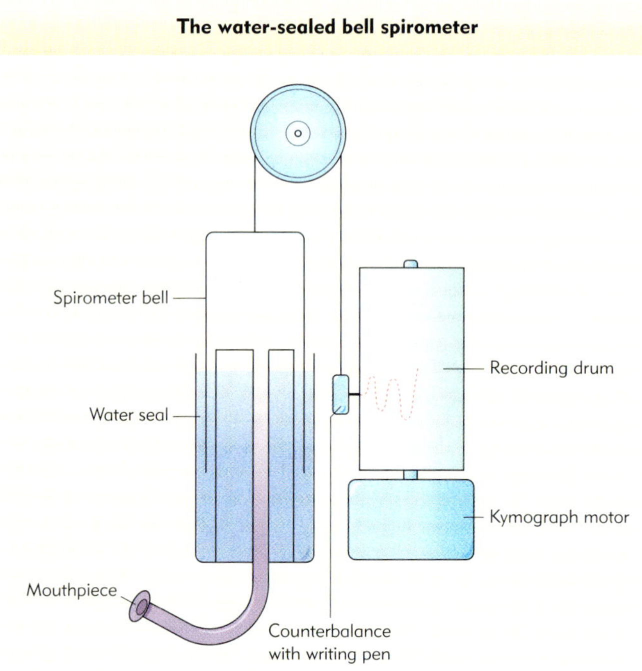

Figure 43.1 The water-sealed bell spirometer. The kymograph indicates rate of change of volume in the spirometer bell and hence the expiratory and inspiratory flow rates.

Water-filled spirometers have the disadvantages that they are heavy, subject to spillage, and electronic outputs are not directly obtained. In attempts to solve these problems, various other devices have been introduced. One widely used device that is convenient and readily transported is the *bellows* or *wedge spirometer*. As gas moves into the bellows, the bellows move about the hinge and a pointer tracks over moving paper to define the expiratory volume–time trace. It does not, however, record tidal volume or inspiratory volumes. Bellows spirometers need to be carefully calibrated, with particular attention paid to the linearity of the readings.

Since spirometry is used to assess the volumes of the gas breathed and flow is derived from the rate of change of volume, an alternative approach is actually to determine flow and then derive volume by integration. Some caution, however, is required with this approach since integration over relatively long time periods, as may occur in patients with severe obstructive lung disease, tends to be unstable. Accurate flow-measuring devices and high-quality electronic circuits are, therefore, required. One widely used and accurate flow-measuring device is the *Fleisch pneumotachograph,* in which flow is determined from the pressure difference across a small resistance. It is based on Poiseuille's equation, which states that the flow through a tube is directly proportional to the pressure difference across it. This relationship applies only to laminar flow, which depends on the critical value of Reynold's number not being exceeded (see Chapter 10). Because Reynold's number is directly related to the diameters of the tubes through which the gas flows, the Fleisch pneumotachograph uses a bundle of tubes of small diameter instead of one large tube to provide the resistance. Condensation in the device is prevented by a heating element.

A very simple lightweight device that determines the peak flow rate is the *Wright peak flowmeter*. The expired gas passes through an orifice and moves a lever against a spring by an amount calibrated to read the peak flow. This device is not as accurate as most other spirometers but it is simple, cheap, and convenient and may be used by patients at home.

Lung volumes

The divisions of the lung volumes (and common abbreviations used for these entities) are illustrated in Figure 43.2. Note that the various subdivisions, by convention, are termed as volumes and combinations of subdivisions are capacities. Spirometry can only determine the volumes and capacities that are actually ventilated: that is, the vital capacity and its subdivisions.

Vital capacity may be determined in three ways: from a single expiratory effort; from a single inspiratory effort; or from the sum of expiratory reserve volume and inspiratory capacity. In healthy subjects, there should be little difference between these methods, but in patients with obstructive disease the measurement from the single expiratory maneuver may be lower, owing to air trapping, and inspiratory measurements provide higher values.

Expiratory reserve volume and inspiratory capacity may be used to derive residual volume and total lung capacity from measurements of FRC.

Maximal flow rates

Flow of any fluid through a tube or system of tubes may be given by Poiseuille's equation:

$$F = \frac{\pi}{8} \times \frac{P_1 - P_2}{\eta\, l} \times r^4$$

where $P_1 - P_2$ is the pressure gradient across the resistance, η is the viscosity of the fluid, and r and l are terms relating to the radius and length of the tube, respectively. Resistance to flow is expressed by analogy with Ohm's law as $(P_1 - P_2)/F$ and is proportional to $1/r^4$. Therefore, changes in r, which in the lung relate to radius of the airways, have a major impact on the flow. Assessments of airways resistance by spirometry are based only on the flow part of the expression and ignore pressure. Patients with fibrotic lung disease, in which the elastic recoil of the lung is exceptionally large, have particularly large expiratory flow rates. It might also be expected that the maximum flow achieved would be critically dependent on the effort made by the subject. However, the flow remains relatively unaffected by effort because high levels of intrathoracic pressure have the effect of compressing the unsplinted intrathoracic airways. As air flows along the system of airways, the pressure falls from maximal at the alveolar end to atmospheric at the mouth. The positive pressure within the thorax compresses the alveoli to drive the air out, but it also compresses the airways and at some stage there will be a point, called the equal pressure point, at which the external and internal airways pressures balance; just beyond this point, airways close and flow is limited. Flow is, therefore, dependent largely on the elastic properties of the lung and the diameters of the airways and only to a smaller extent on the effort made by the subject.

Flow may be assessed from the forced expiratory spirogram. Several measurements may be made from this. The most commonly used is the *forced expiratory volume in the first second,* (FEV_1); other measurements include $FEV_{0.75}$, the volume expired in three-quarters of a second; and the *maximum mid-expiratory flow rate,* the volume expired between 25 and 75% of

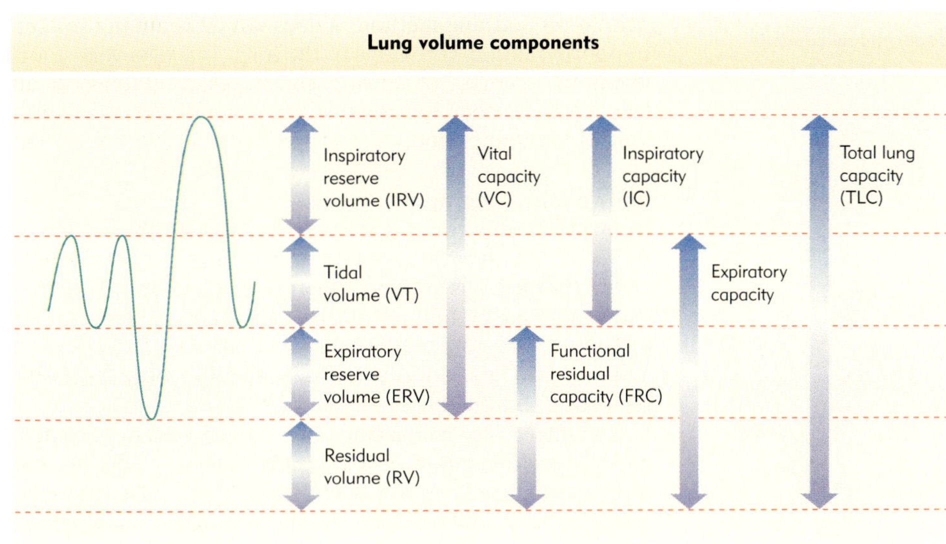

Figure 43.2 Lung volume components. The total lung capacity can be divided into various subdivisions (called volumes) and combinations of subdivisions (called capacities).

vital capacity divided by time. *Peak expiratory flow,* the instantaneous maximum, is sometimes used because it can readily be estimated using Wright's peak flowmeter, and may be abnormal when FEV_1 is relatively normal in people with large airway obstructions (see below).

Flow–volume loops provide an alternative method for evaluating airways resistance. Instead of plotting volume against time, as in the expiratory spirogram, flow is plotted against either absolute lung volume or change in volume. This may be obtained for both expiration and inspiration. The normal expiratory curve (Fig. 43.3) is roughly triangular in shape. The highest flow is at the onset of expiration when the elastic recoil is maximal and diameter of the airways is maximal because of the negative intrathoracic pressure distending the airways. The inspiratory part of the loop is dependent on the inspiratory muscles and is normally more even. Patients with obstructive disease have a lower peak expiratory flow and this declines more rapidly with reducing volume, resulting in a concave shape (Fig. 43.3). This is particularly apparent in patients with emphysema who also have reduced elastic recoil.

In most patients flow–volume loops do not provide much more information than the expiratory spirogram. However, they are of use in assessing the effects of large-airways resistance, such as that occurring in tracheal stenosis or goiter compression. In these conditions, the high peak flow velocities cause the Reynold's number to exceed the critical value and flow becomes turbulent. When flow is turbulent, it becomes a function of the square root of pressure instead of pressure and this effectively limits flow. This causes reduction and flattening of both expiratory and inspiratory flow rates (Fig. 43.3). Inspiratory flow is dependent on inspiratory muscle effort and is reduced when the muscles are weakened: for example, following diaphragmatic paralysis.

FUNCTIONAL RESIDUAL CAPACITY

The FRC is the volume of gas in the lung at the end-expiratory point. It is the sum of residual volume and expiratory reserve volume and cannot be determined by spirometry. Three main methods are available for estimation of FRC: inert gas dilution, nitrogen washout, and body plethysmography.

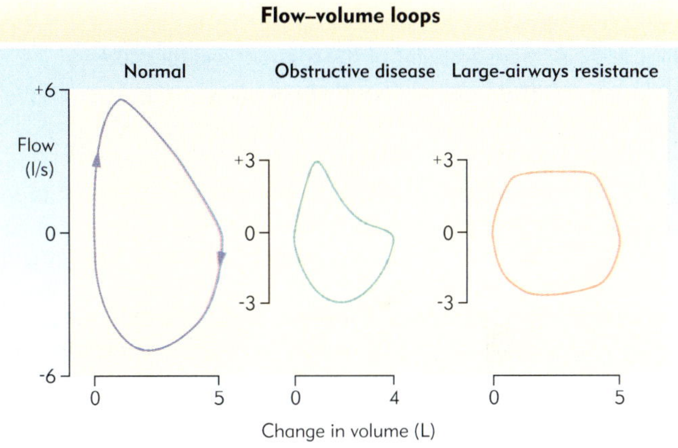

Figure 43.3 Flow–volume loops. Flow (expiration upwards) is plotted against change in volume for normal individuals (left), in obstructive disease (centre), and in patients with diseases such as goiter compression or tracheal stenosis, who have large-airways resistance (right).

Inert gas dilution

An inert, insoluble, readily detectable gas is required. The principle of the method is that the subject breathes from a closed-circuit system containing the gas until there is complete equilibrium between the lungs and the circuit. Assuming that the subject is switched into the circuit (Fig. 43.4) at the end-expiratory point, FRC is calculated from the dilution of the tracer gas. The main constituents are a mouthpiece attached to a tap, a sodalime canister to absorb carbon dioxide, a pump for circulating the gas to prevent a large dead-space effect, a spirometer, a gas analyzer, and an inlet for oxygen to replace that which is taken up from the lungs. Usually helium is used and the circuit is initially filled with a mixture of about 20% helium in air and oxygen, with the tap to the patient closed and the pump turned on to mix the gases thoroughly. The initial helium reading, $F_{He}1$, is taken and the patient then is turned into the circuit at end-expiration.

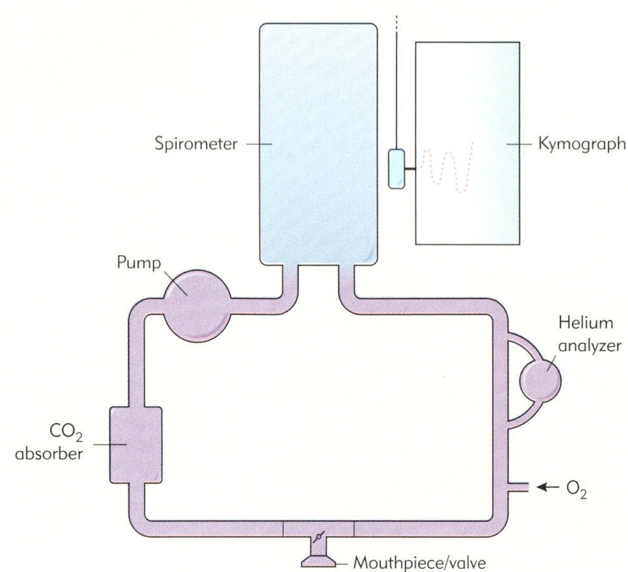

Figure 43.4 Measurement of functional residual capacity (FRC) by the inert gas dilution method.

Rebreathing continues, with replacement of consumed oxygen, until the helium reading becomes stable (FHe2). This may take 3 minutes in healthy subjects but much longer in those with obstructive disease.

After mixing, the volume of helium in the circuit V_{He} is equal to V_C FHe1, where V_C is the volume of circuit. Therefore, $V_C = V_{He}/$ FHe1. After rebreathing, the same volume of helium becomes equilibrated through both circuit and lung so that:

$$V_{He} = (V_C + \text{FRC})\text{FHe2}$$

Solving these equations gives

$$\text{FRC} = V_{He}\left[\frac{\text{FHe1} - \text{FHe2}}{\text{FHe1} \times \text{FHe2}}\right]$$

The main limitation of this method is that in patients with obstructive disease, and especially those with emphysema in which ventilation of regions of the lung is very poor, FRC is likely to be underestimated. The patient may need to rebreathe for up to 10 minutes before a steady value of the helium concentration is obtained, and even then distribution of the gas throughout the lung is likely to be incomplete.

Nitrogen washout

The principle of the nitrogen washout method is that the patient breathes 100% oxygen and expires to a spirometer with monitoring of the nitrogen in the expired gas until all is washed out. Allowance needs to be made for washout of dissolved nitrogen from other body compartments. The estimate of FRC is made from the volume of collected gas and its nitrogen concentration by calculating the volume that would have initially contained the nitrogen washed out. The disadvantages of this method are that washout takes a long time and, like the helium-rebreathing method, it does not estimate the volume of poorly ventilated regions of the lung. It is also very sensitive to the accuracy of the nitrogen analysis and to any small leak that may occur, for example at the mouth, during the prolonged washout period.

Body plethysmography

Body plethysmography applies Boyle's law to the gas in the thorax and derives an estimate of its volume. This is usually called thoracic gas volume (VTG) to distinguish it from the value derived by helium dilution or nitrogen washout. It determines the total gas volume, whether ventilated or not, and may also be used to determine airways resistance (or its reciprocal, conductance).

The subject sits in an airtight box, the plethysmograph (Fig. 43.5), inserts a mouthpiece and applies a nose clip. The mouthpiece is connected to a flowmeter: for example, a Fleisch pneumotachograph, and a shutter. Mouth pressure is recorded. At the end-expiratory point, detected by the flowmeter, the shutter is closed and the subject is asked to pant gently against the shutter. Since no gas enters or leaves at the mouth, the mouth pressure is equal to that in all gas-containing regions of the lung, whether adequately ventilated or not. Since the total mass of gas and its temperature are constant throughout the respiratory efforts, Boyle's law can be applied:

$$P_1V_1 = P_2V_2$$

$$P_B\text{VTG} = (P_B - \Delta P)(\text{VTG} + \Delta V)$$
$$= P_B\text{VTG} + P_B\Delta V - \Delta P_B\text{VTG} - \Delta P\Delta V$$

where P_B is barometric pressure; ΔP and ΔV are the changes in lung pressure and volume, respectively, occurring with the inspiratory effort. Since both ΔP and ΔV are relatively small, their product can be ignored. Thus:

$$\text{VTG} = \frac{P_B\Delta V}{\Delta P}$$

The value of ΔP is determined from the change in mouth pressure and ΔV is determined from the plethysmograph either by use of a very sensitive volume recorder or, usually, by determining changes in plethysmograph pressure and converting that to volume by use of a calibrating pump that induces a measured pressure change for a known volume change.

The body plethysmograph can also assess *airways resistance*. The output from plethysmograph pressure, P_{BOX}, can be plotted against either the mouth pressure or the flowmeter output, F. These alternatives can be switched automatically when the shutter is opened or closed. When the shutter is open and the subject pants, recordings are obtained of F/P_{BOX}. With the shutter closed (as when determining thoracic gas volume), we obtain P_A/P_{BOX}, where PA is alveolar (equal to mouth) pressure. By dividing these two tangents, $(P_A/P_{BOX})/(F/P_{BOX})$, we obtain P_A/F, which is airways resistance. This is often expressed as its reciprocal, airways conductance (F/P_A), or as specific conductance, which is obtained by dividing by thoracic gas volume.

TRANSFER FACTOR

The primary function of the lungs is the transfer of the respiratory gases. The transfer factor test was designed to provide

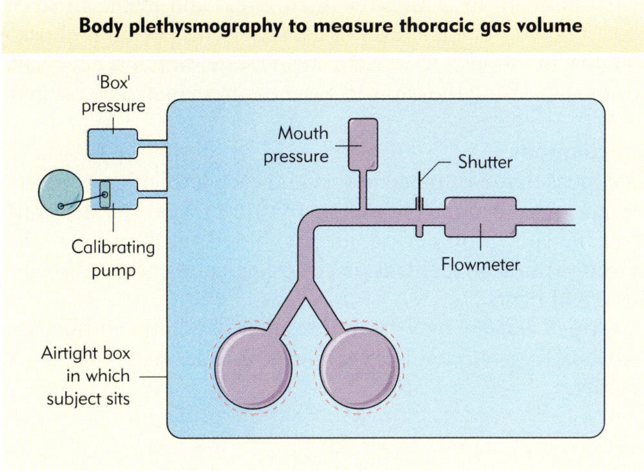

Figure 43.5 Body plethysmography to measure thoracic gas volume. This method measures the thoracic gas volume (VTG) as the total volume, whether ventilated or not. It can also be used to determine airways resistance or conductance. Alveolar volume is shown as spheres with change in inspiration shown by dashed outlines.

a noninvasive method of assessing the efficiency of this process. Carbon dioxide is much more soluble and diffusible than oxygen and the only factor that is likely to prevent its elimination is inadequate alveolar ventilation. Oxygen, however, may not cross the lung at a rate sufficient for full oxygenation of hemoglobin. Information about oxygen transfer requires arterial blood sampling and is discussed in the next section. Information on the likely efficiency of oxygen transfer can be obtained from the rate of transfer of carbon monoxide. Carbon monoxide has similar solubility and diffusibility to oxygen but the affinity of hemoglobin for carbon monoxide is over 200 times greater than that for oxygen, so even at very low concentrations carbon monoxide is readily taken up by the pulmonary capillary blood.

Measurement

Transfer factor may be determined by a steady-state method that assesses the rate of uptake of carbon monoxide by analysis of its inspiratory and end-tidal concentrations. However, more commonly used now is the single breath method. The subject takes a vital capacity breath of a gas containing a small concentration of carbon monoxide, holds it for a known period, then rapidly expires it. The rate of carbon monoxide transfer can be determined from the difference between the volumes of carbon monoxide inspired and expired and the breath-holding time.

In practice, there are a number of complications to this simple concept. To work out the amount of carbon monoxide transferred, we need to know the concentrations and volumes of the gas within the lung at the start and end of breath holding. The concentration at the start is not the same as that in the inspired gas because it is diluted by residual volume. For this reason, an inert indicator such as helium is added to the inspired gas, which would typically consist of 0.3% carbon monoxide, 15% helium, 25% oxygen, and the balance as nitrogen. This gas fills a bag within an airtight box, which has a connection to a spirometer so the spirometer can indirectly record changes in volume in the bag. The subject takes a maximal inspiration from the bag with the volume recorded by the attached spirometer.

After the breath hold (usually 10 seconds), expiration is initially to the spirometer to washout deadspace gas before a mixed alveolar sample is collected and analyzed to determine FAHe and FACO.

Helium is not taken up by the lungs and its dilution would be the same as that of the of carbon monoxide, so that carbon monoxide at the start of the breath hold is FICO(FAHe/FIHe). The alveolar volume, which in healthy subjects is equal to total lung capacity, is VI(FIHe/FAHe). The rate of transfer of carbon monoxide declines during the breath-holding period because its alveolar partial pressure decreases as it is taken up. This introduces a logarithmic function:

$$\text{Transfer factor} = \frac{f \times V\text{I} \times \text{FIHe}}{t \times \text{FeHe}} \times log_{10}\left[\frac{\text{FICO} \times \text{FAHe}}{\text{FACO} \times \text{FIHe}}\right]$$

For units of mL/min per mmHg, f is 160 and for units of mmol/min per kPa, f is 53.6.

Transfer coefficient is sometimes determined. This is simply transfer factor/total lung capacity.

Membrane diffusing capacity and *alveolar capillary volume* are believed to be the two factors determining the total diffusing capacity or transfer factor. The following equation links them:

$$\frac{1}{\text{T}} = \frac{1}{\text{L}D_m} + \frac{1}{(\theta V_c)}$$

where TL is the transfer factor of the lung, D_m is membrane diffusing capacity, V_c is pulmonary capillary volume, and θ is the reaction rate of carbon monoxide with hemoglobin, which depends on the oxygen tension. Transfer factor is determined at normal oxygen tension, then after breathing 100% oxygen and breathing in the test gases mixed with oxygen rather than oxygen and nitrogen. This procedure yields two values for transfer factor. The reaction rates θ are determined knowing the oxygen tensions during both estimates, and TL and D_m can then be solved using simultaneous equations.

Interpretation

The significance of the transfer factor can best be appreciated by considering the stages in the passage of carbon monoxide from alveoli to pulmonary capillary blood. The first and most important consideration is that the alveoli containing the gas should be adequately supplied with capillaries containing blood. Although the gas must diffuse across the alveolar–capillary membrane, this rarely is a limiting factor unless there is very severe thickening or advanced pulmonary congestion and edema. Transfer factor is, therefore, mainly dependent on the quantity of hemoglobin present in the pulmonary capillaries and on the close and even distribution of ventilated alveoli and perfused capillaries. Transfer factor would be expected to be high when pulmonary blood volume is increased, as in the supine compared with the upright posture, and during physical exercise. During pulmonary congestion, the increased blood volume in the lung may result in a very high transfer factor although in advanced disease with lung damage, the transfer factor may become low.

Low values of transfer factor are found in anemia, and correction factors may be applied. Low values are also associated with lung diseases involving pulmonary capillaries and alveoli. These include fibrosing alveolitis, in which there is uneven obstruction of both alveoli and capillaries. Multiple pulmonary microemboli usually cause only a modest reduction in transfer factor unless the degree of embolism is sufficient to cause pulmonary hypertension. Obstructive lung disease, asthma, and bronchitis are not usually associated with marked reductions in transfer factor. However, in emphysema, transfer factor is greatly reduced because of the marked destruction of pulmonary vessels and alveoli and the gross uneveness of ventilation and perfusion.

ASSESSMENT OF PULMONARY FUNCTION DURING EXERCISE

The main symptom in respiratory disease is breathlessness and, except in very severe conditions, this only becomes a problem during exercise. It is, therefore, necessary to study lung function during exercise to make an effective evaluation. Exercise tests may be carried out for several reasons. In some people, exercise may provoke bronchospasm. In the investigation of these patients, a moderately severe bout of exercise is undertaken followed by serial estimates of expiratory flow rates for up to 30 minutes afterwards. Exercise tests may also be used to evaluate a patient's exercise tolerance. For this purpose, an incremental exercise program may be used: for example, the Bruce protocol. Exercise is continued up to either exhaustion or reaching the age-related maximal heart rate. The other purpose of exercise testing is to stress the cardiorespiratory system by causing increases in pulmonary blood flow and decreases in pulmonary arterial oxygen levels. The lungs then have the problem of transfering more oxygen in a shorter time. This stress should unmask defects that may not be apparent at rest.

Procedure for exercise testing

Ideally, a motorized treadmill with controllable speed and gradient or an electrically braked cycle ergometer are used. However, it is possible to exercise using cheaper devices such as a self-powered treadmill, a mechanically braked cycle ergometer, or even a box to step on and off. A method of collecting the gas is essential. Ideally a 120L Tissot spirometer would be used, but an alternative would be a Douglas bag and a gas meter. Arterial blood gas needs to be collected both at rest and during exercise; for this it is necessary to have an arterial catheter. Analysis of arterial blood and the expired gas can be carried out using a suitable analyzer. Some laboratories may be equipped with devices that determine ventilation, expired gas concentrations, oxygen uptake, and carbon dioxide output automatically.

The exercise protocol selected depends on the purpose of the study and the ability of the patient. Initially, after insertion of the arterial catheter and allowing sufficient time for stabilization, the mouthpiece is inserted and after flushing the spirometer (or bag) with expired gas, a timed collection is made. Values obtained at rest tend to be of limited value as the presence of a mouthpiece frequently causes the patient to overbreathe or, occasionally, underbreathe. For this reason, it is useful to take a resting blood sample before inserting the mouthpiece. To assess the various aspects of respiratory function it is not always necessary for the patient to attempt maximal exercise, and much useful information can be obtained from measurements at rest, and in light and moderate exercise – these levels being selected for the particular patient. The calculations assume that the blood and the gas samples are taken at the same time. To achieve this, blood samples should be withdrawn half-way through a gas collection period. Gas collections may be taken for 2 minutes during rest and in the third or fourth minute of each level of exercise. This period is chosen to allow the subject to reach a steady state, which is necessary for the blood and the expired gas measurements to be related.

Calculations

The measurements made at rest and each level of exercise are volume of gas expired per minute ($\dot{V}\text{E}$), average respiratory rate over the collection period, arterial blood gases and pH, and mixed expired concentrations of oxygen and carbon dioxide, $\text{FE}O_2$ and $\text{FE}CO_2$.

Oxygen uptake may be determined from the difference between the volume of oxygen inspired and that expired per minute.

$$\dot{V}\text{E}O_2 = \dot{V}\text{E} \times \text{FE}O_2$$

and

$$\dot{V}\text{I}O_2 = \dot{V}\text{I} \times \text{FI}O_2$$

Inspired volume is not precisely known but may be calculated on the assumption that the volume of nitrogen (and other inert gases) remains unchanged.

$$\dot{V}\text{E}N_2 = \dot{V}\text{E}\,(1 - \text{FE}O_2 - \text{FE}CO_2)$$
$$\dot{V}\text{I}N_2 = \dot{V}\text{E}N_2$$
$$\dot{V}\text{I} = \dot{V}\text{E}N_2/0.79$$

so that

$$\dot{V}\text{I}O_2 = \dot{V}\text{E}N_2 \times 0.265 = \dot{V}\text{E}\,(1 - \text{FE}O_2 - \text{FE}CO_2)\,0.265$$

Subtracting,

$$\dot{V}O_2 = \dot{V}\text{E}\,[(1 - \text{FE}O_2 - \text{FE}CO_2)0.265 - \text{FE}O_2]$$

Note that $\dot{V}\text{E}$ is usually expressed at standard temperature and pressure, dry (STPD).

Carbon dioxide output is a more simple calculation:

$$\dot{V}\text{E}CO_2 = \dot{V}\text{E}\ \ \text{FE}CO_2$$

The *respiratory exchange ratio*, *R*, is $\dot{V}\text{E}CO_2/\dot{V}\text{E}O_2$

Alveolar–arterial oxygen tension difference ($\text{PA}O_2 - \text{Pa}O_2$) is calculated using the alveolar gas equation. The air inspired into the alveoli is saturated with water vapour at body temperature, leaving the tension of oxygen that would exist in the absence of gas exchange as $(P_B - w)\text{FI}O_2$ where $P_B - w$ is barometric pressure less water vapour pressure. As the gas equilibrates in the alveoli, some of the oxygen is replaced by carbon dioxide. This would leave the alveolar oxygen tension as the saturated inspired level minus the alveolar carbon dioxide tension if each oxygen molecule were precisely replaced by one carbon dioxide. This occurs only when $R = 1$. When R does not equal 1, it is necessary to correct for this. The full form of the alveolar gas equation is

$$\text{PA}O_2 = \text{FI}O_2(P_B - w) - \frac{\text{PA}CO_2}{R} + \frac{\text{PA}CO_2}{R} \times \text{FI}O_2(1 - R)$$

The term on the right is relatively small and is often ignored. $\text{PA}CO_2$ may be substituted by $\text{Pa}CO_2$ (partial pressure of carbon dioxide in arterial blood). The alveolar to arterial oxygen tension difference is obtained by subtracting the value of $\text{Pa}O_2$ taken at the same time as the gas collection from the value of $\text{Pa}O_2$ derived above. The alveolar tensions determined using this method assume an 'ideal' lung. Errors are likely to occur in patients with lung disease, particularly those associated with significant amounts of ventilation–perfusion unevenness (mismatch).

Wasted ventilation or *'physiologic' deadspace*, the sum of the anatomic deadspace and the alveolar deadspace (inadequately perfused alveoli), can also be determined from the data obtained in these studies. Deadspace can be defined as that portion of tidal volume which does not take part in gas exchange (i.e. no carbon dioxide is evolved). The volume of carbon dioxide evolved to each breath is assumed to come only from functioning alveoli. Thus, $V_T \times F_{ECO_2} = (T - V_D)F_{ACO_2}$, where V_T and V_D are tidal volume and deadspace volume, respectively. By rearranging this equation and using P_{ECO_2} to substitute for F_{ECO_2}, and P_{ACO_2} (or better Pa_{CO_2}) to substitute for F_{ACO_2}, the equation becomes $V_D/V_T = (Pa_{CO_2} - P_{ECO_2})/Pa_{CO_2}$. The value of V_T is determined from the minute ventilation and the respiratory frequency, and deadspace is calculated by subtracting the deadspace volume of the breathing valve and mouthpiece.

Interpretation

Severe exercise associated with lactic acidosis increases ventilation disproportionately and results in lower values for pH and Pa_{CO_2}. Otherwise, blood gases and pH should be little changed, particularly during mild and moderate exercise. Hyperventilation lowers P_{CO_2} and raises pH. If the patient was hyperventilating chronically before the study, the pH would likely have reverted to near normal by renal compensation. Until the onset of acidosis, minute ventilation normally increases linearly with the increase in $\dot{V}_{O_2}$. Oxygen uptake is approximately 4% of minute ventilation. This may vary to some extent depending on the type of exercise and tends to be less in older subjects. Nevertheless, a significant departure from this value, to less than about 3%, suggests an abnormally high minute ventilation as a consequence of either hyperventilation or an abnormally large deadspace; in the latter, alveolar ventilation would not be abnormally large and Pa_{CO_2} would not be low.

Exercise testing with arterial blood gas analysis can provide information on the evenness of ventilation and perfusion throughout the lungs (Fig. 43.6). Even in healthy subjects in the upright position, there is considerable unevenness of both ventilation and perfusion (see Chapter 44). Because of gravity, pulmonary blood flow increases from the apex to the base of the lung. Gravity also causes the lung to be stretched more at the apical part and, consequently, the compliance also increases from apex to base, with a resulting increase in basal ventilation. Nevertheless, even though both ventilation and perfusion increase from apex to base, the ventilation/perfusion ratio is highest at the apex and decreases progressively towards the base. In patients with diseases involving the alveoli and pulmonary capillaries, there is much more unevenness, with some alveoli inadequately ventilated and others inadequately perfused (Fig. 43.6). Alveoli that are ventilated and not perfused contribute to the wasted ventilation (alveolar deadspace). A pure increase in deadspace would have little effect on the blood gases because normal exchange would take place in functioning alveoli. Alveoli that are perfused but not ventilated have a completely different effect and result in venous admixture. This is effectively an intrapulmonary shunt. Shunting caused by ventilation/perfusion imbalance can be distinguished from permanent shunts, for example caused by cardiac defects, because if the patient with lung disease is given 100% oxygen to breathe the blood becomes fully saturated.

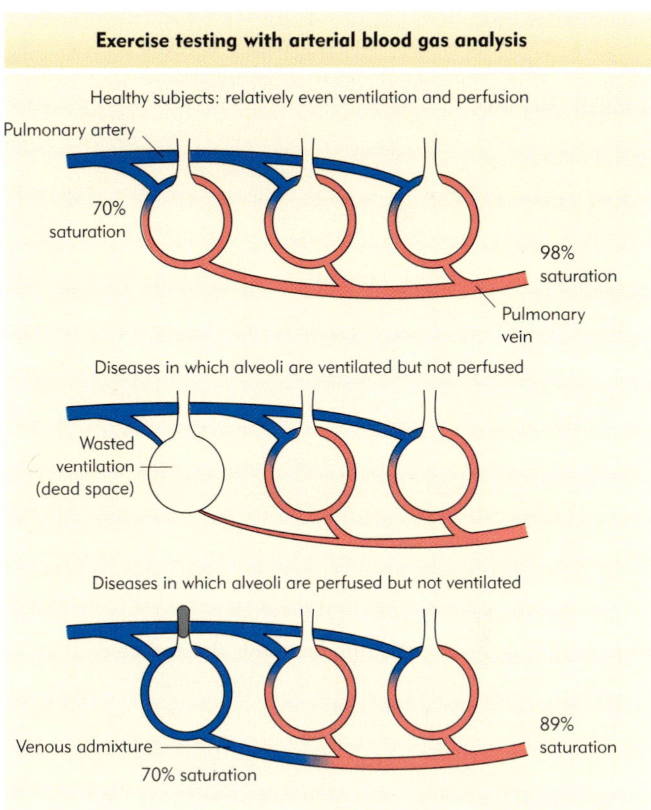

Figure 43.6 Exercise testing with arterial blood gas analysis. Even in normal individuals, there is some unevenness in ventilation and perfusion. In patients with diseases invading the alveoli or the pulmonary capillaries, there is more unevenness, with some alveoli inadequately ventilated and others inadequately perfused. The former results in wasted ventilation (deadspace), the latter in venous admixture.

Normally wasted ventilation is no more than one third of tidal volume at rest, and this proportion decreases with exercise as tidal volume increases. The alveolar–arterial oxygen difference is normally less than 2kPa (15mm/Hg). The difference results from differences in ventilation–perfusion ratios and blood entering the left atrium from the thebesian and bronchial veins.

ANATOMIC DEADSPACE AND CLOSING VOLUME

Anatomic deadspace is defined as the volume of the conducting airways, where no gas exchange takes place (Fig 43.7). *Closing volume* is the volume towards the end of a forced expiration after which some airways have effectively closed and more of the expired gas comes more from the relatively poorly ventilated regions of the lung. *Closing capacity* is the volume of gas within the lungs at the point at which airways closure begins. It is the sum of closing volume and residual volume.

These values can be determined using the technique described by Fowler, which involves a single breath of pure oxygen. The method requires a rapidly responding nitrogen meter, a recording spirometer, and an *X–Y* plotter to relate the expired nitrogen concentration to the expired volume. The procedure is for the subject to make a maximal expiration to atmosphere, then take a vital capacity inspiration of 100% oxygen.

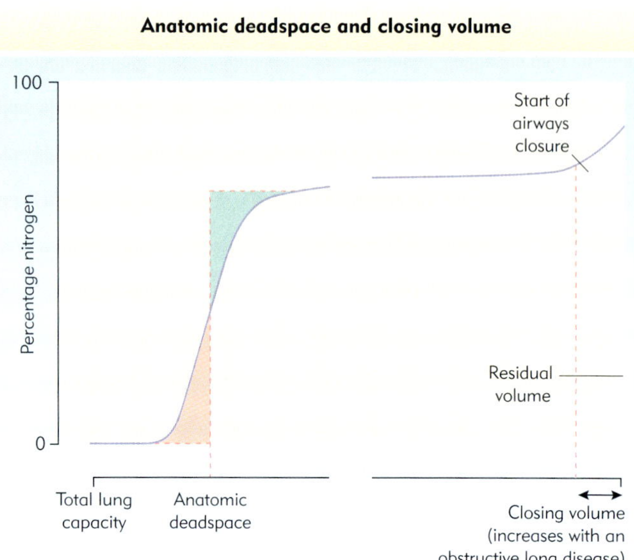

Figure 43.7 Assessment of the anatomic deadspace and closing volume. In Fowler's method, a single vital capacity inspiration of oxygen is followed by expiration into a spirometer with continual measurements of nitrogen concentration (y axis) and volume (x axis). The anatomic deadspace is estimated at the middle of the rising phase of the nitrogen curve, i.e. by equating shaded areas. Closing volume starts when nitrogen level rises again and the total volume in the lung at that time is closing capacity (closing volume + residual volume).

The subject then expires to residual volume into the spirometer during which continous recordings of nitrogen concentration and volume are made. Initially, the expired gas comes from the deadspace and is oxygen free. There is then a mixing phase; anatomic deadspace is determined by bisecting the line of mixing. As the breath continues, alveolar gas is expired; if ventilation is even, the plateau rises only slowly. A more steep rise during the plateau can be used as a measure of uneven ventilation. Towards the end of the expiration, the nitrogen concentration may show a secondary rise. This is because the airways in the more compliant regions of the lung (bases) have closed and the expirate comes from the apical part, which, because of its lower compliance, received less oxygen during the initial inspiration. The volume expired after the start of this secondary increase in nitrogen is the closing volume. It is small in young healthy subjects but increases with age and is particularly large in the presence of obstructive lung disease.

COMPLIANCE

Compliance refers to the relationship between the change in volume of the lungs, chest wall, or both, and the changes in the relevant distending pressure. *Static compliance* is the value obtained when all measurements are made at times when there is no gas flow. *Dynamic compliance* is measured by relating volume and pressure during very slow breathing(see Chapter 42). Dynamic compliance is likely to be less than the static value particularly in patients with obstructive disease, because of the increased pressure gradients required to cause gas flow. Generally, subjects with larger lungs have similar pressure changes; consequently, their compliance is likely to be greater. For this reason we usually normalize compliance by dividing it by total lung capacity. This is the *specific compliance*.

Lung compliance is a measure of the elastic forces acting on the lung and other factors impeding its expansion. It is, therefore, increased when the lung becomes stiff, as in fibrotic disease, and reduced when the fibrous and elastic tissues are destroyed, as in emphysema. It is also influenced by surface tension at the alveoli, so it is low when surfactant is depleted. Compliance is also reduced by bronchial smooth muscle contraction as well as when the pleurae are thickened. Compliance and its measurement are discussed in detail in Chapter 42.

Further Reading

Bates DV. Respiratory function in disease, 3rd edn. Philadelphia, PA: Saunders; 1989.

Cotes JE. Lung function, assessment and application in medicine, 5th edn. Oxford: Blackwell Scientific; 1993.

Forster RE, DuBois AB, Briscoe WA, Fischer AB. The lung. Chicago, IL: Year Book Publishers; 1986.

Nunn JF. Applied respiratory physiology, 4th edn. London: Butterworth, 1993.

Chapter 44 Pulmonary circulation

E Heidi Jerome

Topics covered in this chapter

Pulmonary circulation
Ventilation–perfusion matching
Pulmonary edema

The chief function of the lungs is to provide a large surface area for the exchange of oxygen and carbon dioxide between the air and blood. The pulmonary circulation is uniquely suited to this purpose. This chapter reviews the physiology of the pulmonary circulation, including microvascular dynamics, ventilation–perfusion relationships, and pulmonary edema, a common cause of ventilation–perfusion mismatching.

PULMONARY CIRCULATION

Anatomy

The right and left pulmonary arteries follow the mainstem bronchi into the lung parenchyma. Both the arteries and the bronchi then follow a branching pattern to the level of the respiratory bronchiole, about 17–23 orders or generations. The arteries give rise to arteriolar and capillary networks within the walls of alveolar ducts and alveoli (Fig. 44.1). The pulmonary venules and then veins collect blood from the capillary network and return it to the left atrium, pursuing a course separate from the arteries and bronchi.

The pulmonary arteries and arterioles have three layers: intima, media, and adventitia. The intimal layer is made up of endothelial cells and matrix. Pulmonary endothelium is of the continuous type, with tight intercellular junctions. In the small arterioles, capillaries, and small veins, which collectively make up the microcirculation, endothelial cells have very attenuated cytoplasm overlying basement membrane. The medial layer of arteries and large arterioles contains smooth muscle cells, less prominent than in systemic vessels of comparable size, sandwiched between layers of elastin and collagen. The muscular layer of the arterioles thins as the vessels decrease in size to the microvessel level, where only an occasional pericyte represents the medial layer. The pulmonary veins are rich in elastin and collagen, with minimal smooth muscle. The adventitia of all pulmonary vessels contains fibroblasts and collagen fibers.

These anatomic features allow the pulmonary circulation to receive the full cardiac output from the right ventricle at low pressures and to provide adequate exchange of oxygen and carbon dioxide within the alveolar wall. The low resistance to high-volume flow is made possible by the ability of vessels in the pulmonary circulation to distend and by the vast microvascular network. While the pulmonary arteries and arterioles comprise a surface area of about 2.5m^2, the capillary surface area is estimated at 50–150m^2.

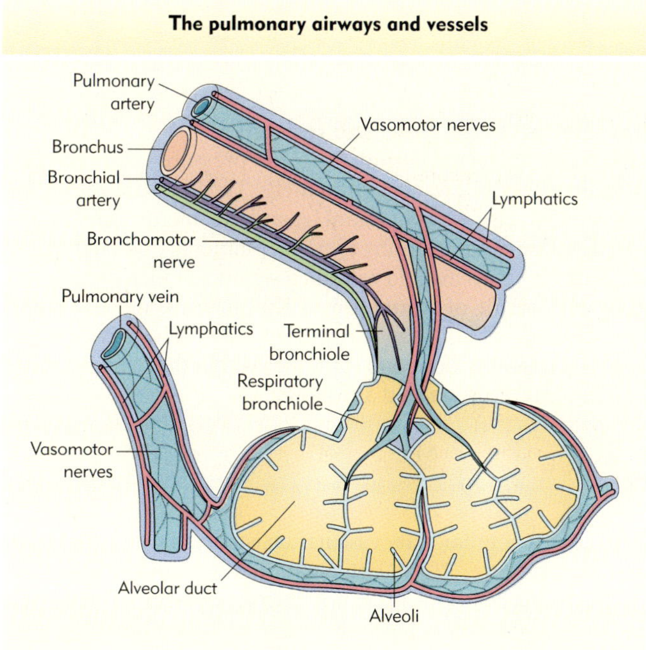

Figure 44.1 Structure of the pulmonary airways and vessels. The bronchus and pulmonary artery branch in parallel to the level of alveoli and capillaries. The pulmonary venous return pursues a separate route through the lung parenchyma. Lymphatic vessels course through the peribronchovascular connective tissue surrounding airways and vessels. The bronchial artery and its branches as well as vasomotor nerves are also contained within the connective tissue.

The venules and veins have nearly the same surface area as the arteries and arterioles. About 150mL of blood is contained in the arteries, only 80mL in the capillaries, and 250–750mL in the distensable veins. The normal capillary transit time of approximately 0.75 seconds allows for adequate exchange of oxygen and carbon dioxide. At very high pulmonary blood flow during exercise, the capillary transit time decreases and may cause a defect in oxygen diffusion across the alveolar–capillary membrane. Because carbon dioxide is a more diffusable gas, its exchange is unaffected at high blood flow.

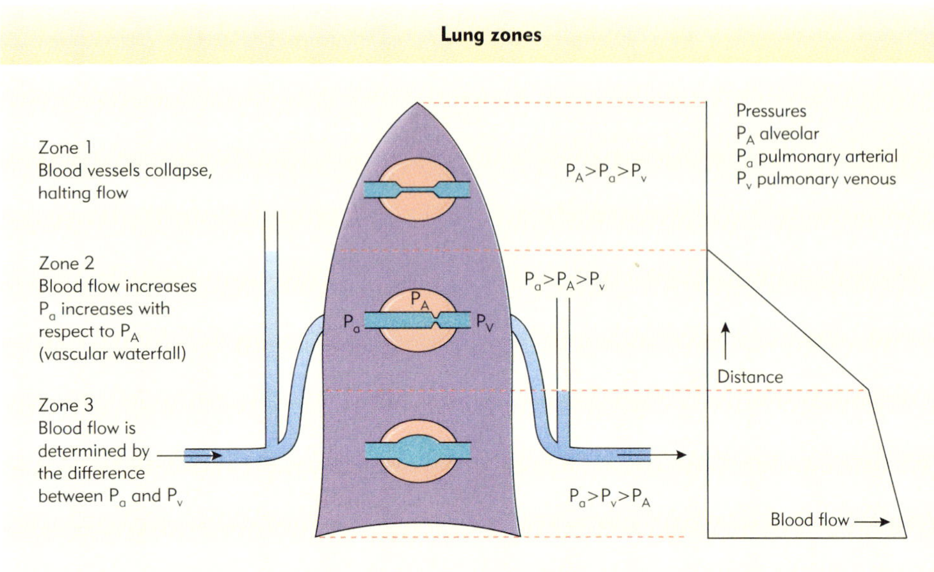

Figure 44.2 Lung zones demonstrating blood flow in relation to vascular and alveolar pressures. In zone 1, alveolar pressure exceeds vascular pressure, collapsing vessels and halting blood flow. Arterial pressure increases down the lung with respect to alveolar pressure (the vascular waterfall) (zone 2) until, in zone 3, the difference between arterial and venous pressures determines blood flow as both are greater than alveolar pressure, distending the vessels. (Adapted with permission from West, 1964.)

Vascular pressure, flow, and resistance

Beyond the neonatal period, the mean pressure within the pulmonary artery is low, about 15mmHg. The pressure within the pulmonary veins is about 5mmHg, and the microvascular pressure is intermediate. During exercise, pulmonary blood flow can increase three- to fivefold without a significant increase in pressure as a result of distention of the arteries and veins and recruitment of additional capillary beds. The relationship between pressure, flow, and resistance within the pulmonary circulation can be described as follows:

$$\text{PVR} = \frac{(\text{P}_{\text{PA}} - \text{P}_{\text{LA}})}{\dot{Q}}$$

where PVR is pulmonary vascular resistance, PPA is pulmonary arterial pressure, PLA is left atrial pressure, and $\dot{Q}$ is cardiac output. This relationship is not entirely correct because pulmonary blood flow is pulsatile and nonlaminar, blood is nonhomogenous, and the geometry of the vascular bed changes during respiration. A Starling resistor model of lung blood flow is helpful in describing the pulmonary circulation. A Starling resistor is a collapsible tube (the microvessels) passing through a rigid box (the alveolar network) with variable upstream (pulmonary arterial) and downstream (pulmonary venous) pressures.

West and colleagues used the Starling resistor model to describe three conditions of lung blood flow (Fig. 44.2). Alveolar pressure (P_A) acts as a Starling resistor to exert a resistance to flow through the collapsible pulmonary vessels. In zone 1, pressure at the pulmonary arterial end of the capillary is lower than alveolar pressure, so that blood flow cannot occur. In zone 2, arterial pressure (Pa) exceeds alveolar pressure, which is greater than venous pressure. Flow through zone 2 depends on the difference between arterial and alveolar pressures. Venous pressure (Pv) does not affect flow through zone 2; blood flow increases with vertical distance as the arterial–alveolar pressure difference increases. In zone 3, both arterial and venous pressures exceed alveolar pressure; as a result, flow is dependent on the difference between arterial and venous pressures and on distention of the microvessels within the alveolar wall. A fourth zone has been added to explain the reduction in flow in the most dependent parts of the lung as a result of increased interstitial pressure (P_i), where arterial pressure exceeds intersititial pressure which exceeds alveolar and venous pressure (Pa > P_i > P_A > Pv).

West used this model to describe the effects of gravity on pulmonary blood flow. Zone 1 represents the uppermost portion of the lung while zone 3 represents the most dependent portion of the lung. However, flow varies not only with gravity but also with resistance caused by branching and with the variable diameter and length of the pulmonary vessels. The central and dorsal portions of human lungs are best perfused, with a gradient of lower flow toward the periphery. Considerable flow heterogeneity exists even within a transverse segment of the lung; consequently, West's zones remain useful descriptors of flow for individual lung units. The additional zone in which interstitial pressures limit blood flow regardless of alveolar pressures highlights the importance of lung gas volume in determining blood flow and resistance. As lung volume increases, the larger, extra-alveolar vessels increase in diameter because they are tethered by the interstitium. At higher lung volumes, alveolar microvessels may be flattened. At low lung volumes, extra-alveolar vessels diminish in diameter while alveolar vessels increase in size. The opposing effects of lung volume on extra-alveolar and alveolar vessel size and resistance are optimally balanced at functional residual capacity (FRC).

Hypoxic pulmonary vasoconstriction

Although vasomotor tone is low in pulmonary vessels under normal conditions, hypoxia increases pulmonary vascular resistance. When hypoxia involves a circumscribed area of lung, as in regional atelectasis, edema, or one-lung ventilation, blood flow is diverted away from this segment to other, better oxygenated alveoli. This physiologic response contrasts to that in vessels elsewhere in the body, which dilate in response to hypoxia. Low oxygen tension in the alveoli and microcirculation is the stimulus for constriction of the small arterioles and venules. Although the effect can be modulated by autonomic innervation and endothelium-derived factors, neither of these are essential for the reflex. Hypoxic pulmonary vasoconstriction (HPV) is present in transplanted lungs. High pulmonary blood flow diminishes the degree of HPV. HPV is also diminished in severe lung injury, such as acute respiratory distress syndrome (ARDS), and by volatile anesthetics, in a dose-dependent fashion.

Effects of oxygen and pH

Global hypoxia, rather than regional hypoxia, causes an increase in pulmonary vascular tone throughout the lung. Therapy with supplemental oxygen counteracts this effect. The hypertensive response to hypoxia is greatest in individuals with increased smooth muscle and collagen content in the medial layers of the arteries (e.g. in normal neonates, people living at high altitudes, and in those with primary pulmonary hypertension).

Both respiratory and metabolic acidosis increase pulmonary vasomotor tone while respiratory and metabolic alkalosis decrease it. The effect is related only to pH, as hypercarbia in the presence of normal pH does not increase tone.

Autonomic control of pulmonary vessels

Pulmonary vessels have sympathetic, parasympathetic, and sensory innervation. At low resting vascular tone, α_1- and α_2-adrenoceptor stimulation results in vasoconstriction, while there is little response to β_2-adrenoceptor stimulation. At increased basal vascular tone, β_2-adrenoceptor stimulation causes vasodilatation and α-adrenoceptor stimulation causes constriction. Muscarinic cholinergic stimulation causes constriction when basal tone is low and vasodilatation when tone is high. Sympathetic and parasympathetic nerve fibers also contain vasoactive intestinal peptide (VIP) and substance P, which are vasodilators. The importance of these neurotransmitters in health and disease is unknown.

Nitric oxide and other endothelium-derived agents

Normal resting pulmonary vascular tone is low; a likely candidate for maintaining this tone is nitric oxide (NO) or related compounds. The endothelial cells lining the pulmonary vessels produce dilating and constricting substances that contribute to the control of pulmonary vascular tone. Endothelium-derived relaxant factor has been identified as NO; it dilates the pulmonary vessels and abolishes HPV. Endothelin 1 is a potent pulmonary vasoconstrictor and a vasodilator, depending on dose and age of the subject. Endothelium-derived hyperpolarizing factor, as yet unidentified, constricts the microvasculature. The complex interactions between NO and endothelin 1 (modulated by other mediators) may be the most important determinants of pulmonary vascular pressure and resistance.

In response to sheer stress or an agonist such as bradykinin, constitutive, endothelial Ca^{2+}/calmodulin-dependent nitric oxide synthase (cNOS or eNOS) forms a NO radical from L-arginine in lung endothelial cells (Fig. 44.3). NO diffuses across the cell membrane into the adjacent smooth muscle where it activates guanylyl cyclase to produce cyclic guanosine 3,5-monophosphate (cGMP) from guanosine 5-triphosphate (GTP). The cGMP interacts with cGMP-dependent protein kinase to cause a decrease in intracellular calcium ion concentration and smooth muscle relaxation. The effect is terminated by a phosphodiesterase that converts cGMP to GMP (Chapter 3).

A second, inducible and calcium-independent nitric oxide synthase (iNOS) is produced in lung smooth muscle cells and macrophages. This isoform can produce large quantities of NO compared with the endothelial cNOS. The cNOS isoform may be responsible for a steady, low rate of NO production and smooth muscle relaxation in the normal pulmonary circulation, while iNOS may produce increased NO in pathologic conditions.

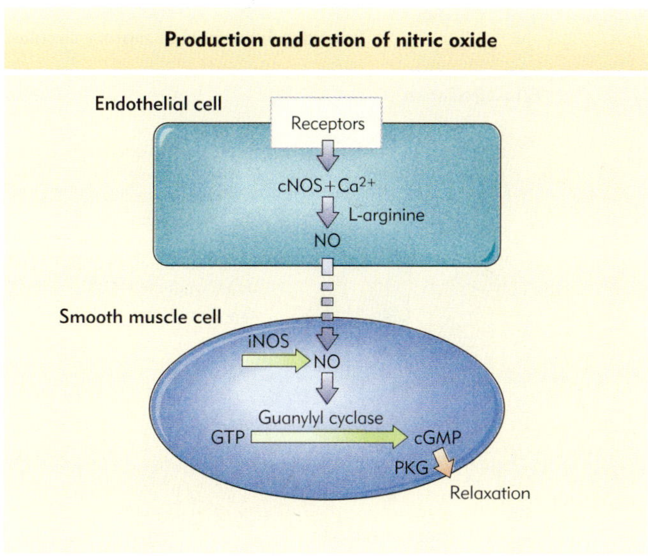

Figure 44.3 Production and action of nitric oxide. Nitric oxide causes relaxation of smooth muscle, giving vasodilatation (see text).

Acetylcholine is known to produce pulmonary vasodilation via a NO-dependent pathway. Nitroglycerin (glyceryl trinitate) and nitroprusside act as dilators in both the systemic and pulmonary circulations through chemical breakdown to NO.

Inhaled NO is used as a selective pulmonary vasodilator. With the exception of hyperoxia and alkalosis, conditions/agents that dilate the pulmonary circulation also cause systemic hypotension. Since inhaled NO is directly delivered to its site of action in pulmonary smooth muscle cells and is then rapidly inactivated by binding to heme, it is effective as a pulmonary dilator without causing systemic dilation. It has been used to treat persistent pulmonary hypertension of the newborn, primary pulmonary hypertension, and acute respiratory distress syndrome, disorders in which basal NO production may be diminished. Inhaled NO may also be useful in treating the pulmonary hypertension of lung transplantation and some types of congenital heart disease. However, the safety of NO administration has not been clearly established. NO is inactivated by binding to the heme moiety of hemoglobin, causing some degree of methemoglobinemia. The reaction of NO with oxygen produces peroxynitrite and nitrogen dioxide, which are toxic to tissues. The extent to which these metabolites are produced during NO inhalation therapy is unclear.

Endothelin 1 is a small peptide of 21 amino acid residues that is cleaved from the larger proendothelin 1 (big endothelin 1) by endothelin-converting enzyme in endothelial cells. The hemodynamic effects of endothelin 1 are mediated by at least two distinct receptors, ET_a and ET_b. The ET_a receptors are located on smooth muscle cells and mediate vasoconstriction, whereas the ET_b receptors on endothelial cells mediate both vasodilation and vasoconstriction. A second subpopulation of ET_b receptors on smooth muscle cells mediates vasoconstriction. The vasodilating effects of endothelin 1 are associated with NO release and potassium channel activation. The vasoconstricting effects are associated with phospholipase activation, hydrolysis of phosphoinositol to inositol

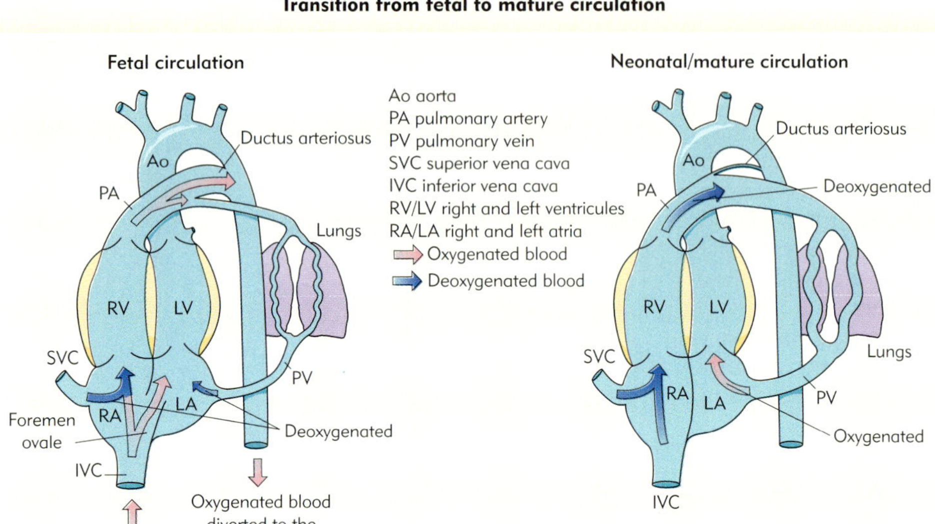

Figure 44.4 Transition from the fetal to the mature circulation. In the fetus (left), oxygenated blood from the placenta passes to the systemic circulation because of the presence of the foramen ovale and the ductus arteriosus. The high pulmonary vascular resistance in the fetus promotes efficient delivery of oxygenated blood to the systemic circulation. After the transition to a mature circulation in the neonate (right), deoxygenated blood entering the right atrium meets lower resistance in the right ventricle and pulmonary artery and so passes into the pulmonary circulation.

trisphosphate and diacylglycerol, and intracellular Ca^{2+} release. Endothelin 1 can produce sustained vasoconstriction, transient vasodilation, or a biphasic combination. In fetal and newborn pulmonary vasculature, the dominant effect is vasodilation, while in juvenile and adult vessels it is vasoconstriction. This developmental difference is probably related to receptor population densities. Interaction with platelet activating factor (PAF), bradykinin, and prostanoids may also modulate the effects of endothelin 1. In chronic pulmonary hypertension, endothelin levels are elevated. Endothelin 1 and NO appear to regulate one another through feedback loops.

The prostaglandins, thromboxane, PAF, and leukotrienes, all lipid-derived mediators, are produced by endothelial cells and other cell types in the lung. Prostaglandins E_2 and $F_{2\alpha}$ are primarily vasoconstrictors but, depending on dose and underlying vascular tone, may have dilating effects. Prostaglandin E_1 is a vasodilator that is used clinically to maintain a patent ductus arteriosus as a bridge to surgery in some children with congenital heart disease. Prostacyclin is used as a vasodilator in the treatment of primary pulmonary hypertension. Thromboxane A_2 is a potent vasoconstrictor. PAF is a proinflammatory agent with vasodilating properties at low concentration and vasoconstricting properties at higher concentrations. The leukotrienes (LTC_4, LTD_4 and LTE_4) are mainly vasoconstrictors; LTB_4 is a neutrophil chemoattractant without vasoactive properties.

Other vasoactive mediators

Bradykinin dilates the pulmonary vasculature by a NO-mediated pathway. Angiotensin I is converted to angiotensin II, a potent vasoconstrictor, by angiotensin-converting enzyme in the pulmonary vasculature. Histamine causes vasoconstriction via H_1 receptors and vasodilation via H_2 receptors. Serotonin causes vasoconstriction. The importance of these substances in maintaining normal tone is unknown but probably limited. Under pathologic conditions, these mediators as well as cytokines, coagulation factors, and oxygen radicals may be important in the perturbation of pulmonary vascular tone.

Vasomotor effects of anesthetics

Both intravenous and inhalational anesthetics may have multiple effects on the autonomic nervous system, humoral mediators, prostanoid production, and the NO pathway. On balance, intravenous anesthetics, except ketamine, do not alter pulmonary vascular tone. Ketamine increases pulmonary vascular tone and resistance in adults while leaving it unchanged in infants. Inhalational anesthetics minimally decrease pulmonary vascular tone, with the exception of nitrous oxide, which slightly increases tone.

Transition from fetal to adult circulation

In the transition from fetal to neonatal life, the pulmonary circulation goes from accepting little blood flow to accepting all of the cardiac output. Prenatally, venous return of oxygenated blood from the placenta to the right atrium is shunted away from the lungs across the foramen ovale into the left atrium, and pulmonary arterial blood is shunted across the patent ductus arteriosus into the aorta (Fig. 44.4). Extensive muscularity of pulmonary arteries in the relatively hypoxic environment of the fetus produces high pulmonary vascular resistance, and the patent foramen ovale and ductus arteriosus provide alternative routes for blood flow. In late gestation, resistance begins to decrease and at birth, with the onset of respiration, pulmonary vascular tone decreases dramatically. The foramen ovale and ductus close functionally. The process occurs rapidly, with pulmonary artery pressure decreasing from systemic levels in the fetus to 50% of systemic pressure at 3 days of life and to low adult pressures by a week of life. The medial smooth muscle of the arteries involutes and the ductus and foramen ovale usually close permanently. An increase in NO production accompanies the decrease in pulmonary vascular resistance.

In addition to increasing pulmonary blood flow at birth, the neonate must clear significant amounts of alveolar and interstitial liquid that is residual from the fetal period. This is accomplished within the first 24 hours of extrauterine life, mainly by absorption into the pulmonary circulation. Other important changes that occur early in life are the continued development of new alveoli and microvessels; this occurs mostly over the first 2 years, being complete by 8 years.

Bronchial circulation

The lungs have a second circulation, the bronchial vasculature, that arises from the systemic circulation and receives about 1% of cardiac output. The bronchial arteries (Fig. 44.1), usually two to four in number, have their origin at the aorta or, occasionally, from the intercostal arteries. At systemic pressures, they perfuse the walls of the bronchi down to respiratory bronchioles as well as the pulmonary arteries and veins, connective tissue, and pleura. Their microvascular surface area is small compared with the pulmonary circulation, but they form extensive anastomoses with the pulmonary microcirculation such that most of the bronchial arterial blood flows through alveolar capillaries and returns to the left atrium via the pulmonary veins. A small amount of bronchial venous blood returns to the right atrium via the bronchial vein and hemiazygos vein. Because the bronchial microvessels surround the airways and pulmonary vessels, they are in a unique position to cause airway and interstitial edema or to remove edema from these sites. The bronchial circulation may contribute to the pathophysiology of asthma or, because of the bronchopulmonary anastomoses, to microvascular lung injury.

VENTILATION–PERFUSION MATCHING

Since gas flow is tidal and blood flow is relatively constant, the degree of matching of these two entities throughout the lung is important in preventing hypoxia and hypercarbia. The ventilation–perfusion ratio ($\dot{V}/\dot{Q}$) describes the degree of matching. Typical resting alveolar ventilation of 4L/min and perfusion of 5L/min gives a ratio of 0.8. More important than the overall quantity is the regional matching of ventilation to perfusion.

A simplified model of gas-exchange units (Fig. 44.5) shows three possible ventilation–perfusion relationships. In the first exchange unit, which shows a situation with no ventilation of the alveolus and good perfusion of the accompanying capillary, a pulmonary shunt is present. The $\dot{V}/\dot{Q}$ is zero. This occurs when closing capacity exceeds FRC. In a well-functioning unit, ventilation of the alveolus is matched to perfusion of the capillary. A third form demonstrates good ventilation of the alveolus but absent perfusion of the capillary; this represents deadspace and has a $\dot{V}/\dot{Q}$ of infinity. Few lung units function at the extremes as complete shunt or deadspace units, but under various pathophysiologic conditions will have varying degrees of $\dot{V}/\dot{Q}$ mismatch.

Both the shunt fraction and the deadspace fraction can be determined from physiologic measurements. The shunt equation is:

$$\frac{\dot{Q}_S}{\dot{Q}_T} = \frac{(Cc'O_2 - CaO_2)}{(Cc'O_2 - C\bar{v}O_2)}$$

where $\dot{Q}_S$ is shunt blood flow; $\dot{Q}_T$ is cardiac output and $Cc'O_2$, CaO_2, and $C\bar{v}O_2$ are pulmonary capillary, systemic arterial, and mixed venous oxygen content, respectively. Capillary oxygen content is determined from the alveolar gas equation (Chapter 45). Shunt fraction is about 5% in healthy, young, upright humans. It increases with age as closing capacity exceeds FRC. Deadspace ventilation is determined as:

$$\frac{V_D}{V_T} = \frac{(P_ACO_2 - P_ECO_2)}{P_ACO_2}$$

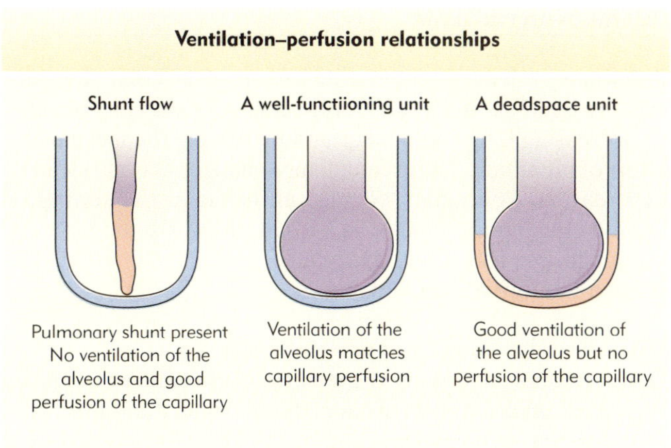

Figure 44.5 Ventilation–perfusion relationships.

where V_D is volume of the deadspace; V_T is tidal volume; P_ACO_2 is partial pressure of carbon dioxide in the alveolus, which can be approximated as $PaCO_2$; and P_ECO_2 is partial pressure of carbon dioxide in mixed expired gas. Deadspace ventilation is normally 25–30% of tidal volume.

As the pulmonary circulation is a low-pressure system, gravity has predictable effects on lung perfusion, with dependent portions of the lung receiving the greatest blood flow (see above). In healthy, spontaneously breathing, awake humans, gravity also causes the dependent portions of the lung to be slightly better ventilated. In supine and lateral positions, there is less vertical distance from top to bottom of the lung; therefore, the effect of gravity is less. However, the decrease in FRC in nonupright positions causes more lung units to be underventilated, increasing shunt. General anesthesia, with or without paralysis, further decreases FRC by relaxing intercostal muscles and the diaphragm. Endotracheal intubation decreases FRC by removing the physiologic end-expiratory pressure normally provided by glottic closure. Although the endotracheal tube decreases the anatomic deadspace by bypassing the upper airway, positive-pressure ventilation increases alveolar deadspace by preferential flow of gas to nondependent portions of the lung, worsening $\dot{V}/\dot{Q}$ mismatch. Surgery involving abdominal or thoracic cavities will further decrease FRC by increasing diaphragmatic, chest wall, or retractor pressure on the lungs. In healthy humans, $\dot{V}/\dot{Q}$ increases from 0.8 before anesthesia, to 1.3 during anesthesia with spontaneous ventilation, to 2.2 during positive-pressure ventilation, and to 3.0 with positive end-expiratory pressure (PEEP). Although PEEP decreases shunt by increasing FRC, it also decreases pulmonary blood flow, thus decreasing the mixed venous oxygen partial pressure ($P\bar{v}O_2$) and barely increasing that in the arteries (PaO_2).

In addition to these effects of anesthesia and ventilation on $\dot{V}/\dot{Q}$ matching, pathologic conditions can dramatically alter pulmonary shunt and deadspace ventilation. Pulmonary embolism of air, thrombus, or amniotic fluid (Chapter 65), or the microemboli that occur in acute respiratory distress syndrome are examples of increased deadspace ventilation. Fluid-filled or atelectatic alveoli, which occur in pulmonary edema and infant respiratory distress syndrome, respectively, are examples of increased pulmonary shunt.

PULMONARY EDEMA

Pulmonary edema in its extreme form of alveolar flooding causes a decrease in $Pa{O_2}$ not only because of shunting but also by decreasing lung compliance and increasing the mechanical effort of breathing. These compliance changes may also lead to hypercarbia. Pulmonary edema can occur in the setting of injured lung parenchyma or as a result of hydrostatic forces in normal lungs. The lungs have several protective features that prevent the formation of edema.

Microvascular liquid and protein exchange

Under normal conditions, the intact endothelial barrier allows passage of small amounts of liquid into the interstitial space surrounding the vessel. Although there is some debate concerning the exit site, it is likely to occur in the small arterioles and capillaries. Filtration occurs because the hydrostatic pressure is greater inside than outside the vessel. This filtrate contains small solutes such as sodium and chloride ions in isotonic (to blood) concentrations. However, the protein content of this liquid is low compared with blood because the endothelial barrier limits the passage of larger molecules. Albumin, a relatively small protein of 64,000Da, is present in normal interstitial liquid at a concentration approximately half that of blood. Larger protein molecules (e.g. globulins) do not significantly cross the endothelial barrier. The liquid that leaves the normal microcirculation is resorbed from the interstitium by the protein osmotic pressure gradient into the microvessels downstream, where intravascular hydrostatic pressure is lower.

The passage of water and protein out of and into the microcirculation can be described by the Starling equation:

$$J_v = L_p S(P_c - P_i) - \sigma(\pi_c - \pi_i)$$

where J_v, the filtration rate across the microvascular endothelium, depends on the surface area (S) and the hydraulic conductivity (L_p) of the endothelium. Recruitment of additional segments of the microcirculation increases the surface area available for filtration. Hydraulic conductivity of a barrier is determined by physical and chemical properties that permit passage of water through the barrier. Solutes freely follow water across the endothelium. The product of hydraulic conductivity and surface area is often referred to as the filtration coefficient (K_f). The difference in hydrostatic pressure between the capillary and the interstitium is given by ($P_c - P_i$). Normally, capillary pressure is higher than interstitial pressure, favoring outward flow of liquid, but a large volume of edema liquid in the interstitium raises interstitial hydrostatic pressure slightly, thus decreasing the value of ($P_c - P_i$) and decreasing outflow. The colloid osmotic reflection coefficient of the barrier (σ) is determined by physical properties that allow or inhibit the passage of protein across the barrier. Large pores or open cell junctions give a low reflection coefficient approaching zero, while small pores or tightly closed junctions give a high reflection coefficient approaching 1. The term ($\pi_c - \pi_i$) represents the difference in osmotic pressure between the capillary and the interstitial space. Under normal conditions π_c is higher than π_i because blood has a higher protein concentration than interstitial liquid. This tends to draw liquid back into the microvessel. However, π_i is dependent on π_c. If π_c is decreased for several hours, π_i decreases to a similar extent and the baseline difference is re-established.

Microvascular liquid exchange

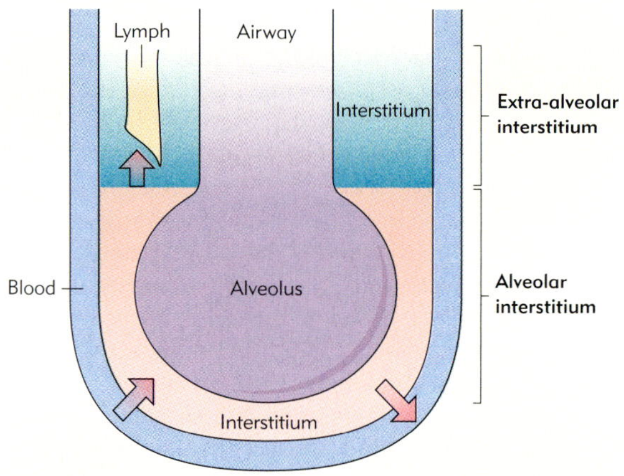

Figure 44.6 Microvascular liquid exchange. Microvascular filtrate leaves the circulation to enter the alveolar interstitium. It is resorbed downstream or cleared to the extra-alveolar interstitium, where it is removed by lymphatics.

Under normal conditions, a small amount of liquid is not resorbed into microvessels and moves from its initial perimicrovascular location in the alveolar wall to the extra-alveolar interstitium (Fig. 44.6), where it is carried away from the lung by lymphatics. Lymphatic protein concentration approximates interstitial protein concentration and, therefore, it is used in calculations of filtration. Lung lymph is returned to the blood via the thoracic duct, which empties into the venous return to the right heart.

Edema formation

The terms of the Starling equation differentiate 'hydrostatic' (which includes hypoproteinemic) edema from 'permeability' edema. In hydrostatic edema, the driving forces [($P_c - P_i$) and ($\pi_c - \pi_i$)] and the available surface area (S) for filtration are increased, favoring outflow of liquid containing little protein into the interstitium. The terms L_p and σ, which describe barrier characteristics, remain constant. In permeability edema, L_p increases and σ decreases, signifying loss of barrier properties, and protein-rich liquid flows into the interstitium.

During hydrostatic pulmonary edema when endothelial and alveolar barriers are intact, microvascular reabsorbtion and lymphatic clearance can remove most of the liquid. Excess liquid that is not removed by these mechanisms moves into the loose interstitial space surrounding bronchi and vessels (Fig. 44.7). The loose interstitium provides an important reservoir for excess liquid. Its matrix contains hyaluron, which absorbs water and keeps interstitial pressure low. The edema liquid can then be cleared by bulk flow along an interstitial pressure gradient, which favors movement away from the alveolar interstitium towards the hilum or the pleural space, where it affects gas exchange minimally. Edema liquid may also be absorbed by osmotic and hydrostatic pressure gradients into bronchial microvessels that surround the bronchi and larger vessels.

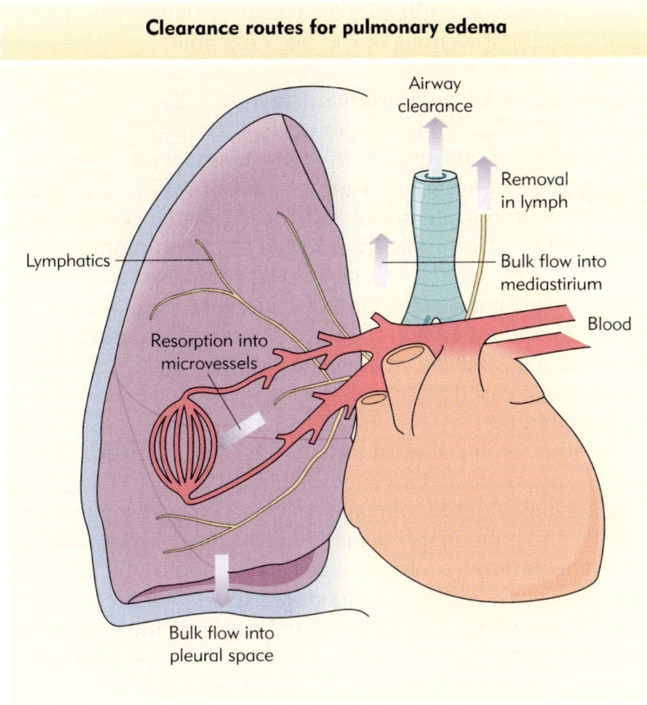

Figure 44.7 Clearance routes of pulmonary edema. The four routes include resorption into microvessels, removal by lymphatics, bulk flow into the pleural space or mediastinum, and airway clearance.

Clearance of protein-poor liquid from the interstitium occurs rapidly, over several hours.

The capacity of the interstitial space has been estimated at 7mL/kg: about 500mL in a 70kg human. This amount of pulmonary edema will be visible on a chest radiogram yet may not affect oxygenation because the alveoli are protected from entry of edema liquid. Oxygenation decreases when liquid enters alveoli and blood passing by the walls of these alveoli cannot take on oxygen (i.e. shunt occurs). The alveoli are protected by the large capacity of the interstitial space and by tight junctions between alveolar epithelial cells.

Under normal conditions, the airway epithelial barrier has very low permeability to both proteins and solutes, about ten times less than the endothelial barrier. In fact, to apply the Starling equation to the normal epithelium one must include solutes as well as proteins in calculating the effect of osmotic pressure. However, when the capacity of the lung interstitium to hold liquid is exceeded, edema liquid enters the alveoli by bulk flow, completely filling some alveoli while adjacent alveoli remain gas filled. The site of liquid entry into the alveolus is not known but may be the terminal or respiratory bronchioles. Edema liquid entering the airways has the same protein concentration as interstitial liquid, confirming bulk flow rather than filtration of liquid. The mechanism of liquid clearance from the alveoli is substantially different and requires more time than clearance from the interstitium.

The scenario of edema liquid movement just described occurs in the setting of intact endothelial (microvascular) and epithelial (alveolar) barriers. When either the endothelial or epithelial barrier becomes more permeable, some protective mechanisms cease to operate. With a low colloid osmotic reflection coefficient, there is no osmotic gradient to draw water back into the microvessels. The consequences of barrier breakdown are magnified when increased microvascular pressures, induced by mediators of lung injury, recruit additional surface area and drive an increased volume of edema liquid into the interstitium and alveoli. Lymphatic clearance, which has a finite capacity, becomes overwhelmed, and interstitial clearance to the hilum or pleural space becomes more important. A damaged epithelium allows easy passage of edema liquid, and the absorptive properties of the interstitium are less protective. Liquid can pass from interstitium to alveoli and back depending on relative pressures in the two sites. Protein-rich edema liquid from the alveolar spaces may move into the larger airways, causing visible airway edema. Oxygenation deteriorates as a result of both alveolar shunting and hypoventilation. Hypoventilation is caused by the increasing work of breathing through edematous, noncompliant lungs.

The barrier function of endothelium and epithelium depends on the tight junction or zona occludens between adjacent cells and the focal adhesions attaching cells to underlying matrix. There is increasing evidence that the function of the zona occludens and focal adhesion in endothelium is an active process involving cell surface receptors that signal protein kinases (Chapter 3). The final step in opening or closing of the zona occludens and focal adhesions is probably mediated by cytoplasmic contractile proteins. The opening of junctions appears as gap formation between cells on electron microscopy. Numerous mediators can increase endothelial cell permeability, including oxygen radicals, cytokines, leukocytes, complement, endotoxin, prostanoids, and leukotrienes. Mechanical stress on endothelial cells from very high intravascular pressures may also contribute to increased permeability. The permeability changes may be permanent, resulting in endothelial cell death, or reversible. The epithelium lining the alveoli and airways may also become leaky in response to mechanical forces, mediators, or direct injury, from acid for example. Before resolution of edema can occur, the integrity of endothelium and epithelium must be re-established.

Once airway epithelial integrity is restored, the process of alveolar clearance can occur. This involves active transport of Na^+ from the airway lumen to the ablumenal side by an ATPase pump, with passive movement of water following the Na^+. Beta-adrenergic agents speed this process. Any protein in the alveolar edema remains in the airway lumen and is concentrated as water leaves. This protein is cleared much more slowly over days, possibly by endocytosis. If the epithelium does not heal and active Na^+ transport does not take place, edema cannot be cleared. After water and electrolytes re-enter the interstitium surrounding the airways, they may be reabsorbed into intact pulmonary microvessels or into the bronchial microvasculature, which lies in the peribronchovascular interstitium. Alternatively, liquid and solutes may be cleared by bulk flow to the pleural space or mediastinum or through lymphatics, although lymphatic clearance is less important during recovery from edema than during formation.

Treatment of pulmonary edema

Because of this sequence of events in formation and recovery from hydrostatic and increased permeability edema, current therapy is directed at lowering intravascular pressures and providing positive airway distending pressures to prevent alveolar shunt and to increase movement of water out of alveoli into the interstitium. Inhaled NO may improve $\dot{V}/\dot{Q}$ mismatch by dilating microvessels in proximity to well-ventilated alveoli. Intravenous vasodilators may improve pulmonary edema by decreasing microvascular pressure or may worsen pulmonary edema by increasing microvascular surface area available for edema formation.

Positive-pressure ventilation has complex effects on edema. It may be life saving in the event of respiratory failure; however, high airway pressures damage alveolar epithelium. Pressure transmitted to the interstitium may help propel liquid through the loose bronchovascular interstitium but may also inhibit movement of liquid from the perimicrovascular sites to the extra-alveolar interstitium and may interfere with cardiac function. Several strategies have been developed to decrease barotrauma from ventilation. They include permissive hypercapnea ($Pa{CO_2}$ = 80–100mmHg), pressure-controlled ventilation, high-frequency ventilation, and extracorporeal membrane oxygenation. Total and partial liquid ventilation also decrease barotrauma to the alveoli while improving oxygen exchange.

As the cascade of mediators causing acute lung injury is elucidated, therapies will be aimed at blocking specific mediators. To date, however, antibodies to specific cytokines have proven ineffective in preventing or treating lung injury.

Classification of pulmonary edema

Clinically, the pulmonary edema associated with cardiac disease and renal failure is hydrostatic edema with low-protein liquid in the lung interstitium and alveoli. Left ventricular muscle weakness and mitral and aortic valvular disease cause increased pressure to be transmitted to the pulmonary circulation. In renal failure, volume overload and hypoproteinemia cause low-protein edema. Gastric acid aspiration, bone marrow or amniotic fluid emboli to the pulmonary circulation, reperfusion injury, and the acute respiratory distress syndrome all cause an increased permeability edema through endothelial or epithelial injury.

Another group of edema states has characteristics of both hydrostatic and increased permeability edema. This group includes high-altitude pulmonary edema, neurogenic pulmonary edema, and pulmonary edema following acute airway obstruction. The pathophysiology is unclear, but important elements include hypoxia, elevated pulmonary arterial pressure, and sympathetic discharge. The edema liquid may contain erythrocytes as well as protein.

Key References

Bhattacharya J, Gropper MA, Staub NA. Interstitial fluid pressure gradient measured by micropuncture in excised dog lung. J Appl Physiol. 1984;56:271–7.

Bindslev LG, Hedenstierna G, Santesson J, Gottlieb I, Carvallhas A. Ventilation–perfusion distribution during inhalation anaesthesia. Acta Anaesth Scand. 1981;25:360–71.

Froese AB, Bryan AC. Effects of anesthesia and paralysis on diaphragmatic mechanics in man. Anesthesiology. 1974;41:242–55.

Furchgott RF, Zawadzki JV. The obligatory role of endothelial cells in the relaxation of arterial smooth muscle by acetylcholine. Nature. 1980;288:373–6.

Hedenstierna G, Strandberg A, Brismar B, et al. Functional residual capacity, thoraco-abdominal dimensions and central blood volume during general anesthesia with muscle paralysis and mechanical ventilation. Anesthesiology. 1985;62:247–54.

Staub NA. Pathophysiology of pulmonary edema. In: Staub NA, Taylor AE, eds. Edema. New York: Raven Press; 1984:719–811.

West JB, Dollery CT, Naimark A. Distribution of blood flow in isolated lung; relation to vascular and alveolar pressures. J Appl Physiol. 1964;19:713–24.

Further Reading

Crystal RG, West JB, eds. The lung: scientific foundations. New York: Raven Press; 1991.

Matthay M, Ingbar D. Pulmonary edema. New York: Marcel Dekker; 1998.

Nunn JF. Applied respiratory physiology, 4th edn. London: Butterworth Heinemann; 1993.

Stanley TH, Sperry RJ. Anesthesia and the lung. Dordrecht: Kluwer Academic;1992.

West JB. Pulmonary pathophysicology – the essentials, 5th edn. Baltimore, MD: Williams & Wilkins; 1997.

West JB. Respiratory physiology – the essentials, 5th edn. Baltimore, MD: Williams & Wilkins; 1994.

Zapol WM, Bloch KD. Nitric oxide and the lung. New York: Marcel Dekker; 1997.

Chapter 45 Gas exchange

Mark C Bellamy and Alan Davey-Quinn

Topics covered in this chapter

Alveolar gas equation
Ventilation–perfusion relationships
Gas transfer between alveolus and capillary
Principles of oxygen transport
Carbon dioxide transport
Altitude and depth

Gas exchange and transport of gases between the lung and tissues is a two-way process: O_2 passes from the atmosphere via the lung, the blood stream, extracellular fluid, and the interstitium into cell cytoplasm and ultimately into mitochondria. Metabolism of O_2 results in production of high-energy phosphates in the cytoplasm and, predominantly, in the mitochondrion. Consumption of O_2 results in water and CO_2 production. The latter is eliminated by reversal of the route outlined for delivery of O_2 to the tissues.

There is a gradient of O_2 partial pressures between atmospheric air, alveoli, and so on, down to the mitochondrion (Fig. 45.1). The traditional term for total O_2 available to tissues passing down this cascade is 'O_2 flux', though the more common term is tissue O_2 delivery (DO_2). Many factors have an impact on tissue DO_2, and these are discussed in physiologic sequence beginning with the alveoli and finishing at the mitochondria.

ALVEOLAR GAS EQUATION

The concentration of O_2 measured in the alveoli differs from that in inspired gas. First, inspired air is warmed and humidified through the upper airway. The nasal conchae and airway mucosa are important in this process. Warming and humidification of inspired gases continues down to the alveolar level. By the time gas reaches the alveoli, water vapor has been added at its saturated vapor pressure at body temperature. This is close to 6.3kPa (1atm = 100kPa = 760mmHg) and this reduces the partial pressure of the components of inhaled gas. Alveolar O_2 is further diluted by the presence of CO_2. These processes can be described by the alveolar gas equation, which allows mathematical expression of the arterial O_2 concentration (PaO_2).

The concept of an alveolar gas equation, permitting calculation of the 'ideal' alveolar gas was first suggested by Benzinger in 1937 and later developed by Rossier (1943). The best-known formulation of the calculation is that suggested by Riley and colleagues (1946). Subsequently, a number of variants have been produced that differ in derivation and form but give similar results. Derivation of ideal alveolar (A) partial pressure of O_2 (PAO_2) is based on a set of common assumptions. First, a wide range of shunt and ventilation/perfusion ($\dot{V}/\dot{Q}$) mismatch is assumed to give rise only to small differences in $PACO_2$ of ideal alveolar gas (i.e. $PACO_2$ always closely

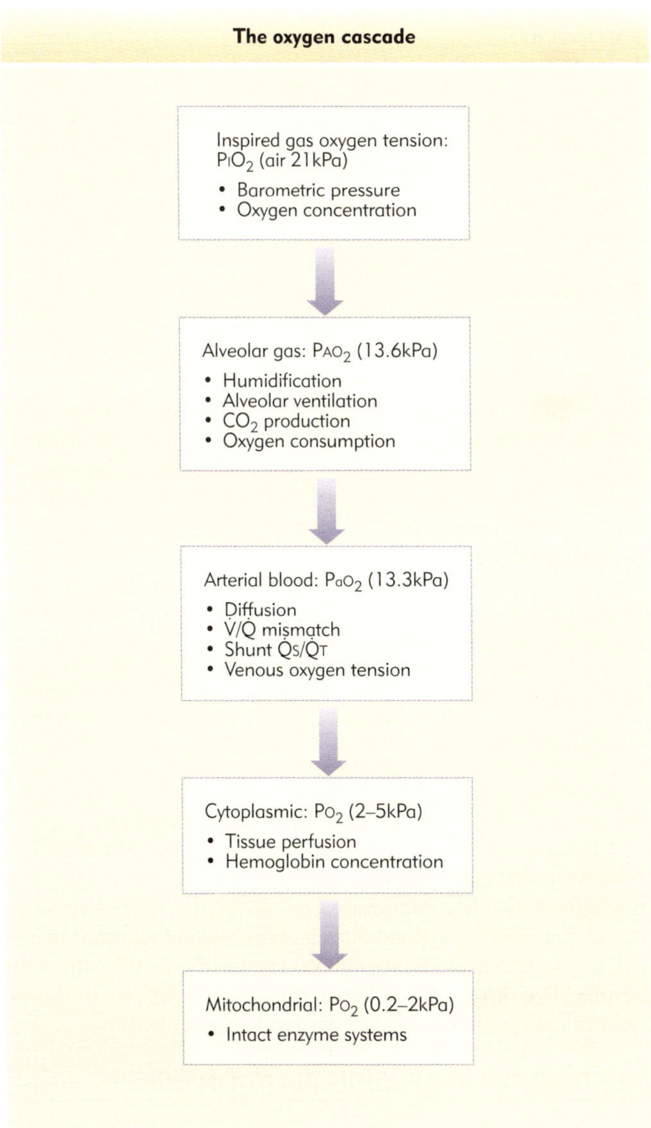

Figure 45.1 The oxygen cascade. Factors that contribute to the typical values are shown. Conversions: 21kPa at sea level = 160mmHg (1atm = 100kPa = 760mmHg).

approximates $PaCO_2$). The second assumption is that the respiratory exchange ratio (RQ) of ideal alveolar gas closely approximates that of mixed expired gas (a measurable entity). Assuming that the O_2 and CO_2 found in the alveoli replace the O_2 present in inspired gas (PIO_2), Riley's equation in its most approximate form is:

Equation 45.1

$$PAO_2 \approx PIO_2 - PaCO_2$$

This is very approximate and inaccurate for a number of reasons. First, the RQ is seldom 1: more O_2 is consumed than CO_2 produced. A second effect of the RQ is that there is a reduction in alveolar gas volume; as a result, expired volume does not equal inspired volume. As discussed above, PAO_2 is further reduced by the presence of water vapor. Benzinger's version of the equation corrects for the effect of RQ but not for the inequality of inspired and expired gas volumes:

Equation 45.2

$$PAO_2 \approx PIO_2 - \frac{PaCO_2}{RQ}$$

This version of the equation is adequate for clinical purposes but insufficiently accurate for precise physiologic estimations. Riley modified the equation to allow for the presence and inequality of exchange of gases not undergoing metabolism (for example, nitrous oxide):

Equation 45.3

$$PAO_2 \approx PIO_2 - \frac{PaCO_2}{RQ}[1 - FIO_2(1 - RQ)]$$

where FIO_2 is the inspired O_2 fraction. This equation is valid only at steady state and not during rapid changes in the concentration of O_2 or inert gases, such as occurs on induction and recovery from anesthesia, or during changes in barometric pressure, as in descent to depth or ascent to altitude.

Perhaps the best-known and most usable form of the alveolar gas equation is that proposed by Filley, MacIntosh, and Wright. Their equation makes no assumptions about inert gases and does not require calculation of the RQ:

Equation 45.4

$$PAO_2 = PIO_2 - PaCO_2\frac{(PIO_2 - P\bar{E}O_2)}{P\bar{E}CO_2}$$

Where $P\bar{E}$ is the partial pressure of mixed expired gas.

Equation 45.3 fails to take account of changes in inert gas concentration. Equation 45.4 makes no assumption about these and automatically compensates; consequently, if both versions of the equation are applied during periods of induction or recovery from nitrous oxide anesthesia they will produce different results. The difference between these results allows theoretic quantification of alveolar nitrous oxide concentration.

VENTILATION–PERFUSION RELATIONSHIPS

Oxygen tension in the alveoli is, in part, determined by alveolar ventilation. This is a function both of alveolar minute ventilation ($\dot{V}A$) and of pulmonary deadspace. Deadspace is volume within the respiratory tract that does not take part in gas exchange. It is made up of 'anatomic' and 'physiologic' deadspace. Anatomic deadspace includes areas such as the upper airway, trachea, and main bronchi – areas that are ventilated but where no gas exchange occurs. Physiologic deadspace additionally includes those areas that are anatomically capable of gas exchange and that may from time to time contribute to it, but which at the time of measurement are not actively involved in gas exchange, although they are still ventilated. Areas contributing to physiologic deadspace include lung tissue that is inadequately perfused. For example, if the vascular supply to one lung were to be completely occluded, while that lung still underwent ventilation, then the entire ventilation to that lung would contribute to the physiologic deadspace. This is an extreme case and might be seen in massive pulmonary embolus, for example. In practice, most lung tissue is normally perfused to a greater or lesser extent. However, the best-ventilated areas of lung are not necessarily the best-perfused areas. This disparity between ventilation and perfusion is known as $\dot{V}/\dot{Q}$ scatter or mismatch (Chapter 44).

The extent to which alveolar oxygenation contributes to arterial oxygenation is also related to the phenomenon of venous admixture. Venous admixture occurs because not all blood returning to the left side of the heart from the pulmonary circulation has been fully oxygenated. While the O_2 tension in the ideal alveolar capillary closely approximates that in the alveoli, venous blood returning from appropriately ventilated and perfused alveoli is diluted by nonoxygenated blood from a number of sources as it reaches the left side of the circulation. Some venous admixture results from normal anatomic flow: for example, venous return from bronchial and thebesian veins. Occasionally, venous admixture may result from abnormal anatomic variants: for example, intracardiac shunting of blood from the right to the left side of the circulation, as is seen in ventricular septal defects and the Eisenmenger syndrome. A further contribution to venous admixture results from $\dot{V}/\dot{Q}$ mismatch. Where areas of lung are well perfused but relatively poorly ventilated, there is, in effect, a right-to-left shunt of deoxygenated venous blood that dilutes the oxygenated venous return to the left heart.

Both deadspace (areas of ventilation not undergoing perfusion) and shunt (deoxygenated venous blood crossing from the right heart circulation to the left heart circulation without adequate exposure to an oxygenated alveolus) contribute to impaired gas exchange. A pure deadspace lesion can theoretically be overcome by increasing $\dot{V}A$ and thereby increasing alveolar ventilation. As can be seen from the alveolar gas equation, a pure deadspace lesion will result in hypoxemia because of accumulation of CO_2 within the alveolus. An alternative approach would be to increase the inspired O_2 concentration. By contrast, a pure shunt lesion is far less responsive to increases in inspired O_2 concentration. In the extreme case of 100% shunt, changes in inspired O_2 concentration would make no difference at all to arterial oxygenation as all the circulation would pass from the right to the left heart without exposure to oxygenated lung. In normal physiology and in most pathologic processes, although the lesion in oxygenation can be described in terms of deadspace and shunt components, the phenomenon of $\dot{V}/\dot{Q}$ mismatching more satisfactorily describes the combination of these two phenomena.

Alveolar ventilation

The anatomic deadspace results in not all inspired gas reaching the alveolus. Approximately one-third of the tidal volume (VT) remains within the upper airway trachea and bronchi and is exhaled unchanged with the next breath. The volume of gas per minute which reaches the alveoli (and is potentially able to undergo respiratory exchange) is known as the alveolar minute ventilation (normally about 5L/min). In theory, the entire volume of gas within the alveoli is available for respiratory exchange for the whole time it is present at this site. This is because of the relatively large alveolar surface area and the rapidity of diffusion of gas through the (small) alveolar volumes. Indeed, so efficient are these processes that mass movement of gas at the alveolar level hardly contributes at all to alveolar O_2 exchange. Any gas reaching terminal respiratory bronchioles rapidly diffuses, which has practical consequences. The phenomenon is thought to be important in facilitating jet ventilation. Moreover, large particulate material may be inhaled and reach small bronchioles but as it is not subject to the same diffusion processes as gas molecules, the particulate material tends to rain out in the smaller airways and does not deposit in alveoli.

During spontaneous respiration, dependent lung regions are better ventilated than the upper zones (Chapter 44). This is true, independent of patient posture. In contrast to this, where breathing occurs at an abnormally low lung volume, the distribution of ventilation is reversed. This pattern of ventilation is seen in patients with chronic obstructive pulmonary disease and in the elderly and is associated with a functional residual capacity (FRC) that is low compared with closing capacity (Chapter 42). The inequality of ventilation is further complicated by inequalities in intrapleural pressure adjacent to different lung regions. There are also regional differences in the size of alveoli. This has been confirmed experimentally using an *in situ* fixation of the lung of a dog, which demonstrated that alveoli at the apex are about four times the volume of basal alveoli. Moving down the lung, most of the change in alveolar volume is seen in the lung apex, and the volume change demonstrates an exponential rate of decline (Fig. 45.2).

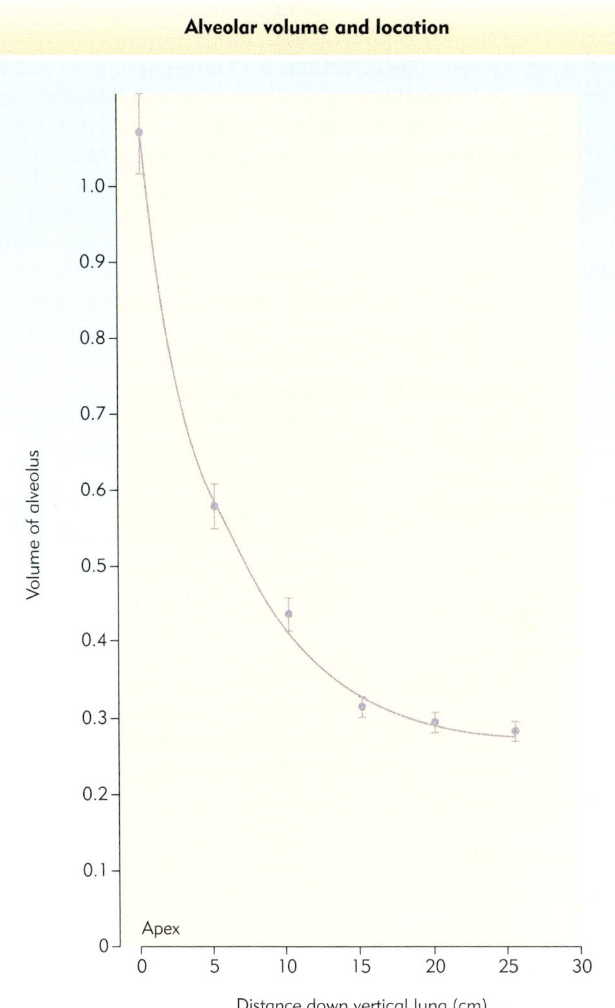

Figure 45.2 Alveolar volume according to location (apical–basal). (With permission from Feldman, 1982.)

Pulmonary blood flow

Just as there are regional inequalities in ventilation, so there are regional inequalities in perfusion. Assuming no major intracardiac shunt, almost all the cardiac output flows through the lungs; therefore pulmonary blood flow closely approximates cardiac output (5L/min). The volume of blood in the capillary bed at any moment is small compared with this (approximately 100mL). As $\dot{V}_A$ and cardiac output at rest are roughly the same, the overall (whole lung) $\dot{V}/\dot{Q}$ ratio is close to 1.

Because of gravitational effects, pulmonary blood flow is usually greater in the lung bases than at the apex. This will be subject to postural change and increases in cardiac output. For example, the elevation in cardiac output consequent on vigorous exercise results in a selectively greater increase in apical than in basal blood flow. Uneven distribution of perfusion results primarily from hydrostatic pressure differences within the lung. This is modified by lung volume; at very low lung volumes, there is a reduction in basal perfusion just as there is a reduction in basal lung ventilation until, in the extreme case, the normal basal to apical perfusion ratio is reversed.

These effects of hydrostatic pressure are greater in lung tissue than in other tissues because of the thinness and extreme delicacy of the membrane separating pulmonary capillary blood from alveolar gas. Pressures within the alveolus and arteriolar and venous systems all play an important part. West has divided the lung into three zones to explain the differential contribution of these components. By convention these are known as West's zones 1, 2, and 3 (Chapter 44).

As we move down the lung, the increase in blood flow from zone 1 to zone 3 is much greater than the increase in ventilation. This means $\dot{V}/\dot{Q}$ is high at the lung apices and low in the bases. Oxygen concentration in the alveolus (C_{AO_2}) is a function both of alveolar ventilation and the rate at which O_2 can be removed by blood flow. Therefore C_{AO_2} and hence O_2 tension in pulmonary capillary blood are a direct function of the $\dot{V}/\dot{Q}$ ratio, giving rise to regional differences in gas exchange through the lung. The calculated value of P_{AO_2} in the apex exceeds that in the base by 5kPa. The same is true of CO_2 excretion into the alveolus; there is a 1.3kPa excess P_{ACO_2} in the apex over that seen in basal alveoli.

Although the lung apex has a higher $\dot{V}/\dot{Q}$ ratio and P_{AO_2} than the base, it contributes less to total oxygenation because of its lower blood flow. This effect is further exacerbated by the sigmoid shape of the oxygen–hemoglobin dissociation curve: as hemoglobin cannot be more than 100% saturated, very high values of P_{AO_2} contribute relatively little to O_2 carriage in the blood compared with more moderate levels of P_{AO_2} (see below). The effects of $\dot{V}/\dot{Q}$ mismatching in health are further compounded by the effects of postural change and positive pressure ventilation during anesthesia. Atelectasis also contributes to $\dot{V}/\dot{Q}$ mismatching, particularly with nitrous oxide anesthesia.

Values for $\dot{V}/\dot{Q}$ ratios can be measured using the multiple inert gas technique, a research procedure that is not widely available. A slightly less precise approach, as mentioned above, is that adopted by Riley (1946), who considered the lung as three compartments: ventilated but unperfused alveoli (deadspace); perfused but unventilated alveoli (shunt); and appropriately perfused and ventilated alveoli ($\dot{V}/\dot{Q}$ ratio 1). This approach does not represent lung physiology but is a mathematical description that may be of some value clinically.

The Bohr equation

The proportion of V_T not reaching perfused alveoli and, therefore, not taking part in respiratory exchange is deadspace volume (V_{DS}):

■ Equation 45.6

$$\dot{V}_A = f(V_T - V_{DS})$$

where $\dot{V}_A$ is the alveolar minute ventilation and f is respiratory frequency. A rearrangement of the above equation yields the deadspace to tidal volume ratio V_{DS}/V_T:

■ Equation 45.7

$$\frac{V_{DS}}{V_T} = 1 - \frac{\dot{V}_A}{f V_T}$$

In other words, the ratio between $\dot{V}_A$ and the minute volume plus the V_{DS}/V_T ratio equals one. Bohr refined this concept when he produced his deadspace equation in 1891. During expiration, all eliminated CO_2 begins as alveolar CO_2 and subsequently becomes the CO_2 of mixed expired gas. Therefore, Equation 45.7 can be refined to the form:

$$\frac{V_D}{V_T} = 1 - \frac{P\bar{E}CO_2}{PaCO_2}$$

The Bohr equation describes the physiologic deadspace (the sum of the anatomic and alveolar deadspace). A preferable terminology is to refer to this as 'Bohr deadspace'.

Shunt equation

The second component of Riley's model is shunt. As described above, this is the element of blood flow that can be considered as passing from the right side of the circulation to the left heart without exposure to an oxygenation alveolus (Fig. 45.3). Again this is a mathematical concept as in reality there are degrees of $\dot{V}/\dot{Q}$ mismatching rather than areas of normal $\dot{V}/\dot{Q}$ ratio interspersed with areas of true shunt. Nevertheless, the approach may have some clinical utility. It is based on the assumption that total O_2 flux through the pulmonary circulation is the sum of capillary and shunt O_2 flux.

$$C_{CO_2}\dot{Q}_C + C\bar{v}O_2\dot{Q}_S = C_{AO_2}\dot{Q}_T$$

This can be rearranged as:

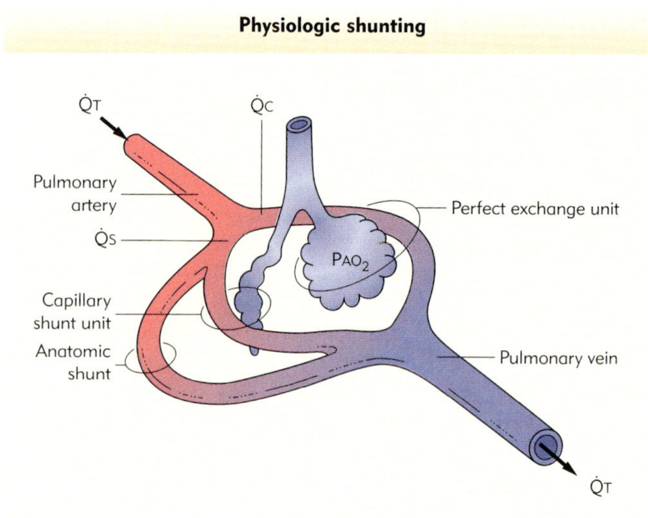

Figure 45.3 The mathematical concept of physiologic shunting. $\dot{Q}_T$ = cardiac output; $\dot{Q}_C$ = proportion of $\dot{Q}_T$ exchanging perfectly with alveolar air; $\dot{Q}_S$ = proportion of $\dot{Q}_T$ not exchanging with alveolar air; P_{AO_2} = partial pressure of O_2. (With permission from Feldman, 1982.)

■ Equation 45.8

$$\frac{\dot{Q}_S}{\dot{Q}_T} = \frac{C_{CO_2} - C_{AO_2}}{C_{CO_2} - C\bar{v}O_2}$$

where $\dot{Q}_S/\dot{Q}_T$ is the shunt fraction, C_{CO_2} is the O_2 content of ideal end capillary blood, C_{AO_2} is the O_2 content of arterial blood and $C\bar{v}O_2$ is the O_2 content of mixed venous blood. In order to use Equation 45.8 clinically, it is necessary to convert P_{AO_2} to C_{CO_2}. This calculation requires reference to the oxygen–hemoglobin dissociation curve (see below) and hemoglobin concentration. In addition, a contribution from O_2 carried in blood in physical solution has to be added.

Shunt and venous admixture can result in arterial hypoxemia; this effect is exacerbated as cardiac output falls and, consequently, whole body O_2 delivery falls. If O_2 extraction remains constant and assuming a constant metabolic rate, $C\bar{v}O_2$ is reduced. Where shunt and venous admixture are large, no matter how high the value of C_{CO_2}, the mixing of venous blood with a low and falling O_2 content will result in reduced C_{AO_2}. This effect is partly offset because a reduction in cardiac output results in a similar reduction in shunt fraction. Many investigators have observed that these two effects almost completely cancel each other, except where shunt is very large, cardiac output is very low, or where shunt is a consequence of regional pulmonary atelectasis. There is reasonable evidence that the observed reduction in shunt is a consequence of hypoxic vasoconstriction. This response is lost in severe acute lung injury; therefore, in this condition, arterial oxygenation is often dependent upon cardiac output.

A number of approaches have been proposed to link inspired O_2 concentration, shunt, and arterial oxygenation. Clearly a bedside estimation of this relationship is clinically useful. Historically, the earliest and most widely used approach was that of Nunn *et al.* (1973), who proposed the iso-shunt diagram (Fig. 45.4). An alternative approach was

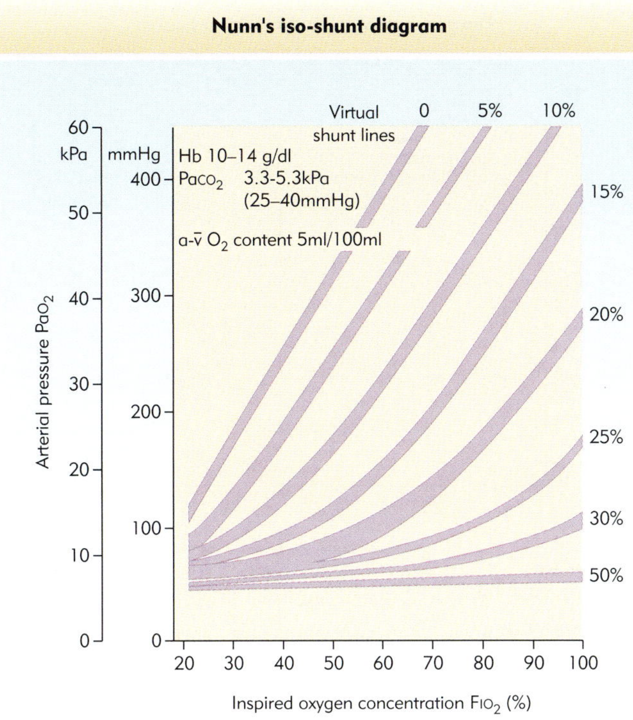

Figure 45.4 Nunn's iso-shunt diagram. The diagram allows estimation of shunt from Fio_2 and Pao_2. Once this has been ascertained, the effect of alterations in Fio_2 can be predicted. (With permission from Nunn, 1993.)

suggested by Severinghaus. To date, the most accurate has been an estimation of shunt and deadspace by an iterative computer method, based on inspired O_2 concentration and arterial O_2 saturation (Sao_2) developed by Sapsford.

GAS TRANSFER BETWEEN ALVEOLUS AND CAPILLARY

Alveolar gases pass into pulmonary capillaries by passive diffusion according to their physicochemical properties. The extent to which this process occurs for O_2 is related to pulmonary capillary transit time. Under normal circumstances, O_2 transfer falls just short of equilibrium. Therefore, pulmonary blood flow, rather than the capacity for O_2 diffusion, normally limits pulmonary capillary oxygenation. This situation may differ in the face of pathologic processes or reduced inspired O_2 concentration (for example at low barometric pressure).

Oxygen in the alveolus is separated from capillary blood by a membrane. Outside the basement membrane are collagen and elastic fibers, though these are absent where alveolus and pulmonary capillary overlap. The capillary is separated from the alveolus only by a small tissue space. A single-cell layer of endothelium with basement membrane has a thickness of 0.2μm, bringing the total thickness of the alveolar capillary membrane to 0.5μm. The mean diameter of the pulmonary capillary is around 7μm (i.e. similar to the diameter of a red blood cell). This arrangement forces red blood cells into close contact with the alveolar capillary membrane, which facilitates rapid uptake of O_2 into the cell.

The diffusing capacity for O_2 is the ratio between O_2 uptake and the alveolus-to-pulmonary capillary tension gradient driving uptake, which is difficult to quantify. In clinical practice, diffusing capacity is generally measured for carbon monoxide (CO). This is because the affinity of hemoglobin for CO is extremely high and the tension of CO in pulmonary capillary blood is, in effect, always zero. The formula for calculating diffusing capacity is thus simplified to:

■ Equation 45.9

$$\text{Diffusing capacity (CO)} = \frac{\text{CO uptake}}{P_{A}\text{CO}}$$

The elements in this equation are much more readily measured than those in the equivalent equation for O_2. A low value for CO diffusing capacity does not necessarily mean that there is thickening of the alveolar capillary membrane or impermeability (e.g. caused by fibrosis or edema formation) at this level. The lesion may be entirely functional. Furthermore, diffusing capacity may become abnormal where there is $\dot{V}/\dot{Q}$ mismatching or a short capillary transit time. A reference value for CO transfer factor at steady state varies from laboratory to laboratory but is around 113mL/min per kPa, of which the most significant component is thought to relate to diffusing capacity across the membrane. The CO transfer factor varies considerably with body size because, although the alveolar-to-capillary tension gradients are similar irrespective of body size, gas volume and alveolar capillary membrane surface area vary enormously with size. Transfer factor (diffusing capacity) is, therefore, substantially greater when lung volume is large. Likewise, advancing age results in reduction of diffusing capacity.

Interestingly, posture is also associated with changes in transfer factor. Diffusing capacity is considerably increased with supine posture. This may, at first, seem paradoxical as supine posture is associated with reduced lung volume and with increased $\dot{V}/\dot{Q}$ mismatching. One explanation is that supine posture is also associated with more uniform pulmonary blood flow and an increase in total pulmonary blood volume. This may also be associated with reduced pulmonary capillary transit time, allowing greater time to equilibrium in those capillary beds where transit time is a limiting factor. Diffusing capacity is increased with exercise (up to a plateau), which again is likely to be related to elevated cardiac output and increases both in total pulmonary blood flow and $\dot{V}_A$.

PRINCIPLES OF OXYGEN TRANSPORT

As can be seen from Fig. 45.1, there is a cascade of O_2 tensions from alveolus to mitochondrion. At this level, O_2 functions as an electron acceptor in the energy-generating processes of oxidative phosphorylation and production of ATP (see Chapter 1). High-energy phosphate bonds in ATP are the fuel source for most biochemical and enzymatic processes of the cell. The delivery of O_2 to the tissues is the product of arterial O_2 content and cardiac output. The O_2 content of arterial blood is principally related to the O_2-carrying capacity of hemoglobin, although there is an additional component from dissolved O_2. Hemoglobin is a tetramer of heme with four globin chains (two α- and two β-chains). Each hemoglobin molecule is capable of binding four molecules of O_2 to heme (Fig. 45.5). From this observation and from the molecular weight of hemoglobin (around 63,500) one can calculate that at 100% saturation

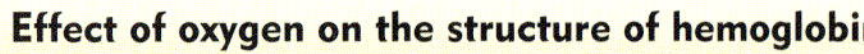

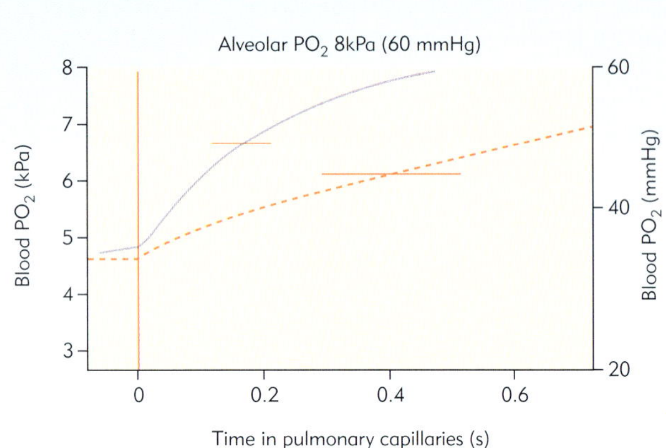

Figure 45.5 A schematic of the effect of oxygen on the structure of hemoglobin. The circles and squares symbolize two conformational states of the α- and β-globin chains of hemoglobin. The circles symbolize a low-affinity state and the squares a high-affinity state. The two states differ significantly in structure and in their subunit interactions, as well as in their O_2 affinities. The binding of one O_2 molecule to one subunit in the tetrameric protein alters the conformation of that subunit and alters subunit interactions. This strains the other subunit structures and induces them to undergo structural changes and assume the high-affinity state. This transition is responsible for the cooperative O_2-binding behavior of hemoglobin, leading to the sigmoid binding curve and cooperative O_2 binding. (With permission from Nunn, 1993.)

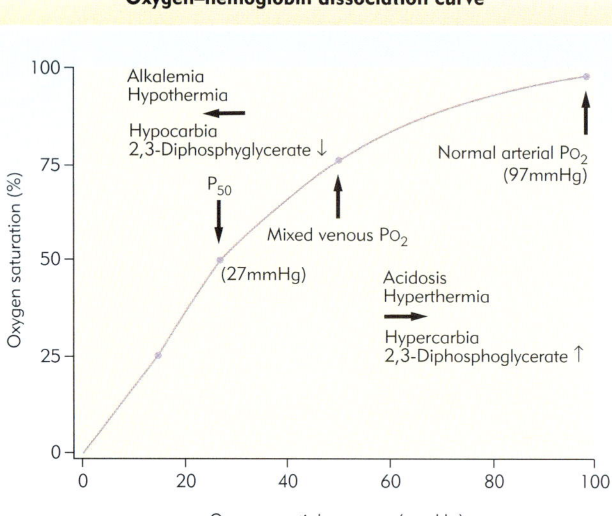

Figure 45.6 The oxygen–hemoglobin dissociation curve.

1.39mL O_2 would combine with 1g hemoglobin. The measured value is slightly less (1.34). Consequently, the bound O_2 in a given volume of blood is:

■ **Equation 45.10**

$$O_2 \text{ bound} = [Hb] \times Sao_2 \times 1.34$$

where [Hb] is hemoglobin concentration and Sao_2 is oxygen saturation. The dissolved O_2 in the same volume of blood can be calculated from Pao_2 and the solubility constant (0.025mL/kPa). Delivery of O_2 to the tissues is then given by the equation:

■ **Equation 45.11**

$$Do_2 = \{([Hb] \times 1.34 \times Sao_2) + (Pao_2 \times 0.025)\} \times Q$$

where Q is cardiac output.

When O_2 is bound to hemoglobin, the conformation of the protein changes and the globin chains slide across each other (see Fig. 45.5). When O_2 is unloaded the β-chains pull apart. This allows the glycolytic metabolite 2,3-diphosphoglycerate (2,3-DPG) to slide between them and bind, resulting in lower affinity of hemoglobin for O_2. The well-known sigmoid shape of the oxygen–hemoglobin dissociation curve results (Fig. 45.6). The partial pressure of O_2 at which hemoglobin is 50% saturated is known as P_{50}, which is normally 3.55kPa (26.6mmHg). As O_2 affinity increases, the sigmoid curve is shifted to the left; in other words P_{50} falls. Correspondingly, when O_2 affinity is reduced, the curve shifts right and P_{50} rises. The normal Po_2 (97mmHg or 13kPa) is typically associated with an O_2 saturation of 98–100%. The O_2 saturation of mixed venous blood is around 75%: approximately 25% of the O_2 delivered to tissues is used for metabolic processes and the remaining 75% is returned to the heart and lungs still in combination with hemoglobin. This corresponds to a mixed venous value ($P\bar{v}o_2$) between 40 and 50mmHg (5.3 and 6.7kPa). Typical whole body O_2 delivery is of the order of 650mL/min per m^2 and typical O_2 extraction is around 160mL/min per m^2.

The oxygen–hemoglobin dissociation curve is shifted to the right by 2,3-DPG, increasing temperature, increasing acidosis, and increasing Pco_2 (the Bohr effect). The reverse of these processes causes a corresponding left shift. The usual stimulus for O_2 to be unloaded from hemoglobin is falling tissue Po_2. The more hypoxic and acidotic a tissue bed becomes, the more O_2 carried on hemoglobin becomes available. This results in a corresponding reduction in O_2 saturation (Fig. 45.7). Conditions associated with tissue hypoxemia bring about right shifting of the curve with reduced oxygen affinity. In the lung and pulmonary capillary bed, opposite conditions pertain, which result in a left shift with increasing O_2 affinity and O_2 uptake. The capacity of P_{50} to change according to physiologic circumstance greatly enhances the ability of hemoglobin to load O_2 in the lung and unload it in (relatively) hypoxic tissues.

The sigmoid shape of the oxygen–hemoglobin dissociation curve has other important physiologic implications. Because the curve is roughly flat above a Po_2 of 80mmHg (10.6kPa), there is a relatively constant O_2 hemoglobin saturation for arterial blood across the normal physiologic range despite considerable variation in PAo_2. The steep part of the O_2 hemoglobin dissociation curve permits unloading of O_2 from hemoglobin even at relatively high Po_2 values. This favors delivery of large amounts of O_2 into the tissues by diffusion.

Fetal hemoglobin differs structurally from adult hemoglobin. The β-chains are absent and are replaced by γ-chains. The fetal oxygen–hemoglobin dissociation curve is of a similar shape to that

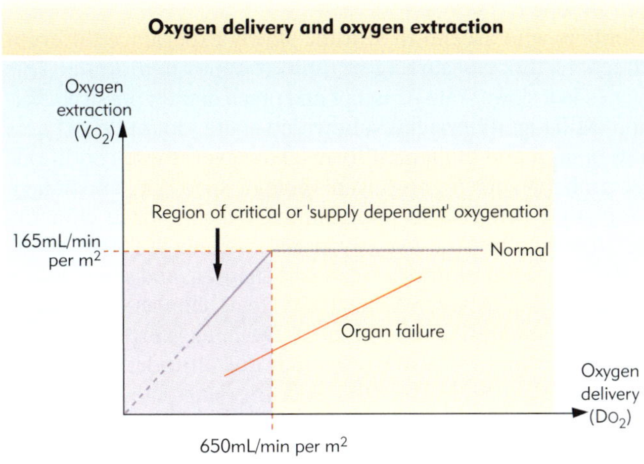

Figure 45.7 Relationship between oxygen delivery and oxygen extraction. See text for explanation.

of the adult but is shifted to the left, resulting in a P_{50} of 20mmHg. This means that fetal hemoglobin will load O_2 preferentially to adult hemoglobin, thus ensuring effective transfer of O_2 across the placenta from maternal to fetal blood. Fetal hemoglobin is rapidly replaced by adult hemoglobin during the first year of life, except in conditions such as sickle cell disease where a high concentration of fetal hemoglobin may persist for many years.

Although the majority of hemoglobin present in the adult is HbA (two α- and two β-chains), a small proportion of abnormal hemoglobin may also be present. Around 2% is represented by HbA_2, which is composed of two α- and two δ-chains.

Hemoglobin can combine with molecules other than O_2; the most important of these is CO, which has an affinity for hemoglobin around 300 times greater than that of O_2. The formation of carboxyhemoglobin (HbCO) gives rise to a functional anemia and tissue hypoxia as it is incapable of binding O_2. This is compounded by displacement of the oxygen–hemoglobin dissociation curve to the left, which further worsens tissue hypoxia by limiting the ability of hemoglobin to unload O_2. Displacement of CO from hemoglobin occurs slowly under normal clinical conditions but can be accelerated by administration of 100% O_2 or by treatment in a hyperbaric O_2 chamber. The criteria for treatment with hyperbaric O_2 include a carboxyhemoglobin concentration of >20%, neurologic dysfunction, or a history of loss of consciousness.

The iron molecules located within the heme ring are normally in the +2 oxidative state (ferrous). Oxidation of hemoglobin to the ferric (+3) oxidative state results in formation of methemoglobin, causing functional anemia because of its poor O_2-binding characteristics. A number of oxidant drugs and stresses may give rise to methemoglobinemia, including paracetamol (acetominophen) toxicity and local anesthetic toxicity, most notably with prilocaine. These result in excess production of methemoglobin, which overwhelms the erythrocyte membrane-bound enzyme methemoglobin reductase. Treatment is with either ascorbic acid or methylene blue (1mg/kg).

Oxygen delivery to the tissues is a function not only of the O_2 content of arterial blood and the physicochemical properties of hemoglobin but also of tissue blood flow. Blood flow depends on the arteriovenous pressure gradient and vascular resistance (see Chapter 38). As arterial and venous pressures are generally constant, the principal determinant of blood flow across a tissue bed is the vascular resistance of the bed. Recent evidence indicates that hemoglobin may also control blood flow by regulating vascular constriction and dilation. A major portion of nitric oxide in the blood binds to thiols of hemoglobin forming *S*-nitrosohemoglobin (SMNO-Hb), which releases NO and *S*-nitrosothiols on deoxygenation in the microcirculation, causing vasodilatation and increased blood flow.

The final stage of O_2 delivery to tissues is diffusion from capillary blood. This process is determined by the partial pressure gradient between the capillary and the cell. Oxygen utilization by tissues will increase the transcapillary O_2 tension gradient and (according to the shape of the oxygen–hemoglobin dissociation curve) the volume of O_2 unloaded to tissues. So long as the metabolic requirements of tissues are met, O_2 extraction is fairly constant, irrespective of DO_2. When DO_2 becomes flow limited, there is a linear relationship between O_2 delivery and O_2 extraction. This principle is known as flow-limited or critical O_2 delivery (see Fig. 45.6). Pathologic disturbances of this relationship may occur in shock states and multisystem organ failure. Critical or inadequate DO_2 results in anaerobic metabolism and the glycolytic pathway terminates in lactate production rather than further metabolism to the TCA cycle.

CARBON DIOXIDE TRANSPORT

As O_2 is consumed, CO_2 is produced. In general, the processes involved in CO_2 elimination are the reverse of those involved in O_2 absorption as the same principles of partial pressure gradients and gas exchange apply. Carbon dioxide is much more soluble than O_2 in water and undergoes much more rapid tissue diffusion. Most CO_2 present in blood occurs as the bicarbonate ion. Generation of free CO_2 by metabolic processes results rapidly in production of carbonic acid through the action of the catalytic enzyme carbonic anhydrase. This enzyme is present in large quantities in red blood cells. Carbon dioxide is transported in the circulation in three forms in dynamic equilibrium: the bicarbonate ion; free in physical solution; and as carbamino compounds (including those resulting from its binding to hemoglobin). As with O_2, physical solution is a relatively unimportant entity, accounting for only about 6% of total CO_2 transfer. The solubility coefficient is around 0.23mmol/L per kPa at body temperature.

Carriage as bicarbonate ion makes the greatest contribution to CO_2 transport (approximately 90%). Under the action of carbonic anhydrase, CO_2 combines with water according to the following equation (Chapter 56):

$$CO_2 + H_2O \rightleftharpoons H_2CO_3 \rightleftharpoons H^+ + HCO_3^-$$

Carbamino compounds are formed by the reversible chemical reaction between CO_2 and terminal amino groups of protein chains or side-chain amino groups of lysine. The predominant site for formation of carbamino compounds in blood is hemoglobin. Reduced hemoglobin is at least three times more capable of binding CO_2 than is oxyhemoglobin. It is also less acidic than oxyhemoglobin. This facilitates its function as a proton acceptor and in this way increases solubility and production of bicarbonate ions. These two processes facilitate uptake of CO_2 in peripheral tissues. The reverse processes occur in the lung, promoting off-loading of CO_2 (Haldane effect). Additionally, CO_2

is transported by dissociation of carbonic acid to bicarbonate and hydrogen ions within red cells. The hydrogen ions are buffered by hemoglobin and the bicarbonate diffuses out of the erythrocyte down a concentration gradient in exchange for chloride ions (the Hamburger shift). The reverse occurs in the lungs.

ALTITUDE AND DEPTH

High altitude

As altitude increases, barometric pressure falls. The concentration of atmospheric O_2 is a constant, 21%. At sea level, this represents 21kPa, but this partial pressure is reduced with increasing altitude. A second phenomenon that comes into play at high altitude is reduced PO_2 secondary to dilution with water vapor. The saturated vapor pressure at body temperature is 6.3kPa. Therefore, the PO_2 of inspired air reaching the lower airway is

Equation 45.12

$$PIO_2 = 0.21(\text{barometric pressure} - 6.3)\text{kPa}$$

Most commercial aircraft fly at an altitude of 9100m (30,000 feet) and military aircraft at much greater altitude. Such aircraft are pressurized and military aircraft use supplemental O_2. This is crucial because at 19,000m (63,000 feet), depending on weather conditions, barometric pressure is only 6.3kPa and, therefore, equals the saturated vapor pressure of water at body temperature. Hence PAO_2 and $PACO_2$ become zero. In practice, asphyxiation would occur at lower altitudes.

Fortunately for mountaineers, there is also an effect of geographical location and latitude. Barometric pressure in the Himalayas is consistently slightly higher than that predicted from altitude alone. At the summit of Mount Everest, barometric pressure has been measured at 2.5kPa greater than expected. This is crucial to the feasibility of ascents without supplemental O_2. At 9100m (30,000 feet), the PIO_2 is predicted to be 4.9kPa. Use of 100% O_2 can restore PIO_2 to the sea-level value up to approximately this height. Lower PIO_2 values will be obtained using supplemental O_2 at heights between 10,000 and 19,000m (33,000 and 63,000 feet). At 19,000m, the saturated vapor pressure of water exceeds atmospheric pressure and, therefore, body fluids (and water at body temperature) will begin to boil.

Rapid ascent to altitude from sea level, for example by an unpressurized aircraft, results in a number of physiologic and ventilatory changes: A rapid reduction in PIO_2 reduces PAO_2. The reduction in PAO_2 is offset by hyperventilation (see Equations 45.1–45.4). This response is suboptimal as the ventilatory response to hypoxia is attenuated by the resulting hypocapnia. Where altitude is sustained for some days, acclimatization begins to occur. During this process, bicarbonate shifts in cerebrospinal fluid restore ventilatory drive. Early signs of hypoxia at altitude include impairment of night vision and impairment of mental performance. This can, in the extreme form, lead to loss of consciousness. This occurs on ascending acutely to altitudes above 6000m (20,000 feet). The time between attaining altitude and loss of consciousness varies according to the altitude reached. This is important to pilots in the event of acute cabin pressure loss. The shortest time to loss of consciousness is one lung-to-brain circulation time (this is similar to the well-known arm-to-brain circulation time in anesthesia) of 15 seconds. At heights below 16,000m (50,000 feet), there is a longer interval before loss of consciousness.

Acute mountain sickness

Climbers who ascend to altitude slowly experience different effects to those occurring in rapid changes in altitude. This relates to a slower rate of ascent and much greater physical exertion. Milledge (1985) has subdivided acute mountain sickness into benign and malignant forms. However, these conditions are probably only points on a pathologic spectrum, and benign forms may progress to malignant. Unacclimatized climbers develop breathlessness or exertional dyspnea at 2000m (6600 feet). At greater altitudes, headache, nausea, and sleep disturbance develop. Above 5000m (16,000 feet), climbers experience dysphoria, amnesia, and dizziness. Dyspnea is experienced at rest. Sleep apnea is also common at this altitude. Most commonly Cheyne–Stokes breathing occurs, punctuated by periods of apnea. This greatly exacerbates hypoxia. Cheyne–Stokes breathing and sleep apnea are related to hypoxic ventilatory drive and are relatively uncommon in those who live habitually at high altitude. There may also be a genetic component to adaptation to altitude, with adaptation differing between Himalayan and South American high-altitude dwellers.

Pulmonary edema can complicate acute altitude exposure. It is more commonly seen in unacclimatized climbers than in those ascending more slowly and allowing full acclimatization; nevertheless it is idiosyncratic. The etiology has not been incontrovertibly established but likely explanations include hypoxic pulmonary vasoconstriction and acute pulmonary hypertension. Mental dysfunction may be further complicated by cerebral edema. Papilledema has been observed.

As acute mountain sickness in its malignant form is often rapidly fatal, treatment should include supplemental O_2, descent from altitude, and treatment of fluid overload (for example with acetazolamide, a carbonic anhydrase inhibitor and diuretic).

Acclimatization at altitude occurs over a period of days or months. Components of acclimatization include bicarbonate shift in the cerebrospinal fluid, which restores hypoxic drive; hemoglobin concentration rises secondary to increasing erythropoietin levels; and a left shift in the oxygen–hemoglobin dissociation curve at altitude (facilitating O_2 uptake) through changes in both pH and 2,3-DPG concentration.

High pressure and diving

Exposure to high pressure has a venerable history. Alexander the Great was lowered to the sea bed in a diving bell in 320BC. Saturation divers and one or two other groups of workers are exposed to environments where the atmospheric pressure approximates that of the sea outside their diving bell or pressure suit. Ventilatory requirements at high barometric pressures are similar to those at standard temperature and pressure provided O_2 consumption is expressed at standard temperature and pressure and minute volume at body temperature and at the barometric pressure to which the diver is exposed. Confusion is best avoided by thinking in terms of the number of molecules – or moles – O_2 consumed or CO_2 produced. These are essentially constant irrespective of depth. However, the volume that a mole of O_2 occupies at standard temperature and pressure is 22.4L whereas at 10atm it is 2.4L. The value for $CACO_2$ is given by its rate of production divided by $\dot{V}A$. Both gas volumes must be measured under the same conditions of temperature and pressure. Therefore, $CACO_2$ at 10atm is about one-tenth of sea level values (i.e. around 0.53%). Likewise, PAO_2 can be calculated from the alveolar gas equation (see above). Hence at 10atm, CIO_2 of 21% reflects a PIO_2 of 210kPa and a PAO_2 of 203kPa.

Effects of increased pressure on breathing mechanics are also significant. The effects of loss of weight that divers experience through buoyancy, together with pressure on the thoracic cage from water, significantly alter respiratory mechanics and distribution of pulmonary blood flow. Gas density increases proportionally with pressure. Therefore, at 10atm, inspired gas is 10 times as dense as it is at sea level. As can be seen from Poiseuille's formula and the Reynolds' number, this will have the effect of increasing resistance to flow while at the same time reducing the tendency to turbulent flow. The maximum breathing capacity at sea level is 200L/min, but this is reduced to 50L/min at 15atm. In practice, at barometric pressures above 6atm it is customary for divers to breathe a helium–oxygen mixture. This reduces the tendency to nitrogen narcosis and restores maximum breathing capacity because the helium has a much lower density than nitrogen (or air). Helium–oxygen mixtures can also allow lower C_{IO_2} values because these are still compatible at depth with an adequate P_{AO_2}.

Key References

Feldman S. Scientific foundations of anesthesia, 3rd edn. London: Heinemann, 1982.

Johnson AO, Page RL, Sapsford DJ, Jones JG. Flying and hypoxaemia at altitude. New method is more precise. Br Med J. 1994;308:474.

Lindberg P, Gunnarsson L, Tokics L, et al. Atelectasis and lung function in the postoperative period. Acta Anesthesiol Scand. 1992;36:546–53.

Milledge JS. Acute mountain sickness: pulmonary and cerebral oedema of high altitude. Intens Care Med. 1985;11:110.

Nunn JF, Benatar SR, Hewlett AM. The use of iso-shunt lines for control of oxygen therapy. Br J Anesth. 1973;45(7):711–8.

Riley RL, Lilienthal JL, Proemmel DD, Franke RE. On the determination of the physiologically effective pressures of oxygen and carbon dioxide in alveolar air. Am J Physiol. 1946;147:191–8.

Rossier PH, Mean H. L'insufficance pulmonaire: ses diverses formes. J Suisse Med. 1943;11:327–32.

Rothen HU, Sporre B, Engberg G, et al. Atelectasis and pulmonary shunting during induction of general anaesthesia – can they be avoided? Acta Anesthesiol Scand. 1996;40:524–9.

Sapsford DJ, Jones JG. The P_{IO_2} vs. SpO_2 diagram: a non-invasive measure of pulmonary oxygen exchange. Eur J Anesthesiol. 1995;12:375–86.

Further Reading

Nunn JF. Nunn's applied respiratory physiology, 4th edn. Oxford: Butterworth Heinemann; 1993.

Stamler JS, Jia L, Eu JP, *et al*. Blood flow regulation by *S*-nitrohemoglobin in the physiological oxygen gradient. Science. 1997;276:2034–7.

West JB. Ventilation: blood flow and gas exchange, 5th edn. Oxford: Blackwell Scientific; 1990.

Chapter 46 Regulation of respiration

John Feiner and John Severinghaus

Topics covered in this chapter

Ventilatory responses
Altitude and acclimatization
Sleep and sleep apnea
Abnormalities of chemoreceptor function

Mammalian pulmonary ventilation is driven by two types of chemoreceptor. Medullary receptors respond to changes in blood partial pressure of carbon dioxide (P_{CO_2}) (and slowly to blood pH). Peripheral carotid body chemoreceptors respond primarily to hypoxia and also to pH and P_{CO_2}. Wakefulness contributes a supratentorial drive to the medullary integrating centers, where the central and peripheral inputs are combined. During sleep, however, humans are largely dependent on chemoreceptor drive, and the absence of these systems can result in profound hypoventilation. During anesthetic care, either under sedation or general anesthesia, ventilation may also become largely determined by chemoreceptor loops. Ventilatory responses also have significant impacts on other areas of human physiology. Hypoxic drive influences performance at high altitude, and performance in underwater and competitive swimming. The course of disease processes such as chronic obstructive pulmonary disease (COPD) and respiratory failure are also affected by ventilatory drive. Ventilatory responsiveness may be an important factor determining the way patients respond to anesthetic drugs.

Anesthesiologists are in a unique position to observe the functioning of the ventilatory control system. We alter ventilatory responses with anesthetics and analgesics then observe and measure these effects directly with pulse oximetry, end-tidal gas monitoring, or blood gas analysis. Anesthesiologists developed an early interest in these ventilatory control systems and contributed much research into this area of physiology. This chapter will focus on human ventilatory control by O_2, CO_2, and H^+. The impact of anesthetic and other drugs used in surgery and intensive care is covered in Chapter 47.

VENTILATORY RESPONSES

Ventilatory responses arise from many sources. The most important are the central and peripheral chemoreceptors. Many other receptors provide input to ventilation, such as airways receptors and intrapulmonary receptors. Most commonly, investigators study the ventilatory response to CO_2 at high arterial partial pressure of O_2 (Pa_{O_2}) (hypercapnic ventilatory response, HCVR), the hypoxic ventilatory response (HVR), and their synergistic (multiplicative) interaction. Other investigators emphasize the separation between the faster peripheral chemoreceptors and the slower central response. The reason for the latter distinction is that HCVR has both central and peripheral components, although studies are usually designed to measure the central chemoreceptor response. The HVR is designed to measure the peripheral chemoreceptor response; however, it may include a component of central response to a depressant effect of hypoxia.

Hypercapnic ventilatory response

When we are awake, P_{CO_2} is closely regulated to near 40mmHg (5.3kPa) by the medullary respiratory center. Exercise increases alveolar ventilation ($\dot{V}_A$, L/min) in proportion to whole body CO_2 production ($\dot{V}_{CO_2}$, L/min), keeping the fraction of CO_2 in expired alveolar air constant: $F_{ECO_2} = \dot{V}_{CO_2}/\dot{V}_A$ or approximately 0.05 [= (200mL/min)/(4000mL/min)]. In anesthesia, $\dot{V}_A$ is often altered without change of CO_2 production, resulting in reciprocal changes of P_{CO_2}. This proportionality we commonly express (omitting factors such as barometric pressure) as:

$$\dot{V}_{CO_2} \approx \dot{V}_A \times P_{CO_2}$$

Central chemoreceptors

While breathing air at sea level, about two-thirds of the ventilatory response to CO_2 arises from stimulus of superficial chemosensitive neurons located near the ventral surface of the medulla, and the rest from the effect of P_{CO_2} (via pH) on the carotid bodies. Even when breathing O_2, small amounts of peripheral stimulation can still be detected. The central chemoreceptors respond primarily to the pH of the extracellular fluid (ECF), which varies (within 1–2 minutes) with arterial P_{CO_2} (Pa_{CO_2}). Cerebrospinal fluid (CSF) and ECF are slowly altered (hours to days) either by primary metabolic acidosis/alkalosis or in compensation for abnormal Pa_{CO_2}, as in COPD hypoventilation or in hypoxic hyperventilation (e.g. altitude). These ECF HCO_3^- changes differ in both timing and magnitude from the blood changes and impact ventilatory control in ways that can be understood only when the HCO_3^- levels of the ECF are determined.

The relationship between Pa_{CO_2} and $\dot{V}_A$ depends on the level of CO_2 studied. When we are awake, reduction of Pa_{CO_2} may not reduce $\dot{V}_A$ and small rises of Pa_{CO_2} may result in little increase in $\dot{V}_A$ because of a 'wakeful drive' partly arising from visual input. This 'flat' portion is referred to as the 'dog leg' of the CO_2 response curve (Fig. 46.1). As CO_2 increases (about 2–3mmHg above normal), the relationship between Pa_{CO_2} and minute ventilation ($\dot{V}_E$) becomes linear, defining HCVR as the slope ($\dot{V}_E/Pa_{CO_2}$). At extremely high CO_2 levels (≥100mmHg), the response flattens as the maximum $\dot{V}_E$ is approached. In addition, in extreme hypercapnia, CO_2 'narcosis' may alter ventilatory responsiveness. Normal HCVR varies widely, from 1 to 4L/min per mmHg even when normalized for body size.

In sleeping or anesthetized normoxic or hyperoxic subjects, if Pa_{CO_2} is reduced about 5mmHg below the resting value, ventilation ceases. This Pa_{CO_2} value is known as the 'apneic threshold'. Hypoxia can drive ventilation to lower Pa_{CO_2}. The HCVR slope is increased by hypoxia, typically being doubled at an arterial blood saturation with O_2 (Sa_{O_2}) of 75% (Fig. 46.1), as the input from carotid bodies interacts in the medulla with stimuli originating in the central CO_2 receptors.

Normal sleep slightly reduces the slope of the CO_2 response but also shifts its position (defined as the intercept on the *x* axis) to a slightly higher Pa_{CO_2} (1–4mmHg). Most anesthetic agents reduce the slope in proportion to the depth of anesthesia and also raise the intercept.

Modification of central chemoreceptor signals

The zero-ventilation intercept of the CO_2-response curve (and, therefore, the apneic threshold) varies with changes in metabolic acid–base status of blood; it also changes slowly as this alters CSF HCO_3^- levels. As acidosis stimulates breathing, the CO_2-response line shifts leftward, reducing the intercept. At lower values of Pa_{CO_2}, changes in P_{CO_2} cause a larger pH fall (because of the log relationship of pH to P_{CO_2}); as a result, HCVR rises by $40/Pa_{CO_2}$ each 1mmHg rise of Pa_{CO_2}. Much of the interest in chemoreceptor physiology in anesthesia arises from the substantial changes in ventilatory responses caused by anesthetics, sedative hypnotics, and opioids (Chapter 47). What little evidence exists suggests that all these agents depress the integrated respiratory center responses rather than the chemoreceptor sensitivities. For example, morphine does not block the activation by high Pa_{CO_2} of the ventral medullary chemoreceptor cells (as shown by a c-*fos* expression method).

Dynamic changes

The central chemoreceptor responses are significantly slower than the carotid body responses. Although the circulatory delay from the lung to the brainstem is on the order of a few seconds, the 'washin' of a step rise of alveolar P_{CO_2} (P_{ACO_2}) into brain tissue is exponential, with a time constant of 1–2 minutes. The CO_2 response will then begin, but it takes a substantial amount of time for the $\dot{V}_E$ to reach its final steady-state value. Figure 46.2 shows the change of $\dot{V}_E$ with time following a step increase in end-tidal P_{CO_2} (P_{ETCO_2}) from 40 to 55mmHg. If this occurs at 21% O_2, both central and peripheral chemoreceptor components are present. At a high fraction of inspired O_2 (F_{IO_2}) (not shown), the response is monoexponential, disclosing both the magnitude (gain) of the central chemoreceptor response and the speed of the response.

Measurement

Two main techniques are used to measure HCVR. The most common technique is the Read rebreathing method. This involves rebreathing for approximately 6–8 minutes from a 5–7L bag containing initially a mixture of 7% CO_2 in O_2; P_{CO_2} immediately jumps to approximately the mixed venous level and then rises at about 2–4 mmHg/min. The value of P_{ETCO_2} is plotted against $\dot{V}_E$, and the slope is then determined by least-squares regression over the linear portion of the plot (see Fig. 46.1). This method cannot be used to determine the intercept. The steady-state technique employs a step increase in P_{ETCO_2}, which is then held constant at the chosen level until steady-state $\dot{V}_E$ is reached, as shown in Figure 46.2. This usually requires about 6 minutes, which is roughly three time constants. Inspired CO_2 must be increased abruptly to produce this step change and must be continuously adjusted to maintain P_{ETCO_2} constant while $\dot{V}_E$ increases. HCVR is the (5–10 minutes) steady-state ratio of change in $\dot{V}_E$ versus change in P_{CO_2}. HCVR should be similar with the two methods.

The rise in P_{ETCO_2} or Pa_{CO_2} produced by anesthetics and adjuvant drugs is a qualitative way to demonstrate ventilatory depression. There are two better techniques that have been used. In the first, P_{CO_2} is elevated to a constant level before drug administration and the fall of ventilation produced by the drug is measured. In the second, the P_{CO_2} needed to drive ventilation to some constant increased value such as 15L/min is determined; the drug effect is measured as the rise in P_{CO_2} at this ventilation.

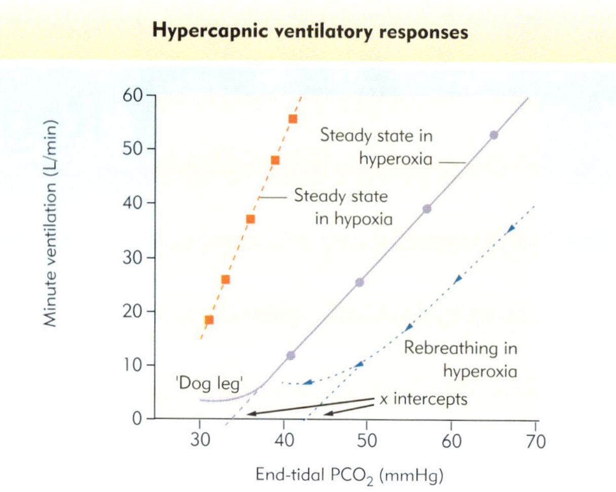

Figure 46.1 Hypercapnic ventilatory responses. Simulation of the relationship between end-tidal partial pressure of CO_2 (P_{ETCO_2}) and minute ventilation ($\dot{V}_E$) under different conditions. Ventilation does not continue to fall as P_{ETCO_2} is lowered in awake subjects because of a wakeful drive to breath; this gives rise to the 'dog leg'. In hypoxia [oxygen saturation (Sa_{O_2}) 75%], the steeper slope (approximately double) is caused by peripheral chemoreceptor stimulation. The CO_2 response obtained from rebreathing in hyperoxia has essentially the same slope as that obtained in the steady-state technique; however, the curve is shifted to the right because of the slow time constant of the central chemoreceptors, which yields a different x intercept, the expected 'apneic' threshold. The slope ($\Delta\dot{V}_E/\Delta P_{ETCO_2}$) is determined from regression in the linear portion of the curve, as shown by the extrapolated line.

Hypoxic ventilatory responses

The HVR is the slope of the increase of $\dot{V}_E$ plotted against the decrease of Sa_{O_2} ($\dot{V}_E/Sa_{O_2}$). Moderate steady hypoxia (e.g. Sa_{O_2} 70–90%) has a dual effect on breathing, stimulating ventilation via the carotid bodies within seconds (HVR); however, after

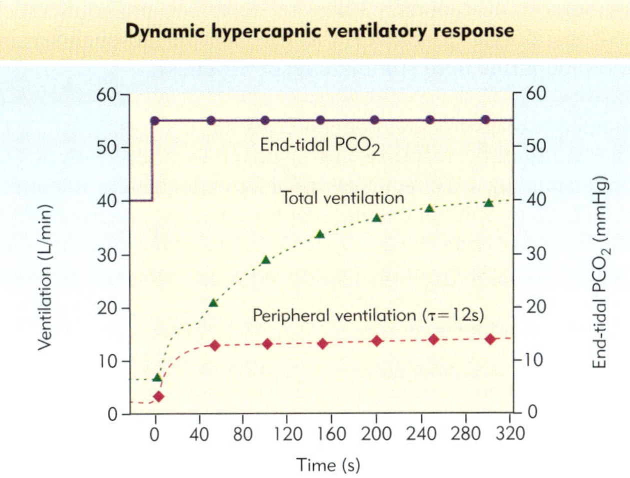

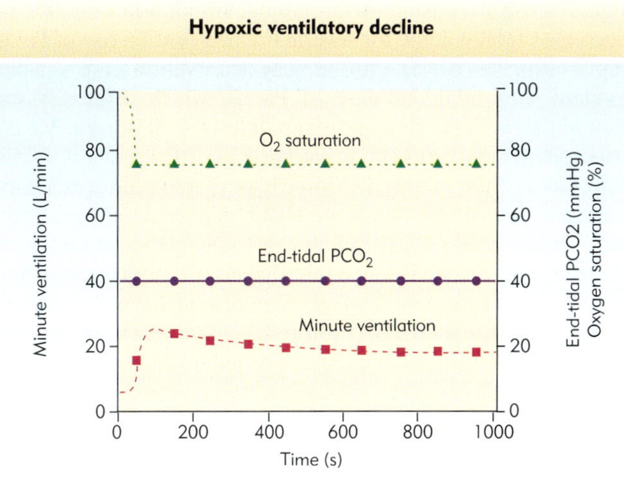

Figure 46.2 Dynamic hypercapnic ventilatory response. In the control period of this simulated response, end-tidal partial pressure of CO_2 (P_{ETCO_2}) was raised slightly above resting to ensure that ventilation was above the 'dog leg' (see Fig. 46.1). It was then abruptly raised to 55mmHg by addition of inspired CO_2. When tested during normoxia, the rise in minute ventilation with a step increase in P_{ETCO_2} has a small rapid component (~12-second time constant) arising in peripheral chemoreceptors (estimated by the dotted line) followed by a slightly delayed slow rise (~2-minute time constant, delay exaggerated here) as P_{CO_2} in the medullary chemoreceptors rises to a new equilibrium above arterial P_{CO_2} (P_aCO_2). Peripheral chemoreceptor stimulation is responsible for approximately one third of the total steady-state response, the slope of which is defined as the change in minute ventilation ($\Delta\dot{V}_E/\Delta P_{ETCO_2}$ (2.0L/min per mmHg in this example).

Figure 46.3 Hypoxic ventilatory decline (HVD). The development of HVD is shown in prolonged hypoxic exposure. After about 5 minutes of step hypoxia, HVD slowly eliminates about half of the hypoxic increase of ventilation. HVD is still poorly understood but is of medullary, not peripheral, chemoreceptor origin. The HVD decrement is variable, eliminating all of the hypoxic response in some individuals.

about 5 minutes, this initial response decays even at constant P_{aCO_2}, and after 20–30 minutes only about half the incremental ventilation persists (Fig. 46.3). This decay, believed to be a consequence of CNS hypoxia, is called hypoxic ventilatory decline (HVD). The absolute decrease in ventilation from peak values is proportional to HVR, the initial response slope. The decline, expressed as a percentage of peak ventilation, is relatively consistent. Little or no decline or depression occurs in subjects with blunted HVR (see below) or in animals after peripheral chemoreceptor denervation. HVD appears to inhibit incoming peripheral drive.

The mechanism of HVD is complex and may be multifactorial. HVD occurs in mild hypoxia without any detectable effect on mental function in normal subjects, precluding any role for ATP production failure. However, in peripherally denervated animals, ventilation is truly depressed by severe hypoxia, especially under anesthesia. At the onset of hypoxia, pH on the central chemoreceptor surface initially rises as a result of increased cerebral blood flow caused by hypoxia, but this is quickly followed by falling pH owing to local lactic acid generation. Increased cerebral blood flow caused by hypoxia reduces the difference between tissue and arterial P_{CO_2}, lowering the P_{CO_2} at the central chemoreceptors. This may explain a portion of HVD but is not sufficient alone. HVD can be nearly eliminated by minimizing hypoxic brain lactic acid generation in both volunteers and animals using the drug dichloroacetate. This acidification seems to be narrowly confined to a region near the location of the central chemoreceptors. A paradox is that acidification is usually associated with stimulated ventilation, whereas in HVD it occurs in the context of ventilatory decrease. One possible theory is that ventilatory reduction occurs if intracellular acidosis exceeds extracellular acidosis; during ventilation stimulated with CO_2, extracellular acidosis is greater than intracellular because intracellular proteins buffer the rising P_{CO_2}. Without knowing both intra- and extracellular acid–base balance, an incomplete picture may be formed, creating an apparent paradox.

Several neurotransmitters and neuromodulators are known to depress ventilation. Endorphins seem a likely source of ventilatory decline; however, naloxone does not modify HVD in adult humans and has only a small inconsistent effect in neonates. Adenosine likely plays some role in the process, since aminophylline partially blocks HVD in humans. Methylxanthines have been used clinically to prevent neonatal apneic episodes, further suggesting an important link between adenosine, HVD, and clinical ventilatory response mechanisms. HVD can also be reduced with γ-aminobutyric acid (GABA) antagonists.

In neonates, both animal and human, HVD is prominent and hypoxia may cause apnea, especially before substantial carotid body response has developed. Understanding the potential of hypoxia to cause ventilatory depression is important in pathophysiology. Anesthetic agents may block HVR and even enhance HVD, contributing further to the depressant effects of hypoxia.

Hypoxia and peripheral chemoreceptors

The carotid bodies are located at the bifurcation of the carotid artery and are entirely responsible for hypoxic ventilatory stimulation in humans. They contain special cells with a very high metabolic rate that are in contact with nerve endings and are supplied with very high blood flow. The peripheral chemoreceptors have significant tone during air breathing. Inhalation of 100% O_2 decreases tidal volume for several breaths (until a rise of $Pa{CO_2}$ replaces the lost drive). Carotid body denervation leads to a permanent ~6mmHg increase of $Pa{CO_2}$, which originally was thought to indicate that approximately 15% of normal $\dot{V}E$ is a consequence of carotid body discharge. Further analysis, taking into account the fact that chronic hypercapnia induces a compensatory rise of CSF and blood HCO_3^- sufficient only to restore CSF and arterial pH about half way to normal, now interprets this observation as evidence that the carotid bodies contribute about 30% of total ventilatory drive in resting normoxic humans.

The chemosensitivity of peripheral chemoreceptors is slowly modulated by chronic hypoxia. A few days to weeks at about 4000m altitude causes a doubling of HVR through unexplained upregulation of responsiveness within the carotid bodies. Longer hypoxia eventually leads to enlargement of carotid bodies (see below).

The carotid bodies are innervated by the carotid sinus nerve, a branch of the glossopharyngeal nerve. Efferent sympathetic and parasympathetic nerves modify chemoreceptor responses by direct effects and by changes in vascular tone, which controls flow through the sinusoids. The carotid sinus nerve also transmits baroreceptor information.

The main functional cell in the carotid body is the type I or glomus cell, which contains many mitochondria, catecholamines, and inhibitory and excitatory neurotransmitters [including dopamine, norepinephrine (noradrenaline), acetylcholine, serotonin, substance P, etc.]. Carotid bodies are characterized by high O_2 consumption and very high blood flow, yielding an unusually small difference between arterial and venous $P{O_2}$. Anemia does not affect carotid body discharge, nor does carbon monoxide. These organs, therefore, 'sense' arterial not tissue $P{O_2}$ and do not sense arterial O_2 content or saturation. The relationship of nerve output rate to $P{O_2}$ is hyperbolic, approaching an asymptote of maximum stimulus at about 30mmHg. This results in the approximately linear relationship of neural output to blood O_2 desaturation rather than to $Pa{O_2}$. The mechanism of detection of hypoxia is very complex, probably involving alteration of oxygen-sensitive K^+ channels. But the high O_2 consumption suggests that a diffusion limitation between blood and the detection mechanism in the type I cells is involved. Hypercapnia and increased H^+ are also important stimuli of the peripheral chemoreceptors. Unlike the central chemoreceptors, the peripheral receptors are immediately accessible to metabolically derived H^+ and are affected by changes in this parameter.

Modification of peripheral chemoreceptor signals

Alteration of the ventilatory response to peripheral chemoreceptor signals may occur in the integrating centers (both medullary and supramedullary). For example, the state of arousal, metabolic rate, and exercise have all been shown to have profound effects on HVR. Long-term hypoxia is thought to downregulate or 'blunt' the central response to incoming stimuli (see below). Most drugs that alter hypoxic responses do so mainly at the integrating centers. An exception is the effect of nondepolarizing muscle relaxants, which have been found to depress carotid chemoreceptor hypoxic sensitivity in proportion to their blockade of neuromuscular transmission.

Catecholamines are important modulators of the carotid body. Dopamine, which is secreted by the glomus cell, inhibits carotid body responses. Exogenously administered dopamine at clinical doses causes significant inhibition of peripheral chemoreceptor responses. Likewise, dopamine antagonists such as droperidol can augment HVR. Epinephrine (adrenaline) and norepinephrine both stimulate responsiveness.

Interaction of central and peripheral inputs

The ventilatory response to hypoxia is altered by CO_2. Understanding this effect is essential for understanding the function of the peripheral chemoreceptors. The interaction of CO_2 with hypoxia occurs in a multiplicative not additive manner. This means that the slope of the hypoxic response is steeper at higher levels of CO_2 and is not simply shifted upward and parallel, which would be an additive response. Conversely, hypoxia increases the slope of the CO_2-response curve in hypoxia (see Fig. 46.1). Most of this interaction resides within the peripheral chemoreceptors. It is possible that central CO_2 responses also interact with peripheral chemoreceptor responses; however, most results indicate that the central hypercapnic response simply adds to the peripheral response. This interaction makes asphyxia the most potent stimulus of the peripheral chemoreceptors. On the other end of the spectrum, profound hypocapnia from hyperventilation can reduce hypoxic responsiveness to nearly zero. Metabolic acid–base changes operate in a similar fashion.

Dynamic changes

One of the most distinguishing features of the peripheral chemoreceptors, compared with the central receptors, is their fast response time. The time constant is approximately 12 seconds, with a delay from lung to carotid body of only a few seconds. Figure 46.4 shows the rapid change of $\dot{V}E$ in response to decreased $Sa{O_2}$. Compare this rapid response with the slow increase in ventilation caused by stimulation of central chemoreceptors in Figure 46.2. The carotid body response is so fast that the output of the peripheral chemoreceptor changes phasically at a frequency equal to that of tidal breathing, corresponding to the slight fluctuations in $Pa{O_2}$ and $Pa{CO_2}$ that occur with tidal breathing. The peripheral chemoreceptors are fast enough and sufficiently sensitive to detect these fluctuations. It is still unclear whether this phasic activity contributes part of the ventilatory response (e.g. in exercise).

Measurement

Peripheral chemoreceptor sensitivity can be measured using a variety of responses. In animal preparations, the activity of nerve fibers from the carotid sinus nerve can be directly measured. In humans and in most animal experiments, $\dot{V}E$ is the most useful response. The hypoxic stimulus may be quantitated by changes in either $Pa{O_2}$ or $Sa{O_2}$, at constant $Pa{CO_2}$ ('isocapnic'). For clinical purposes, $Pa{O_2}$ is estimated from alveolar gas samples, as end-tidal $P{O_2}$ ($PET{O_2}$). Under most circumstances, this should be a close approximation. When expressed relative to $P{O_2}$, the isocapnic hypoxic response appears hyperbolic, with an asymptote at 32mmHg (Fig. 46.5). A common way to measure hypoxic response is to fit the data obtained at low $P{O_2}$ (40–60mmHg) to a hyperbola of form $\dot{V}E = A/(P{O_2} - 32)$, where A is the extrapolated, but not measurable, ventilation at 33mmHg (incorrectly called a shape parameter). More usefully, A is eight times the increase in ventilation at $Pa{O_2}$ 40mmHg, which can be directly measured. With the advent of pulse oximetry, most researchers have used $Sa{O_2}$, with the added convenience of the near linear HVR slope (Fig. 46.6). With this method, the value of HVR may be determined at constant $P{CO_2}$ by a single measurement of the increase of ventilation caused by reduction to any low saturation (preferably between 70 and 85%).

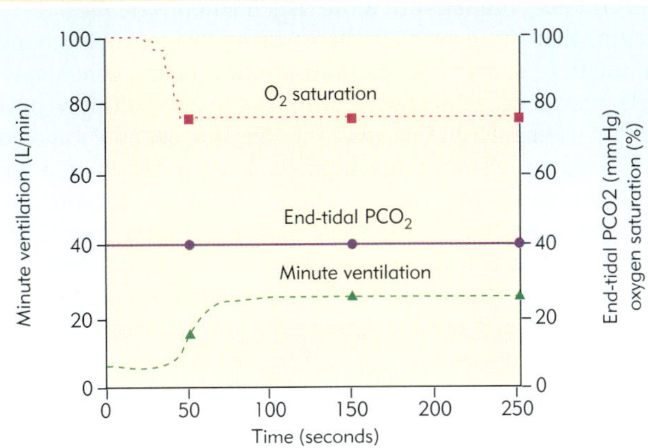

Figure 46.4 Steady-state isocapnic hypoxic ventilatory response. In this simulated example, oxygen saturation is lowered stepwise to 75% and ventilation rises rapidly as a result of stimulation of the carotid bodies. The end-tidal partial pressure of CO_2 (P_{ETCO_2}) is kept constant by addition of CO_2 to the inspired gas mixture (at an above-normal level, as in Fig. 46.2). Ventilation attains a plateau in about 2 minutes.

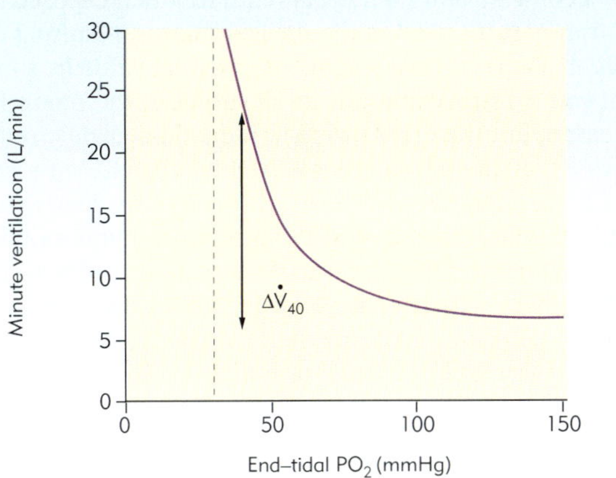

Figure 46.5 Measurement of the hypoxic ventilatory response (HVR) using partial O_2 pressure (Po_2). The hypoxic response expressed relative to Po_2 is hyperbolic and has usually been quantitated using a sensitivity parameter *A*, where the minute ventilation ($\dot{V}_E$) is $A/(Po_2 - 32)$. Another measure of hypoxic response is $\Delta\dot{V}_{E_{40}}$, the increase in ventilation when Po_2 is lowered from 200 to 40mmHg ($A = 8\Delta\dot{V}_{E_{40}}$). Using a rebreathing system with an adjustable CO_2 absorber to hold partial pressure of CO_2 (Pco_2) constant, a response curve similar to this can be obtained as Po_2 falls over about 5–10 minutes, although it may include some hypoxic ventilatory decline (HVD) component.

The pattern of hypoxia has important effects on the values obtained in the measurement of HVR. Some investigators use a technique of rapid desaturation to a predetermined Sao_2 and then hold this level constant until the response reaches equilibrium, over a period of 2–3 minutes. This steady-state technique is distinguished from a 'ramp' technique where progressive hypoxia is produced, usually by rebreathing. During the ramp technique, HVD presumably occurs, yielding a lower value of HVR than a rapid steady-state technique in the same individual. The sudden change in F_{IO_2} required of the steady-state technique is technically more difficult, and holding Sao_2 constant during the increasing ventilation requires continued adjustment. During the rebreathing technique, the decline in Sao_2 occurs naturally through oxygen consumption and makes overshooting to extremely low values of Sao_2 less likely.

Other measurements of peripheral chemoreceptor function may be used. The response to doxapram, a peripheral chemoreceptor stimulant, is simple, but it has not been proven to relate to HVR quantitatively in different subjects or under differing conditions. Carotid body sensitivity has been measured using single breaths of increased CO_2, or of 5% CO_2 in N_2, recording the transient response before central chemoreceptors are stimulated. Another technique has used nonlinear regression to partition the response to a step rise of $Paco_2$ into a fast time-constant component, representing peripheral chemoreceptors, and a slow time-constant component, representing the central chemoreceptor response (see Fig. 46.2). With this technique, both the gains and time constants of the central and peripheral chemoreceptors are determined in a single test.

Failure to control $Paco_2$ perfectly during measurement of HVR is the single most important factor confounding the interpretation of research results on HVR. Because of the interaction between hypoxia and CO_2 within the peripheral chemoreceptors, most investigators consider maintaining isocapnia during measurement of HVR essential. If $Paco_2$ is allowed to fall, both central and peripheral chemoreceptor drives fall, more so in subjects with high HVR, introducing multiplicative error and scatter and minimizing the difference between high and low HVR responses.

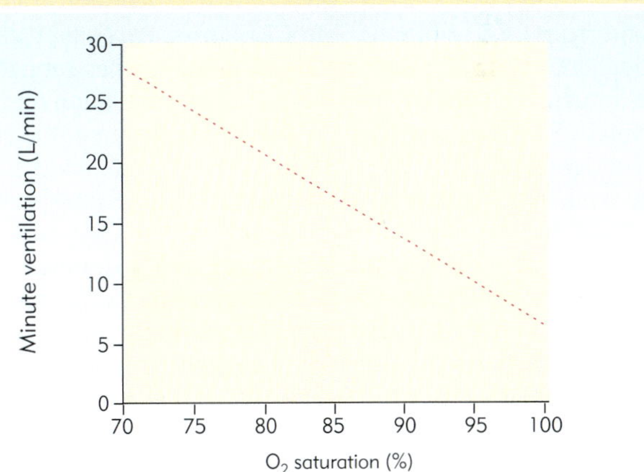

Figure 46.6 Measurement of the hypoxic ventilatory response (HVR) using oxygen saturation (So_2). The acute isocapnic steady-state ventilatory response to a step fall of O_2 saturation is a linear function of desaturation (between 65 and 90%) and may be quantitated by a simple slope, change in minute ventilation $(\Delta\dot{V}_E)/\Delta Sao_2$ (HVR = 0.75L per minute/% O_2 saturation in this simulated example). The normal range of HVR is 0.2–1.0 L per minute/% O_2 saturation. Illustrated slope = 0.7.

The HVR value depends on the exact Pa_{CO_2} held constant. Most work has been done at 'resting' Pa_{CO_2}. However, subjects may become anxious and hyperventilate when exposed to unfamiliar apparatus used in the measurements, resulting in a low HVR. If Pa_{CO_2} is raised above the resting value by some constant but arbitrary amount in all subjects, the mean HVR is increased, but the error owing to individual anxiety remains.

HVR varies considerably between subjects, with values of 0.2–1.5%/L/min. About 10% of individuals have been reported to have very little response. While some of these nonresponders may have been misidentified by use of a test value for Pa_{CO_2} that was too low, there is clearly a wide range of response. It is not known whether such abnormally low sensitivity is central or peripheral, but subjects with low values for both HCVR and HVR may be more likely to have central integrative abnormalities.

ALTITUDE AND ACCLIMATIZATION

Events occurring at altitude help to illustrate the mechanisms of ventilatory control and, therefore, these have been widely studied. Although a low HVR may be the underlying cause of acute mountain sickness and should lead to worse performance at altitude, such correlations have not been adequately confirmed.

At altitude, P_{AO_2}, reduced by lower P_{IO_2} from lower ambient pressure, stimulates peripheral chemoreceptors, causing an increase in $\dot{V}_E$. Increased $\dot{V}_E$ lowers Pa_{CO_2}, which, in turn, reduces central chemoreceptor drive. In the initial new steady state, this central chemoreceptor inhibition limits the rise of ventilation to about 10% at 4000m altitude, and Pa_{CO_2} settles at about 35–36mmHg. Over the first 8 to 24 hours, Pa_{CO_2} gradually falls as the HCO_3^- levels in the CSF are reduced at the central chemoreceptors (by several mechanisms, which may include lactic acid production, active transport pH regulation, and diffusion from CSF to blood). After 24 hours, Pa_{CO_2} typically is about 30mmHg at this altitude. If one then breathes enough O_2 to eliminate the hypoxic drive momentarily, ventilation remains elevated; Pa_{CO_2} rises only about 3–4mmHg, a sign of the compensatory metabolic acidosis of the CSF. Arterial blood at this time is alkaline because renal compensation for the respiratory alkalosis is much slower. Over the subsequent days to weeks at this altitude, the carotid body drive slowly doubles (by 2 weeks), further reducing Pa_{CO_2} and increasing ventilation.

The higher $\dot{V}_E$ has substantial benefits in increasing arterial P_{O_2}. This is particularly true at levels of hypoxia corresponding to the steep portion of the oxyhemoglobin dissociation curve, where a Pa_{O_2} increase of several millimeters of mercury can lead to a significant improvement in oxyhemoglobin saturation. In addition, HVD is present at altitude.

Chronic altitude exposure (months to years) leads to physiologic changes that differ from those occurring in acute exposure. While hypertrophied carotid bodies are believed to continue their intensified rate of stimulus, the integrating portions of the respiratory center appear to become less responsive. Hypoxic responses are depressed; Pa_{CO_2} is elevated, and Pa_{O_2} is lower. In some individuals, O_2 administration may actually increase ventilation through release of HVD, where peripheral chemoreceptor responses are low. Carotid bodies themselves increase in size with prolonged exposure to altitude. Lower ventilatory responsiveness causing lower Pa_{O_2} is also a contributing factor to chronic mountain sickness. This reduced HVR, or blunting, is not reversible even after years at sea level.

SLEEP AND SLEEP APNEA

During sleep, humans are more dependent on chemical drive to breathe than during wakefulness, which provides supplementary stimulation. Subnormal chemoreceptor reflexes, which may be little in evidence while awake, can lead to devastating hypoventilation during sleep. Likewise, the effects of sedatives and analgesics that cause respiratory depression may be far greater during sleep in subjects with abnormally low HVR and HCVR; this is probably a major factor in sleep apnea. Changes in ventilation and ventilatory control during sleep have important clinical consequences. Nighttime disturbances of ventilation can lead to daytime somnolence and dysfunction. In the worst cases, cor pulmonale may develop from chronic hypoxemia.

Differences may exist between ventilatory changes occurring in REM sleep and those occurring during other stages of sleep. One of the main differences between the two states is the irregular breathing patterns seen during REM sleep (Chapter 13). Short apneic episodes may also occur during REM sleep. These patterns are probably mediated through central nonchemical drive and include changes in respiratory rate, tidal volume, and even periods of apnea. It is likely that chemical control of breathing may actually stabilize, not contribute to, this irregular pattern. Despite differences between REM and nonREM sleep, the following are generalizations that probably apply qualitatively to both REM and nonREM sleep.

Loss of wakefulness leads to a fall in $\dot{V}_A$ and rise in Pa_{CO_2}. Without chemoreceptor responses, the decrease in $\dot{V}_A$ with sleep is even more pronounced. The value of Pa_{O_2} may also fall during sleep. Alveolar hypoventilation, as described above, reduces $P_{AO_2}$and Pa_{O_2}. Increased ventilation/perfusion ($\dot{V}/\dot{Q}$) maldistribution may also occur. In periodic breathing with apneic episodes, more profound arterial O_2 desaturation may occur. The extent of desaturation depends on the duration of apnea and the functional residual capacity. Apneic episodes are terminated by partial or complete arousal, resulting from stimulation of chemoreceptors.

Periodic breathing may occur during the early stages of sleep as a result of fluctuations in the state of CNS arousal. Breathing eventually settles into a regular pattern during the deeper stages. Ventilatory responses to the increased Pa_{CO_2}, which occurs during sleep, may exaggerate periodic breathing. The slope of the ventilatory response to CO_2 is reduced during sleep. The curve is also shifted to a higher Pa_{CO_2}; that is, the *x* intercept (apneic threshold) is higher. HVR also appears to be reduced. Although reduced, ventilatory control systems are still active, and abolition of responses may result in absence of breathing.

Sleep apnea, while often a consequence of obesity, is modified by chemoreceptor function. Chemoreceptor tone may affect airway muscle tone. Arousal from obstruction is mediated by chemoreceptor responses. The peripheral chemoreceptors are probably essential for this response, since Pa_{CO_2} rises and Pa_{O_2} falls during apnea. Peripheral chemoreceptor sensitivity may determine how low Sa_{O_2} falls during periods of airway obstruction and apnea.

ABNORMALITIES OF CHEMORECEPTOR FUNCTION

Several abnormalities of chemoreceptor function can be identified in normal individuals, while others are unusual and represent disease states. Alteration in ventilatory control also provides insight into the fundamental working of this regulatory system.

Periodic breathing occurs in a variety of circumstances, even in normal individuals. The best-defined type of periodic breathing is Cheyne–Stokes breathing, which is characterized by sinusoidally rising and falling tidal volumes with or without periods of apnea. Cheyne–Stokes breathing can occur in normal individuals during certain stages of sleep. During sleep at sea level, the periodic breathing is most likely a consequence of changes in the state of arousal, with changing ventilatory response and apneic thresholds. Cheyne–Stokes breathing is also a well-known phenomenon during sleep at high altitude. It may also occur in such pathologic states as congestive heart failure.

Certain conditions predispose to instability in the ventilatory response system, which results in periodic breathing. Hypoxia is one of the most important factors promoting periodic breathing. The hypoxic stimulus on the peripheral chemoreceptors results in increased ventilation. Increased ventilation decreases $Paco_2$, which decreases the slope of the hypoxic response. Because of the shape of the oxyhemoglobin dissociation curve, increased ventilation can also markedly improve oxygenation, which will further change the output of the peripheral chemoreceptors. During sleep, without the separate stimulus from wakefulness, this increase in ventilation can lead to such a sharp drop in peripheral chemoreceptor stimulation that apnea results. Apnea will then lead to an increase in $Paco_2$ and a fall in Sao_2. The resultant increased peripheral chemoreceptor stimulation and ventilation can start this cycle again.

This system is complex, and many factors influence whether these changes will result in a continued unstable breathing pattern or whether the pattern will stabilize with time. The circulatory delay to the chemoreceptors is one of the most significant factors leading to periodic breathing. It is believed that increased delay to both peripheral and central chemoreceptors is the primary reason that heart failure can result in periodic breathing. Higher peripheral chemoreceptor responses also tend to increase periodic breathing. Almitrene, a drug that increases the gain of the peripheral chemoreceptors, increases periodic breathing at high altitude.

Several diseases of chemoreceptor function have been found. Ondine's curse (severe central sleep apnea) was initially described with loss of central chemoreception following surgery near the brainstem. During wakefulness, individuals function well. However, profound hypoventilation or apnea can occur during sleep. Congenital forms have been described as the primary alveolar hypoventilation syndrome. Afflicted individuals appear to lack both peripheral and central chemoreceptor function. The defect most likely resides in areas of the brainstem above the entry of the peripheral and central chemoreceptor signals into the CNS. These individuals may require ventilatory support during sleep and may have significant hypoventilation or apnea during anesthesia and in the perioperative period.

Abnormal chemoreceptor function should also be suspected in individuals with serious neurologic abnormalities. The premature infant up to postconceptual ages of 50–60 weeks is at risk of apnea during anesthesia. The exact problem in chemoreceptor function has not been defined. Abnormal chemoreceptor function has been implicated in sudden infant death syndrome (SIDS).

Key References

Berger A, Mitchell R, Severinghaus JW. Regulation of Respiration. N Eng J Med. 1977;297:92–7, 138–43, 194–201.

Eyzaguirre C, Fidone SJ, Fitzgerald RS, Lahiri S, McDonald DM. Arterial chemoreception. New York: Springer-Verlag; 1990.

Forster HV, Dempsey JA. Ventilatory adaptations. In: Hornbein T ed. Regulation of Breathing, Part II. New York: M Dekker; 1981:845–901.

Hickey RF, Severinghaus JW. Ventilatory adaptations: drug effects. In: Hornbein T ed. Regulation of Breathing, Part II. New York: M Dekker; 1981:1251–312.

Loeschcke HH. Central chemosensitivity and the reaction theory. J Physiol. 1982;332:1–24.

McDonald DM. Peripheral chemoreceptors. In: Hornbein T ed. Regulation of Breathing, Part I. New York: M Dekker; 1981:105–319.

Pietak S, Weenig CS, Hickey RF, Fairley HB. Anesthetic effects on ventilation in patients with chronic obstructive pulmonary disease. Anesthesiol. 1975;45:160–6.

Severinghaus JW. Respiratory control related to altitude and anesthesia. In: Stanley TH, Sperry RJ eds. Anesthesia and the lung, Vol 25. Dordrecht: Kluwer Academic Publishers; 1992:101–15.

Temp JA, Henson LC, Ward DS. Effect of a subanesthetic minimum alveolar concentration of isoflurane on two tests of the hypoxic ventilatory response. Anesthesiol. 1994;80:739–50.

Further Reading

Cherniack NS, Widdicombe JG. The respiratory system. In: Fishman AP ed. Handbook of physiology. Bethesda, MD: American Physiological Society; 1986.

Duffin J. The chemoreflex control of breathing and its measurement. Can J Anesth. 1990;37:933-42.

Neubauer JA., Melton JE, Edelman NH. Modulation of respiration during brain hypoxia. J Appl Physiol. 1990;68:441-51.

Nunn JF. Nunn's Applied Respiratory Physiology, 4th edn. London: Butterworths–Heinmann; 1993.

Chapter 47 Drugs that affect the respiratory system

Keith H Berge and David O Warner

Topics covered in this chapter

Effects on ventilatory function
Effects on airway function
Effects on pulmonary vasculature

Many drugs that are utilized in the conduct of clinical anesthesia have profound effects on respiratory function. These actions have the potential for both benefit (e.g. relief of bronchospasm in asthmatic patients) and harm (e.g. impairment of pulmonary gas exchange). This chapter reviews the actions of anesthetic drugs and adjuvants on the striated skeletal muscles responsible for the bellows function of ventilation, the smooth muscle that determines airway caliber, and the vascular smooth muscle that regulates blood flow within the pulmonary vasculature. Although many of these agents affect more than one of these components, the discussion focuses on that area in which the drug exerts its greatest effect.

EFFECTS ON VENTILATORY FUNCTION

It is fortunate that respiratory muscle function is relatively well-preserved during ether anesthesia; indeed, this property was crucial as it allowed the safe use of inhaled anesthetics before the advent of assisted ventilation. Modern inhaled anesthetic drugs have many advantages, but they profoundly depress the function of both the bellows muscles of the chest wall (e.g. the diaphragm) and the muscles responsible for maintaining upper airway patency. Although anesthetic techniques have evolved to cope with this depression, alterations in respiratory function caused by anesthesia constitute a major source of morbidity and mortality in modern anesthetic practice.

Normal physiology

Although the complexity is often not appreciated, even quiet breathing requires integration of medullary respiratory centers to coordinate the activity of multiple muscle groups. This activity may be voluntarily controlled, but is most often automatically regulated to maintain the partial pressure of arterial carbon dioxide ($Paco_2$) within a very narrow range in response to a wide range of metabolic demands. Respiratory muscles also have other important functions, such as in speech and maintenance of posture. The control systems that regulate this complex system are complicated and highly susceptible to disruption by anesthetic drugs. The level of consciousness itself is an important variable that affects ventilatory control, especially of upper airway muscles.

In awake human subjects, consistent phasic (i.e. intermittent) electromyographic (EMG) activity is observed in the diaphragm, the parasternal intercostal muscles, and the scalene muscles during inspiration. As a result of this phasic activity, the diaphragm descends and the rib cage expands, which generates airflow. Expiration during quiet breathing is primarily passive, caused by relaxation of the diaphragm and the passive recoil of elastic tissues of the respiratory system. Active expiration, utilized during exercise-induced hyperpnea, is produced by contraction of the abdominal muscles, as well as of the transversus thoracis and internal intercostal muscles in the lateral rib cage. In upright postures, abdominal muscles are tonically active to support the abdominal contents against gravity and to prevent shortening of the diaphragm, which would impair its efficiency. Tonic activity has also been reported in the diaphragm and intercostal muscles, but this is unclear.

Several upper airway muscles demonstrate phasic EMG activity during inspiration, which helps maintain upper airway patency throughout the period of negative upper airway pressures generated by inspiratory flow. This activity is of critical importance; in its absence, even modest negative upper airway pressures can markedly narrow the upper airway. To overcome this collapse, active muscle contraction causes the glottis to widen during inspiration in human subjects, and narrow during expiration. Phasic and tonic activity is also present in several other upper airway muscles to maintain airway patency.

Drug effects

General anesthetics

At doses that produce surgical anesthesia, most general anesthetics (with the possible exception of ketamine) decrease resting minute ventilation, and thus increase the $Paco_2$ maintained during spontaneous breathing (Fig. 47.1). Most agents also impair the response of minute ventilation to hypercapnia. These effects are partially offset by surgical stimulation. At equipotent combinations, such effects can also be ameliorated by the substitution of nitrous oxide for a portion of the volatile anesthetic. The difference between the level of $Paco_2$ that supports spontaneous ventilation and the level that results in apnea is only 4–5mmHg (0.5–0.7kPa), regardless of the depth of anesthesia. Thus, efforts to assist ventilation result in only minimal reduction of hypercapnia before apnea results. For this reason, controlled ventilation is commonly used for anesthetized patients if normocapnia is desired. These drugs also have important depressive effects on the activity and coordination of the muscles that surround the upper airway, which may compromise its patency.

The mechanisms by which anesthetics affect breathing are unclear. At high concentrations, all general anesthetics produce

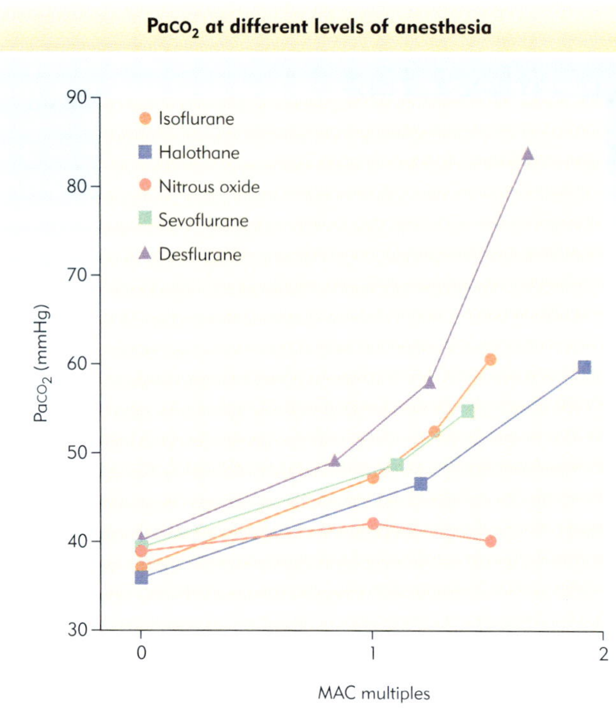

Figure 47.1 Maintenance of Paco$_2$ during spontaneous breathing at different levels of anesthesia as multiples of minimal alveolar concentration (MAC). Note that at equivalent anesthetic depth, desflurane is the most potent and halothane and nitrous oxide are the least potent respiratory depressants.

a global depression of respiratory motoneuron function and apnea, presumably by directly depressing medullary function. However, at surgical levels of anesthesia, these effects are considerably more complex. For example, halothane anesthesia has differential effects on various respiratory muscle groups, depressing activity in the parasternal intercostal muscles, but actually increasing activity in muscles with expiratory actions, such as the transversus abdominis. Halothane anesthesia also enhances the response of neural drive to the diaphragm during carbon dioxide rebreathing. Thus, it appears that at modest depths of surgical anesthesia, halothane and other anesthetics produce respiratory depression by altering the distribution and timing of neural drive to the respiratory muscles, rather than by producing a global depression of activity (Fig. 47.2). Hypoxic ventilatory drive that arises from carotid chemoreceptors is also depressed by the volatile anesthetics. The anesthetic concentration necessary for this effect is unclear – some studies showed a clinically significant effect at very low concentrations, whereas in other studies the depression was significant only at surgical depths of anesthesia. The upper airway muscles appear to be more susceptible to anesthetic-induced depression than those in the diaphragm.

In addition to causing hypoventilation, the actions of general anesthetics on the respiratory muscles have other important consequences. Disruption of normal upper airway muscle activity may produce airway obstruction, and changes in the position and motion of chest wall structures alter the underlying lung function. Lung changes produced by deformation of the chest wall include a decrease in the functional residual capacity of the lungs and the formation of atelectasis in dependent lung regions (Fig. 47.3), changes that significantly impair pulmonary gas exchange (Chapter 44). Although this impairment can usually be overcome by increasing the inspired fraction of oxygen intraoperatively,

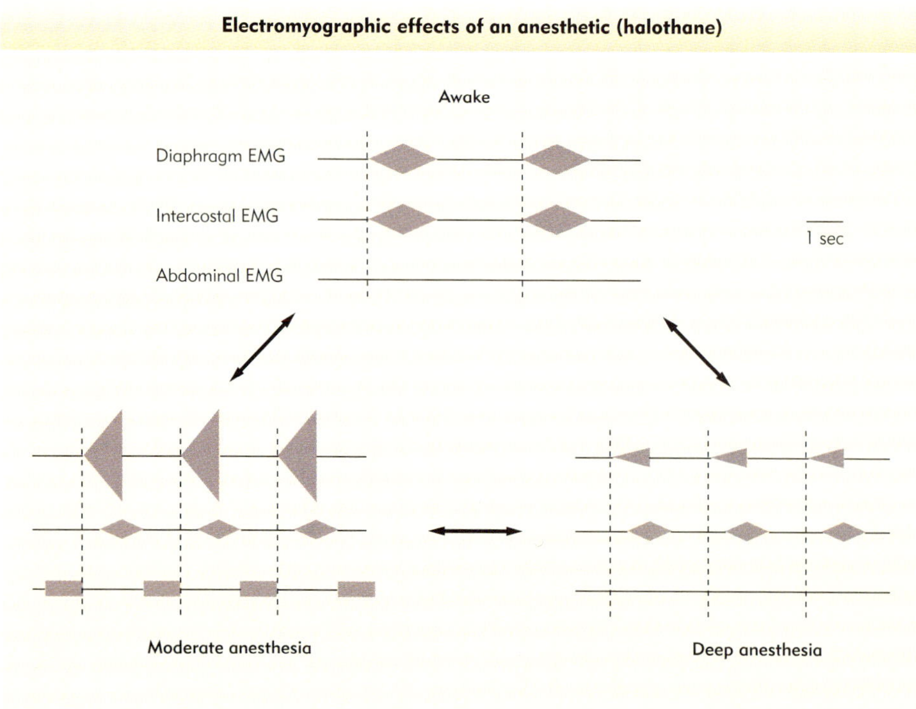

Figure 47.2 Effects of an anesthetic (halothane) on EMG activity. The patterns of EMG activity for three muscles with respiratory actions are given in a supine human subject. While awake, the diaphragm and intercostal muscles are active during inspiration and synchronous, and the abdominal muscles are not active. With moderate anesthesia, the pattern of activity changes in its timing (increased breathing frequency and asynchrony between the diaphragm and intercostals), intensity of activity (decreases in intercostal activity and increases in diaphragm activity), and the appearance of new activity (expiratory activity in the abdominal muscles). Such changes in respiratory muscle coordination promote inefficiency of the bellows function of the chest wall and result in hypoventilation and increases in Paco$_2$. At deep levels of anesthesia, global depression of all respiratory muscle function occurs.

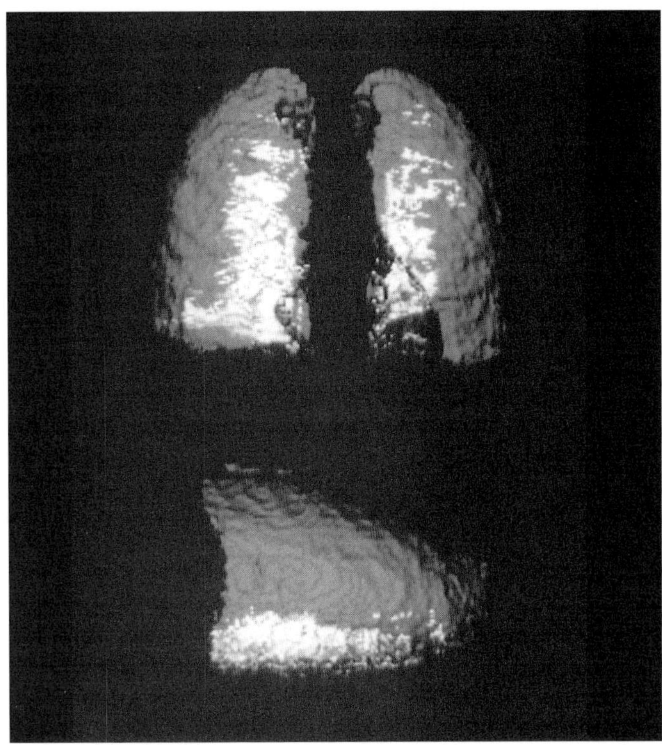

Figure 47.3 Volume image of a halothane-anesthetized subject obtained by a fast three-dimensional CT scan. The surface of the lung is shown in shades of gray and areas of lung atelectasis are shown in white. Conceptually, this represents the view of a gray, transparent, three-dimensional model of lung shape, with a superimposed opaque white model of atelectasis. In the top panel, the anteroposterior view clearly shows the right and left lungs, with a visible cardiac shadow. The lateral view in the bottom panel demonstrates that the atelectatic areas are located in the most dependent lung regions. In this view, posterior is down, and caudad is left. (Reproduced with permission from Warner DO, Warner MA, Ritman EL, 1996.)

changes in chest wall function may persist into the postoperative period and produce significant postoperative morbidity.

Opioids

Opioids cause hypoventilation by dose-dependent depression of the brain stem respiratory centers, which produces a decrease in both respiratory rate and tidal volume. The slope of the ventilatory response to hypercapnia is reduced and the x-intercept is increased. Similar effects are observed after intravenous, intramuscular, epidural, and intrathecal administration, albeit at different doses. As with general anesthetics, opioid effects may be modulated by the level of consciousness. For example, patients may maintain adequate ventilation when aroused, but not when allowed to fall asleep in the postoperative period. The partial agonist or mixed agonist–antagonist agents are associated with profound hypoventilation less commonly, but also have limitations in analgesic properties. Some opioids, such as morphine, can release histamine and thereby exacerbate bronchospasm in susceptible patients. The potent synthetic opioids, such as fentanyl and its derivatives, can produce rigidity of chest wall muscle sufficient to render ventilation of the lungs impossible in the absence of neuromuscular blockade. This rigidity is typically associated with advanced age and rapid administration of large doses (e.g. up to 80% of patients who receive fentanyl 30microg/kg), although it is occasionally seen with much lower doses.

Benzodiazepines

When used alone in modest doses, these drugs generally do not cause significant respiratory depression. Reported effects on hypercapnic responses are variable, with some studies showing moderate effects, and others no effect. Clinically, when combined with fentanyl, benzodiazepines may produce profound depression of resting breathing, although it is of interest that the combination has no greater effect on hypercapnic sensitivity compared with fentanyl alone.

α_2-Agonists

First developed for treatment of hypertension, drugs such as clonidine possess hypnotic and analgesic properties that are now being exploited in clinical anesthesia. When administered either intravenously or into the central neuroaxis, they have only modest effects on resting breathing, similar to those observed during natural sleep, and little effect on hypercapnic responses.

Ventilatory stimulants

Some agents have been employed clinically to stimulate respiratory drive. Doxapram is an analeptic agent that increases the depth and rate of respiration, presumably by stimulation of either brain stem nuclei or carotid body chemoreceptors. While shown to be effective in the short term to promote return to adequate ventilation during recovery from anesthesia, its use in many areas has become uncommon as it is felt that mechanical ventilation, either invasive or noninvasive, is safer and more reliable. Methylxanthine drugs, such as theophylline and caffeine, may increase skeletal muscle performance. At therapeutic concentrations, both of these drugs are reported to improve diaphragmatic contractility, although it is unclear whether this effect is actually responsible for decreases in subjective dyspnea in patients who have chronic obstructive pulmonary disease (COPD) treated who have these compounds. Often considered to be a ventilatory stimulant, theophylline actually has little effect on hypercapnic responses, but may augment hypoxic responses and resting breathing.

EFFECTS ON AIRWAY FUNCTION

Normal physiology

The airways of the respiratory system, from the nasal passages to the terminal alveoli, are highly responsive to neural and humoral input. As such, their functioning can be altered profoundly by drugs, exogenous allergens, and circulating factors such as cytokines. Normal airway reflexes include protective cough reflexes, vasomotor regulation of nasal airflow resistance, and regulation of lower airway resistance via alteration of smooth muscle tone of the conducting airways. Various receptors are distributed liberally throughout the airways to mediate the afferent limb of these responses. Effectors include the skeletal muscles of the chest wall and upper airways, and the smooth muscle that lines the trachea and bronchi. In humans, the predominant innervation of airway smooth muscle is via cholinergic fibers in the vagus nerve that synapse with ganglia in the airway wall (Fig. 47.4). Stimulation of these parasympathetic pathways produces bronchoconstriction, mucus secretion, and vasodilatation of

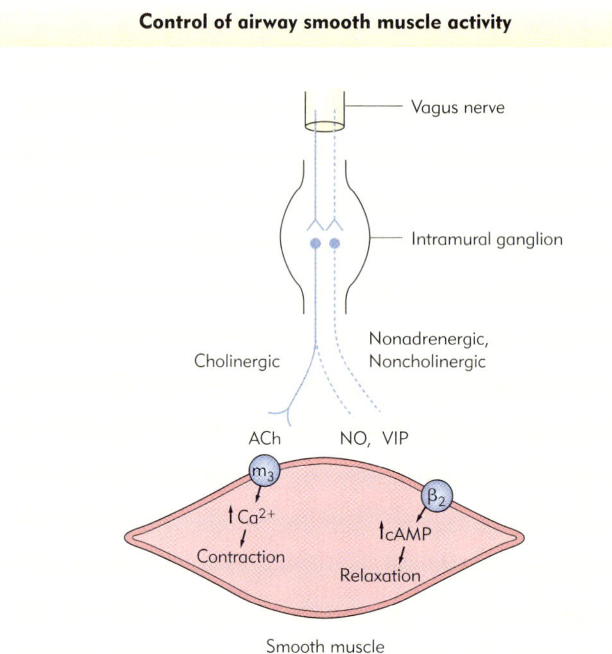

Figure 47.4 Systems that control airway smooth muscle activity in humans. Note that β_2-adrenergic receptors on airway smooth muscle are not innervated. It is not known if the nonadrenergic, noncholinergic system utilizes distinct neural pathways (dashed lines) or whether its putative mediators nitric oxide (NO) or vascoactive intestinal peptide (VIP) are cotransmitters released with acetylcholine (ACh) from postganglionic nerves. (cAMP, cyclic adenosine monophosphate.) (Adapted with permission from Warner DO. Airway pharmacology. In: Benumof J, ed. Airway management: Pri-ciples and practice. St. Louis: Mosby–Yearbook; 1995.)

bronchial vessels. Although there are abundant β_2 adrenoreceptors in the human airway, these receptors are not innervated by sympathetic nerves, but rather are activated by circulating epinephrine (adrenaline). Other neural systems inhibitory to airway smooth muscle, termed nonadrenergic, noncholinergic systems, are less well defined; candidate neurotransmitters include nitric oxide and vasoactive intestinal peptide (VIP). Cholinergic neurotransmission in the vagus nerve can also be modified by a variety of mechanisms, including prejunctional inhibition by muscarinic and opioid receptors.

Pathophysiology

Asthma is one the of the few chronic diseases in the developing world that has an increasing prevalence, which is paradoxic given the increasing knowledge of its pathogenesis and treatment. Theories of pathogenesis have shifted from belief in an underlying defect in smooth muscle reactivity to a view of asthma as a chronic inflammatory disease. Evidence indicates that the histologic alterations seen in the airway of asthma sufferers (i.e. patchy epithelial desquamation, thickening of the collagen layer of the basement membrane, and smooth muscle hypertrophy) are the end result of ongoing inflammatory changes, and arise from chronic airway mucosal infiltration by activated eosinophils, lymphocytes, and mast cells. The characteristic changes in smooth muscle reactivity are thus a consequence of chronic exposure to inflammatory mediators. Therefore, the primary pharmacotherapy of asthma is increasingly aimed at quelling this chronic inflammatory response, and less at attempts to correct the secondary effects by utilizing bronchodilating agents.

Allergic asthma is characterized by airway hyper-responsiveness to a variety of specific and nonspecific stimuli, pulmonary eosinophilia, elevated serum IgE, and excessive airway mucus production by goblet cells. Recent animal data indicate an important role for $CD4^+$ (helper) T lymphocytes producing a type 2 cytokine profile (T_H2) including interleukin (IL)-4, IL-5 and IL-13. The latter cytokine may be a central mediator of allergic asthma.

Drug effects

Glucocorticoids

Based on the understanding of asthma as an inflammatory disease, corticosteroids have assumed a primary role in its treatment. These drugs bind to specific receptors in the cytoplasm and then translocate to the nucleus, where they regulate the function of several genes (Chapter 3), generally decreasing the production of inflammatory mediators such as cytokines. The advent of inhaled corticosteroids, which are poorly absorbed into the systemic circulation, represents a significant advance in asthma therapy and has minimized the undesirable side effects associated with chronic corticosteroid use, such as significant adrenal cortical suppression or osteoporosis. Indeed, few significant adverse side effects result from systemic absorption at dose levels adequate to achieve desired symptom control in the majority of patients. Adverse local side effects include thrush and dysphonia, presumably from deposition of the drug on the oropharynx and vocal cords. Adrenal suppression can be detected by sensitive measures in patients who receive high-dose inhaled therapy, but it is rarely of clinical significance. Patient compliance may be an issue, as there is little patient perception of immediate benefit from treatment and considerable patient concern about the side effects of corticosteroid therapy. In patients who have severe asthma, systemically administered corticosteroids, with their attendant risks of adverse effects, may be required.

Sympathominetic agents

Sympathominetic agents bind to β_2-receptors on the smooth muscle cell membrane, which stimulates adenylyl cyclase and increases the intracellular concentration of cAMP. This action can prevent or reverse the bronchoconstriction that results from provocative substances such as leukotrienes, acetylcholine (ACh), bradykinin, prostaglandin (PG), and histamine. They may also modulate cholinergic neurotransmission, affect inflammatory cells, and stimulate mucociliary transport. Although β_2-agonists are effective when administered systemically via the intravenous or subcutaneous route, inhaled administration is convenient and minimizes undesirable systemic side effects. When administered by this route, the short-acting β_2-agonists, such as albuterol and terbutaline, provide rapid symptomatic relief, while the long-acting agents, such as salmeterol and formoterol (eformoterol), are of slower onset but provide a more sustained effect. This makes these agents particularly useful in those who suffer nocturnal exacerbations of asthma.

Recently, concern has arisen that excessive use of short-acting inhaled β_2-agonists might increase the morbidity and mortality from asthma, although the increased usage noted prior to an adverse event might simply be a marker for increasingly unstable asthma. It has been suggested that chronic use of β_2-agonists only may relieve symptoms but not treat the underlying inflammatory process. For this reason, many physicians recommend that these drugs be used episodically for acute exacerbations of symptoms, rather than as chronic therapy.

Cromolyn (cromoglycate) and nedocromil

Cromolyn and nedocromil inhibit the release of inflammatory mediators from several types of cells. They are generally more effective in the prophylaxis than in treatment of bronchospasm. Efficacy varies widely among patients, but because of the relative safety of these drugs, a therapeutic trial is often indicated.

Methylxanthines

Methylxanthines, including caffeine and theophylline, relieve bronchospasm via multiple mechanisms of action. Classically, theophylline was thought to act by inhibiting phosphodiesterases that metabolize cAMP, which increased intracellular cAMP concentration and caused bronchodilatation. However, drug concentrations *in vitro* necessary to demonstrate this effect exceed therapeutic levels *in vivo*. Other possible mechanisms of action include antagonism of adenosine, stimulation of endogenous catecholamine release, anti-inflammatory actions, and cardiovascular effects. Once the mainstay of chronic asthma therapy, these drugs have been somewhat eclipsed by inhaled corticosteroids. When properly used, these drugs remain safe and efficacious for the management of patients who have asthma and COPD.

Muscarinic antagonists

Drugs such as ipratropium bromide act as competitive antagonists of ACh at the m_3 subtype muscarinic receptor, which mediates parasympathetic bronchoconstriction. They also inhibit mucus secretion in the airway. These drugs generally have limited usefulness in the chronic therapy of asthma, which perhaps reflects a minor role for cholinergic motor tone in the pathogenesis of asthma. They appear to be more effective in the management of patients who have COPD.

Leukotriene receptor antagonists

The use of leukotriene receptor antagonists is the first novel therapeutic strategy for asthma to be brought to market in over 25 years. These agents are the first specific antagonists of an inflammatory mediator that may contribute to airway reactivity in asthma. Pranlukast is the first competitive antagonist of leukotriene receptors to reach the marketplace. The results of several large clinical trials worldwide show pranlukast to be both safe and effective in decreasing concomitant bronchodilator and corticosteroid use while improving peak expiratory flow rate and decreasing symptom severity scores (Fig. 47.5). Although clinical experience is limited, these agents may prove very useful in the chronic therapy of asthma.

Anesthetic drugs and adjuvants

Volatile anesthetics are potent bronchodilators that reduce responses to bronchoconstricting stimuli in both humans and animals, including responses to endotracheal intubation. As a result of these bronchodilating effects, volatile anesthetics have been used to treat status asthmaticus, although their efficacy in this condition is only anecdotal.

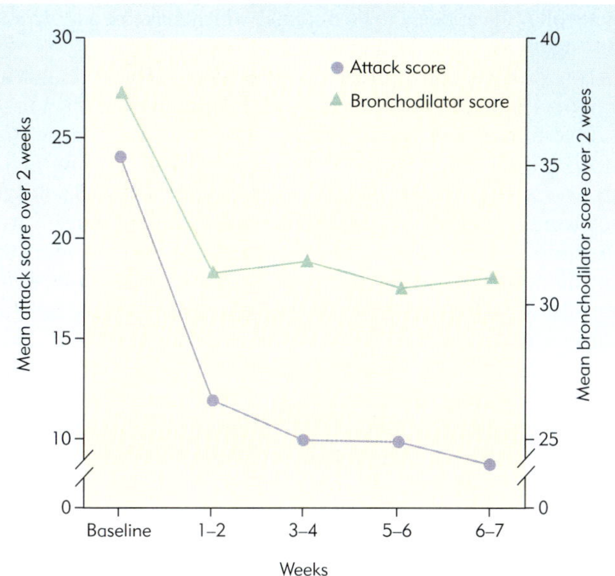

Figure 47.5 Effects of the leukotriene antagonist prankulast on symptom score and bronchodilator use score. Use of prankulast significantly improved these measures of asthma severity during an 8-week clinical trial. (Data taken with permission from Barnes NC, de Jong B, Miyamoto T. Worldwide clinical experience with the first marketed leukotriene receptor antagonist. Chest. 1997;111:52S–60S.)

Volatile anesthetics attenuate reflex bronchoconstriction in part by depressing neural pathways that mediate these reflexes at multiple sites. This action has been localized in the vagal motor pathway to a depression of parasympathetic ganglionic transmission and, at higher concentrations of volatile anesthetic, to attenuation of ACh release from postganglionic nerves. Volatile anesthetics also directly relax airway smooth muscle by at least two mechanisms. They decrease intracellular Ca^{2+} concentration during both the initiation and maintenance of airway smooth muscle contraction, and they may decrease the amount of force developed by the smooth muscle for a given level of intracellular Ca^{2+} (i.e. the 'Ca^{2+} sensitivity'). The relative importance of the bronchodilatory actions contributed by neurally mediated versus direct relaxant effects of volatile anesthetics on smooth muscle depends on the mechanism that produces bronchoconstriction. During reflex bronchoconstriction, such as that produced in response to noxious stimuli (e.g. airway instrumentation), depression of neural pathways is of greatest importance. During bronchoconstriction produced by the release of mediators from inflammatory cells, such as during anaphylactic or anaphylactoid reactions, direct effects assume greater importance.

Although only a few differences among the bronchodilating properties of volatile agents have been identified in experimental studies, in clinical practice isoflurane and desflurane are more irritating to the airway than is halothane. This stimulation of airway receptors may produce coughing, breath holding, and laryngospasm, and limits the usefulness of these agents for the induction of anesthesia by inhalation. For desflurane, stimulation of airway receptors may also be responsible for the hypertension and tachycardia observed after its acute administration. Irritation by sevoflurane appears to be minimal, which makes it a more suitable agent for inhalation induction (Chapter 24).

Intravenous anesthetics also may affect airway reactivity. *In vitro* studies show that thiopental (thiopentone) produces a dose-dependent constriction of isolated trachea by promoting the release of thromboxane A_2. This finding is not observed with oxybarbiturates such as methohexital (methohexitone). Thiopental has also been reported to cause bronchospasm by the release of histamine, but other studies did not demonstrate an association between bronchospasm and barbiturate administration. Although thiopental releases histamine from skin mast cells, this effect has not been demonstrated in the lung. Ketamine also depresses neural airway reflex pathways, and directly relaxes airway smooth muscle by decreasing intracellular Ca^{2+} concentration. Ketamine-induced release of endogenous catecholamines may also contribute to its bronchodilating effects. Propofol apparently blunts airway reflexes, as propofol induction of anesthesia permits insertion of the laryngeal mask airway without reflex responses such as laryngospasm. The incidence of wheezing during induction is reduced for propofol when compared with barbiturates, which suggests its usefulness in patients who have reactive airways.

Perioperative management of asthma

Preoperative preparation is directed toward minimizing airway inflammation and reactivity, with continuation of anti-inflammatory agents and bronchodilators until immediately before surgery. Firm data to support the traditional preference for regional anesthesia in these patients is lacking, although it seems reasonable to avoid the stimulation of airway manipulation when feasible. Volatile anesthetics remain the foundation of general anesthetic techniques, with little difference in clinical outcome observed among the available agents when utilized after intravenous induction. Propofol appears to be the intravenous drug of choice for induction. If airway instrumentation is necessary, prior adequate anesthesia of the airway is essential. This is conveniently provided by a period of ventilation with a volatile anesthetic following intravenous induction. In addition, both β_2-agonists and muscarinic antagonists blunt increases in respiratory system resistance associated with endotracheal intubation. Lidocaine (lignocaine) may also be useful, with intravenous administration preferred, as airway irritation by nebulized lidocaine may actually increase airway resistance in asthmatic subjects.

If bronchospasm develops, it is of primary importance to first firmly establish the diagnosis of bronchospasm, as many other processes, such as mechanical obstruction of the endotracheal tube, may produces signs that mimic bronchospasm. Once the diagnosis is confirmed, anesthesia should be deepened utilizing a volatile anesthetic. Other drugs to deepen anesthesia, such as propofol and fentanyl, may also be useful. The role of intravenous aminophylline is unclear, as in experimental animal models of asthma it has no benefit beyond that provided by volatile anesthetics. In contrast, β_2-agonists provide further bronchodilation under such circumstances, and are definitely indicated. If given via inhalation, repeated doses may be necessary, as the efficiency of nebulized drug delivery is decreased through endotracheal tubes, especially in the setting of severe bronchospasm. In severe cases, intravenous administration of β-adrenergic agonists (e.g. epinephrine) may be necessary.

EFFECTS ON PULMONARY VASCULATURE

Normal physiology

The caliber of the pulmonary vasculature is regulated by several factors, which include the mechanical stresses associated with gravity and changes in lung volume, neural control via autonomic nerves, substances released from the vascular endothelium, and factors intrinsic to vascular smooth muscle, such as those responsible for hypoxic pulmonary vasoconstriction (HPV; Chapter 44). These factors are normally precisely integrated to optimize the balance between regional ventilation and perfusion, and thus gas exchange. That pulmonary vessels comprise a low-pressure system makes gravitational effects relatively important in determining blood flow, according to well-described zones. However, recent evidence suggests that intrinsic regional differences in vascular conductance not related to gravity are also important.

Abundant sympathetic and parasympathetic innervation of pulmonary vessels occurs. Sympathetic stimulation increases pulmonary vascular resistance, primarily via stimulation of α_1-adrenoreceptors. The effect of parasympathetic stimulation varies with species and with the level of pre-existing vascular tone, and its physiologic role remains unclear. A variety of endogenous peptides, amines, and lipid mediators affect vascular tone, including angiotensin II, bradykinin, vasopressin, atrial naturetic peptide, endothelin, ACh, histamine, serotonin, and eicosanoids. Many of these mediators, such as nitric oxide, are produced in the vascular endothelium. As with neural innervation, the exact physiologic role and interactions of these compounds are unknown.

Finally, small pulmonary arteries respond to local hypoxia by increasing their tone (HPV), which serves to direct blood flow away from relatively hypoxic areas of the lung, thus better matching local ventilation to local perfusion and limiting the amount of hypoxemia that results from atelectasis (Chapter 50). Although the mechanisms responsible for HPV remain unknown, it appears to be intrinsic to vascular smooth muscle. As it remains intact in denervated, transplanted lungs, HPV is not neurally mediated.

As a consequence of the large surface area of the pulmonary capillaries (approximately 70m^2 in the adult human lung), a significant amount of fluid and accompanying solutes tend to leave the microcirculation and enter the interstitium by processes dependent on the relative balance of hydrostatic and osmotic forces. Fluid is normally returned to the circulation by lymphatic drainage. A safety factor exists in the system such that pressure in pulmonary capillaries can increase three- to four-fold before lung interstitial volume increases.

Pathophysiology

Several chronic disease states result in hypertension in the pulmonary arterial circulation, including increased pulmonary flow that results from congenital cardiac disease, increased outflow pressure from cardiac failure or valvular disease, increased tone from chronic hypoxia, loss of vascular lumen from thromboembolism, parenchymal disease, or idiopathic disease (e.g. primary pulmonary hypertension). Many of these chronic conditions produce vascular remodeling, characterized by increased concentric airway smooth muscle mass, endothelial cell injury, and intimal proliferation. The overall physiologic result of these responses to lung injury is not only impairment of the gas exchange ability of the lung, but also right ventricular strain (which may ultimately result in heart failure and death).

Acute pulmonary hypertension may result from acute lung injury (ALI), a pathologic lung response sustained by activated inflammatory cells, predominately polymorphonuclear leukocytes. The generalized inflammation of the lung seen in this disorder creates increased pulmonary vascular tone and pulmonary hypertension by altering the reactivity of the pulmonary vasculature to both endogenous and exogenously administered vasoactive substances. As an example of the disruption of normal function, HPV is generally inhibited by ALI. Lung fluid balance is also affected, producing a flooding of the alveoli which is worsened by the increased hydrostatic pressure gradient caused by pulmonary hypertension. Surfactant function, important to maintain the architectural integrity of the lung, is also impaired in ALI. A bewildering variety of inflammatory mediators may be responsible for or contribute to the changes seen in ALI, and the changes produced may be acute (with rapid resolution) or result in chronic impairment from fibrotic changes.

Drug effects

Inhaled anesthetics

Volatile anesthetics, in the absence of underlying pulmonary disease, affect pulmonary vascular pressures to only a small degree. As in the systemic circulation, they appear to interfere with the normal response of the pulmonary vasculature to dilating factors released from the endothelium. Nitrous oxide can increase pulmonary vascular resistance when administered to patients who have coexisting pulmonary hypertension. Inhaled anesthetics directly inhibit HPV in isolated lung models; however, halothane and isoflurane have only minimal further effects on oxygenation in anesthetized patients who undergo one-lung ventilation, presumably as a consequence of other compensatory mechanisms. For example, decreases in cardiac output produced by anesthetics may actually tend to enhance the effectiveness of HPV and offset concurrent direct inhibition.

Respiratory gases

Responses to increases in $Pa{CO_2}$ and $Pa{O_2}$ can be difficult to predict, as both local and systemic factors interact. However, in general, both produce vasodilatation within physiologic ranges in most vascular beds. Carbon dioxide response is particularly notable in the cerebral vasculature, and oxygen response is most notable in the coronary vasculature. Chronic inhaled oxygen therapy has been shown to reverse or at least impede progressive worsening of pulmonary hypertension in patients who suffer from hypoxia – inducing lung diseases such as COPD. Oxygen is a drug with a definite therapeutic window. Too little oxygen in the inspired mixture, or too low an inspired partial pressure ($P{IO_2}$) as may occur at high altitude, results in pulmonary hypertension via HPV, and ultimately in tissue hypoxia. High values of $P{IO_2}$ are directly toxic to the lung parenchyma, as can occur when breathing concentrated oxygen for prolonged periods, or when breathing room air under hyperbaric conditions. High oxygen concentrations overwhelm normal antioxidant defense mechanisms, such as superoxide dismutase, glutathione peroxidase, and catalase, and render tissues susceptible to damage by free radicals such as superoxide, hydroxyl, and singlet oxygen. Although hyperoxia is toxic to all tissue beds, the respiratory system is most at risk because of its exposure to the highest concentrations, and it manifests symptoms and histologic changes after as little as 6 hours of exposure to 100% oxygen at 759mmHg (101kPa). Ultimately, with continued exposure these changes result in systemic hypoxemia as they disrupt efficient gas exchange. Although the best way to decrease the risk of toxicity is to limit inspired oxygen concentration to the minimum concentration beyond the 21% found in room air needed to prevent evidence of tissue hypoxia, it is generally considered safe to provide 50–60% oxygen concentrations for prolonged periods of time.

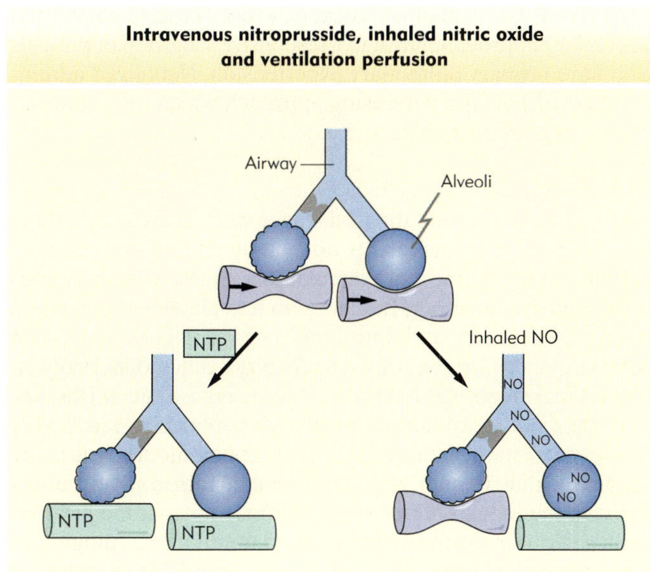

Figure 47.6 Effects of intravenous NTP and inhaled nitric oxide (NO) on ventilation perfusion matching. Two alveoli are shown with accompanying pulmonary capillaries, one with normal ventilation and one with no ventilation because of airway obstruction or atelectasis; nitroprusside (NTP) dilates all pulmonary arteries, which may worsen mismatching of ventilation to perfusion; nitric oxide dilates only arteries associated with ventilated alveoli, which may improve matching of ventilation to perfusion. (Adapted with permission from Lunn RJ. Inhaled nitric oxide therapy. Mayo Clin Proc. 1995.)

Vasodilators

Systemically administered vasodilators, such as the nitrovasodilators, β_1-agonists, Ca^{2+} channel antagonists, or prostacyclin (PGI_2), produce a response in all vascular beds, including the pulmonary vasculature. Unfortunately, all currently available intravenously administered agents tested in dose ranges sufficient to reduce pulmonary pressure result in systemic vasodilatation and hypotension to a degree that renders their use problematic. In addition, intravenous vasodilators such as nitroprusside (NTP), PGI_2, PGE_1, or isoproterenol interfere with HPV to increase venous admixture and further worsen arterial hypoxemia. As a consequence, systemic therapy has little role in the therapy of pulmonary hypertension, except perhaps for the Ca^{2+} channel blockers, which (despite interfering with HPV) improve survival in a responsive subgroup of patients who have primary pulmonary hypertension. Nebulized administration of PGs is a promising approach which may confer a degree of pulmonary selectivity.

Nitric oxide

Nitric oxide is a vasodilating substance with an extremely short half-life, and is principally produced by endothelial cells. In addition to regulating local vascular tone, nitric oxide regulates several other physiologic functions such as platelet aggregation, neurotransmission, and antitumor and antimicrobial activity. Nitric oxide diffuses out of the endothelial cell and into adjoining vascular smooth muscle cells, causing relaxation and vasodilatation via the cyclic guanosine monophosphate (cGMP) messenger system (Chapter 3). The short half-life of nitric oxide (approximately 100ms), and therefore the limitation of its effect to the immediate locale of its formation from arginine by nitric oxide synthesis, results from its rapid binding to hemoglobin. The nitrovasodilators NTP and nitroglycerin (NTG) act by the release of nitric oxide through spontaneous chemical breakdown, although other mechanisms of action may also be important. That NTP is a more potent arteriolar vasodilator and NTG a more potent venodilator most likely reflects regional differences in the uptake or breakdown of these drugs, with subsequent release of nitric oxide.

Inhaled nitric oxide therapy has been advocated as a method to produce selective pulmonary vasodilatation to treat pulmonary hypertension. Although toxic in higher concentrations, inhaled nitric oxide in a concentration range of 60ppb to 60ppm (cigarette smoke contains up to 1000ppm) results in selective pulmonary vasodilatation with minimal systemic vasodilatation. A possible additional benefit of the inhalation route is that nitric oxide is delivered directly to those vascular beds that provide flow to those lung regions that are best ventilated, and therefore does not worsen venous admixture and arterial hypoxemia as do intravenously administered agents (see Fig. 47.6). Nitric oxide has proved useful in improving gas exchange or pulmonary artery pressures in neonates after correction of cardiac anomalies, in persistent pulmonary hypertension of the newborn, and in acute respiratory distress syndrome. Randomized, controlled clinical trials are underway to determine whether inhaled nitric oxide improves outcome or merely improves physiologic parameters such as Pa_{O_2} in the short term.

In summary, many anesthetics and adjuvants have significant effects on the respiratory system. Some of these, such as profound depression of respiratory muscle function, may require active intervention by the anesthesia practitioner, while others, such as bronchodilatation, are fortuitously quite beneficial. Several promising new therapies, such as leukotriene antagonists and inhaled nitric oxide, may soon become integrated into the therapeutic armamentarium.

Key References

Drummond GB. Upper airway reflexes. Br J Anaesth. 1993;70:121–3.

Froese AB, Bryan AC. Effects of anesthesia and paralysis on diaphragmatic mechanics in man. Anesthesiology. 1974;41:242–55.

Greenberger PA. Corticosteroids in asthma. Rationale, use, and problems. Chest. 1992;101:418–21.

Pizov R, Brown RH, Weiss YS, et al. Wheezing during induction of general anesthesia in patients with and without asthma. Anesthesiology. 1995;82:1111–16.

Nandi PR, Charlesworth CH, Taylor SJ, Nunn JF, Doré CJ. Effect of general anaesthesia on the pharynx. Br J Anaesth. 1991;66:157–62.

Warner DO, Warner MA, Ritman EL. Atelectasis and chest wall shape during halothane anesthesia. Anesthesiology. 1996;84:309–21.

Westbrook PR, Stubbs SE, Sessler AD, Rehder K, Hyatt RE. Effects of anesthesia and muscle paralysis on respiratory mechanics in normal man. J Appl Physiol. 1973;34:81–6.

Further Reading

Barnes PJ. Modulation of neurotransmission in airways. Physiol Rev. 1992;72:699–729.

Gal TJ. Bronchial hyperresponsiveness and anesthesia: physiologic and therapeutic perspectives. Anesth Analg. 1994;78:559–73.

Iscoe SD. Central control of the upper airway. In: Mathew OP, Sant'Ambrogio G, eds. Respiratory function of the upper airway. New York: Marcel Dekker, Inc; 1988:125–92.

Lunn RJ. Inhaled nitric oxide therapy. Mayo Clin Proc. 1995;70:247–55.

Warner DO. Airway pharmacology. In: Benumof J, ed. Airway management: principles and practice. St Louis: Mosby–Yearbook; 1995:74–101.

Zapol WM, Bloch KD. Nitric oxide and the lung. New York: Dekker; 1997.

Chapter 48 Hypoxia and oxygen therapy

Brett A Simon

Topics covered in this chapter

Physiology of hypoxemia
Postoperative hypoxemia
Oxygen therapy
Extrapulmonary oxygenation
Hyperbaric oxygen therapy
Oxygen toxicity

Hypoxia is a life-threatening condition in which O_2 delivery is inadequate to meet the metabolic demands of the tissues. Since O_2 delivery is the product of blood flow and O_2 content, hypoxia may result from decreased tissue perfusion (low cardiac output, vascular occlusion), decreased O_2 tension in the blood (hypoxemia), or decreased O_2-carrying capacity (anemia, carbon monoxide poisoning, hemoglobinopathy). In addition, hypoxia may result from a problem in O_2 transport from the microvasculature to the cells (interstitial edema, microvascular injury) or in utilization within the cell (cyanide toxicity). No matter what the cause, an inadequate supply of O_2 ultimately results in the cessation of aerobic metabolism and oxidative phosphorylation, depletion of high-energy compounds, cellular dysfunction, and death. The time course of cellular demise depends on the relative metabolic demands, O_2-storage capacity, and anaerobic capacity of the individual organs. Survival times (the time from the onset of circulatory arrest to significant organ dysfunction) range from 1 minute in the cerebral cortex to approximately 5 minutes in the heart and 10 minutes in the liver and kidneys, while revival times (the duration of anoxia beyond which recovery is no longer possible) are roughly four or five times longer.

This chapter focuses on the pathophysiology of hypoxemia, with special emphasis on perioperative hypoxemia and the therapeutic use of O_2 as treatment. Conventional O_2 therapy is discussed, as well as the indications and principles behind the use of less-common therapies such as heliox, extracorporeal membrane oxygenation (ECMO), the intravascular oxygenator (IVOX), and hyperbaric O_2. Finally, issues that limit the use of high concentrations of O_2 because of toxicity are covered.

PHYSIOLOGY OF HYPOXEMIA

Pulmonary mechanisms of hypoxemia

Hypoxemia generally implies a failure of the respiratory system to oxygenate arterial blood. Classically there are five causes of hypoxemia: low inspired O_2 fraction (F_{IO_2}), increased diffusion barrier, hypoventilation, ventilation/perfusion ($\dot{V}/\dot{Q}$) mismatch, and shunt or venous admixture. The physiology of these mechanisms is discussed in detail in Chapters 45 and 46 and is reviewed here briefly in order to rationalize approaches to O_2 therapy.

Low F_{IO_2} is a cause of hypoxemia only at altitude or in the event of equipment failure (e.g. a mislabeled gas tank or line, or gas blender malfunction). An increase in the barrier to diffusion of O_2 within the lung also rarely causes hypoxemia in a resting patient except in end-stage parenchymal lung disease. Both of these problems may be alleviated with administration of supplemental O_2, the former by definition and the latter by increasing the gradient driving diffusion.

Hypoventilation causes hypoxemia by reducing the alveolar partial pressure of O_2 (P_{AO_2}) in proportion to the build-up of CO_2 (P_{ACO_2}) in the alveoli, as described by the relationship between alveolar ventilation ($\dot{V}_A$) and P_{ACO_2} (Equation 48.1) and in the alveolar gas equation (Equation 48.2, approximation assuming the inspired partial pressure of CO_2 is zero):

Equation 48.1

$$P_{ACO_2} = K\left(\frac{\dot{V}_{CO_2}}{\dot{V}_A}\right)$$

Equation 48.2

$$P_{AO_2} = P_{IO_2} - \frac{P_{ACO_2}}{R}$$

where $\dot{V}_{CO_2}$ is the CO_2 production, P_{IO_2} the partial pressure of O_2 in the inspired gas, R the respiratory exchange ratio, and K a proportionality constant. In essence, during hypoventilation there is decreased delivery of O_2 to the alveoli while its removal by the blood remains the same; this causes its alveolar concentration to fall. The opposite occurs with CO_2. Or more quantitatively, with hypoventilation $\dot{V}_A$ falls and the P_{ACO_2} rises (Equation 48.1); as a result the P_{AO_2} falls (Equation 48.2). Under normal conditions breathing room air at sea level (corrected for the partial pressure of water vapor), the P_{IO_2} is about 150mmHg (20kPa), the P_{ACO_2} about 40mmHg (5.3kPa), R is 0.8, and, therefore, the P_{AO_2} is normally around 100mmHg (13.3kPa). It would require substantial hypoventilation, with the P_{ACO_2} rising to over 70mmHg, for the P_{AO_2} to fall below 60mmHg. This cause of hypoxemia is readily prevented by administration of even small amounts of supplemental O_2.

Shunt and $\dot{V}/\dot{Q}$ mismatch are related causes of hypoxemia, but with an important distinction in their responses to supplemental O_2. As discussed in Chapter 45, optimal gas exchange occurs when blood flow and ventilation are quantitatively matched. As ventilation increases relative to blood flow, the P_{AO_2} increases, but because of the shape of the oxyhemoglobin dissociation curve (see Chapter 45), increasing P_{AO_2} beyond a certain level does not contribute much to the O_2 content of the blood. In addition, lung regions with a high $\dot{V}/\dot{Q}$ have a relatively diminished blood flow, the extreme being regions of pure deadspace, which contribute nothing to the oxygenation of the blood while decreasing the efficiency of CO_2 removal. Conversely, in regions with a low $\dot{V}/\dot{Q}$, perfusion is increased relative to ventilation, and the Pa_{O_2} of the blood leaving these regions is low relative to regions with better matched $\dot{V}/\dot{Q}$. Since at these lower P_{O_2} values the oxyhemoglobin dissociation curve is steep, the O_2 saturation and content of blood leaving these regions falls significantly. At extremely low values for $\dot{V}/\dot{Q}$, there is no ventilation to a perfused region and pure shunt results; the blood leaving the region has the same low P_{O_2} and high P_{CO_2} as mixed venous blood. Thus, regions of high $\dot{V}/\dot{Q}$ do little to improve oxygenation while areas of low $\dot{V}/\dot{Q}$ have a disproportionate effect on reducing arterial oxygenation.

The deleterious effect of $\dot{V}/\dot{Q}$ mismatch on arterial S_{O_2} (Sa_{O_2}) is thus a result of the asymmetry of the oxyhemoglobin dissociation curve. Adding supplemental O_2 will generally make up for the fall in P_{AO_2} in low $\dot{V}/\dot{Q}$ units and thus improve P_{AO_2}. However, since there is no ventilation to units with pure shunt, supplemental O_2 will not be effective in reversing the hypoxemia from this cause. Because of the steep oxyhemoglobin dissociation curve at low P_{O_2}, even moderate amounts of pure shunt will cause significant hypoxemia despite O_2 therapy (Fig. 48.1). For the same reason, factors that decrease mixed venous P_{O_2}, such as decreased cardiac output or increased O_2 consumption, enhance the effects of $\dot{V}/\dot{Q}$ mismatch and shunt in causing hypoxemia.

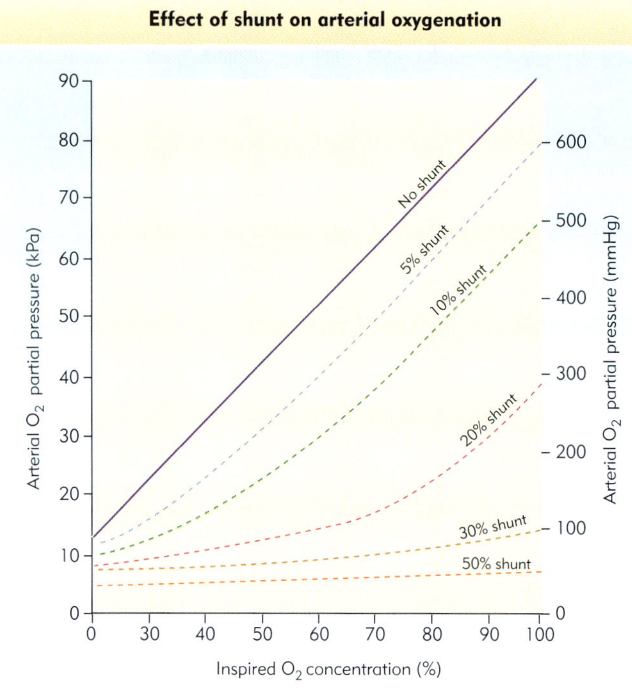

Figure 48.1 The effect of shunt on arterial oxygenation. The effect of increasing degrees of pure shunt on arterial O_2 partial pressure (P_{O_2}) as a function of the inspired O_2 concentration. (With permission from Nunn, 1993.)

Nonpulmonary causes of hypoxia

In addition to failure of the lungs to oxygenate blood adequately (hypoxic hypoxia), there are a number of other factors that can contribute to hypoxia at the tissue level. These may broadly be divided into categories of O_2 delivery and O_2 utilization. Oxygen delivery decreases globally when cardiac output falls or locally when regional blood flow is compromised (stagnant hypoxia), as from a vascular occlusion (stenosis, thrombosis, microvascular occlusion) or increased downstream pressure to flow (compartment syndrome, venous stasis, or venous hypertension). Decreased O_2-carrying capacity of the blood will likewise decrease O_2 delivery, as occurs with anemia (anemic hypoxia), carbon monoxide poisoning, or hemoglobinopathy. Finally, in unusual situations, hypoxia may occur when transport of O_2 from the capillaries to the tissues is decreased (edema) or when utilization of O_2 by the cells is impaired (cyanide toxicity) (histotoxic hypoxia).

POSTOPERATIVE HYPOXEMIA

Postoperative hypoxemia is a common form of hypoxemia of particular interest to anesthesiologists. Hypoxemia is typically defined as an Sa_{O_2} of 90% or below, measured by pulse oximetry, and lasting for a specified amount of time, usually greater than 30 seconds or 1 minute. If Sa_{O_2} falls below 85%, this is termed severe hypoxemia. In the mid-1970s, it became apparent that certain patients recovering from anesthesia were prone to develop unrecognized hypoxemia. With the advent of continuous pulse oximetry in the early 1980s, it was found that postoperative hypoxemia was far more frequent than previously suspected. Depending on the patient population, age, and type of surgery, Sa_{O_2} values below 90% were found to occur in 35–60% of patients in the immediate postoperative period, of which 12–22% experienced severe hypoxemic episodes. This observation prompted the routine use of supplemental O_2 for all postoperative patients. Of note, several later studies still found a significant incidence of hypoxemia in postoperative patients despite supplemental O_2 therapy, a finding thought to be related to the lack of efficacy of some modes of O_2 supplementation.

Risk factors that predispose patients to developing postoperative hypoxemia include obesity, smoking, pre-existing heart and lung disease, and the extremes of age. Incidence is higher after general than after regional anesthesia. Of particular importance is the site of the operation, with thoracic and high abdominal incisions associated with hypoxemia as well as increased risk of respiratory complications in general. In fact, there is a significantly increased incidence of hypoxemic episodes on the second postoperative night in patients having undergone abdominal surgery compared with those having had middle-ear surgery. Finally, as might be expected, a low initial Sa_{O_2} on admission to the postanesthesia care unit (PACU) is a strong risk factor for subsequent desaturations.

Mechanisms of postoperative hypoxemia

There are a number of reasons why patients are at risk of desaturation in the immediate postoperative period. First, there is a reduction in functional residual capacity (FRC), with resultant atelectasis and increased shunting, that persists into the postoperative period. FRC falls as a result of decreased chest wall recoil with muscle relaxation and anesthesia, an effect compounded by the use of 100% O_2 and absorption atelectasis. Second, decreased clearance of secretions, whether because pain prevents deep breathing and coughing or from decreased mucociliary clearance (owing to airway drying, the presence of the endotracheal tube, and anesthetic effects), compounds this effect. Third, increased O_2 consumption during shivering can reduce mixed venous PO_2, contributing to hypoxemia from shunt and $\dot{V}/\dot{Q}$ mismatch. Fourth, inhibition of hypoxic pulmonary vasoconstriction by inhalation anesthetics may contribute to increased shunting and poor $\dot{V}/\dot{Q}$ matching.

In addition, a number of factors contribute to postoperative hypoventilation. Residual anesthetic effects depress respiratory drive and the ventilatory responses to hypoxia and hypercarbia. Residual muscle weakness further contributes to hypoventilation and to an inability to overcome mild airway obstruction. Pain control is important at both extremes: inadequate pain control can inhibit adequate tidal volumes and coughing, while excessive opioid effects depress ventilatory drive. Depletion of total body CO_2 stores from prolonged intraoperative hyperventilation can also exacerbate postoperative hypoventilation.

Finally, diffusion hypoxia, in which the rapid diffusion of nitrous oxide from pulmonary capillary blood into the alveolar compartment dilutes and reduces the partial pressures of O_2 and CO_2, can also contribute to hypoxemia during and immediately after emergence.

Supplemental oxygen in the postoperative period

The use of supplemental O_2 after extubation in the operating theater, during transport, and in the PACU has become routine in recent years. This practice is rationally based on the frequent occurrence of desaturation during this time, the minimal cost, and the perceived harmlessness of O_2 administration. Most of the causes of hypoxemia discussed above are counteracted by supplemental O_2. However, it should be remembered that desaturation can still occur despite O_2 administration. Furthermore, when supplemental O_2 is administered, desaturation occurs at a later time after airways obstruction or hypoventilation, potentially delaying the detection of these critical events. Therefore, whether or not O_2 is administered in the immediate postoperative period, it is essential that both O_2 saturation and adequacy of ventilation be frequently assessed.

OXYGEN THERAPY

The goal of O_2 therapy is to increase PaO_2 or SaO_2 to an appropriate level. In some situations, such as in the immediate postoperative period, this may be simply greater than some minimal value, typically SaO_2 greater than 90%. In other situations, such as in the rare patient with severe chronic obstructive pulmonary disease (COPD) who is dependent upon hypoxic ventilatory drive, it may be necessary to control the FIO_2 more precisely. In patients with impending respiratory failure, it may be necessary to deliver as high an FIO_2 as possible. Consequently, it is important to understand the advantages and limitations of the different O_2 delivery devices available.

Only a closed system with an airtight seal to the patient's airway and complete separation of inspired and expired gases, such as an anesthesia circuit or mechanical ventilator, can precisely control the FIO_2. In other systems, the actual delivered FIO_2 will vary with the ventilatory pattern (rate, tidal volume, inspiration to expiration ratio, inspiratory flow) to varying degrees. Low-flow systems have a limited ability to raise the FIO_2 because they depend on entrained room air to make up the balance of the tidal volume, diluting the inspired O_2. As a result, the FIO_2 delivered by these systems is extremely sensitive to small changes in ventilatory pattern. Deep, slow breathing entrains more room air and lowers the FIO_2, while shallow breathing entrains less, with resultant higher FIO_2. High-flow devices attempt to deliver the entire inspired volume at a controlled FIO_2, either by utilizing a reservoir from which the inspired gas may be drawn on demand or by providing a flow rate in excess of that of the patient. While these systems are better able to control the FIO_2 with different ventilatory patterns, they are still subject to departure from the desired delivered FIO_2. Therefore, in any patient where oxygenation is marginal or close control is required, it is important to monitor arterial O_2 saturation by pulse oximetry or frequent arterial blood gas analysis.

Administration of supplemental O_2 is not without potential complications. High flows of dry O_2 can dry out and irritate mucosal surfaces of the airway and the eyes, as well as decrease mucociliary transport and clearance of secretions. Humidified O_2 should, therefore, be used when therapy for more than 1 hour is required. High O_2 concentrations delivered to poorly ventilated lung regions can promote absorption atelectasis, occasionally resulting in a worsening of shunt and a paradoxical worsening of hypoxemia after a period of O_2 supplementation. It can also mask the consequences of postanesthetic hypoventilation, as discussed above. Any O_2-enriched atmosphere constitutes a fire hazard, and appropriate precautions must be taken in the operating theater, during local/sedation procedures, and for patients on O_2 at home. Finally, in a small group of patients with severe COPD who are dependent on hypoxic ventilatory drive, the provision of too much O_2 can depress this drive and result in hypoventilation. In these cases, supplemental O_2 should be carefully titrated to ensure adequate arterial saturation. If hypoventilation results, then mechanical ventilatory support with or without tracheal intubation should be provided.

Oxygen-delivery systems

Low-flow devices

Devices such as face tents are primarily used for delivering humidified gases to patients and cannot be relied upon for delivery of predictable amounts of supplemental O_2. Nasal cannulae or nasal prongs are twin flexible prongs that sit just inside each naris and deliver 100% O_2 at rates of 1–6L/min. The nasopharynx acts as a reservoir for storing the O_2, and patients may breathe through either their mouth or nose as long as the nasal passages remain patent. Variations in the system exist that allow gas sampling for end-tidal CO_2 monitoring through one prong. This apparatus is simple, comfortable, well tolerated by most patients, and can deliver upwards of 40% FIO_2 under ideal conditions and a flow of 6L/min, although 24–28% would be more typical at 2–3L/min. Higher flow rates are poorly tolerated for more than brief periods because of mucosal drying.

The simple face mask, a clear plastic mask with side holes to allow inspiratory air entrainment and clearance of exhaled gas, is commonly used at flow rates of 6–15L/min in situations when higher concentrations of O_2 without tight control are desired, such as during transport to the PACU after general anesthesia. The tracheostomy mask is similar in principle.

The maximum F_{IO_2} of a face mask may be increased from around 60% to greater than 85% by adding a 600–1000mL reservoir bag, as in a partial rebreathing mask. This device requires O_2 flows of 6–15L/min to prevent the reservoir bag from completely deflating (which would allow entrainment of room air around the edges of the mask) and to flush CO_2 out of the mask. It receives its name because the initial portion of the expiration is captured in the reservoir bag and is rebreathed on the subsequent breath. This rebreathed volume comes mainly from the patient's deadspace and, therefore, contains minimal CO_2. Finally, the T-piece, which is connected to an endotracheal or tracheostomy tube and blows O_2 at low flow rates (4–15L/min) past the tube opening and through a length of expiratory tubing, also relies on the volume of this expiratory tubing to act as a reservoir to provide O_2-enriched gas for the next inspiration. The maximum F_{IO_2} depends on the volume of the expiratory reservoir relative to the tidal volume as well as on the flow rate. It is important that adequate flow rates be used with these devices to prevent significant rebreathing of CO_2. Figure 48.2 presents some actual delivered tracheal O_2 concentrations for several commonly used O_2-delivery devices.

High-flow devices

The most commonly used high-flow O_2-delivery devices employ the Venturi principle (Fig. 48.3a). These devices utilize specially designed mask inserts that reliably entrain room air in a fixed ratio to provide a relatively constant F_{IO_2} at specified flow rates. Lower delivered F_{IO_2} values use greater entrainment ratios, resulting in higher total (O_2 plus entrained air) flows to the patient, ranging from 105L/min for 24% F_{IO_2} to 32L/min at 50% F_{IO_2}. While these flow rates are much higher than those obtained with low-flow devices, they may still be lower than the peak inspiratory flows for patients in respiratory distress and, therefore, the actual delivered O_2 concentration may be lower than the nominal value. Oxygen nebulizers are another type of Venturi device that provide patients with humidified O_2 at 35–100% F_{IO_2} at high flow rates. Again, the patient may still entrain room air with these devices when their minute ventilation is abnormally high.

Oxygen blenders provide high inspired O_2 concentrations at very high flow rates. These devices mix high-pressure compressed air and O_2 to achieve any concentration of O_2 from 21 to 100% at flow rates of up to 100L/min. These same blenders are used to control F_{IO_2} for ventilators, continuous positive airway pressure/biphasic positive airway pressure (CPAP/BiPAP) machines, oxygenators, and other devices with similar requirements. Despite the high flows, the delivery of high F_{IO_2} to an individual patient also depends on maintaining a tight fitting seal to the airway and/or the use of reservoirs to minimize entrainment of diluting room air.

Transtracheal oxygen delivery

In recent years, the use of continuous transtracheal delivery of low flows of O_2 via a minitracheostomy has gained considerable popularity for patients with chronic lung disease, particularly COPD. In addition to reducing O_2 requirements and increasing comfort and convenience for these patients, it has been found that there is also a significant decrease in the inspired minute ventilation for patients, achieved through a reduction in tidal volume at the same respiratory rate. This decrease, and the resultant fall in the work of breathing and increased exercise tolerance, are independent of the Sa_{O_2} and are also found when air is administered in the same manner. Most likely, this improvement is achieved via reduction in the anatomic deadspace, with the tracheal administered flow washing the exhaled gas out of the trachea and providing fresh gas for the next breath.

Estimated inspired O_2 fraction (FIO_2) with low-flow O_2 delivery systems

System	Flow (L/min)	FIO_2
Nasal cannula	1	0.24
	2	0.28
	3	0.32
	4	0.36
	5	0.40
	6	0.44
Mask		
Simple	≥5	0.40±0.60
Partial rebreathing	≥8	≥0.60
Non-rebreathing	≥10	≥0.80

Figure 48.2 Estimated inspired O_2 fraction (F_{IO_2}) with low-flow O_2-delivery systems. Values are based on quiet breathing with tidal volume 500mL, rate 20 breaths/min, inspiratory time 1 second, and an anatomic reservoir of 50mL. (With permission from Kacmarek and Stoller, 1995.)

Continuous positive airway pressure/biphasic positive airway pressure devices and noninvasive ventilation

The CPAP technique was initially used in spontaneously breathing intubated patients to overcome the additional work of breathing imposed by a narrow endotracheal tube as well as to maintain and recruit lung volume to improve oxygenation in the same manner that positive end-expiratory pressure (PEEP) does in mechanically ventilated patients. This approach was successfully extended to nonintubated patients via the use of tight-fitting nasal or full face masks. By adding a second, higher level of pressure support synchronized to the respiratory cycle (BiPAP), nonintubated patients can receive the equivalent of a moderate level of pressure support ventilation. The F_{IO_2} is controlled by use of an O_2 blender, or room air may be used. Conventional ventilators in pressure support/PEEP mode may also be used to control F_{IO_2}. These devices improve both oxygenation, through increased F_{IO_2} and recruitment of lung volume (reduction of shunt), and ventilation, by providing pressure support during inspiration. These techniques can be used to avoid intubation and mechanical ventilation in patients with acute respiratory decompensation while treatment of the underlying cause is undertaken, or to provide intermittent rest to patients prone to respiratory muscle fatigue, such as those with myasthenia gravis or other neuromuscular disorders. In addition, BiPAP has been very useful in maintaining airway patency at night in patients with obstructive sleep apnea.

The Venturi principle

a

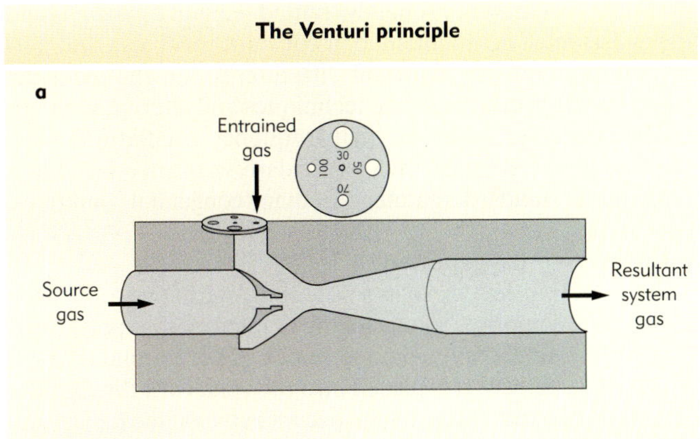

b

Nominal inspired O_2 fraction (FIO_2) (%)	O_2 flow (L/min)	Approximate O_2:air ratio	Total flow to patient (L/min)
24	4	1:25.3	105
28	6	1:10.33	68
31	8	1:6.9	63
35	10	1:4.6	56
40	12	1:3.2	50
50	12	1:1.67	32

Oxygen dilution accuracy ±5% for each manufacturer. Data for the Baxter Airlife Percent O_2 Mask (adult).

Figure 48.3 The Venturi principle. (a) In the Venturi device, the gas source, usually O_2, provides the driving flow. The resultant system gas is a mixture of the source gas and the entrained gas, and its flow rate is the sum of the source gas and the entrained gas flow rates. Many devices operating on the Venturi principle permit selection of the resultant FIO_2 by adjustment of a variable orifice that limits inflow of the entrained gas. (b) The nominal O_2 dilution in the Venturi device is given in the table. [(a) With permission from Kaplan, 1983; (b) with permission from Baxter Healthcare Corp.)].

Heliox

In acute severe airway obstruction, the use of a mixture of helium and O_2 (heliox) to reduce airways resistance, decrease work of breathing, and improve ventilation through increased airflow may be lifesaving until definitive treatment can take effect. Airflow through the larynx and trachea is generally turbulent, as described by the Reynolds' number for flow through a pipe:

$$Re = \frac{(\rho d v)}{\eta}$$

where ρ is density, d is diameter, v is velocity, and η is viscosity. As the dimensionless parameter Re increases, so does the likelihood and intensity of turbulent flow. Flow through a narrow orifice, such as a glottis obstructed by a tumor, increases greatly in velocity and tends to create a jet. Both the increased velocity and the jet tend to increase the turbulence in the flow. In contrast to laminar flow, where pressure drop is proportional to the flow rate and the viscosity of the gas, the pressure drop in turbulent flow is proportional to the square of the flow rate and the gas density. Therefore, for the same flow rate, turbulence greatly increases the pressure that the patient must generate to produce that flow. By changing from air to heliox, a mixture with one-third the density of air, both the Re (and thus the amount of turbulence) and the pressure drop required to support the flow are decreased, allowing increased air flow, decreased work of breathing, and improved ventilation. One drawback to the use of heliox, which usually comes premixed as 79% helium and 21% O_2, is that it limits the FIO_2 since a high concentration of helium must be used in order for there to be a significant effect. Heliox administration may be a useful temporizing measure for acute obstruction of the larynx or large airways while awaiting definitive treatment (surgery, irradiation, reduced swelling) and may be used in the operating theater to facilitate airway management. In addition, heliox has been used successfully to avoid intubation in patients with severe asthma while awaiting the effect of pharmacologic treatment.

EXTRAPULMONARY OXYGENATION

In severe respiratory failure, when high levels of PEEP and peak inspiratory volume are required to support oxygenation and ventilation, furthering of lung injury caused by the extreme mechanical stresses of artificial ventilation becomes a significant factor in the downward spiral of the critically ill patient. Attempts have been made, therefore, to supplement or completely bypass the gas-exchanging functions of the lung through artificial means. The strategy is to support gas exchange partially or completely, reduce or eliminate mechanical ventilatory support, and allow the underlying pathophysiologic process [pneumonia, adult respiratory distress syndrome (ARDS)] to improve or stabilize until other treatment is feasible (surgical correction of congenital heart disease, heart and/or lung transplantation).

Extracorporeal membrane oxygenation/gas exchange

Extracorporeal membrane oxygenation (ECMO) or extracorporeal gas exchange (ECGE) refers to the pumping of blood through an external gas-exchanging device. In one approach veno-venous ECMO/ECGE is utilized, in which blood is withdrawn from the central venous circulation, passed through an oxygenator (which removes CO_2 as well), and returned back to the right atrium whereupon the heart pumps the blood through the pulmonary and systemic circulations. Typically, the lung is ventilated gently with O_2 or an O_2/CO_2 mixture to maintain normal arterial blood gases. Alternatively, veno-arterial bypass, in which the blood is returned to the systemic circulation, and complete 'lung rest' with either static inflation or minimal ventilation may be used.

ECMO was introduced for severe neonatal respiratory failure in the 1970s and became standard care in the mid-1980s. Initial experience with adult veno-arterial ECMO in the late 1970s, however, was discouraging. Changing the approach to veno-venous bypass, with the intention of using ECMO primarily for CO_2 removal and utilizing low-level ventilation of the lungs for oxygenation, significantly improved the outcome for pediatric and adult patients. While ECMO may be lifesaving, its use involves significant risks as well as the application of significant resources. Intravascular access may be difficult, requiring sacrifice of the jugular vein and carotid artery on one side in neonates. Systemic anticoagulation with heparin is required, and bleeding complications and the need to transfuse blood oxygenation in poorly perfused or injured regions. By improving local tissue hypoxia through vasodilatation, increased diffusive flux of O_2, and stimulation of angiogenesis, oxygen free radical-mediated bacterial killing by neutrophils and other phagocytic defenses are enhanced. Hyperbaric O_2 itself is bactericidal for certain anaerobic strains including *Clostridium perfringens,* the agent responsible for gas gangrene. Tissue ischemia promotes the adherence of neutrophils to blood vessel walls with release of proteases and free radicals, causing local tissue destruction; it also inhibits the collagen matrix formation required for wound healing. Both of these effects are reduced with hyperbaric therapy. Finally, hyperbaric O_2 competes with carbon monoxide for binding to both hemoglobin and intracellular metabolic enzymes, reducing the half-life of carboxyhemoglobin from 4–5 hours to approximately 20 minutes at 2.5atm and improving cellular respiratory function.

Indications and use

Administration of hyperbaric O_2 requires the subject to be completely enclosed in a pressurized chamber. The most common device for this purpose is the monoplace chamber, typically a clear acrylic cylinder just large enough to hold a single supine patient. The chamber is pressurized with 100% O_2 and the patient breathes the O_2 freely. The chamber is equipped with access hatches and an intercom for communication. Less common and more elaborate is the multiplace chamber, a free-standing pressurized metal 'room' that can contain several patients as well as medical or technical staff simultaneously. These larger chambers are pressurized with air, and patients breathe 100% O_2 via a mask, hood, or endotracheal tube; critically ill, mechanically ventilated patients requiring close medical monitoring can be accommodated. Single treatment durations range from 45 minutes for carbon monoxide poisoning to up to 5 hours for severe decompression disorders. Chronic therapies, such as for problems with wounds or radiation necrosis, may require 20–30 90-minute sessions over days to weeks. A list of conditions for which hyperbaric O_2 therapy is considered potentially helpful is presented in Figure 48.4. Pure O_2, particularly at superatmospheric pressures, is highly flammable and constitutes a significant fire and explosion hazard.

OXYGEN TOXICITY

Oxygen should be considered to be a drug and the benefits of its administration must be balanced against its risks, primarily toxicity. The mechanism responsible for several aspects of O_2 toxicity involves the formation of highly reactive O_2-derived species that damage cellular structures. These substances include singlet oxygen (O), the superoxide free radical ($O_2^{\bullet -}$), the hydroxyl free radical ($OH^{\bullet}$), and the powerful oxidizing agent hydrogen peroxide (H_2O_2). These substances are naturally occurring and are produced by neutrophils and macrophages for intracellular killing of parasites and other infectious agents. Natural defenses occur in the form of enzymes (such as superoxide dismutase, catalase, and various peroxidases) that rapidly remove or inactivate small amounts of these compounds. However, these reactive species may also be inappropriately generated under conditions of ischemia/reperfusion, in response to ionizing radiation, and by activation of marginating neutrophils during infection and injury. The rate of production is greater when the O_2 concentration is increased, and the body's natural defenses may be overwhelmed. These O_2-

products are common. A highly trained team of physicians and therapists must be maintained in constant readiness, and personnel must be in constant attendance at the bedside. Improvements in critical care techniques and alternative ventilatory strategies (such as high-frequency oscillation) have reduced the need for ECMO, particularly in the neonate, but it remains the standard treatment for many congenital conditions.

Intravascular oxygenation

The IVOX was developed as a potential alternative to ECMO. This device comprises a long bundle of microporous polypropylene hollow fibers and a double-lumen gas feed tube through which O_2 is passed. It is placed into the vena cava through the femoral vein, and gas exchange occurs between the device and the venous blood flow returning to the heart. Systemic heparinization is required. It is capable of transporting 40–70mL/min O_2 and CO_2 depending on the device size, which represents around 25% of basal gas-exchange requirements. Its function is limited by the surface area available for gas exchange and the blood flow past the device; cardiac output tends to fall after placement and increased resistance from its presence in the inferior vena cava may cause blood to shunt around the device through collateral pathways. The ability of IVOX to improve oxygenation is inherently limited by the unfavorable diffusion gradient and nonlinear effect of shunt on arterial oxygenation. However, its ability to remove CO_2 increases with hypercapnia as a result of the increased gradient for diffusion, making it more effective in those situations where it is most needed.

In patients with severe ARDS, the IVOX is able to transfer measurable amounts of O_2 and CO_2 and reduce the intensity of mechanical ventilator support with a minimum of hemodynamic consequences. There is, however, a 25% incidence of IVOX-related complications, including blood loss, thrombotic events, device malfunctions, infection, hemodynamic instability, and vascular injuries. With improvements in heparin-bonded materials (which would reduce the need for anticoagulation) and gas-exchange efficiency, the IVOX may yet prove effective in enabling a reduction in the ventilatory support needed for patients with respiratory failure, particularly those with problems of ventilation and CO_2 removal rather than oxygenation.

HYPERBARIC OXYGEN THERAPY

Physiologic effects

The inhalation of 100% O_2 at 2–3atm results in PaO_2 tensions over 2000mmHg (267kPa) and tissue O_2 tensions up to 400mmHg (53kPa). The amount of O_2 dissolved in blood increases from 0.3mL/dL breathing ambient air at sea level, to 1.5mL/dL breathing 100% O_2, to approximately 6mL/dL breathing 100% O_2 at 3atm: an increase in carrying capacity capable of meeting resting metabolic demands without any contribution from hemoglobin-bound O_2. Hyperbaric O_2 treatment, by virtue of the exposure of the entire body to elevated pressure, reduces the size of inert gas bubbles in blood vessels and additionally hastens their dissolution by replacing the inert gas with O_2, which is metabolized by the tissues. This effect is the basis of the familiar hyperbaric therapy for decompression sickness ('the bends'), an affliction of divers who have ascended too rapidly, and for arterial air embolization.

In addition, hyperbaric O_2 has a number of biochemical and cellular effects, mostly related to improvement of local tissue

Indications for hyperbaric O_2 therapy

Disease for which the weight of scientific evidence supports hyperbaric oxygen as effective therapy

Primary therapy
- Arterial gas embolism
- Decompression sickness
- Exceptional blood-loss anemia
- Severe carbon monoxide poisoning

Adjunctive therapy
- Clostridial myonecrosis
- Compromised skin grafts and flaps
- Osteoradionecrosis prevention

Diseases for which the weight of scientific evidence suggests hyperbaric oxygen may be helpful

Primary therapy
- Less severe carbon monoxide poisoning

Adjunctive therapy
- Acute traumatic ischemic injury
- Osteoradionecrosis
- Refractory osteomyelitis
- Selected problem wounds
- Radiation-induced soft-tissue injury

Diseases for which the weight of scientific evidence does not support the use of hyperbaric oxygen, but for which it may be helpful

Adjunctive therapy
- Necrotizing fasciitis
- Thermal burns

Figure 48.4 Indications for hyperbaric O_2 therapy. (With permission from Tibbles and Edelsberg, 1996.)

derived reactive species cause cellular injury by directly damaging DNA and sulfhydryl-containing proteins and by lipid peroxidation. Protein damage occurs through the formation of disulfide bridges, which may inactivate important enzymes. In lipid peroxidation, a free radical interacts with an unsaturated fatty acid, disrupting the lipid molecule and generating another free radical in the process, thus causing a chain reaction. This process can disrupt cell membranes, particularly of the epithelial layer of the lung and digestive tract.

Pulmonary oxygen toxicity

The highest Po_2 in the body is found in the lung, which is consequently the organ most susceptible to O_2 toxicity. There are great species differences in the tolerance to high concentrations of O_2. An Fio_2 of 1.0 is fatal for most rats after about 3 days, while monkeys can survive for approximately 2 weeks and humans appear even more resistant. Animal studies reveal that the primary change seen in the lung is thinning and vacuolization of the alveolar epithelial lining, resulting in increased permeability and interstitial fluid accumulation. Later, large areas of epithelium are lost, accompanied by proliferation of type II alveolar cells, which are more resistant to injury. The combination of type II cell proliferation and interstitial fluid accumulation results in a greatly thickened alveolar/capillary membrane. This process is accelerated in the presence of compounds that can act as electron donors for the formation of reactive O_2 species, such as paraquat and the chemotherapeutic agent bleomycin.

In human volunteers breathing 100% O_2 at 1atm, the first symptoms of substernal distress occur after about 10 hours. Further exposure results in worsening distress, followed by occasional and then paroxysmal coughing, which is worsened by a deep breath. There is also a measurable decrease in vital capacity, which progresses as the duration of the exposure increases. The time to onset of symptoms appears to be related to the product of exposure time and Po_2, such that 10 hours at 1atm is equivalent to 5 hours at 2atm, and so on. Furthermore, it is the Po_2 and not the concentration of O_2 that matters, since astronauts exposed to 100% O_2 at 0.33atm for extended periods of time (Po_2 255mmHg) showed no signs of toxicity. Finally, there appears to be infinite tolerance to exposure to 0.5atm O_2. While the onset of symptoms in healthy volunteers does not necessarily relate to the production of cellular injury in patients, it provides the basis for the clinical guideline in which it is recommended that the Fio_2 is reduced to below 0.6 as soon as clinical conditions permit.

Oxygen convulsions and retrolental fibroplasia

In addition to pulmonary O_2 toxicity, O_2 convulsions and retrolental fibroplasia (RLF) in the neonate are important clinical conditions related to O_2 exposure. Oxygen convulsions are potentially fatal convulsions that may occur after exposure to O_2 at a partial pressure in excess of 2atm. The convulsions are thought to be related to a reduction in the concentration of the inhibitory neurotransmitter gamma-aminobutyric acid (GABA), possibly as a result of inactivation of sulfhydryl-containing enzymes by O_2 free radicals. RLF or retinopathy of prematurity is an abnormality of the peripheral retinal vessels that occurs mainly in premature infants when the immature retinal vascular bed has been exposed to high O_2 concentrations. Immature retinal vessels appear to be especially sensitive to elevated O_2, which may cause vasoconstriction and retinal hypoxia, although the exact duration or concentration of Pao_2 required for injury is unknown. If severe, neovascularization may occur that can invade the vitreous and cause retinal detachment. While cases of RLF have occurred in premature infants not exposed to high concentrations of O_2, there is increasing incidence with low birth weight (less than 1500g) and with exposure to O_2 concentrations greater than 30%.

Key References

Hall JB, Wood LDH. Oxygen therapy in the critically ill patient. In: Hall JB, Schmidt GA, Wood LDH, eds. Principles of critical care. New York: McGraw-Hill; 1992:165–80.

Hall JR. Techniques of ventilation and oxigenation. In: Kaplan JA, ed. Thoracic Anesthesia, 2nd edn. New York: Churchill Livingstone; 1983.

Nunn JF. Nunn's applied respiratory physiology, 4th edn. Boston, MA: Butterworth–Heinemann, 1993.

Tibbles PM, Edelsberg JS. Hyperbaric-oxygen therapy. N Engl J Med. 1996;334:1642–8.

Further Reading

Kacmarek RM, Stoller JK. Principles of respiratory care. In: Ayers SM, Grenvik A, Holbrook PR, Shoemaker WC, eds. Textbook of Critical Care, 3rd edn. Philadelphia, PA: Saunders;1995:688-9.

Ichiba S, Bartlett RH. Current status of extracorporeal membrane oxygenation for severe respiratory failure. Artif Organ. 1996;20:120–3.

Sim KM, Evans TW, Keogh BF. Clinical strategies in intravascular gas exchange. Artif Organ. 1996;20:807–10.

Chapter 49 Artificial ventilation

Peter J Papadakos

Topics covered in this chapter

Respiratory failure
Indications for mechanical ventilation
Adult respiratory distress syndrome
Modes of ventilation
Ventilator-associated lung injury
Weaning from mechanical ventilation

Artificial ventilatory support is one of the most widely used therapeutic techniques in anesthesiology and critical care. An essential keystone of cardiopulmonary resuscitation, it can be lifesaving during a variety of clinical situations, from routine operating room use to the support of a spectrum of acute and chronic disease states in the intensive-care unit (ICU).

These disease states may be localized to the lung or be systemic in nature. Only through a clear understanding of the mechanisms of respiratory failure and of the technology of ventilatory support can the practitioner properly apply artificial ventilation to the broad spectrum of patients who need it.

RESPIRATORY FAILURE

Mechanical ventilatory support should be instituted whenever a patient's ability to maintain gas exchange has failed. Respiratory failure can be classified as hypoxemic, hypercapnic, or both and can be compensated or uncompensated. Mechanical ventilation is most commonly instituted to treat uncompensated hypercapnic respiratory failure.

Hypercapnic respiratory failure

The natural ventilatory pump consists of the bones and muscles of the chest wall as well as the neural network controling their function. This system is responsible for ensuring adequate alveolar ventilation. Three aspects of the ventilatory pump, either alone or in combination, can result in pump failure and elevation of the arterial partial pressure of carbon dioxide ($Paco_2$) through hypoventilation: inadequate ventilatory muscle function, excessive ventilatory load, or compromised central ventilatory drive.

Drugs of various categories can affect neuromuscular transmission and hence muscle function. The most common class used both in the operating room and the ICU are the neuromuscular blocking agents (see Chapter 32). Long-term use of steroids, calcium channel blockers, and aminoglycoside antibiotics can also impair neuromuscular transmission. Inadequate ventilatory muscle function can occur as a result of inadequate electrolyte balance, malnutrition, inadequate nerve function (neuropathy), and muscle diseases (myopathy). Chronic pulmonary disease, as well as neuromuscular disease, may precipitate respiratory failure because of a decrease in the force–velocity relationship of muscle, which may decrease maximal muscle contraction. The mechanical disadvantage caused by a flattening of the diaphragm, as occurs in severe chronic obstructive pulmonary diseases (COPDs) or kyphoscoliosis can reduce ventilatory muscle strength. In addition, COPD may lead to detraining of muscle, atrophy, or fatigue of ventilatory muscles, all leading to a reduced efficiency of ventilation and carbon dioxide retention.

Excessive ventilatory loading may itself cause respiratory failure, but it is usually associated with other factors that compromise respiratory function. In patients with chronic pulmonary and neuromuscular disease, the increased load can come from the accumulation of secretions, from mucosal edema, or from bronchospasm. These compounding factors, even when mild, may be enough to precipitate respiratory failure. Any factor that elevates minute ventilatory requirements may increase ventilatory load and may precipitate respiratory failure when associated with reduced neuromuscular capability.

Depressed central ventilatory drive caused by closed head injury, drugs (sedatives and opioids), hypothyroidism, or idiopathic central alveolar hypoventilation syndrome can lead to respiratory failure. Increased central drive may also precipitate failure when coupled with a compromise in respiratory function and increased ventilatory load. A good example of this is a patient with metabolic acidosis, increased carbon dioxide production and with a dyspnea-related anxiety, who cannot tolerate the increase in respiratory rate and fatigue.

Hypoxemic respiratory failure

Failure of the lung to maintain adequate oxygenation is referred to as hypoxemic respiratory failure. The five basic mechanisms associated with hypoxemic respiratory failure are ventilation–perfusion mismatch, right-to-left shunt, alveolar hypoventilation, diffusion defect, and inadequate fraction of inspired oxygen (Fio_2).

Hypoxemic respiratory failure can usually be treated with supplemental oxygen and continuous positive airway pressure (CPAP); however, in severe cases of adult respiratory distress syndrome (ARDS), heart failure, or pneumonia, mechanical ventilation may also be necessary.

INDICATIONS FOR MECHANICAL VENTILATION

From a physiologic perspective, indications for mechanical ventilation are apnea, acute ventilatory failure, impending acute ventilatory failure, and severe oxygenation deficit. Acute ventilatory failure requires ventilatory support when the $Paco_2$ is elevated sufficiently to cause an acute acidosis (pH <7.30), although the precise limits on pH and $Paco_2$ cannot be defined globally and must be customized for individual patients. Impending acute ventilatory failure is an indication for mechanical ventilation when the patient's clinical course shows progressive failure despite maximal treatment. Examples may include asthma, neuromuscular fatigue, or COPD.

Oxygenation deficit is not as common an indication for mechanical ventilation but does account for a large proportion of patients in the ICU. The severe hypoxemia of pneumonia and ARDS may drive the ventilatory pump to fail if not corrected. If the patient requires a high Fio_2 (>0.80) and CPAP >10cmH_2O then mechanical ventilation may be required. Reducing the work of the physiologic ventilatory pump with mechanical support usually improves oxygenation by reducing the oxygen cost of breathing, which may be up to 25% of oxygen delivery.

ADULT RESPIRATORY DISTRESS SYNDROME

The term adult respiratory distress syndrome (ARDS) was proposed in 1967 to describe a clinical constellation of signs and symptoms associated with a variety of insults that followed a predictable and consistent clinical course. The features of this syndrome include alveolar collapse and microatelectasis, noncardiogenic pulmonary edema, and hypoxemia. Defining ARDS is problematic because the clinical presentation embraces a continuum of gas exchange and chest radiographic abnormalities. The term acute lung injury (ALI) has been applied to a wide spectrum of pulmonary pathologic processes that result in consistent abnormalities of gas exchange and chest radiography. ARDS is considered the most severe form of ALI.

The accepted international definitions for ALI and ARDS were developed at a 1992 American/European Consensus Conference on ARDS (Fig. 49.1). The diagnosis of ARDS depends on the presence of all criteria defining ALI, except that the degree of deficit of oxygenation is greater; in ARDS the Pao_2/ Fio_2 should be 200mmHg regardless of positive end-expiratory pressure (PEEP) therapy. ALI/ARDS refers to the whole spectrum of lung injury, based on lung physiology. Commonly, ARDS is used to denote a severe degree of ALI associated with significant morbidity and difficulty with ventilatory support.

Definitions of acute lung injury (ALI) and adult respiratory distress syndrome (ARDS)

Factor	ALI	ARDS
Time course	Acute	Acute
Bilateral infiltrates	Diffuse	Diffuse
Partial pressure O_2/fraction of inspired O_2 (Pao_2/Fio_2) (mmHg)	≤300	≤200
Evidence of cardiac failure	None	None
Pulmonary capillary wedge pressure (PCWP) (mmHg)	<18	<18

Figure 49.1 Definitions of acute lung injury (ALI) and adult respiratory distress syndrome (ARDS).

Common causes of adult respiratory distress syndrome (ARDS)

Direct injury risk factors	Indirect risk factors
Aspiration	Sepsis (SIRS)
Diffuse pulmonary infections	Hypotension
Near-drowning	Severe trauma
Toxic gas inhalation	Massive transfusion
Lung contusion	Cardiopulmonary bypass

Figure 49.2 Common causes of adult respiratory distress syndrome (ARDS).

Pathogenesis

Injury to specific cellular elements in the lung produces lung parenchymal changes; the capillary endothelial cell appears to be the most susceptible to injury. Endothelial cell damage results in increased transudation of water and protein into the lung interstitium. Injury to the alveolar epithelium leads to alveolar instability and alveolar flooding, resulting in diffuse microatalectasis. Alveolar injury may also result from damage of the surfactant system. The mechanism for these injuries may be modulated or triggered by the same or similar cytokines that trigger the systemic inflammatory response syndrome (SIRS) (Chapter 70). This diffuse microatelectasis in conjunction with the noncardiogenic edema leads to reduction of compliance, loss of alveolar units, worsening hypoxemia not responsive to increases in Fio_2, and bilateral infiltrates on chest radiography of a mixed alveolar and interstitial pattern.

ARDS is always secondary to some other event or illness; the most common causes of ARDS are either an airway source or a vascular source of injury (Fig. 49.2) although other causes have been reported. These causes lead to activation of multiple cellular elements such as neutrophils and macrophages; these in turn release cytokines (tumor necrosis factor, interleukins 2, 4, 6, 8, etc.), platelet activating factor, compliment (C3a and C5a), arachidonic acid metabolites (prostaglandins, leukotrienes, thromboxane A_2) and oxygen free radicals (see Chapter 70). Alveolar collapse and microatalectasis may further modulate these cellular mechanisms and lead to further injury, both local and systemic.

Management of ALI/ARDS is based on correction of the underlying disease process and optimization of ventilation and oxygenation of the lung. Mechanical ventilation with alveolar recruitment and stabilization along with supplemental oxygen are the keystones of therapy.

MODES OF VENTILATION

Positive pressure inflation can be achieved with ventilators that control either ventilating power (pressure or flow) or termination of inspiration (using pressure, flow, volume, or time limits). The waveforms of both flow and pressure cannot be controlled simultaneously, however, because pressure is developed as a function of flow and the impedance to breathing. Impedance to breathing varies with the patient based on their airway resistance and compliance. Older ventilators offered only a single control variable and single cycling criterion. The new generation of ventilators has multiple control options.

Traditional modes

Flow-controlled, volume-cycled ventilation

For many years, flow-controlled, volume-cycled ventilation has been the prevalent technique for adult patients. Flow can be controlled by selecting a waveform and setting a peak flow valve or by selecting a waveform and setting the combination of tidal volume and inspiratory time (Fig. 49.3). By controlling tidal volume, a certain lower limit for minute ventilation can be guaranteed, but the pressure required varies widely with the impedance to breathing. Also, once chosen, the flow is highly inflexible in response to increased or decreased inspiratory flow demands.

Pressure-preset or targeted ventilation

Newer pressure-cycled ventilators are generations removed from the pressure-cycled ventilators of the late 1950s and 1960s. These new ventilators are high-capacity machines that provide pressure-preset or pressure-targeted ventilatory modes (e.g. pressure control or pressure support as options for full or partial ventilatory assistance). After a breath has been initiated, these modes apply and maintain a targeted amount of pressure at the airway opening until a specified time (pressure control) or flow (pressure support) cycling is met. Maximal pressure is controlled, but tidal volume is a complex function of the applied pressure and its rate of approach to a target pressure, available inspiratory time, and the impedance to breathing (i.e. compliance, inspiratory and expiratory resistance, and auto-PEEP). The ventilation systems with high flow pressures can compensate well for small air leaks; therefore, they are appropriate for use with leaking or uncuffed endotracheal tubes such as those used in neonatal or pediatric patients.

Because of its virtually 'unlimited' ability to deliver flow and its decelerating flow profile, pressure-targeted ventilation is also an appropriate choice for spontaneously breathing patients with high inspiratory flow demands. The decelerating flow tends to improve the distribution of ventilation in a lung with heterogeneous mechanical properties. During pressure-control, as opposed to volume-control, ventilation, no intrapulmonary redistribution of gas that has already participated in gas exchange of another lung unit ('Pendelluft') can occur. The efficiency of gas exchange is, therefore, enhanced. Pressure-control modes also limit lung exposure to high pressure and barotrauma. Many of the new modes of ventilation are pressure-control modes.

Standard modes of positive-pressure ventilation

Controlled mechanical ventilation

In controlled mechanical ventilation, the machine provides a fixed number of breaths per minute and is not influenced by any efforts by the patient to alter frequency. This mode demands constant vigilance to make appropriate adjustments for changes in ventilatory requirements. Most patients require sedation to ensure comfort and ablate breathing efforts.

Assist-control ventilation

In assist-control ventilation, each inspiration triggered by the patient is powered by the ventilator using either volume-cycled or pressure-targeted breaths. As a safety mechanism, a back-up safety rate is set so that if the patient does not initiate a breath

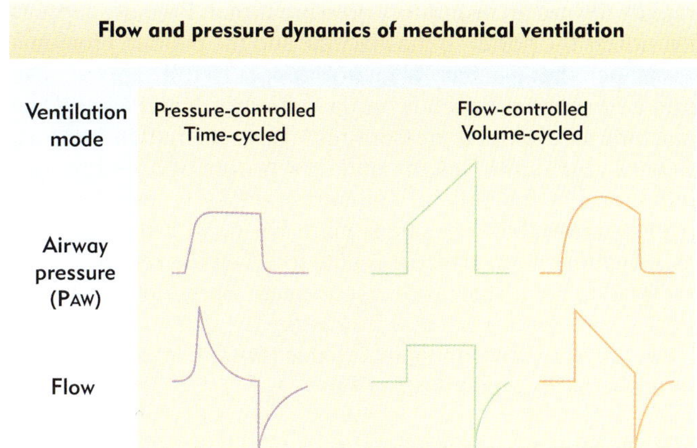

Figure 49.3 Flow and pressure dynamics of mechanical ventilation.

within the number of seconds dictated by the set frequency a machine breath is initiated. Sensitivity to the patient's inspiratory effort, the key controller, can be adjusted to require a small or large negative pressure deflection below the set level of end-expiratory pressure to initiate the inspiratory phase. New machines can be flow triggered; they initiate a cycle when a flow deficit is sensed in the expiratory limb of the circuit relative to the inspiratory limb during the exhalation period.

Synchronized intermittent mandatory ventilation

During intermittent mandatory ventilation (IMV), the patient is connected to a system that allows both spontaneous and machine breaths. Ventilator breaths can be either volume cycled or pressure controlled. Spontaneous breathing cycles can be supported or unsupported. Spontaneous breaths that are supported are usually supported by pressure support. If breaths from the ventilator are preferentially timed to coincide with spontaneous breathing, the mode is termed synchronized IMV (SIMV). SIMV can provide a wide range of support, from full to a weaning mode, depending on the mandatory frequency used and is one of the most common modes of mechanical ventilation available in the late 1990s.

Increased work of breathing can occur with IMV/SIMV. Several factors can be significant contributors to this increased load: inadequate circuit design with high inspiratory resistance, small endotracheal tube diameter, and high resistance valves for CPAP/PEEP. This external imposed workload may lead to weaning failure.

IMV and SIMV are highly popular and are useful in routine patients who will not require an endotracheal tube for long, but should be used with care in complex situations in patients with intrinsic disease. Some of the newer pressure-control modes may be more helpful in these patients.

Pressure-support ventilation

Pressure-support ventilation (PSV) is a method in which each breath taken by a spontaneously breathing patient is boosted by added pressure. After a breath is initiated, pressure builds rapidly toward an inspiratory pressure target. Pressure support hybridizes the power of the machine and the patient, providing assistance that can vary from no support to full support. The range of support depends on the patient's dynamics and the machine's developed pressure relative to the patient's effort. Because the depth, length, and flow profile of breathing are influenced by the patient, well-adjusted PSV tends to be relatively comfortable. Pressure support has its widest application as a weaning mode, since it is able to offset the resistive work required to breath spontaneously through an endotracheal tube. Pressure support is not an ideal mode for patients with unstable ventilatory drive or highly variable thoracic impedance (e.g. bronchospasm, copious secretions).

New modes of ventilation

In recent years, more complex ventilators have been introduced to support better patients with complex disease; these patients include those with ARDS and those requiring weaning from dependence upon a ventilator.

Pressure-controlled inverse ratio ventilation

To prevent gas trapping, at least as much time is allowed for exhalation as for inhalation; however, for certain patients, gas exchange may improve markedly when this ratio is extended to values greater than 1:1. Historically, pressure-controlled inverse ratio ventilation (PCIRV) was first applied to neonates with hyaline membrane disease. Now PCIRV is widely used for adult patients with refractory ARDS and other forms of hypoxemia.

How PCIRV improves oxygenation is a highly debated topic. It may raise mean intrathoracic pressure, increase lung volume, and splint the lungs open. Auto-PEEP is generated in most patients and may be necessary for optimal oxygenation unless an equivalent level of PEEP is applied. Also, sustained tethering forces may be generated and these may recruit lung units that would otherwise remain collapsed secondary to the pressure generated by collapsed lung tissue (counteractive force). Lung units with very long time constants may also benefit in that they are given sufficient time to ventilate.

Although it is commonly used as a technique of last resort in cases of ARDS, PCIRV may have a more rational use in the earliest phase of lung failure when lung units are most recruitable. It may be important, in protecting the lungs, to keep lung units open, thereby decreasing shear forces. Consequently, PCIRV may be most useful in critically ill patients where successful management depends on alveolar recruitment.

Airway pressure-release ventilation and biphasic airway pressure

Airway pressure-release ventilation (APRV) and biphasic airway pressure (BiPAP) can be thought of as variants of IRV intended for use with spontaneously breathing patients. The mechanism is used to provide added ventilatory support for patients who need CPAP for oxygenation but cannot provide adequate ventilatory drive without machine assistance. Both APRV and BiPAP allow ventilatory efforts around CPAP. They also allow for depressurization of the system, either partially or completely, for short periods at a set frequency. After this release, fresh gas enters until pressure equals the set upper limit. BiPAP differs from APRV in that it allows for an option to have the patient breathe for extended periods of time spontaneously at either level of end-expiratory pressure.

As with IRV, these modes may generate sustained higher airway pressures, which may exert traction and improve ventilation in lung units with slow time constants. Unlike IRV, maximal alveolar pressures are more readily controlled. Patients remain conscious and control their alveolar ventilation. In some variations of BiPAP, pressure support can be titrated into spontaneous cycles at either pressure baseline. The BiPAP system can, therefore, provide the entire range of ventilatory support from completely controlled ventilation to unsupported breathing, depending on the frequency and duration of the release cycles. The efficacy of the pressure-release cycle depends on the duration of the release, the mechanical properties of the chest, the level to which airway pressure is allowed to fall, and the cycling frequency between the two pressure baselines.

A problem with these systems is that as ventilatory support increases, mean airway pressure falls, decreasing some of the oxygen-exchange advances of the higher CPAP levels. These modes may not be helpful for patients with significant airflow obstruction or greatly reduced lung compliance.

Pressure-regulated volume control

Pressure-regulated volume control (PRVC) is a mode that is a combination of the decelerating flow of pressure control with a volume guarantee. This mode allows for nearly continuous monitoring of lung mechanics. Inspiratory pressure is regulated to a value based on the volume–pressure calculation of the previous breath compared with the preset target volume. As compliance changes, the pressure is regulated to the lowest possible limit as long as the target pressure is reached.

The ability of pressure-control modes to open collapsed alveoli differs from that of volume-control modes. These observations provide a rationale for a ventilator mode that preserves lung integrity by opening the lung and splinting it open throughout the entire ventilatory cycle. PRVC increases oxygen delivery in patients with ARDS by alveolar recruitment. The work of breathing can be reduced because of the rapid flow-triggering system. PRVC makes it relatively easy to use pressure control without the worry of ongoing adjustments as compliance changes.

Volume support

Volume support (VS) is an automated form of pressure support for a spontaneously breathing patient. The advantage is that the ventilator automatically monitors the mechanical properties of the lung/thorax and, if they change, adapts pressure support levels to secure the desired volume. As the patient improves their efforts, the inspiratory support from the ventilator decreases. This 'auto pressure support' may be useful in weaning.

Permissive hypercapnia

As our knowledge of pulmonary pathophysiology has increased, we are allowing $Paco_2$ levels to rise as a trade-off to preventing barotrauma (see below). Permissive hypercapnia is a ventilatory strategy that assigns higher priority to avoiding injurious pressure than to maintaining normal levels of alveolar ventilation. Allowing $Paco_2$ to rise above baseline normal values is perhaps the simplest technique for reducing ventilatory workload, the pressure cost of breathing, and the number of machine cycles per minute. Gradual increases in $Paco_2$ over several hours are generally well tolerated and are accompanied by minimal shifts in intracellular pH. Permissive hypercapnia is now commonly used in the strategy to protect the sick lung with tidal volumes in the range 5–7mL/kg.

Tracheal gas insufflation

Tracheal gas insufflation (TGI) is the placement of a catheter carrying a constant flow of gas down the endotracheal tube. It is used in conjunction with permissive hypercapnia. A flow rate of 2–4L/min is applied to remove deadspace gas. This technique can help to lower $Paco_2$ nearer to normal levels, which may be helpful in patients with acidosis or head injury. Functional residual capacity (FRC) also increases with higher flow rates, possibly through splinting open of alveolar units. Experience is limited using TGI in the management of respiratory failure. It may, however, offer a relatively simple means of reducing $Paco_2$ when pressure-targeted ventilation results in excessive hypercapnia.

VENTILATOR-ASSOCIATED LUNG INJURY

Mechanical ventilation is not without the risk of lung injury. The cause of injury is usually the use of improper ventilator settings because of a failure to understand basic lung physiology. High levels of inspiratory pressure will, of course, cause alveolar distention. This high-pressure barotrauma can lead to pulmonary interstitial emphysema, pneumomediastium, subcutaneous emphysema, and pneumothorax. Pneumothorax is of the greatest clinical concern in that it can progress rapidly to life-threatening tension pneumothorax.

Another newer concept of lung injury is that the cyclic opening and closing of alveolar units may generate both shear forces and surfactant depletion (Fig. 49.4). If an aerated alveolus is located next to a collapsed one and it is expanded with a transpulmonary pressure of 30cmH_2O, the true pressures acting as shear forces within the interalveolar septum may reach values of approximately 140cmH_2O. In normal lungs during end-expiration, the surfactant molecules are compressed on a small alveolar area, generating a low surface tension or a high surface pressure, thus preventing the alveoli from collapse (see Chapter 42). If the alveoli collapse, the alveolar surface becomes smaller than the total surface of the surfactant molecules; the molecules are squeezed out of the surface, forced toward the airways, and are lost to the alveoli. During the next inflation of the alveoli, the surface is replenished with surfactant that was stored in the hypophase, a space just underneath the active layer. During the following expiration, this mechanism is repeated and again surfactant molecules are forced into the airways. With large tidal volumes and multiple mechanical breaths, surfactant molecules are lost rapidly. This continuous alveolar transgression from high-inspiratory to low-expiratory volumes below a normal FRC not only washes out pulmonary surfactant but also induces high-permeability pulmonary edema, which also inactivates the surfactant. It may be useful to apply adequate levels of PEEP or splint alveoli through PCIRV to assure a sufficient FRC.

Evidence is now being developed that nonoptimal ventilator settings may lead to the release of various interleukins and other cytokines tht may activate the systemic inflammatory response cascade. Also, poorly managed mechanical ventialtion may lead to the transmigration of bacteria into the systemic circulation. this has coined the new concept of biotrauma.

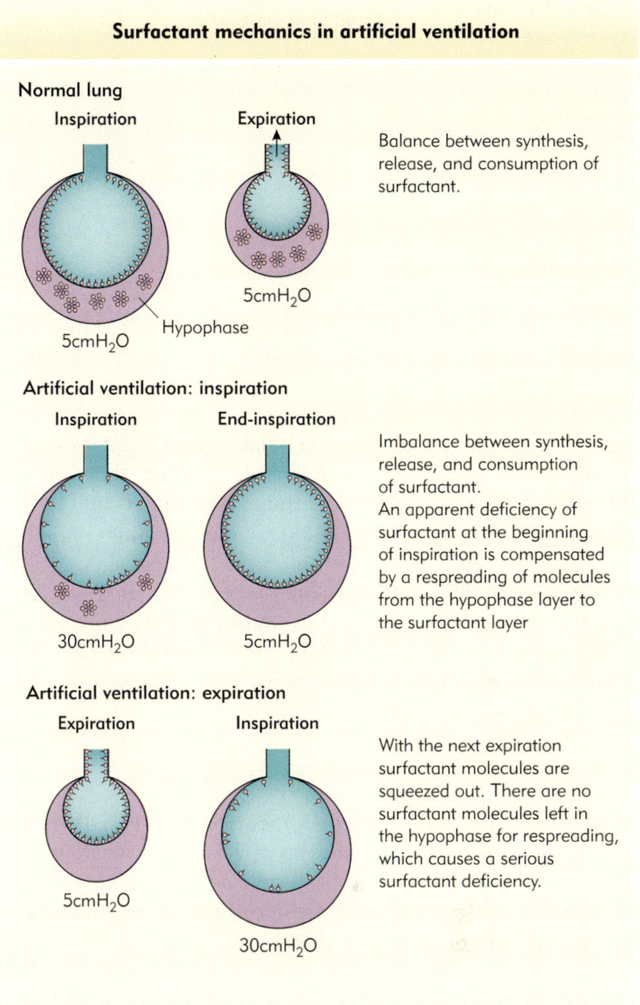

Figure 49.4 Surfactant mechanisms in artificial ventilation.

Evidence is now being developed that nonoptimal ventilator settings may lead to the release of various interleukins and other cytokines that may activate the systemic inflammatory response cascade. Also, poorly managed mechanical ventilation may lead to the transmigration of bacteria into the systemic circulation. This has coined the new concept of biotrauma.

Open lung concept

The law of Laplace links the pressure at the alveolar level to the surface tension and radius (see Chapter 42). In a healthy lung, alveolar surfactant minimizes the surface forces at the air–liquid interface and thus ensures alveolar stability at all alveolar sizes. During lung injury, all lungs present with some degree of dysfunction of the natural surfactant system. The degree of dysfunction determines the amount of pressure needed to expand the alveoli from a state of a small radius (volume) to a larger radius (volume). It can further be derived from the law of Laplace that the pressure necessary to keep alveoli expanded is smaller at a high FRC, since the FRC is directly correlated to the amount of open lung units and their size (Fig. 49.5). If we apply a peak pressure of 40–60cmH_2O for 10 breaths and then splint the lung open during this procedure

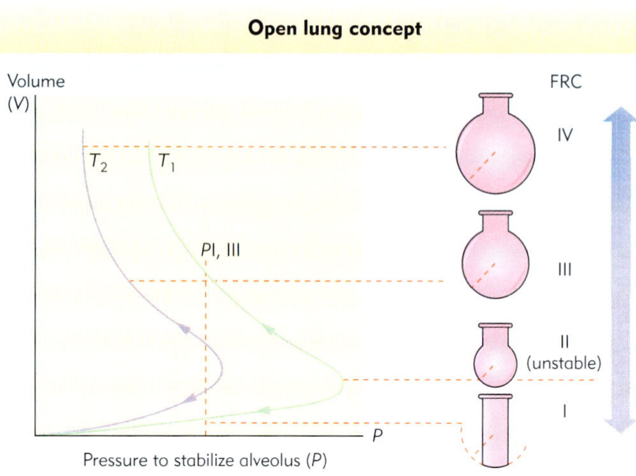

Figure 49.5 The open lung concept. Open lung units are more efficient and function at a lower pressure. The opening pressure is higher when the surface tension is higher. The pressure needed to keep the alveoli open is smaller at a high functional residual capacity (FRC) (IV and III) and is unstable at FRC I and II. T = surface tension of liquid–air interface; R = radius of the alveolus. Law of Laplace: $P = 2T/R$.

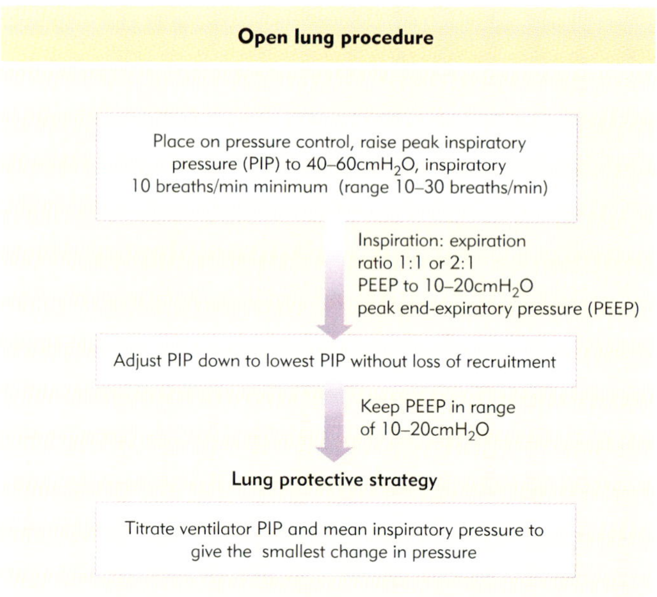

Figure 49.6 Open lung procedure. The goal of the open lung approach is to recruit alveolar beds and maintain them 'open' at the lowest change in pressure in order to minimize alveolar shear forces.

with either elevated PEEP (10–15cmH$_2$O) or PCIRV to give an inspiration-to-expiration ratio of 1:1 or 2:1, we may stabilize the alveoli at a better position on the volume–pressure curve (Fig. 49.6). We can then reduce peak pressure to 30–35cmH$_2$O but splint the alveoli with PEEP or PCIRV and thus decrease both surfactant depletion and shear forces. This may be an important strategy to decrease complications from mechanical ventilation and should be started early in the management of respiratory failure.

Positive end-expiratory pressure

End-expiratory pressure may be applied during continuous mechanical ventilation (PEEP) or spontaneous breathing with or without partial ventilatory support (CPAP). PEEP and CPAP typically are used to reduce or prevent expiratory atelectasis in patients with acute lung injury and to provide splinting in the open lung concept.

PEEP and CPAP reduce inspiratory load in patients with chronic obstructive disease with air trapping secondary to incomplete exhalation. Patients with no lung pathology who require short-term mechanical ventilation may require a PEEP of 5cmH$_2$O. Patients with ALI or ARDS are usually started on levels of 10–15cmH$_2$O PEEP, which is then titrated according to arterial oxygen partial pressure ($Pa{O_2}$) and lung mechanics. An optimum value for PEEP can be calculated by developing a pressure–volume curve and titrating PEEP to an inflection point (Fig. 49.7). With PEEP at or above the inflection point, hysteresis is reduced and the slope is changed. This characteristic pressure–volume loop is observable in early ARDS.

Auto-PEEP is end-expiratory pressure caused by chronic airflow limitations: increased tidal volume, increased rate, reverse inspiration-to-expiration ratio, or inadequate expiratory times. It may be both beneficial in splinting alveolar units open or it may be sometimes detrimental by generating very high peak inspiratory pressures, thereby triggering barotrauma. Auto-PEEP should therefore be routinely followed in clinical practice and adjusted for optimal levels.

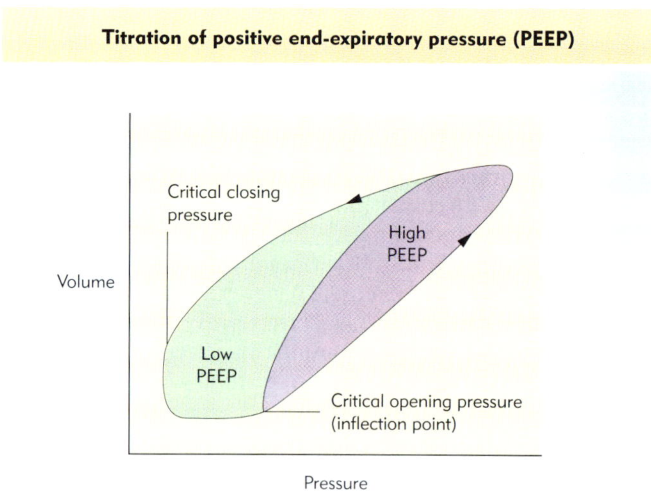

Figure 49.7 Titration of positive end-expiratory pressure (PEEP). With PEEP at or above the inflection point, hysteresis is reduced.

WEANING FROM MECHANICAL VENTILATION

In approximately 75–80% of patients, ventilatory support is easily discontinued when the physiologic indication for it is reversed. Another 10–15% require use of specific weaning protocols, which usually allow discontinuation within 8 to 72 hours. The remaining 5–10% of mechanically ventilated patients require a more gradual weaning.

Techniques for weaning include gradual reduction of pressure/volume support, SIMV, and a trial of breathing with T-piece/CPAP with increasing periods of unsupported breathing (<30–60 minutes). Discontinuation of ventilatory support requires a basic level of physiologic readiness including reversal of indication for ventilation, $Pa{O_2} \geq 60$mmHg (8kPa) with $F{IO_2} \leq 0.50$, PEEP ≤5cmH_2O, intact ventilatory drive, cardiovascular stability, decreased pulmonary secretions, normal electrolytes, normal body temperature, adequate nutritional status, and absence of other major organ failure.

During weaning, predictors of outcome can be assessed, although no predictor has 100% predictive power. Clinical judgment is often more important than reliance on any singular weaning variable. Standard basic criteria include vital capacity ≥ 10mL/kg, negative inspiratory pressure less than –30cmH_2O, and minute ventilation <10L/min. A newer measure is the rapid shallow breathing index, which is respiratory rate divided by tidal volume in liters: a value below 80 is proposed as predicting successful weaning.

Key References

Amato MBP, Barbas CSV, Modeiros DM, et al. Effect of a protective ventilation strategy on mortality in the acute respiratory distress syndrome. N Eng J Med. 1998;338:347–54.

ACCP Consensus Conference. Mechanical ventilation. Chest. 1992;104:1833–59.

Apostolakos, MJ, Papadakos PJ. High-inflation pressure and positive end-expiratory pressure injurious to the lung? Yes. Crit Care Clin. 1996;12:627–34.

Bernard GR, Artigas A, Brigham KL, et al. Report of the American–European Consensus Conference on ARDS: definitions, mechanisms, relevant outcomes and clinical trial coordination. Intens Care Med. 1994;20:225–32.

Gattinoni L, Pesenti A, Bombino N, et al. Relationships between lung-computed tomographic density, gas exchange, and PEEP in acute respiratory failure. Anesthesiology. 1988;69:824–32.

Gattinoni L, Pelosi P, Crotti S, et al. Effects of positive end-expiratory pressure on regional distribution of tidal volume and recruitment in adult respiratory distress syndrome. Am J Respir Crit Care. 1995;151:1807–14.

Marini JJ, Kelsen SG. Re-targeting ventilatory objectives in adult respiratory distress syndrome: new treatment prospects – persistent questions. [Editorial] Am Rev Resp Dis. 1992;146:2–3.

Markström AG, Lichtwarck-Aschoff M, Svensson BJ, Nordgren KA, Sjöstrand UH. Ventilation with constant versus deceleration inspiratory flow in experimentally induced respiratory failure. Anesthesiology. 1996;84:883–9.

Papadakos PJ, Halloran W, Hessney JI, et al. The use of pressure-controlled inverse ratio ventilation in the surgical intensive care unit. J Trauma. 1991;31:1211–15.

Papadakos PJ, Lachmann B, Böhm S. Pressure control ventilation review and new horizons. Clin Pulm Med. 1998;5:120-3

Seneff MG, Zimmerman JE, Knaus WA, et al. Predicting the duration of mechanical ventilation. The importance of disease and patient characteristics. Chest. 1996;110:469–79.

Smith TC, Marini JJ. Impact of PEEP on lung mechanics and work of breathing in severe airflow obstruction. J Appl Physiol. 1988;65:1488–99.

Tharatt RS, Allen RP, Albertson TE. Pressure-controlled inverse ration ventilation in severe adult respiratory failure. Chest. 1988;94:755–62.

Villar J, Petty TL, Slutsky AS. ARDS in its middle age what have we learned. Applied Cardiopulmonary Pathophysiology. 1998;7:167–72.

Yang KL, Tobin MJ. A prospective study of indexes predicting the outcome of trials of weaning from mechanical ventilation. N Eng J Med. 1991;324:1445–50.

Further Reading

Hess DR, Kacmarek RM. Indications and initial settings for mechanical ventilation. In: Hess DR, Kacmarek RM, eds. Essentials of mechanical ventilation. New York: McGraw-Hill; 1996:67–72.

Lachmann, B, Danzmann E, Haendly B, et al. Ventilator setting and gas exchange in respiratory distress syndrome. In: Prakash O, ed. Applied physiology in clinical respiratory care. Boston, MA: Martinus Nijkoff; 1982:141–57.

Sjöstrand UH, Lichtwarck-Aschoff M, Nielsen JB, et al. Different ventilatory approaches to keep the lung open. Intens Care Med. 1995;21:310–18.

Tobin MJ, Alex CG. Discontinuation of mechanical ventilation. In: Tobin MJ, ed. Mechanical ventilation. New York: McGraw-Hill; 1994:1124–77.

Chapter 50 Applied thoracic physiology

Simon C Body and Philip M Hartigan

Topics covered in this chapter

Lung isolation
Physiology of one-lung ventilation
Physiology of end-stage pulmonary disease
Jet ventilation
Anesthesia for specific thoracic surgical procedures

Recent advances in our understanding of the physiology of one-lung ventilation (OLV) and the development of thoracic surgical techniques, such as lung transplantation and lung volume reduction surgery (LVRS), require specialized knowledge of many fields. Developments in surgical therapy of noncancerous lung disease, such as emphysema, have necessitated the provision of anesthesia for thoracic surgery in patients who previously would have been rejected for any surgical procedure; this requires an increased understanding of the pathophysiology of these diseases, as well as the principles of respiratory physiology and the changes brought about by OLV.

LUNG ISOLATION

Indications for lung isolation

The most common indication for OLV is pulmonary surgery, with surgery on other thoracic nonpulmonary structures being less common (Fig. 50.1). Other indications are less frequent. For thoracoscopy, the use of OLV is necessary to obtain good working conditions. A bronchopleural (cutaneous) fistula or open airway can result in inadequate ventilation during two-lung anesthesia because of low resistance to gas flow through the fistula. During sleeve resection, lung transplantation, and pneumonectomy the surgical open bronchus is difficult to manage without OLV. Contamination of an uninfected lung with infected material or blood can result in pneumonia, sepsis, hypoxemia, and physical obstruction to ventilation. Trauma to the tracheobronchial tree or giant unilateral bullous are rare indications for OLV.

Contraindications to lung isolation

Patients with severe ventilatory impairment, who often present for diagnostic lung biopsy, have such poor gas exchange that OLV is frequently impractical. Occasionally, patients are encountered in whom it is impossible to place the required hardware for OLV, such as patients who have upper or lower airway abnormalities. Patients who have lower airway obstruction, frequently tumors, may have such severe obstruction that placement of a double-lumen tube (DLT) or bronchial blocker is difficult, if not impossible, and it can be associated with tumor bleeding, aspiration, or obstruction.

Indications and contraindications to lung isolation

Indications

- To provide a quiet operative field: thoracoscopy, thoracotomy, thoracic nonpulmonary surgery
- To avoid spillage or contamination: infection, massive hemorrhage, unilateral pulmonary lavage (alveolar proteinosis or cystic fibrosis)
- Control of the distribution of ventilation: bronchopleural (cutaneous) fistula, surgery of a major conducting airway, giant unilateral lung cyst or bulla, differential lung ventilation

Contraindications

- Severe ventilatory impairment
- Inability to safely place hardware

Figure 50.1 Indications and contraindications to lung isolation.

Bronchial anatomy

For the anesthesiologist, the important anatomic features of the tracheobronchial tree are the lengths and diameters of the mainstem bronchi. The left and right mainstem bronchi are approximately 48 ± 8mm and 18mm in length, respectively (Fig. 50.2). The correlation between bronchial length and height is clinically useful. Both bronchi are shorter in females because of their reduced height, but males and females of the same height have similar bronchial lengths.

Choice of DLT size primarily depends on endobronchial diameter and length. This is because the correct positioning of a left DLT requires that the endobronchial cuff lies beyond the carina, without herniation, and that ventilation to the contralateral mainstem bronchus and ipsilateral upper lobe bronchus are unobstructed. Accordingly, the most proximal safe position is when the proximal end of the bronchial cuff is level with the carina, and the most distal safe position is when the tip of the endobronchial portion of the DLT is level with the upper lobe bronchus. For a right-sided DLT, the margin of safety is not determined by the length of the bronchus, but by the length of the right upper lobe ventilation slot.

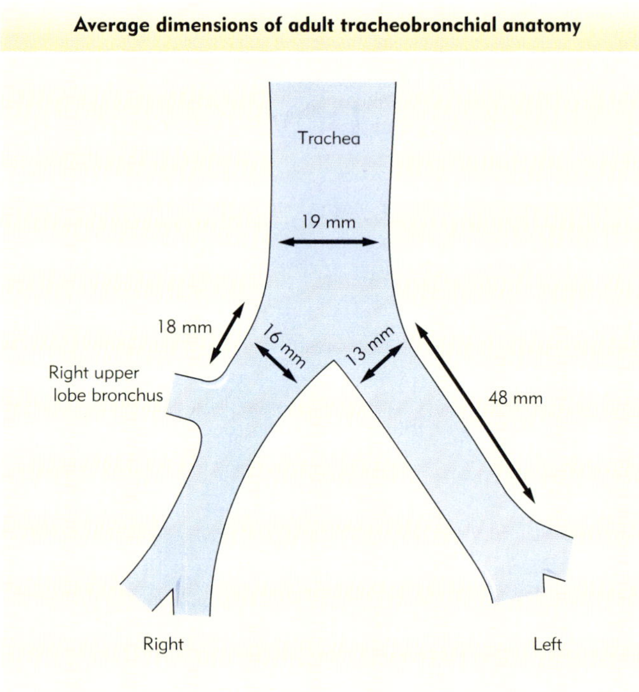

Figure 50.2 Average dimensions of adult tracheobronchial anatomy. Dimensions are for an individual of height approximately 169cm (66.5in). (Modified with permission from Meredino et al., 1954; and Benumof JL et al., 1987.)

PHYSIOLOGY OF ONE-LUNG VENTILATION

Thoracic surgery usually requires unilateral lung deflation and the lateral decubitus position. The open chest causes downward mediastinal shift, which compresses the dependent lung. During spontaneous ventilation, inspiration results in a more negative intrathoracic pressure in the dependent lung and a downward mediastinal displacement that reduces the effective tidal volume (VT). During expiration of the dependent lung, some of the exhaled gas inflates the deflated nondependent lung. For this reason lung isolation and positive pressure ventilation are required. Physiologically, OLV is best understood by reviewing the effects of the lateral decubitus position followed by induction of anesthesia, thoracotomy, and lung isolation.

Lateral decubitus position

In the upright position, the normal gravitational gradient of pulmonary artery pressure and lung compliance results in the greatest blood flow and ventilation in the base of the lung. The gravitational gradient of blood flow exceeds the gradient of ventilation, which results in a spectrum of ventilation/perfusion ratios ($\dot{V}/\dot{Q}$; Chapter 34). Lateral decubitus positioning changes that gradient to a side-to-side gradient, but does not alter its magnitude. Both ventilation and perfusion to the dependent lung are increased. In the upright position, the normal perfusion ratio is a 55:45 (R:L) between the lungs. In the lateral decubitus position, the perfusion ratio is approximately 65:35 (R:L) when the right lung is dependent, and 45:55 (R:L) when the left lung is dependent. Alteration in the distribution of ventilation is less marked than the changes seen with perfusion, and other factors (mode of ventilation, chest opening, lung isolation, and malpositioning) have a greater impact. During spontaneous ventilation the hemidiaphragm dependent undergoes greater excursion than the nondependent hemidiaphragm and ventilation favors the dependent lung, because of greater concavity (doming) of the dependent hemidiaphragm.

Induction of anesthesia, muscle paralysis, and positive pressure ventilation

Induction of anesthesia causes little change in pulmonary blood flow distribution, but functional residual capacity (FRC) is reduced by approximately 500mL (20%). The change in FRC alters the compliance in each lung – the dependent lung compliance decreases slightly, while the nondependent lung compliance increases slightly, such that compliance of the nondependent lung is approximately 30% greater. These compliance changes have a small effect on the distribution of ventilation, increasing that of the nondependent lung and decreasing that of the dependent lung, and thereby slightly increasing $\dot{V}/\dot{Q}$ mismatching. The differences in lung compliance are over-ridden during spontaneous ventilation by greater doming of the dependent hemidiaphragm, allowing greater diaphragmatic excursion and more ventilation to the dependent lung. Contraction of the nondependent hemidiaphragm, by contrast, causes little air movement, but stiffens the mediastinum, increasing ventilation to the dependent lung.

Muscle paralysis and intermittent positive pressure ventilation (IPPV) abolish the advantage of the domed dependent hemidiaphragm and increase nondependent lung ventilation (and thus increased $\dot{V}/\dot{Q}$ mismatch). Alveolar pressure is evenly distributed throughout the lung, but pleural pressure (PPL) is highest in the dependent lung. Ventilation to the dependent lung is impeded by compression of the dependent hemithorax by the mediastinum and abdominal contents (Fig. 50.3). Patient malposition may increase the restriction to dependent lung expansion, which further reduces dependent lung ventilation and increases $\dot{V}/\dot{Q}$ mismatching. In contrast to the distribution of ventilation, muscle paralysis and IPPV have little direct effect on the distribution of perfusion between the two lungs. They may impair venous return and cardiac output, and have small effects on the relative preponderance of zones 1, 2, and 3 in the lung (Chapter 34).

Open chest

Thoracotomy raises the normally negative end-expiratory PPL to atmospheric pressure (PB) in the nondependent chest. The lung partially deflates unless severe emphysematous disease is present. The compliance of the nondependent lung increases because the impedance of chest wall movement is removed during mechanical ventilation. Positive pressure ventilation with an open chest greatly favors the more compliant nondependent lung, while expansion of the dependent lung is restricted on all sides by the mediastinum, the bed and supporting pads, and the abdominal contents pressing up on the diaphragm. As the dependent lung still receives the majority of pulmonary perfusion, $\dot{V}/\dot{Q}$ matching is further impaired.

One-lung ventilation

Initiation of OLV causes considerable change in the distribution of ventilation *and* perfusion. On initiation of OLV, ventilation of the dependent lung is increased, while ventilation of the nondependent lung ceases. Before initiation of OLV, little alteration in the distribution of perfusion occurs despite the described changes in ventilation. With initiation of OLV, and

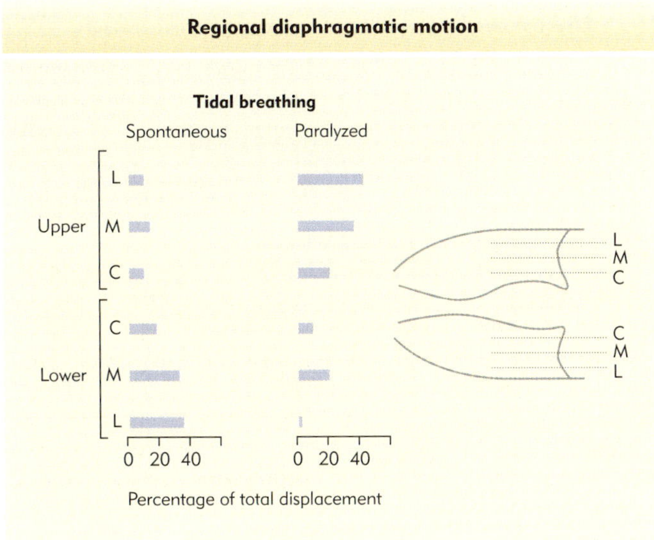

Figure 50.3 Regional diaphragmatic motion. This is shown for anesthetized spontaneous ventilation and for IPPV in the lateral decubitus position. Diaphragmatic motion was recorded in the lateral (L), middle (M), and central (C) positions of the diaphragm. Regional displacement, which reflects ventilation, is expressed as a percentage of total value. Regional lung displacement shifted from dependent (lower) lung predominance to nondependent (upper) lung predominance after initiation of anesthesia and muscle paralysis. (Modified with permission from Froese AB, Bryan AC, 1974.)

consequent nondependent lung atelectasis and alveolar hypoxia, blood flow to the nondependent lung decreases. The primary mechanism for the redirection of blood flow to the nondependent lung is hypoxic pulmonary vasoconstriction (HPV). Lobar atelectasis and lobar ventilation with nitrogen yield the same amount of pulmonary vasoconstriction, and selectively infused vasodilators to the atelectatic lung restore blood flow to normal. Mechanical small-vessel obstruction from lung deflation likely plays only a minor role in the redirection of blood flow, but large-vessel obstruction by surgical manipulation may be important. Usually, HPV decreases the magnitude of blood flow to the nondependent lung, and therefore shunt, by approximately 50%, depending on the amount of lung made atelectatic. Thus, with HPV the effective shunt through the nondependent, nonventilated lung is usually approximately 20%. In addition, a persistent, small physiologic shunt occurs in the dependent ventilated lung.

Without HPV, severe hypoxia would always result from OLV (see Fig. 47.6). The HPV response is immediate, with little potentiation or attenuation of the response over time. Alveolar hypoxia, of any origin, duration, or lung volume, causes localized pulmonary vasoconstriction. Both alveolar partial pressure of carbon dioxide (P_{ACO_2}) and blood pH modulate the HPV response. While hypocapnia and metabolic alkalosis directly antagonize HPV and cause vasodilatation, hypercapnia and metabolic acidosis moderately enhance the vasoconstrictor response. Other gas compositions and other nongas factors affect the extent of HPV. Mixed venous P_{O_2} ($P\bar{v}_{O_2}$) modifies the extent of HPV. High $P\bar{v}_{O_2}$ decreases HPV, low $P\bar{v}_{O_2}$ mildly increases HPV, and HPV is maximal when alveolar P_{O_2} is approximately 20–40mmHg (2.7–5.3kPa).

In the lateral position, during two-lung ventilation the dependent lung may have a low FRC and be poorly ventilated, especially when the chest is open. However, data vary as to the state of the dependent lung during OLV. Depending on the patient's position, lung disease, and pattern of ventilation, FRC may be either high or low. Areas of low FRC may exist in the dependent lung despite the relative increase in ventilation. This can result from absorption atelectasis caused by breathing 100% oxygen or oxygen–nitrous oxide mixtures, decreased FRC because of induction of general anesthesia, and areas of pulmonary pathology. Many patients who undergo OLV have expiratory gas flow halted by the start of the next inspiration, a phenomenon variously known as intrinsic positive end-expiratory pressure ($PEEP_I$), auto-PEEP, or dynamic hyperinflation. This phenomenon raises FRC to a varying degree, depending upon the patient's disease and the ventilator settings. The incidence of $PEEP_I$ is higher with smaller endotracheal tubes and in patients who have emphysematous lung disease. These data imply that extrinsic PEEP ($PEEP_E$) will not improve, or may worsen, oxygenation in many patients, because they already have inspiratory flow-limited expiration and normal or high FRC. Patterns of ventilation that severely increase dependent lung volumes may increase dependent lung pulmonary vascular resistance (PVR), and therefore increase blood flow and shunting to the nondependent lung. Examples of ventilatory techniques that perhaps increase shunt are high peak inflation pressures, using $PEEP_E$, high V_T, and rapid respiratory rates. A minority of patients may have small lung volumes or atelectasis, and may benefit from applying $PEEP_E$ to the dependent lung.

Ventilation of the dependent lung

The aims of ventilation during OLV are avoidance of hypoxemia, hypercapnia and micro or macroscopic barotrauma to the lung. Ventilation with 100% oxygen reduces the likelihood of hypoxemia, the most common complication of OLV. High oxygen concentrations dilate the dependent lung vasculature, thereby decreasing nondependent lung shunt and increase the oxygen content of dependent lung venous blood. Ventilation of the dependent lung with an inspired oxygen fraction (F_{IO_2}) of 1.0 usually results in an arterial partial pressure of oxygen (P_{aO_2}) of 150–210mmHg (20–28kPa) after a period of 10–15 minutes. Reducing the F_{IO_2} to 0.5 yields an average P_{aO_2} of about 80mmHg (10.6kPa) by observation and by calculation. These P_{aO_2} values are safe, but the wide variation in oxygenation between patients and uncertain nature of thoracic anesthesia leave no margin of safety when using an F_{IO_2} of 0.5. For these reasons, the use of an F_{IO_2} of 1.0 is the safest and most reasonable course. Presuming no technical difficulties (i.e. the DLT is correctly positioned and ventilation of the dependent lung is successful with an appropriate V_T and high F_{IO_2}), the physiologic causes of hypoxemia may be generally grouped into the interdependent categories of increased nondependent-lung shunt and impaired dependent-lung gas exchange.

Studies that examine the effect of V_T on oxygenation are not consistent. For two-lung anesthesia, V_Ts <10mL/kg are associated with atelectasis. However, during OLV a V_T of 10mL/kg is often associated with high peak inflation pressures. Patients who have severe chronic obstructive pulmonary disease

(COPD) and limited expiratory flows often need VTs <10mL/kg to avoid PEEPI.

To achieve normocapnia in the face of a reduced VT during OLV, the respiratory rate should be increased. As reductions in VT are not associated with equivalent percentage reductions in dead space (VD) and alveolar ventilation, respiratory rate must usually be increased to a greater extent than any reduction in VT. Although alveolar ventilation can be maintained at the same level as two-lung ventilation in most patients, it is not so for all patients. Despite this, symptomatic hypercapnia is rarely observed, and little change in carbon dioxide excretion occurs.

Some patients have low lung volumes in the dependent lung and desaturate during OLV. A subgroup of those patients who desaturate might be expected to show improvement in oxygenation with PEEPE, because of increased FRC and reduced $\dot{V}/\dot{Q}$ mismatch. In contrast, many patients have worsened oxygenation with dependent lung PEEPE. Two factors limit the efficacy of PEEPE. First, not all patients have low lung volumes, and not all patients who have low lung volumes desaturate, because of differences in pre-existing respiratory disease and FRC during OLV. Second, PEEPE may raise PVR in the dependent lung. If areas of atelectasis and alveolar hypoxia exist, PEEPE would improve oxygenation and decrease PVR in the dependent lung. Although mild-to-moderate PEEPE has no effect on PVR, high levels [>10cmH$_2$O (>1kPa)] of PEEPE may increase vascular resistance in hyperexpanded areas of the lung. Increases in regional vascular resistance may distribute blood away from well-oxygenated (and ventilated) lung segments to areas of low $\dot{V}/\dot{Q}$ ratio and to the nondependent lung, thereby increasing shunt fraction. As a result of pulmonary vascular recruitment, changes in total lung PVR, cardiac output, and systemic vascular resistance (SVR) are not usually seen until PEEPE exceeds 10cmH$_2$O (1kPa).

In some patients who have increased FRC, caused by baseline pulmonary disease or PEEPI, the addition of PEEPE may not improve arterial oxygenation. The critical point at which the gas exchange benefits of dependent lung alveolar recruitment are overwhelmed by increasing nondependent lung shunt varies between patients. Studies have found improvement, no effect, and worsening of arterial oxygenation in individual patients who receive PEEPE (Fig. 50.4a).

Intrinsic PEEP occurs with mechanical ventilation during two- and one-lung ventilation, especially in patients who have severe airways disease. The intraoperative diagnosis of intrinsic PEEPI is best made by examining end-expiratory flow using a pneumotachograph or looking at a mechanical rotary flow sensor in the anesthesia circle system. Patients who have PEEPI most likely will not benefit from PEEPE. Manual hyperinflation, high VT, short expiratory times, or PEEPE are maneuvers that increase lung volumes and may improve oxygenation. As knowledge of the optimal FRC for an individual patient is limited, it is wise to avoid PEEPE unless there has been a failure of nondependent lung continuous positive airway pressure (CPAP) and intermittent lung reinflation, except in patients who are suspected of having a low FRC because of small preoperative lung volumes or obesity.

Several pathologic conditions of the dependent lung that may contribute to hypoxemia are atelectasis, infection, effusion, mucous plugging, pulmonary emboli, and interstitial pulmonary edema. Patient malpositioning, which leads to extrinsic chest compression and atelectasis, may also contribute to hypoxemia. Prior partial resection of the dependent lung reduces the available surface area for gas exchange, although this alone is seldom a limiting factor. Impaired gas exchange also occurs in patients who have advanced COPD as a consequence of capillary bed destruction and disruption of normal alveolar architecture, leading to increased physiologic shunt (as well as VD). Somewhat paradoxically, the degree of hypoxemia during OLV tends to correlate poorly or negatively to the severity of obstructive disease based on preoperative spirometry [forced expiratory volume in 1 second (FEV$_1$)]. This may result from a counterbalancing beneficial degree of dependent

Effect of one-lung ventilation on oxygen partial pressure

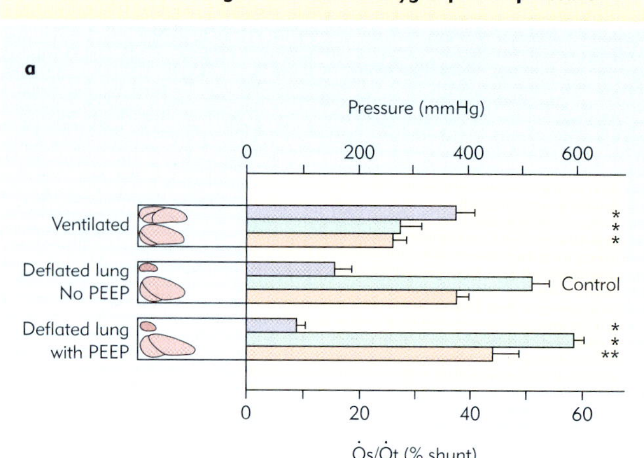

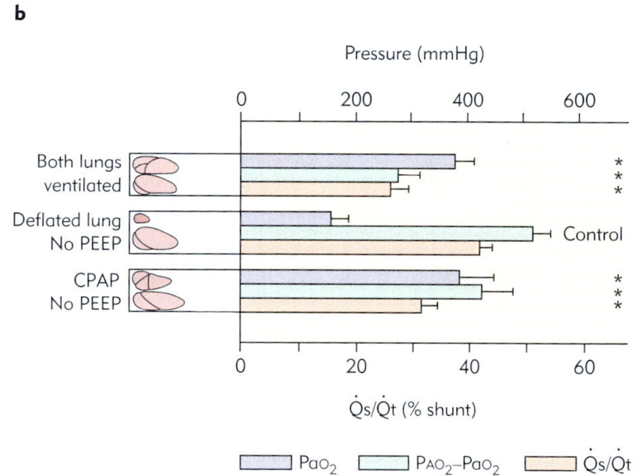

Figure 50.4 Effect of OLV on PaO_2. (a) With dependent lung PEEP [10cm H_2O (1kPa)]. PaO_2, PAO_2 – PaO_2, and shunt fraction (QS/QT) are shown for two-lung ventilation, and OLV with and without PEEP. OLV causes PaO_2 to fall and QS/QT to rise. The introduction of dependent lung PEEP further reduced PaO_2 and increased shunt fraction. (b) With nondependent lung CPAP[10cm H_2O (1kPa)]. PaO_2, PAO_2 – PaO_2, and QS/QT are shown for two-lung ventilation, and OLV with and without CPAP. OLV causes PaO_2 to fall and QS/QT to rise. The introduction of nondependent lung CPAP caused PaO_2 to rise to two-lung ventilation values. (*p <0.05, **p <0.01.) (Modified with permission from Capan LM, Turndorf H, Patel C, et al., 1980.)

lung PEEPI imposed by the limitations to expiratory flow in severe COPD. Gas trapping in the nondependent lung may also transiently reduce nondependent lung shunt in such patients by delaying the collapse of that lung.

Physiology of the nondependent lung

Hypoxemia is the most common complication of OLV. As the predominant cause of hypoxemia during OLV is shunt in the nondependent lung, therapies to improve arterial oxygenation during OLV should be directed toward this lung. Factors that increase blood flow through the nondependent lung or decrease blood flow through the dependent lung increase shunt and worsen hypoxemia. An important exception to this rule is if the nondependent lung is oxygenated. Even though blood flow to the nondependent lung increases due to inhibition of HPV, the effective physiologic shunt is reduced because oxygen uptake occurs. It is possible to oxygenate the nondependent lung without interfering with surgery under most circumstances. Possible methods of oxygenation are oxygen insufflation, intermittent ventilation, CPAP, and high-frequency ventilation.

Oxygen insufflation to the nondependent lung is usually ineffective because lung inflation, and therefore alveolar gas exchange, does not occur. Only rarely is oxygen insufflation rapid or effective enough to be useful. Reinflation of the lung is the most effective and rapid means of improving arterial oxygenation. However, reinflation causes considerable interference with the conduct of surgery. Partial reinflation is often adequate to improve oxygenation without interfering with surgery, provided desaturation is not severe. Initial hypoxia, treated by lung reinflation and then deflation tends not to recur with such severity.

Nondependent lung continuous positive airway pressure

Thoracotomy and effective OLV are invariably followed by nondependent lung deflation and atelectasis. Partial reinflation of the nondependent lung with oxygen reduces the physiologic shunt fraction of the lung. The apt term, CPAP, has been used to describe the use of oxygen to partially reinflate the lung without tidal ventilation. At a low level [5cmH$_2$O (0.5kPa)], CPAP improves oxygenation, but does not interfere with surgery by excessive inflation of the operative lung. The mechanism of CPAP [$\leq$10cmH$_2$O ($\leq$1kPa)] is by partial re-expansion of the lung, and oxygenation of nondependent lung blood flow. Institution of 10cmH$_2$O (1kPa) CPAP has no significant hemodynamic effect, but is more likely to lead to excessive inflation of the operative lung. The lack of a hemodynamic effect is intuitive, as the same level of PEEPE on the dependent lung also has no hemodynamic effect. Higher levels of CPAP [$\geq$15cmH$_2$O ($\geq$1.5kPa)] may also redirect some of the blood flow to the dependent lung by increasing nondependent lung PVR (Fig. 50.4b). Also, CPAP commenced after lung inflation is more effective than CPAP commenced from a fully deflated lung, as the opening pressure of collapsed alveoli is higher than the usual CPAP pressure.

The most effective means of treating hypoxemia during OLV is CPAP. Rarely, patients who do not respond adequately to CPAP can be treated by reinflation of the nondependent lung. If lung volumes in the dependent lung are low, adjustment of dependent lung ventilation (larger VT, higher respiratory rate, shorter expiratory time) may improve oxygenation. In a few remaining individuals, a combination of nondependent lung CPAP and dependent lung PEEPE may improve oxygenation.

Although high-frequency ventilation of the nondependent lung improves oxygenation compared to OLV *without* nondependent lung CPAP, it is usually not more effective than OLV *with* CPAP. Its disadvantages are high equipment cost and considerable interference with surgery because of lung inflation and vibration of the large airways.

Nondependent lung perfusion

It might be possible to further and selectively vasoconstrict the nondependent hypoxic lung, while vasodilating the dependent, ventilated normoxic lung, and thereby decrease blood flow and shunt through the nondependent lung. Administration of inhaled vasodilators alone [e.g. nitric oxide or prostacyclin [prostaglandin I$_2$ (PGI$_2$)] to the dependent lung appears an attractive approach, but has not been found helpful, possibly because the dependent lung is already maximally vasodilated. During OLV, intravenously administered vasoconstrictors alone have not improved oxygenation, probably because they vasoconstrict areas of the lung that are more vasodilated, such as the dependent, oxygenated lung. The combination of an inhaled vasodilator delivered to the ventilated, dependent lung and an intravenous vasoconstrictor may be useful. The intravenous vasoconstrictor almitrine improves oxygenation during OLV, alone and in combination with nitric oxide. Almitrine is a peripheral chemoreceptor agonist and selective pulmonary vasoconstrictor that enhances HPV in low doses and perhaps attenuates HPV in high doses. The use of available vasoconstrictors, such as phenylephrine, along with nitric oxide during OLV has not been investigated.

All volatile agents inhibit HPV at high concentrations, although desflurane, sevoflurane and isoflurane may have less effect than halothane and enflurane. The effect of volatile anesthetic agents on HPV during OLV is complex, because volatile agents depress HPV and cardiac output in a dose-dependent fashion. Low cardiac output may decrease $P\bar{v}O_2$ and pulmonary artery pressure (PPA), which results in increased HPV. However, low $P\bar{v}O_2$ increases the effect of shunt upon PaO_2

The use of volatile anesthetics at less than the minimum alveolar concentration (MAC) is routinely safe and does not significantly worsen hypoxemia. Studies that have compared total intravenous anesthesia and the use of volatile agents during OLV have failed to show significant advantages from total intravenous anesthesia.

PHYSIOLOGY OF END-STAGE PULMONARY DISEASE

Dynamic hyperinflation

Dynamic hyperinflation (PEEPI) results from the commencement of inspiration before termination of expiratory flow. Patients who have COPD have areas of high lung compliance and high airways resistance with resultant long expiratory time constants. Patients who have severe COPD may have maximal expiratory flows of 200mL/s or less at lung volumes between FRC and up to nearly total lung capacity (TLC). Development of PEEPI and hyperinflation is a frequent consequence of the initiation of IPPV in these patients. As end-expiratory pressure increases, expiratory flow increases until a new steady-state lung volume occurs.

High levels of PEEPI during OLV result from severe airflow restriction (due to long expiratory time constants) and deleterious ventilator settings (such as high VT and short expiratory times). In patients with minimal airways disease undergoing OLV, FRC and PEEPI are usually normal or low. In these patients, PEEPE may improve $Pa{O_2}$ and $Pa{CO_2}$ without causing hemodynamic compromise by increasing FRC. By contrst, in patients with severe COPD, FRC and PEEPI are frequently elevated, especially during OLV. In these patients, low levels of PEEPE do not significantly increase total PEEP, yet improve $Pa{O_2}$ and $Pa{CO_2}$, although the effect is unpredictable. Higher levels of PEEPE may excessively increase FRC and PPL. High PPL adversely effects cardiac output, oxygen delivery and gas exchange. The critical levels of PEEPE, above which these adverse effects occur, are difficult to predict. Because hypercapnia sets lower limits to alveolar ventilation, there are limits to adjustments in VT, respiratory rate and I:E ratio to avoid expiratory flow limitation and PEEPI. Intraoperatively, it is difficult to accurately determine the level of PEEPI, although expiratory flow limitation is easy to observe using expiratory flow monitoring. Therefore, PEEPE should be cautiously used, for despite frequently improved gas exchange, its use can cause alveolar-capillary injury and hemodynamic disturbance. Initiaition of IPPV frequently results in a reduction in mean arterial pressure and cardiac output, because of raised intrathoracic pressure, impaired venous return, and worsened right ventricular function.

Pulmonary hypertension

Mild-to-moderate COPD has little effect on the pulmonary circulation and right heart. If hypoxia develops, chronic vasoconstriction and structural changes in small pulmonary arteries ensue by an unclear mechanism. Intimal thickening, medial hypertrophy, and smooth muscle hyperplasia lead to chronic pulmonary hypertension. Although pulmonary vasoconstrictor responses to hypoxia are intact, the predominant cause of pulmonary hypertension is an alteration in the morphology of the pulmonary vasculature caused by chronic hypoxia, and perhaps airways inflammation. Long-term oxygen therapy partially reverses pulmonary hypertension, which implies that alveolar hypoxia is a significant cause. Other contributory causes are a reduction in alveolar-capillary surface area, polycythemia, PEEPI, and impaired endothelium-induced vasodilatation. The rise in pulmonary artery pressures with progression of disease is slow, averaging only 3mmHg/year (0.4kPa/year), but its presence is an adverse sign.

The right ventricle is easily able to cope with acute and chronic increases in filling, because of its compliance, and the extraordinary ability of the pulmonary vasculature to dilate. The low-resistance pulmonary circulation is normally able to cope with large changes in flow without significant changes in pulmonary artery pressure. In contrast, the right ventricle's ability cope with increases in PVR is poor. Even if pulmonary hypertension is absent or mild, in the presence of COPD stressors such as exercise, hypoxia or pulmonary resection may cause significant increases in pulmonary artery pressure. Patients who have COPD rarely have mean pulmonary artery pressures above 40mmHg (5.3kPa) and cardiac output is usually well preserved, but cardiac output and pulmonary artery vasodilator reserves to stressors are reduced, because pulmonary capillary dilatation and recruitment is limited. The response to raised PVR is a reduction in right ventricular stroke volume, cardiac output, and ejection fraction, and an increase in end-diastolic volume. Chronic hypoxemia (because of disease or altitude) and pulmonary hypertension cause right ventricular hypertrophy. The extent of right ventricular hypertrophy is related to the degree of hypoxemia and is present at autopsy in at least 10% of patients who have COPD.

Cor pulmonale can be imprecisely defined as an alteration in the structure and function of the right ventricle as a result of primary pulmonary disease. The diagnosis of cor pulmonale and pulmonary hypertension is difficult because of the need for invasive techniques and the irregular shape of the right ventricle. Diagnosis is difficult by clinical examination alone and is aided by chest radiography, transthoracic echocardiography, electrocardiogram evidence of right-heart hypertrophy, computed tomography (CT), radionuclide assessment, magnetic resonance imaging (MRI), or right heart catheterization. Cor pulmonale also induces changes in left ventricular structure and function. The right and left ventricles are inextricably linked by shared blood supply, encircling musculature, and interventricular septum, and both are encased by the pericardium (Chapters 36, 39). Their shared interventricular septum and pericardium means that diastolic volume overload of either ventricle causes altered diastolic compliance and dimensions of the other ventricle. The presence of the pericardium enforces diastolic ventricular interdependence. Left ventricular hypertrophy and failure have been observed in patients who have cor pulmonale; however for most patients left ventricular dysfunction is not significant. Acute increases in PVR during surgery, perhaps caused by pulmonary artery clamping or OLV, are not well tolerated in patients who have severe COPD. Right ventricular function is impaired, with right ventricular dilation and decreased stroke volume. Acute impairment of left ventricular function may also occur. The impairment in right ventricular function may persist into the postoperative period.

JET VENTILATION

Bernoulli's theorem states that the lateral pressure of a fluid (gas) flowing through a tube of varying diameter is least where the diameter is least, and velocity is consequently greatest. This is the basis of the Venturi principle of jet ventilation. Venturi's principle is utilized in a number of applications in anesthesia and respiratory therapy, such as gas mixing and nebulizers (Chapter 48). If high-pressure gas is injected through a narrow needle, the pressure immediately adjacent to the tip is subatmospheric. The sub-PB at the tip of the injector port results in entrainment of ambient gas in a ratio of 2–3:1 under optimal circumstances, which results in a 'VT' greater than the jet volume and a variable gas composition. The volume and composition of the ventilating gas with jet ventilation depends upon the driving pressure, duration of injection, size of the injection port, airways resistance, and pulmonary compliance. Exhalation occurs because of passive lung deflation. High-pressure [about 345kPa (about 50psi)] 100% oxygen is regulated by a single-stage pressure regulator and the timing of gas injection is achieved by a manual valve actuator. Although automatic jet ventilators are available, they are rarely used during thoracic surgery.

Two modes of jet ventilation exist. Jet ventilation in itself refers to delivery of gas through a narrow orifice at delivery pressures >103.5kPa (>15psi), respiratory frequencies <1Hz (<60min^{-1}), and with VT > VD. High frequency jet ventilation (HFJV) may or may not use the same equipment, but refers to respiratory rates of 1–6Hz (60–360min^{-1}) with VT < VD. Jet ventilation and HFJV have been used for operative laryngoscopic surgery, flexible and rigid bronchoscopy, thoracotomy, thoracoscopy, bronchopleural fistula, and tracheal resection. The predominant advantages of jet ventilation and HFJV for thoracic surgery are the ability to ventilate an open trachea or bronchus, the ability to utilize smaller hardware in the airway, reduced motion in the surgical field, and maintenance of normal gas exchange during endoscopy and OLV. Gas exchange in HFJV occurs as a result of turbulent flow in the major airways. Mixing in the upper airways is enhanced by turbulence at airway branching, radial diffusion, and bulk flow. In smaller airways, laminar flow predominates. In terminal bronchioles and alveoli, gas exchange is mediated by bulk flow of the gas, along with asynchronous filling and emptying of alveoli, as well as cardiac and HFJV oscillations. In jet ventilation gas exchange occurs via similar mechanisms, but with a greater predominance of bulk flow over other mechanisms.

For logistic reasons, the use of jet ventilation during thoracic surgery is usually limited to a few clinical scenarios in which the airway is not intact, either in the bronchial or tracheal tree, or in which the intubation hardware does not provide for a closed airway. Disadvantages are the need for specialized hardware, lack of familiarity with the technique and equipment among anesthesiologists, inability to deliver volatile anesthetic agents, contamination of the airway with blood and secretions, and difficulty in regulating the temperature and humidity of the delivered gas. Patients who have high inspiratory resistance or poor compliance, including the obese, are often poorly ventilated by jet ventilation and HFJV. Care should be taken to avoid hyperinflation during jet ventilation and HFJV.

Ventilation is difficult to monitor during jet ventilation, although this can be performed using a distal sampling port in some situations. Monitoring of V_T is difficult and must rely on clinical signs such as chest and abdominal wall movement. As a result of uncertain V_Ts and the dilution of delivered oxygen by room air, arterial blood gases are the most accurate measurements of ventilation and oxygenation.

Concerns and reports of barotrauma attributable to the use of jet ventilation occur in the literature. Quantification of the pressure and volume stress imposed upon distal airways by jet ventilation is difficult and dependent on the driving pressure, volume of entrained gas, inspiratory time, airway anatomy, compliance and resistance, and other factors. Some authors recommend the use of a pressure-reducing valve so that the initial driving pressure is <345kPa (<50psi), which is then increased to achieve an adequate V_T. Considerable caution should be exercised when the jet outlet is near or distal to the carina.

ANESTHESIA FOR SPECIFIC THORACIC SURGICAL PROCEDURES

Anterior mediastinal masses and extrinsic tracheobronchial obstruction

Anesthetic care for patients who have anterior mediastinal masses has special physiologic considerations. Case reports exist of acute, life-threatening, or fatal compression of the major airways, pulmonary artery, superior vena cava (SVC), and heart by anterior mediastinal masses during general anesthesia. Masses of the anterior mediastinum may compress these structures in a dynamic fashion, depending on thoracic volumes, position, state of muscle relaxation, or (most importantly) the presence or absence of spontaneous ventilation. The central physiologic principle is that upright positioning and spontaneous respiratory efforts tend to relieve obstruction and maintain flow through major airways and vessels extrinsically compressed by anterior mediastinal masses.

Patients who have tumors of the mediastinum may be asymptomatic, or may present with signs or symptoms referable to the structure(s) being compressed (e.g. positional cough, dyspnea, stridor, syncope, SVC syndrome, pulsus paradoxus, etc.). Importantly, the severity of the patient's preoperative symptoms may be unrelated to the degree of respiratory or cardiovascular compromise encountered during anesthesia.

Several mechanisms conspire to exacerbate the degree of extrinsic compression from anterior mediastinal masses during anesthesia. Of these, suppression of spontaneous ventilation is the most important. The negative interpleural pressure created by spontaneous inspiratory efforts tends to increase the caliber of distal airways by radial traction and increases the transmural pressure gradient in favor of expansion of intrathoracic vessels and proximal airways. Even if spontaneous ventilation is preserved, general anesthesia results in a decrease in the anterior–posterior dimensions of the rib cage and reduction in FRC by approximately 500mL. Reduction in FRC causes a decrease in radial traction and a decrease in intrathoracic airways caliber, and thus exacerbates extrinsic compressive effects. The degree of obstruction is worse in the supine position because of a direct gravitational effect and additional decreases in FRC. The compressive weight of the tumor upon hilar and mediastinal structures is more likely to be apparent in the supine position. Muscle paralysis, as an independent variable, may also exacerbate obstruction. Since muscle relaxation does not independently affect the reduction in FRC that occurs with induction of anesthesia, the mechanism by which paralysis independently worsens extrinsic airway compression is not apparent.

There are two mechanisms by which IPPV may worsen airways obstruction. It may raise intrapleural pressure, and thus decrease the airway-stenting action of a negative intrapleural pressure (Fig. 50.5). Also, IPPV may further impair airflow through stenotic airways because higher inspiratory flow rates through the stenotic region of the airway may lead to increased turbulence. This same phenomenon has been proposed to explain the occasional observation of airway obstruction with spontaneous breathing during emergence from anesthesia. Even with spontaneous respirations, if tachypnea occurs the higher velocity may change laminar flow to turbulent, and thus impair airflow. A mixture of helium and oxygen may be advantageous in that its lower density decreases the resistance to flow and increases the critical velocity at which laminar flow begins to become turbulent (Chapter 48). This advantage must be weighed against the decreased F_{IO_2} possible using helium/oxygen mixtures.

The degree of dynamic obstruction of vessels, cardiac structures, or the airway can be assessed by supine and upright echocardiography and flow–volume loops (Fig. 50.5). Static measures, such as CT or MRI scans may be misleading and the degree of obstruction that constitutes high risk is unknown. Tracheomalacia, or distal tracheobronchial compression, is associated with the greater risk, while more proximal, compressible tumors such as retrosternal thyroid masses tend to be more easily managed by forcing a stenting endotracheal tube distal to the affected region of the airway.

Tracheobronchial resection for intrinsic obstruction

The majority of intrinsic obstructive lesions are stenotic, with a few that show chondromalacia. Symptoms are determined by

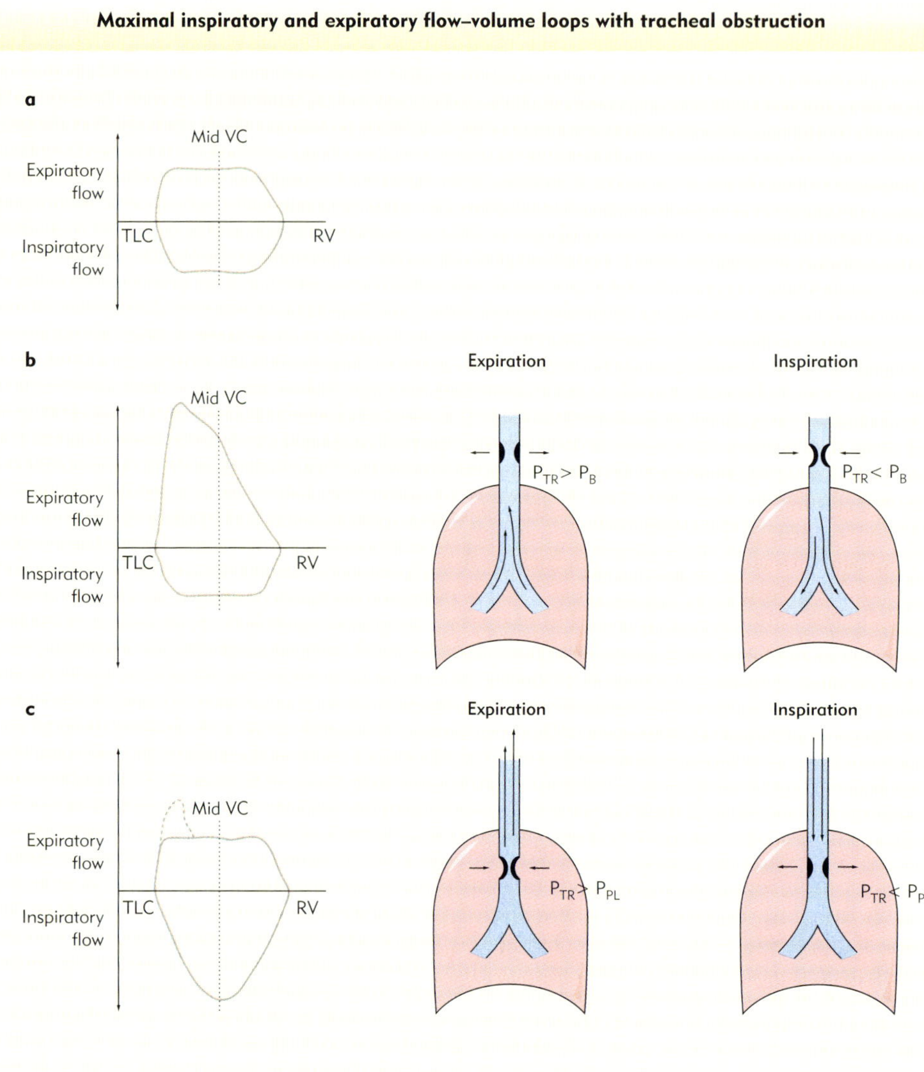

Figure 50.5 Maximal inspiratory and expiratory flow–volume loops with tracheal obstruction. Mid vital capacity (VC) flow ratio of expired:inspired flow (vertical dotted line) is sometimes indicative of the level and fixed nature of the obstruction. (a) The flow–volume loop for fixed tracheal obstruction. In fixed obstruction, airway diameter is unchanged and therefore flow is reduced in both inspiration and expiration. The effort-independent portion of expiration near TLC is markedly limited, whereas there is less reduction in the effort-independent portion near residual volume (RV). Mid-VC flow ratio is approximately 1.0. (b) The flow–volume loop for variable extrathoracic obstruction, which is more limited in inspiration than expiration because intratracheal pressure (P_{TR}) is less than P_B. During expiration, P_{TR} exceeds P_B, and therefore the obstruction is diminished. Mid-VC flow ratio is usually >1.0. (c) The flow–volume loop for variable intrathoracic obstruction (in which the flow transient shown by the dashed line is occasionally observed). Variable intrathoracic obstruction is more limited in expiration than inspiration because P_{PL} exceeds P_{TR}. During inspiration, P_{TR} exceeds P_{PL}, and therefore the obstruction is diminished. Mid-VC flow ratio is usually <1.0. (Modified with permission from Kryger et al., 1976.)

the extent of stenosis, but asymptomatic individuals may have severe obstruction. Dyspnea upon exertion often occurs at a lesional diameter of approximately 5–6mm or 30% of the normal cross-sectional area of the trachea, and stridor at rest is apparent at a diameter of approximately 4mm. Pulmonary function tests can help in the diagnosis and assessment of obstruction. Typically, fixed obstruction results in markedly reduced expiratory and inspiratory flows (see Fig. 50.5). Intrathoracic variable obstruction results in greater expiratory flow limitation than during inspiration. The explanation is that during expiration the raised intrathoracic pressure results in tracheal compression, which worsens the resistance of the stenosis. During inspiration a more negative intrathoracic pressure results in some dilatation of the stenosis, and therefore reduced resistance at the stenosis.

Since IPPV results in higher mean intrathoracic pressures than does spontaneous ventilation, tracheal obstruction may be significantly worsened by IPPV. For this reason spontaneous ventilation is maintained until either control of the distal airway is obtained by intubation or it is shown that IPPV does not worsen the obstruction. As with all obstructive lesions, the potential for dynamic hyperinflation and consequent cardiovascular compromise is present.

Lung transplantation

Patients who have end-stage COPD and other end-stage pulmonary diseases such as cystic fibrosis, primary pulmonary hypertension, and α_1-antitrypsin deficiency have a limited life span. Medical therapies such as domiciliary oxygen therapy, corticosteroids, and bronchodilators have limited success. Two surgical therapies are available – lung transplantation and LVRS (see below) – to small subgroups of patients who have end-stage pulmonary disease. Patients who have COPD and cystic fibrosis are the largest proportion of patients who receive lung transplantation. These patients have similar pathophysiology, of which the most important issues to the anesthesiologist are dynamic hyperinflation (PEEPi), impaired gas exchange, pulmonary hypertension, and right ventricular dysfunction.

Either single- or sequential single- (bilateral-)lung transplantation is performed. Single-lung transplantation is performed for primarily nonsuppurative disease, although emphysema and primary pulmonary hypertension are relative indications. Bilateral-lung transplantation is performed for cystic fibrosis, and has been utilized for emphysematous COPD because of the commonly observed 'crowding' of the donor lung by the emphysematous native lung. Essentially, because compliance and airways resistance of the native lung are greater than those of the donor lung, expansion of the native lung compresses the donor lung. In some situations, LVRS of the native lung after single-lung transplantation has been carried out to reduce 'crowding'. In a smaller proportion of patients who have pulmonary fibrosis, primary pulmonary hypertension and other nonobstructive disorders, pulmonary hypertension and right ventricular failure are pre-eminent. In patients who have poor right heart function and severe pulmonary hypertension, bilateral lung transplantation or heart–lung transplantation has been carried out.

Two physiologic insults are present during lung transplantation that are not found during LVRS – pulmonary artery clamping and reperfusion of the transplanted lung(s). Pulmonary artery clamping for pneumonectomy is a severe physiologic insult to the patient's very limited pulmonary vasodilatory and right heart reserve. Techniques to reduce PVR intraoperatively are 100% oxygen and pulmonary vasodilators, especially nitrovasodilators, PGI_2, Ca^{2+} channel antagonists, and phosphodiesterase inhibitors, in combination with an appropriately increased preload and inotropes. The response to these interventions is variable, with pulmonary vasodilator therapy frequently limited by systemic vasodilatation and hypotension. The exception is with inhaled nitric oxide. A significant percentage of patients who undergo lung transplantation require cardiopulmonary bypass (CPB) to support the circulation, or to improve gas exchange during the pneumonectomy phase of transplantation. Prediction of which patients will require CPB is useful for logistic reasons – to avoid an unexpected precipitous need for CPB and to avoid unnecessary CPB (as the use of CPB is associated with bleeding and worsened postoperative graft function). Factors that increase the likelihood of CPB are poor right-ventricular function and pulmonary hypertension, severe obstructive lung disease, and severely reduced exercise capacity and oxygen uptake. Patients who do not tolerate OLV or pulmonary artery clamping also require CPB, although not all these patients can be identified by pulmonary artery clamping.

Reperfusion of the donor lung is accompanied by occasional brief hypoxemia and frequent systemic hypotension, possibly caused by air embolus, lung-'plegia'(preservation solution)-induced hyperkalemia, hypothermia, PGs, or other vasodilators. These effects are short lived and usually easily treatable. A delayed response, the 'pulmonary reimplantation response', is characterized by poor oxygenation, low compliance, and low-pressure pulmonary edema. Severe early allograft dysfunction occurs in 15–35% of lung transplant recipients. Most likely this represents a form of ischemia–reperfusion injury, but it may be confounded by loss of lymphatic drainage, pulmonary denervation, and occasionally stenosis of the pulmonary venous anastomosis. Although intraoperative fluids have not been shown to be related to postoperative oxygenation, a widespread clinical belief is that fluids should be limited, and that diuretics are therapeutic for improved graft function.

Nitric oxide appears to be a physiologically appropriate drug for pulmonary dysfunction after lung transplantation. The role of nitric oxide in amelioration of allograft dysfunction after lung transplantation is probably more complex than just pulmonary vasodilatation. Nitric oxide is a potent inhibitor of platelet and

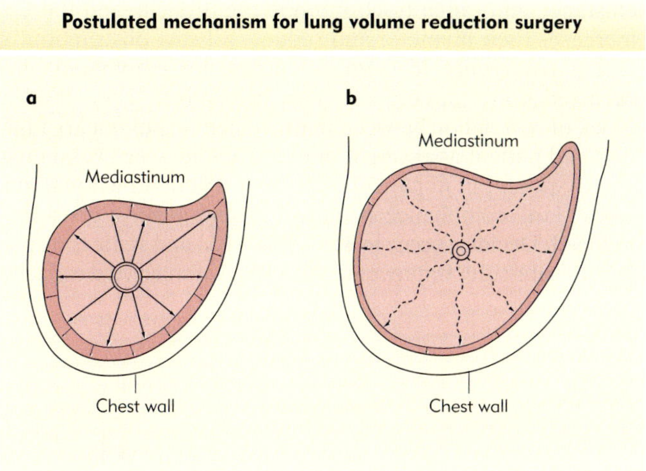

Figure 50.6 Postulated mechanism of effect for LVRS. (a) Normal negative intrapleural pressure is generated by retraction of the chest wall and lung recoil, which results in radial traction on the bronchi. (b) In emphysematous lung disease, loss of lung tissue elastic recoil results in chest wall hyperinflation and reduction in radial traction on the bronchi, and therefore increased airways resistance and increased lung compliance. Reduction in lung volume causes increased lung elastic recoil and increased radial traction on the bronchi, and thus improves lung compliance, reduces chest wall diameter (decreased RV), and perhaps decreases airways resistance. (Modified with permission from Brantigan O, Mueller E, Kress M, 1959.)

neutrophil aggregation and adhesion, modulates vascular permeability and has potent anti-inflammatory actions. Accordingly, inhaled nitric oxide may provide prophylaxis of pulmonary dysfunction and also reduce P_{PA} and improve $\dot{V}/\dot{Q}s$ matching. However, nitric oxide may be cytotoxic, perhaps because nitric oxide–superoxide species may worsen ischemia–reperfusion injury. Several studies show that inhaled nitric oxide or intravenous infusion of nitric oxide donors after transplantation cause improved oxygenation and lower PVR, even if administered for only short periods. A reduction in PVR by lung transplantation causes both immediate and long-term improvement in right ventricular function.

Lung volume reduction surgery

Emphysematous lung disease has a high mortality (10%/year if $FEV_1 < 1.0L$), and patients who have severe COPD who undergo surgery have a very high incidence of postoperative complications and death. Major therapeutic modalities consist of bronchodilators, anti-inflammatory drugs, antibiotics, and supplemental oxygen therapy. Despite medical therapies, the course of the disease is progressive, with increasing limitation and high mortality.

In the late 1950s, Brantigan developed the concepts of lung resection for treatment of emphysema, but had unacceptably high perioperative mortality. He postulated that emphysematous lung disease resulted in a loss of tissue elastance that caused terminal bronchioles to become dynamically obstructed (Fig. 50.6). Resection of emphysematous lung tissue allows the remaining more normal lung to expand within the hyperexpanded chest wall. Lung resection results in improved tissue elastance and radial traction upon the bronchi, and thereby increases their diameter and reduces airways obstruction. A recent resurgence in surgical therapy for emphysema has occurred. Outcomes of LVRS have been mixed. There is often a lack of correlation between improvement in pulmonary function and patient assessment of exercise tolerance, well-being, and dyspnea, but in patients who have a good functional outcome, lung compliance is increased and airways resistance reduced. Declines occur in TLC, FRC, RV, and static transpulmonary pressure. Improvements in FEV_1, forced vital capacity, exercise duration and severity, dyspnea indices, and oxygen uptake occur. Blood gases change little, but oxygen requirements sometimes decrease.

Guiding principles in anesthesia for LVRS are avoidance of dynamic hyperinflation, treatment and avoidance of bronchospasm, prevention of further increases in PVR, optimization of OLV, and early postoperative extubation. PEEPi is deleterious as it may cause bullous rupture, cardiovascular compromise, increased dependent lung shunt, or increased air-leak at surgical staple lines.

Key References

Benumof JL et al. Margin of safety in positioning modern double-lumen endotracheal tubes. Anesthesiology. 1987;67:729-38.

Brantigan O, Mueller E, Kress M. A surgical approach to pulmonary emphysema. Am Rev Respir Dis. 1959;80:194–206.

Capan LM, Turndorf H, Patel C, et al. Optimization of arterial oxygenation during one-lung anesthesia. Anesth Analg. 1980;59:847–51.

Froese AB, Bryan AC. Effects of anesthesia and paralysis on diaphragmatic mechanics in man. Anesthesiology. 1974;41:242–55.

Kryger et al. Diagnosis of obstruction of the upper and central airways. Ann J Med. 1976;61:85-93.

Marshall B, Marshall C. Continuity of response to hypoxic pulmonary vasoconstriction. J Appl Physiol. 1980;59:189–94.

Meredino et al. Human measurements involved in tracheobronchial resection and reconstruction procedures. Surgery. 1954;35:590–7.

Miller FL, Chen L, Malmkvist G, Marshall C, Marshall BE. Mechanical factors do not influence blood flow distribution in atelectasis. Anesthesiology. 1989;70:481–8.

Ranieri VM, Dambrosio M, Brienza N. Intrinsic PEEP and cardiopulmonary interaction in patients with COPD and acute ventilatory failure. Eur Respir J. 1996;9:1283–92.

Solway J, Rossing TH, Saari AF, Drazen JM. Expiratory flow limitation and dynamic pulmonary hyperinflation during high-frequency ventilation. J Appl Physiol. 1986;60:2071–8.

Further Reading

Bardoczky GI, Yernault JC, Engelman EE, et al. Intrinsic positive end-expiratory pressure during one-lung ventilation for thoracic surgery. The influence of preoperative pulmonary function. Chest. 1996;110:180–4.

Cohen E, Eisenkraft J. Positive end-expiratory pressure during one-lung ventilation improves oxygenation in patients with low arterial oxygen tensions. J Cardiothorac Vasc Anesth. 1996;10:578–82.

Cooper JD, Patterson GA, Sundaresan RS, et al. Results of 150 consecutive bilateral lung volume reduction procedures in patients with severe emphysema. J Thorac Cardiovasc Surg. 1996;112:1319–29.

Eppinger MJ, Ward PA, Jones ML, Bolling SF, Deeb GM. Disparate effects of nitric oxide on lung ischemia–reperfusion injury. Ann Thorac Surg. 1995;60:1169–75.

Moutafis M, Liu N, Dalibon N, et al.. The effects of inhaled nitric oxide and its combination with intravenous almitrine on Pao_2 \during one-lung ventialtion in patients undergoing thoracoscopic procedures. Anesth Analg. 1997;85:1130–5.

Nevin M, Van Besouw JP, Williams CW, Pepper JR. A comparative study of conventional versus high-frequency jet ventilation with relation to the incidence of postoperative morbidity in thoracic surgery. Ann Thorac Surg. 1987;44:625–7.

Reed CE, Dorman BH, Spinale FG. Mechanisms of right ventricular dysfunction after pulmonary resection. Ann Thorac Surg. 1996;62:225–31.

Singh H, Bossard RF. Perioperative anaesthetic considerations for patients undergoing lung transplantation. Can J Anaesth. 1997;44:284–99.

Solway J, Rossing TH, Saari AF, Drazen JM. Expiratory flow limitation and dynamic pulmonary hyperinflation during high-frequency ventilation. J Appl Physiol. 1986;60:2071–8.

Chapter 51 Hematology

Mark C Bellamy

Topics covered in this chapter

Bone marrow, blood cells, and plasma constituents
Coagulation
Drugs affecting coagulation and platelet function
Hemostatic defects and bleeding disorders
Evaluation of coagulation
Transfusion therapy
Blood products
Blood groups
Risks of blood transfusion

Patients undergoing surgical operations frequently require blood transfusion and can develop derangement of the hemostatic pathway and fibrinolysis. These changes require active support from the anesthetist, which demands a clear understanding of the pathophysiology and basic clinical principles. This chapter covers elements of transfusion practice, hemostasis, and coagulation disorders.

BONE MARROW, BLOOD CELLS, AND PLASMA CONSTITUENTS

In fetal life, the yolk sac is the main site for hemopoiesis until 6 weeks of gestation. From 6 weeks until 7 months, the liver and spleen play the major role. Both liver and spleen continue to produce red blood cells until 2 weeks after birth, although the principal site of hemopoiesis from 7 months of fetal life onwards throughout normal childhood and adult life is bone marrow. In infants, practically all bones are involved. In adults, hemopoiesis is confined to vertebrae, ribs, sternum, skull, sacrum, pelvis, and proximal femur. Under extreme conditions, there can also be expansion of hemopoiesis into other long bones. The phenomenon of extramedullary hemopoiesis (liver and spleen) is also occasionally seen.

A common, pluripotential stem cell gives rise to all cells of the hemopoietic line. After a number of divisions and early differentiation, the pluripotential stem cell differentiates into progenitor cells for the three main marrow cell lines: erythroid, granulocytic (including monocytes), and megakaryocytic. Progenitor cells are capable of responding to a number of stimuli with increased production of one or other cell lines according to need. Transplanted hemopoietic cells seed successfully to the marrow whereas they fail to survive at other sites. This is the basis for bone marrow transplantation.

Red blood cells

The pronormoblast is the earliest red blood cell recognizable in the marrow. Progressively smaller normoblasts result from cell division. As this process of maturation proceeds, cells develop a progressively greater hemoglobin content. There is progressive loss of RNA and protein-synthesizing apparatus from the cytoplasm, and the cell nucleus is extruded from late normoblasts. This results in a cell known as a reticulocyte, which initially resides within bone marrow and has low levels of cytoplasmic RNA (but is still capable of synthesizing hemoglobin). Hemoglobin-synthesizing capability is lost when the cell enters the circulation as a mature erythrocyte. The mature cell is a biconcave disc with no nucleus. At times of hemopoietic stress, reticulocytes may also appear in the peripheral circulation.

Erythropoiesis is predominantly governed by the hormone erythropoietin. Relative renal hypoxemia gives rise to expression of a nuclear transcription factor that causes increased expression of the erythropoietin gene. Erythropoietin increases the number of stem cells committed to erythropoiesis.

The mature red blood cell has a diameter of 8μm and a lifespan of 120 days. It is extremely flexible and can pass through vessels in the microcirculation with a minimum diameter of only 3.5μm. It is capable of synthesizing adenosine triphosphate (ATP) and the reduced form of nicotinamide adenine dinucleotide (NADH) by the anaerobic glycolytic pathway. The red cell membrane-associated enzyme methemoglobin reductase is associated with the glycolytic pathway and NAD^+/NADH metabolism. Function of this enzyme is important for maintaining the ferrous (Fe^{2+}) oxidative state of iron in hemoglobin. Oxidation to the ferric state (Fe^{3+}) results in methemoglobin, which is ineffective as an oxygen carrier. Many drugs can induce significant oxidative stress and, thus, result in methemoglobin production. These include acetaminophen (paracetamol) and most local anesthetic agents, notably prilocaine.

Red cell production in the marrow is a process requiring many precursors to synthesize the new cells and their proteins, including hemoglobin. Essential substances, known as hematinics, include vitamins [vitamin B_{12}, folate, vitamin C (ascorbic acid), D-α-tocopherol (vitamin E), vitamin B_6, vitamin B_1 (thiamine), vitamin B_2 (riboflavin), pantothenic acid)], metals (iron, manganese, cobalt), and essential amino acids.

Deficiencies can result in failure of erythropoiesis, with characteristic anemias. Megaloblastic (i.e. large, immature cells) anemia results from deficiencies of vitamin B_{12} or folate. Iron-deficiency anemia results in small, hypochromic cells. Anemia may also occur with amino acid or androgen deficiency, although this may be simply an adaptive response to reduced tissue oxygen consumption rather than a direct effect of the 'hematinic' deficiency. The anemias of chronic disease fall into this category.

Hemoglobin

Hemoglobin is a red cell protein that facilitates oxygen and carbon dioxide transport (Chapter 45). There are approximately 640 million molecules of hemoglobin in each red blood cell. Hemoglobin consists of four polypeptide chains (two α- and two β-chains). Each of these chains is associated with a heme prosthetic group. Each hemoglobin chain has a molecular weight of 68,000. Adult blood contains traces both of hemoglobin F (fetal hemoglobin) and hemoglobin A_2. These contain α-chains, but the β-chains are replaced with γ- and δ-chains, respectively. Most hemoglobin (65%) is synthesized at the erythroblastic stage, and the remainder at the reticulocyte stage. Heme synthesis (predominantly in the mitochondrion) begins with the condensation of glycine and succinyl coenzyme A. Vitamin B_6 is a coenzyme for this process. A ring structure is formed (protoporphyrin) that then combines with iron to form heme. Each heme molecule associates with a globin chain manufactured on the polyribosomes. A tetramer forms comprising two α- and two β- chains, each with its associated heme molecule.

White blood cells

Leukocytes may be divided into two broad groups: phagocytes and lymphocytes. Phagocytes include neutrophils (polymorphonuclear cells or polymorphs), eosinophils, basophils, and monocytes. Neutrophils have a diameter of 12–15μm and a characteristic dense multilobular (two to five lobes) nucleus. The cytoplasm is characterized by numerous fine azurophilic granules. Mature polymorphs contain two types of granule, both derived from lysozymes. Primary granules contain myeloperoxidase and acid phosphatase. Secondary granules contain alkaline phosphatase and lysozyme. The earliest recognizable neutrophil precursor is the myeloblast, which is seen in bone marrow but not in peripheral blood; this divides to form myelocytes, with a distinct myelocyte for the eosinophil and the basophil cell lines. The myelocytes divide to form metamyelocytes, which further mature to take on the multilobular form of the mature polymorph. Intermediate nuclear morphologies are known as 'band' or 'juvenile' forms. At times of high neutrophil production (infection), immature band forms may be seen in the peripheral circulation.

Lymphocytes are small cells (7–15μm in diameter) produced in both marrow and thymus. Larger lymphocytes may be seen following antigenic stimulation. The immune response is a function of both T and B lymphocytes (Chapter 52).

Platelets

Platelets are produced in bone marrow from megakaryocytes, which are derived from the pluripotential stem cell. Each megakaryocyte undergoes rapid nuclear replication without cell division. With the addition of further nuclei, there is an increase in cytoplasm and cell size. When the cell reaches the eight-nucleus stage, replication ceases. The cytoplasm becomes progressively more granular and produces microvesicles, which coalesce to form platelet demarcation membranes. Fragmentation of megakaryocyte cytoplasm then follows, with release of platelets. Each megakaryocyte releases about 4000 platelets. Young, immature platelets spend 24 hours in the spleen before entering the circulation. Platelets have a lifetime of 10–15 days.

Plasma

Blood cells are suspended in plasma, a solution of electrolytes; proteins such as albumin, globulins, and clotting factors; lipids; and lipoproteins. Plasma acts as a vehicle for nutrient transport and the immune system and plays a key role in coagulation and hemostasis.

COAGULATION

Coagulation occurs as a consequence of the interaction between damaged tissue, plasma clotting factors, and platelets. The coagulation cascade is balanced by the fibrinolytic cascade, which regulates breakdown of fibrin and fibrinogen and prevents excessive formation of thrombi. Normal clotting and hemostasis represents a dynamic interaction between the coagulation cascade, the fibrinolytic cascade, and platelet function.

Platelet function

The principal role of platelets is formation of mechanical plugs during hemostasis. Key functions in this process include adhesion, release (platelet degranulation), aggregation, fusion, and platelet procoagulant activity. After blood vessel injury, platelets are exposed to subendothelial connective tissues. This promotes platelet adhesion, which is dependent on the presence of the plasma protein von Willebrand factor, part of the main fraction of factor VIII [factor VIII-related antigen (VIIIR:AG)]. The rate of adhesion depends on surface membrane glycoproteins (absent in the Bernard–Soulier syndrome).

Exposure to collagen at sites of vascular injury, or the presence of activated thrombin, results in platelet degranulation. Platelet granules contain adenosine diphosphate (ADP), serotonin, fibrinogen, lysozyme, and heparin-neutralizing factor [also known as platelet factor 4 (PF4)]. The release process is dependent on prostaglandin synthesis (Fig. 51.1). Platelet membrane peroxidation results in the synthesis of thromboxane A_2. Thromboxane A_2 reduces the level of cyclic adenosine monophosphate (cAMP) and initiates the release reaction. Thromboxane A_4 potentiates platelet aggregation and is a potent vasoconstrictor. Hence, compounds affecting levels of platelet cAMP affect the release reaction. The vasodilator prostaglandins, such as prostacyclin, synthesized by vascular endothelium stimulate adenylyl cyclase. Prostacyclin has an important role in limiting clot formation and in preventing platelet adhesion to normal vascular endothelium.

Platelet aggregation requires thromboxane A_2 and follows ADP release. Adenosine diphosphate causes platelet swelling and facilitates a reaction whereby membranes of adjacent platelets stick to each other. This initiates a positive feedback loop in which further ADP and thromboxane A_2 are released, resulting in secondary platelet aggregation. This self-fueling process results in aggregation of a sufficiently large platelet mass to plug the breach in the vascular endothelium.

Platelets have a procoagulant activity. Following aggregation and release, platelet membrane phospholipid, platelet factor 3 (PF3), is exposed. This exposed surface provides a suitable template for concentration and orientation of proteins involved in the coagulation cascade.

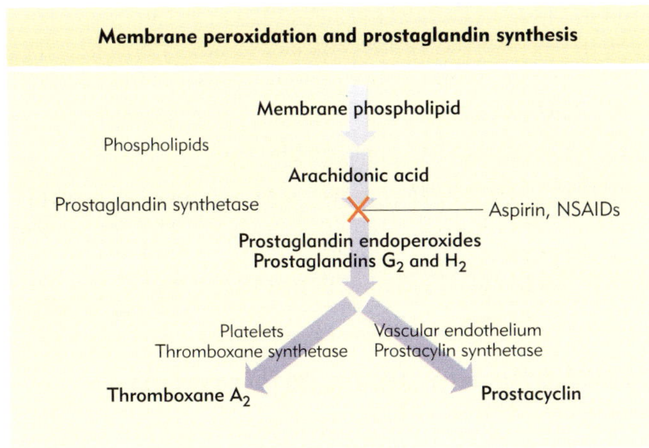

Figure 51.1 Processes involved in membrane peroxidation and prostaglandin synthesis. (PG, prostaglandin.)

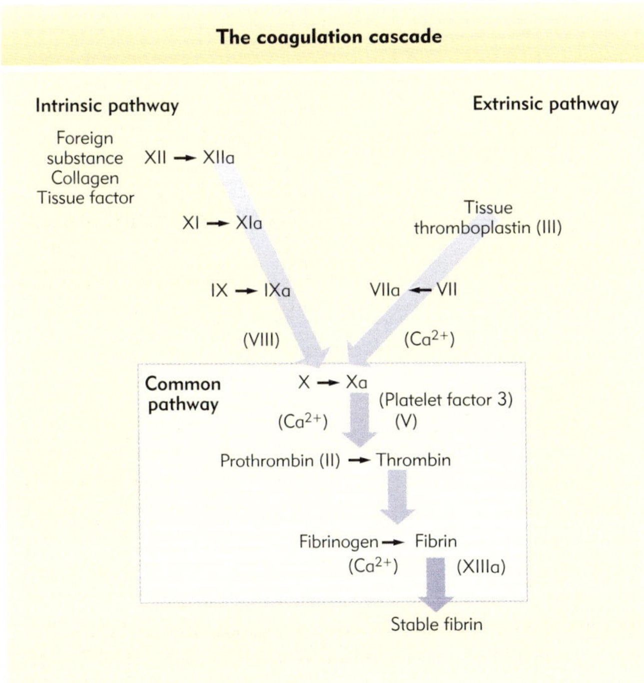

Figure 51.2 The coagulation cascade.

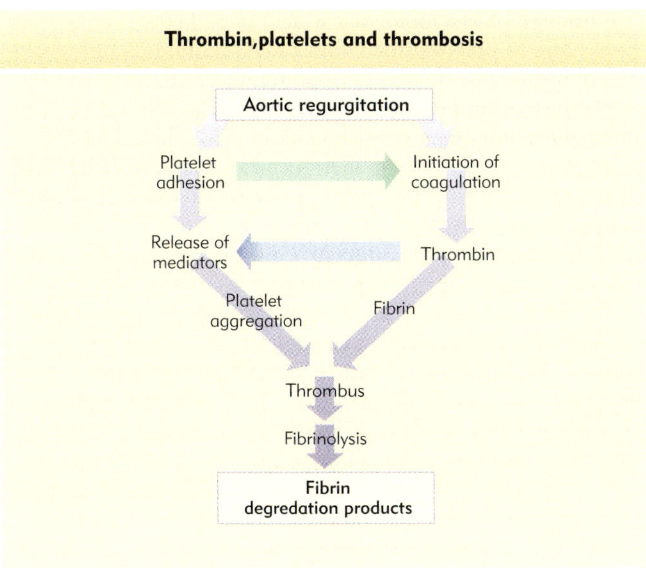

Figure 51.3 Thrombin and platelets and their interaction in thrombosis.

Finally, platelet fusion occurs. The membranes of adjacent platelets fuse in the presence of high concentrations of ADP and enzymes released in the release reaction. This process is further potentiated by thrombin. Fibrin formation reinforces the stability of the evolving platelet plug and eventually results in clot retraction and stabilization. Platelet degranulation (release reaction) may also promote vascular endothelial healing by release of specific growth factors.

The coagulation cascade

The coagulation cascade is a biologic amplification system: relatively few initiating factors sequentially activate a proteolytic cascade (Fig. 51.2) in which each activated component catalyzes the activation of several molecules of the next component, giving an amplified response. The precursor proteins are cleaved sequentially to give activated enzymes culminating in the generation of thrombin. Thrombin converts soluble inactive plasma fibrinogen to fibrin, which becomes cross-linked to produce a stable fibrin plug. This plug combines with platelets to form a clot and undergoes retraction to produce effective hemostasis. The interactions of the coagulation, platelet, and fibrinolytic systems are summarized in Figure 51.3.

Classically, the coagulation cascade is considered in two limbs. The intrinsic pathway is initiated by injury to vascular endothelium, which exposes collagen and other subendothelial components. These result in activation of factor XII, with subsequent activation of factors XI and IX. In combination with factor VIII, PF3, and calcium ions, there is activation by proteolitic cleavage of factor X. Activated factor X (Xa), in the presence of calcium and factor V, cleaves prothrombin to thrombin. Thrombin cleaves fibrinogen to fibrin, which polymerizes to form clot.

Factors XII, XI, IX, X, and VII and prothrombin circulate in the plasma as inactive precursors (zymogen) and are all activated by proteolytic cleavage. The activated clotting factors are themselves serine proteases, that is they have a serine residue at their active centers that is involved in the hydrolysis of peptide bonds.

The intrinsic system of activation is complemented by an alternative pathway, the extrinsic system. Following tissue injury, a number of tissue activators elicit conversion of factor VII to factor VIIa, which produces small amounts of thrombin locally. This thrombin has two effects: it causes fibrin deposition at the site of vascular injury and has a positive feedback loop increasing activated factor VIII and factor V. This amplifies and accelerates the intrinsic pathway.

Factor VIII is a large protein (1.5–2.0MDa), consisting of two components. The larger component (VIIIR:AG) is involved in platelet-related activities, including platelet adhesion to exposed subendothelial connective tissue and platelet aggregation. Von Willebrand factor (VIII:WF) is part of factor VIIIR:AG. The remaining component, factor VIII coagulant (VIII:C), is noncovalently bound to VIIIR:AG.

Fibrinogen has a molecular weight of 340,000. It consists of three pairs of polypeptide chains, α-, β-, and δ-chains, cross-linked by disulfide bonds. Thrombin releases fibrinopeptide A and B from α- and β-chains of fibrinogen by proteolysis. This forms fibrin monomer, consisting of the cross-linked α-, β-, and δ-chains. Hydrogen bonds then form spontaneously between molecules of fibrin monomer, giving rise to fibrin polymer. Factor XIII is activated by thrombin. Activated XIII stabilizes fibrin polymer by introducing Glu–Lys isopeptide bonds between adjacent fibrin monomers.

The hemostatic response results from interaction between the clotting cascade, platelet activity, and the blood vessel wall. Following vascular injury, there is immediate constriction of the damaged vessel, with reflex constriction of adjacent small arteries and arterioles. In massive injury, this immediate reflex prevents exsanguination. Reduction in blood flow velocity permits contact activation of platelets and the coagulation cascade. These processes are accompanied by release of vasoactive amines, thromboxane from platelets, and fibrinopeptides liberated by fibrin formation. These all potentiate local vasoconstriction at the site of injury. This process is potentiated by VIII:WF. Activation of platelets and the coagulation cascade, as described above, results in definitive hemostasis when fibrin formed by coagulation combines with the platelet mass to produce a retractile clot.

However, if coagulation were to continue unchecked, there would be widespread vascular occlusion. Numerous feedback processes control clotting. Activated clotting factors (serine proteases) are inhibited by the circulating serine protease inhibitor antithrombin (previously known as antithrombin III). Antithrombin neutralizes thrombin, as well as factors Xa, VIIa, IXa, and XIa, by formation of peptide bonds with the active serine sites. Activated coagulation factors and other procoagulants are filtered by the reticuloendothelial system, in particular hepatic Küpffer cells. The vitamin K-dependent anticoagulant protein, protein C, is produced in the liver. This combines with protein S to produce protein C–S complex. Activated complex binds to and inhibits factor VIII. Patients who have homozygous protein C deficiency develop widespread intravascular coagulation resulting in blindness through retinal artery occlusion, stroke, and coagulopathy through disseminated intravascular coagulation (DIC). Such patients rarely survive infancy. In the heterozygous form of the disease, patients survive into adult life but may develop multiple systemic thromboses, including pulmonary embolus or the Budd–Chiari syndrome. These complications are exacerbated by pregnancy or the oral contraceptive pill, which reduce circulating levels of protein C. Paradoxically, anticoagulants such as warfarin may increase the tendency of these procoagulant phenomena by inhibition of the formation of vitamin K-containing clotting factors and hence further inhibition of protein C activity.

The fibrinolytic system

In addition to the regulatory mechanisms described above that limit activation of the clotting cascade, there is also a biologic cascade (amplification) system for limitation of clot size and dissolution of stable fibrin, the fibrinolytic cascade (Figs 51.4 & 51.5). Excessive fibrinolysis becomes a clinical problem for anesthetists in the areas of cardiac, vascular, and transplantation surgery; it may also occur during sepsis. Fibrinolysis occurs as a result of digestion of fibrin by proteolytic enzymes.

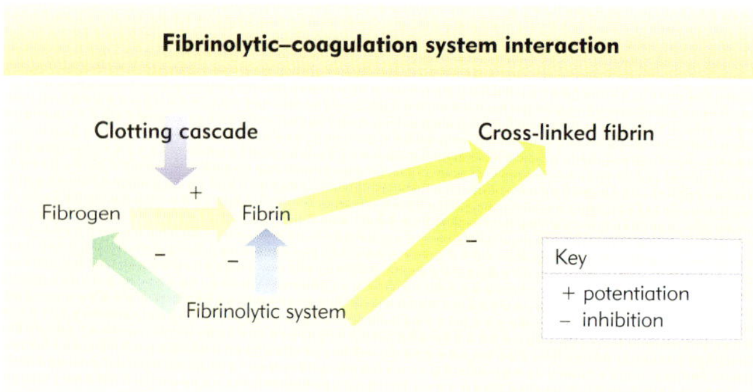

Figure 51.4 Interaction between the fibrinolytic and coagulation systems.

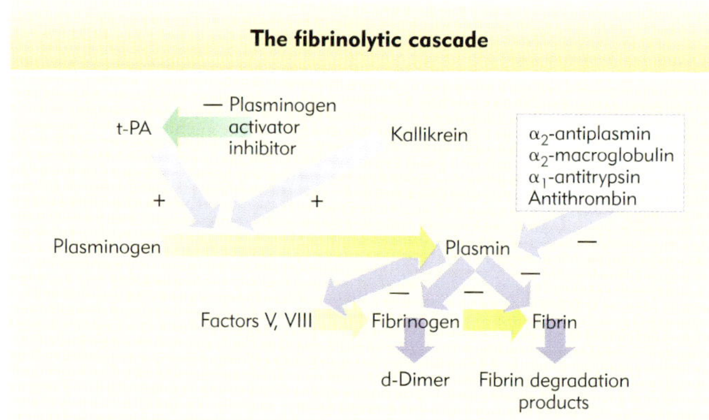

Figure 51.5 The fibrinolytic cascade. t-PA, tissue plaminogen activator.

Plasmin is the key serine protease involved in fibrinolysis. Plasminogen is activated to plasmin by two plasminogen activators: tissue type (t-PA) and urokinase (u-PA); t-PA is active when bound to fibrin. Endothelium also produces a rapid t-PA inactivator, plasminogen activator inhibitor (PAI). There are three subclasses of this inhibitor, although most effects appear to be attributable to PAI_1. Platelets stimulated by thrombin also produce PAI. Consequently platelet aggregation limits fibrinolysis. There are a number of complex interactions. Activated protein C (an anticoagulant in the clotting cascade) also reduces endothelial production of PAI. Hence, protein C is also a promoter of the fibrinolytic process by increasing circulating levels of t-PA. Factor XII activation (secondary to endothelial damage) promotes kallikrein release and hence activation of fibrinolysis. Once plasminogen has been activated to plasmin, it triggers the complement cascade.

Plasminogen is adsorbed onto fibrin at specific lysine-binding sites. Fibrin (but not fibrinogen) also has t-PA-binding sites. The fibrin molecule constitutes an environment that facilitates presentation of t-PA to plasminogen and cleavage of this zymogen to plasmin. Plasmin digests fibrin to fibrin degradation products (FDPs) [fibrin split products (FSPs)]; the plasmin is then released from lysed fibrin and returns to the circulation. Normally, free plasmin is rapidly inactivated by α_2-macroglobulin and antithrombin. When present in excess, free plasmin cleaves fibrinogen producing d-dimer and can inactivate factors V and VIII; this occurs in DIC.

Processes regulating fibrinolysis display anatomic variation. Fibrinolysis is more active in the arterial than in the venous system, in deep than in superficial veins, and in the upper than in the lower limbs. In pregnancy, both fibrinogen and plasminogen levels are increased, but t-PA levels are reduced. At the same time α_2-antiplasmin levels are increased; overall fibrinolysis is reduced. Hormones involved in the neurohumoral stress response (corticosteroids, catecholamines, vasopressin) cause a transient increase in fibrinolytic activity. Hence, there is increased fibrinolysis during surgery, and possibly during venous occlusion. This latter effect may also be as a consequence of reduced PAI. Increased fibrinolysis in venous occlusion may explain the mechanism of action of calf compression devices in preventing deep venous thrombosis during surgery.

DRUGS AFFECTING COAGULATION AND PLATELET FUNCTION

A number of drugs affect coagulation and platelet function. They may exert their effect by potentiating naturally occurring inhibition of coagulation, particularly at the level of factor Xa and thrombin (e.g. the heparins). The venom of the Malayan pit viper *(Ancrod)* promotes intravascular conversion of fibrinogen to fibrin and subsequent breakdown to FDPs, which are in themselves antifibrinolytic. Several anticoagulants (the oral anticoagulants) exert their effect by antagonizing vitamin K and hence suppressing synthesis of vitamin K-dependent clotting factors: factors II, VII, and X (half-lives 60, 80 and 36 hours, respectively), protein C, and other proteins. Fibrinolysis may be either enhanced (t-PA, streptokinase, urokinase), or inhibited (aprotinin, tranexamic acid, ϵ-aminocaproic acid).

Heparin

Unfractionated heparin is a water-soluble mucopolysaccharide organic acid (Fig. 51.6). It is present in high concentrations in liver and in the granules of mast cells and basophils. It exerts its anticoagulant effect by binding with antithrombin. This brings about a change in conformation that substantially enhances antithrombin binding and inhibits factors XIIa, XIa, IXa, and Xa and thrombin (see Fig. 41.3). As heparin is derived from multiple biologic sources, its activity may vary per unit weight; consequently, heparin dose is expressed in standard international units (IUs).

Indications for heparin include anticoagulation during cardiopulmonary bypass (Chapter 41), treatment and prophylaxis of deep vein thrombosis, treatment of pulmonary embolism, and protection of patency of intravascular catheters and extracorporeal systems (e.g. in renal dialysis). Heparin exerts its effect immediately when given intravenously. The peak effect after subcutaneous injection occurs after 30 minutes. Heparin is not active orally and is metabolized in the liver and excreted by the kidney; it has an elimination half-life between 2 and 3 hours. The effect of heparin is monitored by activated partial thromboplastin time (APTT), a measure of the intrinsic coagulation cascade. Therapeutic range of APTT is 60–100 seconds (1.5 to 2.5 times normal).

Adverse effects

Heparin has a number of adverse effects. The most common is hemorrhage. This is unusual where APTT is maintained within the therapeutic range. Some patients are at particular risk for heparin-induced bleeding [e.g. patients who have vitamin K deficiency (antibiotic therapy, liver disease) or who have had recent surgery]. Although therapeutic doses of heparin may represent a relative contraindication to regional anesthetic blockade, low-dose heparin prophylaxis (5000IU twice daily subcutaneously) is not a contraindication to central neural blockade. Patients on long-term heparin therapy may develop a reduction in antithrombin activity to 10–20% of normal levels and may exhibit 'heparin resistance', requiring an increased dose. Heparin resistance can result in paradoxic thrombosis. Antithrombin levels are restored by administration of fresh frozen plasma or antithrombin concentrate.

A complication of prolonged heparin therapy (typically 5 days or more) is heparin-induced thrombocytopenia. This occurs more frequently when bovine lung heparin is used than

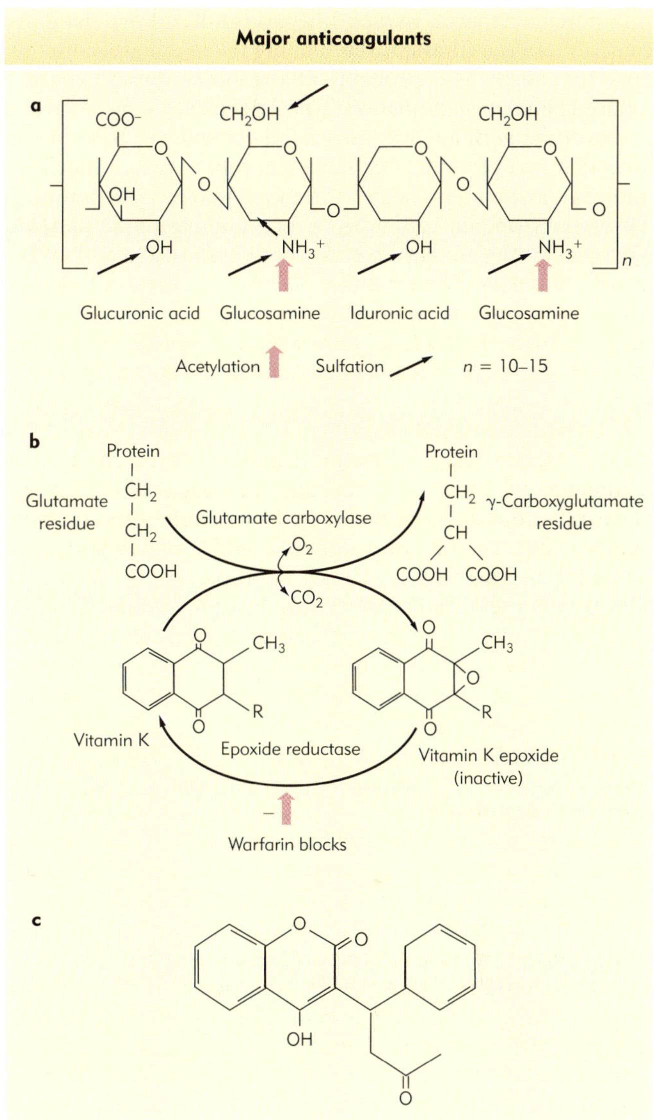

Figure 51.6 Major anticoagulants. (a) The repeating structure of heparin has a high affinity for antithrombin. (b) Vitamin K is involved in the conversion in the liver of glutamate residues in certain plasma proteins to γ-carboxyglutamate (GLA) residues. (c) Warfarin and other coumarin derivatives block the reduction of vitamin K epoxide formed in this reaction back to its active form.

with porcine heparin. In type 1 heparin-induced platelet deficiency, there is a transient self-limiting fall in platelet count to 50×10^9 cells/L. It is probably as a result of direct heparin-induced platelet agglutination. Type 2 deficiency is more severe and overlaps with heparin-associated thrombosis. It occurs in around 6% of patients. Platelet count falls to 10×10^9 cells/L and is associated with thromboembolic phenomena. Thrombocytopenia results from immune-mediated platelet aggregation triggered by immunoglobulins G and M antibodies against platelets. The condition generally resolves rapidly on discontinuation of heparin, although occasionally it may persist for 1–2 months; in this case, intravenous immunoglobulin therapy is used. Reintroduction of heparin can be catastrophic.

Low-molecular-weight heparins

Low-molecular-weight heparins (e.g. enoxaparin) have a relatively specific effect against factor Xa compared with other clotting factors. A 20mg dose of enoxaparin has an effect on factor Xa that is the equivalent of 2000IU of heparin. The low-molecular-weight heparins in clinical doses do not affect prothrombin time (PT), APTT, platelet aggregation, or binding to fibrinogen. They are rapidly absorbed after subcutaneous injection, as maximum activity is seen within 1–4 hours. The half-life of enoxaparin action is between 4 and 5 hours. It is excreted renally (largely intact), although there is some hepatic conjugation.

Oral anticoagulants

The commoner oral anticoagulants are coumarin derivatives that resemble vitamin K in structure. These include warfarin and the dicoumarides (e.g. phenindione) (Fig. 51.6). The anticoagulant effect of these drugs is related to their ability to interfere with production of biologically active vitamin K-dependent clotting factors (II, VII, IX, X). The anticoagulant effect of warfarin is seen 8–12 hours following either oral or intravenous administration, with the peak effect at 3–5 days (this corresponds with the nadir levels of vitamin K-dependent factors). Warfarin has a half-life of 24–36 hours. It is metabolized in the liver to a number of inactive derivatives that are conjugated and excreted both in bile and urine. In clinical practice, warfarin is used principally to reduce the incidence of thromboembolism associated with prosthetic heart valves and atrial fibrillation. Dosage is monitored and adjusted according to PT, which is very sensitive to a reduction in factors VII and X. As factor VII has a very short half-life (7 hours), its concentration falls earliest. A therapeutic PT is 1.5–4 times the normal value. An excessively prolonged PT cannot be easily corrected merely by omitting a dose of warfarin because the drug has a long elimination half-life and synthesis of vitamin K-dependent factors may be delayed. Similarly, a subtherapeutic PT needs correction by several doses of warfarin over a period of 3–4 days.

Warfarin should be discontinued 3–4 days prior to elective surgery to allow the PT to normalize. Clot formation on prosthetic heart valves is life threatening and requires urgent cardiopulmonary bypass. Anticoagulation should, therefore, be maintained perioperatively in patients who have prosthetic valves and others at high risk of thromboembolism. In these patients, intravenous heparin is substituted as the warfarin is tailed off. Heparin is preferable in these circumstances as its effects are more readily controllable because of its shorter half-life and because its effects can be reliably reversed with protamine. Reversal of the effects of warfarin can be attempted prior to emergency surgery using vitamin K (10–20mg intravenous) and fresh frozen plasma. Because warfarin is highly protein bound, many drugs that displace it from its binding sites may substantially potentiate its anticoagulant effect (e.g. co-trimoxazole, metronidazole, amiodarone, quinidine, and tolbutamide). Cimetidine inhibits the cytochrome P450 system and hence reduces hepatic warfarin clearance. Some drugs [e.g. the barbiturates and rifampin (rifampicin)] increase the activity of hepatic microsomal enzymes, which reduces the anticoagulant effect of warfarin. In theory, volatile anesthetic agents may displace warfarin from protein-binding sites and hence prolong its anticoagulant effect; this has been demonstrated for halothane.

Platelet drugs

Many drugs interact with platelets either to potentiate or to inhibit function. Desmopressin [1-deamino-8-D-arginine vasopressin (DDAVP)], an analog of arginine-vasopressin, is frequently used in patients who have platelet dysfunction (e.g. in renal failure) to promote platelet activity. The nature of this effect is not fully understood, although it is probably related to its ability to release von Willebrand factor from vascular endothelium, which then interacts with platelets to promote adhesion.

Antifibrinolytic drugs also potentiate platelet function, in part by promoting cross-linking of fibrin and platelet adhesion to fibrin, and in part by preserving the functional activity of platelet surface glycoproteins, including glycoprotein Ib and IIa. Drugs in this category include tranexamic acid and ϵ-aminocaproic acid. The primary effect of these drugs is inhibition of fibrinolysis, mediated through binding of these molecules to lysine residues on free plasmin. Hence, these drugs function as pharmacologic mimics of α_2-antiplasmin and α_2-macroglobulin.

Another antifibrinolytic drug that potentiates platelet function is aprotinin. This drug is now well established both in cardiac surgery and liver transplantation. Aprotinin is a nonspecific serine protease inhibitor. It is active against kallikrein, plasmin, trypsin, and thrombin. It also has a direct effect on platelet function, enhancing integrity and function of surface glycoproteins and enhancing the platelet release reaction. In cardiac surgery, aprotinin has been shown to reduce blood loss in high-risk patients, particularly where aspirin has been given preoperatively. Its use in liver transplantation is more controversial. Antifibrinolytic drugs have been associated with increased risk of arterial thrombosis.

Nefamostat mesylate is a new synthetic protease inhibitor. It has a short half-life and has been used as an anticoagulant for plasma. Its use in cardiopulmonary bypass significantly reduces blood loss and is associated with platelet preservation and reduced fibrinolysis. Etamsylate (ethamsylate) also promotes enhanced platelet activity, acting by stimulating platelet aggregation.

Drugs that inhibit platelet function include the arachidonic acid derivative prostacyclin (epoprostenol). Prostacyclin is produced by endothelial cells. It inhibits platelet aggregation through activation of adenylyl cyclase and is a potent vasodilator. Nonsteroidal anti-inflammatory drugs (NSAIDs), including aspirin, inhibit cyclo-oxygenase activity and prostacyclin production. Prostacyclin is rapidly degraded to 6-keto-prostaglandin $F_1\alpha$, which is devoid of biologic activity. Ticlopidine, used to treat recurrent stroke, appears to act by selectively blocking platelet responses to ADP.

Aspirin differs from other NSAIDs in that it is an irreversible rather than a reversible enzyme inhibitor (Chapter 27). Nonsteroidal anti-inflammatory drugs block prostaglandin synthesis and production of both thromboxane A_2 and prostacyclin is inhibited. Aspirin has an irreversible effect; consequently, thromboxane synthetase is inhibited for the lifetime of the platelet and there is a prolonged effect on production of the prothrombotic prostaglandin thromboxane A_2. However, its effect on the vascular endothelium is more transient because the nucleated endothelial cells can rapidly regenerate functional enzyme. Overall, the effect of a dose of aspirin is prolonged inhibition of thromboxane A_2 production and an antiplatelet (anticoagulant) effect that may last days or weeks, with only transient inhibition of prostacyclin. By contrast, other NSAID drugs show a reversible effect on prostaglandin synthetase enzymes, and their antiplatelet effect is generally limited to the duration of action of the drug.

Dipyridamole, originally introduced as a vasodilator, acts as a phosphodiesterase inhibitor in vascular smooth muscle, increasing platelet cAMP and inhibiting aggregation. Dipyridamole does not affect cyclo-oxgenase activity directly, and thromboxane A_2 and prostacyclin formation are unchanged. In thromboembolic conditions where platelet lifespan is reduced, dipyridamole tends to restore it.

Protamine, prepared from fish sperm, is currently the only drug available for heparin neutralization (Chapter 41). It has a high arginine content, which makes it strongly basic (cationic) and enables it to form a stable complex with the highly negatively charged heparin molecule. In general, 1–2mg protamine is necessary to neutralize 1mg (100IU) heparin. Protamine has several adverse effects; these include hypotension and flushing, which are probably related to histamine release and which can be minimized by giving protamine very slowly. There is a high incidence of anaphylactic and anaphylactoid reactions to protamine; these are most common in patients who have fish allergy and in diabetics receiving protamine-based insulin. Protamine activates complement and releases platelet thromboxane A_2, which may lead to severe pulmonary vasoconstriction and bronchoconstriction. Pretreatment with a cyclo-oxygenase inhibitor (aspirin) may offset this effect.

HEMOSTATIC DEFECTS AND BLEEDING DISORDERS

Bleeding disorders may result from abnormalities of the vasculature, of platelet function, or from disorders of the coagulation cascade. 'Vascular' bleeding disorders are a mixed group of conditions characterized by easy bruising and spontaneous bleeding from small vessels. The underlying abnormality is either in the vessel wall or in perivascular connective tissue. In general, these conditions are not severe. Standard clotting tests and screening tests are often normal, although the Ivy bleeding time may be prolonged.

Acquired vascular defects may result in abnormal bleeding. These include senile purpura, purpura of infections, Henoch–Schönlein syndrome, steroid purpura, and scurvy.

Abnormal bleeding caused by thrombocytopenia or abnormal platelet function is characterized by mucosal hemorrhage, spontaneous purpura, and prolonged bleeding from surgery or trauma. Causes of thrombocytopenia include failure of platelet production and increased destruction of platelets. Failure of platelet production may result from selective depression of megakaryocytes, for example by drugs (azathioprine, ranitidine), chemical toxicity, or viral infection (e.g. cytomegalovirus). Platelet production may be depressed as part of generalized bone marrow failure (e.g. aplastic anemia, leukemia, myelosclerosis, marrow infiltration by tumor, cytotoxic drugs).

Causes of increased platelet destruction include autoimmune thrombocytopenic purpura (acute or chronic). Idiopathic thrombocytopenic purpura (ITP), seen predominantly in young women, may occur in conjunction with systemic diseases, such as lupus erythematosus. Platelet sensitization with autoantibodies (IgG) results in early clearance of platelets from the circulation by the reticuloendothelial system. In severe disease, mean platelet survival may be reduced to less than 1 hour. Platelet transfusion may be relatively ineffective. Treatment is based around immunosuppression, as fewer than 10% of patients recover spontaneously. Acute thrombocytopenia occurs most frequently in children. Most cases follow viral infection or vaccination. Spontaneous remission is the rule.

Drug-induced immune thrombocytopenia is a cause of increased platelet destruction. Several drugs, including quinine, quinidine, sulfonamides, and rifampacin may produce immune thrombocytopenia. The drug induces formation of antibody directed against a drug–plasma protein hapten. Circulating immune complexes are adsorbed onto the platelet. Consequently, platelet damage is coincidental to the underlying process. The damaged platelet is removed by the reticuloendothelial system. Treatment is discontinuation of suspected drugs. Recovery is generally rapid (see heparin-adverse effects, above).

Disorders of platelet function may be present in patients who have skin or mucous membrane hemorrhage in whom bleeding time is prolonged despite a normal platelet count. Thromboelastography (see below) is likely to reveal a reduced maximum amplitude. Hereditary disorders of platelet function are rare. There is defective platelet adhesion (as well as coagulopathy) in von Willebrand's disease.

Acquired platelet dysfunction may be secondary to drugs (NSAID, aspirin, dipyridamole) or systemic disease. Such conditions include Waldenström's hypogammaglobulinemia associated with multiple myeloma and renal failure (see below).

Disseminated intravascular coagulation (DIC) is a disorder of platelets and clotting factors. It complicates many disease processes including sepsis, trauma, and malignancy (Fig. 51.7). It generally presents as an acute disorder, although there is also a chronic form. Disseminated intravascular coagulation is characterized by activation of the clotting cascade with formation of small thrombi throughout the microcirculation, which leads to vascular occlusion and ischemic damage, particularly in the kidney and splanchnic bed. Fibrinogen, coagulation factors, and platelets are rapidly consumed (consumptive coagulopathy). This leads to rapid worsening of clotting. Platelet plugs and fibrin in the microcirculation trigger the fibrinolytic cascade. These have an anticoagulant effect, prolonging thrombin time. All clotting tests are abnormal (PT, APTT, and thrombin time). Characteristically, fibrinogen levels are reduced and both FDP and d-dimer levels are raised. Perhaps the best laboratory correlate of clinical disease course is the fibrinogen level.

Management of DIC is focused on controlling any predisposing condition. Treatment of the coagulopathy is likely to be ineffective until the underlying disorder has been treated. Fresh frozen plasma, cryoprecipitate, and platelets are used as directed by both laboratory tests and clinical end points (hemorrhage). Historically, heparin was used to prevent consumption of clotting factors. This practice has now largely been abandoned because of the risk of exacerbating bleeding, but

Causes of disseminated intravascular coagulation

Cause	Example
Obstetric	Amniotic fluid embolism, intrauterine death, placental abruption, eclampsia
Infections	
Bacterial	Meningococcus, pneumococcus, systemic Gram-negative sepsis, bacterial endocarditis
Viral	Cytomegalovirus, herpesvirus, varicella
Parasites	*Plasmodium* spp. (malaria), fungal
Major trauma	Burns, major hemorrhage, head injury
Malignancy	Lung, pancreas, prostate
Metabolic	Malignant hyperthermia, liver failure, hemolytic uremic syndrome, anaphylaxis

Figure 51.7 Causes of disseminated intravascular coagulation.

may sometimes be required where arterial thrombosis is a major feature. Antifibrinolytic drugs are not used, as fibrinolysis in DIC is generally a secondary phenomenon.

Coagulation disorders (disorders of the clotting cascade) may either be hereditary or acquired. Hereditary disorders affecting each of the 10 coagulation factors are described. The most common are hemophilia (factor VIII) and Christmas disease (factor IX). Von Willebrand's disease is a disorder of factor VIIIR:AG.

Although all of these conditions are rare, hemophilia A is the least rare. It is an X-linked disorder, although up to one third of patients have no family history and may represent new mutations. The incidence is 1 in 10,000. The lesion is low or absent factor VIII:C activity as a consequence of abnormal structure or absence of the factor. In general, factor VIIIR:AG and von Willebrand factor are quantitatively and qualitatively normal. Perioperative and traumatic hemorrhage is potentially life threatening. Whole blood clotting time is prolonged. Activated partial thromboplastin time is likewise prolonged, and factor VIII is reduced. Bleeding time and PT are normal. Bleeding episodes can be treated with factor VIII concentrates or cryoprecipitate. Fresh frozen plasma contains factor VIII but is rarely used as the increment in factor VIII levels is small for each unit. Spontaneous hemorrhage is uncommon unless factor VIII is below 20% of normal. During major surgery, factor VIII should be maintained between 60 and 100% of normal values.

Christmas disease (hemophilia B) is caused by factor IX deficiency. Its clinical presentation and inheritance closely resemble those of hemophilia A. The incidence is 1 in 50,000. Hemorrhage and surgery are treated with factor IX concentrates. As factor IX is relatively stable, fresh frozen plasma is also effective in the treatment of this condition.

Von Willebrand's disease results from a defect in the synthesis of the major fraction of factor VIII: VIIIR:AG. The platelet effect of von Willebrand factor (promotion of platelet adhesion to subendothelial tissue) results from a specific abnormal configuration of the VIIIR:AG molecule. The condition is characterized by perioperative hemorrhage and bleeding from mucous membranes. Laboratory investigation shows a prolonged bleeding time with low levels of VIII:C and VIIIR:AG. Platelet aggregation in response to ADP is normal but is defective in response to ristocetin (ristomycin). Bleeding episodes are treated with cryoprecipitate or concentrates of factor VIII.

Several disease states lead to acquired bleeding disorders. The coagulopathy of liver disease is multifactorial. Because of biliary obstruction, there may be reduced absorption of fat-soluble vitamins (A, D, E, K) and a selective reduction in synthesis of vitamin K-dependent clotting factors (II, VII, IX, X). Progressive deterioration of hepatocellular function leads to reduced synthesis of the remaining clotting factors, with the exception of factor VIII, which is produced by endothelial cells. Patients who have cirrhotic liver disease show enhanced fibrinolysis. This is because of reduced clearance of t-PA and reduced synthesis of the antifibrinolytic globulins α_2-antiplasmin and α_2-macroglobulin. Platelet function and numbers decline as hepatic synthetic function fails. The liver constitutively produces thrombopoietin, the cytokine responsible for signaling platelet synthesis, and patients who have liver failure and cirrhotic liver disease often suffer portal hypertension and hypersplenism, which lead to abnormal platelet production, sequestration and pooling.

Patients who have renal disease likewise suffer abnormal hemostasis through an acquired disorder of platelet function secondary to uremia. Accumulation of middle molecules and metabolic acids interfere with von Willebrand factor and subsequent platelet aggregation. Platelet dysfunction is proportional to uremia and is restored following dialysis or transplantation. The platelet dysfunction of renal disease may be corrected (at least in part) by desmopressin.

EVALUATION OF COAGULATION

Abnormal bleeding may result from thrombocytopenia, platelet function disorders, or abnormalities of the clotting cascade. The most common cause of abnormal bleeding is thrombocytopenia. Therefore, initial investigation should include a full blood count and blood film examination.

Bleeding time

Bleeding time is one of several measures of platelet plug formation *in vivo* and may detect abnormalities of platelet function where blood count and platelet numbers are normal. The commonly used method uses the Ivy template. Bleeding should stop spontaneously after 3–8 minutes. Bleeding time is prolonged with thrombocytopenia or platelet dysfunction.

Prothrombin time

The PT tests the extrinsic and common pathways (see Fig. 51.3). Both factor VII and factors common to both systems are evaluated. Tissue thromboplastin (extracted from brain) and calcium ions are added to plasma, and a clot should form within 10–14 seconds.

Activated partial thromboplastin time

The APTT is a measure of the intrinsic system. Hence, factors XII, XI, IX, and VIII are tested, in addition to factors common to both systems. A surface activator (e.g. kaolin), phospholipid, and calcium ions are added to plasma, which should produce a clot within 30–40 seconds. Both PT and APTT are normally correctable by adding normal plasma to the plasma being tested. Failure of this maneuver to correct PT or APTT suggests that an inhibitor of coagulation is present (e.g. FDPs, heparinoids).

Thrombin time

Fibrinolysis may be suspected on the basis of a reduced fibrinogen, prolonged thrombin time, or presence of d-dimer or FDPs. Thrombin time is assayed by adding thrombin to plasma and observing the time to fibrin formation, normally 10–12 seconds.

Thromboelastography

In perioperative thromboelastography (TEG), a sample of fresh blood (0.3mL) is placed into a small well at 37°C and is gently rotated. A piston connected to a recorder is suspended in the sample well. As fibrin strands begin to form, the piston begins to oscillate with the movement of the well. The evolving TEG trace produces a dynamic clot fingerprint that progressively describes activation of the clotting cascade, fibrin formation, the fibrin–platelet interaction (clot stability), clot retraction, and fibrinolysis (Fig. 51.8).

Thromboelastography correlates only loosely with results of standard coagulation tests. This reflects the interdependency of TEG variables rather than reliance on independent end points. Thromboelastography is more sensitive than standard tests of clotting at detecting subtle changes in balance between coagulation, fibrinolysis, and related hemostatic pathways. A prolonged reaction time gives evidence of a defect in the early part of the clotting cascade, perhaps implying a need for fresh frozen plasma. A reduced α angle is related to a reduced rate of clot propagation, suggesting a need for fibrinogen (cryoprecipitate). Maximum amplitude relates to clot tensile strength. This reflects platelet numbers and function as well as the effectiveness of fibrin cross-linking.

Specific tests

Most clotting factors may also be assayed by specific tests, including radioimmunoassay, enzyme-linked immunosorbent assay (ELISA), or specific factor assays based on APTT or PT in which all factors except the one to be measured are present in reagent plasma. This requires a supply of plasma from patients who have known hereditary deficiencies of the factor in question. Factor levels in test plasma are assessed by the degree to which test plasma corrects the prolonged clotting time of substrate-deficient plasma.

TRANSFUSION THERAPY

In the 1940s, blood transfusion was considered a surgical procedure. We now live in an era of separate stored products and the future will include bioengineered substitutes. Raw materials for blood transfusion come from a variety of sources: volunteer, paid, or conscripted donors. There has been interest in related blood donors and autologous transfusion (self-donation).

Whole blood is collected from the donor into an anticoagulant solution. Anticoagulant solutions are generally citrate-based, chelating calcium ions and thus interfering with clotting. Donations from different donors can be pooled or apheresis can be used to produce quantities of blood components from a single/few donor(s). Apheresis ('taken away') extracts a portion of the blood, for example plasma or platelets (once or twice weekly), and retransfuses the remainder back into the donor. This technique limits the number of donors to which the recipient of a multiple unit donation is exposed. Donor blood is tested for hepatitis viruses (A, B, and C), for human immunodeficiency virus (HIV) 1 and 2, *Treponema pallidum* (syphilis), ABO and Rhesus compatibility, and cytomegalovirus. Collected samples are processed into red cells, platelets, and plasma. Red cells are stored at 4°C and tested for compatibility prior to release for transfusion. Platelets are pooled into units of four or more, stored at 22°C, and gently agitated through their shelf life to prevent adherence to plastics. Plasma is stored at –20°C and transfused within 2 hours of thawing, or fractionated to make a number of pooled blood products.

Blood-giving sets should normally include a 170μm filter. Microaggregate filters should be avoided and never used for platelet transfusion. Blood products should only be mixed with isotonic saline (avoid solutions such as Hartmann's, Ringer's lactate, and other calcium-containing solutions, as these may cause coagulation of the product). Before administration, the product should be checked for hemolysis within the bag (pink supernatant). Blood products may be presented cold from the fridge; if these are to be transfused rapidly, it is necessary to use appropriate blood-warming devices. It is important to avoid overheating blood, as this results in hemolysis, cytokine release, and serious adverse reactions. There is a risk of bacterial infection in units that have been open for more than 4 hours.

The 'group and save' or 'type and screen' procedure reduces the need for unnecessary expensive cross-matching. It can be performed hours or days in advance and documents the ABO and Rhesus type of the patient's blood. Screening may also be performed for 'unexpected' red cell antibodies. This should mean that a suitable unit of donor blood can be selected and rapidly cross-matched within 10–15 minutes.

The thromboelastogram

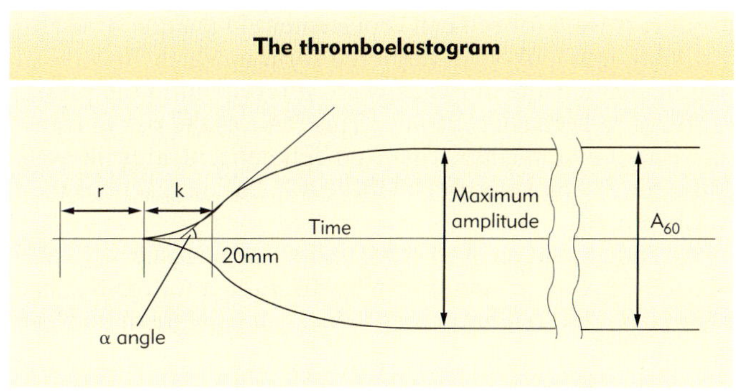

Figure 51.8 Schematic representation of the thromboelastogram. The diagram is discontinuous as A60, the amplitude at 60 minutes, would otherwise be far to the right of the figure.

BLOOD PRODUCTS

Whole blood

Whole blood is prepared from a single donation and consists of 450mL of blood with 63mL anticoagulant (typically citrate). The hematocrit varies between 0.35 and 0.45. It contains no functional platelets and levels of factor V and VIII are 20% of normal. Albumin and other clotting factors are normal. Whole-blood transfusion is indicated for replacement of blood loss where clotting factors are also required. In general, this means hemorrhage exceeding 50% of the patient's blood volume.

Red cell concentrate

Red cell concentrates (packed red cells) are prepared from a single donor and consist of 220mL of packed cells and 80mL of plasma. The hematocrit lies between 0.65 and 0.75. This product is used for red cell replacement in anemia. It is also available in a leukocyte-depleted form in which 70–90% of platelets and white blood cells are filtered out in the preparation of red cell concentrates. This reduces the risk of transmission of cytomegalovirus. Red cell concentrates likewise cause fewer white blood cell febrile transfusion reactions than whole blood.

An added solution of 50–80mL saline adenine glucose (SAG) or SAG-M (with mannitol) can be substituted for the residual plasma as a red cell nutrient, producing a hematocrit between 0.5 and 0.7.

Platelets

Platelets are produced either as single donor or pooled donor (4–6) units. Each donation consists of 40–70mL of plasma with platelet suspension equivalent to 5.5×10^{10} platelets (UK); the exact number of platelets per donation is described by national standards and varies considerably between countries. The ideal platelet transfusion should be ABO and Rhesus compatible, especially in young women. A transfusion of 5–6 units of platelets produces an increment in platelet count of between 20×10^9 and 40×10^9 cells/L. Platelets may also be produced by single donor apheresis. Between 150 and 500mL of plasma are produced with around 3×10^{11} suspended platelets.

Fresh frozen plasma

Fresh frozen plasma (FFP) is produced as a single donor product. Units of FFP consist of 250–500mL of separated plasma frozen at –20°C. It includes both labile and stable factors, albumin, gammaglobulin, fibrinogen, and factor VIII. Fresh frozen plasma can transmit hepatitis viruses and HIV; virologic safety relies on donor screening. Transfused units of FFP should be ABO compatible. The dose is usually between 2 and 5 units according to the results of clotting tests (prothrombin time or TEG). Very occasionally, FFP may cause anaphylaxis.

Cryoprecipitate

Cryoprecipitate is collected in packs containing between 1 and 6 single-donor units. It is collected by harvesting the precipitate that forms during slow thawing of frozen plasma. The resulting precipitate is resuspended in 10–20mL of plasma. Each unit contains 150mg fibrinogen, 150IU factor VIII, and fibronectin. Between 6 and 18 units are required in hemophilia, DIC, and fibrinolytic states to raise plasma fibrinogen level by 1g/L.

Albumin

Albumin is produced by fractionation of a large plasma pool followed by pasteurization at 60°C for over 10 hours, which is thought to produce complete viral inactivation, although it may not inactivate prion proteins. Albumin solutions are presented as 5% solution and 20% sodium-depleted (salt-poor) solution. Albumin is indicated in the treatment of shock states, hypoproteinemia, and liver disease.

Factor concentrates

A number of factor concentrates are available, including separated freeze-dried factor VIII and IX (250IU per vial) and both pure and impure forms of factors VII, IX, and XI. These factors have been associated with viral transmission. In recent years, there has been a shift toward production of factor concentrates by human recombinant techniques. Human recombinant factor VIII is now standard in the treatment of hemophilia in most countries, following experience in the late 1970s and 1980s with hepatitis and HIV transmission.

BLOOD GROUPS

Red blood cells possess over three hundred antigen systems expressed on the cell surface. These antigen systems are genetically determined. They are important in the recognition of 'self' as opposed to 'non-self'. The surface antigens are of clinical relevance in blood transfusion compatibility, and to some extent in compatibility of transplanted organs. The transfusion of cells of a different antigenicity to the patient's can result in lysis by endogenous antibodies, or production of new antibodies with this potential.

The main group of cells involved is the red blood cell. Some antigenic systems are known as blood group systems. A blood group results from expression of alleles at a single locus or at closely linked loci. There are 18 important blood group systems. These, together with their number of potential antigens, include: ABO (4), Rhesus (45), MNS (38), P (1), Lutheran (18), Kell (21), Lewis (3), Duffy (6), Kidd (3), and others. By convention, the genotype is distinguished from the phenotype by the use of italic script. For example, A1 is a genotype, but A1 a phenotype.

Most red blood cell antigens are expressed, and readily detectable, by the age of two years. Thereafter, they remain stable throughout life. Many components of the genotype are inherited together, because of linkage on the same chromosome. However, some degree of re-combination is possible because of the phenomenon of cross-over. This occurs after the first meiotic division. Cross-over is more likely where alleles are remotely located on the chromosome. Most blood group systems follow simple Mendelian inheritance.

ABO And Transfusion

Important among blood group systems is the ABO system. Inheritance of this system is characterised by co-dominance and silent genes (amorphs). Silent genes have no observable phenotypic expression. Many blood group genes result directly in expression of a protein antigen: the Rhesus system is an example of this. Other blood group systems, such as the ABO system, are characterised by a carbohydrate antigen. Expression of the gene encoding for carbohydrate antigens is dependent on the presence of appropriate substrate or enzyme systems. These may, in turn, rely on the presence of another gene. The ABO system relies on the presence of the H gene to produce necessary substrate: in those rare individuals (Bombay) who lack this gene, carbohydrate antigens of the ABO system are not expressed. Red blood cells of these individuals appeared to be group O by phenotype, whereas they may be other blood groups by genotype.

The ABO blood group system is the most important blood group system. It is fully expressed by six months of age, and by this time most individuals have antibodies directed against any antigens of the ABO system which are not present in the host. These antibodies, endogenously present, will destroy incompatible cells *in vivo*. Prior to blood transfusion, grouping using sera against A1, A2, B or A+B as appropriate is used. This results in agglutination in the case of incompatibility.

Because of the presence of antibodies in incompatible transfusion recipients, donor red cells have the potential to be rapidly broken down. Therefore, only red cells against which an endogenous antibody is not present may be transfused. Thus, blood for transfusion must generally be ABO compatible. Possible exceptions to this include the transfusion of group O blood to other blood groups (universal donor) and the ability of patients with group AB blood to receive donations from all other blood groups (universal recipient). During blood cross matching, ABO compatibility is first established. This is accompanied by antibody screening. Once potential suitable donor units have been identified, cross-matching is then possible. Patients who have received a blood transfusion should have a new cross-match performed after 48 hours if further transfusion is required. This is because of the potential of the first transfusion to stimulate new antibody production within this time span. Where massive blood transfusions are administered, for example, an exchange transfusion (10 units or more) within a period of a few hours, further compatibility testing is academic until a 48 hour period has elapsed. This is because of the diversity of antigens present, and wash-out of host derived antibodies.

Rhesus System

The Rhesus system is the second most important blood group system. The antibody against the most important antigen, Rhesus D is not endogenously present. However, it is rapidly formed after exposure to the Rhesus D antigen (for example, following transfusion or during pregnancy). The antibody against Rhesus D is clinically important because of the facility with which it can cross the placenta and cause hemolytic disease of the newborn. Other important antigens in the Rhesus system are the C and E antigens. It is thought that these are encoded at a single locus.

RISKS OF BLOOD TRANSFUSION

The most common risk of blood transfusion is the unavailability of appropriate blood when it is needed. Transfusion of the wrong blood accounts for three quarters of all transfusion-related deaths. This is generally as a result of inaccurate labeling of the patient blood sample or the blood for transfusion, or failure to check patient and product identities. Viral transmission is a real but rare problem. Recent figures suggest that the risk of HIV transmission in the UK is around 1 per million donor exposures. The risk of transmission of hepatitis viruses, particularly hepatitis C and E, is higher than this. As yet, the risk of transmission of prion proteins (causing variant Creutzfeldt–Jacob disease) is unknown but may be lymphocyte dependent. There is much discussion currently about presenting all transfusion products in a leukocyte-depleted form. Remaining risks relate to febrile white cell reactions, hyperkalemia, hemolyzed blood, and bacterial contamination.

Complications of blood transfusion include acid–base and electrolyte changes. Although stored blood is acidic, transfusion rapidly corrects metabolic acidosis in the shocked anemic patient. Hyperkalemia rarely occurs in blood that has been stored for less than 2 weeks. Blood transfusion with citrate-anticoagulated products may cause rapid reduction in plasma ionized calcium, resulting in systemic anticoagulation and myocardial depression. There is a risk of hypothermia when cold blood is transfused rapidly.

Acute transfusion reactions are relatively uncommon. These include hemolytic reactions, 75% of which are caused by ABO incompatibility. Anaphylactic reactions occasionally occur. These are a consequence of antibodies to IgA in IgA-deficient patients. Febrile white blood cell reactions are common and caused by antibodies to leukocyte antigens. These antibodies can also give rise to noncardiogenic pulmonary edema. Approximately 1–2% of transfusions result in histamine release and urticaria. Post-transfusion purpura is an uncommon complication of blood transfusion.

When emergency transfusion is given, there is controversy as to whether group O blood or group-compatible blood should be used. Group O blood has the advantage that there is no risk of ABO incompatibility and errors in patient identification do not pose a problem. It is rapidly available and can be held in a flying squad refrigerator for immediate use. ABO compatible blood has the advantage that it does not deplete stocks of group O blood. There is no problem of changing blood group for follow-on transfusions, and little risk of hemolysis in the patient from antibodies in transfused plasma. The decision on which to use should be based on locally defined protocols.

Transfused blood has the capacity to carry oxygen almost immediately following transfusion. Evidence for this is presented by the fact that exchange transfusions with bank blood do not generally result in massive acidosis, multiple organ failure, or even a reduction in mixed venous oxygen content. Transfused blood has reduced intracellular 2,3-diphosphoglycerate, but this is offset by the effects of local acidosis and hypoxia.

New blood substitutes

For many years there has been a quest for appropriate and effective substitutes for blood transfusion. Traditionally, much reliance has been placed on the use of artificial colloid solutions (modified fluid gelatin, starches, etc.). These are effective as plasma expanders and hence improve tissue oxygen delivery. They do not carry oxygen (apart from in solution). More recently, there has been much interest in the development of oxygen-carrying substances. Initial work on perfluorocarbons appeared promising. However, the oxygen dissociation curve of currently available compounds precludes their use as blood substitutes in clinical practice.

Stroma-free hemoglobin solutions seem much more promising and are currently in phase III clinical trials. The most likely to enter clinical practice are those based on recombinant 'human' blood, although a bovine version has also been produced. Production of human stroma-free hemoglobin is from hemoglobin harvested from expired pooled donor units heat treated for viral inactivation and as a genetically engineered product. As free hemoglobin would pass rapidly across the glomerulus and give rise to renal failure, a larger version of the molecule is required. A number of approaches have been used. The most favored is polymerization (or dimerization) of the molecule using an inorganic cross-link, for example the difumarate bond. The resulting dimer has an oxygen 50% saturation pressure (P_{50}) similar to that of blood and, therefore, has similar oxygen carriage and off-loading characteristics. It differs from blood in that it is less viscous and is stroma free (i.e. has no cellular material). This means that shelf life may be prolonged. There are no surface antigens present, hence there is no need for cross-matching. Stroma-free hemoglobin solutions are effective as oxygen carriers and very effective at delivering oxygen to the tissues. There may be an uncoupling of supply-dependent oxygen extraction, leading to further spectacular improvements in tissue oxygenation. Moreover, these compounds appear to bind nitric oxide and may have a vasopressor effect as well as an effect on limiting tissue ischemia reperfusion injury.

Further Reading

Booth NA. The laboratory investigation of the fibrinolytic system. In: Thomson JM, ed. Blood coagulation and hemostasis, 4th edn. Edinburgh, UK: Churchill Livingstone; 1991:115–49.

Crosby ET. Perioperative hemotherapy: I. Indicators for blood component transfusion. Can J Anaesth. 1992;39:695–707.

Crosby ET. Perioperative hemotherapy: II. Risks and complications of blood transfusion. Can J Anaesth. 1992;39:822–37.

Dzik WH, Arkin CF, Jenkins RL, Stump DC. Fibrinolysis during liver transplantation in humans: role of tissue-type plasminogen activator. Blood. 1988;71:1090–5.

Hoffbrand AV, Pettitt JE. Essential haematology, 3rd edn. Oxford, Blackwell; 1993.

Irving GA. Perioperative blood and blood component therapy. Can J Anaesth. 1992;39:1105–15.

Powell CC, Schultz SC, Malcolm DS. Diaspirin crosslinked hemoglobin (DCLHb): more effective than lactated Ringer's solution in restoring central venous oxygen saturation after hemorrhagic shock in rats. Artif Cell Blood Substit Immobil Biotechnol. 1996;24:197–200.

Reah G, Bodenham AR, Mallick A, Daily EK, Przybelski RJ. Initial evaluation of diaspirin cross-linked hemoglobin (DCLHb) as a vasopressor in critically ill patients. Crit Care Med. 1997;25:1480–8.

Salem MR. Blood conservation in the surgical patient. Baltimore, MD: William & Wilkins; 1996.

Snook NJ, O'Beirne HA, Young Y, Enright S, Bellamy MC. Use of recombinant human erythropoeitin to facilitate liver transplantation in a Jehovah's Witness. Br J Anaesth. 1996;76:740–3.

Yassen KA, Bellamy MC, Sadek SA, Webster NR. Tranexamic acid reduces blood loss during orthotopic liver transplantation. Clin Transplant. 1993;7:453–8.

Chapter 52 The immune system

Helen F Galley and Nigel R Webster

Topics covered in this chapter

- Innate immunity
- Acquired immunity
- Major histocompatibility complex
- Cells of the immune system
- Hypersensitivity reactions
- Transplantation immunology
- Cancer immunology
- Human immunodeficiency virus
- Immune modulation by anesthetics

The extremely adaptive and complex immune system is able to recognize and eliminate a variety of foreign cells and molecules. The immune system has both the function of recognition and that of response. The recognition component is remarkably specific; it can discriminate between self and non-self and also can identify the subtle chemical differences that distinguish one pathogen from another. The *recognition response* is then converted to an appropriate *effector response* to enable the neutralization or elimination of the particular organism, cancer cell, or foreign tissue. Subsequent exposure to the same antigen induces a *memory response*, characterized by a rapid enhancement of immune reactivity.

INNATE IMMUNITY

Immunity is the only state of protection from infectious disease and consists of both specific and nonspecific components. Nonspecific, or *innate immunity*, is the pre-existing resistance to disease and comprises four types of defensive barriers: anatomic, physiologic, phagocytic/endocytic, and inflammatory. Anatomic barriers prevent microorganisms from entering the body and include the skin and mucous secretion. Intact skin prevents the penetration of most pathogens; a low skin pH also inhibits bacterial growth. The conjunctivae and the alimentary, respiratory, and urogenital tracts are covered by mucous membranes, which are protected by saliva, tears, and mucus. In the gastrointestinal tract, for example, organisms trapped in mucus are propelled out of the body by ciliary action. Physiologic barriers include temperature, pH, and a variety of soluble factors, including lysozyme, *interferons* (IFNs), and complement. *Lysozyme*, found in mucus, cleaves the peptidoglycan layer of bacterial cell walls. The IFNs are produced by virus-infected cells and bind to nearby cells inducing a generalized antiviral state. The *complement* system is a multicomponent triggered enzyme cascade that results in membrane-damaging reactions that destroy pathogenic organisms and facilitate their clearance.

Complement

The complement system is a group of serum proteins. activated in a sequential enzymatic cascade; they have an important role in antigen clearance. There are two pathways of complement activation: the *classical pathway*, which is activated by specific immunoglobulin molecules, and the *alternative pathway*, which is activated by a variety of microorganisms and immune complexes. Each pathway involves the activation of different complement proteins but results in a common end point: generation of a *membrane attack complex* (MAC), which is responsible for cell lysis. This complex inserts itself into cell membrane phospholipid and makes large transmembrane channels in the target cell, disrupting the membrane and causing cell lysis. Complement components also amplify antigen–antibody reactions, attract phagocytic cells to sites of infection, augment phagocytosis, and activate B lymphocytes. The complement system is nonspecific and will, in theory, attack host cells as well as foreign cells. To prevent host cell damage, regulatory mechanisms, including spontaneous hydrolysis of complement components and inactivating proteins, restrict complement reactions to designated targets.

Phagocytosis

Ingestion of extracellular macromolecules and particles is achieved via *endocytosis* and *phagocytosis,* respectively. In endocytosis, macromolecules in extracellular fluid are internalized by invagination of the plasma membrane to form endocytic vesicles (Chapter 2). *Pinocytosis* is nonspecific, whereas in *receptor-mediated endocytosis* macromolecules bind selectively to membrane receptors. The ingested material is degraded by enzymes of the endocytic processing pathway. Phagocytosis involves ingestion of particles, including whole microorganisms, via expansion of the plasma membrane to form a *phagosome*. Virtually all cells are capable of endocytosis, but phagocytosis occurs in only a few specialized cells (Fig. 52.1). Dedicated phagocytes include polymorphonuclear neutrophils, mast cells, and macrophages; nonprofessional phagocytes such as endothelial cells and hepatocytes also have phagocytic potential. Cells infected with viruses and parasites are killed by large granular lymphocytes termed natural killer (NK) cells, and by eosinophils.

The inflammatory response

The *inflammatory response* to tissue damage or invasion by pathogenic organisms results in vasodilatation, increased

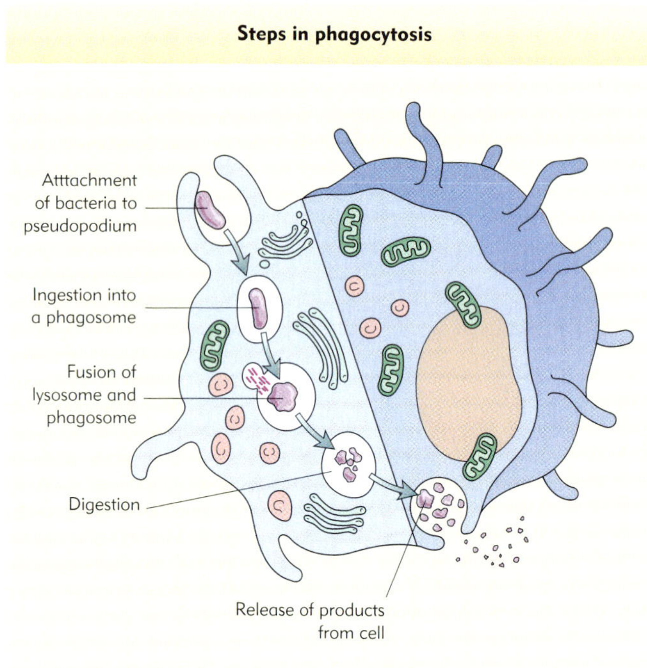

Figure 52.1 Phagocytosis of bacteria. The steps in phagocytosis.

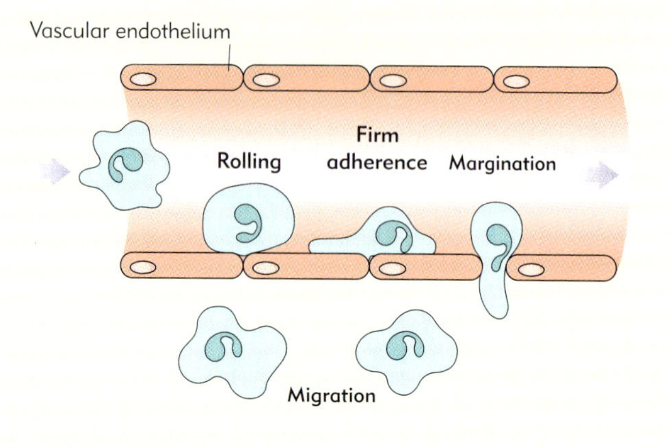

Figure 52.2 Process of neutrophil adherence to, and extravasation across, the vascular endothelium.

capillary permeability, and influx of phagocytic cells. Movement of phagocytic cells involves a complex series of events including *margination*, or adherence of cells in the bloodstream to the endothelial cell wall; *extravasation*, or movement of phagocytes between capillary endothelial cells into the tissue; and *chemotaxis*, the migration of phagocytes through the tissue to the site of inflammation. The process of leukocyte margination is a carefully regulated process involving specific adhesion molecules. These comprise three structurally dissimilar groups of molecules and are located on the extracellular portion of the cell membrane of both endothelial cells and leukocytes. Examples include E-selectin, intercellular cell adhesion molecule (ICAM), and vascular cell adhesion molecule (VCAM). These molecules cause circulating leukocytes to slow down and then roll along the endothelium. Firm adherence and transmigration then occur (Fig. 52.2). The inflammatory response is initiated by a series of interactions that involve several chemical mediators produced by the invading organisms or damaged cells and the cells of the immune system and plasma enzyme systems. These include complement, C-reactive protein and other *acute-phase proteins*, *histamine* and *kinins*, and bacterial cell wall products such as *endotoxin* and *exotoxin*.

ACQUIRED IMMUNITY

Specific or *acquired immunity* targets microorganisms that are not destroyed by the innate immune system. Specificity, diversity, memory, and the ability to discriminate self from non-self are key features of acquired immunity. Acquired immunity is intricately involved with the innate immune response. Cells of the phagocytic system activate specific immune responses and modulate the production of soluble mediators that orchestrate the inflammatory response and the interplay involved in the elimination of a foreign organism.

The immune response can also be classified into humoral (from body fluid) and cell-mediated processes. The humoral component involves interaction of B cells with antigen and the proliferation and differentiation of the B cells into antibody-secreting plasma cells. Antibody is the effector of the humoral response; it binds to antigen, which neutralizes the antigen and facilitates its removal. The complex of antibody and antigen is known as the immune complex. B cell activation also activates the complement system, resulting in lysis of the foreign organism. Effector T cells generated in response to antigen are responsible for cell-mediated immunity. Cytokines secreted by T cells activate various phagocytic cells, enabling killing of intracellular bacteria. Cytotoxic T cells (Tc cells) are important in the recognition of altered self cells (i.e. virus-infected cells or tumor cells).

MAJOR HISTOCOMPATIBILITY COMPLEX

The major histocompatibility complex (MHC) is a tightly linked cluster of genes located on chromosome 6 and associated with intercellular recognition and self/non-self discrimination. MHC molecules play major roles in the acceptance of self (histocompatible) or rejection of non-self (histoincompatible). The MHC complex encodes immune mediators and antigens (human lymphocyte antigens or HLA), which play an important role in antigen recognition by T cells, and determines the response of an individual to infectious antigens and hence their susceptibility to disease. The MHC genes are organized into those encoding three classes of HLA molecule (Fig. 52.3): class I (regions A, B, and C), class II (region D), and class III (regions C4, C2, Bf). Class I genes encode glycoproteins expressed on the surface of most nucleated cells and present antigens for the activation of specific T cells. Class II genes encode glycoproteins expressed mainly on antigen-presenting cells, including macrophages and B cells, where they present antigen to other defined T cell populations. Class III genes

The major histocompatibility complex								
Complex	HLA							
MHC class	II			III		I		
Region	DP	DQ	DR	C4, C2, Bf		B	C	A
Gene products	DPαβ	DQαβ	DRαβ	Complement proteins	Tumor necrosis factors, αTNF, βTNF	HLA-B	HLA-C	HLA-A

Figure 52.3 Simplification of the organization of the major histocompatibility complex (MHC).

encode several different immune products, including complement system components, enzymes, and tumor necrosis factors (TNFs); they have no role in antigen presentation.

CELLS OF THE IMMUNE SYSTEM

Leukocytes (white blood cells) develop from a common pluripotent stem cell during hematopoiesis and proliferate and differentiate into different cells in response to hematopoietic growth factors: a process that is balanced by programmed cell death or *apoptosis*. The *lymphocyte,* the only cell to possess specificity, diversity, memory, and recognition of self/non-self, is the central line of the immune system. *Monocytes, macrophages*, and *neutrophils* are accessory immune cells specialized for phagocytosis. This process is facilitated by *opsonins* (e.g. complement and antibody), which increase attachment of antigen to the membrane of the phagocyte (Fig. 52.4). Macrophages are also important in antigen processing and presentation in association with a class II MHC molecule, and for secretion of interleukin-1 (IL-1). Lymphocytes constantly recirculate between blood, lymph, and tissues, mediated by interactions between cell adhesion molecules on the vascular endothelium and receptors for the adhesion molecules on the lymphocyte surface.

Different maturational stages of lymphocytes can be distinguished by their expression of surface antigens that can be identified by particular monoclonal antibodies. A particular surface molecule that is identifiable by one or more monoclonal antibodies (several different antibodies may bind to one surface antigen, reacting at different parts of the molecule) is called *cluster of differentiation* or CD antigen.

Antigen processing and presentation

Antigens are substances such as proteins, carbohydrates, and glycoproteins that are capable of interacting with the products of a specific immune response. An antigen that is capable of eliciting a specific immune response by itself is called an immunogen. Foreign protein antigens must be degraded into small peptides and complexed with class I or class II MHC molecules in order to be recognized by a T cell. This is called antigen processing. Whether complexing occurs with class I or II MHC molecules seems to be determined by the route by which the antigen enters the cell. Mature immunocompetent animals possess large numbers of antigen-reactive T and B lymphocytes. Their specificities are determined prior to contact with antigen by random gene rearrangements in the bone marrow during cell maturation. When antigen interacts with and activates mature antigenically committed T and B cells, it brings about the expansion of the particular population of cells with the given antigenic specificity for that antigen. This is called *clonal selection* and *expansion*. This process explains both specificity and memory attributes. Specificity is implicit since only those lymphocytes possessing appropriate receptors will be clonally expanded. Memory occurs because there is a larger number of antigen-reactive lymphocytes present after clonal selection and many of these lymphocytes have a longer life span (hence are termed *memory cells*). The initial encounter of antigen-specific lymphocytes with an antigen induces a *primary response*; subsequent encounters are more rapid and intense (*secondary response*). Self/non-self recognition is achieved by clonal elimination during development of lymphocytes bearing self-reactive receptors, or functional suppression of these cells in adults.

Antibody structure

Antibodies or immunoglobulins are lymphocyte-produced protein molecules that combine specifically with antigens. Antibody molecules consist of two identical light chains and two identical heavy chains joined by disulfide bonds. Each heavy and light chain has a variable amino acid sequence region and a constant region. The unique heavy-chain constant region sequences determine the five classes or *isotypes* of immunoglobulins: IgM, IgG, IgD, IgA, and IgE. These isotypes vary in their effector function, serum concentration, and half-life. IgG is the most common isotype and the only immunoglobulin to cross the placenta. IgM exists as a pentamer and is most effective in viral neutralization, bacterial agglutination, and complement activation. IgA is the predominant isotype in external secretions including breast milk and mucus. IgD and IgE are the least abundant isotypes; IgD and IgM are the major isotypes on mature B cells, and IgE mediates mast cell degranulation.

Monoclonal antibodies are laboratory manufactured homogeneous antibodies with identical antigenic specificity. These antibodies are produced by cloned *hybridoma* cells, which are manufactured by fusing normal lymphocytes with myeloma cells. The clone retains the normal antibody functions and receptors of lymphocytes with the immortal growth characteristics of myeloma cells. Monoclonal antibodies provide an indefinite supply of antibody with a highly defined antigenic specificity that recognizes a single antigenic determinant or *epitope*. Monoclonal antibodies are under investigation as therapeutic agents in sepsis (Chapter 70) and immunosuppression (see below).

Cytokines

Orchestration of immune and inflammatory responses depends upon communication between cells by soluble molecules. These molecules are given the generic name cytokines and include chemokines, ILs, growth factors, and IFNs. Cytokines are low-molecular-weight secreted proteins that regulate both the amplitude and duration of the immune inflammatory responses (Fig. 52.5). They have a transient action that is tightly regulated.

Figure 52.4 Cells of the immune system.

Cells of the immune system

Cell type	Function	Mediator production
Monocytes and macrophages	Phagocytosis, antigen presentation, cytokine release, activation of TH cells, secretion of complement proteins, secretion of hydrolytic enzymes, secretion of reactive oxygen species	Interleukin (IL) 1β, IL-6, IL-8, IL-12, interferon (IFN) α, transforming growth factor (TGF) β, tumor necrosis factor (TNF) α
Neutrophils	Phagocytosis, cytokine release, secretion of hydrolytic enzymes, secretion of reactive oxygen species	IL-1β, IL-6, IL-8,
Natural killer cells	Nonspecific tumor cell cytoxicity, antibody-dependent cytotoxicity	IFN-γ, IL-3
T lymphocytes	Antigen recognition on presenting cells, cytokine release	IL-2, IL-3, IL-4, IL-5, IL-9, IL-13, IFN-γ, TNFβ, IL-6, IL-10 IFN-γ, TNFβ
Helper subset 1 (TH1)		
Helper subset 2 (TH2)		
Cytotoxic (Tc)		
B lymphocytes	Antigen recognition, antibody production, cytokine release	IL-1β, IL-12
Eosinophils	Phagocytosis, parasitic killing	IL-1β, IL-3, IL-5, granulocyte–macrophage colony-stimulating factor (GM-CSF)
Basophils	Role in allergic reactions	–
Mast cells	Role in allergic reactions, histamine release, cytokine release	IL-1β, IL-3, IL-6, GM-CSF, TGFβ, TNFα

Cytokines are extremely potent, combining with small numbers of high-affinity cell-surface receptors and producing changes in the patterns of RNA and protein synthesis. They have effects on growth and differentiation in a variety of cell types with considerable overlap and redundancy between them, partially accounted for by the induction of synthesis of common proteins. Interaction may occur in a cascade system in which one cytokine induces another, through modulation of the receptor of another cytokine, and through either synergism or antagonism of two cytokines acting on the same cell. Cytokines should not be categorized as growth stimulators or inhibitors, or pro- or anti-inflammatory. Rather their specific actions depend on the stimulus, the cell type, and the presence of other mediators and receptors (Fig. 52.6).

Chemokines are a family of small, proinflammatory molecules characterized by four conserved cysteine residues. The α-chemokines have two pairs of cysteine residues separated by a variable amino acid sequence and are chemotactic for neutrophils (e.g. IL-8, platelet basic protein, epithelial neutrophil activating peptide) whereas β-chemokines have two adjacent pairs of cysteine residues and are chemotactic for monocytes/macrophages (e.g. platelet factor 4, monocyte chemotactic protein 1, macrophage inflammatory protein 1) and T cells (e.g. RANTES). Chemokines have been described as having more restricted actions than cytokines, but this is more likely to be a consequence of differential expression of receptors. The IFN family, IFN α, β, and γ, are broad-spectrum antiviral agents that also modulate the activity of other cells, particularly IL-8 and platelet activating factor (PAF) production, antibody production by B cells, and activation of cytotoxic macrophages. Growth factors regulate the differentiation, proliferation, activity and function of specific cell types. The best known are colony-stimulating factors, which cause colony formation by hematogenic progenitor cells (e.g. granulocyte-macrophage colony-stimulating factor or GM-CSF). Other examples include factors that regulate the growth of nerve cells (NGF), fibroblasts (FGF), epidermis (EGF), and hepatocytes.

In addition to the low-molecular-weight protein mediators, there are also lipid mediators of inflammation: for example, PAF and arachidonic acid metabolites. PAF is a labile alkyl phospholipid released from a variety of cells in the presence of antigen and leukocytes in response to stimulation by immune complexes. In addition to its platelet effects, the actions of PAF include the priming of macrophages to respond to other inflammatory mediators and alterating microvascular permeability. Arachidonic acid metabolites include the prostaglandins, leukotrienes, and eicosinoids [hydroxyeicosatetraenoic acids (HETEs) and hydroxyperoxyeicosatetraenoic acids (HPETEs)], all of which have profound inflammatory and vascular actions and may regulate, and be regulated by, other cytokines.

TNF α and TNFβ have a vast range of similar effects and are usually referred to as inflammatory cytokines. They have a central role in initiating the cascade of other cytokines and factors that make up the immune response to infection and play a key role in sepsis (Chapter 70). Their wide variety of effects is attributable to the ubiquity of their receptors, their ability to activate multiple signal transduction pathways, and their ability to induce or suppress an array of genes, including those for growth factors, cytokines, transcription factors, receptors, and acute-phase proteins. Although both TNFs have similar biological activities, regulation of their expression and processing is quite different.

Receptors and antagonists

The biological activities of cytokines are mediated by specific cellular receptors. Often these receptors comprise multiple subunits providing phased stages of activation and biological action. For example the IL-2 receptor complex consists of

Sources and effects of biological mediators

Mediator	Source	Biological activity	Effects on other cells
Interferon (IFN) α, β	T cells, B cells, macrophages, fibroblasts	Pyrogenic, cytotoxic	Macrophages: increases class I MHC antigens, IL-1, PAF production; B cells: proliferation, differentiation; T cells: proliferation; chemotactic
IFN-γ	T_H1, Tc, NK cells	Pyrogenic, antiviral, cytotoxic, antitumor effect, mimics septic shock, causes release of NO and ODFRs, upregulates IL-1 and PAF production	Macrophages: increases class I MHC antigens, IL-1, and PAF production, downregulates IL-2-mediated IL-8 mRNA production; B cells: proliferation and differentiation; chemotactic for monocytes; stimulates formation of adhesion molecules
Tumor necrosis factor (TNF) α, β	Neutrophils, lymphocytes, endothelial cells, smooth muscle cells, macrophages, mast cells	Pyrogenic, cytotoxic, antitumor effect, mimics septic shock, promotes angiogenesis, causes release of NO and ODFRs, induces or suppresses gene expression for cytokines, receptors, and acute-phase proteins	Wide variety of effects through ability to regulate gene expression, important role in host resistance to infection as immunostimulant and mediator of the inflammatory response, promotes hematopoiesis
Interleukins IL-1 α, β	Macrophages, endothelial cells, fibroblasts, hepatocytes B cells, mast cells, eosinophils	Pyrogenic, cytotoxic, antitumor effect, promotes angiogenesis, causes release of NO and ODFRs, induces prostaglandin synthesis, initiates the acute-phase response	Macrophages: TNF and IL-6 production; B cells: proliferation, differentiation; T cells: proliferation; chemotaxis; formation of adhesion molecules; hematopoiesis
IL-2	T_H1 cells	Pyrogenic, antitumor effect, mimics septic shock, causes release of ODFRs	B and T cells: proliferation, differentiation, release of IgG from activated B cells; chemotaxis; augments neutrophil and macrophage function; formation of adhesion molecules
IL-4	T_H2 cells	Cytotoxic, antitumor effect, inhibits induction of NOS, inhibits release of superoxide by macrophages, numerous anti-inflammatory effects	Macrophages: suppresses activation, upregulates class II MHC antigens, inhibits IgG receptor expression, inhibits expression of IL-1, IL-6, IL-8, TNF; stimulates IL-1ra expression; B and T cells: proliferation, differentiation, enhances antigen-presenting capacity; chemotaxis; formation of endothelial cell adhesion molecules; hematopoiesis
IL-6	T_H2 cells, macrophages, endothelial cells, fibroblasts, hepatocytes, mast cells	Cytotoxic, antitumor effect, mimics septic shock, causes release of ODFRs, induces hepatic acute-phase proteins	B cells:differentiation, antibody production; T cells: activation, proliferation, differentiation, induces IL-2 production; formation of adhesion molecules; hematopoiesis
IL-8	Macrophages, endothelial cells, hepatocytes, neutrophils, fibroblasts	Angiogenic, leukocyte infiltration in septic shock and adult respiratory distress syndrome (ARDS)	Neutrophils: activation; upregulates cell adhesion molecules; chemotactic for polymorphonuclear neutrophils
IL-10	T_H2 cells	Inhibits induction of NO, suppresses synthesis of ODFRs, may be immunostimulatory or immunosuppressive	Macrophages: inhibits antigen-presenting capacity, downregulates class II MHC antigen expression, suppresses prostaglandin E2, TNF, IL-1, IL-6, IL-8 production; B cells: induces IgA synthesis, enhances survival, upregulates IL-2 receptors; T cells: inhibits IFN; neutrophils: inhibits proinflammatory cytokine synthesis, upregulates IL-1 receptor antagonist expression
Granulocyte colony-stimulating factor (G-CSF)	Macrophages, endothelial cells	Proliferation, differentiation and activation of neutrophils; mimics septic shock; causes release of ODFRs	Neutrophils: proliferation, prolongs survival, enhances antibody-dependent cytotoxicity and superoxide anion production; chemotactic for granulocytes and monocytes
Granulocyte–macrophage colony-stimulating factor (GM–CSF)	T cells, B cells, macrophages, endothelial cells, fibroblasts, mast cells , eosinophils	Proliferation, maturation and function of hematopoietic cells; causes release of ODFRs	Neutrophils: proliferation, differentiation, prolongs survival, increases superoxide, leukotriene, PAF, and arachidonic acid release, enhances phagocytic activity, inhibits IL-8 production and neutrophil migration; monocytes: proliferation, differentiation, induces IL-1, IL-8, and TNF release; chemotaxis; formation of adhesion molecules; angiogenesis; hematopoiesis
Transforming growth factor (TGF) β	Platelets, fibroblasts, monocytes, mast cells	Stimulatory or inhibitory effects on proliferation and differentiation of many cell types, modulates cellular and humoral immune responses, suppresses chemokine-mediated NO release	Lymphocytes: suppresses B- and T-cell proliferation, inhibits NK activity, inhibits IgG and IgM secretion, upregulates B-cell IgA secretion; macrophages: induces secretion of growth factors; chemotactic for macrophages
IL-1 receptor antagonist (IL-1ra)	Macrophages, endothelial cells, neutrophils, fibroblasts	Blocks the biological activity of IL-1 by competing for the IL-1 receptor	–
Platelet activating factor (PAF)	Macrophages, endothelial cells, neutrophils	Activates and aggregates platelets, mimics endothelial alterations of septic shock, induces release of ODRFs	Macrophages (enhances IL-1, IL-2 and TNF production); intracellular messenger in neutrophils; causes release of lysosomal enzymes; chemotactic for neutrophils; formation of adhesion molecules

IgA, immunoglobulin A; IgG, immunoglobulin G; MHC, major histocompatibility complex, NK, natural killer cells; NO, nitric oxide; NOS, nitric oxide synthase; ODFR, oxygen-derived free radicals.

Figure 52.5 Sources and biological effects of immune mediators.

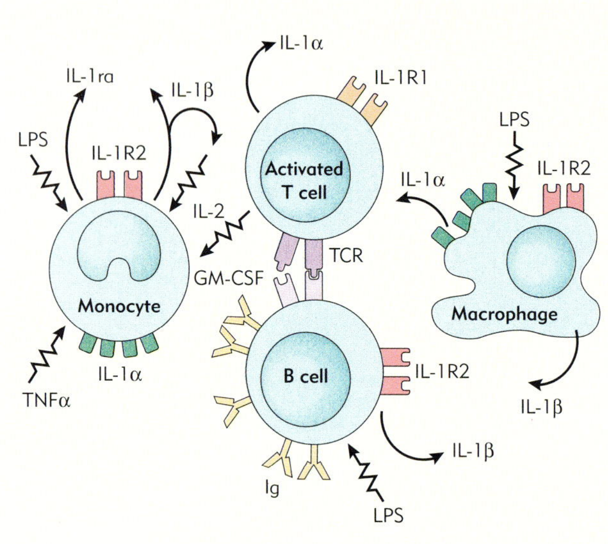

Figure 52.6 The interaction between monocytes, macrophages, and activated T and B cells during the immunoinflammatory response. (Reproduced with permission from Galley et al, 1996.)

three subunits, IL-2Rα, IL-2Rβ, and IL-2Rγ. Although the IL-2Rα/β combination can bind IL-2, IL-2Rγ is also required for high-affinity binding, ligand internalization, and signaling; all of which are required for maximal effect. Other cellular receptors exist in more than one type that act alone but have different binding affinities for different forms of a cytokine protein (e.g. IL-1 receptor type I binds IL-1α better than IL-1β, and IL-1 receptor type II has more affinity for IL-1β). Binding of a cytokine to one type of receptor may result in interactions with another receptor; the two receptors for TNF, for example, use ligand passing in which TNF binds transiently to receptor type I, with full signal transduction, but may then move onto the type II receptor with activation of another signal for apoptosis.

Soluble cytokine receptors have been identified that compete with membrane-bound receptors for cytokines, thus regulating cytokine signals. Exceptions to this are soluble receptors for IL-6 and ciliary neurotropic factor, which act as agonists rather than antagonists. Such soluble receptors may be membrane-bound receptors that are shed into the circulation either intact or as truncated forms (e.g. soluble TNF receptors, sTNF-R) or may begin as related precursor molecules that are enzymatically cleaved (e.g. IL-1R). Soluble receptors may appear in response to stimuli as part of a naturally occurring independent regulatory process to limit the deleterious effects of a mediator (e.g. sTNF-R), but some soluble receptors have little binding activity and may represent superficial and unimportant losses of cellular receptors (e.g. the soluble form of the IL-2Rα). Soluble cytokine receptors not only mediate biological activity but also control desensitization to ligands. This can be achieved by reducing availability of ligands, decreased signaling, and stimulating cellular mechanisms that can prevent activity.

The biological actions of some cytokines are also regulated by receptor antagonists. The receptor antagonist for IL-1 (IL-1ra) competes with receptors for IL-1 but when bound does not induce signaling. IL-1ra binds to cell receptors much more avidly than to soluble receptors; consequently, soluble receptors have little effect on the inhibitory action of IL-Ira. The appearance of IL-1ra is independently regulated by other cytokines as part of the inflammatory process.

Lymphocytes

Acquired immune defenses against specific microorganisms (antigen) form the second component of the immune response. Antibodies activate the complement system, stimulate phagocytic cells and specifically inactivate microorganisms. Lymphocytes, which form the basis of the acquired immune defense system, consist of antibody-producing plasma cells derived from B and T lymphocytes, which control intracellular infections. Binding of microorganisms to antibodies on the cell surface of B cells leads to preferential selection of these antibody-producing cells. This is termed *priming*, and subsequent responses are faster and amplified; this is the basis of vaccination. T cells exploit two main strategies to combat intracellular infections : secretion of soluble mediators that activate other cells to enhance microbial defense mechanisms and production of cytolytic T cells that kill the target organism. The NK cells have an important role in tumor cell destruction. They are large granular lymphocytes that do not exhibit immunologic memory and are nonspecific in their recognition of tumor cells.

Regulation of MHC gene expression [e.g. by cytokines (see Fig. 52.5)] plays a fundamental role in the immune system, since alterations of cell surface expression of class I or II molecules can affect the efficiency of antigen presentation. T lymphocytes consist of two subsets: T helper (TH) cells, which are $CD4^+$, recognize class II MHC molecules and produce IFN-γ and other macrophage-activating factors; Tc cells are $CD8^+$ and recognize both specific antigens and class I MHC molecules on the surface of infected cells.

Circulating TH cells are capable of unrestricted cytokine expression and are prompted into a more restricted and focused pattern of cytokine production depending on signals received at the onset of infection. The cells can be classified according to the pattern of cytokines they produce. TH1 cells secrete a characteristic set of cytokines associated with cellular immunity (cellular cytotoxicity). TH2 cells are associated with humoral or antibody-mediated immunity. Typically TH1 cells secrete IL-2, IFN-γ, TNFβ, and transforming growth factor β (TGFβ), whereas TH2 cells secrete IL-4, IL-5, IL-6, IL-9, IL-10, and IL-13 and also help B cells to produce antibodies. Both cell types produce IL-3, TNFα, and GM-CSF. IL-12 and IL-4 are early inducers of TH1 and TH2 responses, respectively; therefore, the local balance of these cytokines is an important determinant of subsequent immune responses.

HYPERSENSITIVITY REACTIONS

A localized inflammatory reaction called *delayed type hypersensitivity* (DTH) can occur when some subpopulations of activated TH cells encounter certain antigens. Tissue damage is usually limited, and DTH plays an important role in defense against intracellular pathogens and contact antigens. Development of a DTH response requires a prior sensitization

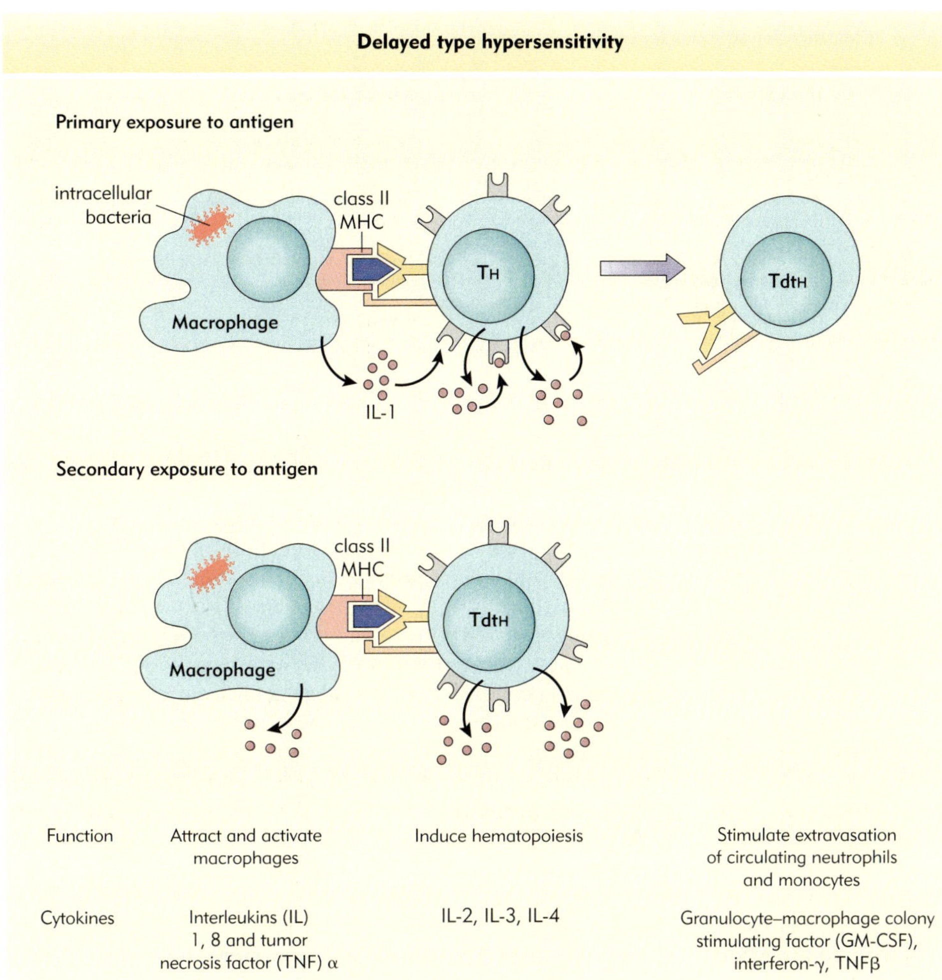

Figure 52 7 Overview of the delayed type hypersensitivity response. In the sensitization phase following primary contact with antigen, TH cells proliferate and differentiate into TdtH cells. Following secondary contact with antigen, TdtH cells secrete a variety of cytokines that have three primary functions.

period when TH cells are activated and clonally expanded by antigen presented along with the required class II MHC molecule on an appropriate antigen-presenting cell. A further antigen contact induces an *effector* response, where the expanded clonal T cell population can respond immediately by producing a variety of cytokines (Fig. 52.7) leading to recruitment and activation of macrophages and other nonspecific inflammatory cells. The activated T cells are generally TH1 cells. A DTH response becomes apparent about 24 hours following secondary antigen contact, peaking at 48–72 hours. The delay occurs because of the time required for cytokines to activate and recruit macrophages. A complex and amplified interaction of many nonspecific cells occurs, with only about 5% of the participating cells being antigen specific. The macrophage is the primary effector cell of DTH responses and the influx and activation of these cells provides an effective host response against intracellular pathogens. Generally, the pathogen is cleared with little tissue damage, but prolonged DTH responses can themselves be damaging, ultimately leading to tissue necrosis in extreme cases.

Immediate hypersensitivity reactions occur within 8 hours of secondary *allergen* exposure and are not cell mediated but humoral in nature and depend on the generation of antibody by secreting plasma cells and memory cells. The hypersensitivity reactions can be classified into type I (IgE dependent), type II (antibody-mediated cytotoxicity), type III (immune-complex-mediated hypersensitivity), and type IV (DTH) (Fig. 52.8). Type I reactions are mediated by IgE antibodies, which bind to receptors on mast cells or basophils leading to degranulation and release of mediators. The principal effects are smooth muscle contraction and vasodilatation; these can result in asthma, hay fever, eczema, and serious life-threatening systemic anaphylaxis,. Type II hypersensitivity reactions occur when antibody reacts with antigenic markers on cell surfaces, leading to cell death through complement-mediated lysis or antibody-dependent cytotoxicity. Type II reactions include hemolytic (Rh) disease of the newborn and autoimmune diseases such as Goodpasture's syndrome and myasthenia gravis. Type III reactions are mediated by antigen–antibody or *immune-complex deposition* and subsequent complement activation. Deposition of immune complexes near the site of antigen entry can cause the release of lytic enzymes from accumulated neutrophils and localized tissue damage. Formation of circulating immune complexes contributes to the pathogenesis of a number of conditions, including allergies to penicillin, infectious diseases (e.g. hepatitis), and autoimmune diseases (e.g. rheumatoid arthritis).

TRANSPLANTATION IMMUNOLOGY

Transplantation is the transfer of cells, tissues, or organs from one site to another. Tissues that are antigenically similar or

Classification of hypersensitivity reactions				
Type	**Name**	**Time**	**Mechanism**	**Manifestations**
I	IgE mediated	2–30min	Antigen binding to IgE induces release of vasoactive mediators	Systemic and local anaphylaxis
II	Antibody-mediated cytotoxic	5–8h	Antibody to cell surface antigens activates complement and antibody-dependent cytotoxicity	Blood transfusion reactions, autoimmune hemolytic anemia
III	Immune-complex mediated	2–8h	Immune-complex deposition induces complement activation	Systemic lupus erythematosus, rheumatoid arthritis, glomerulonephritis
IV (delayed reaction)	Cell mediated	24–72h	Sensitized TdtH cells release cytokines	Contact dermatitis; graft rejection

Figure 52.8 Classification of hypersensitivity reactions.

histocompatible do not elicit rejection; the reverse is termed histoincompatible. There are many antigens that determine histocompatibility, but those loci responsible for the most vigorous rejection reactions are located within the MHC. Graft rejection is an immunologic process involving cell-mediated responses, specifically involving T cells. The immune response is mounted against tissue antigens on the transplanted tissue that differ from those of the host. The most vigorous of these reactions are associated with the MHC (the HLA in humans). However, even with identical HLA antigens, differences in minor histocompatibility loci outside the MHC can contribute to graft rejection. Graft rejection can be divided into the sensitization and the effector stages. During sensitization, leukocytes derived from the donor migrate from the donor tissue into lymph nodes where they are recognized as foreign by TH cells; this stimulates TH cell proliferation. This is followed by migration of the effector TH cells into the graft and rejection. Graft rejection can be suppressed by specific and nonspecific immunosuppressive agents. Nonspecific agents include purine analogs, corticosteriods, cyclosporine (cyclosporin A), total lymphoid irradiation, and antilymphocyte serum. Specific approaches such as blocking proliferation of activated T cells using monoclonal antibodies to the IL-2 receptor or depletion of T cell populations with anti-CD3 or anti-CD4 antibodies have also been used.

CANCER IMMUNOLOGY

Tumor cells display surface structures that are recognized as antigenic and elicit immune responses. Macrophages mediate tumor destruction by lytic enzymes and production of TNFα. NK cells recognize tumor cells by an unknown mechanism. They can either bind to antibody-coated tumor cells, a process known as *antibody-dependent cell-mediated cytotoxicity* (ADCC), or they can secrete a factor that is apparently only cytotoxic for tumor cells. Tumor cell antigens also often elicit the generation of specific serum antibodies, which can activate the complement system, producing the MAC. However, some tumors are able to endocytose the MAC pore and repair the tumor cell membrane before lysis occurs. Complement products can also induce chemotaxis of macrophages and neutrophils and release of toxic mediators. Ironically, antibodies to tumor cells may also enhance tumor growth, possibly by masking tumor antigens and preventing recognition by NK cells.

Cancer immunotherapy

A number of experimental immunotherapy regimens have been used in the treatment of cancer. Injections of cytokines, including IFN-γ and TNFα, are beneficial in some cancers. However, cytokine therapy may also result in unwanted side-effects, including fever, hypotension, and decreased leukocyte counts. *In vitro* activation of lymphocytes with irradiated tumor cells in the presence of IL-2 has also been used. This approach results in the induction of *lymphokine-activated cells* (LAK cells), including cytotoxic lymphocytes and NK cells, which can then be reinfused into the patient, providing enhanced tumor-killing capacity. Monoclonal antibodies to CD3 that activate T lymphocytes *in vitro* and reduce nonspecific T cell activation *in vivo* reduce tumor growth in mice, but human studies have not been performed. Gene therapy in which cells from patients with cancer are genetically altered to increase immune responses are recent developments in cancer immunotherapy. Specifically, trials in patients with melanoma in which melanoma cells are transfected to produce IFN-γ and TNFα are underway. In addition, patients with lung cancer are being given gene therapy to introduce two genes, one that suppresses tumor cell growth and another antisense gene that blocks activation of a gene that allows proliferation of tumor cells. Genetic therapy is likely to be the way forward in cancer immunotherapy.

HUMAN IMMUNODEFICIENCY VIRUS

Human immunodeficiency virus (HIV) is the causative agent for acquired immunodeficiency syndrome (AIDS). The virus infects host cells by binding to CD4 molecules on cell membranes. Upon entry into the cell, the virus copies its RNA into DNA with a viral reverse transcriptase (Chapter 4). The viral DNA then integrates into the host chromosomal DNA forming a provirus, which can remain in a dormant state for varying lengths of time. Activation of an HIV-infected $CD4^+$ T cell triggers activation of the provirus leading to destruction of the host cell plasma membrane and cell death; this leads to severe immunodepression. Since only about 0.01% of the $CD4^+$ T cells are infected by HIV in an HIV-infected individual, the extensive depletion of the TH cell population implies that uninfected $CD4^+$ cells are also destroyed. Several mechanisms have been proposed for this, including complement-mediated lysis, apoptosis, or antibody-mediated cytotoxicity. Early immunologic abnormalities include loss of *in vitro* proliferative responses of TH cells, reduced IgM synthesis, increased cytokine synthesis, and reduced DTH responses. Later abnormalities include loss of germinal centers in lymph nodes, marked decreases in TH cell numbers and functions, lack of proliferation of HIV-specific B cells and lack of anti-HIV antibodies, shift in cytokine production from TH1 to TH2 subsets, and complete absence of DTH responses.

IMMUNE MODULATION BY ANESTHETICS

Increased susceptibility to infection is common in postoperative patients. Although trauma, surgical stress, and endocrine responses modify the immune response, anesthetic agents also modulate immune function, as shown by *in vitro* studies of the responses of immunologically important cells to clinically relevant concentrations of anesthetic agents. Volatile and intravenous anesthetic agents and opioids such as morphine and fentanyl suppress a variety of functions essential to the recruitment and activity of neutrophils, including respiratory burst activity, polarization, chemotaxis, and hydrogen peroxide production. Halothane and sevoflurane also induce leukocyte adhesion to endothelium, shown recently in a sophisticated study using intravital microscopy *in vivo* in rats. In contrast, a similar study found that lidocaine (lignocaine) decreased leukocyte adhesion *in vivo.* Lymphocyte function, as indicated by mitogen stimulation of T-cell proliferation, is attenuated by some intravenous anesthetics. Interferon-stimulated NK cell activity is inhibited by halothane and isoflurane anesthesia in mice. In patients anesthetized with large doses of fentanyl, a prolonged anesthesia-associated suppression of NK cell activity was found.

There have been a few studies on the effect of anesthetic agents on cytokine production. Anesthesia with ketamine decreased TNFα production by peritoneal macrophages in mice, both *in vitro* and *ex vivo*. Propofol and midazolam decrease IL-8 release from stimulated human neutrophils at the post-translational level *in vitro*, probably by altering the way in which the cytokine is transported from the cell. However, a previous *in vitro* study found that propofol and ketamine increased mononuclear cell IL-Iβ, TNFα, IL-4, and IFNγ production. The anti-inflammatory mediator IL-Ira was increased by clinically relevant concentrations of fentanyl in isolated human monocytes. Propofol is formulated in a 10% soybean emulsion (Intralipid), which itself may affect *in vitro* neutrophil respiratory burst activity and chemotaxis and IL-2-dependent lymphocyte responses. However, neutrophil polarization and T-cell proliferation are unaffected. *In vivo* infusion of Intralipid, however, caused increased *ex vivo* T-cell proliferation but decreased chemotactic migration of leukocytes. Consequently, the modulatory effects of anesthetics on cytokine responses remain unclear.

Although many studies have shown marked effects of a variety of anesthetic and analgesic agents on neutrophil, monocyte, and lymphocyte function, and also on cytokine responses to mediator stimulation, the clinical relevance of the observed degrees of immunosuppression in a previously healthy population is likely to be negligible. However, anesthesia-induced effects on specific components of the immune system may be relevant in vulnerable patient populations including the elderly, pediatric patients, the critically ill, and those who are immunocompromised. Further investigations are necessary to determine the contribution of choice of anesthetics on morbidity and mortality.

Key References

Farrar MA, Schreiber RD. The molecular biology of interferon-gamma. Annu Rev Immunol. 1993;11:571–611.

Milstein C. Monoclonal antibodies. Sci Am. 1980;243:66–7.

Rose-John S, Heinrich PC. Soluble receptors for cytokines and growth factors: generation and biological function. Biochem J. 1994;300:281–90.

Sheeran P, Hall GM. Cytokines in anaesthesia. Br J Anaesth. 1997;78:201–19.

Stevenson GW, Hall SC, Rudnick S, Seleny FL, Stevenson HC. The effect of anesthetic agents on the human immune response. Anesthesiology. 1990;72:542–52.

Tami JA, Parr MD, Thompson JS. The immune system. Am J Hosp Pharm. 1986;43:2483–93.

Further Reading

Morisaki H, Suematsu M, Wakabayashi Y, et al. Leukocyte–endothelium interaction in the rat mesenteric microcirculation during halothane or sevoflurane anesthesia. Anesthesiology. 1997;87:591–8.

Galley HF, Webster NR. The immuno-inflammatory cascade. Br J Anaesth. 1996;77:11-6.

Chapter 53 Microbiology

Andrew T Hindle

Topics covered in this chapter

Microorganisms
Antibiotics
Indications for antibiotics
Side effects of antibiotics
Cleaning, disinfection, and sterilization of anesthetic equipment
Infection risk following anesthesia

The care of patients with a microbial infection or at risk for infection relies upon a sound knowledge of the common pathogenic organisms and the ways in which infection may be prevented and treated by nonpharmacologic and pharmacologic methods. In addition, the anesthesiologist must be mindful of the risk that they themselves may be exposed to when caring for such patients. This chapter covers the classification of microbes, the treatment of pathogenic organisms, the principles underlying the cleaning of anesthetic apparatus, and the occupational risk of infection when caring for infected patients.

MICROORGANISMS

Bacteria

Bacteria are single-celled prokaryotic organisms consisting of an outer *cell wall* and a *cell membrane*. Bacteria can be classified by their staining characteristics and their shape (Fig. 53.1). Modern techniques use biochemical and genetic characteristics to extend this classification. The staining pattern of bacteria is affected by the cell wall, which can be classified into one of two main types determined by staining with the Gram stain. Most bacteria are defined as Gram positive or Gram negative.

The cell wall of Gram-positive bacteria contains 90% peptidoglycan arranged in polymeric layers connected by amino acid bridges. The cell wall of Gram-negative bacteria is much thinner, containing only 20% peptidoglycan. Gram-negative bacteria also differ in that they contain a periplasmic space, which surrounds the plasma membrane, and a lipopolysaccharide layer located next to the peptidoglycan layer. The lipopolysaccharide is similar to the cell wall in construction in that it contains phospholipids and is connected to the peptidoglycan layer by lipoproteins. The lipid portion contains lipid A, which is responsible for many of the toxic effects of Gram-negative bacteria.

Fungi

Fungi are simple eukaryotic organisms that can occur as yeasts, single-celled colonies, or molds, a tangle of filaments (attached cells). Fungi are normal inhabitants of the human body but may cause disease when the bacteria that normally keep them in check are compromised by either antibiotic use or a failure in the host immune system These conditions allow proliferation of fungi and development of an *opportunistic infection,* the treatment of which is outlined below.

Classification of bacteria by their staining characteristics

Bacterium type	Staining characteristics	Shape	Names of bacteria
Bacilli	Positive	Rod	*B. antharacis* *C. diptheriae* *Clostridia*
Bacilli	Negative Acid fast	Rod	*Shigella* *E. coli* *Salmonella* *Mycobacterium*
Cocci	Positive	Sphere	*Staphylococcus* *Streptococcus* *Neisseria*
Vibrio	Negative	Comma	*V. cholera*
Spirochete	Negative	Corkscrew	*T. pallidum*
Mycoplasma	Negative		*M. pneumonia*

Figure 53.1 Classification of bacteria by their staining characteristics.

Protozoa

Protozoa are single-celled eukaryotic organisms. They include *Entamoeba histolytica, Giardia lamblia, Toxoplasma gondii,* and the malarial parasites (*Plasmodium* spp.).

Viruses

Viruses contain genetic information in the form of DNA or RNA but must enter a living cell/host to replicate. The virus uses the host protein-synthesizing apparatus and some of the cell's enzymes to generate virus proteins; these assemble to form infectious virus, which can leave the cell to infect other cells.

A virus consists of a capsid core, DNA or RNA, and, sometimes, an envelope (Fig. 53.2). The capsid is the outer shell of the virus that protects the genetic material within. All viruses

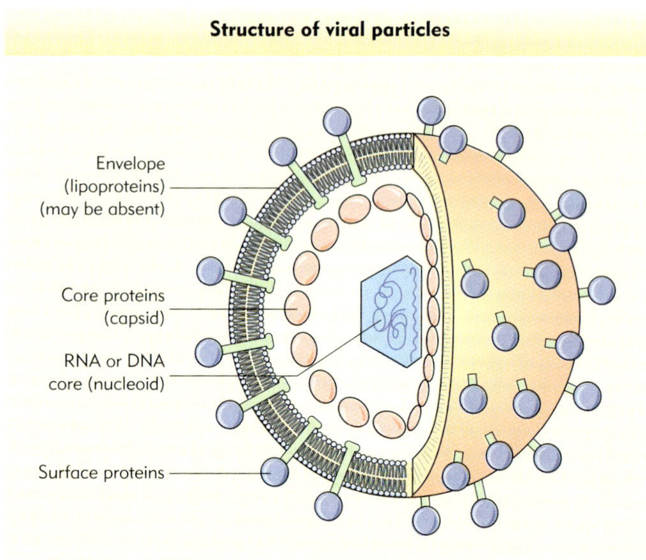

Figure 53.2 Basic components of virus particles.

attach to a specific structure on the host cell surface (adsorption) and subsequently enter the cell. The virus coating is digested and the nucleic acids released. The virus material acts within the cell to synthesize viral parts, which assemble into complete viruses. These leave the cell by one of two processes: budding or lysis.

The arrangement and type of viral genetic material are used for subclassification of viruses. An example of a human double-stranded DNA virus is Epstein–Barr virus (EBV). Influenza virus type A is a human single-stranded RNA virus; the *human immunodeficiency virus (HIV)* is a retrovirus (RNA-based genetic material).

Human cells secrete interferons in response to viral infection; these interact with adjacent cells to make them more resistant to attack by virus. The immune system takes over and begins to fight the infection by removing the virus on the outside of the cells, as well as the virus-infected cells. HIV is an exception to this situation because HIV infects cells of the immune system, leading to an immunocompromised state.

Antiviral drugs are limited in their ability to treat or prevent viral illnesses. No agents actually 'kill' viruses. However, there are drugs that inhibit viral replication. Acyclovir (aciclovir) inhibits the replication of herpes virus by inhibiting DNA polymerase. Azidothymidine (zidovudine, AZT) inhibits HIV replication by inhibiting viral DNA polymerase and by competitive inhibition of viral reverse transcriptase (the latter is probably more important). Dideoxyatidine (zalcitabine, ddC), which acts synergistically with AZT against HIV, inhibits reverse transcriptase and is a DNA chain terminator.

Prions

Prions are thought to be small infectious proteins that are conformational variants of a protein normally found in the brain. Brain prion protein is degraded at a sufficient rate that its concentration does not build up to an unacceptable level. The infectious protein is less amenable to degradation, resulting in accumulation and disease. The diseases most commonly associated with prions are neurologic illnesses resulting from 'slow virus' infection. These include Creutzfeldt–Jacob, kuru, scrapie, and bovine spongiform encephalopathy.

ANTIBIOTICS

The antibiotic era began in the 1940s and antibiotics remain the principal therapy for bacterial diseases. Antibiotics are the most commonly prescribed nonanesthetic drugs given by anesthesiologists, usually as prophylaxis against perioperative infection or in the management of critically ill patients in the intensive-care unit (ICU). Anesthetists must, therefore, be knowledgeable regarding antibiotics, although a recent survey demonstrated a significant lack of knowledge among anesthetists concerning antibiotics and their prescription. Antibiotics have a number of important sites of action to inhibit growth of (bacteriostatic) or kill (bactericidal) bacteria (Fig. 53.3). Synergistic combinations often target multiple sites of action.

Antibiotics affecting cell wall synthesis

Bacteria rely on their cell walls to protect them from a hypotonic environment. The bacterial cell wall is one feature that distinguishes bacteria from mammalian cells and it, therefore, is a potential target for drugs that will only affect the growth of the pathogen. Antibiotics that interfere with cell wall synthesis include the glycopeptides (vancomycin), penicillins, cephalosporins, and teicoplanin.

In order to appreciate the relevant points of attack for individual antibiotics on the cell wall, an understanding of cell wall synthesis is required. The basic building block for cell wall synthesis is *N*-acetylglucosamine (NAG). A series of chemical reactions involving the addition of amino acids terminates in the formation of a precursor molecule that is transported outside the cell membrane and then undergoes subsequent polymerization and cross-linking (Fig. 53.4). Many antibiotics target these steps, resulting in a faulty cell wall and bacterial lysis.

Antibiotics affecting protein synthesis

All bacteria require protein synthesis to function normally. The first stage in the process is the uncoiling of DNA by DNA gyrase. *Quinolones* interfere with this stage by inhibiting DNA gyrase and topoisomerase N. *Rifampin* (rifampicin) binds to RNA polymerase to inhibit messenger RNA (mRNA) synthesis. Subsequent stages rely on the presence of ribosomes (the catalytic complex for protein synthesis in the cell), energy in the form of GTP, mRNA, transfer RNA (tRNA), and amino acids. The bacterial ribosome complex is formed from two subunits, 30S and 50S (S refers to the sedimentation rate of the protein complex), composed of multiple proteins and ribosomal RNA. A number of important antibiotics target the bacterial protein synthesis pathway (Fig. 53.5).

Proteins are synthesized in the ribosomes, a new peptide chain being initiated with messenger RNA (mRNA) binds to a 30S ribosomal subunit. The mRNA contains the code, which determines the amino acid sequence of a peptide chain. In the first step, transfer RNA (tRNA) attaches to a site on the 30S subunit known as the peptidyl (P) site. A 50S ribosome is added to form an 'initiation complex', which starts the transcription process. In the next step, the next molecule of tRNA 'picks up' an appropriate amino acid from the cytoplasm and targets an acceptor (A) site on the 30S subunit. The two amino acids, within the initiation complex, are now joined by an enzyme (peptidyl transferase) to form the first peptide bond. The next step is known as the translocation, where the new dipeptide chain when the second tRNA molecule are moved to the Psite, with the first tRNA molecule dissociating from the complex. At the same time

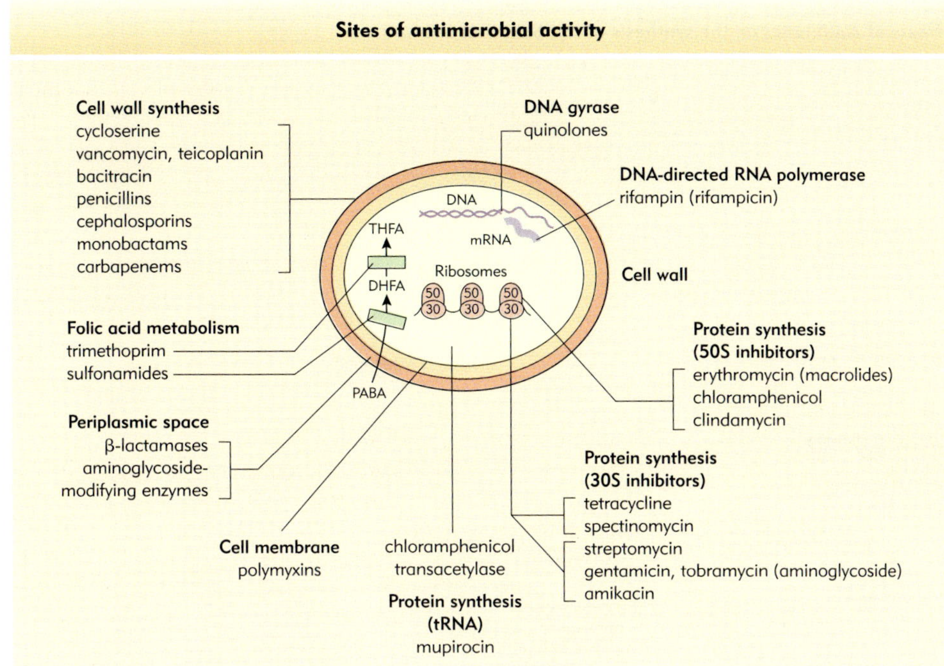

Figure 53.3 Sites of bactericidal or bacteriostatic action on microorganisms. The five general mechanisms of antimicrobial actions are (1) inhibit synthesis of cell wall, (2) damage outer membrane, (3) modify nucleic acid/DNA synthesis, (4) modify protein synthesis (at ribosomes), and (5) modify energy metabolism within the cytoplasm (at folate cycle). DHFA, dihydrofolate; PABA, *p*-aminobenzoic acid; THFA, tetrahydrofolate.

the next coding sequence on the mRNA is aligned with the vacant A site which is ready to receive the next tRNA/amino acid molecule. The lengthening peptide chain becomes attached to the 50S subunit as the process is repeated until a termination code is reached on the mRNA. The peptide chain is then released and the ribosome mRNA complex dissociates. The nascent polypeptide then undergoes various modifications including hydroxylation and phosphorylation of amino acid residues.

Metronidazole, which belongs to the nitroimidazole drug group, is an inactive prodrug; its reduced metabolites act to prevent replication of bacterial DNA, causing strand breakage (Fig. 53.6).

Antibiotics affecting nutrient supply

Bacteria cannot absorb folate and so must use *p*-aminobenzoate to synthesize tetrahydrofolate. The latter is necessary for the ultimate synthesis of DNA, RNA, and bacterial cell wall proteins. The *sulfonamides* and *trimethoprim* interfere with this pathway (Fig. 53.7).

Antibiotics affecting cytoplasmic membranes

Bacteria

Polymyxins (*polymyxin B, colistin*) act by displacing Mg^{2+} and Ca^{2+} from membrane phosphate groups. This disrupts the membrane and essential ions can leak from the cell. Polymyxins have a preferential effect on the cytoplasmic membranes of Gram-negative bacteria and have been used in the selective decontamination of the gut (discussed below).

Fungi

Membranes of fungal cells, unlike bacteria and mammals, contain sterols. Antifungal drugs target these molecules. Polyene antibiotics [*amphotericin B* (amphotericin), *nystatin*] bind to membrane sterols to form a complex that creates a pore in the membrane. Essential constituents of the fungus (sugars, K^+, phosphate esters) leak outwards and cell death rapidly follows. Part of the damage to the cell membrane caused by amphotericin B may occur through inhibition of the Na^+/K^+ ATPase pump and enhancement of nitrite synthesis.

Imidazole compounds (*miconazole, ketoconazole, fluconazole*) inhibit the formation of sterols by blocking the synthesis of ergosterol, probably by interfering with the demethylation of lanosterol, a precursor of ergosterol.

INDICATIONS FOR ANTIBIOTICS

Currently, there are no universally accepted policies regarding the prescription of antibiotics for either prophylaxis or treatment of infection. Common indications for prophylaxis and treatment are outlined below.

Prophylaxis

Prophylaxis is defined as the administration of an antibiotic in order to prevent infective complications in a patient who has no underlying infection. The anesthesiologist is most interested in prophylaxis for surgical procedures. The Canadian Infectious Disease Society has outlined the following requirements for the use of prophylactic antibiotics in surgery:

- high serum levels immediately prior to surgery;
- serum levels sustained throughout the procedure;
- activity against most organisms that can contaminate the operative site.

The decision to use prophylaxis is based upon a risk–benefit strategy. The relative risks of no prophylaxis, in terms of infection risk, are outlined in Fig. 53.8.

Clean low-risk versus high-risk groups

The clean surgical group has been further divided into low- and high-risk groups. The use of prophylaxis is unclear in the lower-risk surgical groups because some studies demonstrate benefit while others do not. More studies are needed to clarify the need for prophylaxis in this area.

There is a high-risk clean group that includes orthopedic and vascular surgery with prosthesis or graft implantation. Patients

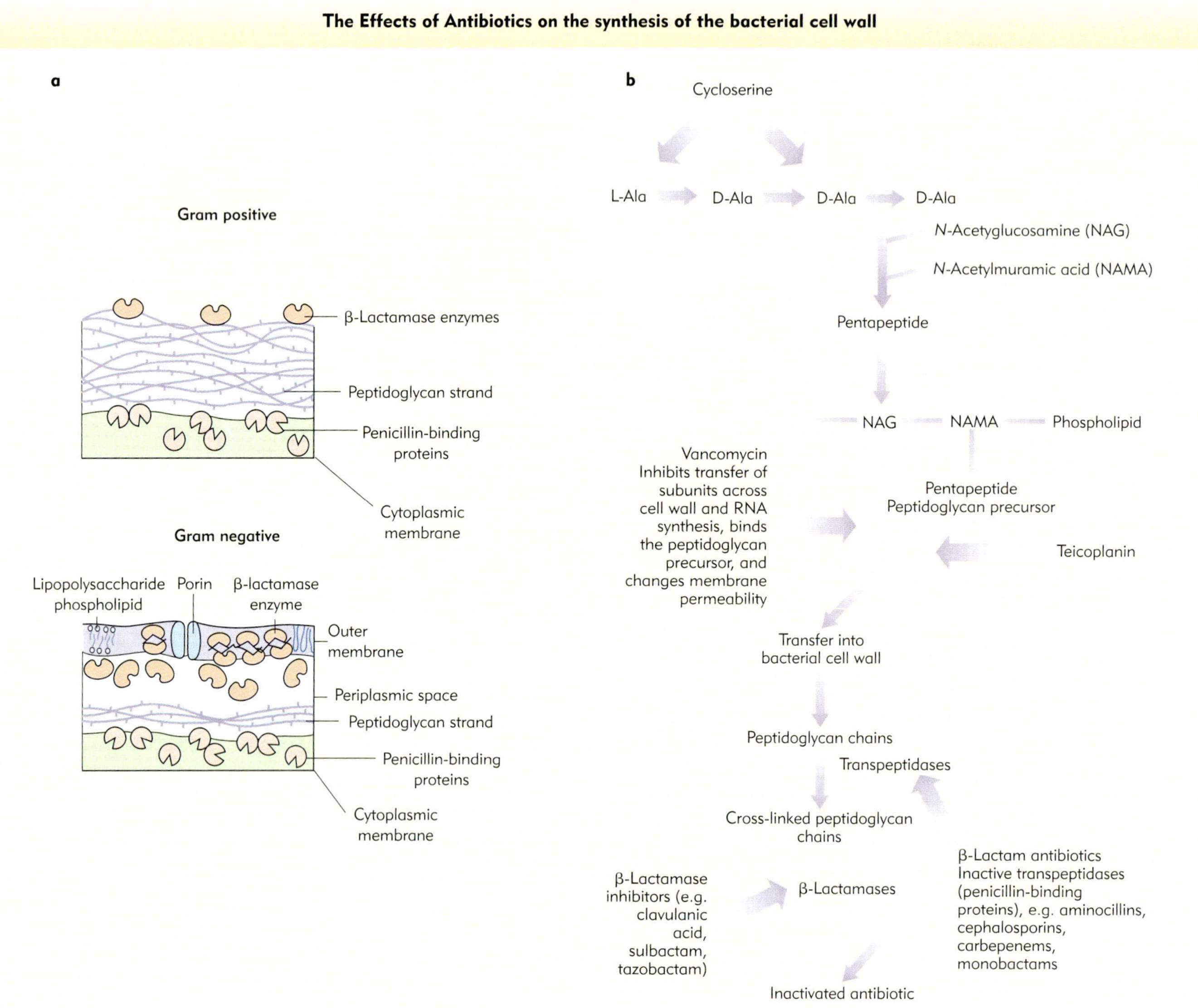

Figure 53.4 The effects of antibiotics on the synthesis. (a) Gram-positive bacteria have a thick outer coating and Gram-negative bacteria have thinner (three to five strands) rigid peptiodoglycan structure with an added outer membrane. (b) The β-lactam drugs act by inhibiting the synthesis of the rigid peptidoglycan part of the cell wall. Other antibiotics have effects on various stages in the synthesis of the bacterial cell wall. The multiplicity of actions of vancomycin is the reason why bacterial resistance to vancomycin is low. Penicillin-binding proteins may signal the induction of β-lactamases, which destroy penicillin and have caused significant problems by increasing the development of resistant bacteria.

undergoing orthopedic hip or knee replacement benefit from the use of antibiotic prophylaxis against staphylococcci and Gram-negative bacteria and from the use of ultraclean-air operating rooms. Gram-negative rods now account for 10–30% of infections after hip replacement because the widespread use of antistaphylococcal drugs has reduced the incidence of staphylococcal infection.

Infection rates are higher in prosthetic knee surgery than in hip surgery because of the complexity of the surgical technology. It is important for prophylaxis to be administered 30 minutes prior to the tourniquet being applied in knee replacement surgery because the cephalosporins take this long to saturate bone.

The choice and duration of antibiotic cover for prevention of graft infection in vascular bypass surgery is debatable. Cephalosporins such as cefuroxime or ceftriaxone are the most popular, but there is no hard evidence to demonstrate that antibiotics prevent graft rejection. However they reduce wound infection from 6–25% without prophylaxis to 0–3% after prophylaxis. The peak time for graft exposure to bacteria occurs at approximately 7–10 days and this may influence the prescribed duration of antibiotic cover. However, prolonging the duration of cover may result in the development of coagulase-negative multiresistant staphylococcal infection. Other high-risk surgical groups that benefit from prophylaxis are outlined in Fig. 53.9. The use of selective decontamination of the digestive tract is discussed below.

Choice of antibiotic

The choice of drug is based upon knowledge of endogenous flora, as the majority of postoperative infections are caused by the presence of endogenous flora at the wound site. Figure 53.10

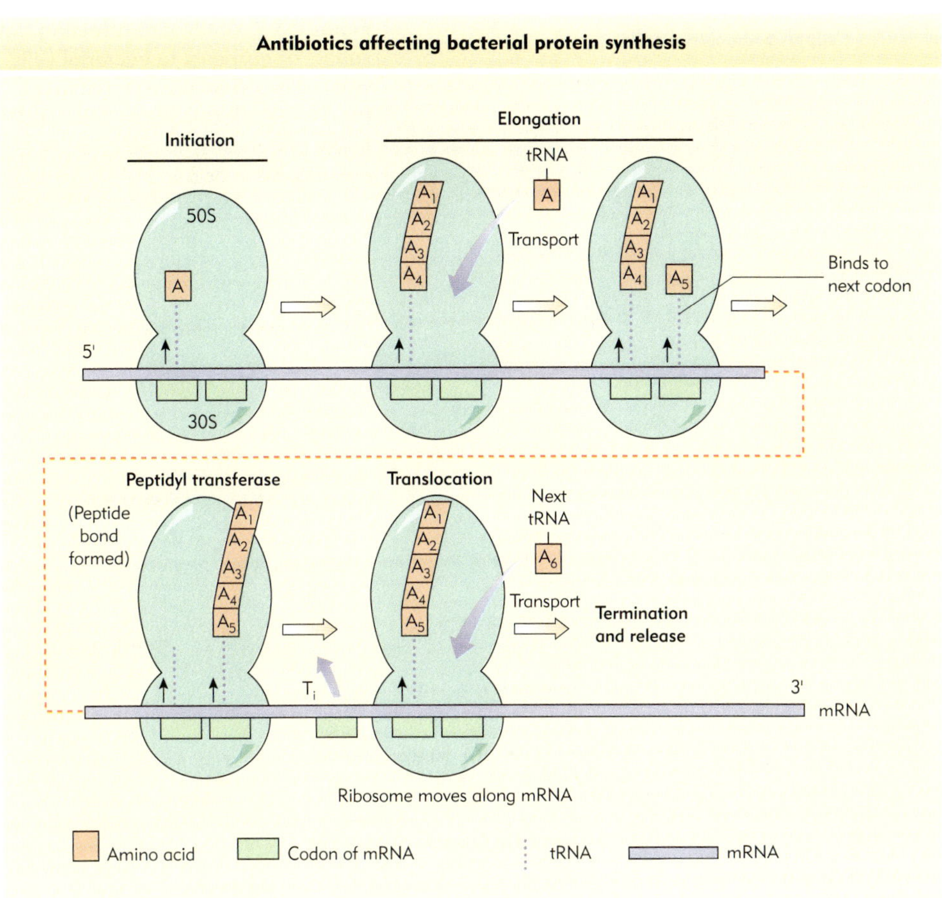

Figure 53.5 Bacterial protein synthesis and points where clinically used antibiotics act.

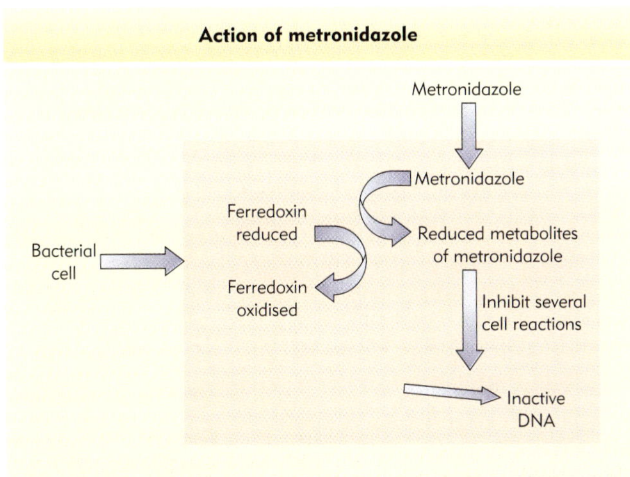

Figure 53.6 Mechanisms of action of metronidazole. The extent of the bacterial reactions inhibited by metronidazole is still uncertain.

presents an overview of recommended prophylactic regimens against endogenous pathogens.

Timing of antibiotic administration

The optimum time for intravenous prophylaxis is approximately 30 minutes before skin incision. The incidence of infection rises proportionally if administration is delayed following the start of surgery. Furthermore, any infusion of antibiotic should be completed 30 minutes before incision. For example, vancomycin requires 1 hour for infusion and, therefore, this should be completed prior to the start of anesthetic induction. Conversely, if antibiotics are administered too early (>2 hours before surgery), there is a sixfold increase in postoperative surgical wound infection. When administration is delayed into the postoperative period, vasoconstriction, inflammation, and the formation of a coagulum prevent delivery of the antibiotic to the wound site, rendering prophylaxis less effective. Prophylactic antibiotics should be administered before the development of a surgical hematoma, as a hematoma is an effective culture media for microorganisms.

Duration of prophylaxis

There is no value in continuing prophylaxis after the period of potential surgical contamination has ended. However, some surgeons would argue that it is justifiable to continue with the antibiotics through the postoperative period if the patient is being monitored invasively or has undergone major complex surgery. It is important that effective concentrations of antibiotic are maintained in the wound for up to 4 hours after the surgical procedure. This is because of the delay in growth of bacteria, known as the lag phase, which can last up to 4 hours.

Single- or multiple-dose prophylaxis

One dose of antibiotic will suffice for most surgical procedures, with multiple doses offering no advantage over single doses for short procedures. There may be value in repeating the dose of antibiotic if a procedure lasts more than 2 hours, if there is blood loss (>1L) sufficient to require transfusion, or if there is sig-

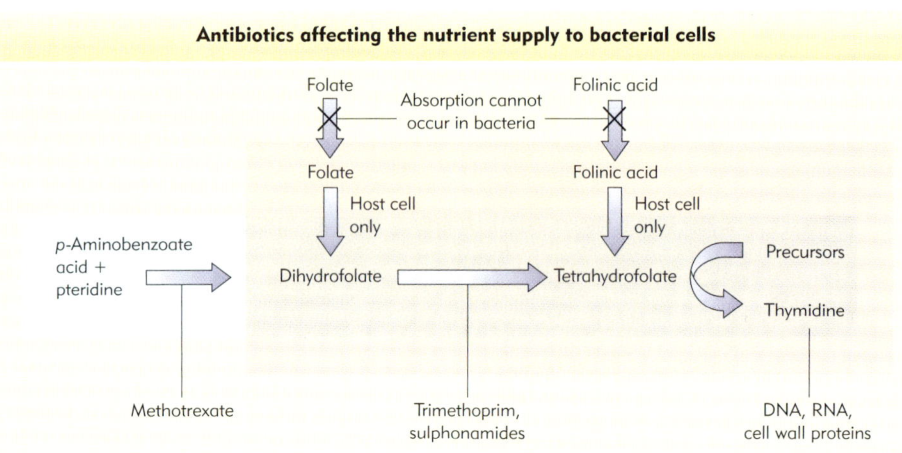

Figure 53.7 Antibiotics affecting the supply of nutrients to bacterial cells. Host cells can produce thymidine from folate. Bacteria cannot absorb folate and must synthesize it from *p*-aminobenzoic acid.

nificant hemodilution from any cause (e.g. coronary artery bypass surgery). Any repeat dose must ensure that the therapeutic effects of antibiotics persist into the lag phase, bearing in mind that the half-lives of most of the antibiotics used in prophylaxis are approximately 2 hours.

Prophylaxis against endocarditis

Anesthesiologists regularly have patients with heart valve lesions who are to undergo cardiac and noncardiac surgery, and they must know when to administer prophylactic antibiotics. These procedures can cause bacteremia, which may infect heart valve lesions with catastrophic consequences. It is extremely difficult to estimate the relative risk of endocarditis developing after a particular procedure just as it is difficult to establish the relative success of prophylaxis within the confines of the current guidelines. The rationale for using antibiotics to prevent endocarditis is not based upon data from well-conducted clinical trials but on a consensus view of what is likely to be effective. The reader is directed to an excellent review on the subject by Dajani *et al.* for the American Heart Association.

Treatment of established infections

This section will be devoted to the principles underpinning the management of infections in the ICU. Patients who are admitted to the ICU acquire their infections from either the community [community-acquired infections (CAI)] or the ICU itself [nosocomial infections (NI)]. The genesis of ICU-acquired infections is related to prolonged stay, cross-infection, immunosuppression, invasive procedures, and multiple antibiotic therapies.

A recent survey of European ICUs showed that 45% of patients were infected and 21% had acquired their infections on the ICU. The source of ICU infection is outlined in Fig. 53.11. The respiratory tract was the most common site of infection (64%), with mortality rates of 30–70%. Ventilator-associated pneumonia, the most common nosocomial infection in the ICU, occurs in 9–25% of patients and causes 35–90% mortality. However, the use of prophylactic antibiotics against ventilator-associated pneumonia causes the development of more virulent bacteria with a higher mortality. The microorganisms most commonly infecting the respiratory tract are outlined in Fig. 53.12.

Risk of infection without antibiotic prophylaxis

Type of wound	Infection risk (%) (no prophylaxis)
Clean (no entry into organ lumen)	1–5
Clean contaminated (controlled entry into organ lumen), e.g. appendix, vagina, biliary tract, oropharynx	3–11
Contaminated (presence of acute inflammation), e.g. spillage from gastrointestinal tract, acute nonpurulent inflammation, fresh accidental wounds	10–17
Dirty (infected), e.g. old traumatic wounds, preoperative presence of microrganisms	⩾27

Figure 53.8 Risk of infection without antibiotic prophylaxis.

The use of prophylactic antibiotics in clean high-risk surgical groups

Clean surgery	Antibiotic
Thoracic – only for chest trauma when tubes placed	Cefamandole Cefuroxime
Neurosurgery – only CSF shunts	Cefazolin
Cardiac	Cefamandole
Breast/hernia	Cefazolin
Ophthalmic	Cefazolin +/– topical aminoglycosides

Figure 53.9 The use of prophylactic antibiotics in clean high-risk surgical groups.

Cross-infection

A significant number of patients acquire their infection on the ICU. This incidence may be reduced with adherence to a strict infection control policy, which may include the following:

- handwashing between patients;

Endogenous pathogens and suggested antibiotics for prophylaxis				
Procedures	**Bacteria at operation site**	**Antibiotic (*penicillin allergy*)**	**Dose**	**Duration**
Cardiac (sternotomy)	*S. aureus* Coagulase negative *S. aureus* Diptheroids Gram negative Enterics	Cefazolin *Vancomycin*[a] *and Gentamicin*[b]	1g preinduction 500mg 8 hourly 1g preinduction[a] 1g 8 hourly[a] 2mg/kg at induction[b]	48 hours
Aortic resection Prosthetic Vascular bypass	As in 1	Cefazolin *Vancomycin*	1g preinduction 500mg 8 hourly 1g preinduction 1g 12 hourly	24 hours
Orthopedic (prosthetic insertions)	*S. aureus* Coagulase negative *S. aureus*	As in 2	As in 2	24 hours
Orthopedic (Other)	As in 3	As above	As above	Single dose
Neurosurgery CSF shunts	As above	As above	As above	Single dose
Head and neck	Oral aerobes and anaerobes *S. aureus* Streptococci	Cefazolin[c] and Metronidazole[d] *Clindamycin*[e] *and Gentamicin*[b]	1g preinduction[c] 500mg 8 hourly[d] 600mg preinduction[e] 600mg 8 hourly[e] 2mg/kg preinduction[b]	48 hours
Thoracic – pulmonary and esophageal	Oral aerobes and anaerobes *S. aureus* Streptococci Gram negative Enterics	Cefazolin *Vancomycin*[a] *and Gentamicin*[b]	1g preinduction 1g preinduction[a] 2mg/kg preinduction[b]	Single dose
Gastroduodenal* Gastric cancer Bleeding DU Genitourinary	Oropharyngeal Flora Gram negative Enterics	As in 7	As in 7	Single dose
Biliary** – open/laparoscopic procedures	Gram negative Enterics *S. aureus* *E. Fecalis* Clostridia	As above	As above	Single dose
Colorectal Appendicectomy Abdominal Trauma	Enteric Aerobes Anaerobes	Cefazolin[c] and Metronidazole[d] *(Vancomycin*[a] *and Gentamicin*[b] *and Metronidazole*[d]*)*	1g preinduction[c] 500mg preinduction[d] 1g preinduction[a] 2mg/kg preinduction[b]	Single dose
Cesarean section	Enteric Aerobes Anaerobes *E. Fecalis* Group B Streptococci	Ampicillin *(Vancomycin*[a] *and Gentamicin*[b] *and Metronidazole*[d]*)*	2g preinduction 1g preinduction[a] 2mg/kg preinduction[b] 500mg preinduction[d]	Single dose
Hysterectomy	Enteric Aerobes Anaerobes	Cefazolin *Vancomycin*[a] *and Gentamicin*[b]	1g preinduction 1g preinduction[a] 2mg/kg preinduction[b]	Single dose

*Absent resident flora. Bacterial translocation from a distal site. The listed organism occurring if the normal environment is compromised either by surgical pathology or antacid therapy (stomach).
**Rarely colonized by bacteria. But prophylaxis required if the patients are either elderly (>60), have a history of obstructive jaundice, a history of biliary tract surgery, gall stones or are about to undergo emergency surgery.

Figure 53.10 Endogenous pathogens and suggested antibiotics for prophylaxis.

- provision of hand-cleansing equipment for each bed space (chlorhexidine 0.2%/alcohol 70%);
- sterilization of reusable equipment;
- daily input and advice from a microbiological consultant.

Incidence and source of infection in the ICU	
Source of infection	**Percentage of patients infected**
Respiratory tract	64
Urinary tract	17.6
Bloodstream	12

Figure 53.11 Incidence and source of infection in the intensive-care unit.

Choice of antibiotic

The source of infection is often unknown on admission of a patient with an infection to the ICU, and 'blind' therapy is commonly instituted in an attempt to cover the most likely infecting organisms. Almost 90% of these patients are prescribed empirical antibiotics on admission to the ICU as 'best guess' cover for the infecting organism. The decision to use an antibiotic at a specified dose is based upon careful consideration of the known local strains of resistant bacteria, the history, clinical findings, radiology, specimen culture, pharmacokinetics of the drug, and the renal and hepatic function of the patient. The identification of the microorganism causing the infection is an essential part in instituting appropriate therapy and avoiding the development of resistant organisms.

Sputum, tracheal aspirate, and pleural fluid analysis are the traditional methods for identification of bacteria but they may be inaccurate. For example, in one study, 45% of the patients with pneumococcal bacteremia had negative cultures from the nasopharynx and trachea. Protected brush specimens and broncheolar lavage may be more reliable in identifying those organisms in the lower respiratory tract because they bypass the contaminant bacteria from the upper respiratory tract. However, prior use of antibiotics in patients before they are admitted to the ICU can make even these methods unreliable. The same methods may be utilized to assess whether the antibiotic is reaching the target tissue. Antibiotics have been assayed in sputum, bronchial mucosa, and epithelial lining. The majority of antibiotics will achieve only low concentrations within sputum samples. However, sputum analysis must be interpreted carefully because the concentration of a drug is subject to a number of variables such as sputum volume. Beta-lactams and gentamicin achieve only 5–20% and 25%, respectively, of their plasma concentrations in sputum, while quinolones enjoy relatively good penetration.

Antibiotic resistance in the intensive-care unit

There is little doubt that a large number of the new and emerging infections in the ICU are the result of the overprescribing of antibiotics by physicians in the ICU. Such infections include the development of methicillin-resistant *Staphylococcus aureus* (MRSA), penicillin-resistant *Streptococcus pneumoniae*, and vancomycin-resistant enterococci. There are a number of possible reasons for this overprescribing, including fear of litigation, fear of withholding treatment in patients with undocumented infections, the perception that an antibiotic with low or no toxicity is harmless, and prophylaxis against ventilator-associated pneumonia.

Mechanisms of resistance

Bacteria can respond quickly to the presence of an antibiotic. They possess a complex and dynamic genetic apparatus that can alter the synthesis of bacterial proteins. This may render the bacteria resistant to an antibiotic. Bacteria can also have access to a pool of antibiotic-resistance genes, which they can pick up and insert into their own genome. Transposable elements of the gene pool, called 'R' plasmids, are known vectors of resistance genes. The indiscriminate exposure of a bacteria to new antibiotics can result in a cascade of gene transfers with devastating consequences in terms of future antimicrobial therapy. Mechanisms by which resistance occurs are outlined in Fig. 53.13.

Incidence of respiratory tract infections in relation to bacterial type	
Organism	**Percentage of patients infected**
Enterobacteraciae	34.4
Staphylococcus aureus[a]	30.1
Pseudomonas aeruginosa	28.7
Coagulase-negative Staphylococci	19.1
Fungi	17.1

[a] 60% of these infections were resistant to methicillin.

Figure 53.12 Incidence of respiratory tract infections in relation to bacterial type.

Mechanisms of resistance to antimicrobials	
Antibiotic	**Mechanism of resistance**
Tetracycline	Active removal from the cell
Erythromycin Fluoroquinolones	Modification of target cell to reduce binding of antibiotic
β-lactams	Hydrolysis (β-lactamases) Alteration in protein binding
Aminoglycosides	Metabolism by phosphorylation, conjugation
Sulfonamides	Overproduction of antibiotic target

Figure 53.13 Mechansims of resistance to antimicrobials.

Candidal infections in the intensive-care unit and antifungals

The least-common infecting organism is the fungus, but the incidence of nosocomial *Candida* spp. infections has risen substantially since the 1980s and, therefore, these infections merit further discussion. Their proportion of all bloodstream infections has risen from 2.5 to 7.1%, with a concomitant rise in pneumonia from 3.9 to 4.4%. Disseminated candidiasis has risen tenfold in patients with HIV and malignancy. Deep candidal infections are difficult to diagnose and carry a mortality of 40%. A heightened clinical acumen, blood cultures, latex serological testing, radiology, and multiple surveillance site

Figure 53.14 Indications for and toxicity of antifungal antibiotics.

Indications for and toxicity of antifungal antibiotics

Antifungal	Indications	Toxicity
Amphotericin	All Candida apart from *chronic disseminated candidiasis*	Nephrotoxic, hypokalemia, chills
Amphotericin (lipid formulation)	As above	Less toxic
Fluconazole	Clinical Candida isolates Good CSF penetration	Minimal toxic profile
Itraconazole	Wide spectrum of activity (covers Aspergillus)	Drug interactions (esp with cyclosporine) Unreliable absorption
Flucytosine	Combination therapy for CNS or endocardial candidiasis Amphotericin treatment failures	Bone marrow and gut toxicity (monitor serum levels) Resistance develops rapidly (never use as sole agent)

testing should all be considered in the appropriate setting. Precise species identification by antifungal sensitivity testing is crucial prior to commencing appropriate antibiotic therapy (Fig. 53.14). Patient groups at risk include both neutropenic and non-neutropenic groups. The administration of fluconazole to the former group, who present with multiple site candidal colonization (nose, oropharynx, rectum, vagina), has been found to reduce the incidence of invasive candidiasis. Patients undergoing general surgery, for example those with recurrent gastrointestinal leaks and perforation, are also at risk from invasive candidiasis, but the risk can be reduced by using fluconazole.

Catheter-related infections

It has been estimated that there is a 10–20% fatality rate in the ICU from intravascular catheter-related infections. While there is no difference in the incidence of infection related to site of insertion, the method of insertion may affect the incidence of infection. Skin should be disinfected using either chlorhexidine or iodine alcohol preparations, although there is a slightly lower incidence of infection with chlorhexidine. The question of wearing gloves, gowns, and a full aseptic technique in terms of reduced risk has not been properly addressed as yet and further studies are needed. The type of catheter may also have an influence upon infection rates. Antibiotic-coated catheters may reduce catheter-related infections.

Selective decontamination of the digestive tract

Selective decontamination of the digestive tract (SDD) involves the use of a combination of antibiotics applied to the gut and systemically to reduce gut colonization with Gram-negative organisms. These are responsible for infections in the ICU that are becoming increasingly resistant to antibiotic treatment. The rationale underlying the use of SDD is to remove these pathogenic bacteria from the gut while leaving the anaerobic indigenous bacteria unaffected. A typical regimen may consist of cefotaxime (systemic), polymyxin E, tobramycin, and amphotericin B. Extensive microbiologic monitoring is required during decontamination; this involves the analysis of throat and rectal swabs for pathogenic organisms. Decontamination may have to be commenced several days before elective surgery if it is to be effective. The type of major surgical procedures involved in this procedure are those in which the normal anatomy is to be disturbed, such as esophageal resection.

The use of SDD in the ICU remains controversial but it remains an effective means by which Gram-negative colonization can be reduced in critically ill patients. However there is no consensus view regarding the use and potential benefits of SDD. There has also been concern raised over the shift in the pattern of microbial populations from Gram-negative to Gram-positive bacteria as a result of SDD.

Antibiotics and renal support therapy

Some patients in the ICU will require modification of the dose of antibiotic in order to achieve effective plasma concentrations. Dosing depends upon the half-life, clearance, and volume of distribution (see Chapter 7). Prescription of drugs in patients with renal failure is aimed at achieving effective plasma concentrations while avoiding toxicity.

Apart from gentamicin and vancomycin, most antibiotics do not require any alteration of dose at creatinine clearance over 50mL/min. These two antibiotics must have their dose reduced when creatinine clearance <50mL/min. In addition, the antitubercular drugs ethambutol, rifampicin, and pyrazinamide need reduced dosing in renal failure.

Some patients in the ICU depend on artificial support in order to maintain fluid and electrolyte balance; methods used include dialysis or one of the various forms of hemofiltration and dialysis.

Hemodialysis/hemofiltration

The dosing of antibiotics can be extremely difficult in patients receiving renal support, with only a few antibiotics being measured on and off dialysis or during hemofiltration. The removal of drugs by dialysis depends on dialysate, drug, and patient factors. Many antibiotics are removed during dialysis; consequently, administration should occur after dialysis. However, for patients with particularly severe infections, it may be advantageous for antibiotics to be administered before dialysis.

Antibiotic kinetics during the various forms of continuous hemofiltration and dialysis are highly variable. The reader is directed to a review by Cotterill for further information on antibiotic dosing schedules during dialytic and hemofiltration techniques.

SIDE EFFECTS OF ANTIBIOTICS

Antibiotics cause a number of side effects, including gastrointestinal, renal, and anaphylactic reactions. It is easier to diagnose side effects in patients not residing in the ICU, but the complexity of the clinical picture in the ICU can make diagnosis of an antibiotic-related side effect extremely difficult.

Anaphylactic and anaphylactoid reactions

Anaphylactic and anaphylactoid reactions are potentially the most serious reactions that anestheologists can expect to see following the administration of antibiotics. Anaphylaxis is mediated by antigen (immunoglobulin E) following prior exposure to the antigen (see Chapter 52). A cephalosporin should not be administered to patients who have a documented hypersensitivity reaction to penicillin, with vancomycin being a suitable alternative (see Fig. 53.10). Cross-reactivity with cephalosporins in people who are allergic to penicillin ranges from 5.4 to 16.5%. There is also significant cross-reactivity between the cephalosporins and the newer carbepenems, such as imipenem. Vancomycin is recommended in patients who are penicillin allergic if dermal testing confirms they are also allergic to cephalosporins. Skin testing is potentially hazardous because it can result in anaphylaxis and may not always diagnose true allergy. Allergic reactions to vancomycin are extremely rare, but a rapid infusion of vancomycin over less than 30–45 minutes may cause reddening of the skin over the face, neck, and hands. This so-called 'red man' syndrome may be distinguished from anaphylaxis by the lack of associated features of anaphylaxis and reversibility on terminating the infusion.

Gastrointestinal side effects

Approximately one third of patients develop gastrointestinal symptoms following antibiotic administration. This may be because of alteration in bowel flora following prolonged antibiotic therapy. Patients receiving single-dose regimens are subject to a lower incidence of morbidity than those receiving multiple doses.

Interactions with other drugs

An increased sensitivity of patients to warfarin has been ascribed to the use of cefamandole (cephamandole) as prophylaxis in cardiac surgery. The mechanism is unknown, as is the case with erythromycin. Penicillins have been reported to decrease the anticoagulant effect of warfarin; again the mechanism is not known.

Hepatic side effects

Penicillins can cause cholestasis while macrolides (erythromycin) and quinolones cause cholestatic hepatitis. Cephalosporins cause little in the way of hepatotoxicity.

Neuromuscular blockade

Antibiotics interacting with the neuromuscular junction or neuromuscular blocking agents include the aminoglycosides, especially neomycin. The neuromuscular blocking effects of these antibiotics appear to be presynaptic as well as postsynaptic. The effects seem to be related, at least in part, to the blockade of Ca^{2+} channels. Both N and P/Q type Ca^{2+} channels are blocked by neomycin, the effects not being reversed by anticholinesterases. Antibiotics interact with neuromuscular blocking drugs and it has been demonstrated that gentamicin and tobramycin prolong recovery from vecuronium.

Renal side effects

Renal toxicity following antibiotics is manifest physiologically by increased renal vascular resistance, reduced renal blood flow, and reduced glomerular filtration rate. Altered tubular function may occur, with increased membrane permeability to K^+, H^+, Ca^{2+}, and Mg^{2+}. Aminoglycosides are selectively concentrated by the kidneys, where they bind to and damage a number of intracellular phospholipid target sites. The β-lactams are also concentrated by the kidney and cause toxicity by lipid peroxidation and depression of mitochondrial function.

CLEANING, DISINFECTION, AND STERILIZATION OF ANESTHETIC EQUIPMENT

The anesthesiologist is responsible for ensuring that equipment is safe and clean. While some of the equipment (endotracheal tubes) is discarded after use by a single patient, there are a significant number of items that are reusable. Cross-contamination between patients as a result of reusing equipment must be prevented. The ways in which anesthetic equipment is cleansed includes decontamination, disinfection, and /or sterilization. There does not appear to be any clear evidence-based guidelines as to which technique is the most effective for specific items of equipment.

Decontamination

Anesthetic equipment, such as laryngeal masks, collect debris as a result of being in contact with patient secretions; this debris should be removed by washing before the item is disinfected or sterilized.

Disinfection

Disinfection involves the removal of nearly all microbes apart from spores. This may be achieved by chemical methods or by *pasteurization*. Pasteurization involves heating to a temperature of 80°C for 10 minutes. This has been shown to cause very little damage to perishable items such as laryngeal masks and red rubber tubes (which are still used in some centers). An alternative to heating is the use of chemical disinfectants.

Chlorhexidine and alcohol solution may be used for cleaning facemasks that may perish during a pasteurization process. Items exposed to a 0.05% solution of chlorhexidine may be left for 30 minutes, but if a 0.5% solution is combined with 70% ethanol, the disinfection time is reduced to only 2 minutes. Facemasks and oropharyngeal airways should be decontaminated and disinfected prior to use. Chlorhexidine and alcohol solution may be used for cleaning the external surfaces of the anesthetic machine and ventilator.

Glutaraldehyde (Cidex) is a very expensive disinfectant and while not recommended for routine use it is very popular for cleaning endoscopic equipment such as fiberoptic laryngoscopes and bronchoscopes. Glutaraldehyde requires bicarbonate (0.3%) to be added for activation. It kills bacteria within a 30-minute immersion, but spores require exposure for 3 hours.

Formaldehyde and paraformaldehyde are relatively inefficient and ineffective as disinfectants. However, the former has been used in combination with a low-pressure autoclave.

Sterilization

Sterilization ensures the killing of all bacteria including spores. The most efficient method of sterilization relies upon the anesthetic equipment being exposed to steam under high pressure and at a temperature in excess of the boiling point of water. The process is called *autoclaving* and cannot be used to sterilize perishable items such as facemasks and plastic items.

Dry heating involves exposing equipment to 150–170°C for 30 minutes. The method is not suitable for plastics or rubber because they can perish at these temperatures.

The use of ethylene oxide or propylene oxide requires a special sterilizer. The process is expensive and prolonged. In addition, when perishable items are exposed to the gas, a period of 5–7 days is required to allow the gas to diffuse out of the items.

Gamma irradiation is an effective method of sterilizing anesthetic equipment but requires significant investment in terms of equipment. It is only suitable for sterilizing large numbers of items.

The use of filters in breathing systems

The use of bacterial filters in breathing systems has become a matter of routine. The perceived advantage of their use includes retention of heat and moisture as well as reduced contamination of the remainder of the breathing circuit. The latter is particularly important when one considers that the same breathing circuits are used for all patients on an operating list. However, patient-to-patient transmission of pulmonary disease has not been demonstrated and the transmission of nonpulmonary disease is even more difficult to detect. There are two types of bacterial filter. Electrostatic filters consist of a single sheet of charged fibers; the charge on the fibers retains small particles. Hydrophobic, pleated filters consist of a membrane with small pores, which retains particles. The filter has to be large in order to have a minimal effect on resistance to air flow, hence the filter is pleated. These filters are also useful heat and moisture exchangers (HMEs). In pediatrics, the deadspace of the hydrophobic filters may be a problem.

Filters should be placed on the inlet and outlet connectors to a circle system. Valves and CO_2 canisters do not have to be disinfected between lists if filters are present. Outlet filters also protect the circuit from soda lime dust, which can damage gas analyzers.

INFECTION RISK FOLLOWING ANESTHESIA

Patient risks

Measures to protect patients against acquiring infections through anesthetic procedures need to address risks related to invasive procedures and risks or potential risks related to airway management. This includes effective disinfection of any equipment that may potentially breach mucosal surfaces, including laryngoscopes, airways, laryngeal masks, and fiberoptic scopes.

Frequent handwashing by the anesthesiologist and the anesthetic assistant is a most important infection-control measure particularly on lists with a high turnover of patients. Hands should be washed before handling a new patient or equipment to be used on a new patient, after leaving a patient, whenever they become contaminated, and before any invasive procedure. Protective gloves should be worn when handling biological materials.

Risk of infection for the anesthesiologist

Infectious hazards for the anesthesiologist come from hepatitis B or C and HIV. The risk of contracting hepatitis B can be reduced by prophylatic immunization. There is no vaccine for hepatitis C or HIV as yet. The take up of vaccination for hepatitis B is in excess of 80%, but there are anxieties that some health care workers do not return for necessary booster doses.

There is a school of thought amongst some anesthesiologists that any patient must be regarded as a potential carrier of HIV or hepatitis B or C. This assumption may have followed from the reticence to adopt hepatitis- or HIV-screening procedures for all patients; such screening has been strongly resisted by health departments. It is also of note that less than 20% of anesthesiologists take any history in order to screen out patients who may constitute a risk for passage of hepatitis or HIV.

The risk of contracting HIV is small (0.4%) following an inoculation injury. However, the risk of seroconversion following exposure to a hepatitis B antigen-positive patient is much higher (30%). The risk of inoculation from patients known to be infected and those whose hepatitis and HIV status is unknown can be reduced if simple precautions are taken. Transmission of infection can be reduced by wearing protective gloves, goggles, not resheathing needles, and the placement of sharps in specified bins that are designated specifically for that purpose.

ACKNOWLEDGMENT

My thanks to Dr M. Ellis, Consultant in Microbiology, for his advice and help in preparing the manuscript.

Key References

Borgers M. Antifungal azole derivatives. In: Greeenwood D, O'Grady F, eds. The scientific basis of antimicrobial therapy. Cambridge: Cambridge University Press; 1985:133–53.

Davies J. Inactivation of antibiotics and the dissemination of resistance genes. Science. 1994;264:375–80.

Marcus R. Surveillance of health care workers exposed to blood from patients infected with the human immunodeficiency virus. N Engl J Med. 1988;319:1118–23.

Further Reading

Allen RM, Dunn WF, Limper AH. Diagnosing ventilator associated pneumonia, the role of bronchoscopy. Mayo Clin Proc. 1994;69:962–8.

Classen DC, Scott Evans R, Pestotnik SI, et al. The timing of prophylactic administration of antibiotics and the risk of surgical wound infection. N Engl J Med. 1992;326:281–6.

Cook D, Randolph A, Kernerman P, et al. Central venous catheter replacement strategies: a systematic review of the literature. Crit Care Med. 1997;25:1417–24.

Cotterill S. Antimicrobial prescribing in patients on hemofiltration. Antimicrob Chemother. 1995;36:773–80.

Dajani AS, Taubert KA, Wilson W, et al. Prevention of baterial endocarditis. Recommendations by the American Heart Association. Am Med Assoc. 1997;277:1794–1801.

Kollef MH. Ventilator associated pneumonia: a multivariate analysis. J Am Med Assoc. 1993;270:1965–70.

Liddwell OM, Lowbury EJ, Whyte W, et al. Effect of ultraclean air in operating rooms on deep sepsis in the joint after total hip or knee replacement: a randomised study. Br Med J. 1982;285:4–10.

Page CP, Bohnen JM, Fletcher JR, et al. Antimicrobial prophylaxis for surgical wounds. Guidelines for clinical care. Arch Surg. 1993;128:79–88.

Rello J, Ausina V, Ricart M, Castella J, Prats G. Impact of previous antimicrobial therapy on the aetiology and outcome of ventilator associated pneumonia. Chest. 1993;104:1230–5.

Van Saene HK, Stoutenbeek CC, Stoller J. Selective decontamination of the digestive tract in the intensive care unit: current status and future prospects. Crit Care Med. 1992;20:691–702.

Vincent JL, Bihari DJ, Suter PM, et al. The prevalence of nosocomial infection in intensive care units in Europe. Results of the European Prevalence of Infection in Intensive Care (EPIC) Study. EPIC International Advisory Committee. J Am Med Assoc. 1995;274:639–44.

Waddell TK, Rotstein OD. Antimicrobial prophylaxis in surgery. Commitee on Antimicrobial Agents Can Med Assoc. 1994;151:925–31.

Chapter 54 Renal physiology

Salim Mujais and Mladen Vidovich

Topics covered in this chapter

Production of a filtrate
Tubular processing of ultrafiltrate
Regulation of urine tonicity
Measurement of renal function
Principles of diuretic therapy
Renal effects of anesthetics

The kidney plays a major role in regulating both the composition and the volume of body fluids. Deviations in body ion content and body fluid volumes are generally corrected by appropriate changes in urinary excretion. The functioning of the kidney can be divided conceptually into two complementary processes: first, production of a plasma ultrafiltrate by the glomerulus; and second, processing of this filtrate by the tubule. The first process is minimally selective in that it separates plasma proteins and cellular elements from plasma water but has no effect on solutes. The second process is the complex but controlled retrieval or excretion of a variety of solutes. This task is accomplished along the length of the tubule, and the varied requirements of the task are met by specialized morphology and function.

Nephrons are the functional units of the kidney; each kidney contains more than one million of these renal tubules. The tubules commence in the cortex of the kidney where a hollow funnel-like structure, Bowman's capsule, surrounds the capillary bed of the glomerulus. The glomerular filtrate captured in Bowman's capsule flows into the proximal convoluted tubule (PCT) from where it goes into a hairpin loop part of the nephron called the loop of Henle. Most nephrons (85%) have a short loop of Henle that passes from the cortex to the outer medulla and returns to the cortex, where it continues as the distal convoluted tubule (DCT). These are the cortical or short-loop nephrons. The remaining 15% of nephrons are juxtamedullary or long-loop nephrons, so called because their Bowman's capsules are closer to the outer medulla than those of the cortical nephrons and the loop of Henle passes through the outer medulla and deep into the medulla before returning, again to form the DCT in the cortex. The collecting tubules penetrate the outer medulla and inner medulla as collecting ducts where they start to coalesce, eventually to form the renal pelvis (Fig. 54.1).

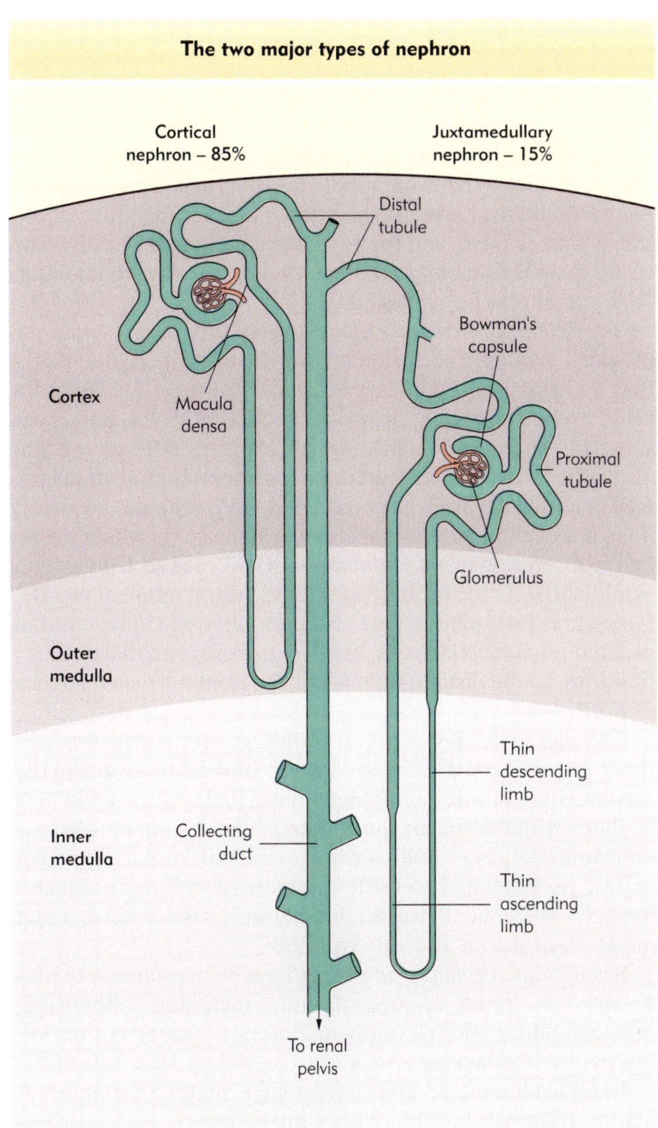

Figure 54.1 The structure and location of the two major types of nephron.

PRODUCTION OF A FILTRATE

Renal blood flow

Under resting conditions in the adult, approximately 20% of cardiac output passes through the kidneys, organs that constitute only about 0.5% of body mass. This rate of blood flow (400mL/min per 100g of tissue) is much greater than that in other vascular beds considered to be well perfused, such as brain, heart, and liver. From this enormous blood flow only a small quantity of urine is formed. Renal blood flow (RBF) in women is slightly lower than in men even when normalized to body surface area, averaging 980 ± 180 (mean ± standard deviation) and 1210 ± 250mL/min per 1.73m^2, respectively.

Autoregulation

Many organs are capable of maintaining relative constancy of blood flow rates during major changes in perfusion pressure, a property termed autoregulation (Chapter 37). For the kidney, the term autoregulation is also used to describe the relative constancy of glomerular filtration rate (GFR) that occurs in response to wide variations in perfusion pressure (Fig. 54.2). The constancy of flow in the face of varying perfusion pressure implies that vascular resistance changes in a direction that matches the perfusion pressure. The changes in renal vascular resistance that accompany graded reductions in renal perfusion pressure are demonstrable in innervated, denervated, and isolated kidneys. This implies that autoregulation of RBF is mediated by events intrinsic to the kidneys. Several hypotheses have been advanced to account for this phenomenon.

According to the *myogenic theory,* arterial smooth muscle contracts and relaxes in response to increases and decreases in vascular wall tension. Consequently, an increase in perfusion pressure, which initially distends the vascular wall, is followed by contraction of resistance vessels, thereby resulting in recovery of blood flow from an initial elevation to a value comparable to the control level. If this theory holds, the nature of the sensing mechanism and the regulatory process that allows the vessel to alter its radius to the exact value necessary to maintain RBF remains to be explained.

The *tubuloglomerular feedback theory* proposes a sequence by which increased perfusion pressure leads to increased blood flow and glomerular capillary hydraulic pressure; this increases GFR and distal tubule flow rate. Increased distal delivery is sensed by the macula densa, which activates effector mechanisms that increase preglomerular resistance, thereby reducing RBF, glomerular pressure, and GFR. This scheme, however, does not explain glomerular–tubular balance, in which proximal reabsorption of Na^+ increases as GFR rises and, therefore, would abrogate the proposed increased distal tubule flow rate. Further, autoregulation persists in nonfiltering kidneys and in isolated renal blood vessels. These factors suggest that delivery of filtrate to the distal tubule is not required for the constancy of RBF.

The *metabolic theory* predicts that, given the constancy of tissue metabolism, a decrease in organ blood flow results in the accumulation of vasodilator metabolites that restore blood flow to its previous level. In the kidney, however, metabolism is determined by Na^+ reabsorption, which, in turn, is approximately proportional to GFR (glomerular–tubular balance). Since GFR frequently varies directly with RBF, it follows that metabolism should also vary with RBF.

Several *autoregulatory substances* have been proposed to play a role in renal autoregulation, including adenosine, prostaglandins, and the renin–angiotensin system, but definitive evidence is lacking.

In all likelihood, several systems participate in the autoregulatory response, but the relative importance of each remains to be defined. The range of perfusion pressures over which RBF is held constant (the autoregulatory range) is reset in hypertension and blood flow will decline at apparently adequate perfusion pressures. In diseased kidneys, this autoregulatory advantage is lost and flow becomes dependent on perfusion pressure, hence the greater vulnerability of the diseased kidneys to declines in perfusion pressure. This highlights the need for careful monitoring and maintenance of blood pressure in patients who have underlying renal disease. It is not uncommon to see intraoperative and postoperative oliguria and azotemia in such patients resolve when blood pressure is increased.

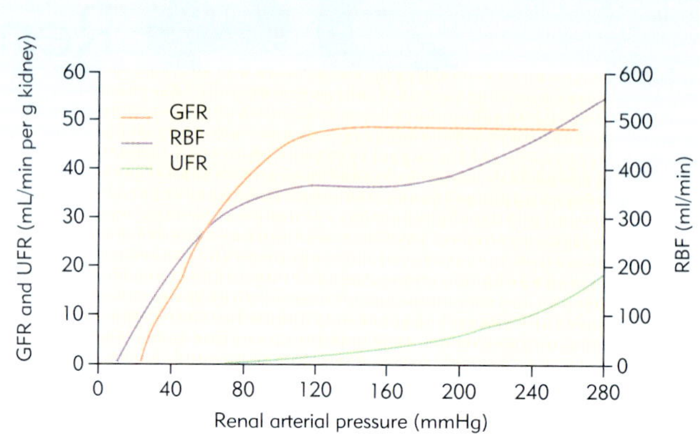

Figure 54.2 Autoregulation of renal blood flow (RBF) and glomerular filtration rate (GFR). Renal arterial pressure in dogs varies from 20 to 280mmHg; autoregulation of RBF and GFR is observed between about 80 and 180mmHg. (UFR, urine flow rate.)

Glomerular filtration

Glomerular filtration is the initial step in renal function. The glomerulus is a specialized capillary bed in that it is located between two arterioles, hence it operates at hydrostatic pressures that are higher and that vary according to the respective resistances of the afferent and efferent arterioles. It also has a very high hydraulic permeability, allowing large volumes to be filtered.

Glomerular filtration rate is determined by three main factors: the balance of pressures acting across the capillary wall, the rate at which plasma flows through the glomeruli, and the permeability and total surface area of the filtering capillaries. These determinants of GFR are, in turn, subject to the influence of a number of physiologic stimuli, including local and circulating hormones. The delivery of Na^+ to the distal tubule may itself modulate GFR by a process of tubuloglomerular feedback, which results in glomerular vasoconstriction when Na^+ delivery to the macula densa is increased and vasorelaxation when Na^+ delivery is decreased.

The glomerular ultrafiltrate compared with plasma is relatively free of large proteins and ions that are partially protein bound (Ca^{2+} and Mg^{2+}) because only the protein-free fraction (around 50%) is filtered.

Determinants of glomerular ultrafiltration

The driving forces that control ultrafiltration of fluid across the glomerular capillary wall are the same as those that determine fluid movement across other capillaries. At any point along the glomerular capillary network, the net forces favoring ultrafiltration (ultrafiltration pressure, PUF) are given by the difference between the transcapillary hydraulic pressure (ΔP), which favors filtration, and the corresponding difference in colloid osmotic pressure ($\Delta\pi$), which opposes it:

Equation 54.1

$$\text{PUF} = \Delta P - \Delta\pi$$

The transcapillary filtration pressure is the difference between the mean hydraulic pressure in the glomerular capillary (P_G) and the mean hydraulic pressure in Bowman's space, which is equal to the pressure in the PCT lumen (P_T):

Equation 54.2

$$\Delta P = P_G - P_T$$

The mean transcapillary oncotic pressure is the difference between the oncotic pressure of plasma in the glomerular capillary (π_G) and that of the filtrate in Bowman's space (π_T). Since the filtrate is practically protein free, π_T is negligible and $\Delta\pi$ is essentially equal to π_G.

The local rate of ultrafiltration is equal to the product of PUF (the net driving pressure) and the local effective hydraulic permeability of the capillary wall (k). For the entire capillary network, a factor (S) would need to be entered to account for the surface area of the glomerulus. The product of the surface area and the hydraulic permeability is termed K_f, the ultrafiltration coefficient. Hence, the single-nephron GFR (SNGFR) can be written:

Equation 54.3

$$\text{SNGFR} = \text{PUF} \times K_f$$
$$\text{SNGFR} = (\Delta P - \Delta\pi)K_f$$
$$\text{SNGFR} = [(P_G - P_T) - (\pi_G - \pi_T)]K_f$$

Single-nephron GFR varies linearly with plasma flow rate up to a plateau, beyond which further increases in flow are without effect. Clinically, this translates into a dependence of GFR on renal plasma flow and renal perfusion pressure within the limits of autoregulation. Ultrafiltration of fluid across the walls of the glomerular capillary occurs only when the local value of ΔP exceeds the opposing difference $\Delta\pi$. Therefore, at mean values of ΔP less than approximately 20mmHg (the normal average value for $\Delta\pi$), the net driving force for filtration is nonexistent, and SNGFR is zero. As ΔP increases above this threshold value, SNGFR also increases, but in a nonlinear manner. This nonlinearity results, in part, from the fact that as ΔP increases the formation of ultrafiltrate causes a concurrent, although smaller, rise in glomerular plasma oncotic pressure that partially offsets the increment in ΔP. A decline in the value of ΔP will lead to a parallel reduction in SNGFR, whereas a rise in ΔP will result in a relatively minor increase in SNGFR.

Afferent and efferent arteriolar resistances

Anatomically, the afferent and efferent arterioles are arranged in series, before and after the glomerular capillaries. Therefore, they are ideally situated to control both P_G and plasma flow rate. Selective alterations in afferent or efferent arteriolar resistance (R_{Aff} or R_{Eff}) are predicted to have specific effects on the various determinants of SNGFR. For example, an increase in R_{Aff} should simultaneously decrease both the glomerular plasma flow rate and P_G, thereby reducing SNGFR, a situation observed in essential hypertension. Conversely, a decline in R_{Aff} would increase both P_G and glomerular plasma flow rate, a situation observed in diabetes mellitus. Selective alterations in R_{Eff} are predicted to have directionally opposite effects on glomerular plasma flow rate and P_G. Therefore, an increase in R_{Eff} would tend to decrease glomerular plasma flow rate but increase P_G. Conversely, glomerular plasma flow rate would be expected to increase and P_G to decrease in response to a selective reduction in R_{Eff}. The control of efferent arteriolar tone is one important mechanism whereby a variety of vasoactive substances alter GFR. Clinically, the most important intervention to manipulate efferent resistance is the use of angiotensin-converting enzyme (ACE) inhibitors or angiotensin II blockers, which reduce the effect of angiotensin II at this site. The renin–angiotensin system is outlined in Figure 54.3 (also see Chapter 55).

Effects of hormones and vasoactive substances

Glomerular ultrafiltration is regulated by the interaction of a variety of hormonal and vasoactive substances either circulating in the plasma or produced locally within the kidney at or near their sites of action (Fig. 54.4). The arcuate arteries, interlobular arteries, and the afferent and efferent arterioles are all influenced by such substances, which can regulate preglomerular and postglomerular resistance and thus RBF, as well as P_G.

During extracellular fluid (ECF) volume expansion, values for whole kidney GFR and SNGFR increase. Urinary Na^+ excretion also increases as filtered load increases in response to both short-term and long-term administration of saline. Conversely, the antinatriuretic response to Na^+ deprivation is frequently associated with a significant reduction in GFR. Although the foregoing suggests a positive correlation between GFR and urinary Na^+ excretion, several key studies question the primacy of GFR in the physiologic regulation of Na^+ excretion, particularly in states of ECF volume expansion. These studies have shown that the natriuresis attending volume expansion may persist even when the filtered load of Na^+ is held constant or is reduced.

The constancy of fractional Na^+ excretion during increases and decreases in GFR is known as glomerular–tubular balance. The balance is maintained provided that tubule fluid and salt transport vary proportionately with changes in GFR. As a corollary, adjustments in Na^+ excretion during volume expansion and contraction represent a disruption of glomerular–tubular balance.

TUBULAR PROCESSING OF ULTRAFILTRATE

The human kidney produces 150–180L of protein-free filtrate per day. The renal tubules process this large volume of filtrate to conserve essential nutrients (glucose, amino acids, etc.), to eliminate potentially toxic substances (organic bases and acids, excess K^+), and to reduce the quantity of salt and water excreted in the final urine to less than 1% of that filtered. The tubule portion of each nephron is divided into segments arranged in series; each segment has unique morphologic characteristics and transport functions (Fig. 54.5)

Proximal tubule

Overall function of the segment

The main function of the PCT is bulk conservation of water and necessary solutes in a selective fashion. It is a very-high-capacity segment that responds to changes in delivery. Several passive transport functions are linked to a single active process to utilize energy expenditure most effectively (Fig. 54.6); in spite of this, oxygen consumption is still high.

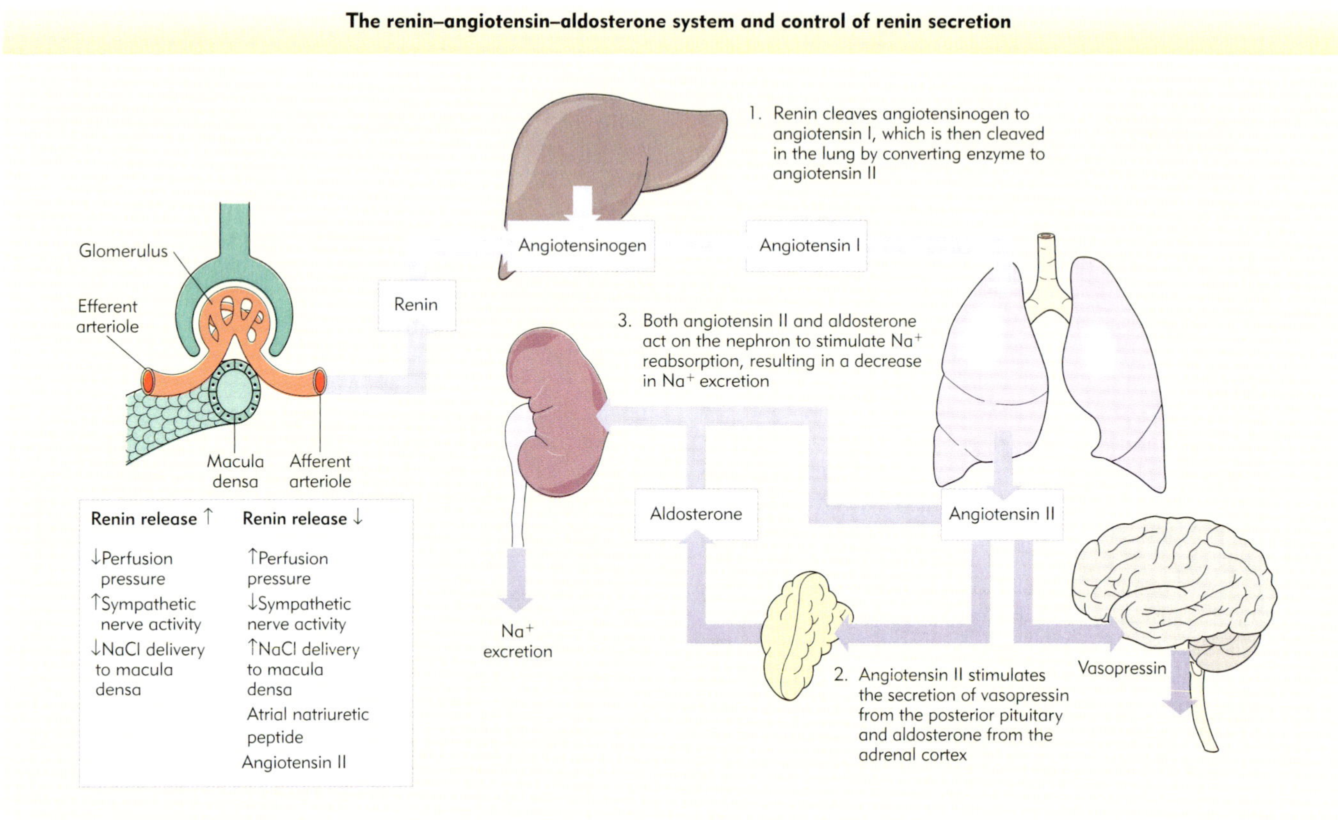

Figure 54.3 The renin–angiotensin–aldosterone system, and factors that control the secretion of renin. (With permission from Berne and Levy.)

The single active process is the Na^+/K^+ pump (Na^+/K^+-AtPase) located at the basolateral membrane of all renal segments. This pump lowers intracellular Na^+ concentration to levels of 10–20mmol/L and creates a gradient between luminal Na^+ concentration and intracellular concentration. By positioning passive transporters that are driven by a Na^+ gradient at the luminal side of the cell, this segment can effect several transport processes. Passive transporters driven by the Na^+ gradient include a glucose/Na^+ co-transporter, an amino acid/Na^+ co-transporter, and Na^+/H^+ exchangers. The above processes create an osmotic gradient between the lumen and the hyperosmotic intercellular space, thereby driving water reabsorption via water channels (aquaporins).

The PCT can be functionally and morphologically divided into three distinct segments, S1, S2, and S3. These are characterized by reducing mitochondrial density, luminal surface area, and endoplasmic reticulum development. This morphologic simplification parallels decreasing contribution to fluid absorption and glucose and amino acid reclamation.

Specific proximal tubule functions

Transport of Na^+ in the PCT can be divided into two phases: entry into the cell via the luminal membrane and exit via the basolateral membrane. The latter process is effected primarily by the Na^+/K^+ pump. At the luminal side, Na^+ is involved in a series of co-transport (symport) and exchange (antiport) with many solutes. The transport of glucose, phosphate, sulfate, carboxylic acid, and amino acids is intimately linked to luminal Na^+ entry. In addition to these co-transport mechanisms, Na^+ also

Hormone receptors present in glomeruli

Adenosine	Insulin-like growth factor
Angiotensin II	Leukotrienes
Atrial natriuretic factor	Norepinephrine (noradrenaline)
Dexamethasone	Platelet-activatlng factor
Dopamine	Platelet-derived growth factor
Endothelin	Prostaglandins
Epinephrine (adrenaline)	Parathyroid hormone
Epidermal growth factor	Serotonin
Histamine (H_1 and H_2)	Vasopressin
Insulin	

Figure 54.4 Hormone receptors present in glomeruli.

enters the proximal tubular cell in a 1:1 exchange for H^+ by a carrier termed the Na^+/H^+ antiporter (see Fig. 54.6).

Glucose reabsorption

Luminal entry of glucose is mediated by a glucose/Na^+ co-transporter with 1:1 coupling. It is driven by the Na^+ gradient, is delivery responsive, but is saturable with a tubular maximum. When this is exceeded glucosuria occurs.

Amino acid reabsorption

Luminal entry of amino acids is mediated by an amino acid/Na^+ transporter with 1:1 coupling. It is driven by the Na^+ gradient,

Segment	Reabsorption as % of filtered			HCO_3^-	Ca^{2+}	PO_4^{3-}
	Na^+ normal	Na^+ high ECV	Na^+ low ECV			
Proximal tubule	67	50	80	85	70	80
Thick ascending limb	20	30	14	10	20	–
Distal convoluted tubule	7	12	4	–	5–10	10
Collecting duct	5	2	2	5	5	–
Urine	1	6	0	0	1	10

Figure 54.5 Segmental distribution of reabsorption along the nephron. (ECV, extracellular volume.)

is delivery responsive but saturable, with a tubular maximum much higher than the corresponding glucose tubular maximum. Hence amino aciduria is not readily observed even with very high plasma levels of amino acids. Detection of amino aciduria is an indication of proximal tubular damage, such as that occurring in Fanconi's syndrome.

Bicarbonate reclamation

The glomerular ultrafiltrate has a pH of 7.25, a partial pressure of carbon dioxide of 60mmHg, and an HCO_3^- concentration of 24mmol/L. In the PCT, tubule fluid is acidified to approximately pH 6.7. This acidification is accompanied by a decrease in the HCO_3^- concentration to 8mmol/L. Because of the removal of 50% of the filtered water in the PCT, this decrease in HCO_3^- concentration reflects reabsorption of approximately 75% of filtered HCO_3^-. Thus, the PCT reclaims the majority of filtered HCO_3^-. Further HCO_3^- reabsorption occurs in the proximal straight tubule (S3). The proton-secretory capacity, however, is far less in this segment than in the PCT. In addition, as a consequence of the decline in luminal pH in the PCT, titratable buffers take their acid form, and ammonia is trapped in the tubule fluid. Hydrogen ions enter the lumen in exchange for Na^+. This process is carrier mediated by the Na^+/H^+ antiporter, is Na^+ dependent (high affinity), and is driven solely by combined gradients of the two cations. The process has an apparent tubular maximum dependent on volume status.

Water transport

Water transport in the PCT occurs mainly via transcellular pathways. Fluid reabsorption is iso-osmotic and driven by solute gradients. Because of the 'leakiness' of the epithelium in this nephron segment, most volume reabsorption can be driven by osmotic pressure differences of 2–3mOsm. Water flow occurs mainly through arginine-vasopressin-independent water channels traversing the membrane.

Calcium transport

Approximately 10g Ca^{2+} (250mmol) is filtered across the glomerulus every day. This amount is many times greater than the total ECF Ca^{2+} content. Of the 10g that is filtered, more than 98% is reabsorbed at various sites in the renal tubules: 70% of filtered Ca^{2+} is reabsorbed in PCT of the kidney. At this site, Ca^{2+} reabsorption does not appear to be under hormonal regulation. The reabsorption is linked to Na^+ reabsorption and is determined at least in part by volume status. When volume is depleted, Na^+ and Ca^{2+} reabsorption at this site is enhanced. Approximately 20% of the filtered Ca^{2+} is reabsorbed in the ascending limb of the loop of Henle.

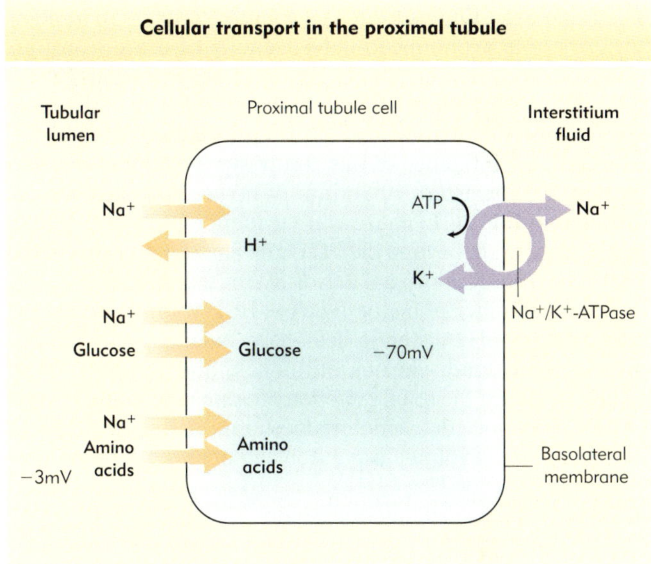

Figure 54.6 Cellular transport model for the proximal tubule. The Na^+/K^+-ATPase transports Na^+ from the interior of the cell across the basolateral membrane, creating a low intracellular Na^+ concentration and a negative intracellular electrical potential, which cause Na^+ to diffuse from the tubular lumen into the cell through the brush border. Glucose or amino acids are co-transported with Na^+ through the brush border of the tubular epithelial cells, followed by facilitated diffusion through the basolateral membranes. Hydrogen ions are antitransported with Na^+ from the interior of the cell across the brush border membrane and into the tubular lumen. Movement of Na^+ into the cell, down an electrochemical gradient established by the Na^+/K^+-ATPase on the basolateral membrane, provides the energy for transport.

Phosphate transport

Approximately 85% of serum phosphate is filtered from the glomerulus. The sites of phosphate reabsorption from the tubule fluid are located along the entire nephron but are concentrated in the PCT. Under conditions of normal phosphate intake, approximately 85% of the filtered load of phosphate can be reabsorbed; this occurs in the PCT. Phosphate/Na^+ co-transport in the brush border membrane is energized by the electrochemical gradient for Na^+ and appears to be the rate-limiting step in reabsorption of phosphate. A large number of factors, such as ECF volume, systemic acid–base balance, plasma phosphate, various hormones (parathyroid hormone, growth hormone, calcitonin, vitamin D), and pharmacologic agents, influence the renal excretion of phosphate.

Magnesium transport

The renal handling of Mg^{2+} involves filtration and partial tubular reabsorption. In humans, 146mmol Mg^{2+} is filtered over a 24-hour period, and only 3% of this amount is excreted in urine (4.2–6.2mmol per day), an amount equal to the daily net intestinal absorption. Of the filtered Mg^{2+}, 20–30% is reabsorbed in the PCT. Although the fractional reabsorption of Mg^{2+} is only half that of Na^+, it changes in parallel with that of Na^+ in response to changes ECF volume.

Urate transport

The renal excretion of urate is a complex process in humans since there is pronounced heterogeneity of urate transport within the PCT. Bidirectional transport (reabsorption and secretion) occurs simultaneously within the PCT. Urate is absorbed by a process that extends along the entire length of the PCT. However, the influence of this absorptive movement is modified by the coexistent operation of a secretory mechanism throughout the PCT. There is no evidence for active tubule transport of urate beyond the PCT. The amount excreted in the final urine is only approximately 6–8% of that filtered.

A large number of factors, such as ECF volume, urine flow rate, urinary pH, systemic acid–base balance, endogenous plasma urate load, various hormones, and pharmacologic agents, influence the renal excretion of urate in humans. Plasma and ECF volume contraction reduce urate clearance, whereas ECF and plasma volume expansion augment urate excretion.

Regulation of proximal tubule transport

The PCT accounts for the reabsorption of two thirds of the filtered Na^+ and is, therefore, a prominent regulator of body Na^+. This segment performs in a delivery-responsive mode.

The effect of physical factors on PCT reabsorption is governed by the principle of glomerular–tubular balance. Volume reabsorption in the PCT is related to GFR. A disruption of glomerular–tubular balance is required in order to initiate natriuresis in response to volume expansion at the whole kidney level. This disruption occurs at least in part at the level of the PCT. The peritubular capillary network is connected in series with the glomerular capillary bed through the efferent arteriole in such a way that changes in the physical determinants of GFR critically influence the hydraulic and oncotic pressures in the peritubular capillaries. The hydraulic pressure in peritubular capillary is significantly lower than that in the glomerular capillary. Also, because the peritubular capillary receives blood from the glomerulus, the plasma oncotic pressure is high at the outset as a result of prior filtration of protein-free fluid. It follows that the greater the GFR is relative to renal plasma flow (the filtration fraction), the greater will be the efferent arteriolar plasma protein concentration. Therefore, the peritubular capillary is characterized by a large oncotic pressure gradient, which greatly exceeds the hydrostatic gradient, resulting in net reabsorption of fluid. The absorptive oncotic pressure gradient normally remains greater than the opposing filtration pressure throughout the capillary length.

Angiotensin II is the main hormonal regulator of Na^+ reabsorption in the PCT by its control of the Na^+/H^+ antiporter. High levels of angiotensin II in the physiologic range enhance Na^+ and fluid reabsorption in this segment. *Parathyroid hormone* inhibits fluid volume and HCO_3^- reabsorption. The decrease in fluid volume reabsorption is a consequence of the decrease in HCO_3^- transport. The primary effect of the hormone is likely to be an inhibition of the Na^+/H^+ exchanger by a cyclic adenosine monophosphate (cAMP) -dependent mechanism. *Catecholamines* increase reabsorption directly. The rich innervation of the PCT and this direct effect highlight the importance of renal nerves in regulating volume absorption. *Dopamine* inhibits proximal Na^+ and Cl^- reabsorption. Renal denervation induces a natriuresis and renal nerve stimulation leads to Na^+ conservation. Alpha-adrenoceptors are responsible for increased Na^+ reabsorption during renal nerve stimulation. Stimulation of dopaminergic receptors decreases PCT Na^+ reabsorption. The effects of renal nerves on volume homeostasis are expected to be most critical in states of extreme salt depletion.

Thin limbs of the loop of Henle

The thin limbs of Henle's loop are composed of the thin descending limb and the thin ascending limb. These make an important contribution to the process of urinary concentration and dilution, primarily by passive water and NaCl transport, respectively. The remarkable separation of passive water reabsorption in the descending loop of Henle and passive NaCl reabsorption in the ascending loop of Henle is attributed to the abrupt change of the passive permeability properties of these segments at the tip of the loop of Henle.

The thin descending limb begins at the end of the PCT at the junction of the outer and inner stripes of the outer medulla. It is permeable to water but impermeable to Na^+ and Cl^-. This leads to water exit into a hypertonic interstitium and gradual concentration of the luminal solutes as the water fraction is progressively reduced.

Ascending thin limbs begin at the bend of the loop in long-looped nephrons. Short-loop nephrons have no ascending loop of Henle. The ascending limb of the loop of Henle is similar to the descending limb in that it has a flat endothelial-like epithelium with minimal Na^+/K^+-ATPase activity. Therefore, it does not transport solutes actively. In contrast to the descending limb, the ascending limb is impermeable to water, moderately permeable to urea, and highly permeable to NaCl. As a result of these differences in permeability, the osmolarity of the tubular fluid can be passively decreased as the fluid moves from the bend of Henle's loop toward the medullary thick ascending limb.

Thick ascending limb of Henle's loop

Overall function of the segment

The thick ascending limb of Henle's loop reabsorbs approximately 30% of NaCl filtered at the glomerulus. This segment is responsible for the ability of mammals to dissociate the excretion of salt and water. It permits the dilution of urine by its ability to reabsorb solutes while being water impermeable, and it assists the concentration of urine by its contribution to the creation of a hypertonic interstitium.

Mechanism of sodium reabsorption

The basic mechanisms of Na^+ transport are similar in the medullary and cortical sections of the thick ascending limb of Henle's loop despite morphologic and permeability differences. Thick ascending limbs reabsorb NaCl at a rapid rate. The mechanism can again be best understood by separating this reabsorptive process into luminal plasma membrane entry and basolateral exit phases (Fig. 54.7). At the latter membrane, the

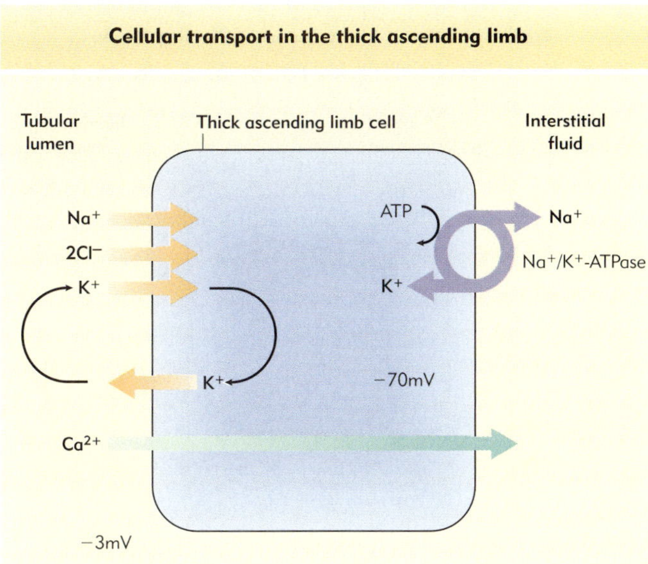

Figure 54.7 Cellular transport model for the thick ascending limb of the loop of Henle. The Na^+/ K^+/2Cl^- co-transporter in the luminal membrane transports these ions into the tubular lumen using the potential energy provided by the Na^+/K^+-ATPase. Calcium ions are reabsorbed by all nephron segments by transcellular and paracellular routes.

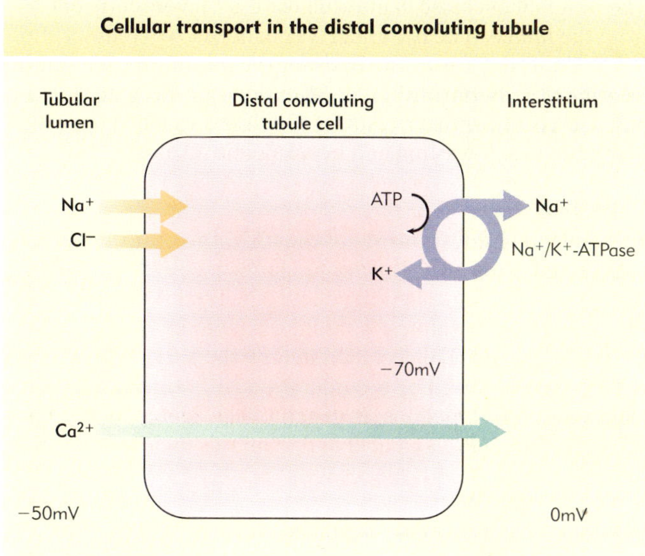

Figure 54.8 Cellular transport model for the distal convoluted tubule (DCT). The basolateral membrane Na^+/K^+-ATPase maintains a low intracellular Na^+ concentration; Na^+ is absorbed from the lumen through a luminal membrane Na^+/Cl^- co-transporter. Active Ca^{2+} reabsorption occurs in this segment.

mechanism of Na^+ exit is again mediated by Na^+/K^+-ATPase as in other nephron segments.

At the luminal side, Na^+ entry is effected by means of a transporter that couples the entry of one Na^+ and one K^+ to two Cl^-. This co-transporter is electroneutral and is driven by the concentration gradient for Na^+ created by the active transport of Na^+ at the basolateral membrane by Na^+/K^+-ATPase. The transported Cl^- exits from the cell via a basolateral Cl^- channel or K^+/Cl^- co-transporter. The K^+ re-enters the lumen via conductive pathways along the luminal membrane. The recycling of K^+ (positive charge) back to the lumen and the basolateral negative Cl^- current create a positive voltage inside the lumen. This positive transepithelial voltage differential, together with high permeability for cations, drives the passive transport of Ca^{2+}, Mg^{2+}, and ammonia. The large reabsorptive fluxes for Ca^{2+} and Mg^{2+} in this region of the nephron account for a major part of their total renal tubular reabsorption. The reabsorption of Na^+ along these segments has another role: it dilutes the tubular fluid by the removal of solute while water remains within the lumen because of low water permeability. The ascending limb also provides the driving force for the generation of the osmotic gradient that is maintained by the countercurrent mechanism and, thus, is responsible for the ability to concentrate the urine. Consequently, interference with Na^+ transport in the thick limbs can alter water handling by the kidneys. The Na^+/K^+/2Cl^- co-transporter is the target protein for loop diuretics. Mutations in its gene lead to Bartter's syndrome, with hypokalemic alkalosis.

Regulation of sodium transport in different segments

The capacity for Na^+ transport varies along the nephron with segments capable of high transport rates being followed by segments with lower transport capacity. The high transport rates of the early segments allows them to react rapidly to changes in the filtered load of Na^+ and leads to effective stabilization of Na^+ delivery to the later nephron segments, where the final concentration of urine Na^+ is determined. This stabilization of distal delivery of Na^+ is required to allow more efficient transport by segments with low transport capacity. Stabilization of distal delivery also sets ideal conditions for hormonal modulation of transport in the final nephron segments. This continuity and interdependence of nephron segments is also exemplified by the observation that transport in many segments is altered by the composition and the rate of tubular fluid delivery from more proximal segments. Hence, alterations in Na^+ transport in proximal segments affect distal transport and may be offset by those alterations.

Increased delivery of fluid from the PCT is associated with increased Na^+ reabsorption in the loop of Henle. Thus, the loop of Henle is capable of reabsorbing most of the increase in load delivered from the PCT. The effect of such increases in reabsorptive capacity minimize increases in delivery to the distal tubule and collecting duct.

Distal convoluted tubule

The DCT is a morphologically and functionally heterogeneous segment that extends from the macula densa to the early branching of the cortical collecting tubule (CCT). The DCT possesses the highest activity of the basolateral Na^+/K^+-ATPase of any of the nephron segments. At the luminal membrane, a thiazide-sensitive Na^+/Cl^- co-transport is responsible for Na^+ transport. The reabsorption of Na^+ in the DCT is mineralocorticoid independent and results in a luminal negative potential difference. Active Ca^{2+} reabsorption occurs in this segment and is modulated by parathyroid hormone (Fig. 54.8). By inhibiting Na^+ reabsorption in the DCT, thiazides lower cellular Na^+ concentration and inhibit the lumen negative potential. This enhances Na^+ entry into the cell by Na^+/Ca^{2+} exchange across the basolateral membrane, favoring basolateral Ca^{2+} exit.

The resultant decrease in intracellular Ca^{2+} favors entry of Ca^{2+} from the lumen. The net effect is enhanced Ca^{2+} reabsorption by the DCT; this forms the basis for the use of thiazides in the treatment of nephrolithiasis. Mutations in the gene for the Na^+/Cl^- co-transporter result in Gitelman's syndrome, which manifests as salt wasting and hypokalemic alkalosis.

Collecting duct

The collecting duct consists of the CCT, the outer medullary collecting tubule (MCT), and the inner medullary collecting duct (IMCD). The collecting duct is the final regulator of the excretion of many solutes. It finetunes the functions of the preceding segments. This is facilitated by the small volume that is delivered to it and by the operations of multiple cell types with specialized functions. In general, this segment determines the excretion of K^+ and acid and regulates the concentration of urine.

Heterogeneity of the collecting tubule

The collecting duct is the most heterogenous part of the nephron. This heterogeneity is both topographic (cortical, medullary, and inner medullary) and cellular (principal cells and two types of intercalated cell: α and β cells). In the CCT and MCT, 60% of cells are of the principal type with the balance being intercalated, whereas in the IMCD 99% of cells are of the principal type. The α intercalated cells are present thoughout the collecting duct, but β cells are present only in the CCT. This morphologic heterogeneity translates into functional differences between the different sections. Reabsorption of Na^+ and secretion of K^+ occurs predominantly in the CCT and IMCD. Secretion of H^+ (a function of α cells) occurs throughout the collecting duct, whereas HCO_3^- secretion (a function of β cells) is observed only in the CCT. The entire collecting duct has a low basal water permeability that is responsive to vasopressin.

Mechanisms of transport

Transport in the CCT is driven primarily by basolateral Na^+/K^+-ATPase. Entry of Na^+ occurs through amiloride-sensitive conductive channels at the luminal membrane. The reabsorption of Na^+ is mineralocorticoid sensitive and generates a negative voltage in the lumen that enhances K^+ exit (via K^+-conductive pathways in the luminal membrane) and H^+ secretion (via a proton-translocating ATPase located at the luminal membrane). Secretion of K^+ and H^+ in the CCT can be enhanced by increased Na^+ delivery and inhibited by blockade of Na^+ transport (Fig. 54.9). The MCT has no appreciable Na^+ transport and, therefore, its transport function is mostly related to H^+ secretion and water transport. The IMCD reabsorb NaCl through amiloride-sensitive conductive channels at the luminal membrane. The reabsorption of Na^+ is mineralocorticoid sensitive and is probably inhibited by atrial natriuretic factor.

The CCT is the major site of K^+ secretion in the nephron. Since most of the filtered K^+ is reabsorbed in proximal portions of the tubule, K^+ secretion in the CCT becomes the major determinant of external K^+ balance. The secretion of K^+ in this segment is achieved by a series of interlocked processes that can be best visualized by following their workings from the basolateral to the luminal membranes. Entry of K^+ at the basolateral membrane is achieved through Na^+/K^+-ATPase. This maintains a high intracellular level of K^+. Exit of K^+ at the luminal membrane occurs through K^+ channels and is dependent

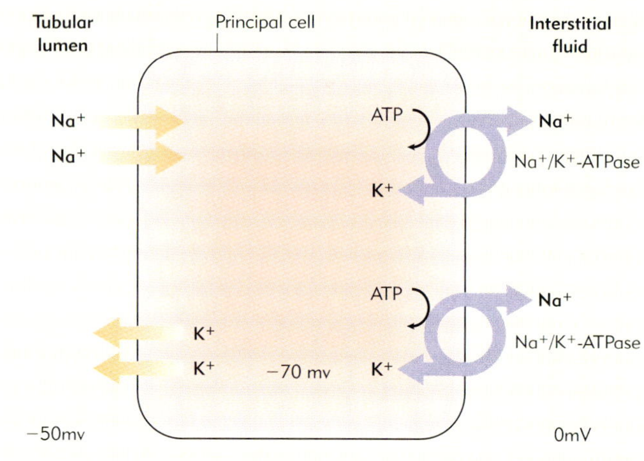

Figure 54.9 Cellular transport model for the cortical collecting tubule. The Na^+/K^+-ATPase maintains high intracellular K^+ and low intracellular Na^+, favoring their passive diffusion across the luminal membrane through specific channels.

on the luminal voltage charge and luminal flow. Luminal voltage is dependent on Na^+ reabsorption, which creates a negative charge. Consequently, enhanced K^+ excretion is dependent on increased activity of Na^+/K^+-ATPase, enhancement of K^+ channels, and increased luminal negativity. All of these changes occur when there is a need to excrete greater amounts of K^+. The increase in Na^+/K^+-ATPase in the CCT described above is the crucial mechanism of K^+ adaptation. This increase in enzyme activity is aldosterone dependent and does not develop if the levels of this hormone are prevented from rising.

Hormonal effects

Binding sites for aldosterone have been identified in the CCT and IMCD, and the direct effects of the hormone are generally restricted to these segments. At the level of the CCT, aldosterone has three major effects: it enhances Na^+ permeability of the luminal membrane by increasing the synthesis of Na^+ conductive pathways; it stimulates the basolateral Na^+/K^+-ATPase when administration of aldosterone is chronic; and it increases the production of ATP. All of these effects appear to be geared to optimize Na^+ transport in this segment. The net physiologic effect of aldosterone at this segment is to enhance Na^+ reabsorption. This leads to an increase in the lumen negative potential difference, which potentiates the secretion of K^+ and H^+. At the level of the IMCD, aldosterone leads to an enhancement of acidification that is Na^+ independent and may be facilitated chronically by stimulation of H^+-ATPase.

Approximately 85% of ingested K^+ is eliminated in the urine and the remainder is excreted in the stool. A number of factors have been shown to modify K^+ transport by the distal nephron, and these act in an integrated fashion to alter the rate of K^+ excretion. High plasma K^+ stimulates K^+ secretion by the distal nephron and low concentrations impair it. Secretion of K^+ by the CCT varies directly with the rate of fluid delivery to these sites. Vasopressin stimulates Na^+ reabsorption and K^+ secretion by both the DCT and the CCT. Aldosterone stimulates K^+

secretion by the CCT by altering the conductance of the apical membrane to both Na^+ and K^+ and by increasing the number of Na^+/K^+ pumps in the basolateral membrane. Increased excretion of poorly permeant anions such as sulfate is accompanied by kaliuresis. Acute acidosis inhibits K^+ secretion by the distal nephron and alkalosis stimulates it.

In response to persistent alterations in dietary K^+ intake, all the K^+ regulatory mechanisms are altered in a manner designed to maintain K^+ homeostasis. An increase in the renal capacity for K^+ secretion occurs following ingestion of a high-potassium diet. Full expression of the adaptive capacity for K^+ secretion is contingent upon the increase in aldosterone. The adapted kidney has from 10 to 20 times the K^+-secretory capacity of the kidney under conditions of a normal K^+ intake.

Acidification

Fluid delivered to the distal nephron is normally low in HCO_3^- (5–7mmol/L) and has a pH of 6.5 to 6.7. The distal nephron reabsorbs the remaining HCO_3^- and further lowers the luminal pH; this permits the titration of filtered buffers and traps ammonia. Acidity of the urine finally excreted depends largely on the distal secretory mechanism, which titrates the nonreabsorbed inorganic phosphate anions to a pH as low as 4.5. This process is limited by the availability of phosphate in the urine. The larger portion of the total acid excretion results, however, from titration of available ammonia to ammonium ion, a process that can be modulated more flexibly and is increased in the presence of acidosis. Acidification is enhanced in the presence of systemic acidosis, hypokalemia, and increased mineralocorticoid activity; it can be decreased by alkalosis, low mineralocorticoid activity, and reduced luminal buffer availability.

REGULATION OF URINE TONICITY

Formation of dilute urine

The tubular fluid presented to the loop of Henle is isosmotic with plasma, as water is reabsorbed passively down the osmotic gradient caused by active reabsorption of solute. In the thick ascending limb of the loop of Henle and the DCT, however, solute is still actively reabsorbed, but water does not follow because these segments are almost impermeable to water. The tubular fluid here is, therefore, hypotonic (see Fig. 54.8). In the absence of vasopressin, the final part of the DCT, the connecting tubule, and the collecting tubules are impermeable to water, and the tubular fluid remains hypotonic, producing a dilute urine.

Production of concentrated urine

The production of concentrated urine depends on the presence of long loops of Henle of the juxtamedullary nephrons passing through the increasingly hypertonic renal medulla (Fig. 54.10). The generation of the increasing solute concentration gradient through the medulla is dependent on the differential permeabilities to urea and NaCl of the thin ascending limb of the loop of Henle and the collecting tubule. Because of the low permeability to urea of the thin ascending limb of the loop of Henle, the tubular fluid presented to the collecting tubule has a high concentration of urea relative to interstitial fluid. The collecting tubule is permeable to urea, which passes out of the collecting tubule in its course through the medulla. This raises the osmolarity of the interstitium of the medulla, and hence water passes passively out of the descending limb of the loop of Henle. As fluid passes down the descending limb, less water passes from the tubule to the interstitium because the tubular fluid becomes progressively concentrated as the water leaves. This generates a concentration gradient down the medulla as the interstitial solutes become less diluted by water leaving the descending limb as it progresses from the outer to the inner medulla. When the tubular fluid reaches the thin ascending limb of the loop of Henle, which is permeable to NaCl, NaCl passes out of the tubule down its concentration gradient, which becomes progressively smaller from inner to outer medulla as the fluid ascends the loop of Henle. This differential reabsorption of NaCl up the ascending limb serves to increase the concentration gradient down the medulla, and hence the loop of Henle has been termed a countercurrent multiplier. In the presence of vasopressin, the collecting tubules are permeable to water. Water will, therefore, flow out of the tubules down the concentration gradient as they pass through the medulla, thus producing a concentrated urine.

Another countercurrent mechanism is crucial for the provision of blood supply to the medulla without destroying the concentration gradient necessary for the production of concentrated urine. The vasa recta are the peritubular capillaries that accompany the loops of Henle as they penetrate and then return through the medulla. The capillary loops of the vasa recta allow passive countercurrent exchange of solute and water between descending and ascending blood as it follows the hairpin course of the loops of Henle.

MEASUREMENT OF RENAL FUNCTION

The concept of renal clearance is a clinically valuable tool. Renal clearance is the volume of plasma completely cleared of a substance by the kidney per unit time (units are mL/min). The clearance of a substance can be calculated from the equation $C = UV/P$, where U and P are the concentrations of the substance in urine and plasma, respectively, and V is the rate at which urine is produced. For a substance that it is relatively filtered at the glomeruli and that is neither secreted nor absorbed by the renal tubules, the clearance will equal the GFR. Such a substance is inulin, which is a plant polysaccharide. An endogenous alternative to inulin is creatinine, a metabolite of muscle creatine. Creatinine is not reabsorbed or metabolized by the kidney and its rate of secretion by the tubules is clinically negligible. Clearance of these substances gives a measure of GFR. The renal plasma flow can be estimated from the renal clearance of a substance that is completely eliminated in its first pass through the kidney. This requires that the substance must be filtered at the glomeruli and secreted extremely efficiently by the tubules. *para*-Aminohippuric acid (PAH) meets these criteria. Like creatinine, it is an endogenous substance, being the end-product of metabolism of aromatic amino acids. Having calculated the renal plasma flow, the RBF can be calculated from the hematocrit. Another measure that is sometimes of interest is the *filtration fraction*, which is the ratio of the GFR to the renal plasma flow. The filtration fraction can be calculated from the creatinine and PAH clearances.

PRINCIPLES OF DIURETIC THERAPY

Sites and mechanisms of action of diuretics

The segment of the nephron affected by diuretics is determined by their specific mechanisms and the distribution of their target sites along the nephron (Fig. 54.11). For example,

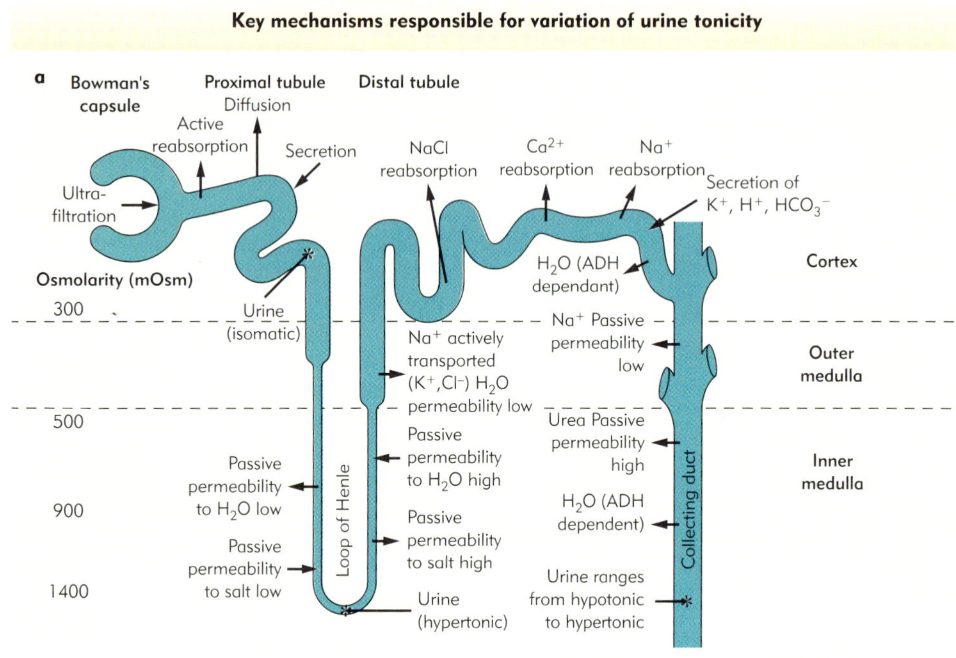

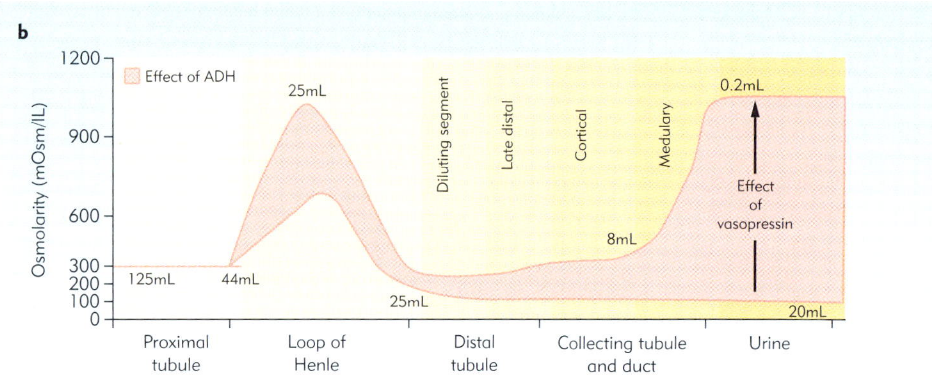

Figure 54.10 Key mechanisms responsible for variation of urine tonicity. Differences in permeability to NaCl, urea, and water in the loop of Henle and collecting duct (a) generate an increasing osmotic gradient from cortex to medulla and produce hypotonic urine in the distal convoluted tubule (b). In the presence of vasopressin, water is reabsorbed from the terminal distal convoluted tubule and collecting ducts, concentrating the urine. In the absence of vasopressin, the permeability of the distal convoluted tubule and collecting ducts to water is low and the urine remains hypotonic. Volumes indicate approximate flow through each tubular segment (in mL/min). (ADH, antidiuretic hormone.)

the site of action of carbonic anhydrase inhibitors is dependent on the distribution of the enzyme along the nephron and the role played by the enzyme in Na^+ transport. Similarly, the site of action of diuretics that inhibit the $Na^+/K^+/2Cl^-$ co-transporter is the segment where this transporter is localized, namely the luminal membrane of the thick ascending limb of Henle's loop. The sites of action of diuretics also determine the degree of natriuresis achieved and the compensatory responses. Thiazides, for example, act at a segment where only 8% of the filtered load of Na^+ is reabsorbed. The resultant diuresis is decidedly modest.

Loop diuretics [furosemide (frusemide), ethacrynic acid, piretanide and bumetanide] inhibit NaCl transport in the thick ascending limb of the loop of Henle by binding specifically and reversibly to the Cl^--binding site of the luminal transporter responsible for the coupled entry of $Na^+/K^+/Cl^-$. The primary site of action of thiazides is in the DCT, where they inhibit Na^+/Cl^- co-transport. Amiloride and triamterene block Na^+ channels in the CCT. The resulting decrease in Na^+ reabsorption reduces the transepithelial electrical potential, the factor that normally favors K^+ secretion. This is the basis for the K^+-sparing effect of these drugs.

Access to the site of action

With the exception of carbonic anhydrase inhibitors and aldosterone antagonists, the major diuretics act from the tubular lumen directly to inhibit transport mechanisms in the luminal membrane. Depending on the degree of protein binding, some diuretics will reach the lumen by glomerular filtration. Since only the unbound fraction is freely filterable, only a small percentage of highly protein-bound diuretics will reach the tubular lumen through filtration. More important, by virtue of their chemical nature, many diuretics are secreted into the lumen by either the organic acid or organic base transport system of the PCT. This mode of entry to the lumen is also affected to a certain degree by protein binding. There is an inverse interplay between the effect of protein binding and the affinity of the tubular transporter for the diuretic. The affinity of the transporter for thiazides is very high and the excretion of the diuretic cannot be increased by a change in protein binding. In contrast to glomerular filtration, renal tubular secretion is a saturable process. Consequently, tubular secretion of a diuretic can be reduced by competitive inhibition from endogenous (as in renal failure) or exogenous (other drugs) organic acids.

Diuretic family	Target	Nephron segment
Osmotic	Filtration	Glomerulus
Carbonic anhydrase inhibitors	Luminal carbonic anhydrase	Proximal convoluted tubule
Loop diuretics	$Na^+/K^+/2Cl^-$ co-transporter	Thick ascending limb
Thiazides	Na^+/Cl^- co-transporter	Distal convoluted tubule
Spironolactone	Aldosterone receptors	Cortical collecting tubule
K^+-sparing diuretics	Na^+ channel	Cortical collecting tubule
Vasopressin inhibitors	Vasopressin receptors	Distal convoluted tubule, collecting tubule and duct

Sites of action of various diuretic families

Figure 54.11 Sites of action of various types of diuretic.

Factors that modify diuresis

Several factors can modify the therapeutic response expected from the administration of a diuretic. First, inhibition of solute transport in one portion of the nephron can be nullified by compensatory changes in transport by other nephron segments. Second, delivery of an inadequate quantity of the drug to its site of action can modify the expected effect of a diuretic. Third, attainment of an appreciable diuretic response requires adequate delivery of solute and fluid to the tubule. If renal perfusion or glomerular filtration is compromised, the degree of diuresis will be markedly blunted.

Renal compensatory responses to diuretics

Drug-induced diuresis is inherently self-limited. Intrarenal adjustments to the reduction in ECF volume occur to prevent the development of severe depletion. Solute and water reabsorption increase in segments of the nephron not altered pharmacologically. This enhancement in reabsorption can occur in unaltered segments either proximal or distal to the site of action of the drug. In the case of proximally acting diuretics, the increase in salt delivery is met very proficiently by the ascending limb of Henle to obliterate the diuretic response almost completely. A notable conserving mechanism that operates with many diuretics is secondary hyperaldosteronism, which increases Na^+ reabsorption in the collecting tubule. The intra- and extrarenal adjustments made in response to the action of diuretics slow down the urinary excretion of salt and water. This phenomenon has been labeled the 'braking phenomenon' and may be the converse of the 'escape phenomenon' observed with mineralocorticoid excess. This is a conceptually and practically very appealing concept that describes the occurrence of a new steady state at a new level of total body sodium. The mechanism for 'braking' varies with different diuretics depending on their site of action. For proximal diuretics, it is mediated by enhanced reabsorption in the loop and the distal segments. For loop diuretics, the braking is brought about by enhanced reabsorption in the PCT secondary to decreased GFR and renal plasma flow and by increased distal mineralocorticoid effect.

Combined diuretic therapy

The segmental localization of the effects of diuretics endows each agent with particular properties and side effects. It may also limit the effectiveness of a diuretic in altering Na^+ balance. It has already been noted how a proximal inhibition of Na^+ transport can be compensated by reabsorption downstream. The segmental peculiarity of diuretic effects can, however, be utilized to enhance natriuresis by combining diuretics that work at different sites. A popular form of this combination therapy is that of using loop agents and thiazides or thiazide-like drugs. This combination prevents the compensatory distal increases in Na^+ reabsorption that limit the effectiveness of loop agents. The overall result can be a profound diuretic effect that is greater than that achieved with either agent alone. By enhancing diuresis, this form of therapy also increases the side effects of diuretic therapy and can lead to volume depletion, severe hypokalemia, and metabolic alkalosis. Careful monitoring and judicious dose adjustment are required to avoid serious complications.

Combination therapy can also be used to limit the kaliuretic effects of diuretics. A major mechanism of K^+ wasting with diuretic therapy is enhanced K^+ secretion by the CCT. This occurs through the interplay of increased Na^+ delivery to this segment, increased Na^+ reabsorption, and increased circulating levels of aldosterone. Addition of a Na^+ channel blocker to a diuretic regimen will block Na^+ reabsorption and hence decrease the secretion of K^+. Similarly, addition of an aldosterone antagonist will block the effect of the hormone at this segment and reduce the kaliuresis. These combinations are very useful in clinical practice and are commonly available in fixed dosage forms.

Resistance to diuretics

The list of clinical conditions in which resistance to diuretics has been described is similar to a list of the most common indications for the use of diuretics. This paradox invites examination of the concept of resistance to diuretics and elucidation of the factors responsible for true resistance and those leading to pseudoresistance. True resistance to diuretics can be defined as a state where administration of a diuretic in proper dosage and with proper attention to pharmacokinetic principles fails to elicit the expected diuretic response in a patient who has a condition usually responsive to this form of therapy. Such a true resistance is fortunately rare and the vast majority of patients who have 'resistance' to diuretics have a pseudoresistance. Clinically, however, uncovering the causes of pseudoresistance can be a challenging undertaking for the physician. The approach to resistance to diuretics resides in posing the question: 'Is it the patient, the physician, or the kidney that is resistant to diuretic therapy?'.

The most common patient-related resistance factors are noncompliance and excessive salt intake. The former is the most common form of pseudoresistance to all known drugs and therapies. The latter is of particular importance in diuretic therapy because the effectiveness of these drugs can be blunted by high salt intake and the severity of their side effects, particularly hypokalemia, can be worsened.

Physician-related resistance factors include use of inappropriate dosage forms or the simultaneous prescription of drugs that blunt the diuretic effect. An example of the former is the use of hydrochlorothiazide alone in a patient who has a GFR below 30mL/min. An example of the latter is simultaneous prescription of furosemide and a nonsteroidal anti-inflammatory drug for an elderly patient who has congestive heart failure and low back pain.

Kidney-related resistance can be divided into two categories: impaired access of the diuretic to its site of action (pharmacokinetic resistance) and blunted organ responsiveness to the diuretic (pharmacodynamic resistance). The factors affecting access of a diuretic to its site of action have been described above. An important issue relates to the quantitative aspects of diuretic access. The degree of diuresis elicited by a diuretic agent is determined by the amount of drug reaching the site of action. Of equal importance is the time course of that delivery to the site of action. Attention to pharmacokinetic principles is clearly of great importance in dissecting the cause of diuretic resistance. Disease states requiring diuretic therapy often lead to modification of drug access to tubular sites of action and of the quantitative aspects of this delivery. Diuretic resistance can be encountered in azotemia because endogenous organic acids compete with diuretics for the active secretory mechanisms in the PCT and larger doses of diuretics are required to achieve a response. In other disease states, the dose–response relationship may be altered because the disease may induce altered transport characteristics in the kidney that thwart the effect of diuretics: decreased solute delivery to the site of diuretic action by reduction of GFR or enhanced reabsorption by segments proximal to that site or distal to it. Finally, intestinal absorption of diuretics may be impaired in severely edematous patients.

An attempt to define the mechanism of resistance to a diuretic should be undertaken before changes in therapy are made. Correcting patient noncompliance, dietary indiscretion, or dose to be administered will solve many cases of pseudoresistance. Attention to drug interference will further reduce the number of cases. When resistance is still encountered, the approach should be to determine first whether adequate amounts of the drug are reaching the target organ. This can be done empirically by attempting gradual increases in dose until a satisfactory response is achieved, or a ceiling dose is reached. This, however, carries a risk of drug toxicity and should be attempted with caution if one is contemplating using large doses of toxic drugs. Alternatively, one can measure drug concentrations in the urine and assess whether adequate amounts are reaching the site of action. This avoids potential toxicity from unnecessarily increasing the dose. If it is determined that adequate amounts of drug are available, then the next step is to determine which disease mechanism is responsible for the blunted diuresis. If hyperaldosteronism is present, then use of aldosterone antagonists or Na^+ channel blockers can be successful. In some cases, modifying the disease-related renal changes will improve the response to diuretics. Use of dopamine, for example, will increase RBF and GFR and restore some of the response to diuretics in patients who have liver cirrhosis and ascites.

Diuretic therapy for most patients should be carried out in a deliberate manner with individualization of care. Such individualization should allow proper consideration of the condition being treated, the goal to be achieved, and the proper means to achieve it.

RENAL EFFECTS OF ANESTHETICS

In the clinical setting, there is a complex interplay of direct and indirect effects of anesthetics at the renal and extrarenal levels. The resultant picture is a composite of the effects on the organ and on the host. Some of the evidence is conflicting; this is likely to reflect the use of different species and models for experiments.

Transport effects of anesthetics

In vitro studies indicate direct effects of anesthetics leading to inhibition of Na^+ and organic anion transport. The effect on Na^+ transport appears to be mediated through inhibition of the Na^+/K^+-ATPase. There is a little effect on water transport.

Changes secondary to cardiac output and regional blood flow charges

Changes in renal hemodynamics may, in part, be the consequence of generalized circulatory effects of anesthetics. Anesthetics cause a redistribution of cardiac output to different organs, with an increased proportion going to the brain and reduced fractions to the myocardium, the splanchnic bed, and skeletal muscle.

Renal function

Most inhalational anesthetics do not appear to lower RBF whereas most barbiturates cause a decrease. Glomerular filtration rate is decreased by all anesthetics, as is the ability of the kidney to excrete a Na^+ load. Many factors can be invoked in these renal changes: reduction in blood pressure and cardiac output, increased sympathetic outflow by the renal nerves, stimulation of the renin–angiotensin system, augmented vasopressin release, and direct renal effects of anesthetics. The relative contribution of each of these factors depends on the physiologic state of the organism and the anesthetic used.

Key References

Berne RM, Levy MN. Principles of physiology. St Louis, MO: Mosby; 1990:416–76.

Jackson EK. Diuretics In: Goodman and Gilman's The Pharmacological Basis of Therapeutics, 9th edn. New York: McGraw-Hill; 1996:685–713.

Chapter 55 Regulation of blood volume and electrolytes

Abhiram Mallick and Andrew R Bodenham

Topics covered in this chapter

Body fluid compartments
Regulation of extracellular fluid volume and blood volume
Measurement of fluid compartments
Disturbances of volume
Assessment and monitoring of fluid status
Maintenance of fluid requirements
Electrolytes

Regulation of the composition and volume of body fluids is fundamental to physiology. Disturbances or adaptation of normal mechanisms are commonly seen in disease or under conditions of physiologic stress. A basic understanding of the body fluids is fundamental to the correct management of patients undergoing surgery or requiring intensive care. In clinical practice, it is impossible to separate the management of fluids from the individual electrolyte disorders, but for the purpose of learning it is convenient to do so.

BODY FLUID COMPARTMENTS

There are three principal body fluid compartments (Fig. 55.1): *intracellular fluid* (ICF), *interstitial fluid* (ISF), and *intravascular fluid* (IVF) or circulating blood volume. The volume of each compartment is determined by the quantities, concentrations, and movements between compartments of water, plasma proteins, and electrolytes, especially Na^+. Total body water (TBW), the distribution volume of Na^+-free water, approximates 60% of total body weight (i.e. 42L in a 70kg person). Intracellular fluid constitutes two thirds of TBW (28L) and ISF, the compartment between the capillaries and cells, constitutes approximately 11L. Intravascular fluid (IVF), or blood volume, is approximately 5L, of which 3L is plasma volume (PV) and 2L is red cell volume. Although intravascular, the red cell volume is technically a part of the ICF. *Extracellular fluid* (ECF) includes both ISF and PV and, therefore, comprises a third of TBW (14L). Sodium balance primarily regulates ECF volume, whereas water balance regulates the ICF volume. Women and obese individuals have reduced ECF volume. In infants and young children, TBW is 80% of the body weight, of which ECF volume is up to 40%, almost half of the TBW.

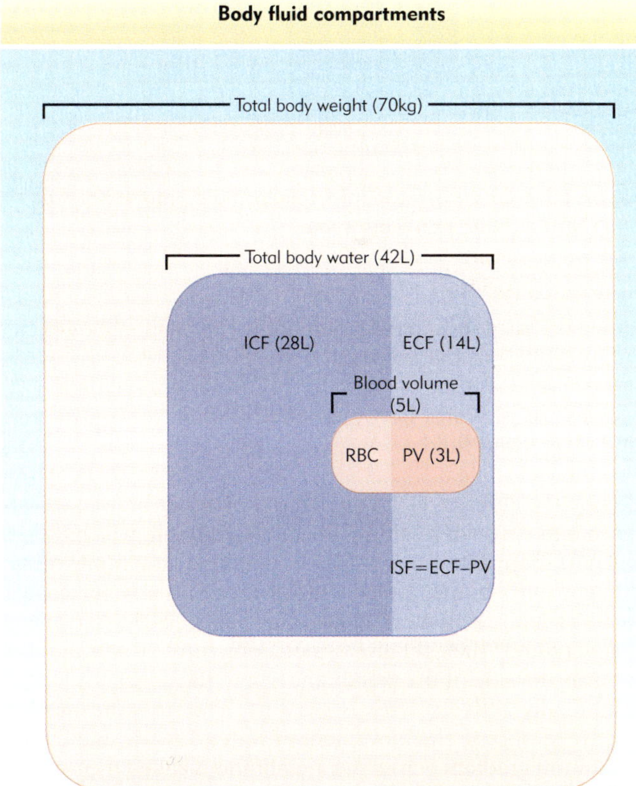

Figure 55.1 Schematic diagram of body fluid compartments. The interstitial fluid (ISF) volume is calculated as the difference between the extracellular fluid volume(ECF) and the plasma volume (PV).

Composition of fluid compartments

Electrolyte and protein concentrations differ markedly in the fluid compartments (Fig. 55.2). The composition of ICF varies somewhat depending on the nature and the function of the cell. The primary determinant of tonicity and osmolality is Na^+, which is distributed predominantly in the ECF with nearly equal concentrations in both ISF and PV, while the ICF contains virtually no Na^+. The plasma proteins, albumin and gamma globulins, determine the plasma colloid oncotic pressure, which in turn maintains adequate PV. There are other osmotically active constituents such as urea but they are equally distributed throughout the TBW. Albumin does not pass easily across the capillaries into the ISF despite a significant concentration gradient because of its large size compared with electrolytes. It is highly concentrated within the circulating blood volume. The protein gradient between IVF

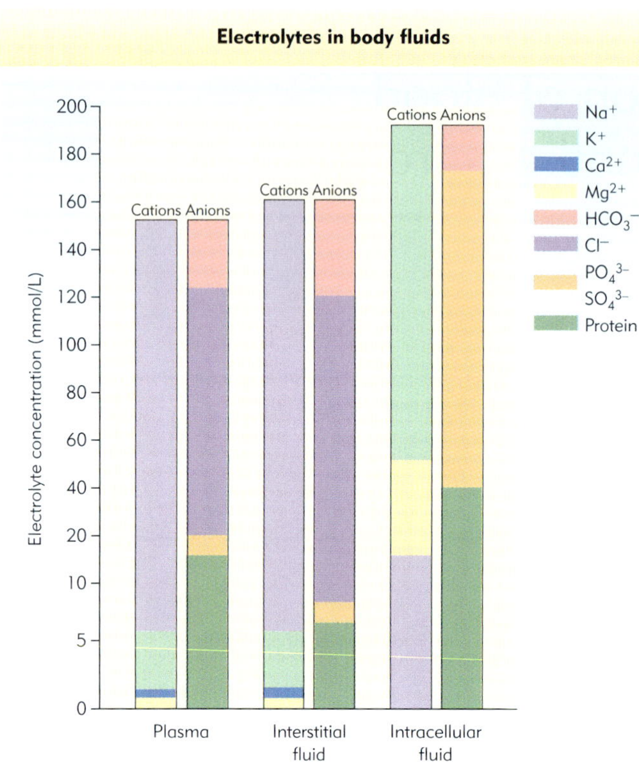

Figure 55.2 Electrolytes in intracellular fluid, interstitial fluid, and plasma. Note nonlinear scale.

and ISF is responsible for maintaining the proportions of circulating PV and ISF volume.

Movement of water between intracellular and interstitial fluid

Osmosis

Osmosis is defined as the movement of water between compartments through a semipermeable membrane which occurs when the concentrations of solutes on either side of the membrane are not equal. The cell membrane is freely permeable to water and the movement of water between compartments is governed by their relative osmotic pressures. Water diffuses towards the side of the membrane where the concentration of osmotically active solutes is greatest. The pressure needed exactly to oppose the movement of water down a solute concentration gradient across the membrane is called the *osmotic pressure*. Each molecule dissolved in water causes osmosis of water directly proportional to the concentration of that molecule. The osmotic pressure is proportional to the number of molecules, and not to their molecular weight.

Osmolarity and osmolality

The osmolarity of a solution quantitates the forces determining the distribution of water and refers to the number of osmotically active particles per liter of solution. In contrast, osmolality is a measurement of the number of osmotically active particles per kilogram of solvent. Therefore, the osmolarity is affected by the volume of the solution and temperature, whereas osmolality is not. Osmotically active solutes depress the freezing point of fluids. The freezing point of normal human plasma is about −0.54°C, which corresponds to an osmolality of 290mosmol/L. All the body fluid compartments have the same osmolality as plasma and hence they are in equilibrium. The osmolality of plasma can be calculated approximately according to the following formula.

Equation 55.1

$$\text{Osmolality} = (\text{Serum Na}^{+} \times 2) + \text{blood glucose} + \text{blood urea}$$
(mosmol/kg)

where Na^+, glucose and urea are expressed in mmol/L. Sugars, alcohols, and radiographic dyes may increase the osmolality but falsely lower the calculated value, generating an increased osmolal gap between the calculated and measured values. A hyperosmolar state occurs when the concentration of osmotically active particles is high. For example, uremia [increased blood urea nitrogen (BUN)], hyperglycemia, and hypernatremia increase serum osmolality.

Tonicity

Tonicity is a term used to describe the osmolality of a solution relative to plasma. Solutions that have the same osmolality as plasma are said to be isotonic; those with greater osmolality are hypertonic, and those with lesser osmolality are hypotonic. All solutions that are initially iso-osmotic with plasma would remain isotonic if it were not for the fact that some solutes diffuse into cells and others are metabolized. Thus, a 0.9% saline solution remains isotonic because there is no net movement of osmotically active particles into the cells. By comparison, a 5% dextrose solution is isotonic when initially infused but as dextrose is metabolized the net longer-term effect is that of infusing a hypotonic solution.

Movement of water between plasma and interstitial fluid

Colloid oncotic pressure

The capillary endothelium has pore sizes of 6.5nm and is freely permeable to small molecules and electrolytes but not to large protein molecules. Plasma proteins, especially albumin, are largely confined to the IVF and exert a colloid osmotic pressure (COP) of about 25mmHg or 1.2mosmol/kg. Fluid filtration across the capillary membrane as a result of the hydrostatic pressure in the vascular system is opposed by the plasma COP.

Starling forces

It is at the capillary level that fluid interchange between the IVF and the ISF takes place. The major determinants of fluid movement are the so-called Starling forces (Fig. 55.3). The net fluid movement is proportional to the difference between the hydrostatic pressure gradient and the osmotic pressure gradient across the capillary wall.

The reflection coefficient (σ) indicates the capillary permeability to albumin with a value of zero representing free permeability and a value of 1 complete impermeability. The reflection coefficient for albumin ranges normally from 0.6 to 0.9 in various capillary beds. As a result, fluid moves into the tissues whenever the hydrostatic gradient increases or when the osmotic gradient decreases. If COP is reduced, fluid accumulates in the ISF, and if the lymphatic clearance is exceeded, edema develops. The effects of Starling forces can be seen during surgery: the face and eyes of patients placed in the head-down position for long periods become edematous [i.e. through increase in capillary hydrostatic pressure (P_c)], while more generalized edema is common in patients given large volumes of crystalloid [low plasma COP

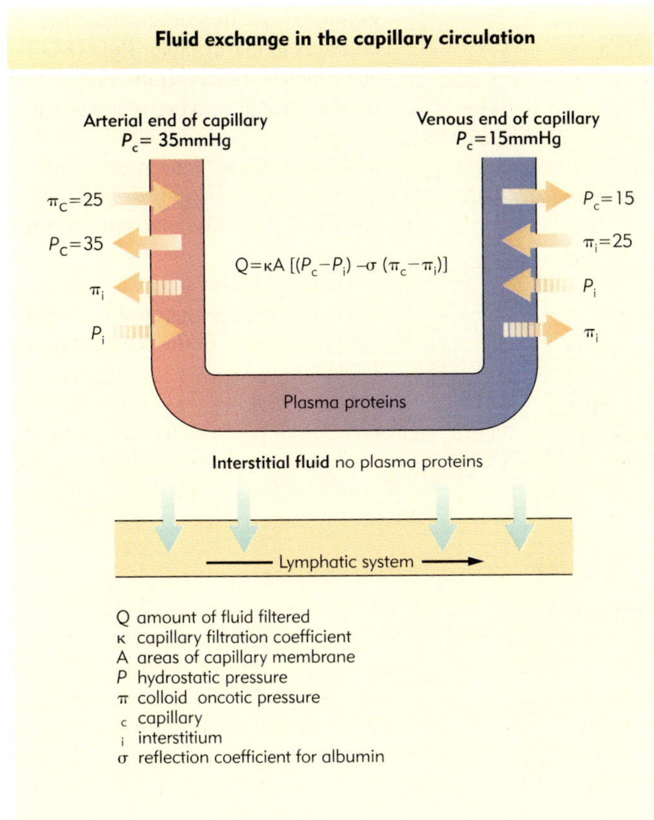

Figure 55.3 Fluid exchange in the capillary circulation. A schematic representation of the Starling forces.

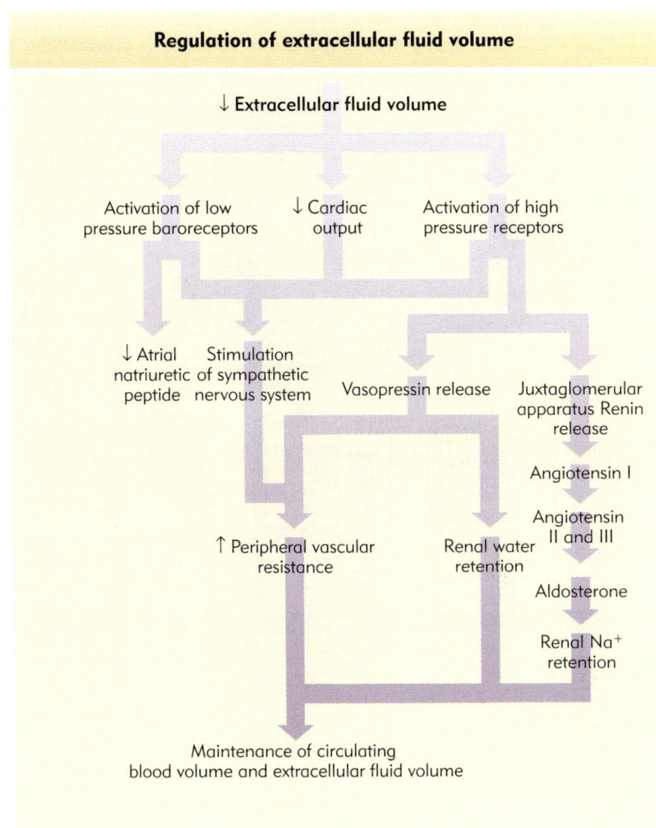

Figure 55.4 Regulation of extracellular fluid volume.

(π_c)]. The value of π_c is equal at arterial and venous ends of the capillary bed while the P_c results in fluid being forced out of the arterial end of the capillary and reabsorbed in the venous end. Overall there is a net efflux of fluid out of capillaries into the ISF, which is removed by the lymphatic circulation.

The ISF volume is determined by capillary filtration and lymphatic drainage (approximately 2L/day); homeostatic mechanisms accommodate only a limited amount of excess fluid. The P_c, the most powerful factor favoring fluid filtration, is determined by capillary flow, arteriolar resistance, venous resistance, and venous pressure. Increased capillary filtration can alter the balance of Starling forces at equilibrium. When coupled with increased lymphatic drainage, preservation of the oncotic pressure gradient limits accumulation of ISF. As increasing ISF volume results in decreasing concentration of proteoglycans and glycosaminoglycans, fluid drains more freely into the lymphatics. If P_c is increased when lymphatic drainage is maximal, edema is formed.

REGULATION OF EXTRACELLULAR FLUID VOLUME AND BLOOD VOLUME

The composition and volume of each fluid compartment are controlled through complex mechanisms that include reflexes mediated by the sympathetic nervous system (Chapter 29), renal mechanisms (Chapter 54), and humoral factors such as vasopressin [antidiuretic hormone (ADH)], natriuretic peptides, and the renin–angiotensin–aldosterone axis (Fig. 55.4).

Circulating blood volume is maintained by renal mechanisms that modulate renal blood flow, glomerular fltration, and tubular reabsorption of Na^+ and water. The integrated responses to increased and decreased ECF volume are summarized in Figure 55.5.

Renin–angiotensin–aldosterone axis

Renin is a protease released from the juxtaglomerular apparatus of the kidney in response to renal hypoperfusion caused by hypovolemia or hypotension (Chapter 54). Renin catalyzes the conversion of angiotensinogen to angiotensin I. The angiotensin-converting enzyme in pulmonary capillaries converts angiotensin I to angiotensin II. Angiotensin II is destroyed rapidly (half-life 1–2 minutes). The development of highly selective angiotensin II receptor ligands allowed the identification of angiotensin II receptor subtypes, designated AT_1, AT_2, AT_3, and AT_4. Most of the known effects of angiotensin II, including vasoconstriction and aldosterone and vasopressin release, can be attributed to the AT_1 receptor. The AT_1 receptor is coupled to a G protein that activates phospholipase C or inhibits adenylyl cyclase. Angiotensin II is a potent vasoconstrictor that produces a rise in systolic and diastolic pressure. Angiotensin III, a metabolite of angiotensin II, also acts directly on the adrenal cortex to increase the secretion of aldosterone.

Regulation of Na^+ reabsorption is mainly achieved in the distal nephron by the mineralocorticoid aldosterone; high concentrations of aldosterone may reduce urinary Na^+ excretion nearly to zero. Aldosterone is the most important hormonal regulator of total extracellular Na^+ and, therefore, of ECF volume. Aldosterone is a steroid hormone that acts primarily in renal collecting ducts to stimulate reabsorption of Na^+ and secretion of

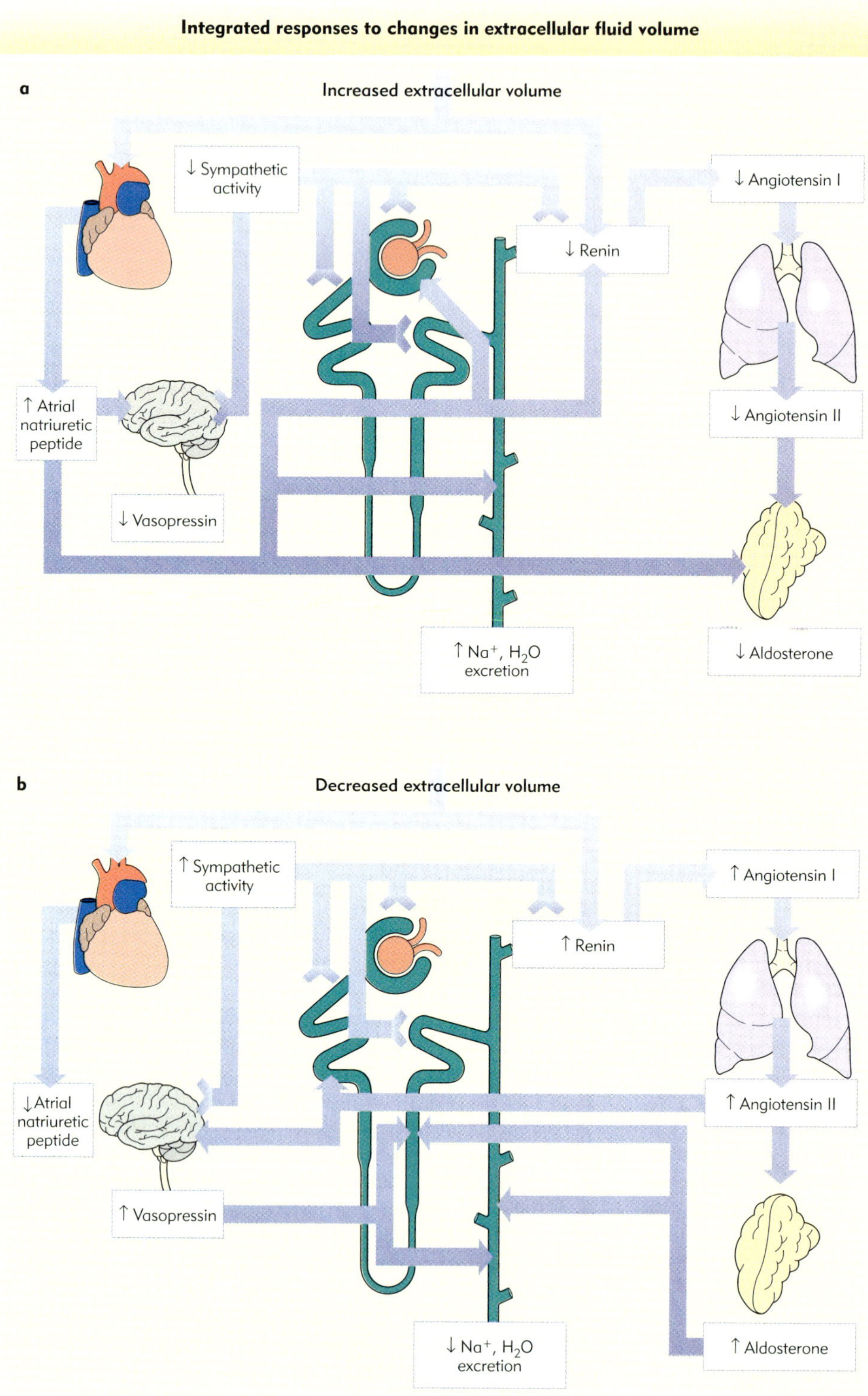

Figure 55.5 Integrated responses to changes in extracellular fluid (ECF) volume. The renal responses to increased ECF volume (a) include an increase in glomerular filtration rate and reduced Na^+ reabsorption in the proximal tubule, loop of Henle, and collecting duct. The mechanisms for reduced Na^+ and water excretion in response to decreased ECF volume are essentially the opposite (b). (With permission from Berne and Levy, 1990.)

K^+ and H^+ (Chapter 54). It binds with intracellular receptors in the nucleus that stimulate the expression of several genes that modulate the activity of ionic transport systems located in the apical and basolateral membranes of target epithelial cells.

Vasopressin

Osmoreceptors are located on the wall of the third ventricle in the hypothalamus. A rise in osmolality as small as 1–2% is sensed by osmoreceptors, which stimulate vasopressin release from the posterior pituitary. Acute arterial hypotension and hypovolemia (a 10% decrease in blood volume) increase vasopressin secretion. Vasopressin directly stimulates constriction of both veins and arteries, thereby increasing total peripheral resistance, right heart filling pressure, and cardiac output. To preserve PV, vasopressin acts primarily on the collecting ducts to increase water permeability, apparently by increasing the expression of water channels (aquaporins); this results in greater water reabsorbtion and excretion of small volumes of highly concentrated urine. The importance of vasopressin is seen when the pituitary or hypothalamus is damaged, leading to failure to secrete vasopressin. Diabetes insipidus follows, with excretion of up to 20L of dilute urine daily. Both aldosterone and vasopressin levels can increase during anesthesia and surgery independent of blood volume, which reduces the usefulness of urine flow as an indicator of volume status and renal perfusion.

Natriuretic peptides

Natriuretic peptides act as endocrine and paracrine hormones to regulate ECF volume and blood pressure at all levels of the circulation. Although the importance of natriuretic peptides is still being assessed, animal studies strongly support an important role for these hormones in body fluid homeostasis.

Atrial natriuretic peptide

Atrial natriuretic peptide (ANP) is a polypeptide hormone of 28 amino acid residues secreted mainly by the cardiac myocytes in response to atrial stretch. It also appears to be present in neurons in hypothalamic and brain stem areas involved in regulation of body fluid volume and blood pressure. Most, if not all, actions of ANP are mediated by activation of particulate guanylyl cyclase with generation of cyclic guanosine monophosphate (cGMP), which mediates its actions in the brain and in periphery. Atrial natriuretic peptide acts on renal tubules to increase Na^+ excretion and glomerular filtration rate, to antagonize renal vasoconstriction, and to inhibit renin secretion. In the adrenal gland, ANP release is a powerful inhibitor of aldosterone synthesis. In the cardiovascular system, ANP induces vasodilatation and shifts fluid from the IVF to the ISF compartment to buffer against excessive PV expansion in the face of an increased total ECF volume. Furthermore, ANP neurons inhibit vasopressin release, leading to a diuresis.

Brain natriuretic peptide

Brain natriuretic peptide (BNP) was initially thought to be released from the brain, hence its name. It is primarily a cardiac hormone in humans. It is synthesized and released into the circulation by the left ventricle in response to increased cardiac volume or arterial pressure. It has a spectrum of activities similar to those of ANP, including diuretic, natriuretic, hypotensive, and smooth muscle relaxant properties. It also inhibits renin and aldosterone release. It appears to be a part of the central mechanism for control of blood volume, blood pressure, and electrolyte and body fluid homeostasis. Brain natriuretic peptide also appears to be responsible for salt wasting and hyponatremia in patients who have subarachnoid hemorrhage.

MEASUREMENT OF FLUID COMPARTMENTS

It is possible to measure the size of the body fluid compartments by injecting a known quantity of substance that will stay in only one compartment. Measurement of its concentration in the compartment allows its volume of distribution to be calculated. This volume is equal to the amount of substance injected (minus any that has been metabolized or excreted during the time allowed for mixing) divided by the concentration of the substance in the sample. Although the principle appears simple, there are a number of factors that must be considered: the material injected must be nontoxic, it must mix evenly throughout the compartment being measured, it should remain unchanged in the body during the mixing period, and its concentration should be relatively easy to measure. Such techniques are used as research tools but are too cumbersome for use in clinical practice.

Blood volume

Plasma volume can be measured by using dyes that bind to plasma proteins, such as Evans blue, or by injecting serum albumin labeled with radioactive iodine. The average PV in a normal 70kg adult is approximately 3.5L (50–55mL/kg). If the PV and hematocrit are known, the total blood (intravascular) volume can be calculated as PV/(1 – hematocrit). Total blood volume is approximately 70–80mL/kg in adults. Infants by the age of 1 year have a blood volume of 85–90mL/kg. The blood volume of a neonate is relatively more: 95–105mL/kg depending on whether the cord is clamped late or early. The red cell volume can be measured by injecting labeled red cells and, after mixing has occurred, measuring the fraction of the red cells that are labeled. A commonly used label for red cells is chromium-51.

Extracellular volume

Extracellular fluid volume is difficult to measure because the limits of this space are ill defined and few substances mix rapidly in all parts of the space while remaining exclusively extracellular. The lymphatic system cannot be separated from the ECF and is measured with it. Many substances enter the cerebrospinal fluid slowly because of the blood–brain barrier. The equilibration is slow with joint fluid, aqueous humor, and in relatively avascular tissues such as dense connective tissue, cartilage, and bone. Substances that distribute in ECF appear in glandular secretions and in the contents of the gastrointestinal tract. As they are separated from the rest of the ECF, these fluids are called transcellular fluids. However, their volume is relatively small compared with the total volume of the ECF.

The most accurate measurement of ECF volume is obtained by using [^{14}C]inulin, a plant polysaccharide. Mannitol and sucrose have also been used for measuring ECF volume. A generally accepted value for ECF volume is about one third of TBW (i.e. 14L in a 70kg person).

Interstitial volume

The ISF volume cannot be measured directly because it is difficult to sample ISF and substances that equilibrate in it also equilibrate in plasma. Its volume can be calculated by subtracting the PV from the total ECF volume.

Intracellular volume

The ICF cannot be measured directly but can be calculated by subtracting the ECF volume from the TBW. Total body water is measured by the dilution technique used to measure the other fluid compartments. Deuterium oxide (D_2O, heavy water) is most frequently used. Tritium oxide and aminopyrine can also been used for this purpose.

DISTURBANCES OF VOLUME

Hypovolemia

Hypovolemia is defined as a depletion of effective circulating volume. It results either from losses from the body, absolute hypovolemia, or from sequestration of fluid within the body, relative hypovolemia (Fig. 55.6). The effective circulating volume may be

Causes of hypovolemia	
Absolute hypovolemia: fluids leave body	
Gastrointestinal	Bleeding
	Vomiting
	Diarrhea
	Fistula
	Tube drainage
Renal	Diuresis
	Osmotic diuresis
	Diabetes insipidus
Skin	Burns
	Large exudative lesions
Trauma	Fracture long bones
	Ruptured spleen
	Hemothorax
Surgical	Blood loss
Relative hypovolemia: fluids redistribute within body	
Internal fluid shift	Third space loss
	Nephrotic syndrome
	Cirrhosis
Capillary leak	Anaphylaxis
	Sepsis or sepsis syndrome
Sequestration	Intestinal obstruction
	Peritonitis

Figure 55.6 Causes of hypovolemia.

low in the presence of expanded ECF volume in many conditions such as sepsis or sepsis syndrome, liver disease, and anaphylaxis. Absolute or relative hypovolemia can be accentuated during anesthesia because sympathetic reflexes are blunted. Anesthetic drugs themselves, including volatile and intravenous agents, may contribute to relative hypovolemia by causing further vasodilatation. Spinal and epidural anesthesia produce relative hypovolemia by blocking efferent sympathetic vasomotor signals.

Edema

Edema, a clinical sign of accumulation of fluid within body tissues, manifests as subcutaneous edema or pulmonary edema. It can occur with fluid overload, decreased fluid excretion (as in renal failure), and expansion of the ISF owing to increased capillary permeability and/or reduced plasma COP. Retention of salt and water by the kidneys in response to body regulatory mechanisms contributes to edema seen in chronic conditions such as congestive heart failure and liver disease. Consideration of the variables of the Starling equation (Fig. 55.3) allows the mechanisms of edema formation to be characterized as related to hydrostatic pressure, to increased capillary permeability, or to lowered COP (Fig. 55.7). In clinical practice, more than one of the mechanisms may operate at the same time.

Hypoalbuminemia

Albumin is a naturally occurring plasma protein with a molecular weight of 69,000 and a degradation half-life of about 18

Causes of edema	
Hydrostatic pressure effect	Fluid overload, cardiac failure, neurogenic pulmonary edema, loss of autoregulation, renal failure
Reduced oncotic pressure (low albumin)	Malnutrition, critical illness, pre-eclampsia, nephrotic syndrome, cirrhosis
Increased capillary permeability	Acute lung injury, brain injury, sepsis or sepsis syndrome, burns, reperfusion injury

Figure 55.7 Causes of edema.

days. Hepatocytes synthesize albumin at a rate of 9–12g/day to maintain a normal plasma concentration of 40g/L. Albumin accounts for 60–80% of plasma COP. The albumin concentration of the ISF is variable depending on the capillary permeability. Albumin from the ISF returns to the circulation via lympatic vessels.

Marked alterations of the concentrations of albumin can occur after major surgery, trauma, burns, and in septic states as a consequence of losses or leakage secondary to increased capillary permeability. Preoperative hypoalbuminemia is a marker of malnutrition or liver disease. Dilutional hypoalbuminemia is frequently secondary to the administration of fluids. Renal loss of albumin is significant in pregnancy-induced hypertension and nephrotic syndrome. In most patients, low albumin levels should be considered as a marker of disease severity rather than as a pathology in its own right.

The threshold for replacing albumin losses is contentious. Most clinicians administer albumin when the serum concentration is less than 20g/L or when there are continuing losses. Low serum albumin is a common finding in critically ill patients. Exogenous albumin administration does not confer any clinical benefit in terms of morbidity and mortality. The lack of benefit appears to be the result of continued extravascular leak of albumin.

ASSESSMENT AND MONITORING OF FLUID STATUS

The gold standard for the diagnosis of hypovolemia is the measurement of blood volume. Surrogate markers of IVF volume are usually used for clinical assessment as labeled red cell dilution techniques are impractical.

Clinical assessment

Conventional clinical assessment and laboratory findings of fluid status can help to identify hypovolemia and hypervolemia. Physical examination includes assessment of skin turgor, urine output, heart rate, and blood pressure. The physical signs of hypovolemia such as oliguria, supine hypotension, and tachycardia are nonspecific and insensitive. Oliguria suggests the presence of hypovolemia, although hypovolemic patients may have urine output within normal limits. Similarly, normovolemic patients may be oliguric because of renal failure or stress-induced endocrine responses. Clinical assessment is also dependent on patient position. Supine hypotension implies a blood volume deficit greater than 30%; orthostatic hypotension indicates a greater than 20% depletion of blood volume. Arterial pressure changes are not always suggestive of volume deficits as there can be hypovolemia in the presence of normal arterial blood pressure. Moreover, arterial blood pressure within the normal range could represent relative hypotension in an elderly or hypertensive patient.

In the tilt test, one of the traditional methods of assessing IVF depletion, a positive response is defined as an increase in heart rate by 20 beats/min and decrease in systolic pressure by 20mmHg when the subject assumes the upright position. However, there is a high incidence of false-positive and false-negative findings and this limits the value of the test. Young healthy subjects can withstand acute blood loss of 20% of blood volume while exhibiting only postural tachycardia and variable postural hypotension, while 20–30% of elderly patients may demonstrate orthostatic changes in blood pressure despite a normal blood volume.

Biochemical markers

Physical signs of intravascular volume may be further confirmed by laboratory tests demonstrating high levels of BUN and creatinine, low urinary Na^+, high urinary osmolality, and metabolic acidosis (Fig. 55.8). Blood urea nitrogen is raised in hypovolemia but may be elevated by high protein intake, gastrointestinal bleeding, accelerated catabolism, and renal failure. Oliguria secondary to hypovolemia is suggested by low urinary Na^+ and high urinary osmolality, caused by increased water absorption. Severe hypovolemia may result in lactic acidosis owing to compromised tissue perfusion.

Laboratory findings of hypovolemia

Test	Normal range	Suggests hypovolemia
Blood urea nitrogen (mmol/L)	2–14	>15
Serum creatinine [mmol/L (mg/L)]	<150 (<17)	<150 (<17)
Urinary sodium [mmol/L (mg/L)]	>30 (>690)	< 15 (<345)
Urinary osmolality (mosmol/kg)	400–800	>800
Serum lactate [mmol/L (mg/L)]	<1.5 (<135)	> 2.0 (>180)

Figure 55.8 Laboratory findings of hypovolemia

Central venous pressure

Central venous pressure (CVP) is commonly measured in critically ill and postoperative patients as an indicator of circulating blood volume. There are a number of pitfalls. Central venous pressure is normally dependent on venous return to the heart, right ventricular compliance, peripheral venous tone, and posture. A normal CVP does not always exclude hypovolemia. It is not particularly reliable in the presence of pulmonary vascular disease and valvular heart disease. The absolute value of CVP is sometimes difficult to interpret as CVP may be maintained through peripheral venoconstriction. It is unreliable in the presence of right ventricular dysfunction or chronic airflow limitation.

Pulmonary artery occlusion pressure

The pulmonary artery catheter has become a popular technique for measurement of pulmonary artery occlusion pressure (PAOP) as an indicator of circulating blood volume and left ventricular preload. Like CVP, the absolute level of PAOP does not confirm or exclude hypovolemia. Impairment of left ventricular function may increase PAOP even in the presence of adequate circulating volume. The interpretation of PAOP also requires caution in mechanically ventilated patients. Measurement of right ventricular end-diastolic volume index with the pulmonary artery catheter fitted with a fast response thermistor appears to be a more accurate predictor of the effect of fluid therapy on cardiac index.

Cardiac output

Cardiac output can be measured by a thermodilution technique utilizing a pulmonary artery catheter. There are also noninvasive techniques for determining cardiac output using Doppler and bioimpedence principles. The absolute value of cardiac output does not confirm hypovolemia, but the response of cardiac output to fluid therapy may indicate IVF volume status. Likewise, changes in stroke volume monitored with esophageal Doppler in response to fluid therapy may help in restoring the circulating blood volume. Small volumes of fluid (e.g. 200mL of a colloid) are administered to produce a small and rapid increase in PV, with assessment of changes in cardiac output, CVP, and PAOP at each addition. A rise in CVP or PAOP of more than 3mmHg represents a significant increase and is probably indicative of an adequate circulatory volume. It is more appropriate to monitor the stroke volume than cardiac output during this technique because of the decrease in heart rate that may occur in response to fluid challenge.

Tissue perfusion

Restoration of depleted IVF volume improves tissue perfusion. Global tissue perfusion may be assessed using the absence of anaerobic metabolism (which gives rise to falling arterial pH and production of lactate) as an indicator of good perfusion. Assessment of regional perfusion is more difficult, but urine output is one simple measurement that is widely used. Monitoring gastric mucosal CO_2 using a tonometer and mucosal blood flow with laser Doppler may help to assess regional gut perfusion, one of the earliest tissues to be compromised in hypovolemia. Normalizing splanchnic perfusion may be one of the goals of fluid resuscitation in patients in intensive care.

MAINTENANCE OF FLUID REQUIREMENTS

Water

In healthy adults, sufficient water is required to balance gastrointestinal losses of 100–200mL/day, insensible losses of 500–1000mL/day (half of which is respiratory and half cutaneous), and urinary losses of 1500mL/day. When deciding whether to replace urinary losses exceeding 1500mL/day, it is prudent to consider whether increased urinary output represents an appropriate physiologic response to ECF expansion or an inability to conserve salt or water.

Electrolytes

Renal Na^+ conservation is highly efficient, resulting in an average daily adult requirement of 1.73g (75mmol). Normal kidneys can reduce daily Na^+ excretion to less than 230mg (10mmol) during chronic Na^+ depletion. The kidneys can also excrete excess Na^+ efficiently; consequently, patients who have normal cardiac and renal reserve may tolerate intravenous administration of Na^+ far in excess of normal daily requirements. Renal conservation and excretion of K^+ is less efficient. The daily K^+

requirement slightly exceeds 1.6g (40mmol). A diuresis typically induces an obligate K^+ loss of at least 400mg (10mmol) for every liter of urine. Other electrolytes, such as Cl^-, Ca^{2+}, and Mg^{2+}, require no short-term replacement but must be supplemented during chronic intravenous fluid maintenance. Combining the daily maintenance requirements for water, Na^+, and K^+ results in a predicted maintenance fluid for a healthy 70kg adult of 2500mL/day with Na^+ 69mg/dL (30mmol/L) and K^+ of 59–78mg/dL (15–20mmol/L). In the perioperative period, fluids containing free water are rarely employed in adults largely because of the necessity for replacing losses of PV and losses into ISF, both of which are Na^+ rich.

Glucose

Glucose-containing intravenous solutions are traditionally used in an effort to limit Na^+ load, to prevent hypoglycemia, and to limit catabolism. However because of the hyperglycemic response associated with surgical stress, only infants and patients receiving insulin or drugs that interfere with glucose synthesis are at risk of hypoglycemia. Iatrogenic hyperglycemia can limit the effectiveness of fluid resuscitation by inducing an osmotic diuresis and may aggravate global and focal neurologic ischemic injury. Glucose administration is indicated during clinical situations where hypoglycemia is likely to occur and in hypernatremic hypovolemia to replace water deficits.

Intraoperative fluid requirements

Surgical patients require replacement of losses of PV and ECF secondary to wound edema, ascites, evaporative losses, and gastrointestinal losses. Replacement must also compensate for the acute reduction of ECF that accompanies hemorrhage and tissue manipulation. Tissue manipulation leads to loss of a proportion of ECF into a space that is slow to equilibrate with plasma and not easily available for mobilization back into the vascular compartment; this is known as 'third space loss'. The anatomic location of third space includes tissue edema and increased extracellular tissue water. During upper abdominal surgery, there may be a movement of up to 15% of ECF into this space. In more extensive surgical procedures, the decrease in ECF presumably may be much greater. It has been shown that in the postoperative period total body weight increases as a result of increase in ISF. In most patients, mobilization and return of accumulated fluid to the PV occurs on approximately the third postoperative day. It may occur sooner or later, depending on patient characteristics, the severity and duration of initial insult, and the development of postoperative complications such as acute renal failure or sepsis.

Guidelines have been developed for replacement of third-space losses during high-risk surgical procedures. In addition to maintenance fluid requirements and replacement of estimated blood loss, the simplest formula provides 4mL/kg per hour for procedures involving minimal trauma, 6mL/kg per hour for moderate trauma, and 8mL/kg per hour for extreme trauma. In present clinical practice, the fluid replacement is usually guided by invasive monitoring during high-risk surgical procedures and in the immediate postoperative period.

Intravenous fluids

The goals of fluid therapy are to meet the basal fluid requirements, to replace the losses, to restore or maintain hemodynamic stability, to enhance microvascular blood flow so that oxygen is delivered to the tissues, and to maintain aerobic cellular metabolism. There are a large number of intravenous fluid preparations, including crystalloids and colloids (Fig. 55.9). Although most fluid replacement is given intravenously or enterally, fluid can be absorbed from subcutaneous, peritoneal, or intraosseous routes. Aside from basic replacement of fluid and electrolyte losses and any daily requirements, there is considerable controversy as to the optimum choice of fluid in any particular clinical situation. It appears crucial to detect hypovolemia at an early stage and to start fluid resuscitation. Early restoration of circulating volume is important rather than the choice of individual fluid. The so-called 'golden hour of resuscitation' infers that there is a short window of time when it is important to correct hypovolemia, not just maintain blood pressure, so that the 'nonvital' organs, especially splanchnic organs, are well perfused. Splanchnic hypoperfusion has been shown to predispose to multiple organ dysfunction syndrome.

Choice of fluids

Intravenous fluids are typically divided into blood, blood products, colloids, and crystalloids. Such fluids can be isotonic or hypertonic. Crystalloids are isotonic fluids with electrolyte composition similar to that of ECF (Fig. 55.9). Such fluids rapidly distribute throughout the ECF; hence large volumes are required to expand the IVF. Approximately 3–4L of fluid will be required to expand the intravascular compartment by 1L. Glucose is rapidly metabolized, leaving water with or without electrolytes depending on the solution. For 5% dextrose, this equates to the administration of water that will equilibrate through both the ICF and the ECF, that is the TBW. It is, therefore, a suitable solution to provide daily water requirement or replace water deficits. However, it should not be used for resuscitation or rapid volume replacement. Gastrointestinal losses and third-space losses should be replaced with isotonic saline or Hartmann's (Ringer's) solution.

Colloids

Colloid solutions contain larger molecules that are retained within the intravascular space if capillary membrane function is intact. They typically have electrolyte concentrations similar to those of crystalloid solutions. The duration of effect of such solutions depends on the size of the molecules, their overall osmotic effect, and their plasma half-lives.

Albumin

Albumin is relatively expensive compared with the synthetic colloids. Albumin 4.5% is iso-oncotic, while 20% albumin, so-called 'salt poor' albumin [Na^+ 138mg/dL (60mmol/L)], provides a very high COP and when infused expands the IVF volume to up to five times the volume administered by drawing fluid in from the ISF. The intravascular persistence of albumin is variable because of leakage into the interstitial space and varies greatly with changes in the patient's condition. In normal individuals, approximately 4–5% of infused albumin escapes from the intravascular space per hour, equivalent to a plasma half-life of about 16 hours. Albumin is currently overused and it is estimated that up to 75% of all albumin usage may be inappropriate.

Gelatins

Gelatins are polypeptides, molecular weight approximately 35,000, prepared from chemically modified bovine collagen. A number of preparations of modified gelatin, either succinylated (Gelofusine) or urea cross-linked (Haemaccel), are commercially

Composition of some intravenous fluids

Fluid	Constituents				Osmolality (mosmol/kg)
	Glucose [mmol/L (g/L)]	Na^+ [mmol/L (g/L)]	Cl^- [mmol/L (g/L)]	Lactate [mmol/L (g/L)]	
Dextrose 5% (D5W)	50 (278)	0	0	0	252
Dextrose 10% (D10W)	100 (555)	0	0	0	505
Hartmann's/Ringer's	0	3.0 (130)	3.87 (109)	2.52 (28)	273
Saline 0.9%	0	3.54 (154)	5.47 (154)	0	308
D5W/0.33% saline	50 (278)	1.3 (56)	1.99 (56)	0	365
Hydroxyethyl starch 6%	0	3.54 (154)	5.47 (154)	0	310
Gelofusine 3.5%	0	3.45 (150)	4.44 (125)	0	310
Albumin 5%	0	3.54 (154)	5.33 (150)	0	310
Dextran 10%	0	3.45 (150)	5.33 (150)	0	310
Albumin 25% (salt poor)	0	1.38 (60)	2.13 (60)	0	1200
Hypertonic saline 7.5%	0	29.4 (1280)	45.4 (1280)	0	2560
$NaHCO_3$ 8.4%	0	23.0 (1000)	0	0	2000

Figure 55.9 Composition of some intravenous fluids.

available. The only major difference between these preparations is in ionic composition, especially Ca^{2+}. Gelatins provide isovolemic volume substitution. They have poor intravascular persistence, with plasma half-lives of 1–2 hours. Therefore, reinfusions are necessary for prolonged volume support. Gelatins do not appear to influence hemostatic mechanisms apart from a dose-dependent dilution of clotting factors. The incidence of severe anaphylactoid reactions does not appear to be a problem any longer, probably because of a reduction in the amount of urea cross-linkage in the preparations.

Dextrans

Dextrans are linear polysaccharide molecules that are not metabolized in the body. A number of preparations are available, including 6% dextran 70 (70kDa), 3% dextran 60 (60kDa), and 10% dextran 40 (40kDa). Smaller fractions are eliminated by the kidneys while the larger fractions pass into tissues and undergo hydrolysis. Dextran 70 has more intravascular volume-supporting effects than dextran 40. Dextran 40 increases microcirculatory flow through reduced red cell and platelet sludging, volume expansion, and hemodilution-induced reduction in whole blood viscosity. Beneficial effects on the microcirculation make them suitable for patients undergoing vascular surgery and graft reconstruction procedures. In the past, the clinical use of dextrans has been associated with severe hypersensitivity reactions and deterioration in coagulation. The risk of such rare hypersensitivy reactions (1 in 2500) has been reduced to less than 1 in 70,000 with the hapten (monovalent dextran) prophylaxis to block circulating antibodies to dextran.

Hydroxyethyl starch

Hydroxyethyl starches (HES) are derived from amylopectin with hydroxyethyl groups introduced into the glucose sections to retard degradation by serum amylase. The degree of substitution, expressed as a number between 0 and 1, indicates the fraction of glucose sections bearing a hydroxyethyl group. A number of preparations of HES with different concentrations (3, 6, and 10%), different average molecular weights (40,000, 200,000, 270,000, and 450,000), and different degrees of substitution (0.45, 0.5, 0.62, and 0.7) are used for volume-replacement therapy. The duration of plasma expansion depends on the physical and chemical characteristics of particular HES solutions and is approximately 24 hours, with 30–40% of the colloid still present in circulation after this period. Hydroxyethyl starch has comparable volume-expanding properties to 4.5% albumin, but there is a concern over the use of larger volumes of HES because of adverse effects on the coagulation process, platelet function, and reticuloendothelial function.

Crystalloid versus colloid debate

There is continuing controversy over the uses and indications for crystalloids versus colloids. The argument in favor of crystalloid is based on the fact that acute changes take place in the blood volume and ECF following trauma or major surgery and the resulting deficit can be corrected by infusing crystalloids, such as Ringer's. Administration of large volumes of crystalloids may be required to maintain PV, and as crystalloids readily leak out of the intravascular compartment, expansion of ISF volume is likely. The pro-colloid argument is based on the view that colloids provide a greater hemodynamic response and PV expansion as most of them remain in circulating blood volume in the absence of increased capillary permeability. Colloids can leak out of the circulation in critically ill patients who have loss of capillary integrity. Pooled data from numerous studies comparing crystalloids and colloids could not demonstrate a difference between them. It has been recommended that crystalloids remain the initial fluid of choice in resuscitation; colloids would be appropriate if resuscitation of the vascular space is the primary aim.

Hypertonic saline

The need to deliver fluid resuscitation in prehospital settings led to the development of hypertonic–hyperoncotic solutions. For a liter of blood loss, 250mL of hypertonic saline can provide the same resuscitation as 3L of isotonic saline (0.9%). In comparison with conventional fluids, hypertonic saline up to 6mL/kg appears to restore systolic blood pressure and cardiac output rapidly with minimal tissue edema. Therefore, such fluid resuscitation is called 'small volume resuscitation'. There are three predominant mechanisms by which hypertonic saline acts: PV expansion secondary to extracellular translocation of ICF and intravascular translocation of ISF, increased cardiac contractility, and vasodilatation. Hypertonic saline plus colloid (6% HES) is claimed to sustain hemodynamic stability for longer than hypertonic saline alone.

Future resuscitative fluids: hemoglobin solutions

As a result of the risks and side effects of homologous blood transfusion, various hemoglobin-based blood substitutes from human and other nonhuman sources have been developed and are currently under clinical evaluation (Chapter 51). Improvement in regional blood flow and enhancement of oxygen transport have been shown with infusion of these solutions. Hemoglobin solutions restore the vascular reactivity to vasopressors by partially scavenging excessive nitric oxide in patients who have progressive severe sepsis. The use of these solutions as an adjunct to conventional fluid therapy of severe hypovolemia and hemorrhagic shock needs further evaluation.

Risks of fluid therapy

Hazards, both documented and theoretical, are associated with the use of colloids, including dose-related alterations in hemostasis, renal complications, adverse effects on transplanted organs, and allergic and anaphylactoid reactions. Dextran may be associated with rare severe anaphylactic reactions. Dextrans appear to decrease the levels of both the components of factor VIII: VIIIR:Ag (factor VIII-related antigen) and VIII:C (factor VIII coagulant). With reduced VIII:C, there is reduced binding to platelet membrane receptor proteins GPIb and GPIIb/IIIa, which results in decreased platelet adhesion (Chapter 51). The effects of various preparations of HES on platelet function have not been well defined. Both normal and abnormal platelet aggregation have been reported. After large doses of high-molecular-weight HES, platelets appear swollen and platelet adhesion is reduced with an increased risk of postoperative bleeding. High-molecular-weight HES appears to diminish the concentrations of factor VIII components VIIIR:Ag and VIII:C more than low-molecular-weight HES. Hypernatremia is inevitable with hypertonic saline resuscitation and appears to increase the incidence of renal failure and failure of other organs.

ELECTROLYTES

Sodium

Sodium is the principal extracellular cation and solute. Serum Na^+ concentration is an index of TBW rather than total body Na^+ under normal conditions. This ion principally maintains serum osmolality and ECF volume. Its role in generation of cell membrane action potentials means that it is essential for proper function of nerve tissue and muscles, especially the myocardium. Disorders of Na^+ concentration – hypernatremia or hyponatremia – usually result from a relative deficit or excess of water, respectively.

Sodium regulation

Serum Na^+ concentration (135–145mmol/L) and body stores of Na^+ are regulated primarily by endocrine and renal functions. The hormones aldosterone, ANP, and vasopressin are involved in normal regulation of total body Na^+. Aldosterone is responsible for renal Na^+ reabsorption in exchange for K^+ and H^+. Atrial naturiuretic peptide has an opposing effect by increasing renal excretion of Na^+; it tends to decrease PV. Normally changes in serum Na^+ lead to an appropriate change in vasopressin release, which in turn can vary renal free water excretion (urine osmolality 50–1400mosmol/kg) in order to maintain serum Na^+ within normal range. Increased vasopressin secretion in response to either raised plasma osmolality or hemodynamic stimuli results in reabsorption of water by the kidney and subsequent dilution of serum Na^+. Inadequate vasopressin release results in renal free water excretion, which can produce hypernatremia in the absence of adequate water intake. The end result of these physiologic processes is that in situations with Na^+ loss, for example diarrhea or excessive sweating, renal Na^+ conservation is high and urinary Na^+ concentration falls to extremely low levels. However, when Na^+ intake is excessive, renal compensation results in a high urinary Na^+ concentration.

Potassium

Potassium, the predominant intracellular cation, normally has an intracellular concentration of 150mmol/L, while the extracellular concentration is only 3.5–5 mmol/L. Total body K^+ in a 70kg adult is approximately 4256mmol (166g) of which 4200mmol (164g) is intracellular (98%) and 56mmol (2g) is extracellular (2%). Potassium plays an important role in cell membrane physiology, especially that of excitable membranes in the CNS and heart (Chapter 5). It is an essential cation in maintenance of resting membrane potentials. Consequently, changes in extracellular K^+ strongly influence excitation of cardiac tissue.

Potassium regulation

Total body K^+ and serum K^+ concentrations are primarily regulated by three hormones: aldosterone, epinephrine (adrenaline), and insulin. Aldosterone increases renal excretion of K^+. Epinephrine and insulin regulate the circulating K^+ concentration by shifting K^+ into cells. Serum K^+ is also regulated by intrinsic renal mechanisms. Assuming a plasma K^+ of 4mmol/L and a normal glomerular filtration rate of 180L/day, a total of 720mmol (28g) K^+ is filtered daily. Most is reabsorbed in the proximal tubules, but only the amount ingested [normally 40–120mmol (1.5–4.7g) daily] is lost in urine. Excretion of K^+ is primarily dependent on secretion into the distal nephron and is increased by aldosterone, hyperkalemia, high urinary flow rates, and the presence in tubular fluid of nonreabsorbable anions such as phosphates and sulfates.

Calcium

Calcium is a divalent cation found primarily in bone (99%) and the ECF. Circulating Ca^{2+} consists of a protein-bound fraction (40%), an anion-bound fraction (10%), and a free 'ionized' fraction (50%). Normal free Ca^{2+} in the ECF is 1.0–1.5mmol/L while that in ICF is about 50nmol/L. The free ionized fraction is the physiologically active portion responsible for vital cellular functions. Calcium is involved in coupling of receptor-stimulated cellular events to cellular responses, neuromuscular transmission and excitation–contraction coupling in muscles, release of hormones and neurotransmitters, enzyme activation, and blood coagulation. Phosphoinositides and cyclic adenosine monophosphate (cAMP), major second messengers regulating cellular metabolism, function through regulation of Ca^{2+} movement. Calcium is also primarily responsible for generation of the plateau phase of the cardiac action potential.

Alterations in serum albumin, common in critically ill patients, can change total serum Ca^{2+} concentration by as much as 30%. The binding of Ca^{2+} is also affected by blood pH. Free fatty acids, raised in response to increases exogenous catecholamines and intravenous lipids in the critically ill, may increase Ca^{2+} binding by forming additional Ca^{2+}-binding sites. Although there are formulae to correct total serum Ca^{2+} for albumin concentration and pH, they are poor predictors of free Ca^{2+}. It is, therefore, essential to measure free Ca^{2+} in critically ill patients.

Calcium regulation

Calcium is regulated through two primary hormones: parathyroid hormone (PTH) and vitamin D (Chapter 63). Both of these hormones are secreted when serum free Ca^{2+} decreases. Metabolites of vitamin D exert a major role in long-term control of circulating Ca^{2+}. Vitamin D, following ingestion or manufacture in the skin under the stimulus of ultraviolet light, is hydroxylated at the 25-position in the liver and the 1-position in the kidney, giving the active metabolite 1,25-dihydroxy-vitamin D. Both PTH and 1,25-dihydroxy-vitamin D stimulate Ca^{2+} release from bone and Ca^{2+} absorption from renal tubules and the intestine; hence, they can maintain a normal circulating Ca^{2+} within narrow limits even in the absence of dietary intake.

Phosphate

Phosphorous, in the form of phosphate, is distributed in similar concentrations throughout intracellular and extracellular fluid. Bone accounts for 85% of body phosphate. Phosphate circulates as the free ion (55%), complexed ion (33%), and in a protein-bound form (12%). The normal total serum phosphate level ranges from 1.3–0.8mmoL (12.3mg to 7.6 dL) in adults. Phosphate plays a vital role in energy storage and is responsible for the primary energy bond in adenosine triphosphate and creatine phosphate. It is also an essential element of second messenger systems, including cAMP and phosphatidoinositol, and is a major component of nucleic acids, phospholipids, and the cell membrane. As a part of 2,3-diphosphoglycerate, it is important for offloading oxygen from hemoglobin.

Magnesium

Magnesium is the second most abundant cation of the intracellular space after K^+. Of total body Mg^{2+}, 99% is intracellular or in the skeleton and only 1% is extracellular. Of the normal total circulating Mg^{2+} [0.8–1.2mmol/L (1.9–2.9mg/dL)], free 'ionized' Mg^{2+} (50%) is physiologically active. Serum Mg^{2+} is regulated primarily by intrinsic renal mechanisms. Free Mg^{2+} is an essential cofactor in more than 300 cellular enzymatic reactions, including most of the enzymes involved in energy metabolism and the Na^+/K^+-ATPase pump. Magnesium affects vascular tone by modulating the vasoconstrictive effects of norepinephrine (noradrenaline) and angiotensin II so that as the Mg^{2+}/Ca^{2+} ratio falls, the vasoconstrictive effect is enhanced. It also acts as an endogenous Ca^{2+} antagonist through effects on Ca^{2+} channels.

Key References

Berne RM, Levy MN. Principles of physiology. St Louis, IL: Mosby; 1990.

Guyton AC. The microcirculation and the lymphatic system: capillary fluid exchange, interstitial fluid, and lymph flow. In: Guyton AC, Hall JE, eds. Textbook of medical physiology, 9th edn. Philadelphia, PA: Saunders; 1996:183–97.

Traylor RJ, Pearl RG. Crystalloid versus colloid: all colloids are not created equal. Anesth Analg. 1996;83:209–12.

Vermeulen LC Jr, Ratko TA, Erstad BL, et al. A paradigm for consensus: the University Hospital Consortium guidelines for the use of albumin, nonprotein colloid and crystalloid solutions. Arch Intern Med. 1995;155:373–9.

Wilkins MR, Redondo J, Brown LA. The natriuretic-peptide family. Lancet. 1997;349:1307–10.

Willatts SM. Normal water balance and body fluid compartments. In: Willatts SM, ed. Lecture notes on fluid and electrolyte balance. Oxford: Blackwell Scientific; 1984:1–27.

Further Reading

Berendes E, Walter M, Cullen P, et al. Secretion of brain natriuretic peptide in patients with aneurysmal subarachnoid haemorrhage. Lancet. 1997;349:245–9.

Gutkowska J, Antunes-Rodrigues J, McCann SM. Atrial natriuretic peptide in brain and pituitary gland. Physiol Rev. 1997;77:465–515.

Huang PP, Stucky FS, Dimick AR, et al. Hypertonic sodium resuscitation is associated with renal failure and death. Ann Surg. 1995;221:543–57.

Mallick A, Bodenham AR. Modified haemoglobins as oxygen transporting blood substitutes. Br J Hosp Med. 1996;55:443–8.

Mclean RM. Magnesium and its therapeutic uses: a review. Am J Med. 1994;96:63–76.

Mortelmans YJ, Vermaut G, Verbruggen AM, et al. Effects of 6% hydroxyethyl starch and 3% modified fluid gelatin on intravascular volume and coagulation during intraoperative haemodilution. Anesth Analg. 1995;81:1235–42.

Skajaa K. Established role of magnesium sulfate as a prophylactic anticonvulsant agent in preeclampsia/eclampsia. Acta Obstet Gynecol Scand. 1996;75:313–15.

Soni N. Wonderful albumin? Br Med J. 1995;310:887–8.

Warren BB, Durieux ME. Hydroxyethyl starch: safe or not? Anesth Analg. 1997;84:206–12.

Zaloga GP, Eisenach JC. Magnesium, anesthesia, and hemodynamic control. Anesthesiology. 1991;74:1–2.

Chapter 56 Acid–base homeostasis

Simon M Enright and Philip M Hopkins

Topics covered in this chapter

Intracellular and extracellular hydrogen ion (H^+) concentrations are normally kept within narrow limits. However, disturbances in the homeostatic mechanisms that maintain a normal H^+ environment are commonly encountered in anesthesia and in intensive care. In this chapter both the basic science of acid–base physiology in normal and abnormal situations and a reasoned approach to the interpretation of arterial blood gas analysis are described.

DEFINITIONS

Acid and base

According to the Brönsted–Lowry concept, an acid is a compound that dissolves in water to release H^+ (protons), (Equation 56.1). A base is a compound that can accept H^+, (Equation 56.2).

Equation 56.1

$$HA \rightleftharpoons H^+ + A^-$$

Equation 56.2

$$B + H^+ \rightleftharpoons BH^+$$

pH and pK_a

pH is a useful means of expressing H^+ concentration ($[H^+]$, where the square brackets denote 'concentration of') – pH is the negative logarithm to the base 10 of $[H^+]$ in moles/liter. As acidity increases, the pH decreases. Neutral pH is the pH at which the concentrations of H^+ and OH^- are equal ($[H^+] = [OH^-]$). Water is more ionized at body temperature than at room temperature, so neutral pH at body temperature is 6.8; this is the average intracellular pH. Normal extracellular pH (7.4) is slightly alkaline. pK_a is the pH at which a compound is 50% ionized.

Buffer

A buffer is a substance with the capacity to bind or release H^+ and thus minimize changes in $[H^+]$ and pH. Buffers consist of mixtures of a weak acid and its conjugate base. A buffer is most effective at its pK_a, at which it is 50% ionized. Most of the buffering capacity (80%) occurs in the range of –1 to +1 pH units around the pK_a. The most important physiologic buffers have their pK_a values close to physiologic pH. The effectiveness of a buffer also depends on the ability of the body to remove potential H^+, for example as CO_2 in the bicarbonate system.

Anion gap

On the basis of electroneutrality, the total serum cation concentration is equal to the total serum anion concentration (Equation 56.3).

Equation 56.3

$$[Na^+] + [K^+] + [Ca^{2+}] + [Mg^{2+}] = [HCO_3^-] + Cl^- + [PO_4^{3-}] + [SO_4^{2-}] + [\text{Protein}] + \text{organic acid anions}$$

To simplify Equation 56.3, the minor serum cations (K^+, Ca^{2+}, and Mg^{2+}) are considered unmeasured cations (UCs) and the minor serum anions (PO_4^{3-}, SO_4^{2-}, protein, and organic acids) are considered unmeasured anions (UA); this gives Equation 56.4.

Equation 56.4

$$Na^+ + UC = HCO_3^- + Cl^- + UA$$

The anion gap (AG) is the difference between the unmeasured anions and cations (Equation 56.5). The normal range for the anion gap is 12 ± 4mmol/L, which is of use in classifying different types of metabolic acidosis.

Equation 56.5

$$AG = UA - UC = Na^+ - HCO_3^- - Cl^-$$

Acidosis and acidemia

Acidosis is an abnormal condition that tends to decrease blood pH. Acidemia is a blood pH <7.35.

Alkalosis and alkalemia

Alkalosis is an abnormal condition that tends to increase blood pH. Alkalemia is a blood pH >7.45.

NORMAL PHYSIOLOGY

Henderson–Hasselbalch equation

The relationship between pH and buffer pK_a may be calculated by the Henderson–Hasselbalch equation.

Equation 56.6

$$pH = pK_a + \log_{10}\frac{[base]}{[acid]}$$

The most important buffering system in extracellular fluids is the carbonic acid–bicarbonate system, and so extracellular pH can be described by Equation 56.7.

Equation 56.7

$$pH = pK_a + \log_{10}\frac{[HCO_3^-]}{[H_2CO_3]}$$

As H_2CO_3 is in equilibrium with the amount of dissolved CO_2 and is dependent on the partial pressure of CO_2 (Pco_2), this equation can be rewritten as the modified Henderson–Hasselbalch equation (Equation 56.8), in which the pK_a of the system is 6.1 and S is the solubility coefficient of CO_2 in plasma.

Equation 56.8

$$pH = 6.1 + \log_{10}\frac{[HCO_3^-]}{(S \times Pco_2)}$$

When Pco_2 is expressed as mmHg, $S = 0.03$; when Pco_2 is expressed in kPa, $S = 0.23$. The Henderson–Hasselbalch equation can be transformed into the Henderson equation (Kassirer–Bleich modification), which has no logarithms (Equation 56.9).

Equation 56.9

$$[H^+] = 23.9 \times \frac{Pco_2}{[HCO_3^-]}$$

It is the ratio of Pco_2 to HCO_3^-, and not the absolute values of either, that determines the extracellular $[H^+]$ and pH. Intracellular pH is maintained at 6.8 ($[H]^+$ = 160nmol/L). The normal range of pH in extracellular fluids is pH 7.35–7.45 (35–45nmol/L of H^+). Thus, a four-fold concentration gradient occurs for H^+ from inside to outside the cell. This is counterbalanced by the intracellular potential of –70mV, which tends to attract H^+ into the cell. In clinical practice we are unable to measure or manipulate intracellular pH.

Production of acids

Normal metabolism produces H^+ and CO_2. Around 50–100mmol/day of H^+ are released from cells into the extracellular fluid. Aerobic metabolism of organic compounds produces water and CO_2. The latter is an essential component of the extracellular buffering system and control of CO_2 depends on normal lung function. The main sources of H^+ are:

- metabolism of amino acids – conversion of amino nitrogen into urea in the liver, or of sulfydryl groups of some amino acids into sulfate (e.g. methionine and cysteine), releases equimolar concentrations of H^+; and
- incomplete metabolism of carbon skeletons of organic compounds – anaerobic carbohydrate metabolism produces lactate and anaerobic metabolism of fatty acids and ketogenic amino acids produces acetoacetate; both processes release equimolar concentrations of H^+ either directly or indirectly.

Buffering systems

Buffering systems are present in both extra- and intracellular fluids (extracellular groups are discussed herein, as these can be measured and manipulated). The main extracellular buffers in blood are H_2CO_3/HCO_3^-, the hemoglobin (Hb) system (HHb/Hb^- and $HHbO_2/HbO_2^-$), proteins (histidine residues), and phosphate ($H_2PO_4^-/HPO_4^{2-}$). The main intracellular buffers are proteins, phosphate, organic phosphate, and HCO_3^-.

The efficacy of a buffer system depends on:

- concentration of the buffer;
- pK_a of system (80% of buffering activity occurs within pK_a ±1 unit; Fig. 56.1); and
- whether the system is 'open' or 'closed'.

Open (physiologic) and closed (chemical) buffering systems

The bicarbonate system has the advantage of being an open system, which means that the system is not constrained by the pK_a and a limited amount of buffer; the result is relatively independent control of CO_2. Thus, altering minute volumes gives the flexibility to adjust CO_2 concentrations back to normal levels. This gives the system up to 20 times the buffering capacity of a closed system, in which the total amount of buffer remains constant.

The major extracellular systems can be divided into the bicarbonate buffer system and the nonbicarbonate buffer system.

Bicarbonate buffer system

Most CO_2, a potentially toxic product of aerobic metabolism, is lost via the lungs, but some is converted into bicarbonate that contributes to the total extracellular buffering capacity. An ideal physiologic buffer has a pK_a around 7.4, but the pK_a of the H_2CO_3/HCO_3^- system is only 6.1. This may seem disadvantageous, but HCO_3^- is still the most important extracellular buffer for the following reasons:

- it accounts for around 60% of the total blood buffering capacity;
- its presence is necessary for efficient buffering by Hb, which accounts for most of the rest of the total capacity; and
- it is necessary for H^+ secretion by the kidneys.

Normally, Pco_2 is kept within narrow limits at about 40mmHg (5.3kPa). This value depends on the balance between the rate of CO_2 production and its removal, and is controlled by chemoreceptors in the respiratory center in the medulla of the brain stem and in the carotid and aortic bodies (Chapter 46).

The components of the bicarbonate buffer system are in equilibrium (Equation 56.10). The initial step is catalyzed by the enzyme carbonic anhydrase, which is present in high concentrations in erythrocytes and renal tubular cells. As these cells have the ability to remove H^+, this reaction favors the production of HCO_3^-. The generation of HCO_3^- is accelerated if $[CO_2]$ rises, $[HCO_3^-]$ falls, or $[H^+]$ falls because it is buffered by erythrocytes or excreted by renal tubular cells. Therefore, an increase in intracellular Pco_2 or a decrease in intracellular $[HCO_3^-]$ in erythrocytes and renal tubular cells maintains extracellular $[HCO_3^-]$ by accelerating the production of HCO_3^-. This minimizes changes in the HCO_3^-/Pco_2 ratio and therefore changes in pH.

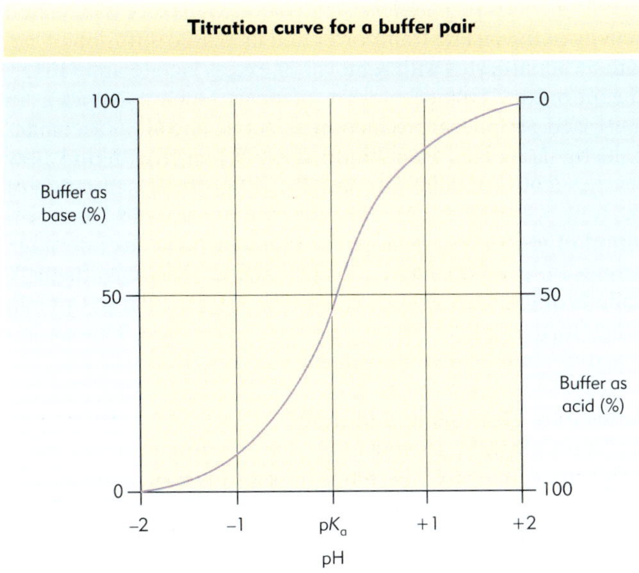

Figure 56.1 Titration curve for a buffer pair. Around 80% of the buffering capacity occurs within –1 to +1 pH units of the pK_a. The pK_a of the bicarbonate system is 6.1, so its buffering capacity within the physiologic range is limited.

Equation 56.10

$$CO_2 + H_2O \rightleftharpoons H_2CO_3 \rightleftharpoons H^+ + HCO_3^-$$

Hemoglobin

Hemoglobin is an important blood buffer, but only works effectively with the bicarbonate buffer system. Buffering by hemoglobin depends on the imidazole group of histidine, which dissociates less (pK_a increases) when hemoglobin is deoxygenated. Thus, oxygenated hemoglobin is a stronger acid than deoxygenated hemoglobin. Deoxygenated hemoglobin is a better buffer than oxygenated hemoglobin and each molecule can accept 0.7mmol of H^+ for 1mmol of oxygen (O_2) released without a change in pH. Intracellular metabolism in erythrocytes does not produce CO_2, which enters from the plasma along a concentration gradient. Inside the cell, carbonic anhydrase catalyzes the production of carbonic acid, which dissociates into H^+ and HCO_3^-.

Most of the H^+ produced is buffered by hemoglobin and the HCO_3^- diffuses out of the cell along a concentration gradient – electrochemical neutrality is maintained by inward diffusion of chloride ions ('chloride shift'). The increase in P_{CO_2} in venous blood is accompanied by an increase in HCO_3^- production in erythrocytes, which thus minimizes change in the HCO_3^-/P_{CO_2} ratio and changes in pH.

Nonbicarbonate buffer systems

The phosphate system (HPO_4^{2-} and $H_2PO_4^-$) has a pK_a of 6.8 and so has theoretic advantages over the bicarbonate system. However, its concentration is only around 1mmol/L (3.1mg/dL) and it can only operate as a closed system. It is of greatest importance in the intracellular compartment and in urine.

Plasma proteins contain titratable groups (primarily histidine) and have the ability to buffer H^+. Plasma proteins only have around 15% of the buffering power of hemoglobin, and therefore buffer only around 5% of all extracellular H^+.

THE ROLE OF THE LUNGS

The lungs are responsible for the excretion of respiratory acid (CO_2). Around 16mol of CO_2 is produced per day (360L). Unless respiratory depression or disease is present, the lungs are able to rapidly compensate for changes in acid–base status (especially acidosis) with changes in minute volume. Stimulation and limitation of minute volume is controlled by neurons in the medulla oblongata and pons which form the respiratory centre. Chemosensitive areas of the centre are able to detect blood concentrations of CO_2 and H^+. Acidosis and increase in CO_2 both cause stimulation and the effect is to increase minute volume, thus CO_2 is eliminated, bringing pH back towards normal.

THE ROLE OF THE KIDNEY

The H^+ produced by the body is mostly removed by ventilation, since it reacts with HCO_3^- to form CO_2 which is exhaled. Therefore, HCO_3^- is lost from the body as CO_2 and the main function of the kidney in acid–base homeostasis is to conserve and produce additional HCO_3^-. The normal plasma concentration of HCO_3^- is 22–30mmol/L, which this is freely filtered at the glomerulus. The transport maximum for HCO_3^- reabsorption is close to the amount filtered at normal plasma concentration. Therefore the response to a high HCO_3^- is continued excretion until the plasma concentration falls to normal levels.

From the renal tubular cells, H^+ is secreted into the lumina, where it is buffered by constituents of the glomerular filtrate. Urinary buffers are constantly replenished by continuous glomerular filtration and reabsorption. Other buffering systems are only useful in the short term, and the kidneys provide the only route for the elimination of most of the excess acid produced. The two renal mechanisms that control HCO_3^- are bicarbonate reabsorption and bicarbonate generation.

Bicarbonate reabsorption

Normal urine is almost free of HCO_3^-. Bicarbonate is filtered at a concentration of about 25mmol/L and an amount equivalent to that filtered is returned to the body by tubular cells. The filtered HCO_3^- combines with H^+, which is secreted by tubular cells, to form H_2CO_3. The H_2CO_3 dissociates to form water and CO_2 (catalyzed by carbonic anhydrase in the brush border); CO_2 diffuses into tubular cells along its concentration gradient and, once intracellular, combines with water to form H^+ and HCO_3^- (again under the influence of carbonic anhydrase). The H^+ is secreted into the tubular lumen in exchange for Na^+. As the intracellular concentration of HCO_3^- rises, it diffuses into the extracellular fluid accompanied by Na^+.

Most of the reabsorption occurs in the proximal tubule (around 90%). No direct transport of HCO_3^- occurs, but there is luminal conversion of HCO_3^- into CO_2. This cycle reclaims buffering power that would be lost by glomerular filtration. The secreted H^+ is derived from cellular water and is incorporated into water in the lumen, with no net loss of H^+. As such, this mechanism only preserves the status quo.

Bicarbonate generation

This process helps to correct acidosis and involves increased activity of carbonic anhydrase with loss of H^+ and generation of HCO_3^-. Carbonic anhydrase is stimulated by:

- a rise in P_{CO_2}, which is caused indirectly by a rise in extracellular P_{CO_2} and a reduction in the CO_2 concentration gradient between inside and outside the tubular cell; and
- a fall of extracellular HCO_3^-, which causes an increase in concentration gradient between inside and outside the cells and leads to a fall in intracellular bicarbonate.

The ability of the kidneys to excrete excess H^+ depends on the presence of filtered buffer bases other than bicarbonate (which is totally reclaimed). Loss of H^+ and buffer base (as Hb) occurs. Bicarbonate formed in the tubular cells diffuses into the extracellular fluid, and therefore a net gain of bicarbonate results.

Urinary buffers

The two important urinary buffers are phosphate and ammonia/ammonium (NH_3/NH_4^+ are considered in the role of the liver).

The pK_a of the phosphate buffer system is 6.8, so at pH 7.4 most is in the form HPO_4^{2-}. Phosphate is the most important urinary buffer because the pK_a is similar to the pH of urine and the concentration of phosphate increases from 1.2 to 25mmol/L (3.7 to 77mg/dL) as water is reabsorbed in the tubular lumen. In mild acidosis, phosphate is released from bone to allow this buffering activity. At a urinary pH of 5.5, most of the filtered phosphate is converted into the dihydrogen phosphate and, therefore, at low pH phosphate cannot maintain the essential buffering of continued H^+ secretion.

THE ROLE OF THE LIVER

The liver is no longer seen as the passive 'slave' to the kidney in acid–base homeostasis, and may have a co-ordinating role. Its main effects are via lactate metabolism and NH_3–glutamine–urea metabolism.

Lactate

Normal production of lactate is around 1400mmol/day from the skin, gut, muscle, brain, and erythrocytes. The protons produced titrate local HCO_3^- and most of the lactate (70%) is removed by the liver (30% via the kidneys and heart), in which it is converted into CO_2 and water by oxidation and gluconeogenesis. Bicarbonate is reformed by gluconeogenesis, which replaces that lost to titration in the periphery. Production and removal of lactate is therefore normally in balance. Lactate enters hepatocytes via two main routes:

- Semispecific monocarboxylate transporter, which is pH sensitive and activated by a pH gradient of acid (outside) to alkaline (inside). Increased activity occurs in starvation and diabetes. Normal lactate concentration in the blood is 0.5–1mmol/L. The transporter becomes saturated at serum lactate >2.5mmol/L.
- Simple diffusion of un-ionized lactic acid, which takes over from the above route at higher serum lactate concentrations. Simple diffusion is not limited by saturation.

Once inside the hepatocyte, the main pathway of lactate disposal is via gluconeogenesis with concomitant bicarbonate regeneration (Equation 56.11). The H^+ is provided by ionization of water ($2H_2O \rightleftharpoons 2H^+ + 2OH^-$), and the hydroxyl ion produces bicarbonate ($2OH^- + 2CO_2 \rightleftharpoons 2HCO_3^-$). Glucose is produced via the intermediates pyruvate and oxaloacetate (intracellular acidosis inhibits the formation of oxaloacetate from pyruvate).

Equation 56.11

$$\underset{\text{(lactate)}}{2CH_3CHOCOO^-} + 2H^+ \rightleftharpoons \underset{\text{(glucose)}}{C_6H_{12}O_6}$$

In mild acidosis (e.g. exercise, mild blood loss) there is increased activity of the lactate transporter and increased diffusion of lactate to hepatocytes with removal of excess lactate and HCO_3^- regeneration. In more severe acidosis (such as shock), an increased peripheral production of lactate and H^+ is accompanied by decreased liver blood flow. When liver blood flow reaches a critical point (around 25% of normal), saturation of the transporter (at lactate concentration of 2mmol/L) and inhibition of gluconeogenesis at the pyruvate–oxaloacetate stage cannot be overcome by increased lactate entry into the cell. Failure of gluconeogenesis causes the intracellular pH to fall, which further inhibits lactate uptake and removal. This sets up a vicious circle of increasing lactic acidosis.

Ammonia, glutamine, and urea

As blood pH falls, urine pH falls and the urine contains more NH_4^+. Increased NH_4^+ excretion appears to allow continued H^+ excretion after urinary buffers such as phosphate have been depleted in acidosis. Normally, around 40mmol/day of NH_4^+ is excreted, but this may increase to 400mmol/day in severe acidosis.

The traditional model is that glutamine is taken up by renal tubular cells and deaminated by glutaminase to produce NH_3. This diffuses into the tubular fluid, where it buffers H^+, secreted by the tubular cells, to form NH_4^+, which is excreted in the urine. The drawback of this model is that cellular deamination of glutamine leads not to NH_3 but to NH_4^+ production, which is unable to buffer further H^+. Consequently, a new theory has emerged in which the liver has a central regulatory role, NH_4^+ is not a buffer, and the kidneys do not simply act as proton excretors.

The liver performs three interrelated functions that affect acid–base homeostasis:

- deamination–oxidation of amino acids;
- urea production; and
- glutamine production.

Amino acids are dipolar molecules at physiologic pH and contain an amino group ($-NH_3^+$) and a carboxyl group ($-COO^-$). Deamination and oxidation in the liver leads to production of NH_4^+ and bicarbonate (100g of neutral amino acid yields 1000mmol of HCO_3^- and 1000mmol of NH_4^+). This bicarbonate load cannot be excreted by the kidney and would rapidly lead to alkalosis. However, oxidation–deamination is closely linked to the energy-dependent formation of urea in the urea cycle, which occurs exclusively in the liver (Equation 56.12).

Equation 56.12

$$CO_2 + 2NH_4^+ \rightleftharpoons \underset{\text{(urea)}}{CO(NH_2)_2} + H_2O + 2H^+$$

Most of the NH_4^+ formed by deamination of amino acids is converted into urea, which is excreted in the urine. For each mole of urea produced, 2 moles of H^+ are formed. This H^+ titrates the bicarbonate formed from deamination of amino acids. Conversion of the NH_4^+ from neutral amino acids (containing one carboxyl and one amino group) into urea leads to H^+ production, which exactly neutralizes HCO_3^- production from deamination. In addition, another pathway is available for the disposal of NH_4^+, in which NH_4^+ is incorporated into glutamine by the enzyme glutamine synthetase. The glutamine route for NH_4^+ disposal does not carry the physiologic penalty of proton production, and therefore leads to a net production of HCO_3^-.

Urea synthesis occurs mainly in the periportal cells of the liver sinusoid (Fig. 56.2). Glutamine synthesis is located in one or two cells at the end of the sinusoid, which are close to the centrilobular vein. These cells have no urea cycle activity and are the only ones that contain glutamine synthetase. Any NH_4^+ not converted into urea by the periportal cells passes to perivenous cells and is vigorously 'scavenged' to produce glutamine. At normal pH a net uptake of glutamine by the liver occurs, but in acidotic conditions there is net production and release of glutamine. Glutamine therefore serves as a nontoxic transport form of NH_3 to the kidneys. It is now obvious that the extent to which bicarbonate (produced by amino acid metabolism) is titrated by H^+ produced during urea synthesis depends on the proportion of amino nitrogen that is converted into either urea or glutamine. By switching the urea cycle on and off, the liver can exert control over acid–base homeostasis. For example, in acidosis the urea cycle is inhibited, net bicarbonate is generated from amino acid metabolism, and NH_4^+ excretion by the kidneys is increased.

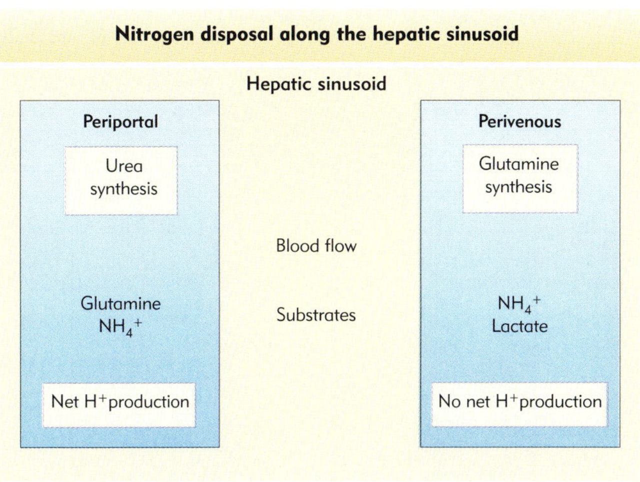

Figure 56.2 Organization of nitrogen disposal mechanisms along the hepatic sinusoid.

DISTURBANCES OF HYDROGEN ION HOMEOSTASIS

Normal $[H^+]$ is low (35–45nmol/L) compared with that of other ions (e.g. $[Na^+]$ is 140mmol/L). However, the small size of H^+ permits high reactivity with binding sites of proteins and small changes in $[H^+]$ can have significant effects on protein function (e.g. enzyme activity). When there is an imbalance between H^+ production and removal, $[H^+]$ and pH deviate from normal, but the range of extracellular pH compatible with life is narrow (6.8–7.7 which corresponds to $[H^+]$ 20–160nmol/L).

The clinical effects of acidemia and alkalemia may be direct or indirect (alterations in blood flow or humoral effects). The principal effects of acidemia include:

- generalized depression of function;
- decreased myocardial contractility, cardiac output, blood pressure;
- dilatation of blood vessels (not responsive to constrictors);
- tendency to fibrillation and other arrhythmias (especially in presence of hypercapnia); and
- depression of central nervous system that leads to coma.

The principal effects of alkalemia include:

- lower plasma $[K^+]$ and arrhythmias;
- reduction in cardiac output and cerebral blood flow; and
- lowered unbound $[Ca^{2+}]$, neuronal irritability, and tetanus.

The four major types of primary acid–base disturbance are now considered – metabolic acidosis, metabolic alkalosis, respiratory acidosis, and respiratory alkalosis.

Metabolic acidosis

Metabolic acidosis occurs when a primary decrease in extracellular bicarbonate causes a fall in pH below 7.35. The causes of metabolic acidosis can be divided into those with a normal anion gap (hyperchloremic) and those with an increased anion gap (Fig. 56.3). Some important causes of metabolic acidosis are given in Figure 56.4.

Normal anion gap (<12mmol/L)

If the anion gap is normal, loss of bicarbonate has occurred, usually via the gastrointestinal tract or kidneys. The result is concentration of the other major measured extracellular anion, chloride, which leads to hyperchloremia.

Increased anion gap (>12mmol/L)

If the anion gap is increased, strong acids have been added to the system that buffer bicarbonate. This may result from retention of endogenous acids produced in excess, such as lactic acid (from tissue hypoxia), or by the addition of exogenous acids.

Lactic acidosis

Lactic acidosis is of importance to anesthetic and intensive care practice and occurs because of tissue hypoxia caused by hypotension, hypovolemia, or sepsis. Lactic acidosis should be suspected when an increased anion gap acidosis occurs and cannot be accounted for by renal failure or ketone production. The normal lactate level is around 1mmol/L. Severe lactic acidosis is associated with levels >5mmol/L.

Compensation in metabolic acidosis

The compensatory response to metabolic acidosis is an increase in ventilation (usually via an increased tidal volume – 'Kussmaul' breathing), but this is only partial and does not return the pH to normal.

Treatment of metabolic acidosis

Treatment of metabolic acidosis includes correction of the underlying disorder and specific alkali therapy. Initial therapy is directed against the cause of the disorder (e.g. improved oxygen delivery and tissue perfusion in lactic acidosis, insulin therapy in diabetic ketoacidosis, and fluid therapy in hypovolemia). Alkali therapy is reserved for severe acidosis (pH <7.25) that is not responsive to general measures, especially when cardiovascular instability is present. Sodium bicarbonate is most commonly used, but has potential drawbacks that include CO_2 production, which leads to hypercapnia and worsening of intracellular acidosis, hypernatremia, and hyperosmolality. Bicarbonate is thus used with caution and only with reference to arterial blood gas status. A simple method to correct the acidosis is based on a half-correction of the base excess. The amount of bicarbonate to be given is calculated by Equation 56.13, in which 0.3 × body weight represents the extracellular fluid volume.

Equation 56.13

$$\underset{(mmol)}{HCO_3^-\ dose} = 0.3 \times \underset{(kg)}{body\ weight} \times \underset{(mmol/L)}{base\ excess} \times 0.5$$

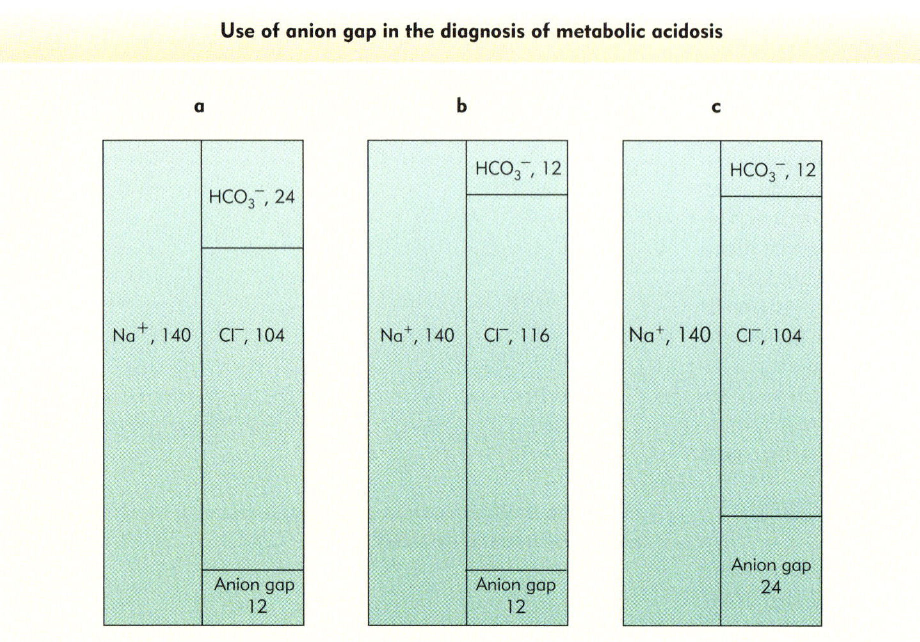

Figure 56.3 Gamble diagram showing the use of anion gap in the diagnosis of metabolic acidosis. (a) Normal pH. (b) Metabolic acidosis – normal anion gap. (c) Metabolic acidosis – increased anion gap. (All concentrations in mmol/L.)

Causes of metabolic acidosis

Cause	Examples
Normal Anion Gap	
Gastrointestinal loss of bicarbonate	Diarrhea, fistulae, uretero-sigmoidostomy
Renal loss of bicarbonate	Renal tubular acidsosis (types I - IV) Carbonic anhydrase inhibitors
Other	Administration of NH_4Cl and other Cl^- containing compounds, hyperalimentation, dilution
Increased Anion Gap	
Cause	**Examples**
Increased acid production	Diabetic ketoacidosis, starvation
Exogenous acid	Methanol, salicylate, ethylene glycol
Lactic acidosis	Shock, sepsis, exercise, inborn errors of metabolism
Decreased acid secretion	Acute and chronic renal failure

Figure 56.4 Causes of metabolic acidosis.

Bicarbonate is given slowly, especially when impairment of ventilation is present, and via a central intravenous catheter. Newer agents such as tromethamine (THAM) and carbicarb (Na_2CO_3 and $NaHCO_3$) have not been shown to reduce mortality in metabolic acidosis.

Metabolic alkalosis

A primary increase in bicarbonate that leads to a pH above 7.45 results in metabolic alkalosis. This can develop in conditions that cause loss of H^+ or gain of HCO_3^-. The special case of pyloric stenosis is considered in detail below. Some important causes of metabolic alkalosis are given in Figure 56.5.

Compensation occurs by hypoventilation, but this is limited by the presence of hypoxic drive at lower PaO_2.

Pyloric stenosis

Pyloric stenosis is a relatively common cause of metabolic alkalosis, and is of prime importance to the pediatric anesthesiologist. The condition occurs mainly in male babies, typically within 2–4 weeks of birth. Unexplained pyloric hypertrophy leads to gastric outlet obstruction that results in repetitive vomiting. There is loss of H^+ (accompanied by Cl^-), which is secreted into the gastric lumen by parietal cells, while bicarbonate formed by these cells returns via venous blood leading to systemic alkalosis. The response of the kidneys is a bicarbonate diuresis with accompanying urinary loss of Na^+ and K^+, which leads to hypovolemia and hypokalemia. As extracellular fluid volume continues to fall, hyperaldosteronism promotes further loss of K^+ and H^+, and worsens the hypokalemia and alkalosis. Treatment consists of slow rehydration with intravenous fluids (saline solution with K^+) and gradual correction of the metabolic alkalosis and electrolyte disturbances, prior to definitive surgery (Ramstedt's procedure).

Treatment of metabolic alkalosis

For diagnostic and therapeutic purposes it is useful to classify the causes of metabolic alkalosis into two groups – chloride responsive and chloride resistant (Fig. 56.6).

Treatment of the majority of metabolic alkaloses (chloride sensitive) is by administration of saline solution. Alkalosis is usually accompanied by hypokalemia, which may be severe; therefore K^+ supplementation (10–40mmol/h) is given with the saline, and frequent electrolyte determination is carried out. For more severe forms of alkalosis (chloride resistant), therapeutic options include carbonic anhydrase inhibition (causing a brisk bicarbonate diuresis), intravenous NH_4Cl (not recommended in hepatic failure because of release of NH_3), or HCl (0.1 or 0.2mol/L in saline given via a central catheter slowly with reference to the base excess). The most effective

Causes of metabolic alkalosis	
Cause	Examples
Loss of H^+	Gastrointestinal : persistent vomiting, nasogastric suction Renal: diuretics (thiazides, loops), excess mineralocorticoid (exogenous - steroid therapy, endogenous - Cushing's disease)
Gain of HCO_3^-	Exogenous alkali (HCO_3^-, citrate, lactate)
Maintenance	Renal failure, hypokalemia, chloride depletion

Figure 56.5 Causes of metabolic alkalosis.

treatment of metabolic alkalosis caused by renal impairment is dialysis.

Respiratory acidosis

Respiratory acidosis occurs when an acute or chronic rise in arterial CO_2 decreases pH to <7.35.

Acute respiratory acidosis

The major causes of acute respiratory acidosis are given in Figure 56.7. In acute respiratory acidosis a compensatory increase in serum bicarbonate may or may not occur, depending on the duration of the precipitating event. Therapy consists of treatment of the underlying cause and improvement in alveolar ventilation (by either respiratory stimulation or, more commonly, artificial ventilation). An inverse relationship exists between arterial $P\text{CO}_2$ ($Pa\text{CO}_2$) and alveolar ventilation (Equation 56.14).

Equation 56.14

$$Pa\text{CO}_2 = \text{metabolic rate/effective alveolar ventilation}$$

The decision to instigate mechanical ventilation is based on clinical grounds (duration of illness, exhaustion, prognosis) and laboratory investigations [arterial blood gases (ABGs)]. Unless significant cardiovascular failure and tissue hypoxia are present, sodium bicarbonate is not required. Some evidence indicates that bicarbonate therapy may improve the efficacy of bronchodilating drugs (such as β_2-receptor agonists) in bronchospastic disorders.

Chronic respiratory acidosis

With chronic respiratory acidosis, such as in a patient who has chronic obstructive airways disease, renal compensation results in an increased reabsorption of bicarbonate, which leads to increased plasma levels, increased base excess, and a return of plasma pH toward normal. These patients may present with acute-on-chronic respiratory acidosis from infective exacerbations, and artificial ventilation may be required because of ventilatory failure from exhaustion or CO_2 narcosis (loss of hypoxic drive with excess O_2 administration). These patients may also develop a metabolic alkalosis as a result of diuretic therapy, which leads to depression of ventilation and further increases in $Pa\text{CO}_2$.

Respiratory alkalosis

Respiratory alkalosis is caused by a primary decrease in $Pa\text{CO}_2$ that leads to pH >7.45. The major causes are given in Figure 56.7.

Respiratory alkalosis caused by overzealous intermittent positive pressure ventilation under anesthesia can result in a decrease in cardiac output and hypotension, left shift of the oxyhemoglobin dissociation curve, hypokalemia and myocardial irritability, decreased cerebral blood flow, bronchoconstriction, posthyperventilation hypoxia, and loss of central respiratory drive. Treatment of respiratory alkalosis is directed at the underlying cause. Long-standing respiratory alkalosis leads to renal compensation via increased excretion of bicarbonate, which results in lower plasma levels and a decrease in pH.

Chloride-sensitive and chloride-resistant metabolic alkalosis	
Cause	Examples
Chloride-sensitive (urinary Cl^- < 10 mmol/L^{-1})	Gastric losses Diuretic therapy Low Cl^- intake Intestinal losses
Chloride-resistant (urinary Cl^- > 10 mmol/L^{-1})	Renal artery stenosis Cushing's syndrome Primary aldosteronism Exogenous mineralocorticoids Severe K^+ deficiency

Figure 56.6 Chloride-sensitive and chloride-resistant metabolic alkalosis.

Causes of respiratory acid-base disturbances	
Respiratory Acidosis	
Cause	**Examples**
Pulmonary disease	COAD, asthma, chest trauma
Central nervous depression	Drugs-opioids, trauma, tumor, infection
Peripheral nervous depression	Myesthenia, polio, neuromuscular blockers
Respiratory Alkalosis	
Cause	**Examples**
Psychological	Hysteria, pain, anxiety
Respiratory	Pulmonary embolus, asthma, pneumonia
Shock	Sepsis, cardiac, hypovolaemic
Central Nervous System	Cardiovascular event, tumor
Drugs	Aspirin, aminophylline
Miscellaneous	Positive pressure ventilation, pregnancy, altitude

Figure 56.7 Causes of respiratory acid–base disturbances.

INTERPRETATION OF LABORATORY VALUES

The mainstay of assessment of acid–base status of a patient is analysis of ABGs (Fig. 56.8). The blood gas analyzer directly measures $P\text{O}_2$, $P\text{CO}_2$, and pH. Other variables are derived from the Henderson equation and from graphic representations such as the Siggaard–Andersen nomogram.

When faced with a set of ABGs it is important to have a scheme for interpretation:

- pH (normal, acidosis, or alkalosis);

Normal values of acid-base variables

Variable	Normal range
pH	7.4 (7.35–7.45)
PaO_2	75–100mmHg (10–13.3 kPa)
$PaCO_2$	35–45mmHg (4.7–6 kPa)
$[HCO_3^-]$	22–26mmol/L
Base excess	–2 to +2mmol/L
[Lactate]	0.7–2.1mmol/L

Standard HCO3– and base excess assume a PaCO2 of 40mmHg (5.3 kPa)

Figure 56.8 Significant values of ABGs and other variables in acid–base status.

- primary disorder (either metabolic, respiratory, or both, determined by assessing PCO_2 and HCO_3^-); and
- compensation, which occurs via respiratory mechanisms (changes in ventilation) in a primary metabolic disorder, or via a metabolic mechanism (renal excretion and/or retention of HCO_3^-) in a primary respiratory disorder. In general, compensation is never complete and overcompensation does not occur.

Acid–base diagrams

In mixed disorders an acid–base diagram can be used to aid diagnosis. These represent the behavior of the whole body during acid–base disturbances and show responses to therapeutic intervention or compensation. They generally involve a graphic representation in which two parameters (from pH, PCO_2, and HCO_3^-) are plotted on the *x*- and *y*-axes, and the third is represented by isobars.

An example is the Davenport diagram (Fig. 56.9), on which pH is plotted against plasma $[HCO_3^-]$. The normal buffer curve shows changes in normal blood when PCO_2 is altered. In uncompensated respiratory disorders, patients move up (acidosis) or down (alkalosis) the normal buffer curve. Patients who have uncompensated metabolic disorder move down (acidosis) or up (alkalosis) the 40mmHg isobar. The diagrams can be used to show compensations for primary acid–base disturbances.

Siggaard–Andersen nomograms use measured values of pH and PCO_2 to calculate the bicarbonate concentration, base excess or deficit, and total buffer base. The Siggaard–Andersen curve nomogram (Fig. 56.10) has pH on the *x*-axis and log PCO_2 on the *y*-axis. Points to the right of a vertical line through pH 7.4 represent alkalosis, and points the left of that line represent acidosis. Points above and below the horizontal line through PCO_2 40mmHg represent hypo- and hyperventilation. The CO_2 titration line passes from the point at which PCO_2 = 40mmHg and pH = 7.4 to the 15g/dL point on the hemoglobin scale. As hemoglobin decreases, the slope of this titration line decreases, which illustrates a reduction in total buffering power of the blood. The CO_2 titration line is plotted for a given blood sample after measuring the pH and then equilibration of the sample with gas mixtures of known PCO_2. Standard bicarbonate (bicarbonate concentration after removal of any respiratory component) is read from the point at which the CO_2 titration line crosses the standard bicarbonate line (horizontal from PCO_2 = 40mmHg). The point at which the CO_2 titration line crosses the lower curved scale is the base excess, and the point where the line crosses the

Davenport diagram

a

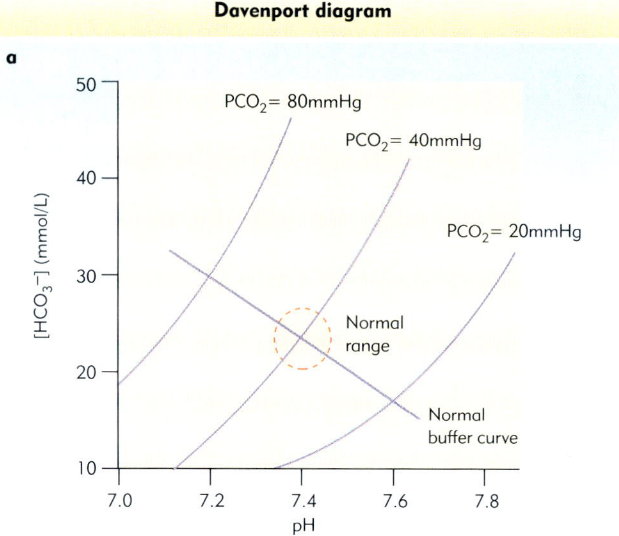

b

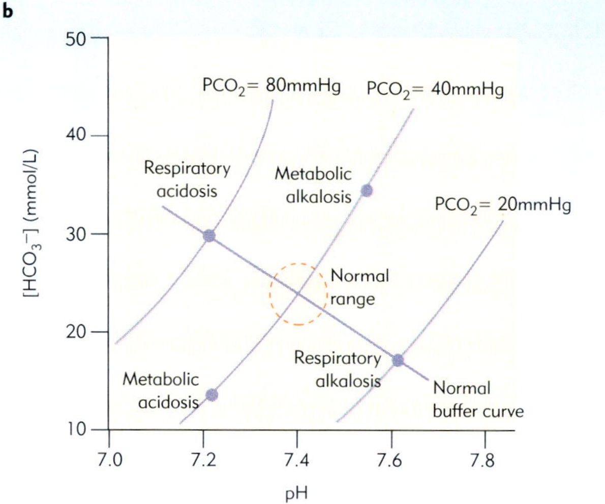

c

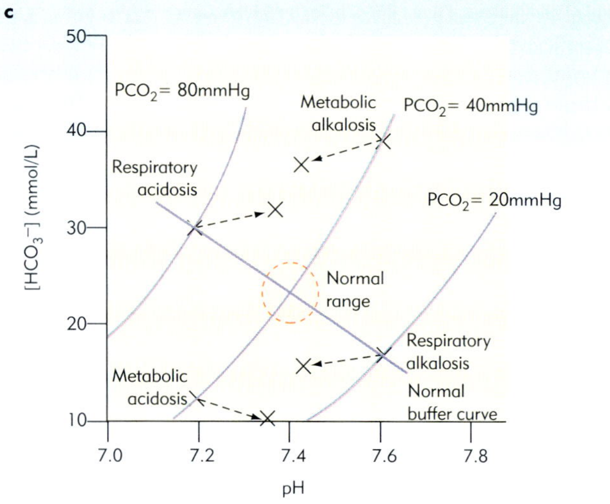

Figure 56.9 Davenport diagrams. (a) For normal changes with altered PCO_2. (b) For primary respiratory disorders (shown along the normal buffer curve), and primary metabolic disorders [shown along the PCO_2 40mmHg (5.3kPa) isobar]. (c) For compensation for primary disorders. (*x*) represents lines of compensation. Modified with permission from Textbook of Critical Care, 1989, Shoemaker et al (Figures 126-10,126-11,126-12) Saunders.

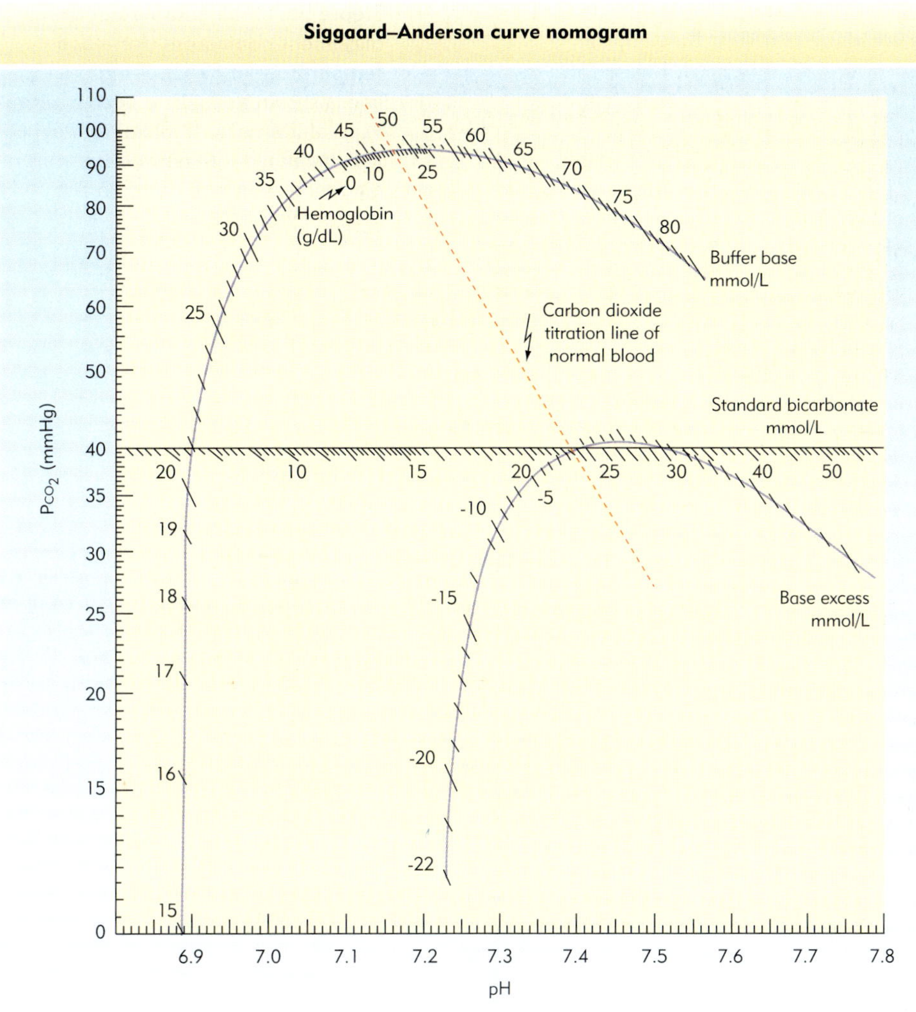

Figure 56.10 The Siggaard–Andersen curve nomogram. This shows the carbon dioxide titration line, which is constructed from equilibration of arterial blood with two gas mixtures of known P_{CO_2} and the hemoglobin concentration. Standard bicarbonate, base excess, and total buffer base are read from the nomogram. (Reproduced with permission of O. Siggard Andersen and Radiometer, Copenhagen, Denmark.)

upper curved scale shows total buffer base concentration (which includes bicarbonate, hemoglobin, and protein buffers).

The Siggaard–Andersen alignment nomogram is shown in Figure 56.11. The pH and P_{CO_2} are measured directly and a line is drawn between these points on the nomogram. The base excess, standard bicarbonate, and total plasma CO_2 are read from the intersection of this line with the relevant scales. The base excess scale is dependent on the hemoglobin concentration.

THE EFFECT OF TEMPERATURE – AN ARTERIAL BLOOD GAS INTERPRETATION

Temperature affects both P_{CO_2} and pH of blood. As blood is cooled, CO_2 becomes more soluble, which results in a reduction of P_{CO_2} by around 4.5% per °C. The pH of blood varies inversely with temperature, the coefficient being –0.015 units per °C (the pH of *in vitro* human blood at 77°F (25°C) would be around 7.6). The reasons for this include the increased dissociation of water at higher temperature (H^+ increases and pH decreases) and the increased buffering of H^+ by the a-imidazole of hemoglobin as temperature falls. These pH changes are seen in human blood *in vitro* and also when the temperature in poikilothermic ('cold-blooded') animals changes *in vivo*. Within the range of normal practice [body temperature 95–104°F (35–40°C)], these small changes are unlikely to affect acid–base management significantly, and temperature correction is of limited value. However, in clinical situations in which body temperature is far from normal [although blood gas analysis is carried out at 98.6°F (37°C)], for example extreme hypothermia associated with drowning or active cooling during cardiopulmonary bypass [with reduction of temperature to around 82.4°F (28°C)], corrections are necessary. There are two types of management of acid–base status in these situations, 'α-stat' and 'pH-stat' (Chapter 41).

Alpha-stat

Alpha-stat management seeks blood pH of 7.4 when measured at 37°C, independent of patient temperature. This means that the actual pH would be much higher (e.g. if temperature was 25°C the actual pH must be 7.58 to have a pH of 7.4 at 37°C). This type of management is simple because no temperature correction is necessary when interpreting a set of blood gases, as these are always measured at 37°C. The alpha-stat hypothesis of pH control is based upon the findings that *in vivo* blood pH of ectothermic animals varies inversely with temperature. However, ectotherms and endotherms have basically similar enzymes, receptors, and transport proteins.

pH-stat

pH-stat regulation aims for a pH of 7.4 when expressed at patient temperature. Thus, a pH of 7.4 at 25°C, when measured at 37°C, would appear extremely acidotic.

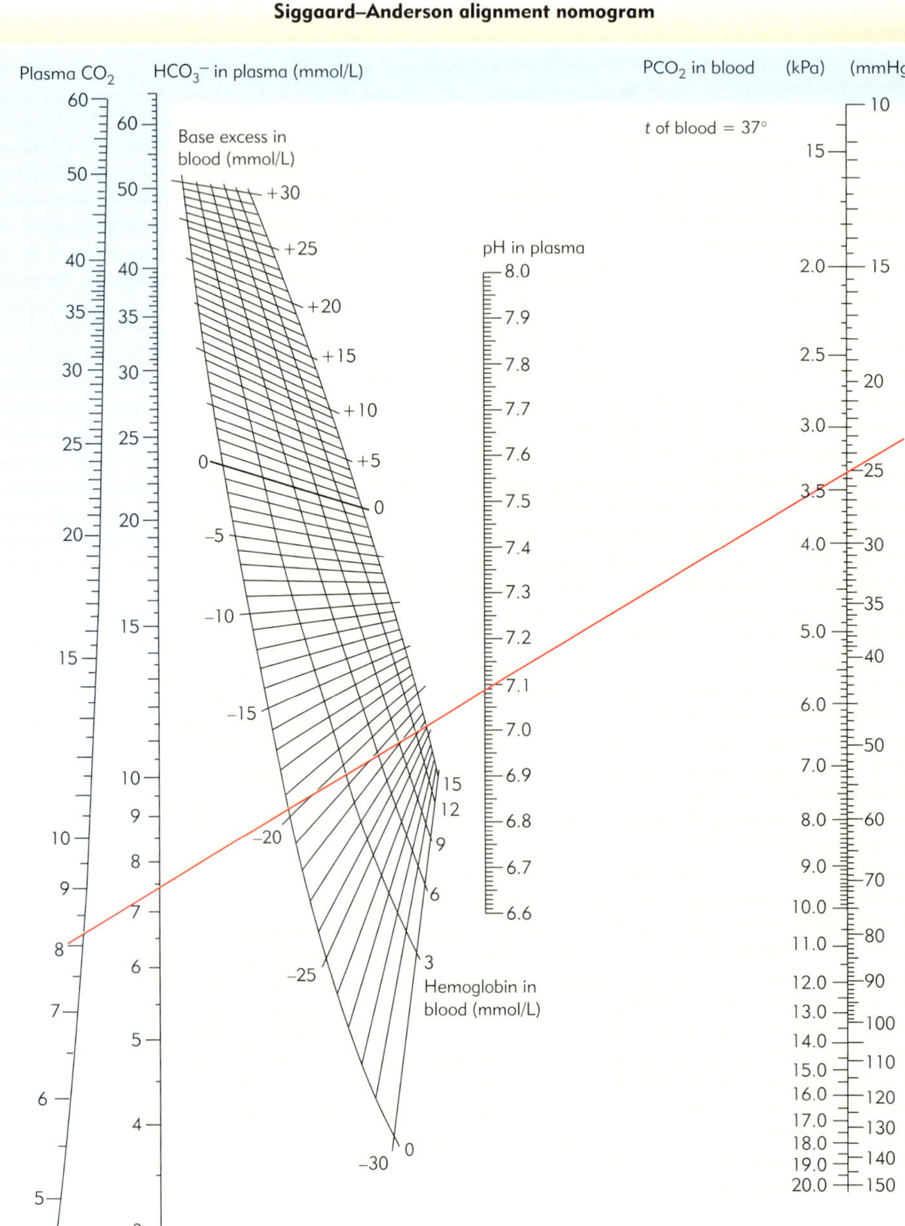

Figure 56.11 Siggaard–Andersen alignment nomogram (for blood temperature of 37°C). A red (—) line is shown to depict a patient with Pco_2 of 25mmHg (3.3kPa) and pH of 7.1. (Adapted with permission from Siggaard–Anderson O. J Clin Lab Invest. 1963;15:211.)

Key References

Astrup PB, Severinghaus JW. The History of Blood Gases, Acids, and Bases. Munsgaard, Copenhagen. 1986.

Cohen RD. Roles of the liver and kidney in acid-base regulation and its disorders. Br J Anaeth. 1991;67:154–64.

Davenport HW. The ABC of acid-base chemistry, 6th edn. Chicago: University of Chicago Press; 1974.

Grogono AW. Acid-base balance. International Anesthesiology Clinics, Spring 1986. 1986;24(1).

Rose BD. Clinical physiology of acid-base and electrolyte Disorders, 4th edn. New York: McGraw-Hill; 1984.

Siggaard-Andersen O. An acid-base chart for arterial blood with normal and pathophysiological reference areas. Scan J Clin Lab Invest. 1971;27:239–45.

Siggaard-Andersen O, Engel K. A new acid-base nomogram. An improved method for the calculation of the relevant blood acid-base data. Scan J Clin Lab Invest. 1960;12:177.

Further Reading

Cohen RD, Simpson R. Lactate metabolism. Anesthesiology. 1975;43:661–73.

Nattie EE. The alphastat hypothesis in respiratory control and acid-base balance. J Appl Physiol. 1990;69(4):1201–7.

Williams JJ, Marshall BE. Editorial: A fresh look at an old question. Anesthesiology. 1982;56:1.

Chapter 57 Renal pathophysiology

Solomon Aronson

Topics covered in this chapter

Acute renal failure
Chronic renal failure
Hypertensive renal disease
Diabetic renal disease
Renal function and anesthesia
Anesthesia in renal failure

In patients who have renal disease, the challenge of optimal perioperative management is demanding because recognition of subtle change is difficult. As our understanding of renal disease evolves, traditional answers have turned into new questions. In the late 1990s, we have gained great insight into the intrarenal actions of intrinsically produced substances and extrinsically administered agents. Overall, however, symptoms of renal failure typically are not detected until less than 40% of normal functioning nephrons remains, and uremic symptoms do not occur until less than 5% of normal functioning nephrons remains (Fig. 57.1).

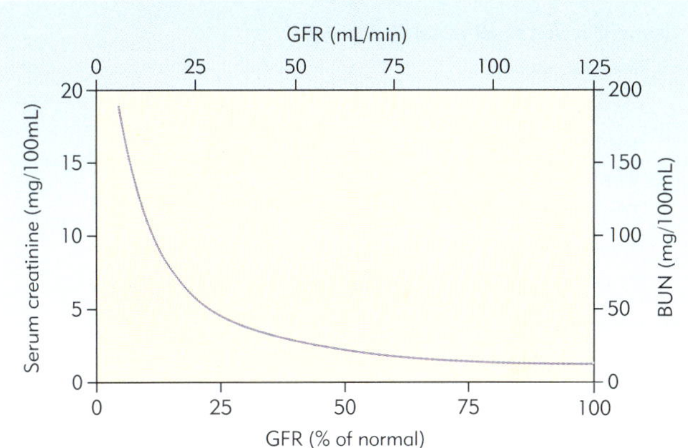

Figure 57.1 Relationship between the rate of glomerular filtration (GFR) and the serum creatinine concentration or the blood urea nitrogen (BUN) concentration. Absolute values for the GFR, as determined by inulin clearance, refer to measurements in healthy adults and from patients who are in nitrogen balance on a normal protein intake. Although there is considerable scatter of these values among individuals, a single average curve has been drawn; however, for a particular person whose GFR has been reduced by, for example, 50%, the serum creatinine concentration could lie anywhere between about 1.4 and 3.0mg/dL.

ACUTE RENAL FAILURE

Acute renal failure (ARF) has been attributed to several mechanisms involving tubular, vascular, and/or glomerular effects. Typically, an early compensatory phase of normal renal adaptation (e.g. pre-prerenal failure) progresses to become decompensatory as prerenal failure ensues. Depending on pre-existing renal function reserve capacity, this stage may occur over a period of hours to days. At this point, the decline in renal function is sufficient to result in retention of nitrogenous end-products of metabolism and an inability to maintain fluid and electrolyte homeostasis. These events are not reversed by modifying nonrenal factors.

There are wide variations in the use of the term 'acute renal failure' in the literature. It is not surprising, therefore, to learn that the reported frequency of ARF among patients admitted to the hospital is 1% and is 2–5% during hospitalization. Perioperative renal failure has been defined clinically as the need for postoperative dialysis or, in some cases, a postoperative serum creatinine level exceeding a predetermined preoperative value [e.g. increase of 0.5mg/dL (440μmol/L) or increase of 50% or greater]. It is estimated that approximately 5% of the general population has renal disease severe enough to affect surgical outcomes adversely.

The onset of ARF following any surgical procedure portends a poor prognosis because of the loss of renal function and because of the life-threatening complications that typically accompany renal failure, including sepsis, gastrointestinal hemorrhage, and CNS dysfunction. The overall reported incidence of renal dysfunction following certain high-risk surgical procedures is as high as 50% (depending on the population analyzed and the methods used to define ARF). The mortality rate of ARF after diagnosis is reported to be 20–90%. Perioperative renal failure accounts for one half of all patients requiring acute dialysis.

The grave significance of ARF was first recognized during the Second World War as a consequence of crush injuries and prolonged hypotension. Since then, it has become clear that ARF can result from decreased renal blood flow from a myriad of causes (Fig. 57.2), a direct insult to the renal tubule, a tubulointerstitial process, or a primary reduction in the filtering capacity of the glomerulus. If clearance is limited by factors that

Causes of renal hypoperfusion associated with acute renal failure

Intravascular volume depletion (hypovolemia)
- Major trauma, burns, crush syndrome
- Fever
- Hemorrhage
- Diuretic use
- Pancreatitis, vomiting, diarrhea, peritonitis, dehydration, bowel preparation

Decreased cardiac output
- Congestive heart failure or low output syndrome
- Pulmonary hypertension, massive pulmonary embolism
- Positive-pressure mechanical ventilation

Increased renal/systemic vascular resistance ratio
- Renal vasoconstriction: α-adrenoceptor agonists, hypercalcemia, amphotericin B (amphotericin), cyclosporine (cyclosporin A)
- System vasodilatation: afterload reduction (vasodilators), antihypertensive medications, anaphylactic shock, anesthesia, sepsis

Renovascular obstruction
- Renal artery: atherosclerosis, embolism, thrombosis, dissecting aneurysm, vasculitis
- Renal vein: thrombosis, compression

Glomerular and small vessel obstruction
- Glomerulonephritis
- Vasculitis
- Toxemia of pregnancy
- Hemolytic uremic syndrome
- Disseminated intravascular coagulation
- Malignant hypertension
- Radiation injury

Increased blood viscosity
- Multiple myeloma
- Macroglobulinemia
- Polycythemia

Interference with renal antoregulation
- Prostaglandin inhibitors with congestive heart failure, nephrotic syndrome, cirrhosis, hypovolemia
- Angiotensin-converting enzyme (ACE) inhibition in presence of renal artery stenosis or congestive heart failure

Figure 57.2 Causes of renal hypoperfusion associated with acute renal failure.

decrease renal perfusion, the etiology is classified as prerenal failure or prerenal azotemia. If renal dysfunction is a consequence of obstruction of the urinary outflow tract, then it is classified as postrenal failure. Intrinsic renal failure is used to describe intrarenal causes. Prerenal azotemia accounts for 70% of general community-acquired ARF and over 90% of perioperative ARF. When prerenal azotemia progresses to renal failure, the terms acute tubular necrosis, vasomotor nephropathy, or ischemic tubular injury are often used interchangeably in the literature.

In patients who have inadequate blood flow (prerenal), injury is commonly caused by the use of drugs that alter intrarenal distribution of blood flow, abnormal hemodynamics, or pre-existing disease. Patients who have pre-existing renal insufficiency, for example, are especially prone to develop ARF during cardiovascular surgery. Patients who have diabetes mellitus and renal insufficiency are especially vulnerable to radiocontrast agents.

The greater the magnitude and duration of the surgical procedure and the number of risk factors (Fig. 57.3) the greater the likelihood of perioperative renal compromise. Risk factors augment rather than induce the risk of ARF. The combined interaction of various acute risk factors appears to be central in the pathogenesis of ARF. The most critical determinants of postoperative renal function are preoperative renal function, the maintenance of appropriate intravascular volume, and normal myocardial function. Under normal physiologic conditions, homeostasis may be maintained despite substantially reduced renal function. Impaired functional reserve capacity becomes evident only when perioperative stress severely comprises renal function.

Intrinsic renal causes of ARF are described according to the primary lesion (i.e. tubules, interstitium, vessels, or glomerulus). Tubular injury is the most common dysfunction seen during the perioperative period and is usually ischemic in origin. Prerenal azotemia and acute tubular necrosis represent extreme examples of the same problem (i.e. insufficient renal blood flow). Most cases of ischemic renal failure are reversible, although irreversible critical necrosis can occur if ischemia is prolonged and severe.

Direct toxicity is the second most common cause of perioperative ARF. Ischemia and toxicity often combine to cause ARF in high-risk patients. Common toxins encountered during the perioperative period include aminoglycoside antibiotics, radiocontrast agents, and various chemotherapeutic agents (e.g. cisplatin). Acute interstitial nephritis, secondary to an acute allergic reaction, is another less frequent cause of perioperative renal failure.

Pathogenesis of acute renal failure

Normally the amount of blood the kidneys receive (1–1.25L/min) far exceeds that needed for their intrinsic oxygen requirement. Essentially all blood passes through the glomeruli, and about 10% of renal blood flow is filtered [a glomerular filtration rate (GFR) of 125mL/min in the normal adult]. The basal normal renal blood flow is 300–500mL/min per 100g tissue, which is greater than that in most other organs (Fig. 57.4). This primarily reflects blood flow to the cortical glomeruli, as perfusion to the inner medulla and papilla is only about 10% of the total flow.

Because the renal cortex contains most of the glomeruli and depends on oxidative metabolism for energy, ischemic hypoxia will initially injure the renal cortical structures, particularly the pars recta of the proximal tubules. As ischemia persists, glucose, glycogen, and other energy substrates are consumed, and the medulla, which depends to a greater extent on glycolysis for its energy sources, is also affected.

Renal clearance is determined by the delivery of waste products to the kidney (i.e. renal blood flow) and the ability of the kidneys to extract them (GFR). A series of systemic and renal compensatory responses are activated initially to preserve ultrafiltration and renal clearance. The hallmark of experimental models of hemodynamically mediated ARF is a reduction of renal blood flow (generally greater than 50%) for at least 40–60 minutes. Once a decrease in renal perfusion is established, then GFR is disproportionately depressed compared with the decline in blood flow. It has been observed that when renal blood flow is decreased sufficiently to depress GFR to less than 5% of

Risk factors for the development of acute renal failure

Acute

- Volume depletion
- Aminoglycosides
- Radiocontrast dye exposure
- Nonsteroidal anti-inflammatory drugs
- Septic shock
- Hemoglobinuria or myoglobinuria

Chronic

- Pre-existing renal disease
- Hypertension
- Congestive heart failure
- Diabetes mellitus
- Advanced age
- Cirrhosis of the liver

Intraoperative

- Aortovascular surgery
- Biliary tract surgery
- Cardiopulmonary bypass and cardiac surgery
- Unstable hemodynamics
- Aorto/renal vascular resistance maldistribution

Figure 57.3 Risk factors for the development of acute renal failure.

normal, blood flow may only be depressed by 25–50% of normal. Hence, although decreased renal blood flow is the initiating event, most of the time there are clearly other factors (tubular pathology) that account for abnormal filtration.

In general, the response to renal hypoperfusion involves three major regulatory mechanisms that support renal function in the setting of decreased renal blood flow: afferent arteriolar dilatation increases the proportion of cardiac output that perfuses the kidney; efferent arteriolar resistance increases the filtration fraction; and hormonal and neural responses improve renal perfusion pressure by increasing intravascular volume, thereby indirectly increasing cardiac output (Fig. 57.5). Some agents involved in regulating afferent and efferent arteriolar tone are shown in Figure 57.2. The afferent arterioles react to reductions in perfusion pressure by smooth muscle relaxation to decrease renal vascular resistance. This property represents a relaxation response or myogenic reflex to reduced transmural pressure across the arteriolar wall. Changes in renal blood flow and GFR that occur with salt loading and aortic constriction are shown in Figure 57.6.

The kidney also possesses a tubuloglomerular feedback system, which is designed to maintain the homeostasis of salt and water excretion. Decreased solute delivery to the macula densa in the cortical portion of the thick ascending limb of the loop of Henle results in relaxation of the juxtaposed afferent arteriolar smooth muscle cells, thus improving glomerular perfusion and filtration.

Reduced delivery of sodium to the macula densa also causes release of renin from the granular cells of the juxtaglomerular apparatus (see Chapter 54). Renin catalyzes the cleavage of angiotensin I from angiotensinogen. Angiotensin I is then transformed into angiotensin II in the lungs by angiotensin-converting enzyme (ACE). Angiotensin II stimulates the production of aldosterone. High concentrations of aldosterone stimulate reabsorption of sodium and water, primarily in the distal tubule and collecting ducts. Initially, angiotensin II exerts a selective vasoconstrictive effect on the efferent arteriole. This occurs, in part, because the kidney synthesizes prostaglandins during hemodynamic instability and increased adrenergic stimulation. Prostaglandin E_2 (PGE_2) specifically decreases the vasoconstrictive effect of angiotensin II (a very potent vasoconstrictor) on the afferent arteriole and, thereby, preserves renal blood flow. Prostaglandin synthesis is inhibited when hydration, renal perfusion, and sodium balance are normal; in these circumstances it will not impact on renal function.

A selective increase in efferent arteriole resistance decreases glomerular plasma flow, thereby preserving GFR. Glomerular filtration is augmented because capillary pressure upstream from the site of vasoconstriction tends to rise. This mechanism enables the kidney to offer high vascular resistance to contribute to the maintenance of systemic blood pressure without compromising its function of filtration. Efferent arteriolar resistance is largely changed through the action of angiotensin II. At low concentration, norepinephrine (noradrenaline) constricts efferent arterioles, indicating that the adrenergic system may also be important for maintaining the renal compensatory response.

Vasopressin [antidiuretic hormone (ADH)] acts primarily on the collecting ducts to increase water reabsorption and results in the excretion of small volumes of concentrated urine. Vasopressin is released from the posterior pituitary gland in response to increased blood osmolarity, which stimulates osmoreceptors in the hypothalamus. Its release is inhibited by stimulation of the atrial baroreceptors or increased atrial volume and is also influenced by stress and increased carbon dioxide partial pressure.

Oxygen delivery and consumption in several organs

Region or organ	Blood flow rate (mL/min per 100g)	O_2 delivery (mL/min per 100g)	O_2 consumption (mL/min per 100g)	O_2 consumption/ O_2 delivery (%)
Hepatoportal	58	11.6	2.2	18
Kidney	420	84.0	6.8	8
Brain	54	10.8	3.7	34
Skin	13	2.6	0.38	15
Skeletal muscle	2.7	0.5	0.18	34
Heart	84	16.8	11.0	65

Figure 57.4 Comparison of the balance of O_2 delivery and O_2 consumption in several organs.

Compensatory responses to impending renal failure

Figure 57.5 Compensatory responses to impending acute renal failure.

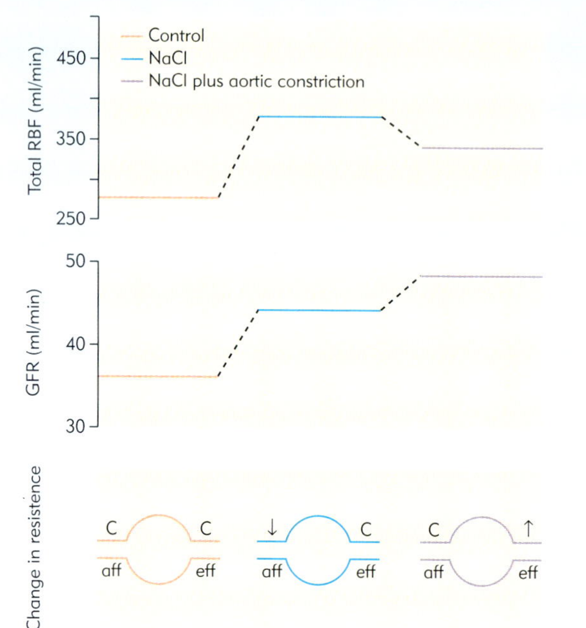

Figure 57.6 Changes in total renal blood flow (RBF) and glomerular filtration rate (GFR) under varying conditions. Under some circumstances, RBF and GFR shift in the same direction, whereas under other conditions they undergo divergent changes. The variations in resistance in the gradient across the glomeruli could be brought about by resistance changes in one or both arterioles; the diagrams merely indicate the predominant alterations. (aff, afferent; eff, efferent.)

Atrial natriuretic peptide (ANP) causes systemic vasodilatation and promotes renal excretion of sodium and water by increasing glomerular filtration. It is secreted by the cardiac atria and other organs in response to increased intravascular volume. It decreases systemic blood pressure by relaxing vascular smooth muscle, reducing sympathetic stimulation, and inhibiting the renin–angiotensin–aldosterone system.

The common denominator of these regulatory mechanisms in the preservation of renal blood flow is salt and water conservation. The control of blood delivery to the kidney, the fraction of plasma filtered, and the amount of volume returned to the systemic circulation are all determined by regulatory mechanisms within the kidney that attempt to preserve filtration function during compromised circulation. These compensatory mechanisms, however, have limits. Excess vasoconstrictive forces may eventually induce a decrease in filtration function.

The mechanisms that influence efferent arteriolar vasoconstriction ultimately will overwhelm the system and cause afferent arteriolar vasoconstriction as well. The resulting decrease in filtration fraction is the hallmark of ischemic ARF. Histopathologic data indicate that the proximal tubules bear the brunt of the initial injury. As renal blood flow decreases and compensatory mechanisms fail, necrotic tubular cell debris is incorporated into occluding casts that lodge within the tubule lumen and cause obstruction. This obstruction causes an increase in tubular pressure, which, in turn, further decreases filtration fraction and promotes backleak upstream. Early cell changes are reversible, such as the swelling of cell organelles, especially in the mitochondria. As ischemia progresses, lack of adenosine triphosphate (ATP) inhibits the sodium pump; water, sodium, and chloride accumulate in tubular cells; potassium levels fall; and the cells begin to swell (Fig. 57.7). In experimental models of ARF, the following pathologic changes occur. Swelling of tubular epithelial cells leads to formation of bullae, which protrude into the tubular lumen distal to the cell. Necrosis of tubular cells results in abnormal membrane permeability. Structural changes in the glomerular epithelium may decrease glomerular filtration. Finally, constriction of intrarenal arteries and arterioles further reduces glomerular blood flow.

The onset of tubular damage in experimental models of ARF is usually within 25 minutes of ischemia; at this point the microvilli of the proximal tubular cell brush borders begin to change. Within an hour, they slough off into the tubular lumen, and membrane bullae protrude into the straight portion of the proximal tubule. After a few hours, intratubular pressure rises and tubular fluid backflows passively. Within 24 hours, obstructing casts appear in the distal tubular lumen. Even if renal blood flow is completely restored after 60–120 minutes of ischemia, the GFR may not immediately improve. Ischemic tubular damage may be exacerbated further by an imbalance between oxygen supply and demand. Most vulnerable to the imbalance are the cells of the thick ascending tubule of the loop of Henle in the medulla. In ischemic-induced ARF, lesions are unevenly distributed among the nephrons, probably reflecting variability in blood flow.

In the clinical setting of hypotension, the kidney has a distinct susceptibility to injury. The reason for this susceptibility is not readily apparent, since renal blood flow is normally high and oxygen supply far exceeds requirements. Although the kidneys receive nearly 25% of the cardiac output and extract relatively little oxygen, the discrepancy between cortical and medullary blood flow and oxygen consumption is marked. The apparent abundance of blood flow to the cortex maximizes flow-dependent

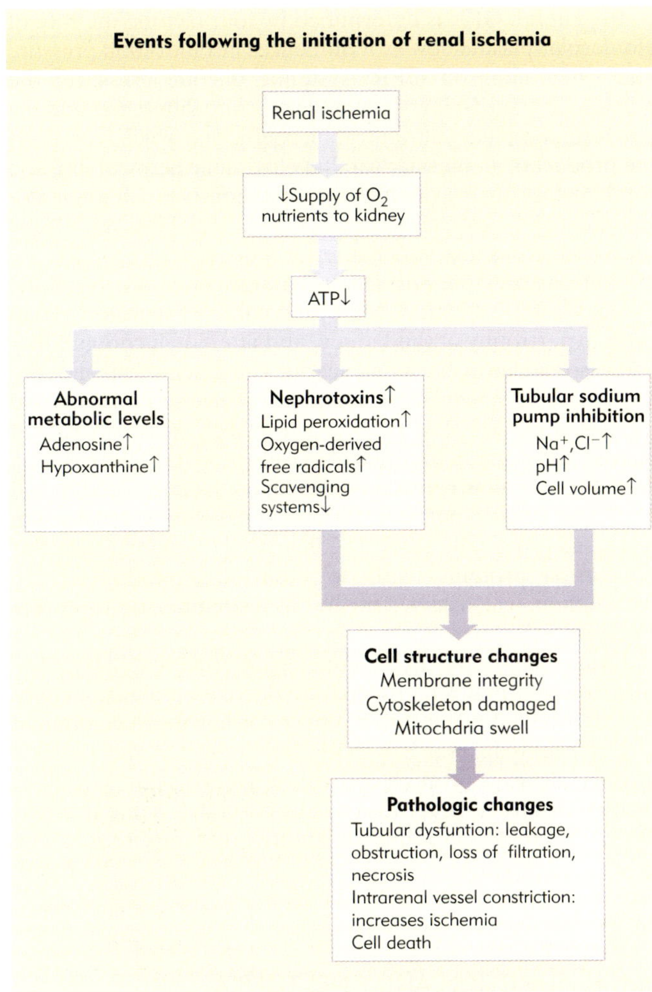

Figure 57.7 Sequence of events following the initiation of renal ischemia.

functions, such as glomerular filtration and tubular reabsorption. In the medulla, blood flow and oxygen supply are restricted by a tubular vascular anatomy specifically designed for urinary concentration. Normally, 90–95% of blood flow is delivered to the cortex compared with 5–10% delivered to the medulla. The selective vulnerability of cells in the thick ascending limb of the loop of Henle is thought to result from their high oxygen consumption. Average blood flow is 500 and 3mL/min per 100g of tissue for the cortex and medulla, respectively, while the oxygen extraction ratio (i.e. oxygen consumption over oxygen delivery) is 0.18 and 0.79 for the cortex and medulla, respectively. Normally the partial pressure of oxygen is about 55mmHg in the cortex and 8–15mmHg in the medulla, making the medullary thick ascending limb of the loop of Henle the most vulnerable to tissue hypoxia. Therefore, severe hypoxia may easily develop in the medulla with what otherwise would seem to be adequate total renal blood flow.

The initial response to decreased renal blood flow is increased sodium absorption in the ascending limb of the loop of Henle, which coincidentally increases oxygen demand in the region most vulnerable to decreased oxygen delivery. To compensate for this, sympathoadrenal mechanisms cause cortical vasoconstriction and oliguria, which tend to redistribute blood flow away from the outer cortex to the inner cortex and medulla. This cortical-to-medullary redistribution of renal blood flow protects the vulnerable medullary oxygen balance. At the same time, decreased sodium delivery to the macula densa causes afferent arterial constriction. With afferent arterial vasoconstriction, glomerular filtration decreases, after which solute reabsorption in the loop of Henle and oxygen consumption are reduced. The severity of cellular injury appears to be related to the degree of imbalance between cellular oxygen supply and demand. In the hypoperfused kidney preparation, oxygen-enriched perfusion reduced cellular damage and hypoxic perfusion increased it; complete cessation of perfusion (GFR zero, preventing ultrafiltration) was associated with less cellular injury than hypoxic perfusion. Modulation by various drugs or compensatory mechanisms can reduce tubular work load and prevent medullary hypoxic cellular injury. Among the compensatory mechanisms that reduce cellular injury are reduced tubular transport or reduced glomerular filtration. Afferent arterial vasoconstriction and consequent oliguria may be a protective response to acute tubular injury. By reducing ultrafiltration, energy-dependent ischemic injury to medullary tubular cells is prevented, even at the cost of retaining nitrogenous waste. Thus, in some cases the oliguria may protect against ARF.

CHRONIC RENAL FAILURE

Hypertensive nephrosclerosis and diabetic nephropathy continue to be the most common causes of end-stage renal disease (ESRD), each contributing about 30% of new cases each year. Cardiovascular complications remain the leading cause of morbidity and mortality in these patients. Among other causes of ESRD are primary glomerular disease (20%) and ARF (5%). The remaining 15% is a combination of unknown etiologies and uncommon causes. Approximately 14 new cases of ESRD per 100,000 are reported each year in the USA by Medicare. Although not necessarily the primary cause for ESRD, hypertension occurs in up to 85% of patients who have chronic renal failure (CRF) and is a major risk factor for their high cardiovascular morbidity.

HYPERTENSIVE RENAL DISEASE

Elevated serum creatinine [1.5–2.9mg/dL (133–257μmol/L)] is a risk factor for decreased survival when associated with essential hypertension. Control of hypertension is critical in modifying the rate of progression of renal insufficiency. Hypertension associated with CRF may be accompanied by reversible sympathetic activation, which appears to be mediated by an afferent signal arising in the failing kidneys. The increased sympathetic nerve discharge is unrelated to age, antihypertensive medication, total body volume, erythropoietin levels, or norepinephrine levels.

Although antihypertensive therapy has reduced mortality and morbidity from congestive heart failure and stroke, a reduction in the development of ESRD has not been clearly established. There is no conclusive evidence regarding the best type of antihypertensive medication (β blocker, clonidine, prazosin) in this regard. The progression of renal insufficiency is accelerated, however, if hypertension is treated only with a diuretic. Among the reasons for failure of antihypertensive treatment regimens to prevent ESRD caused by hypertension is the possibility that control of blood pressure is inadequate (i.e. target pressure may be too high). Another possibility is that antihypertensive drugs reduce systemic blood pressure but not intraglomerular blood pressure, because the preglomerular resistance vessels are dilated.

Therapy with ACE inhibitors can decrease proteinuria and preserve GFR in patients who have diabetes. These effects occur independently of changes in systemic blood pressure. It should be noted that calcium channel antagonists may have a similar effect to that of ACE inhibitors on the progression of CRF. The long-term influence of calcium antagonists on the rate of progression of renal failure in chronic renal disease is not known.

Implications of these findings for the anesthesiologist include the effect on risk stratification of renal insufficiency in the presence of mild versus severe hypertensive disease. The question remains whether primary renal disease has a worse prognosis than hypertensive renal disease for preservation of renal reserve. Studies that have considered perioperative morbidity and mortality in patients who have controlled hypertension compared with uncontrolled hypertension may need repeating with evaluation at lower target blood pressure levels. Calcium channel antagonists and ACE inhibitors both appear to have potential long-term advantages in delaying or preventing the progression of renal disease in essential hypertension as they are capable of a sustained reversal of renal vasoconstriction.

DIABETIC RENAL DISEASE

Between 30 and 45% of patients who have insulin-dependent diabetes mellitus ultimately develop diabetic nephropathy. This injury is preceded typically by glomerular hyperfiltration followed by progressive increase in urinary albumin excretion. Initial microalbuminuria and an associated increase in GFR progress to proteinuria (macroalbuminuria) and decreased in GFR. The decreased GFR is accompanied by histologic evidence of diffuse nodular glomerular sclerosis and heralds overt diabetic nephropathy, which leads eventually to ESRD. Noninsulin-dependent diabetes mellitus is characterized by glomerular hyperfiltration except in the presence of macroalbuminuria, which supports a hypothesis that hyperfiltration causes progressive glomerular damage. Increased protein flux across the glomerular capillary wall, decreased permeability, and a lower ultrafiltration coefficient at the glomerular basement membrane are contributing factors in the progression of diabetic nephropathy. Once macroalbuminuria develops, deterioration in renal function is rapid despite tight control of blood pressure. It is hypothesized that hyperfiltration (in early stages of diabetic renal disease) compensates for decreasing ultrafiltration capacity, which becomes overwhelming when macroalbuminuria becomes clinically evident.

Although control of associated hypertension in patients who have diabetes mellitus slows the progression of renal dysfunction, several other factors are implicated in renal function deterioration. The hyperfiltration seen in early stages of diabetic renal disease is related to metabolic status. Reduction in blood glucose with insulin infusion will cause the GFR to return to normal within hours. Besides hyperglycemia, other factors have been associated with the augmented GFR in incipient diabetic renal disease including increased levels of glucagon, growth hormone, and vasoactive hormones such as angiotensin II, catecholamines, and prostaglandins. In addition the response to circulating catecholamines is modified.

In general, GFR is determined by four factors: the rate of glomerular plasma flow as it influences ultrafiltration pressure and single-nephron GFR; systemic oncotic pressure; the glomerular transcapillary hydraulic pressure difference; and the glomerular capillary ultrafiltration coefficient, which represents the product of glomerular capillary hydraulic permeability and total surface area available for filtration (see Chapter 54). Initiation of the glomerulopathic process in diabetes most likely involves all four factors together or independently to increase glomerular pressure and flow. Hyperglycemia, for example, induces a state of extracellular fluid volume expansion, structural hypertrophy of the kidney, and altered glucoregulatory and vasoregulatory hormone action. These hemodynamic consequences of hyperglycemia lead to renal vasodilatation and increased plasma flow rate, which in turn causes increased glomerular transcapillary flux of plasma proteins. The elevation in glomerular flow (pressure) also alters the permeability and selectivity of the glomerular basement membrane, resulting in increased protein filtration. The increased transglomerular flux of plasma proteins leads to their accumulation in the mesangium, which serves further as a stimulus to proliferate glomerulosclerosis.

Drugs that inhibit ACE reduce glomerular capillary pressure, inhibit renal cell growth, and decrease glomerular capillary permeability to protein, thus retarding the development of glomerulosclerosis. It is thought that the beneficial effects of these drugs is through control of hypertension as well as through a direct effect on the glomerular basement membrane that results in reduced urinary protein excretion. The postulated mechanism is a reduction in mesangial cell protein flux, a decrease in serum lipid concentration, and decreased platelet stickiness.

RENAL FUNCTION AND ANESTHESIA

Anesthetic agents

All anesthetic agents, whether volatile or intravenous, can alter renal function by changing blood pressure and cardiac output so that intrarenal blood flow is redistributed. The redistribution is accompanied by sodium and water conservation and decreased urine formation. Inhalation anesthesia influences renal function primarily by affecting filtration and reabsorption and generally decreases GFR and renal blood flow. These changes are dose dependent and can be blunted by preoperative hydration. One typically observes a decrease in renal blood flow that is greater than the observed reduction in GFR, resulting in an observed increase in filtration fraction. The effect of any particular agent on autoregulation and intrarenal blood flow distribution is specific and dependent on renal perfusion pressure. The autoregulatory mechanism normally preserving renal blood flow includes the efferent arteriolar vasodilatation and vasoconstriction.

The renal nephrotoxic effects of older fluorinated inhalation anesthetics are attributed to increased levels of serum fluoride ions, which cause polyuric renal insufficiency. Prolonged use [9.6 minimum alveolar concentrations-hour (MAC)] of methoxyflurane (which is no longer used clinically) and enflurane cause an increase in serum free fluoride ions. Approximately 5% of sevoflurane is metabolized, a process that generates fluoride ions (see Chapter 24). A recent study has compared urine-concentrating ability after 9.5 MAC-hours of sevoflurane or enflurane anesthesia. Mean plasma fluoride levels were approximately twice as high in volunteers receiving sevoflurane than in those receiving enflurane; 43% of volunteers receiving sevoflurane had plasma fluoride levels that exceeded 95μg/dL (50μmol/L). However, the volunteers receiving sevoflurane did not show any impairment in the ability of the kidneys to concentrate the urine, whereas 20% of volunteers receiving enflurane had transient concentrating deficits on day 1.

The controversy that has arisen concerning the relationship between sevoflurane, nephrotoxicity, and compound A also deserves mention. Carbon dioxide absorbents degrade sevoflurane, resulting in detectable concentrations of the vinyl ether known as compound A, which is nephrotoxic in rats. The nephrotoxicity of compound A in rats involves degradation products that are conjugated in the liver with glutathione. Cysteine conjugates are formed in the bile ducts and kidney by cleavage of two amino acid residues. These conjugates are then metabolized in the kidney by cysteine-conjugate β-lyase to form end-products that cause renal injury characterized by diuresis, glucosuria, proteinuria, and elevated serum blood urea nitrogen (BUN) and creatinine. The degree of renal injury in rats is a function of the concentration of compound A and the duration of exposure. Humans have 10- to 30-fold less renal β-lyase enzyme activity compared with rats. In over 385 patients undergoing elective surgery with fresh gas flow <2L/min (duration of 2–8 hours), sevoflurane did not affect urine albumin, glucose, protein, and osmolality compared with values seen in those undergoing isoflurane anesthesia. In addition, there was no significant correlation in humans between compound A levels and sensitive markers of renal function.

Intraoperative events

A rare intraoperative event that may induce renal failure is hemoglobinuria. Hemoglobin is normally filtered at the glomerulus and enters the urine when the serum concentration is high (50–140mg/dL). If an acute hemolytic transfusion reaction occurs, a high hemoglobin load presented to the kidney can cause dysfunction. Myoglobin is filtered at the glomerulus at serum concentrations above 15mg/dL. Rhabdomyolysis, leading to myoglobinemia and myoglobinuria, may occur with or without renal dysfunction. In the operating room, rhabdomyolysis is most commonly a consequence of muscle ischemia resulting from, for example, arterial embolization or compartment syndrome following trauma. On occasion, myoglobinuria can be seen in the operating room after a traumatic crush injury. Intraoperative rhabdomyolysis may rarely be caused by hypokalemia, hypophosphatemia, myxedema, ethanol abuse, or malignant hyperthermia.

Intraoperative drugs

Gentamicin therapy exacerbates postischemic renal failure. The precise mechanism for exacerbating ischemic-induced reperfusion injury is important, because the timing of administration may affect the degree of renal injury. Gentamicin increased the severity of ARF to the same degree whether it was given before or after the ischemic event, indicating that gentamicin exacerbates postischemic ARF by adversely affecting reperfusion and postischemic compensatory mechanisms, not the ischemic injury process itself. In the normal kidney, gentamicin preferentially accumulates in the cortex, whereas in the postischemic kidney, it appears in the cortex and medulla. Among the commonly prescribed medications used in patients undergoing anesthesia, two in particular should be mentioned because of their ability to induce perioperative renal failure. Nonsteroidal anti-inflammatory drugs (NSAIDs) can induce renal insufficiency because of their action as potent afferent vasoconstrictors in the kidney. Glomerular filtration rate falls because renal blood flow is decreased. Anticholinesterase inhibitors may cause renal insufficiency in patients who have bilateral renal artery stenosis because of their vasodilator effect on the afferent and efferent arteriole, which decreases GFR (Fig. 57.8).

ANESTHESIA IN RENAL FAILURE

Maintenance of adequate blood flow to the kidney is determined by the ratio of renal artery vascular resistance to systemic vascular resistance. Indeed, norepinephrine, despite its vasoconstricting effect, has no deleterious renal effects in patients who have low systemic vascular resistance. Interventions to prevent ischemic renal failure should be designed to preserve the balance between renal blood flow and oxygen delivery, on one hand, and oxygen demand, on the other. There is a physiologically important reason for the paucity of blood flow and, consequently, oxygenation in the medulla. The vasa recta carrying blood to the medulla are arranged in a 'hairpin loop' pattern to allow a countercurrent exchange of solute to maintain the medullary osmotic gradient. A limited blood flow through the vasa recta allows equilibration between the blood and interstitium; this prevents wash-out of solute from the medulla but also limits the medullary partial oxygen pressure to 10–15mmHg. The high metabolic requirement of the thick ascending limb of the loop of Henle in an hypoxic environment makes it especially vulnerable to injury associated with an imbalance in oxygen supply and demand.

Important considerations for the anesthesiologist treating patients who have CRF include extracellular volume status, anemia, acid–base and electrolyte abnormalities, platelet dysfunction, susceptibility to infection, hypertension, left ventricular dysfunction, pericarditis, and neurologic dysfunction. Most of the fluid, electrolyte, acid–base, neurologic, and platelet abnormalities improve with dialysis. Anemia is well-tolerated because tissue blood flow increases with decreased blood viscosity and increased cardiac output. Rightward shift of the oxyhemoglobin dissociation curve as a result of metabolic acidosis and an increased concentration of diphosphoglycerate also aid tissue oxygenation. Adverse drug reactions occur in renal failure through decreased renal excretion, decreased renal metabolism, decreased hepatic metabolism, and altered volume of distribution owing to decreased protein binding and lipid solubility. Reduced protein binding and uremia-induced alterations in the blood–brain barrier in renal disease may result in the need for lower induction doses of intravenous drugs. Accumulation of morphine glucuronides may account for the prolonged depression of ventilation observed in some patients who have renal failure. Drug interactions and altered end-organ responses also contribute to abnormal drug reactions.

Dopamine

Dopamine was first synthesized chemically in the early 1900s. However, its unique renal effects were not appreciated until the 1960s when Goldberg and colleagues demonstrated that low-dose dopamine, in contrast to other catecholamines, increased renal plasma flow, GFR, and urinary sodium

Drugs altering the glomerular blood supply		
Vessels	**Vasodilators**	**Vasoconstrictors**
Afferent arteriole	β_2-Adrenergic agonists, dopamine agonists, acetylcholine, prostaglandin E_2, angiotensin-converting enzyme (ACE) inhibitors	Renin, thromboxane, nonsteroidal anti-inflammatory agents, vecuronium
Efferent arteriole	ACE inhibitors, acetylcholine	Angiotensin II

Figure 57.8 Drugs affecting glomerular blood supply.

excretion. Consequently it has been suggested that this agent would be useful therapy in acute perioperative renal failure. Dopamine dose-dependently activates a wide range of receptors. Low-dose dopamine causes activation of dopamine receptors and as the dose is increased β- and then α-adrenoceptors are activated. The multiplicity of receptors activated and the wide interpatient variability of responses have made it difficult to predict the precise infusion rate required for each patient. Consequently, the maximum dose at which dopamine affects only dopamine receptors must be individually determined. In addition, up- and downregulation of receptors occur; as a result, in any one patient the appropriate dose for a given action can vary over time.

Two peripheral dopamine receptor subtypes have been identified: D_{1A} and D_{2A}. These receptors are primarily responsible for the actions observed when 'renal dose' (low-dose) dopamine is administered. Low doses of dopamine increase renal blood flow and GFR and directly inhibit proximal tubular sodium reabsorption. This results in increased sodium excretion in euvolemic subjects who have normal renal function, although dopamine is not always natriuretic in critically ill patients. Importantly, this response diminishes with prolonged infusion. Regulation of renal sodium excretion depends on an intricate interaction between natriuretic vasodilatory and antinatriuretic vasoconstrictive influences. The use of a single natriuretic vasodilatory agent such as dopamine is unlikely to countermand the effects of the multiple mediators that may be activated to conserve sodium.

Although dopamine causes an increase in glomerular filtration in patients who have normal renal function, patients who have a baseline GFR of less than 70mL/min have no increase in glomerular filtration with low-dose dopamine infusions. This lack of response may be attributed to exhaustion of the renal reserve capacity in patients who have depressed renal function. For example, in chronic renal disease, blood flow has already been shifted to the inner cortex as an adaptive response to the loss of nephron function; consequently, dopamine will have minimal additional effect. There is considerable disagreement concerning the effect of low-dose dopamine on urine output. Despite the limitations in obtaining accurate data regarding changes in urine output, it appears that low-dose dopamine increases urine output in some oliguric patients and in patients with good renal function who are adequately hydrated.

Until definitive studies are available, it would be premature to conclude that dopamine is advantageous in the treatment of oliguric renal failure. The use of low-dose dopamine to protect the kidney from ischemic or toxic insult is based on even more dubious data. Although dopamine has been shown to preserve blood flow in animals treated with norepinephrine, the implication of this finding for critically ill hypotensive humans is unclear. Even in animal models, dopamine appears to be no better than saline in preserving renal function. In the few studies that have examined the effects of dopamine in patients who have ARF, there is no evidence that dopamine preserves or improves renal function. If dopamine-induced natriuresis produces intravascular volume depletion, the kidney may actually be made more susceptible to ischemic injury. There is little evidence as yet to support the theoretic advantages of routinely using prophylactic low-dose dopamine. Furthermore, dopamine may increase the potential for ventricular arrhythmias and myocardial ischemia by causing a deleterious shift in the myocardial oxygen supply-and-demand balance. Respiratory depression by intravenous dopamine has been described in animals as well as in humans. Apparently, low-dose dopamine can reduce arterial oxygen partial pressure through effects on peripheral chemoreceptors.

Mannitol

Mannitol is an osmotic diuretic that promotes free water diuresis by acting as a nonreabsorbable solute (primarily in the proximal tubule). Mannitol effectively causes an expansion of extracellular volume by shifting fluid from the intracellular to the extracellular compartment, with consequent increases in renal blood flow, GFR, and renal tubular flow. Recently, it has been demonstrated that mannitol affects the pressure–flow relationship in the kidney such that higher renal blood flow occurs at similar (or lower) levels of renal perfusion pressures. However, the mechanism by which mannitol increases renal blood flow is not known, or its exact consequence. The effect of mannitol on renal blood flow is thought to be secondary to release of intrarenal prostaglandins or ANP, decreased intravascular cell swelling or decreased renin production, and/or an increase in intravascular volume. Although it is tempting to presume that increasing renal blood flow is beneficial, especially when oxygen and nutrient delivery is compromised, it may not necessarily be so. Another critical unanswered question is what effect mannitol has on intrarenal blood flow distribution. The inner cortex and medulla would stand to benefit the most from increases in oxygen and nutrient delivery when the kidney is susceptible to hypoxic injury, whereas increases in renal blood flow to the outer cortex may tax the kidney at a time that it can least afford.

Theoretic benefits of mannitol can be predicted from its other actions coupled with an understanding of the pathophysiology associated with acute perioperative renal failure. As mentioned previously, mannitol reduces reabsorption of sodium chloride, potassium, phosphate, and water in the proximal tubule, sodium chloride in the thick ascending limb of the loop of Henle, and water in the collecting duct. These are all energy-consuming processes. In addition to preserving oxygen balance by decreasing demand, mannitol may relieve vascular congestion and the endothelial cell edema that may result from hypoperfusion of the medulla. Given the paucity of clinical data demonstrating the benefit of mannitol in preserving renal function, one must carefully weigh its risks (i.e. intravascular volume depletion following acute volume overload, hyperosmolarity, hypokalemia, and hyponatremia) with its theoretic benefit.

Mannitol has been administered with the rationale that preventing cell swelling and increasing intratubular flow might decrease intratubular obstruction and mitigate renal dysfunction. Furosemide (frusemide) and bumetanide have also been used to increase intratubular flow rates. Mannitol and other osmotic agents help to preserve transplanted kidneys *ex vivo* and prevent delayed graft dysfunction, which is most often caused by ischemia. Mannitol is recommended, along with vigorous volume replacement and sodium bicarbonate, for the prevention and treatment of early myoglobinemic ARF and is used with adequate hydration to prevent the nephrotoxic effects of cisplatin.

Although mannitol and furosemide have been shown to help to protect the kidney against ischemic injury in animals, most studies in humans have failed to demonstrate their efficacy in the prevention or treatment of ischemic or toxic ARF. Both mannitol and loop diuretics, if administered early in the course of ischemic ARF, can convert an oliguric to a nonoliguric state, although there is little evidence that this decreases the mortality rate. Patients who respond to diuretics may have less severe renal damage at baseline than those who have no response. Finally, diuretics can be detrimental in ARF induced by radiocontrast agents. At this time, the use of loop diuretics can only be justified to increase urine output for fluid management, with no expectation that these agents will improve outcome.

Calcium channel blockers and other agents

Calcium channel blockers have been advocated as renovascular vasodilators. Vasoconstriction occurs, in part, as a consequence of increased free calcium levels within vascular smooth muscle, causing increased vascular tone. In renal transplantation, calcium channel blockers reduce the incidence of tubular necrosis and delayed graft dysfunction. Calcium channel blockers reduce the vasoconstrictive effect of cyclosporine (cyclosporin A) and may prevent the vasoconstrictive consequences of radiocontrast agents. However, caution should be exercised because the indiscriminate use of calcium channel blockers may be associated with systemic hypotension and low renal perfusion. Calcium channel blockers are, therefore, not recommended or justified in most forms of ARF.

Other agents

Nitric oxide reduces vascular tone in both preglomerular and postglomerular arterioles. At renal perfusion pressure at the lower end of the normal range for autoregulation, nitric oxide is essential to maintain autoregulation.

The effects of adenosine on the kidney are complex. Under conditions of low blood flow, it appears that endogenous adenosine is produced by the kidney. This increases medullary oxygenation at the expense of the cortex, thereby protecting the more vulnerable inner cortical and medullary cells from anoxic damage. Interestingly, systemic administration of exogenous adenosine compromises oxygenation throughout the kidney.

Perioperative oliguria

Premedication and anesthetic drugs may increase or decrease catecholamines, alter renal vascular resistance, depress the myocardium and, therefore, renal blood flow, or have a direct nephrotoxic effect on renal tubular function. Surgery in general, aortic cross-clamping and declamping in particular, trauma, and stress also may influence urine formation by changing myocardial function, sympathetic activity, neuronal or hormonal activity, intravascular volume, or systemic vascular resistance. During general anesthesia, ureteral peristalsis may affect the rate of urine output measured with a Foley catheter. Basal peristalsis within the ureter is influenced by the autonomic nervous system. All of the general anesthetic agents decrease the frequency and force of ureteral contraction and, thus, urine formation. All anesthetic agents alter renal function by changing blood pressure and cardiac output so that renal blood flow in the inner cortex is redistributed, causing sodium and water conservation (i.e. decreased urine formation). Regional anesthesia above level T4 reduces sympathetic tone to the kidney, making renal blood flow and filtration depend directly on perfusion pressure.

Monitoring urine output as a sign of the adequacy of renal perfusion is based on the assumption that patients who have diminished renal perfusion excrete a low volume of concentrated urine. Urinary flow rate and volume are indirect markers of renal function because of the many nonrenal factors that also influence renal function. Urine flow (regardless of the amount) indicates blood flow to the kidney because glomerular filtration and the generation of urine can only occur if perfusion occurs. However, many studies have shown no correlation between urine volume and histologic evidence of acute tubular necrosis; reduction in GFR or creatinine clearance; or changes from preoperative to postoperative levels of blood urea, BUN, or creatinine in patients who have burn injuries, trauma, cardiovascular surgery, or shock states.

Decreased renal perfusion initiates a series of systemic and renal compensatory responses that preserve ultrafiltration. At this stage, glomerular filtration and renal blood flow are maintained by increased distribution of blood flow to the kidney, selective afferent vasodilatation, efferent vasoconstriction, and increased sodium and water conservation. If these protective mechanisms fail and renal blood flow decreases further, afferent arterial vasoconstriction ensues and causes a consequent decrease in capillary hydrostatic pressure and ultrafiltration. As this happens, blood flow and glomerular filtration in the outer cortical nephrons decline because redistribution of renal blood flow protects the vulnerable medullary oxygen balance. Decreased glomerular filtration during compromised flow, therefore, appears to be protective because decreased urine delivery to the tubules requires less reabsorptive work and prevents further oxygen supply-and-demand imbalance.

Modulation by various drugs or compensatory mechanisms can reduce tubular work load and prevent medullary hypoxic cellular injury. Among the compensatory mechanisms that reduce cellular injury are reduced tubular transport and glomerular filtration. Consequently, in some patients selective vasoconstriction may protect against ARF. The beneficial effect of renal vasodilators depends on the regional effects these agents have within the kidney in each specific patient, which is currently unknown. For example, whether low-dose dopamine (a known renal vasodilator) is beneficial remains uncertain since the answer depends on its primary site of action (i.e. an increase in outer cortical flow or vasodilatation of the inner cortex). If vasodilatation causes an increase in renal blood flow and consequent glomerular filtration at a time when the kidney can least afford it because of reduced oxygen delivery, then damage can be potentiated rather than diminished. This paradox underscores the difficulties of renal failure management and may indicate why our management record is so dismal.

Key References

Badr KF, Ichikawa I. Prerenal failure: a deleterious shift from renal compensation to decompensation. N Engl J Med. 1988;319:623–9.

Charlson ME, MacKenzie CR, Gold JP, Shires GT. Postoperative changes in serum creatinine. When do they occur and how much is important? Ann Surg. 1989;209:328–33.

Alpen SL, Lodish HF. Molecular Biology of Renal Function. In:Brenner BM, Rector FC Jr, eds. The kidney, 4th edn. Philadelphia, PA: Saunders; 1991:132-163

Myers BD, Moran SM. Hemodynamically mediated acute renal failure. N Engl J Med. 1986;314:97–105.

Novis BK, Roizen MF, Aronson S, Thisted RA. Association of preoperative risk factors with postoperative acute renal failure. Anesth Analg. 1994;78:143–9.

Shusterman N, Strom BL, Murray TG, et al. Risk factors and outcome of hospital-acquired acute renal failure. Clinical epidemiologic study. Am J Med. 1987;83:65–71.

Valtin H. Renal dysfunction: mechanisms involved in fluid and solute inbalance. Boston, Ma: Little Brown; 1979.

Further Reading

Kellen M, Aronson S, Roizen MF, Barnard J, Thisted RA. Predictive and diagnostic tests of renal failure: a review. Anesth Analg. 1994;78:134–42.

Kharasch ED. Metabolism and toxicity of the new anesthetic agents. (Review) Acta Anaesthesiol Belg. 1996;47:7–14.

Sladen RN. Effect of anesthesia and surgery on renal function. Crit Care Clin. 1987;3:373–93.

Thadhani R, Pascual M, Bonventre JV. Acute renal failure. (Review) N Engl J Med. 1996;334:1448–60.

Chapter 58 Gut motility and secretions

Howard M Thompson and David J Rowbotham

Topics covered in this chapter

Basic anatomy
Regulation and integration of gut function
Peristalsis
Swallowing
Gastric motility and secretions
Motility patterns in the small intestine
Motility patterns in the large intestine

The primary function of the gut is to extract water and nutrients from food. This involves the processes of *digestion*, whereby food is broken down, and *absorption* of its constituents by the intestinal mucosa into the portal circulation.

Both chemical and physical factors are important in digestion. Food is chewed and mixed with salivary amylase in the mouth prior to swallowing. In the stomach, it is softened and disintegrated into smaller particles first by the action of gastric acid and enzymes, and second by mechanical churning through muscular contractions of the stomach wall. Salivary amylase and gastric pepsin start the enzymatic breakdown of nutrients, which continues in the small intestine with the addition of pancreatic enzymes. The end result is the formation of a liquefied residue called chyme.

Gastric chyme is ejected incrementally through the pylorus into the duodenum. Biliary and pancreatic secretions are added and mixed thoroughly with the intraluminal contents by gut wall contractions. Eventually, the products of digestion are brought into contact with the absorptive surfaces of the small intestine. Undigested matter is passed into the large intestine prior to voiding by defecation.

A high degree of control is required to allow the secretory processes and various motility patterns to occur in an orderly and efficient manner. Such control and coordination is achieved by a complex interplay of neural and humoral influences that occur as food passes through the gut.

BASIC ANATOMY

Essentially, the gut is a long muscular tube, lined with epithelial mucosa, that extends from the oropharynx to the anal sphincter. Although the structure of the gut wall varies in different regions of the tract, generally it comprises an outer longitudinal and an inner circular layer of smooth muscle (Fig. 58.1). Anatomically and physiologically it is divided into four distinct regions – esophagus, stomach, small intestine (duodenum, jejunum, and ileum), and large intestine (cecum, colon, and rectum).

REGULATION AND INTEGRATION OF GUT FUNCTION

The function of the gut is coordinated by a complex interplay between the autonomic nervous system (neurocrine secretion), paracrine secretion, and endocrine (hormonal) activity.

Nervous system

The gut is innervated by the autonomic nervous system, which comprises extrinsic (to the gut), sympathetic, and parasympathetic elements together with an intrinsic network called the enteric nervous system (ENS). The ENS is organized into a number of anatomically distinct networks, of which the best described are the *myenteric (Auerbach's) plexus* and *submucosal (Meissner's) plexus* (see Fig. 58.1). The myenteric plexus is located between the circular and longitudinal layers of smooth muscle, and extends the length of the gut, including the upper esophagus where the muscle is striated. The myenteric plexus has an essential role in the generation of peristaltic activity. The submucosal plexus is located between the circular smooth muscle layer and the mucosa. It is most developed in the small intestine, where it is involved in secretory control.

Extensive afferent and efferent communication occurs between the sympathetic and parasympathetic systems and the ENS. Activity in the ENS results in the release of neurotransmitters (neurocrines), which have effects on other nerve cells, smooth muscle cells, paracrine cells, and endocrine cells. The number of identified neurotransmitters of the ENS continues to rise (Fig. 58.2) – more than 20 have now been identified in enteric neurons with most neurons containing several of them. *Acetylcholine* (ACh) and *tachykinins*, such as *substance P*, cause smooth muscle contraction. *Vasoactive intestinal peptide* (VIP), *nitric oxide* (NO), and *adenosine triphosphate* (ATP) are inhibitory to smooth muscle. *5-Hydroxytryptamine* (5-HT) is released by stimulation of the mucosa and involved in the initiation of the peristaltic reflex.

Paracrines

Paracrines are chemicals that diffuse through interstitial fluid to exert an effect close to their site of release. Although paracrines

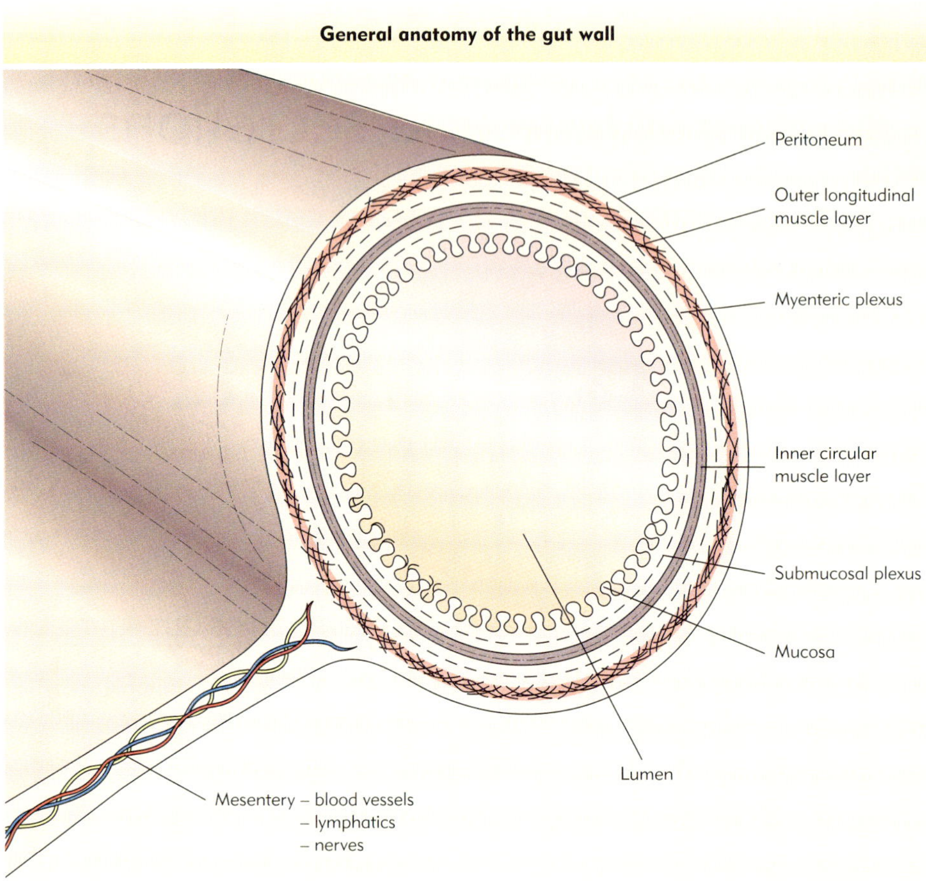

Figure 58.1 General anatomy of the gut wall. The gut is a muscular tube that extends from the oropharynx to the anus and consists of two muscle layers – an inner layer of circular muscle and an outer layer of longitudinally arranged fibers. The luminal surface is lined with mucosa and the outer surface is invested with visceral peritoneum. The ENS consists of two main networks – the myenteric plexus lies between the longitudinal and circular layers of smooth muscle, and the submucosal plexus lies between the circular smooth muscle layer and the mucosa. Blood vessels, lymphatics, and nerves reach the gut by means of the mesentery.

exert only a direct local action, they may bring about more widespread effects, either because the cells from which they are secreted are scattered over a wide area of mucosa, or because they influence the release of gut hormones from endocrine cells. Histamine and somatostatin are important gut paracrines. Enterochromaffin-like (ECL) cells secrete histamine by decarboxylation of histidine; histamine is involved in the control of gastric acid secretion. Somatostatin is found throughout the gastric and duodenal mucosa and in the pancreas. It reduces gut secretions by exerting an inhibitory effect on all of the gut hormones and a direct inhibitory effect on parietal cells.

Hormones

Gut hormones are released from endocrine cells into the bloodstream to exert remote actions by means of specific receptor interaction in a target tissue. Like the neurocrines, many substances have been identified with potential gut hormone activity. Five peptide hormones are recognized as being most important (see Fig. 58.2) – gastrin, cholecystokinin (CCK), secretin, gastric inhibitory peptide (GIP), and motilin.

Gastrin and CCK share the same sequence of five C-terminal amino acids (-Gly-Trp-Met-Asp-Phe), which results in a degree of cross receptor activity. Some gut hormones demonstrate heterogeneity – gastrin, CCK, and secretin exist in more than one molecular form. Many factors influence the release of these hormones, of which vagal stimulation, gut distention, and the presence of intraluminal acid and nutrients are physiologically the most important (Fig. 58.3).

Gut endocrine cells are widely distributed throughout the gastrointestinal mucosa, and belong to the group of secretory cells known as *amine precursor uptake* and *decarboxylation cells*. Gastrin is released from G cells located in the gastric antral mucosa and to a lesser extent in the duodenum. Cells that secrete CCK, secretin, GIP, and motilin are located in the small intestine, particularly in the duodenum and jejunum.

Gastrin

The main role of gastrin is stimulation of gastric acid and pepsin secretion. Acid itself has an inhibitory influence on gastrin release, thus providing a negative feedback system. Gastric distention, the presence of products of protein digestion in the stomach, and vagal stimulation cause gastrin release. Vagal innervation of the G cell is unusual in that it is not cholinergic, but involves *gastrin-releasing peptide (GRP)*.

Cholecystokinin

Not only does CCK cause contraction of the gallbladder and stimulate secretion of enzymes and alkaline fluid by the exocrine pancreas, but also it inhibits the rate of gastric emptying. The main stimulus for CCK secretion is the presence of peptides, amino acids, and fatty acids (chain length >10 carbon groups) in the duodenal lumen.

Secretin

Secretin is released when duodenal pH falls below 4–5. It inhibits gastric acid secretion and at the same time promotes secretion

Chemical mediators in the gut and their physiologic actions

Neurotransmitter	Main Physiologic Functions
Gastrin-releasing peptide (GRP)	Vagal stimulation of gastrin secretion
Acetylcholine (ACh)	Smooth muscle contraction, peristalsis
Substance P	Smooth muscle contraction, peristalsis Possible visceral nociception
Vasoactive intestinal peptide (VIP)	Smooth muscle relaxation, peristalsis Relaxation of sphincters, vasodilatation
Nitric oxide (NO)	Smooth muscle relaxation, peristalsis
Adenosine triphosphate (ATP)	Smooth muscle relaxation, peristalsis
5-hydroxytryptamine (5-HT)	Activation of peristalsis, generation of nausea
Calcitonin gene-related peptide	Possible role in visceral nociception
Somatostatin	Inhibition of release of gut hormones Inhibition of gut secretions
Paracrine	**Main Physiologic Functions**
Histamine	Stimulation of gastric acid secretion
Somatostatin	Inhibition of release of gut hormones Inhibition of gut secretions
Gut Hormone	**Main Physiologic Functions**
Gastrin	Stimulation of gastric acid secretion Stimulation of pepsin secretion Maintenance of gastrointestinal mucosal integrity
Cholecystokinin (CCK)	Stimulation of gallbladder contraction Stimulation of pancreatic exocrine secretion Inhibition of gastric emptying Trophic action on exocrine pancreas
Secretin	Inhibition of gastric acid secretion Stimulation of pepsin Stimulation of pancreatic alkaline secretion Stimulation of biliary alkaline secretion Trophic action on exocrine pancreas
Gastric inhibitory peptide (GIP)	Stimulation of insulin release Inhibition of gastric acid secretion
Motilin	Generation of the migrating motor complex

Figure 58.2 Chemical mediators in the gut and their physiologic actions. Several chemical mediators [neurotransmitters (neurocrines), paracrines, and gut hormones (endocrines)] identified in gastrointestinal nerve, paracrine, and endocrine cells have established physiologic actions. Many other potential mediators have been identified, but as yet their physiologic effects are not fully elucidated.

of biliary and pancreatic alkaline fluid. In this way, secretin neutralizes the acidity of gastric fluid as it enters the duodenum.

Gastric inhibitory peptide

When GIP was first identified it appeared to cause inhibition of gastric secretions and was therefore named 'gastric inhibitory peptide'. This inhibitory effect is now thought to be less important at normal physiologic concentrations of GIP. Carbohydrate and fat in the duodenum cause its release, after which it acts as a stimulus for insulin release in preparation for the imminent arrival of absorbed substrate from the gut.

Motilin

Motilin is involved in the regulation of interdigestive gut motility. It is released in a cyclic manner during fasting with a periodicity of 1–2 hours. It stimulates a burst of peristalsis, the migrating motor complex, which starts in the stomach and then sweeps through the small intestine, clearing it of undigested matter and other debris in preparation for the next meal.

Trophic effects

In addition to their influence on gut motility and secretions, some gut hormones also exert important *trophic* effects. Gastrin is an essential factor in maintaining gastrointestinal mucosal integrity, and CCK and secretin are involved in growth of the exocrine pancreas.

PERISTALSIS

Peristalsis is the reflex propagation of a wave of muscular contraction along the gut wall. It is an important component of gut motility as it creates a tendency for the intraluminal contents to be propelled along in the normal anterograde manner. Peristalsis is an inherent property of the gut that continues even when the gut is denervated from its extrinsic autonomic connections. The ENS, particularly the myenteric plexus, has a pivotal role in the generation of peristaltic waves. Extrinsic autonomic influence modulates activity – parasympathetic activity tends to increase peristalsis and sympathetic activity to inhibit it.

Distention of the gut wall and release of 5-HT (because of mucosal stimulation) initiate the peristaltic reflex (Fig. 58.4). Activity in sensory afferents stimulates cholinergic interneurons that pass both proximally and distally in the myenteric plexus. Proximally, the release of ACh and substance P from excitatory motoneurons mediates contraction of circular smooth muscle. At the same time, distal smooth muscle relaxation is brought about by the release of VIP, NO, and ATP from inhibitory motoneurons. A 'ring' of contraction develops behind the food bolus to propel it along the gut. The same pattern of reflex activity is then activated in a more distal segment of gut, and thus the wave of peristalsis is propagated forward.

SWALLOWING

Swallowing, or deglutition, occurs after food has been chewed, or masticated, in the mouth. Saliva, secreted from the parotid, submandibular, and sublingual glands during chewing, is mixed with food to act as a lubricant. Saliva also has an antibacterial action, helps buffer any gastric acid that may regurgitate into the esophagus, and initiates carbohydrate digestion by way of its amylase content.

The esophagus is a continuation of the pharynx. In its proximal third it comprises striated muscle and in this region innervation of the motor end plate by efferents from the myenteric plexus is uniquely mediated by NO. Striated muscle is replaced gradually by smooth muscle such that by the distal third of the esophagus all the muscle is smooth. There is the typical arrangement of outer longitudinal and inner circular muscle layers. At the pharyngoesophageal junction, the muscle is thickened to form the upper esophageal sphincter (UES). At the gastro-esophageal

Physiologic Stimulants for the Release of Gut Hormones

	Vagal stimulation	Peptides, amino acids	Fatty acids	Carbohydrate	Hydrogen ions	Gastric distension
Gastrin	Stimulation	Stimulation			Inhibition	Stimulation
CCK		Stimulation	Stimulation			
Secretin					Stimulation	
GIP			Stimulation	Stimulation		
Motilin	Stimulation					

Figure 58.3 Physiologic stimulants for the release of gut hormones.

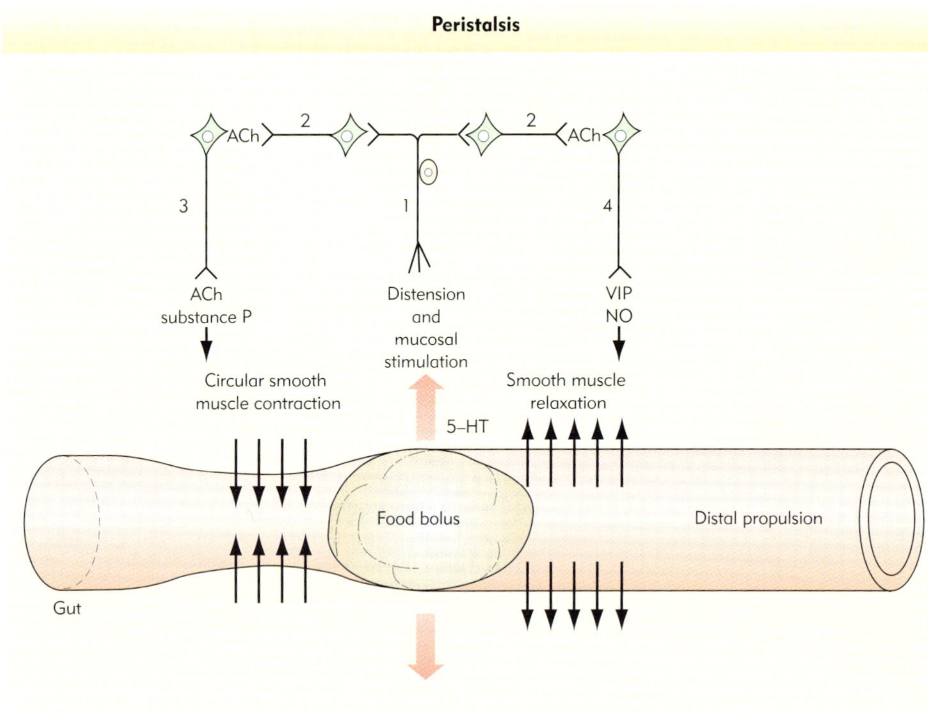

Figure 58.4 Peristalsis. The peristaltic reflex is initiated by distention of the gut wall and the release of 5-HT by mucosal stimulation. Elements of the ENS are involved in the coordination of this reflex. Stimulation of sensory afferents (1) causes a biphasic response in fibers of the myenteric plexus. Proximal to the site of stimulus, cholinergic interneurons (2) relay the signal to excitatory motorneurons (3) which cause ACh- and substance P-mediated contraction of the circular muscle layer. Simultaneously, other cholinergic interneurons (2) relay the signal to distal inhibitory motoneurons (4). Here, the release of VIP, NO, and ATP mediates relaxation of smooth muscle. In this way, the food bolus is propelled forward to initiate the same pattern of neuronal activity distally, thus propagating the peristaltic wave.

junction, the lower esophageal sphincter (LES) is found. In the resting state, both the UES and LES are closed with resting tone considerably higher than in the adjacent esophagus.

Swallowing can be initiated by voluntary action, but once underway proceeds as an involuntary reflex. It is triggered by afferent impulses in the trigeminal (V), glossopharyngeal (IX), and vagus (X) cranial nerves. Integration of the reflex takes place in the nucleus ambiguus and the nucleus of the tractus solitarius with efferent innervation via the trigeminal (V), facial (VII), vagus (X), and hypoglossal (XII) nerves. Chewed food is formed into a bolus and propelled backward into the oropharynx by the tongue. Upward displacement of the soft palate and contraction of the superior constrictor muscle prevent retrograde passage of food into the nasopharynx. Sequential contraction of the superior, middle, and inferior constrictor muscles propels the food bolus into the esophagus. As the food passes through the oropharynx reflex closure of the larynx and inhibition of respiration occurs. Upward movement of the larynx and folding back of the epiglottis protect the laryngeal inlet.

A peristaltic ring of contraction transports the food bolus distally down the esophagus at a velocity of 2–4cm/s. Thus, it takes approximately 10–15s to pass through the 30cm esophagus and enter the stomach. Coordinated relaxation of the UES and LES occurs as the food bolus passes. This sphincteric relaxation may be mediated by NO.

Any food that fails to be swept into the stomach with the *primary peristaltic wave* causes *secondary peristalsis* by way of mechanical stimulation of the esophagus. Secondary peristalsis also occurs whenever esophageal reflux of gastric juice occurs.

GASTRIC MOTILITY AND SECRETIONS

In the stomach, food is temporarily stored while the process of digestion begins. Digestion is achieved by the action of acid and enzymes together with gastric motility patterns that churn up the food and break it down into smaller particles, which eventually become liquefied into gastric chyme.

Gastric juice

The normal stomach secretes approximately 2 liters of gastric juice per day. It is comprised of four main components: hydrochloric acid, pepsin, mucus, and intrinsic factor.

Hydrochloric acid is necessary to activate *pepsin*, from its proenzyme *pepsinogen*; pepsin initiates protein digestion. Low gastric pH is also important to prevent microbial growth. *Mucus* is an essential component in mucosal cytoprotection against the effects of acid, pepsin, and mechanical damage. *Intrinsic factor* is required for the efficient absorption of vitamin B_{12} in the terminal ileum.

Oxyntic glands (Fig. 58.5) play a central role in the production of gastric juice and are located in the main body and fundus of the stomach. These complex structures contain several cell types, including *parietal cells, peptic (or chief) cells*, and *mucus secreting cells*. The parietal cells secrete hydrochloric acid and intrinsic factor, and the peptic cells secrete pepsinogen.

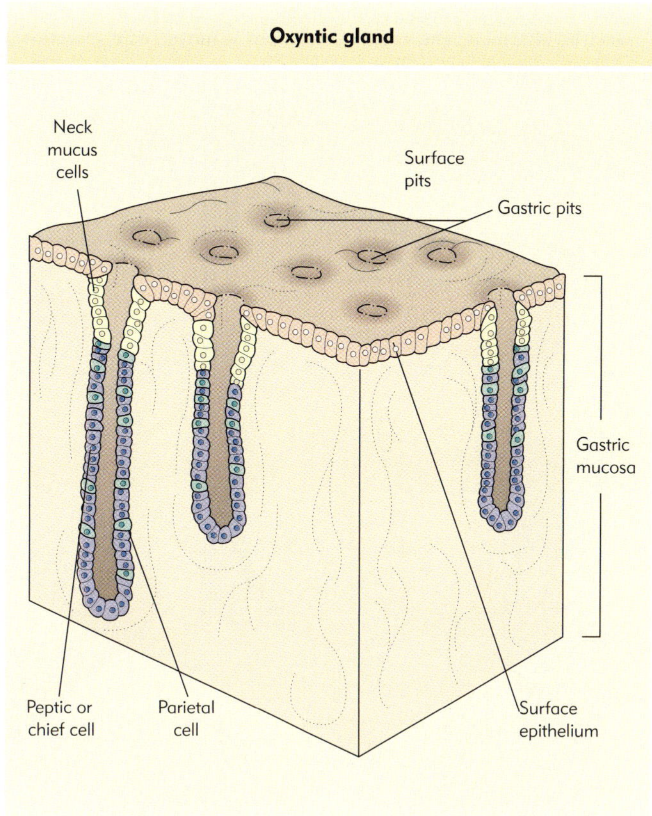

Figure 58.5 Oxyntic gland. Oxyntic glands are found in the main body and fundus of the stomach. They are complex structures that contain several specialized epithelial cell types. Parietal cells secrete hydrochloric acid and intrinsic factor. Peptic (or chief) cells secrete pepsinogen, which is converted into pepsin in the gastric lumen. Mucus cells at the neck of the gland secrete soluble mucus, which mixes with the gastric chyme to act as a lubricant. Oxyntic glands open onto the luminal surface of the stomach to form gastric pits.

Control of gastric acid secretion

The human stomach contains one billion parietal cells, each one capable of secreting three billion hydrogen ions (H^+) per second to produce gastric acid with a pH <1. At the cellular level three chemical mediators are important in the control of gastric acid secretion (Fig. 58.6) – blood-borne *gastrin* from G cells, *ACh* from vagal efferents, and *histamine* from ECL cells.

G-cell derived gastrin is secreted into the bloodstream, in which it equilibrates with interstitial fluid. In the gastric mucosa, gastrin binds to specific surface receptors on both parietal and histamine-secreting ECL cells. Thus, gastrin has two actions – it stimulates directly the parietal cell to secrete acid and it simulates the release of histamine from ECL cells. The histamine has as a paracrine effect and diffuses through interstitial fluid to nearby parietal cells, at which interaction with H_2 receptors activates acid secretion.

Increased *vagal tone* causes acid secretion by stimulation of G cell, ECL cell, and parietal cell types. The neurotransmitter at the ECL cell and parietal cell is ACh, via an M_3 receptor, whereas GRP serves this role at the G cell. Thus vagally mediated acid secretion is brought about directly by stimulation of the parietal cell, and indirectly by gastrin and histamine release.

In the parietal cell, two second-messenger systems are activated to bring about the synthesis and release of H^+. Gastrin and ACh activate the phospholipase C–inositol trisphosphate (PLC–IP_3) system, whereas histamine activates the adenylyl cyclase–cyclic adenosine monophosphate (AC–cAMP) system.

The final common pathway is activation of the luminal membrane H^+,K^+-ATPase, the so-called 'proton pump', which actively transports H^+ into the gastric lumen in exchange for extracellular K^+. The energy required to pump H^+ against the four million-fold concentration gradient (parietal cytoplasm pH is 7.3 versus the luminal pH of <1) is provided by mitochondria that occupy a high proportion of the cytoplasmic volume in the parietal cell. In the resting state, H^+,K^+-ATPase is not in the apical membrane, but in the membranes of tubulovesicles contained within the cytoplasm. When the parietal cell is stimulated to secrete acid, these tubulovesicles fuse with the apical membrane, which increases its surface area greatly and exposes H^+,K^+-ATPase to the gastric lumen.

Generation of H^+ within the parietal cell (see Fig. 58.6) starts with the formation of carbonic acid (H_2CO_2) from carbon dioxide (CO_2) and water (H_2O) catalyzed by carbonic anhydrase (CA). Carbonic acid disassociates into bicarbonate (HCO_3^-) and H^+.

The physiologic influences that control gastric acid production (Fig. 58.7) may be considered in terms of cephalic factors (those that involve the brain), gastric factors (those produced by the presence of food in the stomach), and intestinal factors (those that arise from the transit of food into the duodenum).

Gastric acid secretion starts before food enters the stomach as a consequence of *cephalic factors*. Anticipation, sight, smell, taste, and the acts of chewing and swallowing all initiate, and then perpetuate, acid secretion by stimulation of vagal efferents via the vagal nuclei in the brainstem.

In the *gastric phase*, entry of food into the stomach results in acid secretion in a number of ways. In the empty stomach, low gastric pH (<3) reduces gastrin release from G cells by a direct inhibitory action. Food buffers the low pH and arrests this inhibition. Distention of the stomach by ingested food results in a number of neuronally mediated reflexes to increase acid secretion. Mechanoreceptor activation in the stomach wall sends sensory information via vagal afferents to the brainstem. Stimulation of the vagal nuclei results in efferent vagal activity that leads to acid secretion. As both afferent and efferent limbs of this reflex are vagal, it has been called the *vagovagal reflex*. In addition, two local distention reflexes occur. Localized stretching of the stomach causes gastrin release from G cells (*pyloropyloric reflex*) and acid secretion from parietal cells (*pyloro-oxyntic reflex*). Finally, peptides and amino acids from protein digestion have a direct effect on G cells in both the gastric antrum and duodenum to stimulate gastrin secretion. This intestinal factor is of relatively minor importance compared with cephalic and gastric factors.

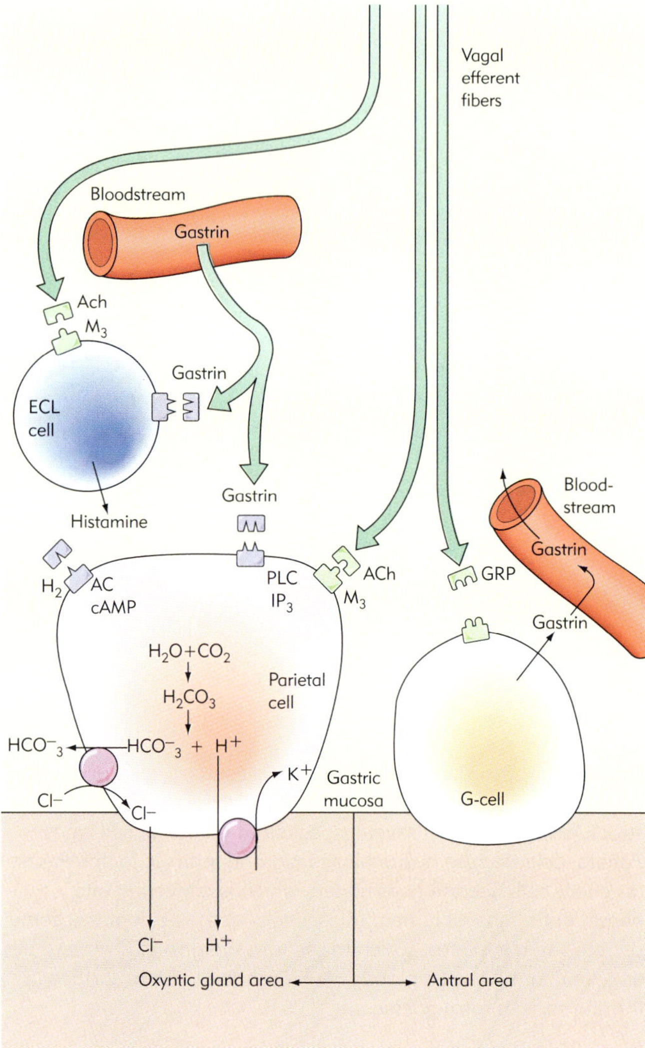

Figure 58.6 Gastrin, histamine, and vagal stimulation in gastric acid secretion. Several factors, including vagal stimulation, activate G cells to secrete gastrin into the bloodstream to act as a gut hormone. Gastrin interacts with receptors on the parietal cell and histamine-secreting ECL cell surface membranes. In this way, gastrin stimulates acid secretion directly from the parietal cell, and indirectly via histamine release. Histamine acts as a paracrine effector by binding to nearby parietal cells at histamine type 2 (H_2) receptors to cause acid secretion. Both the parietal cell and ECL cell are stimulated by ACh from vagal efferents. Vagal stimulation is mediated by GRP at the G cell. Thus, increased vagal tone brings about acid secretion by stimulating all elements of this system. Carbonic anhydrase (CA) catalyzes the formation of carbonic acid (H_2CO_2) from carbon dioxide and water in the parietal cell. This dissociates to liberate H^+, which are 'pumped' into the gastric lumen by membrane H^+,K^+-ATPase. Bicarbonate is extruded from the cell in exchange for chloride, which diffuses into the gastric lumen down its concentration gradient. (AC, adenylyl cyclase; cAMP, cyclic adenosine monophosphate; PLC, phospholipase C; IP_3, inositol trisphosphate.)

Physiologic inhibition of acid secretion

As gastric emptying proceeds and during the interdigestive phase, several factors reduce gastric acid secretion to basal levels. The loss of cephalic factors at the end of a meal reduces vagally mediated acid secretion. As the stomach empties, 'gastric factors' diminish. The pH is buffered less, which allows it to fall with consequent G-cell inhibition. Mechanoreceptor activation is also less and so G-cell and parietal cell activation by neural reflexes is reduced.

Specific paracrine and endocrine factors slow gastric acid secretion. The primary paracrine inhibitor of acid secretion is somatostatin, which is released when gastric pH falls below 3. Somatostatin-secreting D cells are located in close proximity to gastrin cells and thus exert a continuous inhibitory restraint on the secretion of gastrin. Release of the gut hormones secretin and, to a lesser extent, GIP reduces acid secretion by inhibition of parietal and G cells. Secretin release occurs in response to the acidification of duodenal chyme as gastric emptying progresses. The presence of carbohydrate and fatty acids in the duodenal lumen releases GIP. Secretin also stimulates pancreatic and biliary alkaline secretion to neutralize duodenal luminal pH. Some prostaglandins (e.g. PGE_1, PGE_2) inhibit acid secretion as part of the mucosal cytoprotection mechanism.

Antacid drugs

The most widely used antacid drugs are the *H_2 receptor antagonists* (H_2RAs; e.g. cimetidine, ranitidine) and the *proton pump inhibitors* (PPIs; e.g. omeprazole, lansoprazole). Another group, the *prostaglandin analogs* (e.g. misoprostol), also inhibits gastric acid secretion and in addition increases mucosal blood flow and enhances mucus and bicarbonate production. These are not usually used as primary antacids, but rather in association with nonsteroidal anti-inflammatory drugs in an attempt to prevent the antiprostaglandin gastric side effects (e.g. peptic ulceration) associated with their use (Chapter 27).

H_2 receptor antagonists

Since their introduction, H_2RAs have become among the most widely prescribed of all drugs and have revolutionized the management of peptic ulceration. They inhibit acid secretion by competitive and reversible inhibition of H_2 receptors on the parietal cell surface membrane (Fig. 58.8). In this way they directly block the action of histamine in acid secretion and indirectly inhibit the synergistic influences of gastrin and cholinergic vagal stimulation on acid secretion normally mediated via histamine release.

Prompt symptomatic relief is provided by H_2RAs, and they heal 80–95% of peptic ulcers within 6–8 weeks of initiating treatment. Unfortunately, the relapse rate is high, with 80% of patients suffering a recurrence of the ulcer in the first year after treatment. The overall 5-year relapse rate falls to around 20% with half-dose maintenance therapy. The circadian rhythm of acid secretion has a peak secretion in the early hours after midnight, which is a critical time for peptic ulcer formation as the buffering effects of saliva and food are absent; hence maintenance therapy is administered in the evening.

Proton pump inhibitors

The final common pathway of acid secretion is blocked by PPIs through inhibition of H^+,K^+-ATPase in the apical membrane of the parietal cell. Therefore, PPIs have the potential to achieve a greater degree of acid inhibition than H_2RAs, which is reflected in their clinical efficacy. Two subunits form H^+,K^+-

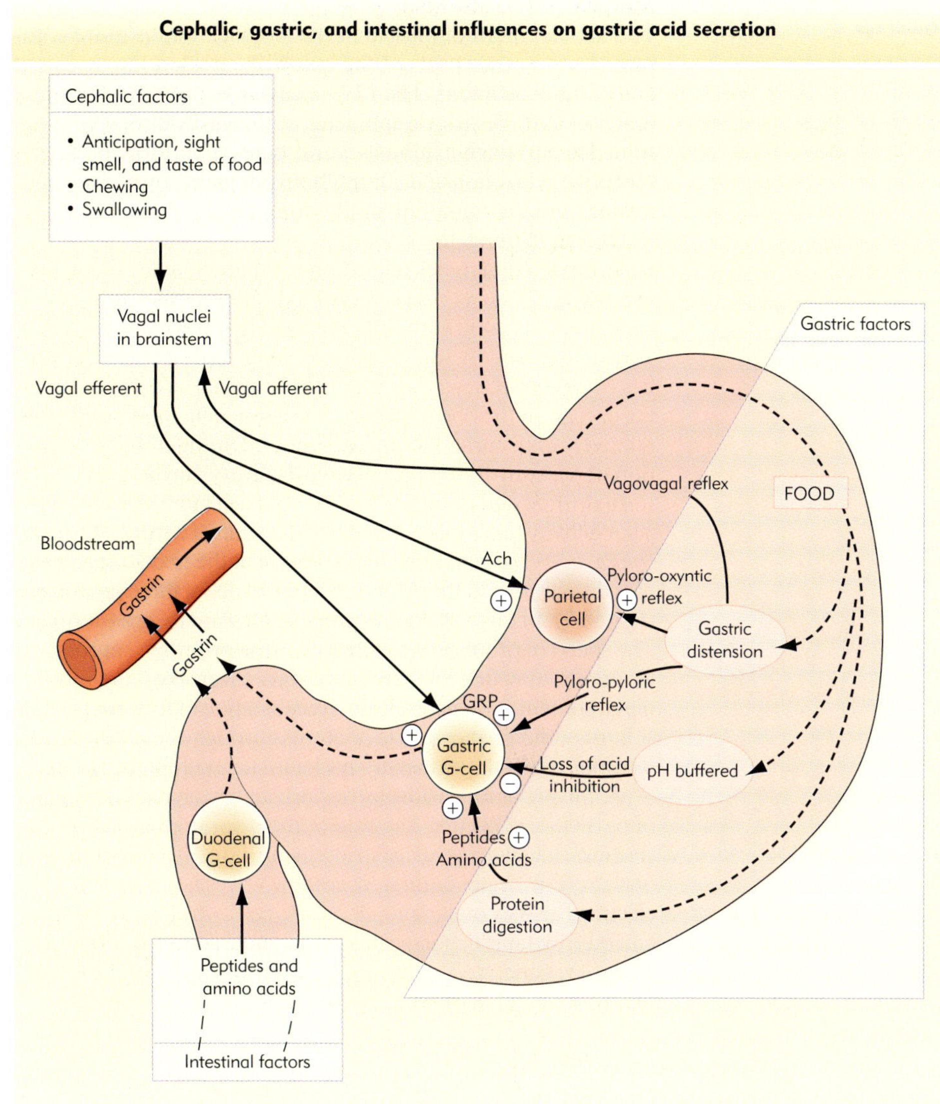

Figure 58.7 Cephalic, gastric, and intestinal influences on gastric acid secretion. *Cephalic factors* – anticipation, sight, smell, and taste of food together with the acts of chewing and swallowing result in vagally mediated acid secretion. *Gastric factors* – buffering of acidic gastric pH stops the inhibition of gastrin release from G cells at pH <3; distention of the stomach wall initiates vagovagal, pyloropyloric, and pylorooxyntic reflexes, which results in activation of G cells and parietal cells; peptides and amino acids directly stimulate G cells in the stomach. *Intestinal factors* – protein digestion products directly stimulate G cells in the duodenum.

ATPase – the α-subunit has 8–10 membrane-spanning domains and is the site of energy-producing phosphorylation, and a smaller β-subunit of unknown function. The PPIs, such as omeprazole and lansoprazole, are benzimidazole sulfoxides, which inactivate H^+,K^+-ATPase by irreversible covalent binding to cysteine groups on the extracellular face of the α-subunit (see Fig 58.8). Thus, it is necessary for the drug to diffuse out of the parietal cell to exert its pharmacologic effect. On the luminal side of the parietal cell apical membrane, the drug is converted in the acid medium from sulfoxide into sulfenamide, which is the active form of the drug. Deactivation of the enzyme is total and permanent; synthesis of new H^+,K^+-ATPase is required for further acid secretion.

Omeprazole provides significantly faster ulcer healing in the first 2 weeks of therapy compared with H_2RAs, as well as better symptomatic relief. Of the antacid drugs, PPIs are the most effective for refractory peptic ulcers, reflux esophagitis, and the Zollinger–Ellison syndrome.

It is now recognized that many peptic ulcers are caused by the growth of the organism *Helicobacter pylori* in the gastroduodenal mucosa. Both H_2RAs and PPIs suppress the growth of this organism, which may be a factor in their ability to heal peptic ulcers. Curative treatment for peptic ulcer disease is now possible by antibiotic eradication of *H. pylori* with very low recurrence rates.

Pepsin

Pepsinogen is secreted from peptic (or chief) cells in the oxyntic gland. Some pepsinogen is also secreted from mucosal cells in the gastric antrum and the duodenum. In the presence of gastric acid, this proenzyme is converted into active pepsin which itself catalyzes further conversion from pepsinogen. The main stimulus for pepsinogen release is the increased vagal activity seen in the cephalic and gastric phases of acid secretion. Gastric acid itself initiates a local cholinergic reflex that triggers pepsinogen secretion from peptic cells. Entry of acidic gastric chyme into the duodenum stimulates the release of secretin. This, together with gastrin, causes further pepsinogen secretion.

Mucus

Two forms of mucus are secreted by the gastric mucosa – soluble and insoluble. Surface mucus cells secrete *insoluble mucus* and bicarbonate, which together with sloughed mucosal cells form a protective barrier over the mucosal surface. Insoluble

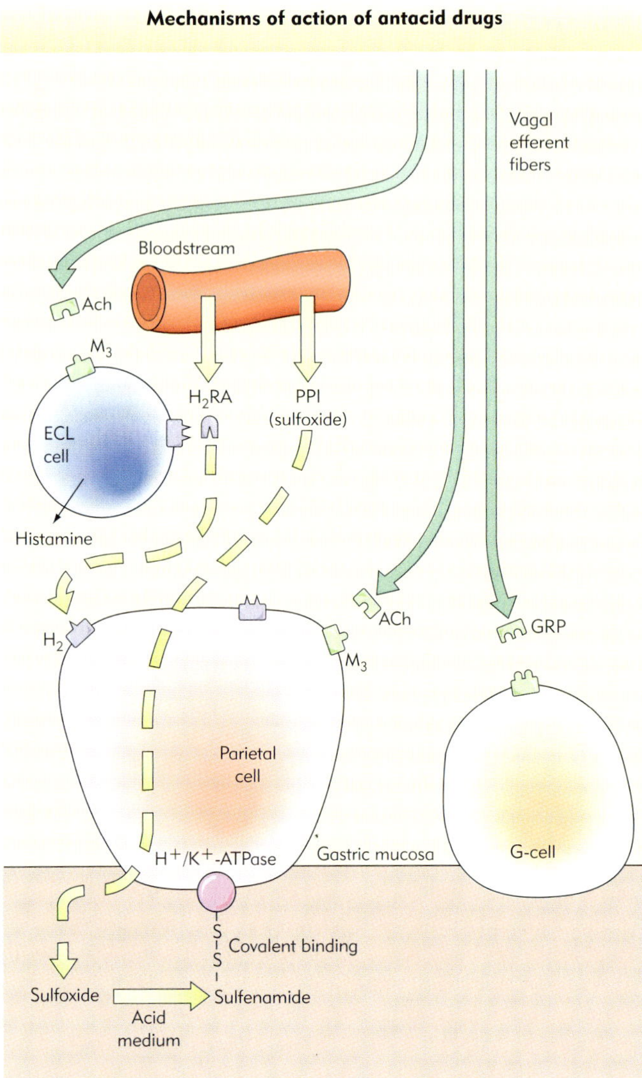

Figure 58.8 Mechanisms of action of antacid drugs. Acid secretion is inhibited by H_2RAs through competitive and reversible inhibition of H_2 receptors on the parietal cell surface membrane (see Fig. 58.7). In this way they directly block the action of histamine in acid secretion, and indirectly inhibit the synergistic influences of gastrin and cholinergic vagal stimulation, normally mediated via histamine release. An acid environment is required for the conversion of PPIs into active sulfenamide before they can irreversibly inactivate H^+,K^+-ATPase. This is achieved by diffusion across the parietal cell into the gastric lumen. Covalent bonds develop between the sulfenamide and cysteine groups on the extracellular face of the α-subunit of the enzyme.

mucus has an important role in the protection of the mucosal surface against acid, pepsin, and mechanical damage. Prostaglandins stimulate this secretion as part of the mucosal cytoprotection. *Soluble mucus* is a mucoprotein secretion from oxyntic neck mucus cells and occurs in response to vagal stimulation. It mixes with gastric contents and functions primarily as a lubricant.

Motility of the stomach

The arrangement of muscle in the stomach wall is more complex than in other parts of the gut, with circular, longitudinal, and oblique elements. The LES occurs at the gastroesophageal junction and the pyloric sphincter at the gastroduodenal junction. The stomach exhibits several types of motility pattern – receptive relaxation and contraction, peristaltic propulsion and mixing, and the migrating motor complex.

During feeding, the smooth muscle in the wall of the proximal stomach undergoes relaxation to make room for the incoming meal. This *receptive relaxation* allows the stomach to accommodate food with little increase in intragastric pressure. This is followed by low amplitude, long-lasting rhythmic contractions that reduce the size of the stomach as gastric emptying occurs. In the proximal part of the stomach, food can remain relatively undisturbed for up to an hour. During this time, digestion of carbohydrate takes place by salivary amylase.

In the mid and distal parts of the stomach more vigorous muscular activity takes place following ingestion of a meal. *Peristaltic contractions* are generated in the region of the mid-stomach and pass distally toward the pylorus at a rate of about three per minute (Fig. 58.9). In this way, food is propelled toward the gastric outlet. The speed of propagation increases as the pylorus is approached to a point at which the peristaltic wave 'overtakes' the intraluminal contents, which results in a combination of forward propulsion of some of the gastric contents through the pylorus, and retropulsion of the remainder back into the body of the stomach. Thus, mixing of food with gastric juice and mechanical reduction of particle size occurs. The role of the pyloric sphincter in controlling the passage of gastric chyme into the duodenum is unclear. The origin of these peristaltic waves lies in the intrinsic electrical activity of the smooth muscle cells, which undergo spontaneous rhythmic depolarization to generate so-called slow waves. These are generated in the mid stomach and pass distally toward the pylorus, but do not necessarily generate peristaltic waves of contraction. Only when the amplitude of these waves reaches a certain threshold does muscular contraction begin. The greater the slow wave potential above the threshold, the greater is the force of muscular contraction. Vagal stimulation and gastrin increase gastric peristalsis, whereas sympathetic stimulation, secretin, GIP, and somatostatin depress activity.

It normally takes several hours for the stomach to empty following a meal. The speed at which substances empty from the stomach depends on their physical state and chemical composition. Liquids rapidly empty, whereas solids take longer (during which time they are broken down and liquefied in gastric juice). The delivery of nutrients to the duodenum from the stomach results in a negative feedback inhibition on gastric emptying. This 'duodenal brake' allows time for further digestion and absorption in the small intestine. Chemoreceptors in the duodenum are sensitive to the chemical composition of the chyme being ejected from the stomach. Hypertonicity, fatty acids, and H^+ activate the secretion of CCK, secretin, and GIP, which inhibit gastric emptying. During the interdigestive period, the *migrating motor complex* is initiated in the proximal stomach.

Several factors can delay gastric emptying in the perioperative period, as summarized in Figure 58.10.

Drugs enhancing gastric emptying

Metoclopramide and *domperidone* are antidopaminergics and effective gastric prokinetics. However, at doses used commonly they do not effectively reverse opioid-induced delay. *Cisapride*

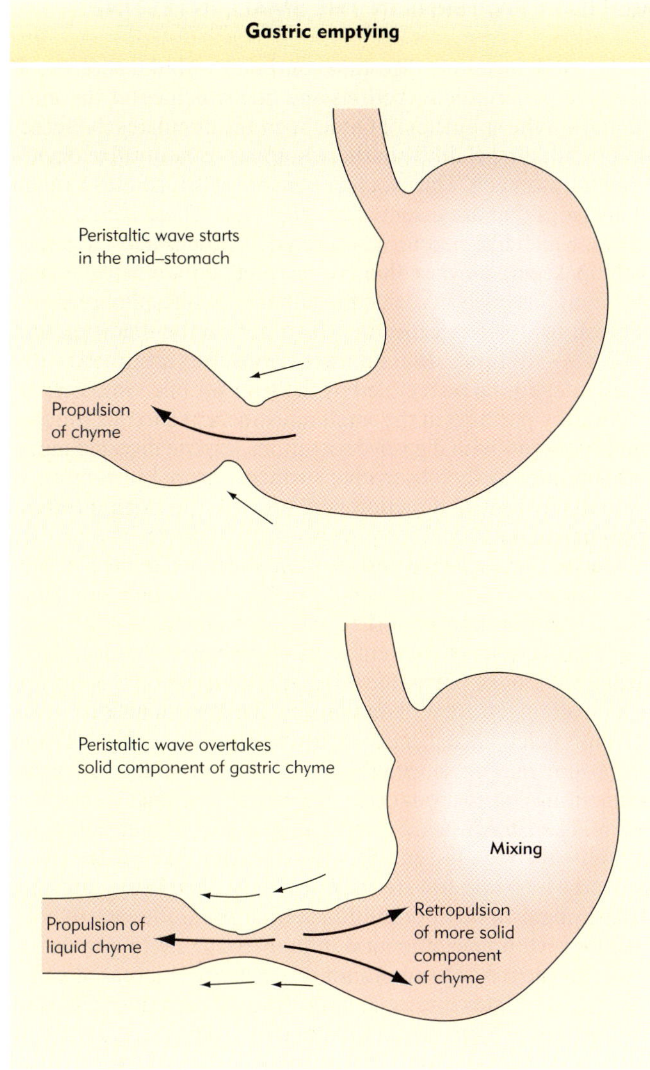

Figure 58.9 Gastric emptying. Food is disintegrated into smaller particles and eventually liquefied into gastric chyme by the actions of acid, enzymes, and muscular activity. The contractions involved are peristaltic in nature and pass from the mid-stomach distally. As the wave of contraction approaches the pylorus, its rate of propagation increases. In this way it overtakes the more solid component of chyme, which undergoes 'retropulsion' back into the body of the stomach. Liquid chyme stays ahead of the contractile wave and is transported into the duodenum.

is more effective in this regard; its mechanism of action is thought to be enhancement of release of ACh at the myenteric plexus. Cisapride is a 5-HT_4 receptor agonist as well, which may also result in increased gastrointestinal motility and cardiac effects. *Erythromycin* promotes gastric motility. Erythromycin analogs that have agonistic activity at the motilin receptor but no antibacterial action are now available and undergoing clinical trial.

Gastroesophageal reflux disease

Reflux of gastric fluid into the esophagus is common, occurring in normal individuals about once an hour without signs or symptoms of tissue damage. Such reflux is cleared rapidly by stimulation of esophageal peristalsis. In some circumstances reflux becomes pathologic, causing symptoms and leading to complications from chronic esophageal injury. Classically, the sensations of 'heartburn' and 'dyspepsia' occur, which may be associated with 'acid' regurgitation into the pharynx. In severe cases, persistent pulmonary aspiration of gastric fluid results in the development of respiratory symptoms and disease. Not infrequently, esophageal chest pain mimics myocardial ischemia; this causes anxiety in the patient and diagnostic difficulties for the clinician. In the early stages of the disease endoscopic and histologic findings may be normal despite significant symptomatology. In such patients, however, 24-hour esophageal pH monitoring demonstrates increased exposure of the mucosa to gastric juice.

Perioperative causes of delayed gastric emptying	
Physiologic	**Pharmacologic**
Pain	Opioids
Anxiety	μ agonists
Elderly (liquids only)	partial agonists
Pregnancy (some patients only)	mixed agonist/antagonists
Pathologic	Anticholinergics
Gastrointestinal tract obstruction	Sympathomimetics
Acute gastritis	Dopamine
Migraine	Ganglion blockers
Electrolyte imbalance	Aluminium and magnesium hydroxides
Diabetes	
Raised intracranial pressure	
Certain muscle disorders	
polymyositis	
dermatomyositis	
systemic sclerosis	

Figure 58.10 Perioperative causes of delayed gastric emptying.

The LES normally provides a barrier between the esophagus and the stomach. The sphincter-like function is related to the architecture of the muscle fibers as the esophagus enters the gastric pouch. Under normal circumstances, the LES remains closed and relaxation occurs only as part of the swallowing reflex as the wave of esophageal peristalsis approaches. Several neural and humoral factors modulate the inherent myogenic tone of the LES. α-Adrenergic stimulation, gastrin, motilin, enkephalin, and substance P increase tone, whereas β-adrenergic stimulation, CCK, secretin, GIP, and VIP decrease it. Metoclopramide, domperidone, cisapride, neostigmine, succinylcholine, and metoprolol increase tone; anticholinergics [e.g. atropine, glycopyrrolate (glycopyrronium)], volatile anesthetic agents, opioids, dopamine, sympathomimetics, Ca^{2+} channel blockers, diazepam, theophylline, caffeine, glyceryltrinitrate (GTN), and alcohol tend to decrease tone.

The causes of gastroesophageal reflux disease (GERD) may be categorized as mechanical incompetence of the LES, inappropriate relaxation of the LES, inefficient clearing of refluxed gastric juice, and abnormalities of the gastric reservoir.

Mechanical incompetence is the most common cause of GERD (accounts for about two thirds of cases). Such incompetence occurs when the anatomy of the LES becomes distorted, as occurs with hiatus hernias and gastric dilation, or when a primary abnormality of myogenic function causes low sphincter pressure.

In some patients increased episodes of reflux occur because of *inappropriate relaxation of the LES*. Abnormal coordination of the components of the swallowing reflex, upon which the vagus nerve has an important controlling influence, may be a significant factor. Hence, if a pharyngeal swallow is not followed by a wave of esophageal peristalsis, reflex relaxation of the LES may occur and allow reflux of gastric juice into the esophagus.

Esophageal clearance is an important component of the human antireflux mechanism. Under normal circumstances swallowing clears any refluxed gastric fluid by means of the primary peristaltic wave. Any residual refluxate stimulates secondary peristaltic waves by distending the esophagus. Acid in the esophagus also stimulates smooth muscle contraction, but this is less organized than the peristalsis initiated by distention. Thus, acid in the esophagus may disrupt normal peristalsis and so impede clearance of refluxate.

Abnormalities of the gastric reservoir may contribute to pathologic reflux, including elevated intragastric pressure, delayed gastric emptying, and increased acid production. Elevated intragastric pressure may result from gastric outlet obstruction or backing up from a more distal intestinal obstruction. In diabetic autonomic neuropathy, failure of active relaxation of the stomach causes raised intragastric pressure. Subsequent dilation of the stomach distorts the anatomy of the LES, shortening its effective length and reducing its resistance to reflux. Delayed gastric emptying that results in a persistent gastric reservoir may occur in conditions such as gastric atony caused by myotonic abnormalities (e.g. advanced diabetes). Gastric hypersecretion exacerbates the disruption of esophageal motility because of acid reflux, as discussed above.

Several components of the refluxate may cause damage to the esophageal mucosa – gastric acid and pepsin are the main injurious agents in gastric juice. If an element of duodenogastric reflux is also present, the situation becomes more complex. In a patient who has high gastric acid production, reflux of alkaline duodenal fluid may have a beneficial effect by neutralizing gastric acidity. In addition, bile salts inhibit pepsin and gastric acid inhibits pancreatic trypsin. However, in a patient who has low gastric acid secretion or who has a high degree of duodenogastric reflux, alkaline duodenal fluid and pancreatic enzymes become injurious agents in their own right. In such patients antacid therapy may worsen the situation.

Persistent pathologic reflux causes recurrent damage and repair cycling with the eventual development of the complications of GERD. This usually takes the form of a benign stricture formation that causes dysphagia or metaplastic transformation of native squamous epithelium into columnar epithelium, characteristic of the so-called Barrett's esophagus. This columnar epithelium is more resistant to acid and associated with a reduction in symptoms of heartburn. Peptic ulcer or malignant disease may further complicate Barrett's esophagus. Pulmonary complications may also follow chronic regurgitation and pulmonary aspiration. Nocturnal cough, wheezing, recurrent infections, and progressive pulmonary fibrosis can all occur.

The aim of treatment is to prevent the tendency to reflux by the suppression of acid production (e.g. H_2 antagonists, PPIs) and surgical correction of a mechanically defective LES (e.g. Nissen fundoplication). Symptomatic relief may be achieved using antacids, alginate, and prokinetic drugs. The most effective antacid drugs, in terms of both symptom relief and healing of esophagitis, are PPIs. Treatment of complications includes dilation of strictures and surveillance for neoplastic change

MOTILITY PATTERNS IN THE SMALL INTESTINE

In the small intestine, digestion continues with the addition of exocrine pancreatic secretions and bile which enter the duodenum via the sphincter of Oddi. Secretin stimulates the secretion of alkaline fluid from these sources to neutralize chyme from the stomach. The exocrine pancreas also secretes a range of enzymes that are essential for digestion. These include proteases, which like pepsin are secreted as proenzymes, together with lipase and amylase that are secreted in their active forms. Bile contains bile salts, which together with phospholipids and cholesterol form micelles that take part in the digestion and absorption of lipids. Bile salts are themselves absorbed in the small intestine to be recycled by the liver for bile synthesis.

Motility patterns in the small intestine serve to mix intraluminal contents with digestive secretions, expose digested nutrient subunits to the absorptive surfaces, propel intraluminal contents in a distal direction, and prepare the small intestine for the next meal.

During the digestive period, *stationary segmenting contractions* occur to divide the small intestine into segments (Fig. 58.11). After a short period, relaxation occurs followed by further contractions in adjacent parts of the gut wall to form new segments. Unlike peristaltic waves, the contraction is not propagated along the gut wall. In this way, the intraluminal contents are pummeled, mixed, and exposed to mucosal surfaces. Distal propulsion may occur with this motility pattern if the stationary segmenting contractions occur in a proximal to distal sequence. Normal *peristalsis* (see Fig. 58.4) also transports intraluminal contents through the gut. Slow waves occur in both the small and large intestine and are similar to those seen in the stomach. They appear to be important in setting the frequency of contractions, with neurohumoral influences interacting to determine the degree of smooth muscle activity. Increased vagal activity stimulates intestinal motility, as do gastrin, CCK, and insulin. Sympathetic stimulation, secretin, and glucagon inhibit smooth muscle activity. The exact role of each of these mediators in the control of motility is unclear. During the interdigestive phase, migrating motor complexes sweep through the small intestine to clear it of undigested matter in preparation for the next meal (see above).

MOTILITY PATTERNS IN THE LARGE INTESTINE

In the large intestine, water and electrolytes are extracted from the intraluminal contents so that semisolid feces are formed as the distal colon and rectum are approached. Storage takes place in the distal colon until voluntary emptying occurs by defecation.

The large intestine consists of the cecum, the ascending, transverse, descending, and sigmoid colon, and the rectum. It is anatomically distinct from the small intestine in that the outer longitudinal muscle is concentrated into three flat bands, called teniae coli. The parasympathetic supply to the descending colon, sigmoid colon, and rectum is from cholinergic parasympathetic elements in the pelvic nerves that originate from sacral roots 2, 3, and 4. As the anal canal is approached, the circular smooth muscle layer thickens to form the internal anal sphincter. Overlapping and slightly distal to the internal anal sphincter are layers of striated muscle that comprise the external anal sphincter.

Passage of intraluminal contents from the small to the large intestine occurs intermittently and is regulated in part by a sphincteric mechanism at the ileocecal junction. The restriction

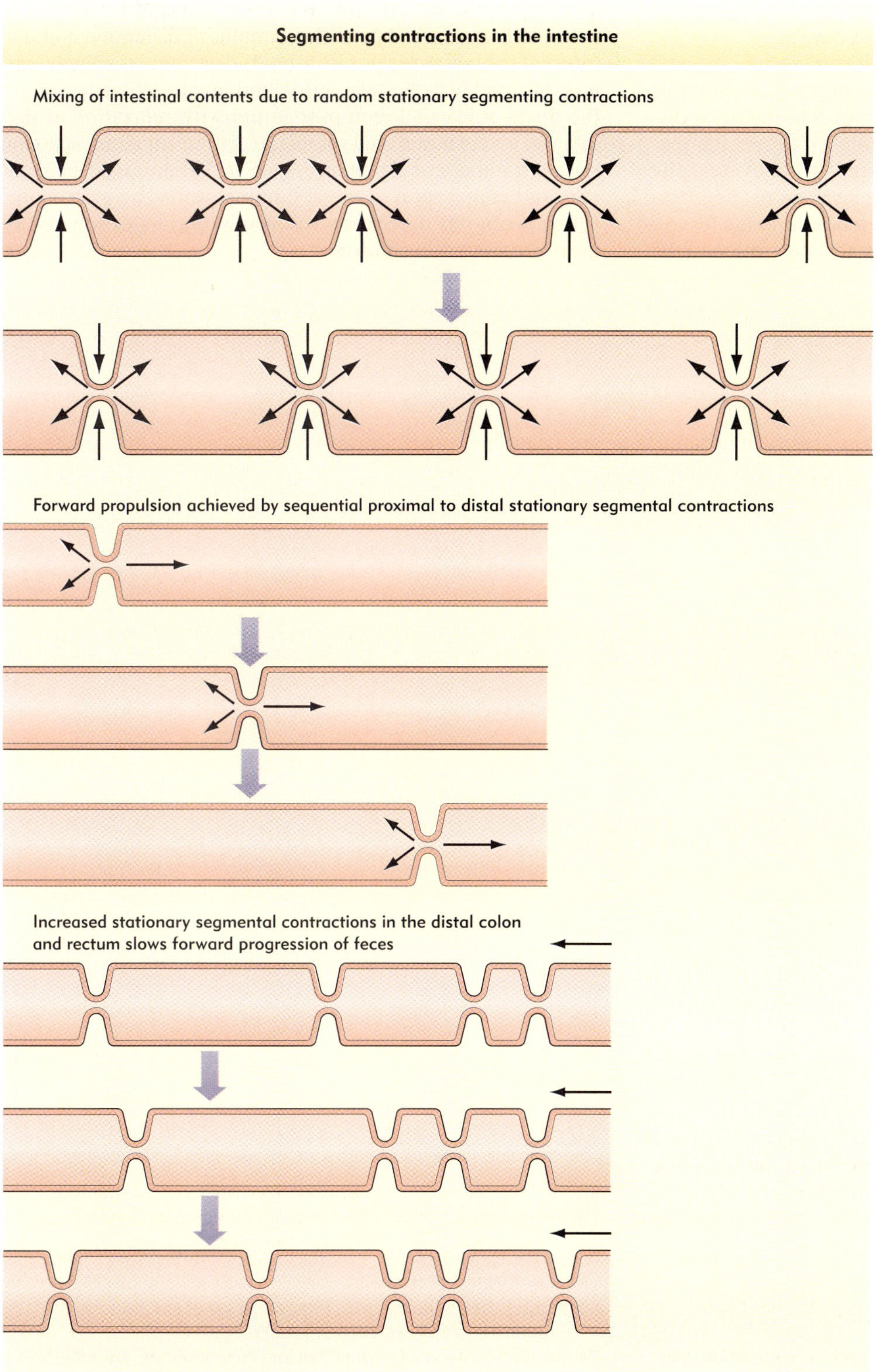

Segmenting contractions in the intestine

Mixing of intestinal contents due to random stationary segmenting contractions

Forward propulsion achieved by sequential proximal to distal stationary segmental contractions

Increased stationary segmental contractions in the distal colon and rectum slows forward progression of feces

Figure 58.11 Segmenting contractions in the intestine. Stationary segmenting contractions divide the small intestine up into short lengths. Subsequent relaxation is followed by a new set of ring contractions that create new segments. Thus, intraluminal contents are mixed with digestive fluids and exposed to the absorptive mucosal surfaces. In the small intestine, sequential patterns of segmenting contractions serve to propel intraluminal contents distally. In the distal large intestine, an increase in frequency of segmenting contractions acts as a brake on the transport of feces as the rectum is approached.

to flow imposed by this periodically relaxes to allow ileal peristalsis and migrating motor complexes to propel intraluminal contents through. Several motility patterns occur in the large intestine – stationary segmental contractions, mass movement, and defecation.

Stationary segmental contractions similar to those in the small intestine occur throughout the colon and rectum. They last about a minute, which is considerably longer than those in the small intestine, and are probably responsible for the haustrations in the large intestine. Functionally, these contractions expose intraluminal contents to the mucosal surface for efficient extraction of water and electrolytes. In the descending colon, sigmoid colon, and rectum the frequency of segmenting contractions increases. This acts as a brake on distal flow as feces approach the rectum. Passage through the colon is slow (normally several days). This passage occurs intermittently in a motility sequence that drives feces distally, called *mass movement*, which occurs about three times per day.

The rectum is normally empty or nearly empty and the anal canal closed due to internal sphincter contraction. Entry of feces into the rectum during a mass movement causes distention. Rectal distention has two effects – it causes the sensation of the urge to defecate, and it activates the *rectosphincteric reflex*, which causes relaxation of the internal sphincter. The urge to defecate can be overcome by voluntary contraction of the external sphincter. Relaxation of the internal sphincter is transient as stretch receptors within the rectal wall accommodate to the stimulus of distention and the internal sphincter regains its tone. If *defecation* is convenient it is initiated by voluntary action and involves contraction of the distal colon and rectum together with relaxation of the internal and external anal sphincters. Often voluntary acts can raise intra-abdominal pressure, such as 'Valsalva type' maneuvers and contraction of the abdominal wall. The gastrocolic reflex promotes defecation following food ingestion and is most prominent in children.

Key References

Ching CK, Lam SK. Drug therapy of peptic ulcer disease. Br J Hosp Med. 1995;54:101–6.

Johnson LR. Gastric secretion. In: Johnson LR, ed. Gastrointestinal physiology, 5th edn. Mosby; 1997: 69–87.

Goyal RK, Hirano I. The enteric nervous system. N Engl J Med. 1996;334:1106–15.

Helander HF, Keeling DJ. Cell biology of gastric acid secretion. Clin Gastroenterol. 1993;7:1–22.

Hellström PM. Motility of the small intestine: a case of pattern recognition. J Intern Med. 1995;237:391–4.

Peters JH, DeMeester TR. Gastroesophageal reflux. Surg Clin North Am. 1993;73:1119–44.

Shamburek RD, Schubert ML. Pharmacology of gastric acid inhibition. Clin Gastroenterol. 1993;7:23–54.

Weisbrodt NW. Motility of the small and large intestine. In: Johnson LR, ed. Gastrointestinal physiology, 5th edn. Mosby; 1997: 43–58.

Further Reading

Ogilvy AJ, Smith G. The gastrointestinal tract after anaesthesia. Eur J Anaesthesiol. 1995;12(Suppl.10):35–42.

Chapter 59 Nutrition, digestion, and absorption

Iain T Campbell

Topics covered in this chapter

DIGESTION AND ABSORPTION

Nutrients are absorbed from the gastrointestinal tract, which consists of the mouth, pharynx, esophagus, stomach, and the small and large intestines. Accessory structures outside the digestive system, but associated with digestion and absorption, are the salivary glands, pancreas, liver, and gallbladder (Fig. 59.1). Their secretions pass into the digestive tract via their ducts. Blood that drains the gastrointestinal tract passes via the portal vein and carries the absorbed products of digestion and metabolism to the liver before circulation to the cells of the rest of the body. The splanchnic circulation receives about 25% of the cardiac output and is at its maximum after a meal.

Various substances and enzymes are secreted by the wall of the gut and the exocrine glands that empty into it. They include a variety of inorganic molecules – hydrochloric acid in the stomach and bicarbonate from the pancreas. Amylase is synthesized and secreted by the salivary glands, pepsin by the stomach, amylase, proteases and a variety of other digestive enzymes by the pancreas, and bile by the liver. The various enzymes are secreted in response to a stimulus; water and inorganic ions follow passively. The nature of the secretion may be modified by the epithelium of the duct as it passes on into the intestine.

Digestion

The large complex molecules of carbohydrates, proteins, and triglycerides are degraded for absorption into simple sugars, small peptides, amino acids, free fatty acids (FFAs), and monoglycerides. Digestion starts with the saliva and continues in the stomach and small intestine, where it is completed and most absorption takes place. Some secretory components, such as water and inorganic ions, pass from the bloodstream through the enterocyte by a variety of transport mechanisms, while others are synthesized in the cells and are stored there until an appropriate nervous or hormonal signal stimulates secretion. Significant amounts of water and inorganic salts are absorbed by the large intestine. A variety of specialized transport systems function in the wall of the gut and transfer specific products of digestion from the lumen into the bloodstream. Others move passively along concentration gradients, and are affected mainly by molecular size and lipid solubility.

Motility and secretion are highly regulated functions, with regulation by a variety of stimuli, from the site and smell of food that stimulate secretion to the vestibular apparatus that induces vomiting via the vomiting center. In contrast, few mechanisms affect digestion and absorption other than the food itself.

The *nervous innervation of the gastrointestinal tract* is via 'short' and 'long' nerves. The short nerves make up the plexi contained within the walls of the digestive tract and give it a degree of autonomous function. The long nerves control function via the central nervous system; the parasympathetic vagus nerve is the major motor nerve and its impulses are excitatory and cholinergic. The parasympathetic sacral outflow (S_{2-4}) supplies the motor nerves for the rectum and lower colon. The sympathetic nerves provide the principal sensory input via the splanchnic nerves. Sympathetic stimulation is mainly inhibitory.

Four hormones – gastrin, cholecystokinin, secretin, and gastric inhibitory peptide – are released in the gastrointestinal tract in response to intraluminal stimuli that act directly on endocrine cells in the luminal lining.

The *salivary glands* contain three types of secretory cell. Serous cells secrete a watery solution, which mixes with mucin from mucous cells to form the mucus that lubricates the bolus of food. Amylase is secreted in response to parasympathetic stimuli. It digests starch to produce maltose and oligosaccharides. Digestion by salivary amylase continues for some time after the swallowed bolus enters the stomach.

The *stomach* produces hydrochloric acid secreted by exocrine glands in the body and the fundus of the stomach. The three types of secretory cells are chief cells, parietal cells, and mucous cells. Chief cells secrete pepsinogen, the inactive precursor of pepsin, and parietal cells secrete hydrochloric acid, which converts pepsinogen into pepsin and provides the optimum pH for pepsin activity. It also kills ingested bacteria and contributes to the breakdown of ingested connective tissue by denaturing protein. The mucus provides a protective covering for gastric mucosa.

Hydrochloric acid is secreted by a H^+,K^+-ATPase in the luminal membrane and Na^+/Cl^- cotransport in the basolateral membrane of parietal cells (Chapter 58). Its secretion is stimulated by vagal mechanisms. These vagal stimuli act also via the nerve plexi within the stomach wall to stimulate gastrin-secreting cells in the wall of the antrum. The gastrin in turn stimulates the body and the fundus of the stomach via the blood to secrete more hydrochloric acid. Histamine is also involved in hydrochloric acid release. The secretion of hydrochloric acid is inhibited when it contacts the antral mucosa and when food passes into the duodenum.

Pepsinogen secretion by the chief cells is stimulated by acetylcholine, which is converted into the active enzyme pepsin by

The digestive processes

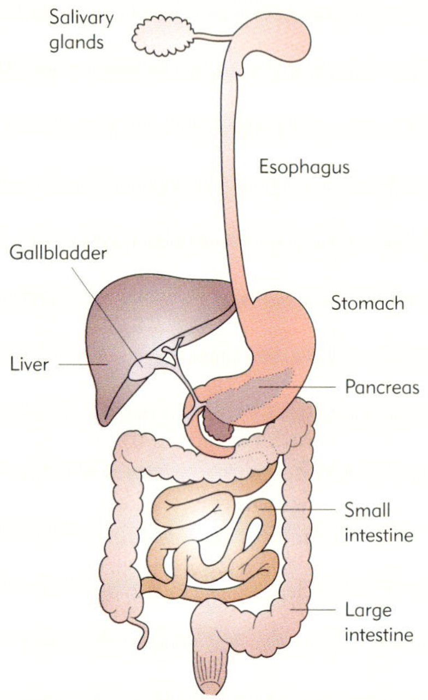

Organ gland	Secretion function	Substrate function	Products
Salivary glands	Salivary amylase	Starch	Oligo-and disaccharides
	Mucous		
Stomach	Hydrochloric acid	Antibacterial	Denatured protein
	Pepsinogen → pepsin	Denatures protein	Polypeptides peptides
		Denatured protein	
Gallbladder	Bile salts	Lipids	Emulsion
Pancreas	Trypsinogen → trypsin	Proteins	Peptides and amino acids
	Chymotrypsinogen → chymotrypsin	Polypeptides	Dextrins and disaccharides
	Amylase	Starch	Free fatty acids and monoglyceride
	Phospholipase, lipase	Phospholipiase, lipids	
Small intestine brush border	Aminopeptidase	Polypeptides	Amino acids
	Dipeptidase	Dipeptides	Monosaccharides
	Disaccharidase	Disaccharides	
Large intestine	Digestion/absorption of endogenous proteins, cellular debris, plasma		

Figure 59.1 The digestive processes.

hydrochloric acid and by pepsin itself. Pepsin is a protease that hydrolyzes protein into amino acids and short-chain peptides.

The *exocrine pancreas* consists of clusters of cells or acini that secrete digestive enzymes into intercalated ducts, which converge into one duct that opens into the duodenum. The epithelial cells lining the ducts secrete a relatively large volume of fluid rich in bicarbonate, which neutralize the acid that enters the duodenum from the stomach, and thus provide the optimum pH for pancreatic digestive enzymes to work.

The pancreas secretes a rich mixture of digestive enzymes that are adequate to digest the whole diet. They include the proteolytic enzymes trypsinogen and chymotrypsinogen. Enterokinase is secreted from the epithelial lining of the small intestine and activates trypsinogen to give trypsin, which itself activates both chymotrypsinogen and trypsinogen. Procarboxypeptidase excreted by the pancreas is converted into carboxykinase by trypsin and hydrolyzes terminal amino acids from proteins and peptides.

The lipid digestive enzymes are lipase (which hydrolyzes triglycerides into FFAs and monoglycerides), phospholipase, and cholesterol esterase. Amylase, similar to salivary amylase, degrades starch to give oligosaccharides (principally maltose), and ribonuclease and deoxyribonuclease hydrolyze nucleic acids.

Secretin and cholecystokinin are hormones released from the duodenal mucosa. Secretin stimulates the secretion of bicarbonate from the duct cells of the pancreas. Cholecystokinin stimulates both the secretion of pancreatic digestive enzymes and contraction of the gallbladder.

Bile salts are intimately involved in the digestion and absorption of fat. The stimulus to the secretion of bile is the absorption of bile salts from the terminal ileum via the portal vein – the enterohepatic circulation. Secretin also stimulates the secretion of water and inorganic ions, principally bicarbonate, into the duodenum. Bile salts help in the digestion of lipid in that they convert large lipid droplets that enter the small intestine into micelles to form an emulsion. Micelles, each of which contains about 20 lipid molecules, diffuse in aqueous solution and are thus more susceptible to the action of lipase, which breaks them down to give FFAs and monoglycerides. These are absorbed along the length of the intestine. Cholesterol and fat-soluble vitamins are also absorbed by the same mechanisms.

Small intestine

When the gastric contents move into the small intestine and are broken down further they become hyperosmotic. Water moves into the gut from the bloodstream and from the various mucosal endocrine glands, and the small intestinal contents become iso-osmotic with blood. Absorption occurs along the small intestine and is normally complete by halfway, so there is a significant reserve of absorptive area. Some water and sodium chloride enters the large intestine, where their absorption is completed.

The absorptive surface of the small intestine is highly folded and convoluted, with finger-like projections or villi that greatly increase the absorptive area (Fig. 59.2). Each villus has its own lymph drainage and arterial and venous supply. In addition, the

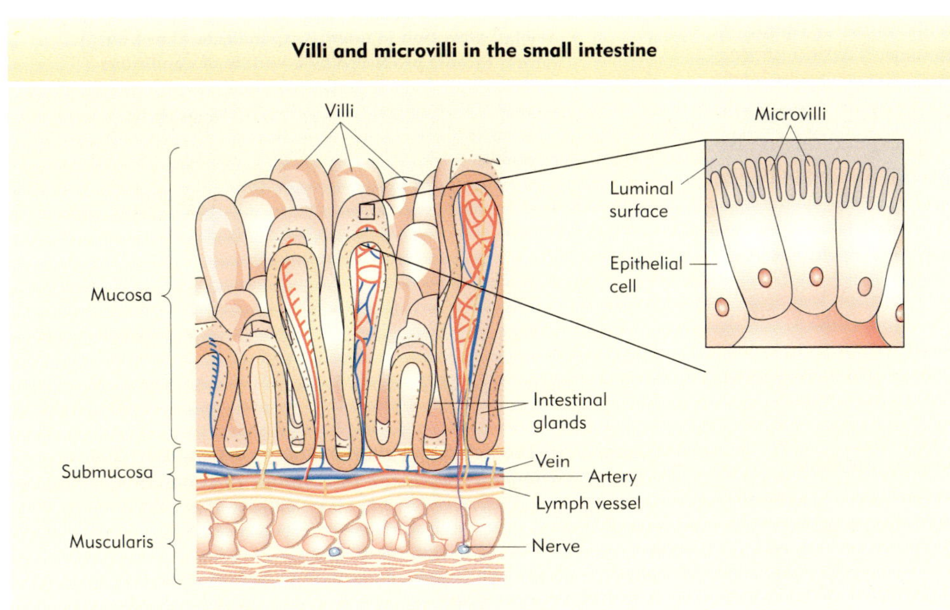

Figure 59.2 Villi and microvilli in the small intestine.

luminal surface of the cells of the intestinal epithelium consist of a series of projections, the so-called brush border, which contains a number of enzymes and transport systems involved in the movement of the products of digestion from the lumen into the circulation. Some molecules also pass down concentration gradients that depend on their lipid solubility.

About 2L of water enters the small bowel each day from the stomach, and another 7L from the various secretions in the bowel, of which about 500mL enter the large intestine and 100mL are excreted in the feces. Water absorption occurs mostly by osmosis following the various products of digestion. Sodium plays a major role in this process; it diffuses through the brush border into the enterocyte and is actively pumped into the circulation by a Na^+,K^+-ATPase in the basal membrane of the cell. Other ions are absorbed by a mixture of active and passive processes, but there are specific transport mechanisms for iron and Ca^{2+}.

Absorption of nutrients

Carbohydrate absorption

Starch is hydrolyzed into oligosaccharides by salivary and pancreatic amylase, and broken down by oligosaccharidases in the brush border of the enterocyte to give monosaccharides. Cellulose, or fiber, is excreted in the feces. The various monosaccharides are absorbed by a variety of mechanisms – fructose is passed by facilitated diffusion, and glucose and galactose by a carrier-mediated mechanism coupled with Na^+ that requires energy.

Protein absorption

Protein in the digestive tract consists not only of dietary protein, but also endogenous peptides derived from digestive enzymes, epithelial cells, and plasma proteins that leak into the tract. The peptides are hydrolyzed by brush border peptidases and the amino acids are absorbed by carrier-mediated transport systems coupled with Na^+ that consume energy. There are specific carriers for different groups of amino acids. Some absorption of di- and tri-peptides occurs.

Lipid absorption

The degradation of triglyceride into monoglyceride and FFAs and the formation of micelles are discussed above, along with the role of bile salts in the absorption of these substances into the enterocyte. Once in the enterocyte, monoglycerides and FFAs are resynthesized into triglycerides. These are aggregated, phospholipid and protein added, and a chylomicron formed, which enters the lymphatic system and the general circulation.

The colon

The principal absorptive function of the large intestine is to absorb Na^+, accompanied normally by about 400mL of the 500mL of water that enters it from the ileum. Some vitamins are also synthesized in the large bowel and the bacterial fermentation of indigestible carbohydrates produce flatus, which consists of nitrogen, carbon dioxide, hydrogen sulfide, and methane. The colonic mucosa also produces mucus and excretes K^+ and bicarbonate. The mucus protects the epithelium from trauma and the bicarbonate neutralizes acids, but when large volumes of fluid are lost in the feces significant K^+ depletion can occur.

NUTRITIONAL (MACRONUTRIENT) REQUIREMENTS

Protein and energy requirements are met by oxidation of carbohydrate, fat, and protein. The principal hormones that control the metabolism of these substances are insulin and glucagon. Insulin is an anabolic hormone; its secretion is stimulated by glucose, but also by some amino acids. When insulin falls, secondary to a decrease in blood glucose, glucagon rises. It stimulates glycogenolysis and lipolysis, which releases glucose from glycogen and FFAs from adipose tissue to use as oxidative fuels. Insulin stimulates the storage of glucose as glycogen, inhibits lipolysis, and stimulates protein synthesis. A lack of insulin, as is seen in diabetes mellitus or in the acute response to trauma, results in a breakdown of body protein.

Assessment of protein and energy requirements

Basal energy expenditure can be calculated from age, height, and weight and sex using one of the standard formulae (Chapter 62), and the value increased by a percentage to take into account activity and, in hospital patients, severity of illness and temperature. Alternatively, basal or resting expenditure can be measured by indirect calorimetry. Unless the calorimeter is part of a ventilator, in which case energy expenditure may be measured throughout 24 hours, basal expenditure is normally measured over a limited period of up to 30 minutes and the results extrapolated to 24 hours, with an appropriate percentage added to allow for activity as described above. In acute illness, energy expenditure is also elevated in a relatively predictable fashion, the precise percentage being dependent on the type of illness (Fig. 59.3).

Predicted elevation in energy expenditure above basal (stress factor) produced by a variety of conditions

Condition	Stress factor
Postoperative	1.00–1.05
Cancer	1.10–1.45
Peritonitis	1.05–1.25
Long bone fracture	1.15–1.30
Severe infection/multiple trauma	1.30–1.55
Burns – proportional to surface area	1.50–2.00

Figure 59.3 Predicted elevation in energy expenditure above basal (stress factor) produced by a variety of conditions. (Adapted with permission from MacBurney M, Wilmore DW, 1981.)

Provision of macronutrient requirements

In a healthy individual about 10–15% of energy requirements are provided by protein and the remainder split roughly 50–50 between carbohydrate and fat. The precise proportions in health are unclear, the concerns being the long-term effects on health of higher or lower percentages provided as fat. In clinical practice it is a common convention to ignore the energy provided by protein and to describe nutritional regimens in terms of non-protein calorie nitrogen (protein) ratios. A relatively healthy individual oxidizes energy and protein with an approximate non-protein calorie:nitrogen ratio of 200:1, an injured patient with a ratio of 150:1, and a critically ill patient with one of 100:1.

Protein

In health, lean body mass is relatively constant and the protein ingested equals that oxidized and excreted as various waste products in the urine, principally urea, plus that lost in feces and in shed skin. This stability of lean body mass is a dynamic one in which protein synthesis and protein breakdown occur simultaneously. For a stable body mass these are in equilibrium, with a proportion equal to the protein intake being oxidized. During the consumption of a protein-free diet, with energy requirements met by carbohydrate and fat, obligatory protein loss is about 0.5g/kg per day – the minimum required to maintain protein balance. A recommendation of 1g/kg per day therefore covers the requirements of a healthy individual.

The standard method used to assess protein metabolism is the measurement of urinary nitrogen excretion and nitrogen balance. However, outside of a metabolic ward, a 24-hour urine collection is extremely difficult to make accurately. Another method used to assess protein metabolism is with tracers; isotopes of various amino acids labeled with ^{13}C or ^{15}N are infused and their appearance is tracked in blood, tissue, urine, and expired air. From the rates of appearance and disappearance of the isotopes and their metabolites in blood, urine, tissue, and expired air, rates of protein synthesis, breakdown, and oxidation are quantified. Using these different techniques, the maximum protein intake is estimated at about 1.5–1.7g/kg per day. Provided energy requirements are covered by carbohydrate and fat, this rate of protein provision stimulates protein synthetic rate to its maximum. Any protein taken in over and above this is catabolized.

In sepsis and trauma, the relationship between protein synthesis and protein breakdown is disturbed. After a relatively minor stimulus, such as elective surgery, protein synthesis is depressed and protein breakdown unaltered, but the net result is a breakdown of protein and a loss of lean tissue. In severe trauma, sepsis, and multiple organ failure, both synthesis and breakdown are elevated (breakdown more than synthesis), so that net protein catabolism still occurs. In severe sepsis, an increase in protein intake to 1.5g/kg per day decreases net protein catabolism, but a further increase in intake (to 2.2g/kg per day) causes the rate of net protein breakdown to increase.

The cause of this net catabolism in trauma and sepsis is gluconeogenesis, which persists despite an apparently adequate nutrient intake. Why this occurs is unclear, but it is certainly caused in part by elevation in levels of the classical counter-regulatory hormones – glucagon, cortisol, and the catecholamines – but the inability to reproduce negative nitrogen balance of this severity by infusing these hormones into normal volunteers indicates that other factors must also be involved. The most obvious ones are the cytokines, probably with an action on hepatic metabolism. Persistence in feeding a septic or injured individual at rates much above 1.5–1.7g/kg per day results only in the excess intake being oxidized, which places an undesirable metabolic and respiratory (CO_2 production) load on a system already strained by illness. In severe catabolic illness, nutritional support alone does not preserve lean tissue. To preserve lean tissue in these patients, it is probable that pharmacologic methods are necessary.

Nature of the protein intake

Proteins differ in their composition depending on the amino acids that are present. The 'standard' protein has usually been taken as whole egg protein, but evidence is now accumulating that in critical illness amino acid requirements differ from this standard. Amino acid solutions enriched or supplemented with glutamine, arginine, and branch chain amino acids are beneficial in trauma and sepsis. This is possibly because of their actions in stimulating immune function, regulating protein metabolism, and providing energy substrate for the enterocyte and the lymphocyte, and because of the pivotal role that glutamine and the branch chain amino acids have in interorgan substrate transfer.

Glucose

Glucose intake or infusion stimulates insulin secretion. Insulin stimulates glucose oxidation, glucose storage, and protein synthesis, and inhibits lipolysis. At lower rates of glucose provision (and insulin response), most of the glucose is oxidized to provide energy. At higher rates (and a higher insulin response), a greater percentage of the glucose provided is stored as glycogen. The amount oxidized does not increase at intakes beyond 4–5mg/kg per minute. When the glycogen stores have been filled, infused, or ingested glucose is converted into fat. For a 70kg (154lb) adult, this maximum rate of glucose intake or infusion corresponds to a daily glucose intake of about 500g, which amounts to 2000kcal (8.4MJ).

In trauma and sepsis, in the stage immediately after injury, insulin secretion is inhibited by catecholamines, but glycogenolysis is stimulated. There is a surfeit of available circulating glucose, but an impairment in the ability to use it. In the recovery phase, insulin concentrations are high relative to blood glucose levels, which indicates a degree of insulin resistance. Some evidence indicates this resistance arises from the inability to store glucose rather than an impairment of the ability to oxidize it.

Lipid

Fat is presented to peripheral tissues as chylomicrons, triglycerides, and lipoproteins, and is metabolized as FFAs. Some fats – linoleic and linolenic acid – are 'essential', but the predominant role of fat in metabolism is to provide the energy requirements not covered by glucose. The rate of fatty acid oxidation is proportional to its concentration in the blood, which in turn is controlled by the lipolytic hormones glucagon (with a reciprocal action to insulin) and, under stress, catecholamines. Following injury, insulin secretion is inhibited and the intense adrenergic discharge stimulates lipolysis, which raises the circulating concentrations of FFAs; the healthy tissues of the body then derive a greater percentage of their energy requirements from fat oxidation.

Provision of fat in artificial nutritional support has traditionally been as long-chain fatty acids (16–18C), but over the past decade it has been recognized that medium-chain fatty acids (8–12C) have significant advantages. They are absorbed by the portal blood, as opposed to the lymphatics, when taken orally and are metabolized more rapidly than long-chain fatty acids as they do not need carnitine to enter the mitochondria. Long chain n-3 fatty acids in fish oil also have certain biologic advantages over the more commonly used n-6 fatty acids, with a dampening effect on inflammatory responses, less thromboxane, and more prostacyclin (prostaglandin I_3) production, reduced blood viscosity, and enhanced immune function, and are now starting to be included in artificial feeding preparations.

ARTIFICIAL NUTRITIONAL SUPPORT – PARENTERAL AND ENTERAL FEEDING

Nutritional support may be enteral via a nasogastric or nasoenteral tube, or via a feeding enterostomy, which can be inserted at operation or via an endoscope. If the gastrointestinal tract is not functioning the nutritional support may be given intravenously (parenterally). The biochemical and physiologic implications of the two routes are quite different, and the use of the gastrointestinal tract is now considered to have certain advantages in terms of its affect on the metabolic response to trauma.

Enteral feeding

Enteral feeding is the preferred route of nutritional support as it is cheaper and more physiologic than parenteral. Food is absorbed via the portal vein and passes through the liver, which has a close association with the pancreas, whose two hormones glucagon and insulin have such fundamental effects on anabolism and catabolism. These are released directly into portal vein blood, so the liver is exposed to higher concentrations of insulin and glucagon than other tissues.

One advantage of enteral feeding is that more 'natural' food can be given, with polypeptides or even whole protein with all the vitamins and minerals – substances that have to be added to parenteral feeds under strict sterile conditions. Another advantage is the potential to maintain the integrity of the gastro-intestinal tract. The intestinal mucosa normally obtains its nutrient requirements from the lumen. Its nutritional and immunologic health depends on its continued exposure to various nutrients and substances presented by the luminal contents, such as food antigens. In starvation, but to an extent with elemental diets, and also in response to hypoperfusion states such as shock, hemorrhage, and sepsis, the wall of the intestinal mucosa becomes permeable and bacteria and endotoxin translocate to the regional lymph nodes and to the portal and systemic circulations. In shock the mucosa is actually disrupted. Some evidence from animal studies indicates that this mechanism may be the cause of the 'systemic inflammatory reaction syndrome'. Inflammatory mediators are released, particularly from macrophages in the liver (Kupffer cells), and multiple organ dysfunction and organ failure may ensue. Little direct evidence supports this contention in humans, but early postoperative enteral feeding after severe abdominal injury, and even after elective abdominal surgery, is associated with fewer postoperative complications than in patients treated conventionally by initial abstention from food and a gradual resumption of spontaneous intake.

The main disadvantages of enteral feeding are mechanical, with the unpredictable ability of the gastrointestinal tract to tolerate and absorb enough nutrients to fulfil nutritional requirements. It is common practice to infuse nutrients continuously, as this facilitates the tolerance of large volumes, but if the infusion is into the stomach the normal mechanisms of gastric acidity maintenance are overwhelmed and the upper gastrointestinal tract, including the esophagus and pharynx, can become colonized with commensals. This may be associated with a higher incidence of nosocomial pneumonia. Aspiration pneumonia is also a potential problem. Diarrhea is a common complication, along with nausea, vomiting, and abdominal distension. In severe illness gastric emptying may also be delayed, which predisposes to the dangers of vomiting and aspiration. Direct infusion of nutrients into the jejunum may solve this problem, but the procedure itself has complications.

Parenteral feeding

The principal difference metabolically between parenteral and enteral feeding is that the gastrointestinal tract and the liver are bypassed, so the regulatory, buffering, and protective effects of these organs on the absorption of nutrients are missing. Nutrients are placed directly into the bloodstream so the patient is exposed to a variety of complications and problems that do not exist when nutritional support is given via the gastrointestinal tract.

Traditionally, intravenous feeding has been given via a central vein because of the hyperosmolar nature of the solutions and the danger of thrombosis. Peripheral intravenous feeding has, however, been carried out successfully in many centers, often with the help of nitroglycerin patches to promote vasodilatation and thus maintain patency of the vein. Direct delivery of nutrient solutions into the venous system also predisposes to infection. Dilute feeds (e.g. 20% dextrose instead of 50%) tend to avoid the problem of thrombosis, but larger volumes have to be given and problems of fluid overload may arise, particularly in critically ill patients. The morbidity and mortality associated with intravenous feeding maintained for less than a week, or given to well-nourished individuals (i.e. essentially people who do not need it), is greater than the benefit gained.

More metabolic problems occur with intravenous than with enteral feeding. Substances administered intravenously have to be well defined chemically and pharmaceutically, so the patient's requirements must be extremely well defined also. Since the advent of parenteral feeding the importance of many substances now given routinely has come to be appreciated, after patients developed signs of deficiency. Examples are the essential fatty acids, phosphates, zinc, copper, selenium, chromium, etc.

Other complications of intravenous feeding result mostly from the consequences of glucose placed directly into the vascular system. Intravenous infusion bypasses the regulatory and buffering functions of gastrointestinal absorption and the liver, and control of blood glucose is more fragile. The insulinemic response may be less than adequate for the prescribed amount of glucose, particularly in septic and injured patients, such that exogenous insulin is needed. This is given into the venous system, whereas normally it would appear in the portal vein. Similarly, if a glucose infusion prompts a vigorous insulin response (or exogenous insulin is given) and the glucose infusion is stopped abruptly the excess insulin in the circulation can produce hypoglycemia.

Hyperglycemia itself can induce a hyperosmolar nonketotic diuresis and, in severe cases, coma. Malnourished patients who are nutritionally replete with glucose, and particularly with added insulin, shift their extracellular phosphate into cells as lean tissue is laid down, which may produce hypophosphatemia unless adequate supplementation is given. Symptoms include paresthesia, confusion, and coma. The same applies to K^+ and Mg^{2+}.

Excessive quantities of glucose raise carbon dioxide production and the respiratory quotient and so increase ventilation, which can be a problem in the presence of respiratory impairment. High levels of glucose and insulin also stimulate the sympathetic nervous system via an action on the hypothalamus, which affects blood pressure, and heart rate and rhythm. The potential for this when these substances are infused directly into the circulation is obviously greater than that with enteral feeding.

Complications from the intravenous infusion of fat include the deposition of lipid in the lungs and reticuloendothelial system, and impaired leukocyte function, but with modern lipid emulsions these are unlikely. Hypertriglyceridemia is sometimes a problem, but usually clears when feeding is slowed or stopped for a while. Administration of heparin and insulin has been suggested if lipemia persists. Heparin stimulates lipoprotein lipase and the release of FFAs, while insulin encourages their deposition in adipose tissue stores.

Hepatic dysfunction and the elevation of liver transaminases is a feature of parenteral feeding. Administration of excessive quantities of intravenous feed, usually glucose based, is associated with deposition of fat in the liver. The precise cause of these abnormalities is not known, although it may be related to lack of enteral stimulation. Inhibition of gallbladder emptying, commonly seen with intravenous feeding, certainly is, and in many patients biliary sludge may form.

When amino acids are given at rates greater than they can be utilized in protein synthesis, the excess is deaminated and the patient may become uremic. This should be monitored for and the rate of amino acid provision adjusted accordingly. The advantages and disadvantages of the enteral and parenteral routes are summarized in Figure 59.4.

STARVATION

Starvation is defined as an inadequacy or absence of exogenous energy substrate depending on whether the starvation is partial or complete. The work of Keys and colleagues in the latter part of the Second World War – the so called Minnesota Study – on normal volunteers provided most of what is known about the whole-body physiologic aspects of starvation. The endocrine–substrate relationships seen in starvation were defined in the 1960s, and in the past 20 years we have come to appreciate that many hospital patients are malnourished, that admission to hospital often results in a decline in nutritional status, and that this may have an adverse effect on outcome.

Adaptation to starvation

Apart from its mineral and water content the body is composed of carbohydrate, fat, and protein. The oxidation of these endogenous nutrients provides the starving individual with energy, but the stores of these energy substrates are finite. There are no 'stores' of protein, so protein loss is associated with a decline in function, be it muscle strength, immune function, or the ability to digest normal food if and when intake is resumed.

The adaptive responses to starvation have two overriding themes – conservation of energy and conservation of protein (nitrogen).

Energy conservation

The body conserves energy in two ways, one behavioral and the other biochemical. Behaviorally, voluntary and spontaneous activity decrease. The individual does not move unless he or she has to. Responses to external stimuli are diminished and in extreme cases responses may be elicited only if survival itself is threatened. Biochemically, basal or resting metabolic rate declines. In absolute terms, a decline in metabolic rate of 30% was described in the Minnesota study, but when normalized to body size (to take account of the loss of body mass) the real decrease was 15%. This decrease in energy expenditure arises partly from a decrease in mass of the most metabolically active tissues – the liver decreases in size by 40%, the gastrointestinal tract by 30%, and the kidneys and heart by 20% each. The mucosa of the gastrointestinal tract decreases in mass and in function, such that if refeeding is started with a normal diet after a prolonged period of adaptation to starvation, the diet is not tolerated and the subject is unable to digest it. In addition, a decrease in sympathetic nervous activity and a decline in thyroid activity occur, both of which lead to a decrease in metabolic rate.

Protein and nitrogen conservation

The basic problem is the ongoing needs of some tissues for glucose and their inability, at least initially, to metabolize anything else. Glucose stores are limited and, when they are exhausted within the first 2 days, the principal alternative source of glucose is synthesis from the gluconeogenic amino acids that make up the body protein. The main consumer of glucose is the brain, but red blood cells and the renal medulla also need it. In the injured or septic individual, the wounded and septic tissue obtain their energy from glucose via glycolysis.

The biochemical changes that occur in starvation keep the brain supplied with glucose, but at the same time minimize the rate at which lean tissue is lost. Adaptation of substrate utilization and oxidation in starvation follows three well recognized sequential phases – the glycogenolytic phase, the gluconeogenic phase, and the ketogenic phase

Glycogenolysis

Glucose is stored as glycogen in liver and muscle. Glycogen acts as a store or buffer of glucose to cover the relatively brief periods (8–12 hours in humans) when the organism does not eat. Glucose is released from glycogen into the bloodstream, and enough

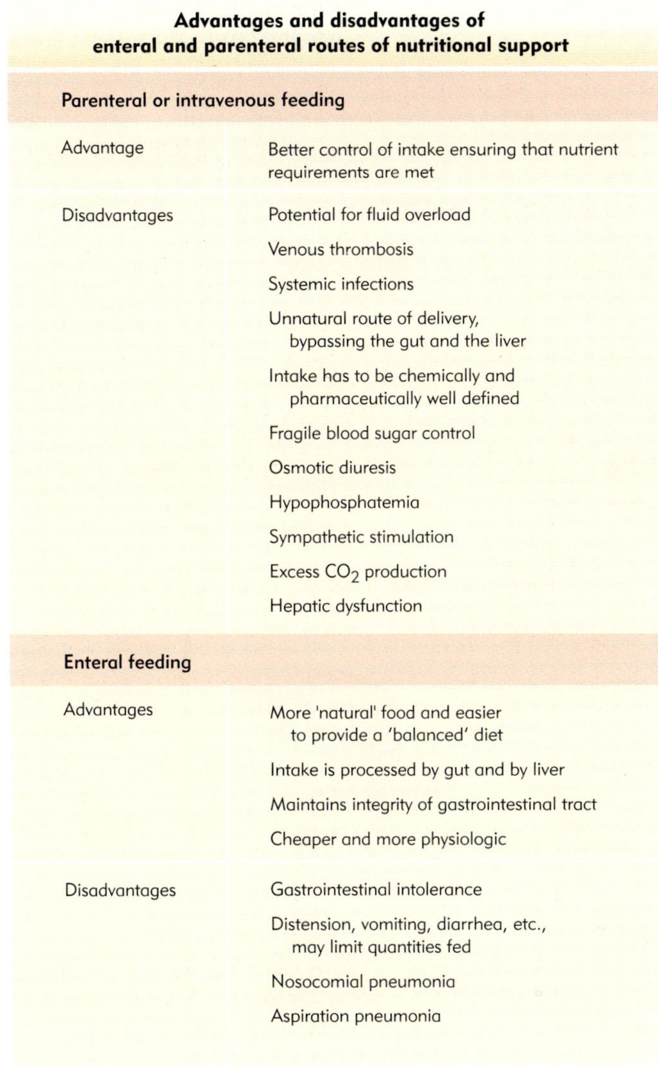

Advantages and disadvantages of enteral and parenteral routes of nutritional support

Parenteral or intravenous feeding	
Advantage	Better control of intake ensuring that nutrient requirements are met
Disadvantages	Potential for fluid overload Venous thrombosis Systemic infections Unnatural route of delivery, bypassing the gut and the liver Intake has to be chemically and pharmaceutically well defined Fragile blood sugar control Osmotic diuresis Hypophosphatemia Sympathetic stimulation Excess CO_2 production Hepatic dysfunction
Enteral feeding	
Advantages	More 'natural' food and easier to provide a 'balanced' diet Intake is processed by gut and by liver Maintains integrity of gastrointestinal tract Cheaper and more physiologic
Disadvantages	Gastrointestinal intolerance Distension, vomiting, diarrhea, etc., may limit quantities fed Nosocomial pneumonia Aspiration pneumonia

Figure 59.4 Advantages and disadvantages of enteral and parenteral routes of nutritional support.

glycogen is present to maintain blood glucose for about 24 hours. Glycogen is also stored in muscle in quantities greater than that in liver, because of the greater muscle mass. Muscle glycogen does not contribute to blood glucose, as muscle lacks glucose-6-phosphatase, but normally provides energy for muscle contraction. However, when oxygen (and energy) demand outstrips supply, such as in severe exercise, or in shock when glycolysis is stimulated by epinephrine (adrenaline), glucose is metabolized to pyruvate and converted into lactate. Lactate can pass into the circulation and, as a gluconeogenic precursor, is synthesized into glucose by the liver.

Gluconeogenesis

When glucose stores run out, the glucose requirements of the brain, erythrocytes, and renal medulla are obtained from gluconeogenesis, the precursors being lactate, glycerol, and the gluconeogenetic amino acids obtained from body protein. Nitrogen passes to the liver and kidney; in starvation, the kidney is also a site of gluconeogenesis. Nitrogen is transferred largely as alanine and glutamine. Branch-chain amino acids have a specific role in this; they are deaminated to their corresponding oxo (keto) acids, which are oxidized in muscle. The amino group is transferred to either pyruvate, the end product of glycolysis, to form alanine or to 2-oxoglutarate (α-ketoglutarate) to form glutamate. Glutamate may combine with a further amino group to form glutamine. About 50% of the amino groups leave muscle as alanine and glutamine, which pass to the liver and kidney for gluconeogenesis.

Ketogenesis

The largest energy store in the body is adipose tissue, in which fat is stored as triglycerides. Ultimately, in prolonged starvation the body obtains most of its energy from fat metabolism. Ketones are synthesized in the liver from fatty acids and substitute for glucose in the peripheral tissues. The brain continues to metabolize glucose, but some metabolic adaptation occurs and eventually the brain derives about half its energy requirements from ketones. As it does so, the rate of consumption of amino acids diminishes; nitrogen excretion, the ultimate index of protein oxidation, declines from 10–12g/day to about 2–6g/day.

Fat is oxidized and ketones are synthesized in the mitochondria. To enter the mitochondrion, the long-chain fatty acids require carnitine and its associated enzymes. The synthesis of carnitine requires a methyl group obtained from the amino acid methionine so that, even for fat to be used as fuel, an ongoing requirement is for the breakdown of lean tissue.

When the fat stores eventually run out a 'premortal' rise in nitrogen excretion occurs as protein oxidation increases just before death. The time an individual can survive without food depends on his or her energy (fat) stores. Some pathologically obese individuals have fasted under medical supervision, receiving mineral and vitamin supplements, for over a year, but in people of normal size and composition death usually occurs at 60–70 days.

Hormonal control of substrate utilization in starvation

The stimulus to gluconeogenesis, and ultimately to ketoadaptation, arises mainly from the decline in blood glucose, followed by a decrease in insulin and a rise in glucagon. Glucagon stimulates hepatic gluconeogenesis as well as lipolysis and the release of FFAs from adipose tissue. The decline in insulin results in the release of amino acids from lean tissue, and ultimately from muscle. Glucagon increases over the first 4 days (the gluconeogenetic phase) and declines toward days 7–10 as the ketogenic phase develops, after which glucagon is stable, but circulating concentrations are higher than normal.

The other hormone involved in protein breakdown is cortisol, but this does not alter in starvation. Its normal diurnal variation disappears and in starvation it is thought to have a permissive role. As starvation continues, tri-iodothyronine decreases in parallel with the decline in energy expenditure and the decrease in protein breakdown. Long-term starvation is accompanied by a decrease in sympathetic activity. These changes are summarized in Figures 59.5 & 59.6.

Recovery from starvation

When weight is regained after a period of semistarvation, adipose tissue is regained at first and by 6 months has increased to quantities greater than those seen before the period of starvation started. Over the ensuing 6 months this excess adipose tissue diminishes to prestarvation amounts and lean body mass also recovers. This type of pattern is seen in patients recovering from major surgery, an episode in which a period of semistarvation is accompanied by a traumatic insult (albeit a controlled one).

Metabolic adaptations to starvation

Energy conservation	Protein conservation
Decrease in spontaneous activity	Glucose required for brain, red cells, renal medulla, wound tissue
Decrease in metabolic rate	Glycogen stores exhausted after 24–48h
Loss of metabolically active tissue	Glucose normally obtained from glucogenic amino acids with loss of lean tissue
Decrease in sympathetic activity	Ketones synthesised by liver from free fatty acids
	Peripheral tissues adapt to using ketones instead of glucos

Figure 59.5 Metabolic adaptations to starvation.

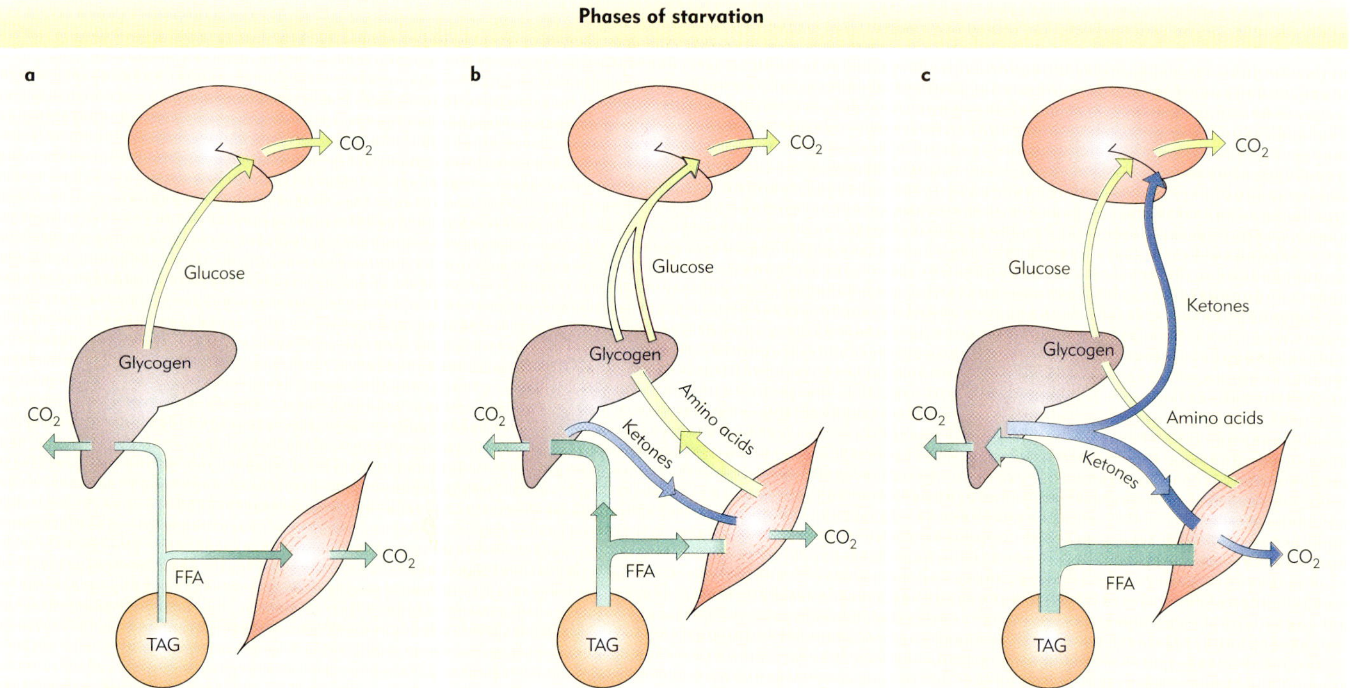

Figure 59.6 Glycogenolytic, gluconeogenetic, and the ketogenic phases of starvation. (a) Glycogen stores in the liver provide glucose for the brain. Peripheral tissues oxidize both FFAs from adipose tissue [triglyceride (TAG)] and glucose from glycogen stores. Glycogen is still present in the muscle, but does not contribute to blood sugar other than indirectly as lactate. (b) In the gluconeogenetic phase, glucose is obtained from amino acids in lean tissue, and the use of FFAs by peripheral tissue is increased. (c) In the ketogenic phase (fully adapted), the brain derives about 50% of its energy requirements from ketones and gluconeogenesis from lean tissue is diminished.

Key References

Carr C, Ling EKD, Boulos P, Singer M. Randomised trial of safety and efficacy of immediate postoperative enteral feeding in patients undergoing gastrointestinal resection. Br Med J. 1996;312:869–71.

Moore FA, Moore EE, Jones TN, McCroskey BL, Peterson VM. TEN versus TPN following major abdominal trauma – reduced septic morbidity. Trauma. 1989;29:916–23.

MacBurney M, Wilmore DW. Rational decision making in nutritional care. Surg Clin North Am. 1981;61:571–82.

Shaw JHF, Wolfe RR. Alanine, urea and glucose interrelationships in normal subjects and patients with sepsis with stable isotope tracers. Surgery. 1986;97:557–67.

Shaw JHF, Wilbore M, Wolfe RR. Whole body protein kinetics in severely septic patients. Ann Surg. 1987;205:288–94.

Streat SJ, Beddoe AH, Hill GL. Aggressive nutritional support does not prevent protein loss despite fat gain in septic intensive care patients. J Trauma. 1987;27:262–6.

Further Reading

Frayn KN. Metabolic regulation. A human perspective. London: Portland Press; 1996.

Hill GL. Disorders of nutrition and metabolism in clinical surgery. Edinburgh: Churchill Livingstone; 1992.

Payne-James J, Grimble G, Silk D, eds. Artificial nutrition support in clinical practice. London: Edward Arnold; 1995.

Chapter 60 Physiology and pharmacology of nausea and vomiting

Karen H Simpson and Louise Lynch

Topics covered in this chapter

Initiation and control of vomiting
Mechanics of vomiting
Mediators of emesis
Postoperative nausea and vomiting

The advantage in the elimination of ingested toxins by emesis is clear, but the role of emesis in perioperative situations is less obvious. Research concerning neuronal pathways and transmitters involved in emesis may facilitate development of therapies for the effective control of emesis. However, there are limitations to animal studies; for example, nausea in animals is impossible to confirm and not all animals can vomit. Animals incapable of vomiting may have developed an adequate system of preingestion toxin detection, which may involve nausea. The feeding habits of many animals that can vomit suggest that a postingestion toxin detection system linked to a means of eliminating the contents of the upper gastrointestinal tract (GIT) is needed. However, there are species differences between animals that vomit, in neuroanatomy and in susceptibility to emetogens (e.g. apomorphine). Humans have both preingestion and postingestion systems for detecting toxins. Higher cognitive activity can recruit nausea and vomiting as a response to many circumstances.

Definitions

Nausea is a subjectively unpleasant sensation associated with awareness of the urge to vomit. Retching refers to the laboured rhythmic activity of the respiratory musculature that usually precedes vomiting. Vomiting or emesis is the forceful expulsion of upper gastrointestinal contents via the mouth, caused by the powerful sustained contraction of the abdominal muscles. Nausea, retching, and vomiting are often, but not invariably, related. An emetogen is a stimulus to emesis, and an emetic is a chemical capable of inducing emesis.

INITIATION AND CONTROL OF VOMITING

Initiation of vomiting

Vomiting can be triggered by a variety of physical, pharmacologic, physiologic, and pathophysiologic stimuli:

- dilatation of the stomach (e.g. obstruction or overeating);
- gastric mucosal irritation (e.g. alcohol or drugs);
- higher cognitive activity (e.g. unpleasant sights, smells, or ideas);
- pharyngeal mucosal stimulation;
- vestibulocochlear stimulation (e.g. motion sickness);
- pregnancy;
- pain;
- poisons, toxins, and medications (e.g. chemotherapy, analgesic, and anesthetic drugs);
- therapeutic radiation;
- raised intracranial pressure, intracerebral hemorrhage, and tumors.

Neurophysiology of vomiting

A toxin recognized by color, smell, or taste causes rejection of the food and development of a learned aversion, which may include nausea. Postingestion detection may occur before or after absorption of the toxin into the blood. Preabsorption detection is mediated by the vagus nerve, particularly in the upper GIT (Figs 60.1 & 60.2). Splanchnic afferent stimulation may play a role, particularly after vagotomy. There are bare vagal nerve endings in the gut wall, most of which terminate in the nucleus of the tractus solitarius (NTS). A few fibers end in the area postrema (AP) and dorsal motor vagal nucleus (DMVN). The NTS has connections with the AP. Most information from the gut probably takes this route. Potential neurotransmitters at this level include thyrotropin-releasing hormone, catecholamines, enkephalin, substance P, vasopressin, and somatostatin.

Mucosal afferents are responsible for the emetic response to luminal toxins. Stimuli to mucosal afferents include hypertonic solutions, copper sulfate, 5-hydroxytryptamine (5-HT), cholecystokinin (CCK), plant alkaloids, and invertebrate toxins. Secondary sensory cells in the gut mucosa may respond to changes in the luminal environment and release a transmitter that causes discharge of afferent fibers. Irradiation, cytotoxic agents, and gut ischemia may produce emesis by releasing 5-HT from the gut mucosa and stimulating vagal afferents. Antagonism of 5-HT_3 and CCK_A receptors does not prevent mucosal afferents from responding to stimuli such as hypertonic saline or luminal acid. Therefore, although the mucosal afferents are sensitive to both 5-HT and CCK, these are not essential mediators in the emetic pathway. Muscular afferents are tension receptors in the gut wall that respond to distention and contraction. They monitor gut content and propagation, to facilitate smooth digestion. Abnormal gut distention or contractility can stimulate vomiting.

Postabsorption detection occurs in the AP (chemoreceptor trigger zone, CTZ). This a vascular area on the surface of the

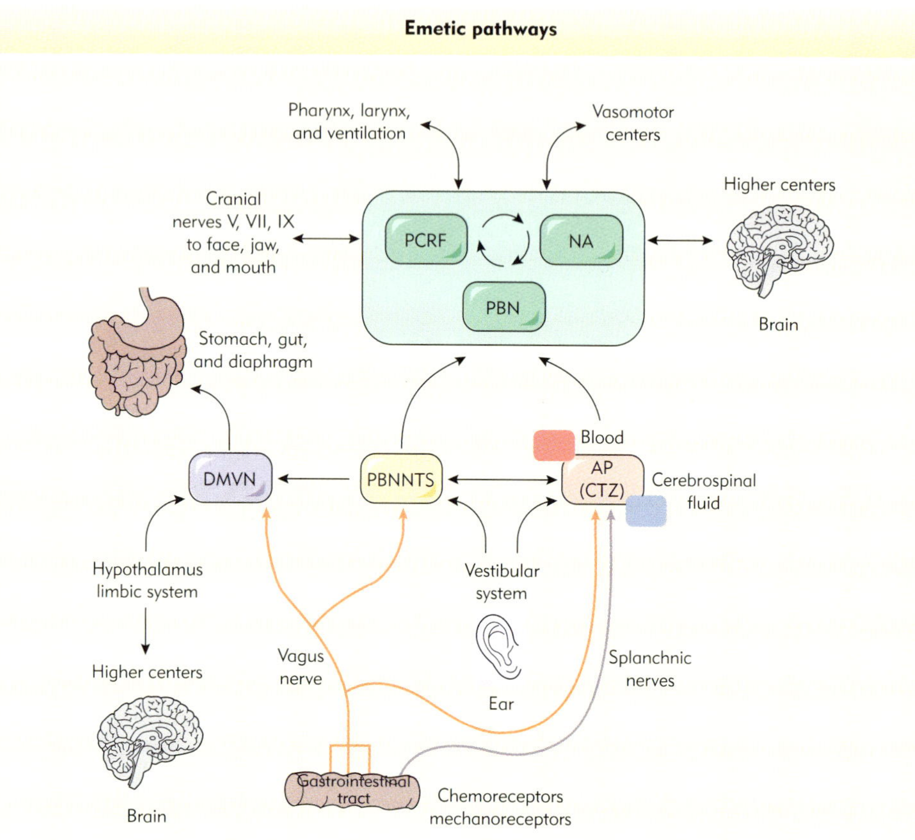

Figure 60.1 Emetic pathways. The control of emesis within the brain and gastrointestinal tract. AP (CTZ), area postrema (chemoreceptor trigger zone); DMVN, dorsal motor vagal nucleus; NA, nucleus ambiguus; NTS, nucleus of tractus solitarius; PBN, parabrachial nucleus; PCRF, parvicellular reticular formation.

caudal end of the floor of the fourth ventricle As the blood–brain barrier is incomplete in this area, the AP has access to agents in both blood and cerebrospinal fluid. The AP receives afferents from the NTS, vagus nerve, splanchnic nerves, and vestibular labyrinth. If the AP is destroyed, vomiting can still occur.

Emesis is mediated by what was previously called the 'vomiting center' (VC), although no such single brain area has ever been identified. The VC should be regarded as a central pattern generator or medullary control system. It coordinates the action of various autonomic and somatic nuclei, which collectively mediate vomiting. A number of brainstem nuclei are involved.

The NTS receives afferents from the vagus and AP. It sends efferents to all nuclei involved in vomiting and to the hypothalamus and limbic system. The parvicellular reticular formation (PCRF) may regulate ventilation during vomiting via connections with the parabrachial nucleus (PBN) and nucleus ambiguus (NA). The PCRF interconnects with trigeminal (V), facial (VII), and hypoglossal (IX) cranial nerve nuclei, controlling the tongue, mouth, and jaws. The NA controls laryngeal and pharyngeal musculature, and some aspects of ventilation. It interconnects with the PBN. The interaction between the two, possibly regulated by the PCRF, may be the mechanism responsible for retching and vomiting. The DMVN receives inputs from the vagus, hypothalamic, and limbic systems, to which it sends afferents. This may be how cortical activity can influence the processing of gastrointestinal afferent information or can initiate vomiting. The DMVN is responsible for motor outputs to the GIT. The efferent limb of the vagal reflex in the vomiting pathway originates from the DMVN. It is mediated by both excitatory cholinergic and inhibitory nonadrenergic noncholinergic (NANC) pathways back to the GIT. Nuclei in the ventrolateral medulla regulate sympathetic outflow from the spinal cord.

MECHANICS OF VOMITING

The motor components of vomiting are integrated by brainstem nuclei. Prodromal phenomena include nausea, salivation, tachycardia, altered breathing, pallor, sweating, and pupillary dilatation.

Visceral events

The contents of the small intestine are returned to the stomach and the gastric contents are confined by a number of visceral events. Gastrointestinal motility in the proximal bowel is inhibited by reduction in electrical control activity. There is relaxation of the proximal stomach followed by initiation of a retrograde giant contraction (RGC) or antiperistalsis in the jejunum. This returns small intestinal contents to the relaxed stomach. Phasic contractions occur in the antrum and small intestine, with inhibition of small intestinal activity, lasting for several minutes.

Striated esophageal muscles contract, shortening the intra-abdominal esophagus toward the diaphragm. Dilatation of the cardia and gastroesophageal sphincter occurs. This enables the gastric contents to pass easily into the esophagus once retching commences. Once active vomiting has ceased, residual esophageal contents are cleared by secondary peristalsis and closure of the lower esophageal sphincter.

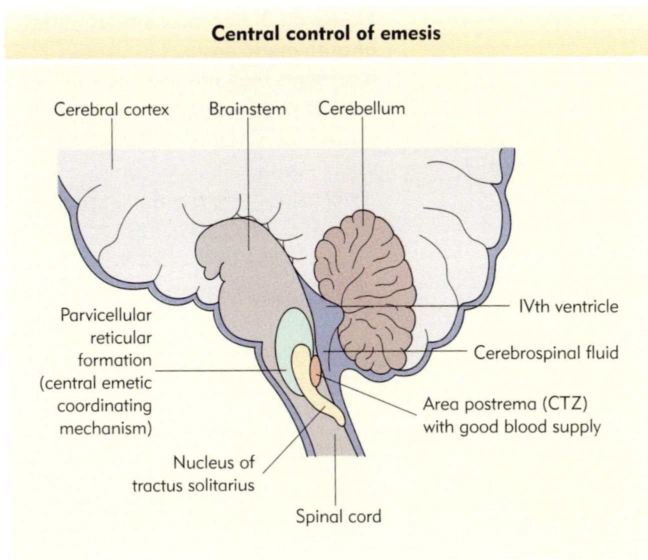

Figure 60.2 Central control of emesis. The structures within the brain involved in the control of emesis.

Somatic events

Retching is characterized by rhythmic inspiratory movements against a closed glottis. This overcomes mechanisms designed to limit gastroesophageal reflux. The diaphragm, abdominal muscles, and internal intercostal muscles contract synchronously. This causes simultaneous large pressure changes (100mmHg): negative intrathoracic and positive intra-abdominal. The upper esophageal sphincter relaxes during a retch and is pulled open by raising of the hyoid bone and larynx, allowing gastric contents to reflux upwards. The esophageal sphincter contracts again between retches to prevent expulsion. During vomiting, the diaphragm does not contract but is fixed in the inspiratory position. The glottis is closed, and the soft palate lifts to close the posterior nares. Contraction of the abdominal muscles produces a pulse of positive pressure, transmitted from abdomen to thorax. This is accompanied by relaxation of the cardia and esophagopharyngeal sphincter and elevation of the soft palate. This allows gastric contents to pass from the stomach to the mouth.

MEDIATORS OF EMESIS

Investigating the emetic pathway

Many neurotransmitters have been implicated in emesis. Identification of agonist and antagonist ligands influences development of therapeutic agents. Animal preparations and human studies have been used to assess the emetic pathway, including vagotomy studies and ablation of the AP.

Known ligands have been used to clarify the actions of unknown substances or receptors. For example, apomorphine is a dopamine (D_2) receptor agonist acting in the AP. Any drug inhibiting apomorphine-induced vomiting is presumably a D_2 antagonist. Intracerebroventricular (ICV) injections of agonist and antagonist ligands have also been used to investigate the site of action of different compounds, and radioligand binding studies have been used to identify central and peripheral receptors involved in emesis.

The c-*fos* gene is rapidly expressed in response to neuronal activation. Mapping of central neuronal circuitry responsible for vomiting has been investigated by administering multiple potent emetic agents and then looking for expression of the c-*fos* protein product throughout the brain. Mapping can also be performed using electrical stimulation, usually in decerebrate cats, to identify anatomic areas responsible for vomiting.

Antiemetics and receptors

Known antiemetics (Fig. 60.3) and emetics can be classified by their interactions with various neurotransmitter receptors.

Dopamine

The classic AP receptor involved in emesis is the D_2 dopamine receptor. Other receptors in the AP may exert their effects by releasing dopamine (e.g. 5-HT_3 receptors). Dopamine receptors are also present in the NTS and DMVN. Dopamine agonists, such as bromocriptine and apomorphine, produce emesis. Dopamine antagonists, such as metoclopramide, droperidol, and prochlorperazine, are antiemetics useful in the management of emesis. Extrapyramidal side effects limit their use, particularly in children. Domperidone is a D_2 antagonist with reduced brain penetrance

5-Hydroxytryptamine

The development of 5-HT_3 receptor antagonists has improved the prevention and treatment of nausea and vomiting associated with chemotherapy and radiotherapy, and these agents may also be useful in the treatment of postoperative nausea and vomiting (PONV). The 5-HT_3 receptors are distributed centrally (AP, NTS, cerebral cortex, hippocampus) and peripherally (gut mucosa, nerve endings, primary afferent nerve fibers). They are ligand-gated, cation-selective ion channels (see Chapters 3 & 19). Activation allows ion channel opening, increasing the conductance to Na^+ and K^+ and resulting in membrane depolarization and neuronal excitation. Agonists include 2-methyl-5-HT and phenyl biguanide, both of which are relatively nonselective. Antagonists include ondansetron, granisetron, zacopride, MDL 7222, and ICS 205930, which are all highly selective. These agents have no effect on apomorphine-induced vomiting. Animal studies show that 5-HT causes emesis by acting on 5-HT_3 receptors located centrally and within the small intestine. Cisplatin damages the intestinal mucosa, releasing 5-HT from enterochromaffin cells and causing emesis. This increased release of 5-HT is reflected by increased plasma and urinary 5-hydroxyindoleacetic acid (5-HIAA) concentrations, its principal metabolite. 5-HT from the gut undergoes extensive first-pass metabolism and does not produce more generalized sequelae. Cytotoxic drugs may release 5-HT from neurons near the hindbrain structures involved in the emetic reflex. The emetic effect of cisplatin is mainly at the gut receptor, rather than at the AP. Antagonism of 5-HT_3 receptors can prevent the emesis that follows increased local 5-HT concentrations. Consequently, reducing 5-HT production might have a similar effect. This can be achieved by inhibiting 5-HT synthesis and depleting endogenous stores. Tryptophan hydroxylase is the rate-limiting enzyme in the synthesis of 5-HT. It can be inhibited by *p*-chlorophenylalanine (*p*-CPA). Animal and patient studies using this agent are in progress. Treatment with *p*-CPA reduces basal and cisplatin-evoked increases in urinary excretion of 5-HIAA and attenuates emesis.

The 5-HT_{1A} receptors are located primarily on presynaptic nerve terminals in the cerebral cortex, raphe nucleus, NTS, and hippocampus and in arterioles. Activation leads to a reduction in cyclic AMP (cAMP) and hyperpolarization of the cell membrane. This inhibits neuronal firing. Agonists such as 8-OH DPAT [8-

Receptor site affinities of antiemetic drugs

Drug group	Receptor site affinity			
	Dopamine (D_2)	Muscarinic (cholinergic)	Histamine (H_2)	Serotonin (5-HT_3)
Phenothiazine				
fluphenazine	++++	+	++	–
chlorpromazine	++++	++	++++	+
prochlorperazine	++++			
Butyrophenone				
droperidol	++++	–	+	+
haloperidol	++++	–	+	–
domperidone	++++			
Antihistamine				
diphenhydramine	+	++	++++	–
promethazine	++	++	++++	–
Anticholinergic				
scopolamine	+	++++	+	–
Benzamide				
metoclopramide	+++	–	+	++
Antiserotonin				
ondansetron	–	–	–	++++
granisetron	–	–	–	++++
zacopride	–	–	–	++++
RG 12145	–	–	–	++++

Figure 60.3 Receptor site affinities of antiemetic drugs. (++++ represents high affinity, and – represents low affinity.

hydroxy-2-(di-*N*-propylamino)tetralin], flesinoxan, and buspirone produce anxiolysis and hypotension. Antagonists include pindolol, cyanpindol, and spiperone. Animal studies have revealed that 5-HT_{1A} agonists antagonize the effects of different classes of emetogen, including cisplatin, morphine, and oral copper sulfate, and are active in motion and conditioned-vomiting models. The precise mechanism of antiemetic action is speculative, but because of the broad spectrum of activity, it is presumably on a convergent structure in the CNS. Preclinical data suggest that behavioral side effects may limit acceptability. Buspirone is an anxiolytic but is only a weak partial agonist at 5-HT_{1A} receptors and has little antiemetic potential.

Characterization of the 5-HT_4 receptor is derived from cumulative evidence from several sources rather than from identification of any particular ligand. The absence of a suitable radioligand has hampered studies of this receptor, but a pharmacologic profile is available. The 5-HT_4 receptor is widely distributed within the cerebral cortex, superior colliculi, GIT, and myocardium. Activation results in membrane depolarization via an increase in intracellular cAMP. Receptor activation in the gut causes release of acetylcholine in the myenteric plexus. This results in relaxation of the esophagus and sphincter, with increased gastric motility and emptying. Receptor activation also causes cerebral activation and tachycardia. Agonists include the benzamides (metoclopramide and cisapride), the benzimidazolones (BIMU-1 and BIMU-8), and some indole derivatives (5-methoxytryptamine). Antagonists include the benzamide SDZ 205,557, the benzimidazolone DAU 6215, and the indole GR113808. The 5-HT_4 receptor does seem to influence emesis, but animal studies have produced conflicting results. Oral agonists (zacopride and 5-methoxytryptamine) provoke vomiting, but administration of the highly potent, selective antagonist GR125487 does not prevent emesis.

Acetylcholine

Acetylcholine is the agonist at muscarinic and nicotinic cholinergic receptors in the parasympathetic nervous system (see Chapter 29). Muscarinic cholinergic receptors are found in the NA, NTS, and DMVN. The vestibular initiation of motion sickness acts via central acetylcholine receptors and can, therefore, only be alleviated by drugs that penetrate the blood–brain barrier. Acetylcholine receptors are also found peripherally, where they mediate the gastrointestinal motor correlates of vomiting. Anticholinergic drugs commonly used in anesthetic practise include atropine, scopolamine (hyoscine), and glycopyrrolate (glycopyrronium). Glycopyrrolate is a quaternary ammonium compound that does not cross the blood–brain barrier and has no useful antiemetic activity. The antiemetic action of anticholinergic drugs results from a combination of central blocking of motion sickness, peripheral reduction of salivary and gastric secretions, motor (antispasmodic) activity, and prevention of relaxation of sphincters. The central potency of scopolamine is around 10 times that of atropine. This probably accounts for its success in the prophylaxis and management of motion sickness. Scopolamine is poorly absorbed enterally but can be absorbed transdermally and after sublingual administration. Side effects include drowsiness and confusion, a particular problem in the elderly.

Opioids

Opioids have both emetic and antiemetic actions. The emetic effect may be via stimulation of opioid (probably μ) receptors in the AP. Ablation of the AP abolishes the emetic response. The receptors responsible for the antiemetic effect of opioids, particularly in high dosage, may be either μ or δ type. The existence of an 'antiemetic' center in the brainstem awaits further investigation.

Adrenergic agents

Alpha-adrenoceptor agonists initiate vomiting in many animal studies. Agonists such as xylazine, epinephrine (adrenaline), and norepinephrine (noradrenaline) evoke vomiting in cats and dogs by their action at α_2-adrenoceptors in the AP. This effect is blocked by antagonists such as yohimbine, tolazoline, and phentolamine. In humans clonidine (an α_2-agonist) may be antiemetic. Methoxamine-induced vomiting is probably mediated by central α_1-adrenoceptors, most likely on postsynaptic cells in the AP. In conditions where adrenoceptors are a factor in causing vomiting, α_2-adrenoceptor antagonists may have a role as antiemetics, for example in pheochromocytoma and endotoxic shock.

Enkephalin

The AP is rich in enkephalin receptors. Local tissue concentrations of enkephalin seem to alter the susceptibility of the AP to excitatory stimuli. Enkephalin also increases dopamine release.

Cholecystokinin

The gastrointestinal mucosa contains CCK, which causes activation of vagal afferents in a similar manner to 5-HT. This effect can be blocked by a specific CCK_A receptor antagonist, devazepide.

Neurokinins

Animal studies have shown that an antagonist of substance P at a neurokinin (NK_1) receptor, CP99,994 [(+)-(2*S*,3*S*)-3-(2-methoxybenzylamino)-2-phenylpiperidine], is effective against a broad range of emetogens. It acts against agents working through a number of mechanisms: release of 5-HT, vagal stimulation (radiation and cisplatin), dopamine D_2 receptors (apomorphine), and opioid receptors (morphine). It is also active against nicotine (a centrally acting emetogen), agents causing gastric irritation (copper sulfate), and a clinically used emetogen (ipecacuanha). In cisplatin-induced vomiting, it was most successful if given following the first vomit, rather than as a prophylactic. It may have a central site of action, which may be the AP. There are no adverse effects in animal studies; human trials are awaited

Sigma receptor modulators

The sigma (σ) receptors are distributed throughout the brain, including the cranial nerve nuclei, hypothalamus, hippocampus, red nucleus, septum, and cerebellum. The role of σ receptors remains poorly defined because of lack of a selective ligand. A large and chemically diverse range of compounds bind to σ receptors (benzomorphan opioids, steroids, and antipsychotic drugs). The ligand usually used to study σ activity (*N*-allylnormetazocine) is not specific and produces many of its effects via interactions with other receptors. More selective σ agonists have been described, including 1,3-ditolylguanidine (DTG), amitriptyline, and *cis*-*N*-[2-(3,4-dichlorophenyl)ethyl]-*N*-methyl-2-(1-pyrrolidinyl)cyclohexylamine (BD737). Antagonists include haloperidol and the putative antipsychotic agent α-(4-fluorophenyl)-4-(5-fluoro-2-pyrimidinyl)-1-piperazinobutanol (BMY 14802). Agonists like DTG produce emesis, which is blocked by antagonists such as haloperidol and BMY 14802. Animal studies in pigeons have shown that antagonists with higher affinity for the σ site have a higher potency in blocking agonist-induced emesis, but studies in rats have produced conflicting results.

Gamma-aminobutyric acid

Benzodiazepines potentiate the inhibitory gamma-aminobutyric acid (GABAergic) interneurons, which are most densely located in the hippocampus, cerebellum, and cortex. Some studies have suggested that benzodiazepines decrease the incidence of PONV and chemotherapy-induced emesis. The mechanism of action may be by anxiolysis, hypnosis, retrograde amnesia, or a specific effect on GABAergic pathways involved in emesis.

Calcitonin

Calcitonin is a polypeptide hormone derived from thyroid C cells that regulates plasma Ca^{2+} concentration (see Chapter 63). Treatment with synthetic calcitonin is associated with nausea and vomiting; the mechanism by which this occurs is unclear. There is some evidence in dogs that suggests that calcitonin is capable of central vagal blockade, which may be relevant.

Histamine

Histamine (H_1) receptors are concentrated in the NTS and DMVN. Centrally acting antihistamines (which often possess anticholinergic activity), for example cyclizine and diphenhydramine, are used in the management of motion sickness and PONV. They have a relatively high therapeutic index and few side effects (drowsiness and anticholinergic effects). It is not clear if their antiemetic effects are mediated via H_1 receptors or acetylcholine.

Cannabinoids

Cannabis is derived from resin of the plant *Cannabis sativa*. The major active constituent is a Δ^9-tetrahydrocannabinol. The body has its own endogenous cannabinoid system, with central and peripheral receptors. An endogenous ligand exists, anandamide, which is a derivative of arachidonic acid. The antiemetic activity of cannabis may be related to psychotropic effects in the forebrain inhibiting the emetic pattern generator via descending pathways. The synthetic derivative nabilone has antiemetic effects and has been used in cancer chemotherapy. The psychoactive nature of the drug has limited research into its therapeutic potential. Adverse effects include euphoria, dysphoria, sedation, incoordination, and fetal toxicity.

Capsaicin

Capsaicin is a sensory neurotoxin causing desensitization of vagal afferent C fibers (see Chapter 21). Resinferatoxin (RTX), a naturally occurring analog, is 1000 times more potent than capsaicin and has none of its profound cardiorespiratory side effects. In animal experiments, RTX has been shown to block emesis induced by copper sulfate (gastric irritation), irradiation (5-HT release and vagal stimulation), and loperamide (a centrally acting emetogen). RTX may induce depletion of a neurotransmitter, possibly substance P or calcitonin gene-related peptide at a central point in the emetic pathway, possibly in the NTS.

Glutamate

Animal studies have shown that glutamate antagonists [in particular non-NMDA (*N*-methyl-D-aspartate) receptor antagonists NBQX and CNQX] can block cisplatin-induced emesis. A site of action in the AP has been postulated.

Antiemetics with unknown mechanism of action

Ginger

The powdered rhizome of *Zingiber officinale* (the common ginger root) is a traditional treatment for gastrointestinal complaints, being regarded as a carminative and spasmolytic agent. Its efficacy in the treatment of nausea and vomiting is unproved.

Some studies have demonstrated that oral premedication with ginger is as successful as metoclopramide for PONV. However, metoclopramide is not always efficacious. The active ingredient in ginger root and its mechanism of action are unknown; a local effect on the GIT has been proposed.

Acupuncture

The traditional Chinese method of acupuncture or acupressure at the P6 (Nei Guan) point is an effective treatment for nausea and vomiting. It is only useful in the conscious patient; it is ineffective if administered during anesthesia. The mechanism by which acupuncture achieves an antiemetic effect is unclear.

Steroids

In chemotherapy-induced emesis where the 5-HT_3 antagonists are not completely successful, the addition of dexamethasone is efficacious. The same is true for PONV. Dexamethasone as a single dose has infrequent side effects. The mechanism of antiemetic action of corticosteroids is unknown. Possibilities include decreased central and peripheral prostaglandin production and an anti-inflammatory action to reduce stimuli from the operative site and/or reduced 5-HT release from the gut.

POSTOPERATIVE NAUSEA AND VOMITING

PONV has been called 'the big little problem'. In the 'ether era', 75–80% of patients experienced PONV. With modern anesthesia and novel antiemetics, PONV still occurs in 20–30%, and intractable PONV occurs in 0.1%. PONV varies between the patients of individual (experienced) anesthetists, between different institutions, and between countries. The United Kingdom has the highest incidence of PONV in Western Europe and Germany the lowest. Patients are often more worried about PONV than pain. Emesis was responsible for dissatisfaction in 71% of patients in a survey of patients undergoing day-case (ambulatory) surgery. Complications can occur from PONV; for example, inhalation of gastric contents, wound dehiscence, bleeding, hematomas, dehydration, and electrolyte disturbances.

Predisposing factors

Risk factors that predispose to PONV include the patient, anesthetic regimen, surgical procedures, and postoperative factors (Fig. 60.4).

Risk factors for developing postoperative nausea and vomiting (PONV)

Predisposing patient factors
- Female gender (perimenstrual > preovulatory)
- Motion sickness
- Vestibular problems
- Morbid obesity
- Early pregnancy

Increased gastric volume
- Excessive anxiety
- Ingestion of solid food
- Delayed gastric emptying

Anesthetic agents
- Inhalational – volatiles, nitrous oxide
- Intravenous – ketamine, etomidate, thiopental
- Opioid analgesics – agonists, agonist–antagonists

Surgical procedures
- Laparoscopy
- Lithotripsy
- Strabismus correction
- Tonsillectomy (and/or adenoidectomy)
- Middle ear operations
- Orchidopexy

Postoperative factors
- Severe pain
- Hypotension/dehydration
- Premature ambulation
- Forcing oral fluid intake

Figure 60.4 Risk factors for developing postoperative nausea and vomiting (PONV).

Patient factors

There are a number of patient-related factors that affect the degree of PONV.

- Anesthetic history. Previous PONV increases the risk of emesis threefold.
- Gender. There is no difference between the sexes in childhood (<11 years) or late adulthood (>70 years); otherwise, the incidence of PONV is two to three times greater in females than in males and the severity of vomiting is greater. The incidence peaks during the third and fourth weeks (luteal phase) of the menstrual cycle.
- Age. PONV is least in infants (<1 year), with an incidence of approximately 5%; it increases to 20% in children (<5 years) and reaches a maximum of 35–50% in late childhood (6–16 years). It decreases throughout adulthood and is lowest by the eighth decade.
- Delayed gastric emptying. PONV increases when gastric motility and emptying are retarded.
- Motion sickness. A history of motion sickness may predispose to PONV.
- ASA status. ASA levels 1 and 2 are at greater risk than 3 and 4.
- Smoking. Smoking seems to confer some protection.
- Anxiety. The influence of mood is not confirmed.
- Body habitus. Obese patients may be more susceptible.

Anesthetic factors

A number of studies have examined the particular effects of different anesthetic agents. The use of benzodiazepines for premedication may reduce PONV. Of the induction agents, thiopental (thiopentone), etomidate, and ketamine are emetogens. Propofol may be antiemetic. A meta-analysis of 84 randomized controlled trials involving 6069 patients showed that use of propofol for maintenance of anesthesia reduced the incidence of PONV by 20%, but only for the first few postoperative hours. The effect was observed only in patients with a high incidence of PONV, such as those having pediatric strabismus and major gynecologic surgery. When used as an induction agent alone, propofol had a statistically significant, but less clinically relevant, effect on PONV. Propofol has been used in low dose (1mg/h per kg body weight) as an antiemetic for chemotherapy previously resistant to 5-HT_3 antagonists. Its mechanism of action is not clear. Propofol has little effect on endogenous 5-HT_3 receptors; it has no antidopaminergic activity and it does not alter apomorphine-induced vomiting. It may act by suppression of the AP, vagal nuclei, and/or other central sites.

The use of nitrous oxide for the maintenance of anesthesia has been suspected of contributing to PONV because nitrous oxide increases gut distention and middle ear pressure, but this is not proven. If it is omitted as part of a standard anesthetic technique, the risk of awareness may outweigh the potential problem of PONV. Most volatile anesthetics have been implicated in emesis. It has been suggested that sevoflurane with propofol infusion produces less immediate PONV than occurs with halothane.

A number of other factors related to the anesthetic procedure can also be influential on PONV.

- Opioid analgesics. Intraoperative opioids are a major cause of PONV.
- Reversal of neuromuscular blockade. The use of neostigmine may be associated with more PONV than if neuromuscular block is allowed to reverse spontaneously.
- Postoperative analgesia. Opioids are associated with higher rates of PONV. Local anesthetic procedures and adequate doses of acetominophen (paracetamol) or nonsteroidal anti-inflammatory drugs reduce opioid requirements and PONV.
- Perioperative fluid regimen. Adequate hydration reduces PONV.
- Experience of the anesthetist. Inexperienced anesthetists have more cases of PONV.

Preoperative surgical factors

Patients presenting for emergency procedures with a full stomach or with GIT obstruction or stasis have a higher risk of PONV. Other emergency patients seem to have a lower risk of emesis than elective patients. Vomiting often accompanies some surgical conditions, notably peritonitis, bowel obstruction, and raised intracranial pressure. Gastric decompression using a nasogastric tube may relieve the nausea associated with gastric distention but can replace it with nausea resulting from stimulation by the tube. The use of a perioperative nasogastric tube to empty the stomach does not alter the incidence of PONV, even if the tube is inserted and removed while the patient is anesthetized.

Operative procedure

Some procedures are emetogenic. PONV has an incidence of 36–76% after adenotonsillectomy, which may be a consequence of blood in the esophagus and stomach stimulating vagal afferents, trigeminal nerve stimulation, and the use of opioids. Other surgery associated with a high risk of PONV includes otoplasty, middle-ear surgery, strabismus surgery, and gynecologic procedures. Intra-abdominal operations often involve direct stimulation of gut vagal afferents, causing emesis. Gut ischemia leads to 5-HT release and PONV. Surgery of increasing duration may lead to increased emesis. In a study of more than 6000 patients, anesthesia lasting less than 60 minutes had an odds ratio of 1.0 for patients developing PONV; surgery of between 60 and 120 minutes had an odds ratio of 1.5, and surgery of more than 120 minutes had an odds ratio of 2.04.

Postoperative factors

There are a number of postoperative factors associated with PONV.

- Relief of postoperative pain reduces PONV. Antagonism of opioid analgesia by naloxone increases PONV.
- Hypotension. Hypotensive patients often feel nauseated, perhaps as a result of reduced medullary blood flow to the AP. Treatment of hypotension with volume replacement, vasoconstrictors, or inotropes cures nausea.
- Ambulation. Motion and changes in position, such as the turning of a supine patient into the recovery position, can precipitate PONV via cholinergic and, perhaps, histaminergic input to the AP from the vestibular apparatus. Opioids may sensitize the vestibular system to motion-induced nausea and vomiting.
- Oral intake. Early oral fluid intake can increase PONV. Day-case patients who are required to ingest fluids prior to discharge have significantly more emesis than patients on a fluid-restricted regimen.
- Opioids. Opioids are the major culprit in PONV. There is little difference in emetogenicity between intramuscular, intravenous patient-controlled analgesia (PCA), intrathecal, and epidural routes.

Studies of postoperative nausea and vomiting

There are many studies on PONV, but poor study design often compromises their interpretation. Various patient, anesthetic, surgical, and postoperative factors must be considered within the design of the research, and appropriate exclusion criteria should be used. Studies should be of double-blind, randomized, controlled design, with a sample size large enough to detect a significant difference in groups, if one exists. The required number of subjects for a clinical trial is related to power, significance, and the size of the difference between the success criteria of the two treatment groups, which should be determined before the trial (see Chapter 17). Logistic regression analysis has been used to identify the relative contribution of individual factors and combinations of factors. This is expressed by the relative odds of developing PONV for a particular factor or combination. Gender, history of PONV, opioids, and interaction between gender and history of PONV are significant independent fixed patient factors that have been identified (history of motion sickness was only weakly associated).

The measured events must be defined. Vomiting is relatively straightforward to assess. Most studies use the number of episodes of vomiting to grade severity. Assessment of nausea is more difficult: duration of symptoms, subjective assessments, or a visual analog score can be used. The data obtained are non-parametric and appropriate statistical analysis is required. The timing of assessment must be standardized. It is often performed in the postanesthesia care unit and then on the ward for inpatients. In day surgery, the time intervals are necessarily different and should include telephone follow-up or a postal questionnaire. Important end points in day surgery include time to first fluid intake, time to discharge, and unanticipated re-admissions to hospital. The decision when to administer rescue antiemetic, an important end point, and which drug to choose may be based on duration of nausea, occurrence of vomiting, and patient request.

Treatment

Despite many studies of PONV, the 'antiemetic for all seasons' remains elusive. This is presumably related to the multifactorial nature of the problem. The results of trials comparing antiemetics are difficult to interpret. Seemingly similar studies often reach different conclusions. Meta-analysis of comparable studies may be of value. The combination of a 5-HT_3 antagonist (e.g. 4mg ondansetron) and a steroid (8mg dexamethasone) has consistently been shown to be effective antiemetic prophylaxis. The 5-HT_3

antagonists are also useful in treating established emesis caused by opioids. Adverse effects associated with low-dose droperidol (0.125–0.5mg) are apparent. It should, perhaps, not be used in day-case anesthesia. It is effective in reducing PONV associated with morphine for PCA, although adverse effects such as dysphoria and akathisia need further assessment. Metoclopramide does not perform well in a large proportion of clinical trials. Antihistamines remain first-line drugs in many centers for safety reasons and their low cost. Cyclizine is as effective as droperidol when mixed with morphine for PCA.. Prochlorperazine, a dopamine D_2 antagonist, is a common second-line choice, with the 5-HT_3 antagonists often used as third-line agents. Nonpharmacologic techniques are not in widespread usage.

No currently available drug blocks all the receptor types involved in the initiation and mediation of PONV. Rather than having departmental protocols determining standard first- and second-line antiemetics, it is more appropriate to give high-risk patients a prophylactic drug to antagonize the proposed mechanism of emesis, or to use a combination with the same aim. The same is true of treatment of established PONV. Pediatric patients deserve special consideration, since PONV is common and often disregarded in this group. Prophylactic antiemetics are effective in children. The cost of prophylactic treatment of all patients has to be weighed against the benefits. All currently available drugs have side effects, which limits their indiscriminate use. Many patients accept pain rather than have the emesis associated with opioids or the dysphoria that can occur with the treatment of opioid-induced nausea. The time of administration of prophylactic antiemetics may be important. Many drugs give better results when given near the end of surgery rather than before anesthesia.

Key References

Costall B, Naylor RJ. Neuropharmacology of emesis in relation to clinicalresponse. Br J Cancer. 1992;66(Suppl. 1):52–88.
Grundy D, Reid K. The physiology of nausea and vomiting. In: Johnson LR, ed. Physiology of the Gastrointestinal Tract, 3rd edn. New York: Raven Press; 1994:879–901.
Smith G, Rowbotham DJ. Postoperative nausea and vomiting. Br J Anaesth. 1992;69:7(Suppl.1).
Watcha MF, White PF. Postoperative nausea and vomiting, its etiology, treatment, and prevention. Anesthesiology. 1992;77:162–84.

Further Reading

Kapur PA. The big ‘little problem’. Anesth Analges. 1991;73:243–5.
Koivuranta M, Laara E, Snare L, Alahuhta S. A survey of postoperative nausea and vomiting. Anaesthesia. 1997;52:443–9.
Lerman J. Are antiemetics cost effective for children. Can J Anaesth. 1995;42:263–6.
Miller AD, Nonaka S, Jakus J. Brain areas essential and non-essential to emesis. Brain Res. 1994;647:255–64.
Strunin L, Rowbotham D, Miles A, eds. Effective management of PONV. UEL centre for Health Services Research and Royal College of Anaesthetists Publication, London. 1999.
Toner CC, Broomhead CJ, Littlejohn IH, et al. Prediction of postoperative nausea and vomiting. Br J Anaesth. 1996;76:347–51.

Chapter 61 Physiology and pharmacology of the liver

Michael Zwillman and Jose Melendez

Topics covered in this chapter

Anatomy
Hepatic hemodynamics
Evaluation of liver function
Pathophysiology of liver injury
Anesthetic considerations
Physiologic aspects of liver transplant
Chemically induced hepatic failure

ANATOMY

Formation of the human liver begins during the third week of gestation as an endodermal thickening, which grows into a hollow sphere lined with columnar epithelium. This sphere grows into the septum transversum and separates into a hepatic portion, a cystic portion, and a ventral portion (Fig. 61.1). The hepatic portion gives rise to the liver proper and intrahepatic bile ducts; the cystic portion forms the cystic duct, gallbladder, and common bile duct; and the ventral portion contributes to the head of the pancreas.

The basic functional unit of the liver is the lobule. The human liver consists of approximately 100,000 lobules, each of which is cylindrical and several millimeters in length (0.8–2.0mm in diameter). The lobule is composed of cellular plates approximately two hepatocytes thick. Between the hepatocytes are bile canaliculi that drain into bile ducts. Each lobule is separated by a fibrous septum and venous sinusoids. The sinusoids receive arterial blood from hepatic arterioles and venous blood from hepatic venules. The sinusoids eventually drain into the central vein. The sinusoids are lined by tissue macrophages (Kuppfer cells) and endothelial cells.

Grossly, the liver is divided into two main lobes, the larger right and the left, and two accessory lobes, the quadrate and the caudate. The falciform ligament and the umbilical fissure separate the right and left lobes. The accessory lobes are themselves subdivisions of the right lobe. The transverse hilar fissure located on the inferior surface of the right lobe divides the quadrate and caudate lobes. The quadrate lobe is bounded on the left by the umbilical fissure and on the right by the gallbladder. The caudate is posterior to the transverse hilar fissure.

The division of the liver is based on the location of hepatic veins called portal scissurae. The main scissura, which contains the middle hepatic vein, divides the liver into two 'functional livers' (right and left), which are further subdivided by portal scissurae that correspond to the right and left hepatic veins. The right portal scissura divides the right liver into two sectors, the anterior and posterior. The left portal scissura divides the left liver into the

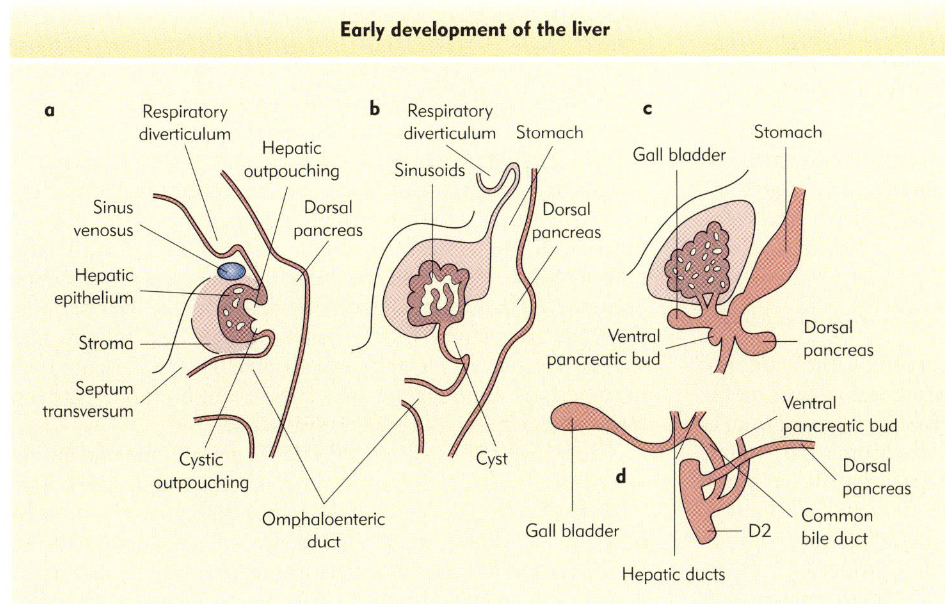

Figure 61.1 Early development of the liver. (a) Hepatic and cystic separations as hepatic epithelium and stroma grow into the septum transversum before 4.5 weeks gestation. (b) Continued growth and presence of liver sinusoids and stomach at 4.5 weeks gestation. (c) Gall bladder and ventral pancreatic bud are clearly defined at 5 weeks. (d) Further development of biliary tract, with hepatic ducts, common bile duct, and second part of the duodenum (D2) present at 6 weeks gestation. (Modified with permission from O'Rahilly R, Müller F. Human embryology and teratology, 2nd edn. New York: John Wiley; 1996.)

superior and posterior sectors. The right anterior sector is divided into segment V inferiorly and segment VIII superiorly (Fig. 61.2). The right posterior sector is divided into segment VI inferiorly and segment VII superiorly. The left portal scissura divides the left liver into two sectors, the anterior and posterior. The umbilical fissure divides the anterior sector into a medial segment IV and a lateral segment III. The left posterior sector corresponds to segment II. The caudate lobe corresponds to segment I.

HEPATIC HEMODYNAMICS

The normal human liver receives approximately 25% of the cardiac output via the hepatic artery and the portal vein and at rest consumes 20% of the body's total oxygen demand. The hepatic artery provides approximately 30–40% of hepatic oxygen requirements at a flow rate of 30mL/min per 100g of liver tissue. The portal vein drains the splanchnic beds, lower esophagus, pancreas, rectum, and spleen, and accounts for the remaining volume of hepatic blood flow. Hence, the portal vein with its large blood volume provides the liver with the majority of its oxygen requirement. The hepatic vein drains the liver sinusoids.

Hepatic arterial flow buffers against portal hypoperfusion by offsetting any acute decreases. Total liver flow decreases in similar proportions to hypotension. Portal venous flow decreases in parallel to that of decreased cardiac output, but not until low systemic pressures are reached. Ischemic hepatitis or 'shock liver' can occur following cardiogenic or hemorrhagic shock with resultant centrilobular necrosis.

Portal hypertension is defined as an intraluminal pressure >12mmHg (>1.6kPa) in the portal vein and its collaterals. Portal hypertension can result from prehepatic, posthepatic, or intrahepatic causes. Prehepatic portal hypertension is exemplified by thrombosis of the portal vein, posthepatic by right heart failure, and intrahepatic by cirrhosis of the liver. Cirrhotic liver disease is the most prevalent cause of portal hypertension.

Volatile anesthetics cause changes in blood flow systemically as well as in specific vascular beds. Halothane increases cerebral blood flow while decreasing myocardial, hepatic, splanchnic, and skeletal muscle blood flows. Isoflurane causes vasodilation in the brain, heart, gastrointestinal tract, spleen, skin, and skeletal muscle. Vasodilation, in both animal models and human isolated vascular specimens, is produced by endothelium-releasing factor, thought to be nitrous oxide (NO). It has been suggested that volatile anesthetics enhance the effects of NO.

Mechanical ventilation also alters hepatic blood flow. Positive pressure ventilation decreases cardiac output and subsequently portal venous flow. Positive pressure ventilation may also increase hepatic vascular resistance as a result of increased intra-abdominal pressure. Whether or not descent of the diaphragm compresses the liver and increases hepatic resistance remains unclear.

EVALUATION OF LIVER FUNCTION

Although not routinely used in the clinical setting, the aminopyrine breath test (ABT) is the most accurate test of liver metabolic function. Aminopyrine, an antipyretic and analgesic, is metabolized exclusively by the hepatic cytochrome 450 system. Acute hepatic insult as well as chronic hepatic insufficiency can be quantitated by ABT. Aminopyrine contains two methyl groups, the carbon atoms of which can be labeled with either ^{14}C or ^{13}C, which allows the metabolic end-product, $^{14}CO_2$ or $^{13}CO_2$, to be measured in exhaled breath. Labeled aminopyrine is given intravenously or orally, and exhaled breath collected and analyzed by scintillation or mass spectrometry. The 2-hour collection of labeled CO_2 is indicative of hepatic metabolic function, although previous investigators have used intermittent collection. Systems are now being tested using nonradioactive ^{13}C label with 'real-time' monitoring of $^{13}CO_2$ production. This technology has great promise, as it is a nonradioactive, minimally invasive, 'real-time' measurement of hepatic function.

Liver enzyme tests on serum, such as for aspartate aminotransferase (AST) and alanine aminotransferase (ALT), assess liver injury, and those for alkaline phosphatase and γ-glutamyl transpeptidase (GGT) reflect localized obstruction and nonspecific biliary disease.

The enzyme ALT is primarily a liver enzyme, while AST is located in heart, skeletal muscle, kidney, brain, and liver. Especially high levels of serum aminotransferase are not necessarily negative signs, since they reflect the existence of functioning hepatocytes. Likewise, acute decreases in aminotransferase levels are not necessarily good, since they may reflect death of the few functioning hepatocytes.

The alkaline phosphatases are a group of four isoenzymes coded for by distinct gene loci, and expressed in different tissues. One gene codes for alkaline phosphatase found in liver, bone, and first-trimester placenta. Others code for alkaline phosphatase found in fetal and adult intestine, and the placenta. Serum levels in healthy subjects originate from the liver or bone. Concentrations vary widely based on age, sex, height, and weight. The highest elevations of alkaline phosphatase are seen in cholestasis, although the level does not differentiate between intra- and extrahepatic biliary obstruction.

The transfer of γ-glutamyl groups to glutathione and amino acids, with the exception of proline, is catalyzed by GGT. This enzyme is located throughout the biliary tract, as well as in seminal vesicles, kidney, pancreas, and spleen. The mean half-life of GGT is 26 days. Serum concentration of GGT is sensitive for detecting biliary tract disease, but lacks specificity for a number

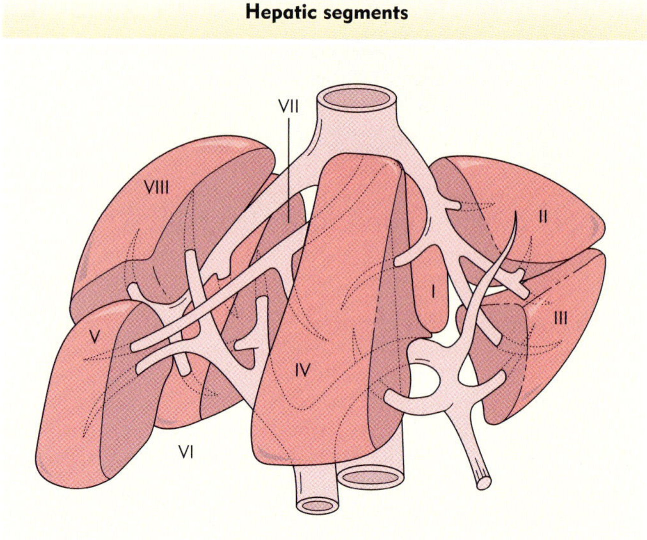

Figure 61.2 Hepatic segments. (Modified with permission from Bismuth H, Chiche L. Surgical anatomy and anatomical surgery of the liver. In: Blumgart L. Surgery of the liver and biliary tract 1st edn. New York: Churchill Livingstone; 1988.)

of reasons. Enzyme production is induced by alcohol and phenytoin. Like alkaline phosphatase, 'normal' serum concentrations vary with age and sex. Despite these limitations, GGT has been used in toxicology screens for the documentation of alcohol use. Its main function is to confirm elevated alkaline phosphatase, especially in children and pregnant women who have physiologically elevated serum alkaline phosphatase concentrations. Concentration of GGT does not increase with pregnancy or during childhood, but that of alkaline phosphatase does.

5´-Nucleotidase catalyzes hydrolysis of inorganic phosphate from the 5´-position on the nucleotide ribose ring. This enzyme is found in the intestine, brain, heart, blood vessels, and endocrine pancreas. In the liver, it is associated with the biliary tree and liver sinusoids. Although 5´-nucleotidase is found throughout the body, it is only released into the serum from hepatobiliary sources. 5´-Nucleotidase is also used to verify the hepatic origin of elevated alkaline phosphatase in pregnant women and in those with concomitant bone disease.

Bilirubin is derived from degradation of heme released from senescent red blood cells. Bilirubin is classified as direct or conjugated (water soluble) and indirect or unconjugated (water insoluble). Bilirubin metabolism involves hepatic uptake, conjugation, and excretion into bile. Bilirubin excretion appears to be the rate-limiting step, as well as the step most likely to go awry. When conjugated bilirubin appears in the blood in greater than usual concentration, biliary obstruction is the likely cause. When unconjugated bilirubin appears in greater than usual concentration intra- or extravascular hemolysis is likely, but genetic dysfunction or toxin should not be overlooked.

In chronic liver disease, albumin and prothrombin time (PT) are useful markers of synthetic activity, but albumin is not a reliable indicator of acute hepatic injury. The total body albumin pool is approximately 500g with a half-life of 20 days. Albumin synthesis is sensitive to external forces as well, notably nutritional status. Decreases in the amino acid tryptophan lead to decreases in serum albumin concentrations. Like albumin, PT is not a sensitive indicator of liver function. The coagulation factors involved in PT have relatively long half-lives, and are all vitamin K dependent. Decreases in vitamin K concentrations and in factor concentrations prolong PT.

The modified Child's-Pugh classification was devised to assess functional hepatic reserve for patients considered for surgery (Fig. 61.3). However, Child's-Pugh Class A and B did not predict postoperative mortality, which was attributed to the subjective nature of the degree of neurologic disorder, nutritional status, and management of ascites in computing the class. The remaining criteria, albumin and PT, are poor indicators of hepatic function at the time of evaluation. As a result, the criteria are rife with observer bias. Despite its limitations, the classification is useful when patients with chronic liver disease are considered for surgery, for which albumin and PT half-lives play less of a role.

Indocyanin green (ICG) is a dye that has favorable characteristics for measuring hepatic blood flow:

- extrahepatic removal is minimal;
- it is avidly protein bound, which results in a consistent volume of distribution;
- hepatic metabolism is nil as it is secreted unchanged in the bile;
- it is removed from the circulation by the liver after intravenous injection; and
- it is nontoxic.

Modified Child's–Pugh classification

Class	A	B	C
Serum bilirubin (mg/dL)	<2.0	2.0–3.0	>3.0
Serum albumin (mg/dL)	>3.5	3.0–3.5	<3.0
Ascites	none	well controlled	poorly controlled
Neurologic disorder	none	minimal	advanced – coma
Nutrition status	excellent	good	poor – wasting
Prothrombin time (seconds prolonged)	1–4	4–6	>6

Figure 61.3 Modified Child's–Pugh classification.

The dye is given intravenously and a single blood level is obtained 20 minutes later. A half-life of >5 minutes, a fractional disappearance of <16%/min, or >4% retention at 20 minutes is considered abnormal. ICG uptake may help detect early hepatic graft rejection.

Phosphorylation of galactose by hepatocyte galactokinase, and final metabolism to CO_2, or removal of galactose from the blood is the basis for the galactose elimination test. Like aminopyrine, galactose can be labeled with ^{14}C with the $^{14}CO_2$ being released in exhaled breath. In a healthy adult the maximal hepatic removal is approximately 500mg/min at a plasma concentration of 50mg/dL. ^{14}C-Galactose clearance is affected by changes in volume of distribution (e.g. dehydration) and appears to be no better than serum albumin concentrations in differentiating cirrhotic patients from normal patients.

Lidocaine (lignocaine) undergoes *N*-demethylation by cytochrome P450 enzymes, in particular P450 3A4, to give monoethylglycinexilide (MEGX) which can be measured in serum. The correlations between lidocaine metabolism, liver transplant rejection, and patient mortality are unclear, but studies that evaluated the outcome in cirrhotic patients are encouraging. Serum levels of MEGX >30ng/mL correlate with good prognosis, while serum concentrations <10ng/mL are associated with poor outcome.

PATHOPHYSIOLOGY OF LIVER INJURY

Hepatitis describes inflammation of the liver caused by chemicals, drugs, alcohol, as well as infectious agents, notably hepatotropic viruses. No clinical features distinguish hepatitis of different etiologies. The presence of viral antigens and their subsequent antibodies and a history of exposure confirm a viral cause. The diagnosis is made by the pattern of hepatic enzyme elevation [i.e. AST, ALT, alkaline phosphatase, lactate dehydrogenase (LDH), 5´-nucelotidase, and GGT]. Bilirubin is invariably elevated with equal fractions of both the direct and indirect forms. The AST:ALT ratio in acute viral hepatitis is usually <1, while it is >1.5 in alcohol-related liver injury. The relative decrease in ALT versus AST in alcoholic liver disease is attributed to the decrease in vitamin B_6, which appears to affect ALT more than AST.

Cirrhosis, regardless of cause, is characterized by the presence of fibrous scars, which consist of collagen Type I and III, proteoglycans, fibronectin, and hyaluronic acid. The consistency of the scar does not vary, yet its location does. Periportal scars are more likely to be caused by a viral etiology, and pericentral deposition is more likely with alcohol-related injury. Grossly, parenchymal and vascular architecture is rearranged by fibrous scarring. Efforts at hepatic regeneration result in the formation of nodules, arbitrarily divided as macronodules (>3mm) and micronodules (<3mm), which have no bearing on disease outcome. Hepatitis B (HBV), C, and D are capable of progressing to chronic disease and cirrhosis.

In intrahepatic portal hypertension, a sequela of cirrhosis, increased portal pressure occurs in the sinusoids as the result of perisinusoidal deposition of collagen with narrowing of sinusoidal channels and compression of the central vein by fibrous scars. As a result of increasing pressure, portal vein bypasses develop wherever the systemic and portal circulations share common capillary beds. Notable sites are veins around the rectum (hemorrhoids), the cardioesophageal junction (esophageal varices), retroperitoneum, and falciform ligament (periumbilical or abdominal collaterals).

Cirrhosis can be classified as compensated or decompensated. The presence of prolonged PT, encephalopathy, ascites, or portal hypertension suggests decompensation. The compensated cirrhotic may have low or normal concentrations of coagulation factors. More importantly, compensated cirrhotics may have neither enzyme changes nor physical symptoms that indicate hepatic dysfunction.

Bleeding in the patient with liver disease is a complicated affair, as both hypercoagulable and hypocoagulable states can exist. Portal hypertension induces splenomegaly and platelet sequestration, which leads to thrombocytopenia. Thrombocytopenia can result from alcohol-related folate deficiency and/or direct platelet toxicity. Profound thrombocytopenia can be seen in patients with aplastic anemia, secondary to hepatitis C (HCV). Liver transplant eliminates this state. Thrombocytopenic patients, particularly those in whom surgery is contemplated, should be transfused with platelets to a perioperative target of 100,000μL.

Cholestasis, which often accompanies cirrhosis, inhibits absorption of vitamin K, as well as decreasing hepatic vitamin K stores. The liver synthesizes vitamin K dependent factors II (prothrombin), VII, IX, and X, protein S, and protein C, and is therefore sensitive to fluctuations in hepatic vitamin K stores. Improvements in coagulation may be achieved with supplementation (10mg/day). If this fails to correct prolonged international normalized ratio (INR) or PT after 2–3 days, vitamin K administration should be stopped and additional causes sought. In addition to vitamin K dependent factors, the liver also synthesizes antithrombin III and factor I (fibrinogen). The main cause of cirrhosis-related bleeding is decreased synthesis of all these factors. In this setting, fresh frozen plasma (FFP) may be administered with the goal of decreasing the PT to within 3 seconds of control. If coagulopathy persists, dysfibrinoginemia should be considered. The cirrhotic liver not only has decreased synthetic capacity but also decreased clearance of activated clotting factors, notably tissue plasminogen activator. The result is systemic fibrinolysis, which further inhibits clot formation, and continued bleeding. Decreased serum concentrations of protein S, protein C, and antithrombin III result in hypercoagulable states. Deficiency of these factors can lead to disseminated intravascular coagulation (DIC). Although heparin is recommended for the treatment of DIC, it should be used with caution in patients with cirrhotic liver disease since it may exacerbate bleeding as clotting factor supplies are exhausted. The patient with liver disease that fails to respond to standard corrective measures may be given 1-desamino-8-D-arginine vasopressin (DDAVP), a synthetic peptide that increases factor VIII concentrations and shortens PT. Both DDAVP and FFP may be used in concert.

In the cirrhotic patient, encephalopathy and ascites account for significant morbidity and mortality. The exact pathogenesis of encephalopathy is unknown. It was previously thought to result entirely from the accumulation of endogenous ammonia, but research shows this not to be the case. Other etiologies have been suggested:

- changes in blood–brain barrier permeability;
- abnormal neurotransmitter balance;
- altered cerebral metabolism;
- impairment of neuronal Na^+ K^+-adenosine triphosphatase (Na^+ K^+-ATPase) activity; and
- increase in endogenous benzodiazepines.

Treatment of encephalopathy is primarily geared toward the reduction of ammonia, although short-term benefit from flumazenil administration has been reported.

Ascites occurs as a result of:

- increased hydrostatic pressure in hepatic sinusoids and splanchnic capillaries;
- overproduction of hepatic and splanchnic lymph leading to a transudation of lymph into the peritoneal space;
- limited or reduced reabsorption of water and protein by peritoneal lymphatics;
- Na^+ retention by the kidney secondary to hyperaldosteronism, increased sympathetic stimulation, alterations in metabolism of prostaglandins, and kinins; and
- impaired renal water excretion, partially caused by increased concentrations of antidiuretic hormone.

Treatment for ascites is geared toward fluid reduction without compromise of intravascular volume.

Hepatorenal syndrome is the occurrence of progressive renal insufficiency without any obvious cause in patients with advanced liver disease. The typical scenario is one of rapidly progressive renal failure over 1–2 weeks. Spontaneous recovery has been reported, but the vast majority of patients die. The differential diagnosis includes acute tubular necrosis and prerenal azotemia. In hepatorenal syndrome, urine Na^+ is typically <10mmol/L with hyperosmolar urine, oliguria (≤ 400ml/24h), fractional excretion of sodium ($FeNa^+$) <1, and a ratio of urine creatinine to plasma creatinine >30:1. The pathophysiology of hepatorenal syndrome is based on the pooling of blood in splanchnic beds and decreasing plasma volume. The kidney perceives a decreased glomerular filtration rate and vasoconstricts, shunting blood away from the renal cortex. Animal models with induced cirrhosis demonstrate increased production of NO. Inhibition of NO synthesis benefits renal function in cirrhotic rats by increasing both arterial and perfusion pressure. This improves systemic hemodynamics and downregulates baroreceptor tone. Human cirrhotics have increased synthesis of NO when compared with noncirrhotics. Although further investigation in humans is required, hepatorenal syndrome may be reversed by inhibition of NO synthesis. After 1 year of cirrhosis, the incidence of hepatorenal syndrome is 18%, and after 5 years, 39%.

Hepatopulmonary syndrome is defined by a triad of signs:

- liver disease;
- increased alveolar arterial O_2 gradients; and
- evidence of reduced intrapulmonary vascular resistance.

Autopsy specimens of human and animal lungs show precapillary pulmonary dilatations and direct arteriovenous communications. These types of lesions have been documented in patients having chronic cirrhosis, postacetaminophen overdose, or after halothane-induced liver failure. Animal and limited human studies show the putative mechanism for pulmonary dilatation to be an endogenous circulating pulmonary vasodilator, NO. Increased NO concentrations have been measured in exhaled breath from cirrhotic patients prior to liver transplant, only to be significantly decreased post-transplant.

Infectious hepatitis

Hepatitis A, an RNA virus of the picornavirus family, is responsible for both epidemic and sporadic outbreaks. The incubation period is 2–6 weeks, during which time blood and feces are infectious and may persist until the onset of jaundice. Transmission of the virus is via the fecal–oral route, there are no carrier states, and chronic hepatitis does not occur. IgM and IgG antihepatitis A antibodies appear early and subsequently provide evidence of exposure and immunity to future hepatitis A infection. The time course of infection is divided into four phases. The incubation phase is characterized by onset of viral replication and peaking at the onset of the pre-icteric phase, in which serum viral antibody is first detected. Aminotransferase, bilirubin, and symptoms reach their peaks during the icteric phase. Often, AST and ALT are eight times the normal levels, with the remaining enzymes and bilirubin only mildly elevated. The convalescent phase is characterized by an increased sense of wellbeing with disappearance of jaundice and abdominal pain.

Worldwide, hepatitis B virus (HBV) is most frequently transmitted by vertical transmission from infected mother to fetus, by sexual contact, and by addicts sharing infected needles. A hepadnavirus, HBV has a genome of partially double-stranded DNA, an inner core nucleocapsid, a DNA polymerase, and an outer envelope that consists of protein, lipid, and carbohydrate. The viral constituents provide antigens to which specific antibodies are generated. These antigens and antibodies reflect the course of infection, and are used as treatment for acute infection and vaccination against future exposure (Fig. 61.4). The incubation period of HBV is long, 50 to 180 days. The appearance of HBV surface antigen (HBsAg) is the first serologic evidence of infection, and occurs before the onset of symptoms and elevation of hepatic enzymes. The concentration of HBsAg peaks during overt disease and declines to undetectable levels in 3–6 months. Persistence of HBVsAg for more than 6 months along with elevated aminotransferase levels is indicative of chronicity. Chronic states progress to cirrhosis and eventual liver failure. Patients with cirrhosis and concurrent or post-HBV infection are at risk for hepatocellular carcinoma, usually after a latent period of 25–30 years postinfection.

Hepatitis D (delta, or HDV) is an RNA virus that requires the presence of HBsAg to replicate. Like HBV, HDV occurs most frequently in intravenous drug users and recipients of multiple blood-product transfusions. The virus has an external coat donated by HBV and an inner coat synthesized by HDV. Delta infection occurs in two forms:

- coinfection, which describes simultaneous infection with acute HDV and acute HBV; and
- superinfection, describing a state of chronic HBV and acute HDV.

The two groups have different morbidities and mortalities. Coinfection is usually self-limited and has a mortality of 1–10%. Superinfection becomes chronic in approximately 75% of cases and cirrhosis develops in up to 70% of affected patients with a mortality of 5–20%.

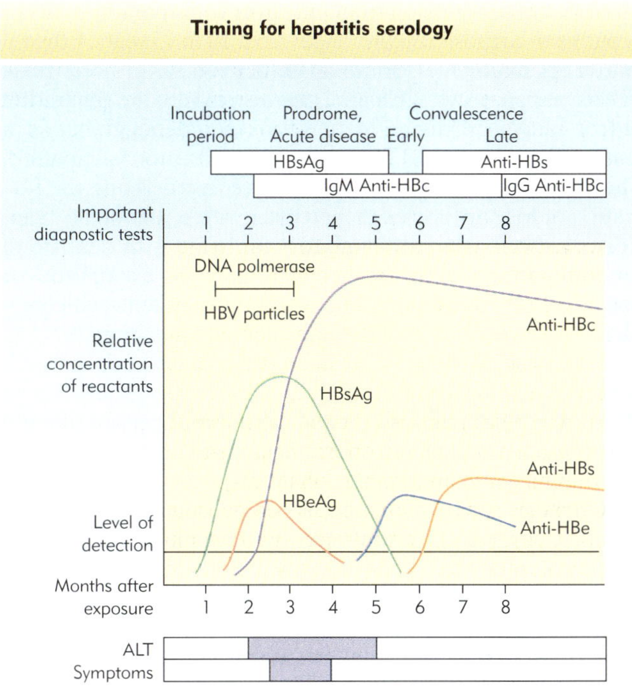

Figure 61.4 Timing for hepatitis serology. HBV, hepatitis B virus; HBsAg, HBV surface antigen; HBc, HBV core; HBe, HBV envelope. (Modified with permission from Hollinger FB, Dienstag JL. Hepatitis B and D viruses. In: Baron EE, Tenover FL, Yolken RH, eds. Manual of clinical microbiology, 6th edn. Washington: ASM Press; 1995.)

Previously called non-A, non-B hepatitis, HCV is a member of the Flaviviridae family, and consists of single-stranded RNA genome, capsid, and envelope. It is the most common cause of post-transfusion hepatitis, but with serologic screening its occurrence is on the wane. In the US, HCV-related liver disease is the leading indication for liver transplant. The largest population at risk is intravenous drug users; however, for a large population of HCV-positive patients no cause can be identified. Vertical transmission is less frequent than for HBV. The average incubation for HCV is 6–7 weeks, and it is a disease of chronicity rather than of acute presentation. Only 20–30% of patients have symptoms, with 50% developing jaundice; >50% of infected individuals develop chronic hepatitis. Serum aminotransferase response is variable, with viremia occurring several weeks before serum levels increase. Factors that appear to favor progression to chronic HCV are male sex, old age, and infection by transfusion and large viral dose. Sequelae of chronic disease are cirrhosis and hepatocellular carcinoma.

Hepatitis E is a single-stranded RNA virus similar to calcivirus. The mean incubation period is 40 days with a range of 2 to 9 weeks. It is the leading cause of sporadic outbreaks of hepatitis in developing nations. Spread is via the fecal–oral route.

Chemical hepatitis

Ethanol

Ethanol abuse leads to three pathologic states: alcoholic steatosis or 'fatty liver', alcoholic hepatitis, and alcoholic cirrhosis. The time frame for progression from one state to another is variable, but progression from fatty liver with sporadic bouts of hepatitis to cirrhosis usually ranges from 10 to 15 years. Ethanol and/or its major metabolite acetaldehyde have direct toxic effects on hepatocytes. Ethanol may also induce the generation of free radicals. Ethanol increases oxygen demand, but as a result of perisinusoidal fibrosis, oxygen diffusion is impaired. These factors contribute to hepatocyte necrosis and the formation of Mallory bodies (hepatocytes with eosinophilic inclusions), as well as an inflammatory infiltrate with neutrophil predominance. Alcoholic hepatitis may be asymptotic or progress to hepatic failure. The syndrome may abate with complete cessation of alcohol use and adequate nutrition.

Alcoholism is the most common cause of cirrhosis in North America and Western Europe, and has increasing incidence in South America. The amount and duration of chronic alcohol abuse before development of cirrhosis remain unclear. Alcoholic cirrhosis may remain clinically silent, discovered incidentally or at autopsy. Metabolic and organ system dysfunction result from alcoholic cirrhosis. Overt diabetes is uncommon, although glucose intolerance secondary to endogenous insulin resistance occurs, a decreased clearance of androstenedione (an estrogen precursor) results in gynecomastia and testicular atrophy in men, and cardiac dysfunction manifests as cardiomyopathy.

Alcoholic cardiomyopathy classically occurs in men aged 30–55 years who have been alcohol abusers for more than 10 years. Putative mechanisms are direct toxic effects of ethanol and its metabolite acetaldehyde; nutritional deficiencies, particularly thiamine (beriberi); and additives in legitimate commercial manufacture (cobalt in beer). Alcohol and acetaldehyde have been shown to decrease Ca^{2+} binding and transport, myocardial lipid metabolism, and myocardial ATPase activity. Two basic patterns of cardiac dysfunction have been demonstrated – left ventricular dilation with impaired systolic function and left ventricular hypertrophy with diminished compliance and normal or increased contractile performance. Presenting manifestations range from insidious onset to catastrophic left-sided failure. Anginal chest pain does not occur without concomitant coronary artery disease or aortic stenosis.

Isoniazid

The exact mechanism of isoniazid (isonicotonic acid hydrazide, INH) toxicity is unclear, but the metabolite acetylhydrazine causes hepatic damage in adults. Age appears to be the most important factor in INH hepatotoxicity. Patients <20 years of age have an incidence of 0.3%, those of 20–34 years 1.2%, and those >35 years 2.3%. Hepatitis presents 4–8 weeks after onset of therapy. Two forms of untoward reactions occur – the first is self-limited and mild, and the second involves focal hepatic necrosis and (rarely) fatal hepatic necrosis.

Methyldopa

The incidence of methyldopa-induced hepatitis is approximately 1%. Hepatic dysfunction can occur after long-term use, but hepatitis is likely to appear within 3 months of treatment onset. An autoimmune reaction is the likely etiology with liver granuloma formation. Methyldopa has also been associated with massive hepatic necrosis.

Carbon tetrachloride

Chronic exposure to carbon tetrachloride was common in years past as it was a solvent in commercial laundries; exposure now is rare. Liver injury appears to be mediated by trichloromethyl or trichloromethylperoxy free radicals formed by cytochrome P450 action. These radicals are believed to react with lipids and proteins, specifically polyenoic lipids, of the endoplasmic reticulum.

Obstructive causes of liver injury

Jaundice caused by obstruction of the common bile duct occurs early with carcinoma of the head of the pancreas or cholangiocarcinoma. Pancreatic carcinoma of the body and tail does not present with early jaundice, and when presentation does occur this is usually an indication of hepatic metastasis. Bile duct obstruction also affects hepatic hemodynamics. Acute biliary obstruction is associated with an increase in liver blood flow, but blood flow is decreased with chronic obstruction. Relief of long-term obstruction is not associated with a return to normal pressures and may even be associated with hemodynamic deterioration and shock. The etiology of hemodynamic derangement in the face of biliary obstruction is not known, but may involve increased portal resistance.

Charcot's triad characterizes cholangitis – biliary pain, jaundice, and fever with chills. Laboratory findings consistent with the diagnosis are leukocytosis, hyperbilirubinemia, and elevated alkaline phosphatase and aminotransferases. Ascending cholangitis is a particularly severe complication because of the complete obstruction of the common duct with purulent accumulation proximal to the obstruction. Sepsis and septic shock may supervene. As a result 'shock liver' may ensue, which causes ischemic hepatitis and centrolobular necrosis.

Primary biliary cirrhosis is a disease of female predominance (9:1) with the average age of onset during the fifth decade. This disease is insidious, progressive, and often fatal. The etiology is unclear, but an autoimmune basis is currently favored. There are four stages:

- the first stage is characterized by extensive septal and intralobular bile duct destruction with profound inflammatory infiltrate;
- the second stage entails proliferation of bile ducts with deranged architecture;
- the third stage involves fibrosis with decreasing severity of inflammatory infiltrate; and
- lastly, the fourth stage, cirrhosis.

Hepatocellular carcinoma results in approximately 3–4%.

Genetic causes of liver injury

Cirrhosis can also manifest as an end-stage complication of genetic diseases (Fig. 61.5).

ANESTHETIC CONSIDERATIONS

Operative outcome is clearly linked to severity of hepatic parenchymal disease. In patients with mild or well-compensated chronic hepatic disease, operative outcome is unchanged from normal. However, the unexpected diagnosis of viral hepatitis during laparotomy carries a mortality of 9.5%. In some studies mortality of inpatients with acute viral or alcoholic hepatic failure approaches 100%. In patients for shunt operations, mortality correlates with the Child's-Pugh classification, ranging from 10% to 76%. Figure 61.6 depicts other variables that increase operative and postoperative mortality in cirrhotic patients. In 104 patients with cirrhosis who underwent operations ranging from herniorrhaphy to thoracotomy, the incidence of complications was 25%. Noncompensated cirrhotics fared worse with an incidence of complications of 35%, while well-compensated cirrhotics

Cirrhosis and genetic syndromes		
Disease	**Inheritance**	**Hepatic manifestations**
Hemochromatosis (iron metabolism)	Autosomal recessive HLA-H on chromosome 6	Fibrous septa resembling alcoholic cirrhosis, progressing to micronodular cirrhosis
Wilson's disease (copper metabolism)	Autosomal recessive, Chromosome 13	Steatosis, acute hepatitis, chronic active hepatitis, cirrhosis possibly massive necrosis
Type IIIa Glycogen storage disease (muscle and liver debranching enzyme deficiency) Type IIIb – liver debranching enzyme deficiency	Autosomal recessive	Periportal fibrosis, micronodular cirrhosis. In Japanese, overt cirrhosis frequent
Type IV glycogen storage disease (branching enzyme deficiency)	Autosomal recessive	Cirrhosis, ascites, hepatic failure. Onset in first year of life, death by age 5 years
Hepatorenal tyrosinema (enzyme deficiency, fumaryl-acetoacetate hydrolase)	Autosomal recessive	Cirrhosis, hepatic failure
Galactosemia (enzyme deficiency, galactose-1-phosphate uridyl transferase)	Autosomal recessive	Jaundice, hepatomegaly, cirrhosis
α-1-antitrypsin deficiency	Autosomal dominant	Fibrous scarring, macronodular cirrhosis, frequently piecemeal necrosis

Figure 61.5 Cirrhosis and genetic syndromes.

experienced a 16% complication rate. The rapid postoperative reaccumulation of ascites was the largest contributor to postoperative complications, with dehiscence, infection, and liver failure secondary to intravascular hypovolemia.

Surgical stimulation and manipulation of the liver markedly increase hepatic oxygen extraction in connection with splanchnic vasoconstriction. A 16% drop in hepatic blood flow is associated with general anesthesia and mechanical ventilation, a further 10% decrease with peripheral surgery, and a 40% decrease with splanchnic surgery. This may be a direct effect of catecholamines on local vascular tone or a combination of unknown factors affecting the blood flow and metabolic state of the liver. Reductions of systemic pressure and cardiac output, such as induced hypotension, hypovolemia, and anesthetic overdoses, reduce hepatic blood flow.

Volatile anesthetics

Hepatic effects of volatile anesthetics have been widely studied. Halothane has a range of hepatic effects. Fulminant hepatic failure has been described in patients undergoing multiple halothane anesthetics (incidence 1:35000), and no safe exposure interval has been demonstrated (Chapter 24). Halothane hepatitis has been linked to obesity, age, sex, level of enzyme induction, and genetic predisposition (see below). In some series, halothane antibodies have been demonstrated in up to 75% of patients. Hepatic necrosis may ensue with 10–80% mortality. Death occurs 1–2 weeks after the initiation of symptoms, which include fever and rash. In addition, a mild transaminase elevation after halothane exposure has been documented in close to 50% of cases. A significant increase in aminopyrine half-life has been shown to occur after halothane exposure, which is not seen with other agents. This pattern precludes the repeated use of halothane.

Volatile anesthetics reduce hepatic blood flow in a dose-dependent fashion because of their effects on cardiac output and systemic pressure. Halothane, owing to its potent myocardial depressive effect, produces the greatest reduction in hepatic blood flow. In addition, halothane reduces oxygen delivery to a greater extent than it reduces systemic pressure. Animal studies

Operative and postoperative variables	
Variable	**Mortality (if present) (%)**
Pulmonary failure	100
Cardiac failure	92
Gastrointestinal bleeding	86
Requirement for more than two antibiotics	82
Required second operation	81
Renal failure	73
More than two units of blood required	69
Hepatic failure	66
Positive blood/urine culture	61
Less than two units of blood required	22

Figure 61.6 Operative and postoperative variables that increase mortality in cirrhotics and percentage mortality. (Adapted with permission from both Brown BR. Risk determination for surgery in patients with parenchymal liver disease. In: Brown BR, ed. Anesthesia in hepatic and biliary tract disease. Philadelphia: FA Davies; 1998;115–23; and Garrison RN, Cryer HM, Howard DA, Polk HC. Clarification of risk factors for abdominal operations in patients with hepatic cirrhosis. Ann Surg. 1984;199:648–55.)

indicate that a 30% reduction in systolic pressure after a halothane anesthetic leads to a 50% reduction in hepatic blood flow and a concomitant increase in oxygen extraction.

Enflurane hepatitis, if real, has an incidence well below 1:800,000. No documentation of antibodies nor of increased incidence with repeated anesthetics or cross-reactivity with halothane has been published. As a result of its increased molecular stability and rapid egress from fatty tissues, enflurane does not undergo as extensive a reductive metabolism as does halothane.

The creation of free radicals and/or toxic products is almost completely eliminated. For equipotent doses, enflurane reduces hepatic blood flow to a lesser extent than does halothane.

Isoflurane and desflurane both undergo negligible hepatic metabolism. As a result, isoflurane anesthesia is not accompanied by free radical formation, and no conclusive association has been made between isoflurane exposure and postoperative hepatitis. Isoflurane produces less dose-dependent reduction in hepatic blood flow and oxygen delivery than do either enflurane or halothane. Isoflurane (one minimal alveolar concentration) preserves the hepatic blood flow buffer effect, which results in a minimal effect on total liver perfusion. In addition, isoflurane attenuates the increases in hepatic oxygen consumption associated with surgery and liver manipulation. Currently, isoflurane is the anesthetic agent of choice during liver surgery and transplantation, although early studies demonstrate that desflurane has no deleterious effects on liver function and hepatocyte integrity, and preserves hepatic blood flow better than does isoflurane.

Extensively used in patients with hepatic disease, nitrous oxide has not been shown to contribute to hepatic disease exacerbation. The sympathomimetic effects of nitrous oxide may increase hepatic metabolic requirements.

Intravenous anesthetics and muscle relaxants

The unpredictability of the response to drugs metabolized by the liver results mainly from altered pharmacokinetics in the presence of liver dysfunction. Alterations of drug availability depend on liver blood flow, extent of protein binding and drug metabolism, and the etiology and stage of liver dysfunction. The elimination of drugs with low hepatic clearance depends more on the metabolic capacity of the liver and less on the hepatic blood flow. In patients with impaired liver function, such drugs experience a prolonged duration of action with no increase in peak levels. In contrast, elimination of drugs with a high hepatic clearance depends on liver blood flow. Reductions in metabolic clearance result in increases of peak drug level with minimal change in elimination half-life. Protein binding, enzymatic induction, intrahepatic shunting, and effects of anesthetics on liver blood flow may also affect the elimination of drugs with a high extraction rate. Chronic alcohol usage can increase anesthetic requirements, owing to increases in drug metabolism.

The safety of barbiturate administration in patients with hepatic disease is well documented, and reports of hepatitis following barbiturates are rare. These have been associated with fever, rash, and eosinophilia, with an onset of symptoms within 5 weeks and lasting several months. Barbiturates increase cytochrome P450 reduction, which may increase toxic metabolite formation. The clearance of thiopental and methohexital is preserved in cirrhotics. Decompensated cirrhotics have reduced serum albumin, which can result in a decrease in the volume of distribution of drugs and protein binding. Consequently, free thiopental is increased in cirrhotics, and dosage should be reduced.

Hepatic injury, ranging from cholestasis to centrolobular necrosis, has been reported following prolonged usage of benzodiazepines. Benzodiazepines have low hepatic clearance and hence have prolonged effects in patients with liver insufficiency. The decrease in diazepam clearance in chronic liver disease correlates with the level of serum albumin. Attention must be paid to active metabolites, which further increase the duration of action. In compensated alcoholic cirrhotics, metabolism of midazolam normal. Uncompensated cirrhotics can have prolonged pharmacologic effects. Electroencephalogram-response differences between cirrhotics and normals at similar drug concentrations suggest alterations in cerebral sensitivity or increased endogenous benzodiazepines

In poorly compensated liver disease, both synthetic and natural opioids exhibit accentuated CNS depression. Patients with chronic liver disease have a normal volume of distribution and elimination half-life. Morphine has been reported to have both unaltered and reduced clearance. Conjugation of morphine is unchanged in cirrhotics, possibly as a result of extrahepatic conjugation. Hypoalbuminemia and hyperbilirubinemia result in decreases in protein binding of morphine with increased free morphine and increased drug availability. Alfentanil has a prolonged duration in patients with liver disease, with a doubling of elimination half-life. The reduction in clearance seems to be related to the etiology of liver disease. Also, an increase in the free fraction of alfentanil results from the reduction of α-1-glycoprotein in cirrhotics. H_2 blockers may further prolong the duration of action. Well-compensated cirrhotic patients do not experience a change in fentanyl elimination half-life, total plasma clearance, or volume of distribution. Fentanyl has a high extraction ratio and hence is more dependent on hepatic blood flow and less on metabolic activity. Sufentanil clearance is unaffected by liver disease. Consistent with its minimal effect on cardiac output and systemic pressure, fentanyl has no effect on liver blood flow and oxygen delivery. In combination with isoflurane, fentanyl has the least effect on hepatic hemodynamics of any opioid, making it a good choice for anesthesia. Opioids may cause biliary spasm, which can be relieved with glucagon or naloxone.

Not enough information is available on the effects of propofol on decompensated cirrhotics. Protein binding is unchanged. Although propofol is metabolized in the liver, the pharmacokinetics are unchanged in uncomplicated cirrhotics. Nonhepatic, possibly pulmonary, metabolism of propofol has been documented during liver transplantation. Propofol causes reductions in systemic pressure, which may decrease liver blood flow. When administered to well-compensated cirrhotics, propofol has been well tolerated.

Etomidate is hydrolyzed by hepatic esterases into carboxylic acid. Terminal half-life is doubled in cirrhotics, but this is only important in prolonged infusions, for which the dosage should be decreased to prevent a cumulative effect. The intermediate distribution phase is responsible for the short pharmacodynamic effect and is unchanged in cirrhotics.

Ketamine is tolerated well in cirrhotics and has no hepatotoxic effects in short procedures. Serum transaminase increase may result after prolonged continuous usage. Ketamine does not alter portal or hepatic artery blood flow but decreases oxygen delivery by increasing oxygen consumption of preportal organs. Increased intracranial pressure in comatose patients is a contraindication to its use.

Patients with cirrhosis have an apparent resistance to muscle relaxants, as a result of an increase in volume of distribution. However, many muscle relaxants exhibit a prolonged duration of action because of a decreased hepatic metabolic function. Thus, the initial dose of pancuronium or D-tubocurarine required to achieve a specific degree of muscle relaxation is higher than expected, but this same dose has an unexpectedly prolonged duration of action. In patients with cirrhosis, protein binding of curare, pancuronium, and vecuronium is similar to that of controls. Single-dose vecuronium pharmacokinetics are not affected in patients with alcoholic liver disease, but large doses may behave in the same way as pancuronium. Time to 50% twitch recovery was doubled in cirrhotic patients who received vecuronium. Sustained usage of vecuronium in patients with cholestasis may lead to prolonged duration of action. Time to maximal neuromuscular blockade was unchanged for rocuronium, but reduced plasma clearance and increased volume of distribution combined to increase elimination half-life. No difference occurs in the volume of distribution, plasma clearance, and elimination half-life of doxacurium.

Reductions in protein synthesis result in decreased plasma pseudocholinesterase activity. However, there is no clinically significant increase in succinylcholine action. The action of mivacurium may be prolonged in patients with decreased pseudocholinesterase activity. Since atracurium is metabolized by Hoffman elimination, independent of liver and renal dysfunction, it is considered the muscle relaxant of choice. Despite an increase in its volume of distribution, atracurium has an unchanged elimination half-life. The drug has been shown to maintain its predictable pharmacokinetic profile in patients *in extremis*. There is also no change in laudanosine clearance.

Amide-linked local anesthetics are metabolized by the liver, so caution should be used in patients with severe liver disease. Local anesthetic pharmacokinetics can be substantially affected (e.g. the half-life of lidocaine may be increased by 300%).

PHYSIOLOGIC ASPECTS OF LIVER TRANSPLANT

The transplant process is divided into three stages – preanhepatic, anhepatic, and neohepatic. Each stage has characteristic physiologic changes that must be managed in a rapid but controlled fashion (Fig. 61.7).

The preanhepatic stage begins with skin incision and mobilization of the native liver. During this stage cardiovascular hemodynamics are the focus of concern. In the cirrhotic patient extensive collaterals have formed that must be dissected as part of liver mobilization and, as a result, significant bleeding may occur. Large-volume ascites may be drained, which causes extensive fluid shifts that further contribute to hemodynamic instability. Manipulation of the inferior vena cava decreases venous return, which reduces cardiac output. Attention must also be paid to electrolytes, maintenance of normothermia, and acid–base status.

The anhepatic stage begins with complete transection of the hepatic artery and portal vein, and occlusion of the inferior vena cava. Cardiovascular stability continues to be an issue along with the addition of pulmonary and metabolic compromise. Venovenous bypass reroutes femoral and portal venous blood, through heparin-coated tubing, to the axillary or internal jugular vein in an attempt to minimize decreased venous return. The alternative is to cross-clamp both the inferior vena cava and portal vein, which definitely decreases venous return. Bypass has its own risks, namely air thromboembolism and hypothermia. Aside from the risks of endotracheal intubation and anesthesia, exposing the surgical field requires extensive and prolonged abdominal wall retraction which leads to atelectasis and decreased pulmonary compliance. Multiple transfusions can cause citrate intoxication, hypocalcemia, and hyperkalemia.

Reanastamosis of the great vessels marks the onset of the neohepatic stage. Portal blood is used to flush the graft prior to reanastamosis. In spite of this, accumulated metabolic acids and K^+ can still be released into the circulation after release of the vascular clamps. The typical reperfusion scenario has no cardiac dysrhythmias, but systemic hypotension manifests for 30 minutes or less. Proper planning prior to vascular clamp removal is paramount, and blood pressure support is frequently necessary. Clearance of metabolic acids (improvement in metabolic acidemia), no exogenous Ca^{2+} requirement, yellow bile production, and hemodynamic stability are signs of a functioning graft.

Liver transplant stages and physiologic changes

Stage	Surgical Maneuvers	Physiologic alterations
Preanhepatic	Dissect porta hepatis Mobilize liver	Acute decompression of ascites Hemmorage (venous congestion)
Anhepatic	Portal venous clamp IVC, hepatic arterial clamp Venovenous bypass (adults) Retraction on diaphragm	Obstruction of venous return Oliguria (venous congestion) Atelectasis, decreased compliance Citrate intoxication
Neohepatic	IVC anastomosis Flush allograft Portal venous, hepatic arterial anastomoses Biliary drainage	Hemmorage, coagulopathy Hyperkalemia Hypothermia Metabolic acidosis

Figure 61.7 Liver transplant stages and physiologic changes. (Adapted with permission from Firestone L, Firestone S. Organ transplantation. In: Miller RD, ed. Anesthesia, Vol. II, 6th edn. New York: Churchill Livingstone; 1998.)

CHEMICALLY INDUCED HEPATIC FAILURE

Hepatic failure can result from infectious hepatitis as well as from intoxication with salicylates, acetaminophen, and idiosyncratic response to halothane.

Halothane

Halothane-induced hepatic dysfunction has an unclear etiology. Metabolic theory suggests that the hepatic cytochrome 450 system, under hypoxic conditions, causes reductive metabolism of halothane rather than the usual oxidative pathway. The reductive metabolism produces various fluoride-containing compounds (Chapter 8). Yet, when the liver is directly challenged with these compounds hepatic dysfunction fails to occur. Other evidence suggests that halothane toxicity occurs during the initial exposure rather than during metabolism. The suggestion that toxicity occurs prior to metabolism may involve hypoxia during anesthetic induction and not after reductive metabolism of halothane – hence the origin of the hypoxic theory. However, the likelihood that hypoxia accounts for fulminant hepatic failure is not convincing. The strongest evidence supports an immunologic mechanism. Hepatic damage is associated with multiple halothane exposures, which suggests a possible sensitization. Other signs of allergy are present, such as eosinophilia, fever after first exposure, and jaundice upon second exposure. Trifluoroacetyl halide, a metabolic product of halothane, has been linked with a humoral antibody response when bound to liver protein. Also, no reason has been found to discount a cell-mediated response.

Salicylates (Reye's syndrome)

Reye's syndrome is a form of hepatic insult that occurs in childhood and is commonly associated with varicella or influenza infection. Reye's syndrome is characterized initially by lethargy with normal bilirubin, ammonia, and aminotransferases, and 75% of patients progress no further. The remainder experience increasing aminotransferases, serum ammonia, hyperbilirubinemia, and CNS compromise. Fatalities range from 10 to 40% and are related to CNS depression and (rarely) hepatic failure. Salicylate use with concurrent childhood influenza or varicella infection is contraindicated. Rare cases have been reported in adults.

Acetaminophen (paracetamol)

Intentional and unintentional overdose with acetaminophen commonly results from its combination with other analgesics and 'over-the-counter' availability. In the adult, 10–15g can be toxic (even fatal). The liver is the major target organ affected by toxic serum concentrations. Acetaminophen is metabolized through glucuronidation, sulfonation, and oxidation by cytochrome P450 2E1. When serum concentrations overwhelm the P450 system, a highly electrophilic compound *N*-acetyl-*p*-benzoquinoneimine (NAPQ1) is formed. This forms a covalent bond with cell proteins and DNA to produce a centrolobular necrosis of the liver. Acetaminophen toxicity occurs in four phases:

- phase one occurs within the first 24 hours of ingestion – nausea, vomiting, anorexia, and diaphoresis may be the only symptoms if any are manifest at all;
- phase two is marked by the onset of right upper quadrant pain, possible hepatomegaly, increased bilirubin, AST and ALT concentrations, prolongation of PT, and oliguria;
- phase three, between 2–5 days postingestion, is characterized by progressive hepatic necrosis with increase in PT, peak elevation of liver enzymes (AST and ALT may rise to 100 times normal), jaundice and encephalopathy; and
- symptom resolution with treatment describes phase four.

Patients who present within 4 hours of ingestion should undergo charcoal lavage pending serum acetaminophen levels. A nomogram correlates serum acetaminophen with probability of hepatotoxicity (Fig 61.8). For serum acetaminophen levels <100mg/kg no treatment is required. Acetylcysteine is the treatment of choice if acetaminophen ingestion is within 24 hours of presentation, and may well be of benefit after 24 hours. Acetylcysteine regenerates glutathione, which combines with acetaminophen to form mercaptopuric acid that is harmlessly excreted by the kidneys.

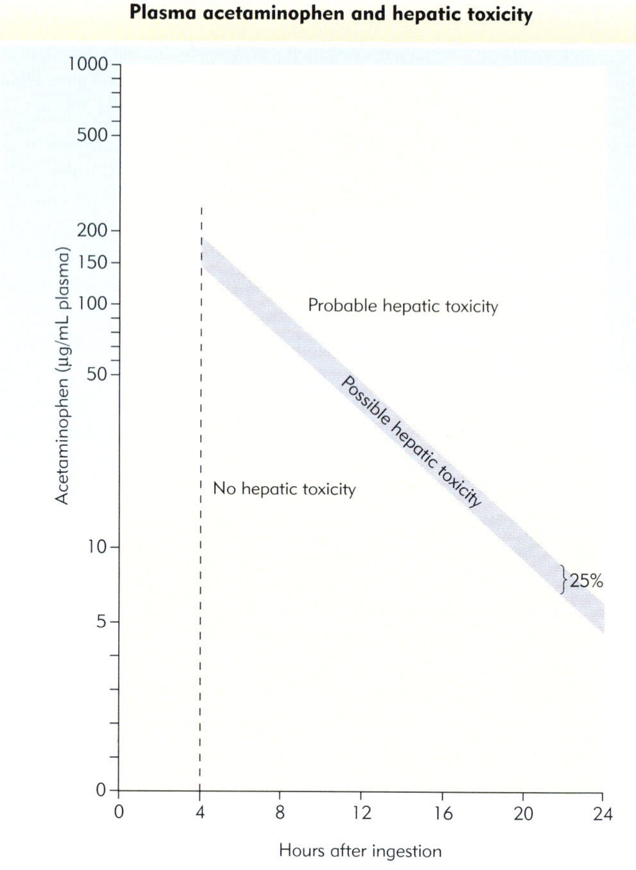

Figure 61.8 Nomogram correlating plasma acetaminophen level after initial exposure and likelihood of developing hepatic damage. (Modified with permission from Rumack B, Matthew H. Acetaminophen poisoning and toxicity. Pediatrics. 1975;55:871–6.)

Key References

Brophy MT, Fiore LD, Deykin D. Hemostasis. In: Zakim D, Boyer TD, eds. Hepatology: a textbook of liver disease, 3rd edn. Philadelphia: WB Saunders; 1998:691–715.

Brown BR. Risk determination for surgery patients with parenchymal liver disease. In: Brown BR, ed. Anesthesia in hepatic and biliary tract disease. Philadelphia: FA Davies; 1998;115–23.

Gelman S. Anesthesia and the liver. In: Barash PG, Cullen BF, Stoelting RK, eds, Clinical anesthesia, 2nd edn. Baltimore: JP Lippincott; 1992;1185–214.

Friedman LS, Martin P, Munoz S. Liver function tests and the objective evaluation of the patient with liver disease. In: Zakim D, Boyer TD, eds. Hepatology: a textbook of liver disease, 3rd edn. Philadelphia: WB Saunders; 1998:791–832.

Mathie RT, Wheatley AM, Blumgart LH. Liver blood flow: physiology, measurement and clinical relevance. In: Blumgart LH, ed. Surgery of the liver and biliary tract, 2nd edn. New York: Churchill Livingstone; 1998;95–110.

Maze M. Anesthesia and the liver. In: Miller RD, ed. Anesthesia, Vol. II, 4th edn. New York: Churchill Livingstone; 1994;1969–79.

Further Reading

Arden JR, Lynman DR, Castagnoli KP. Vecuronium in alcoholic liver disease: a pharmacokinetic and pharmacodynamic analysis. Anesthesiology. 1998;68:771–6.

Couderc E, Ferrier C, Haberer JP. Thiopentone pharmacokinetics in patients with chronic alcoholism. Br J Anaesth. 1984;56:1393–7.

Duvaldestin P, Lebrault C, Chauvin M. Pharmacokinetics of muscle relaxants in patients with liver disease. Clin Anesth. 1985;3:293–306.

Gelman S. General anesthesia and hepatic circulation. Can J Physiol Pharmacol. 1987;65:1762–79.

Elliot RH, Strunin L. Hepatoxicity of volatile anesthetics. Implications for halothane, enflurane, isoflurane, sevoflurane, and desflurane. Br J Anaesth. 1993;70:339–48.

Chapter 62 Regulation of intermediary metabolism

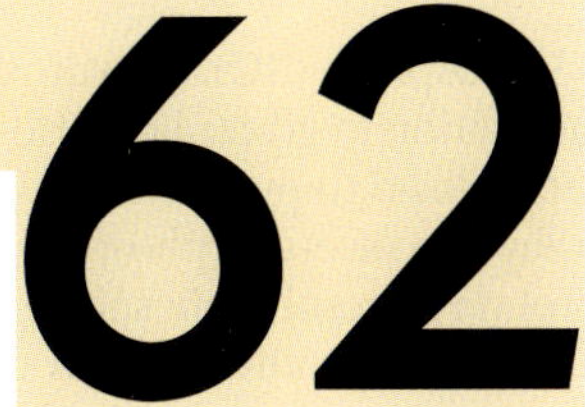

Iain T Campbell

Topics covered in this chapter

BIOENERGETICS

The body obtains its energy from oxidation of carbohydrate, fat, and protein. Glucose is an immediate source of energy, fat the major store, and protein forms the structure of the body itself. Fat and carbohydrate are the principal energy substrates, but 10–15% of energy is normally derived from protein oxidation. Protein synthesis and breakdown take place simultaneously so that lean tissue mass is in a dynamic equilibrium. In the healthy individual, protein oxidation occurs at a rate equal to that of protein intake, usually around 1g/kg per day.

Adenosine triphosphate

The energy derived from oxidation of these complex organic molecules is taken up by the formation of high-energy phosphate bonds, mainly in adenosine triphosphate (ATP). This ubiquitous molecule is the immediate energy supply for most energy-requiring processes in the body. The hydrolysis of ATP into adenosine diphosphate (ADP) releases energy for immediate use in processes such as muscle contraction, membrane transport, protein synthesis, etc. At any one moment the body contains only about 1g of ATP, but the 24-hour turnover rate is in the region of 45kg. Thus, mechanisms for the replenishment of ATP need to be integrated intimately with those of ATP utilization.

Some ATP is formed directly by chemical reactions that incorporate a phosphate group. This is known as *substrate-level phosphorylation* and does not involve oxygen, but most ATP is created by a more complex process known as *oxidative phosphorylation* (Fig. 62.1).

'Oxidation' means loss of electrons, but organic molecules do not give up electrons easily and oxidation of a complex molecule like glucose involves the loss of an entire atom, usually hydrogen. Thus oxidation (dehydrogenation) of a compound such as glucose involves production of the low-energy compound carbon dioxide, acceptance of electrons (H atoms) ultimately by oxygen to produce water, and the release of energy which is 'captured' in ATP.

Highly reduced compounds such as glucose (i.e. containing many hydrogen atoms) are high-energy compounds, whereas oxidized compounds with few hydrogen atoms are of relatively low

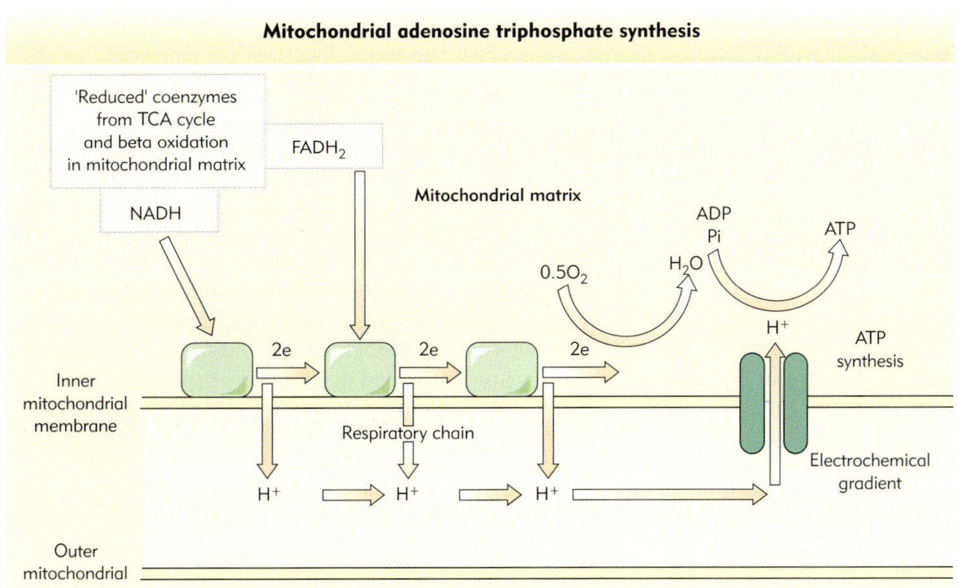

Figure 62.1 Mitochondrial ATP synthesis. Hydrogen atoms are transferred onto the flavoprotein–cytochrome (respiratory) chain, which moves protons through the inner mitochondrial membrane and subsequently generates ATP. (TCA, tricarboxylic acid; NADH, reduced nicotinamide adenine dinucleotide; FADH$_2$, reduced flavine adenine dinucleotide, Pi, inorganic phosphate)

energy. As hydrogen ions are released in various parts of the glucose oxidation pathway, they are taken up temporarily by *coenzymes*, most commonly nicotinamide–adenine dinucleotide (NAD^+) and flavine adenine dinucleotide (FAD), which are converted into NADH and $FADH_2$, respectively. They are then passed on to the flavoprotein–cytochrome system, a series of enzymes situated in the inner membrane of the mitochondrion, known also as the respiratory chain (see Fig. 62.1). Each enzyme in the respiratory chain has a greater affinity for electrons than the one before, which facilitates the passage of electrons from one enzyme to the next, with the release of free energy at each step. Each enzyme is reduced and then reoxidized as electrons pass down the chain. The final enzyme in the chain is cytochrome oxidase, which transfers hydrogen to oxygen to form water.

Enough free energy is released to synthesize a molecule of ATP at three sites in the respiratory chain, and three molecules of ATP are synthesized for each molecule of NADH that is oxidized. The electrons from $FADH_2$ enter the chain at the second electron transfer step; two molecules of ATP are thus synthesized for each hydrogen atom donated, which makes four for each molecule of $FADH_2$ oxidized (see Fig. 62.1).

ATP is not synthesized directly; the energy released drives hydrogen ions (protons) across the inner mitochondrial membrane into the intermembrane space to create an electrochemical gradient across the inner membrane. The protons then pass back down this gradient, passively, into the mitochondrion and drive a reversible ATPase in the membrane; it is this protein ATPase that generates ATP from ADP.

CARBOHYDRATE METABOLISM

The principal product of the digestion and absorption of complex carbohydrate is glucose, but other monosaccharides include fructose and galactose. Glucose passes via the portal system through the liver (where some is stored as glycogen) into the systemic circulation, where it may also be stored as glycogen in muscle or it is metabolized to give carbon dioxide and water with the release of energy and the synthesis of ATP.

Carbohydrate normally provides about 40–50% of the body's energy requirements. Some tissues (such as skeletal and cardiac muscle) can function without glucose, and obtain their energy from fatty acid oxidation should their supply of glucose cease, but others (such as nervous tissue and blood cells) are obligatory users of glucose and cannot survive without it.

Glucose metabolism

Glucose is metabolized via two sequential metabolic pathways, the Embden–Meyerhof pathway (or glycolysis) and the Krebs or tricarboxylic acid (TCA) cycle (Fig. 62.2).

Glycolysis is the first stage of glucose breakdown; most of the steps in this pathway are reversible. Glucose (6C) is metabolized via six discrete steps to give two molecules of pyruvic acid (3C). At the start of the glycolytic pathway glucose is phosphorylated by hexokinase to give glucose-6-phosphate (not shown in Fig. 62.2); this step, in contrast to most others, is irreversible. Glucose-6-phosphate in liver or muscle can either be converted into glycogen (see later) or enter the glycolytic pathway. In the third step of the pathway, a second phosphorylation occurs by phosphofructokinase to give fructose-1,6-bisphosphate. This step is also irreversible; its regulation is related to the energy status of the cell (i.e. the availability of ATP). Fructose-1,6-bisphosphate (6C) is split into dihydroxyacetone phosphate (3C) and glyceraldehyde-3-phosphate (3C). Dihydroxyacetone phosphate undergoes isomerization to glyceraldehyde-3-phosphate, which is eventually metabolized to pyruvate.

In the liver, dihydroxyacetone phosphate can also be synthesized from glycerol via glycerol-3-phosphate, thus providing a link with fat metabolism and a route whereby glycerol from triglycerides can enter the glycolytic pathway. Two molecules of ATP are used in glycolysis and four are produced. In addition, two molecules of NAD^+ are reduced to NADH, which provides the potential for ATP production in the respiratory chain within the mitochondrion. The net gain of ATP to the cell directly from glycolysis of one molecule of glucose is thus only two molecules of ATP, which is not very efficient, but as substrate-level oxidation it occurs in the absence of oxygen. The free-energy yield from glucose at this stage is about 84kJ/mol (20kcal/mol), compared with 2827kJ/mol (673kcal/mol) when glucose is fully oxidized to carbon dioxide and water. The former amounts to only 3% of the total energy available in the molecule.

When NADH is oxidized in the mitochondrion, three molecules of ATP are produced for each molecule of NADH that enters the respiratory chain. The mitochondrial membrane, however, is impermeable to NADH; when NADH is produced in the cytosol by glycolysis, as described above, a shuttle mechanism transfers protons and electrons to FAD within the mitochondrion. For each hydrogen ion, FAD produces only two molecules of ATP, so the two molecules of NADH produced in glycolysis result eventually in a gain of four molecules of ATP instead of six, and this only in the presence of oxygen.

Tricarboxylic acid cycle

Under aerobic conditions, pyruvate now crosses from the cytosol into the mitochondrial matrix and enters the TCA cycle. In a reaction catalyzed by pyruvate dehydrogenase, a 2-carbon acetyl group is transferred from pyruvate to the reduced form of coenzyme A (CoA). The third carbon of pyruvate is lost as carbon dioxide via the lungs. It is as acetyl CoA that the two atoms from pyruvate enter the TCA cycle, which is the final common pathway for the breakdown of all intracellular substrate molecules. All two-carbon acetyl groups (CH_3COO–) enter the TCA cycle in this fashion, coupled to the terminal –SH group of CoA as acetyl CoA ($CH_3COOCoA$).

In the first part of the cycle the acetyl group is transferred to oxaloacetic acid (4C) to form citric acid and free CoA (see Fig. 62.2). There are a further eight steps in the cycle, which generate a number of other intermediate compounds, such as 2-oxoglutarate (5C) and malate (4C), before the regeneration of oxaloacetic acid ready for another round. Two molecules of carbon dioxide are produced for every (2C) acetyl group that enters the cycle; the carbon atoms lost as carbon dioxide in one round of the cycle are those that entered as an acetyl group in the previous round. The oxidation of each of these acetyl groups to carbon dioxide is coupled to the reduction of NAD and FAD, and each round of the cycle generates three molecules of NADH and one of $FADH_2$, as well as one high-energy phosphate bond in guanosine triphosphate (GTP), which is used to phosphorylate a molecule of ADP to give ATP.

The adenosine triphosphate balance sheet

The net gain during glycolysis is two molecules of ATP, and a further four are gained from the NAD^+–FAD mitochondrial shuttle mechanism. Conversion of pyruvic acid into acetyl CoA yields two molecules of NADH per molecule of glucose (i.e. one per molecule of pyruvate – six ATP molecules altogether) and a further six

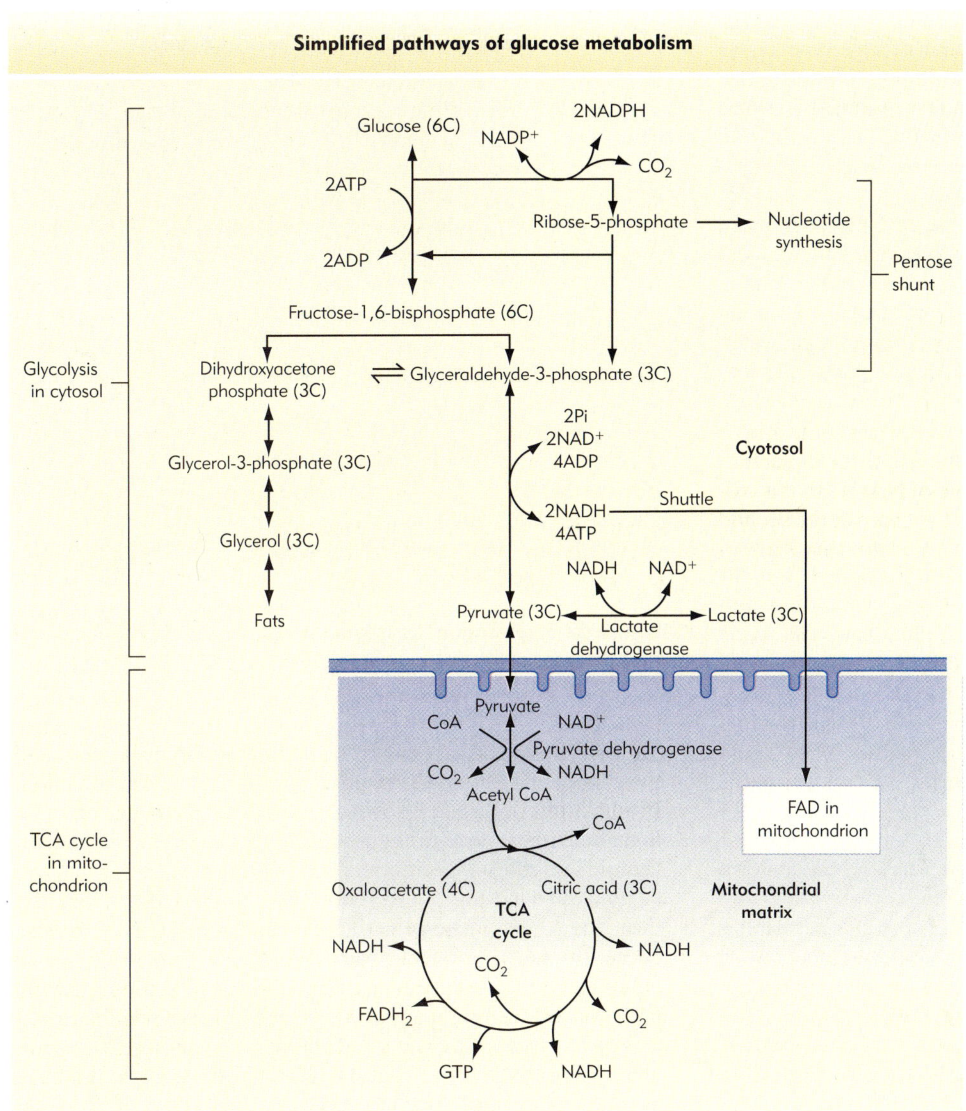

Figure 62.2 Simplified pathways of glucose metabolism. Reduced coenzymes and some ATP are generated by glycolysis. Most ATP is generated in the TCA cycle.

NADH (18 ATP) molecules are produced by two rounds of the TCA cycle, along with two $FADH_2$ (four ATP) molecules and two ATP molecules via GTP. Thus, 36 molecules of ATP are produced from the complete oxidation of one glucose molecule.

Aerobic and anaerobic metabolism

Molecular oxygen is not needed in the TCA cycle itself, but it is essential for the oxidation of reduced coenzymes in the mitochondrial electron-transport chain. The regeneration (reduction) of oxidized coenzyme is vital and requires oxygen. Metabolism in the absence of oxygen stops in the cytosol. Available NAD is converted into NADH, so NAD is not available, and hence glycolysis and ATP production cease. Pyruvate, however, can accept hydrogen from NADH to form lactic acid and release some NAD^+, a reaction catalyzed by lactate dehydrogenase. This allows glycolysis to continue until NAD really is exhausted. When the oxygen supply resumes and NAD once more becomes available, lactic acid is converted back into pyruvic NADH, which ultimately transfers its hydrogen to the cytochrome chain.

The pentose monophosphate shunt

An alternative pathway to glycolysis is the pentose monophosphate pathway or shunt (see Fig. 62.2), which is also situated in the cytosol. Its main function is to provide a supply of pentose sugars, essential in the synthesis of nucleotides and nucleic acids, and the reduced form of nicotinamide–adenine dinucleotide phosphate (NADPH), a phosphorylated form of NADH used in a variety of biosynthetic pathways. The pathway starts with glucose-6-phosphate and ultimately forms two molecules of NADPH and one molecule of ribose-5-phosphate. Excess ribose-5-phosphate, not needed in nucleotide synthesis, is shunted back into the glycolytic pathway as fructose-6-phosphate and glyceraldehyde-3-phosphate. The pentose phosphate pathway does not use ATP or oxygen; whether glucose is metabolized by this route or via the glycolytic pathway seems to depend on whether the cell is engaged in biosynthesis. It is particularly important in the liver.

Glycogen metabolism

Liver

Glucose is absorbed, via the portal vein, from the gastrointestinal tract into the liver. Systemic glucose concentrations average 5mmol/L (90mg/100ml), but after a meal portal blood glucose can rise to 10mmol/L(180mg/100ml). Glucose enters cells by carrier-mediated diffusion via specialized proteins in the membrane. The glucose transporter for the liver is GLUT-2, which is not responsive to insulin. Glucose is absorbed into the liver down a diffusion gradient. Hexokinase phosphorylates the glucose to give glucose-6-phosphate, which is also normally independent of insulin. When more glucose is present than required, it is stored as glycogen, a process stimulated and controlled by insulin and by the presence of glucose itself, and mediated by glycogen synthase via glucose-1-phosphate (Fig. 62.3).

Hepatic glycogen is the body's glucose buffer. Glucose is stored in the liver at times of excess – normally following a meal – and maintains blood glucose in the absence of glucose intake. With a prolonged fast, hepatic glycogen stores become exhausted within 24–48 hours. Glucose can be mobilized from liver glycogen when required. Glycogen is broken down via glucose-1-phosphate into glucose-6-phosphate and glucose is formed from glucose-6-phosphate by glucose-6-phosphatase. The usual stimulus to glycogen breakdown is a fall in blood glucose, and it is mediated by glycogen phosphorylase and brought about by a change in the balance of the hormones insulin and glucagon; insulin secretion falls and glucagon secretion rises. This stimulates phosphorylation of glycogen phosphorylase by phosphorylase kinase, changing it from its inactive *b* form into its active *a* form, which acts on glycogen to release one molecule of glucose as glucose-1-phosphate. The action of glucagon is mediated by cyclic AMP. Other hormones that stimulate glycogenolysis are the catecholamines epinephrine (adrenaline) and norepinephrine (noradrenaline). Their role is important in stress, with the acute mobilization of energy substrate, but probably not in the day-to-day control of blood glucose concentration.

Muscle

Muscle is the other major store of glycogen, which is broken down into glucose-6-phosphate with activation of phosphorylase *b* into phosphorylase *a*, as it is in liver. The stimulus on this occasion is usually a nerve impulse that releases Ca^{2+} from the sarcoplasmic reticulum, which results ultimately in the activation of phosphorylase and the formation of glucose-6-phosphate. The other stimulus to glycogenolysis is epinephrine, a process that occurs in stress, such as 'shock' or severe exercise. Muscle does not express glucose-6-phosphatase so glucose is not released into the blood stream, but is metabolized via the glycolytic pathway. If the demand for oxygen is greater than the supply, as it often is in 'shock' or severe exercise, lactic acid accumulates and diffuses into the general circulation. This produces a metabolic acidosis, usually buffered by hyperventilation and corrected when the balance of oxygen demand and delivery is restored. Lactate also passes to the liver, where it is synthesized to give glucose via gluconeogenesis.

The endocrine pancreas

Glucose metabolism is largely under the control of insulin and glucagon, hormones secreted by the pancreas. Most of the pancreatic cells are concerned with the exocrine functions of digestion in the small intestine, but insulin and glucagon are both secreted by the islets of Langerhans, little groups of cells that are scattered throughout the pancreas. About a million islets constitute around 1–2% of the pancreatic mass and consist of three cell types – A, B, and D. The A cells secrete glucagon, the B cells insulin, and the D cells somatostatin. Each islet is supplied by a branch of the pancreatic artery and the venous drainage, via the pancreatic vein, enters into the portal vein just before it enters the liver. Thus, the liver is the first organ on which insulin and glucagon exert their effects before being diluted by the general circulation.

Insulin consists of two peptide chains linked by two disulfide bonds (Fig. 62.4). The A chain has 21 amino acids and the B chain 30. It is synthesized as a single polypeptide chain (proinsulin) and the connecting peptide, C peptide, is removed before secretion. Insulin is internalized and hydrolyzed by the cells it acts upon, so that circulating concentrations are a function of both rates of utilization and rates of secretion. As C peptide is not utilized it can be used as an indicator of secretion. The stimulus to insulin secretion, and to its synthesis, is the plasma glucose concentration. Secretion is stimulated when plasma glucose rises above 5mmol/L(90mg/100ml). It circulates freely in the blood stream, not attached to any carrier proteins, and binds to specific receptors on its target cells. The intracellular action of insulin is mediated ultimately by dephosphorylation or sometimes phosphorylation of specific enzymes. Only about 50% of the insulin secreted by the pancreas reaches the general circulation – the rest is taken up by the liver after its initial secretion into the portal vein. This close relationship with the liver is a major regulatory factor in the control of glucose metabolism.

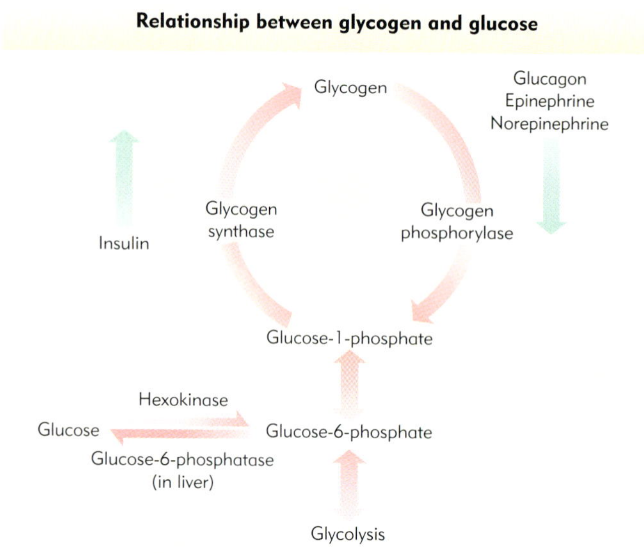

Figure 62.3 Glycogen, its relation to glucose, and the factors that drive its synthesis and breakdown.

Glucagon is a polypeptide of 29 amino acids. Its major action is to elevate blood glucose by stimulating glycogenolysis in the liver. Secretion is stimulated by a fall and suppressed by an increase in blood glucose. Glucagon, like insulin, is also partially removed on its first pass through the liver, but in smaller quantities. It acts on receptors in the membrane of its target cells; the receptors are coupled to stimulation of adenylyl cyclase via G proteins. Glucagon and insulin thus have reciprocal roles in glucose homeostasis.

In addition, glucagon and insulin secretion are both controlled by the sympathetic nervous system. β-Adrenergic stimulation of the islets of Langerhans stimulates insulin secretion, whereas α-adrenergic stimulation inhibits it. Following a stressful stimulus, such as trauma, the α or inhibiting effect is predominant. Sympathetic activation stimulates glucagon secretion.

FAT METABOLISM

Fat is an integral part of the cell membrane and lipids of various sorts are fundamental to the structure of the central nervous system. It is as adipose tissue, however, that fat

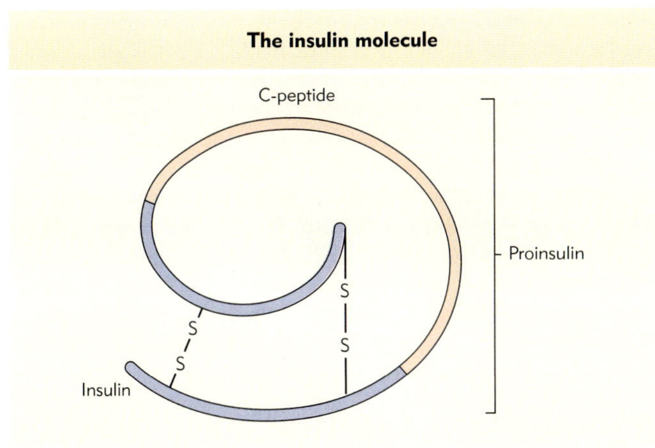

Figure 62.4 The insulin molecule. Insulin is synthesized as proinsulin, which is cleaved to insulin and C peptide.

[triacylglycerol (TAG) or triglyceride] forms the major energy store of the body. Formed of glycerol and three fatty acids, TAG is absorbed from the gastrointestinal tract via the lymphatics in chylomicrons, the largest of the lipoprotein particles that transport lipids in the plasma, and so it does not pass through the liver. In the tissues, lipoprotein lipase hydrolyzes TAG in the chylomicron to release free fatty acids, which mostly pass into adipose tissue (Fig. 62.5). Lipoprotein lipase is synthesized in adipocytes, but in adipose tissue it is attached to the capillary endothelium. It is activated by insulin, which rises rapidly after a meal in response to glucose, but the maximum action of insulin on lipoprotein lipase is 2–3 hours after the meal.

The mobilization of FFAs from adipose tissue is known as *lipolysis*, which releases them (bound to albumin) into the circulation for use as energy substrate. The hydrolysis of TAG to give FFAs and glycerol is controlled by the enzyme hormone-sensitive lipase, situated within the adipocyte, which is stimulated by the catecholamines epinephrine and norepinephrine and inhibited by insulin. Glucagon stimulates lipolysis *in vitro*, but it is unclear whether it is active *in vivo*. It may have a role by virtue of its reciprocal activity with insulin, rising and stimulating lipolysis when blood glucose and insulin levels fall.

Fat as a metabolic fuel

Fatty acids are used as a metabolic fuel by peripheral tissues including skeletal muscle and myocardium. They arise from lipolysis of TAG in adipose tissue in the form of FFAs or from TAG circulating in lipoprotein particles. As TAG cannot be taken up directly by the cell, it is firstly hydrolyzed to FFAs and glycerol. This is carried out by lipoprotein lipase attached to the capillary endothelium, as described previously in relation to fatty acid uptake (see Fig. 62.5). The FFAs are taken up across the cell membrane, possibly by a specific transport mechanism, at a rate closely related to their concentration in the plasma, and oxidized in the cell in accordance with their rate of uptake. The glycerol moiety is transported to the liver, where it is converted into dihydroxyacetone phosphate, a component of the glycolysis pathway, and is either oxidized via pyruvate and acetyl CoA or converted into glucose.

Beta oxidation and carnitine

Fatty acids are oxidized in mitochondria by beta oxidation, which results in the formation of acetyl CoA. Two carbon fragments are cleaved from the end of the fatty acid molecule by a process that involves dehydrogenation, and hydration with hydrogen atoms transferred to a flavoprotein to form acetyl CoA. Most of the metabolically important fatty acids have an even number of carbon atoms, so the whole molecule is converted into acetyl CoA, which can then enter the TCA cycle. The longer-chain fatty acids, however, are unable to penetrate mitochondria unless linked to carnitine, a substance synthesized from methionine and lysine in the liver and kidneys. It is only as acyl carnitine that the longer-chain FFAs gain access to the beta oxidation system in mitochondria.

Ketone bodies

In the absence of exogenous energy substrate, glycogen stores are exhausted within 24–48 hours. The glucose requirements of those tissues that can oxidize nothing else are met initially by glucose formed by gluconeogenesis, which inevitably involves

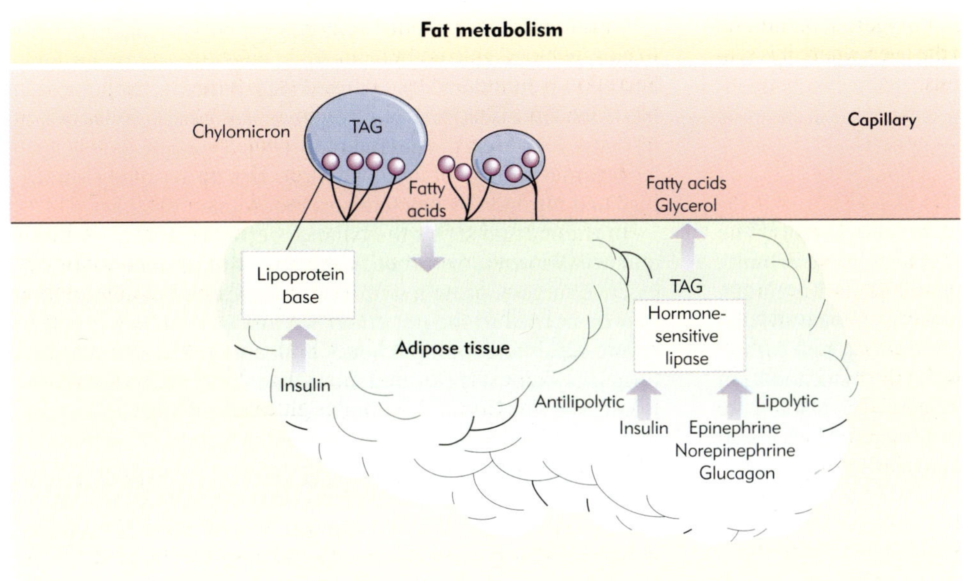

Figure 62.5 Fat metabolism. The take-up of free fatty acids (FFAs) into adipose tissue and the factors that control their release into the circulation. Lipoprotein lipase hydrolyzes TAG molecules in the chylomicron to release fatty acids and glycerol. The process is stimulated by insulin and reversed by hormone-sensitive lipase, which is stimulated by the 'stress' or counter-regulatory hormones.

an undesirable breakdown of lean tissue (see later). After 4–10 days of simple starvation, these tissues adapt (at least in part) to using ketones instead of glucose. The brain adapts to obtain about a half to two thirds of its requirements from ketone bodies. These substances – acetoacetate and β-hydroxybutyrate – are synthesized in the liver from FFAs. Acetone is formed from acetoacetate by loss of carbon dioxide, but it is not metabolized further and is excreted on the breath.

PROTEIN METABOLISM

Proteins are made up of amino acid chains connected by amide bonds (Chapter 1), and are digested in the small intestine and absorbed as amino acids and dipeptides. They are incorporated into different proteins in the body in a continual cycle of replacement and renewal, but in the process some are oxidized and about 10–15% of the body's energy requirements are derived from protein oxidation. The nitrogen in proteins is excreted as urea.

Amino acid metabolism

The first step in the catabolism of an amino acid is removal of the NH_2 group and its replacement with a C=O group (deamination) to form a keto or oxo acid. The various oxo acids are metabolic intermediates in, or closely related to, the metabolic pathways already described (glycolysis, TCA cycle, etc.) and can be oxidized to give carbon dioxide and water. Thirteen of them, derived from the so-called glucogenic amino acids, can be synthesized into glucose only (a process called gluconeogenesis), one can be synthesized into fat (ketogenic), and the remainder can be synthesized into either glucose or fat.

The conversion of amino acids into glucose is important in the absence of glucose intake, particularly as a means of maintaining a supply of glucose for the CNS. Gluconeogenesis occurs in both the liver and the kidney. The removal of the NH_2 group from an amino acid produces ammonia, which is toxic. It is metabolized, however, as soon as it is formed and blood concentrations of ammonia itself are normally very low. In the liver, ammonia forms urea via the urea cycle (see below), but in peripheral tissues NH_2 groups are transferred (transaminated) to keto acids, principally α-ketoglutarate, an intermediate in the TCA cycle, to form glutamate (one NH_2 group) and glutamine (two NH_2 groups). They are also transferred to pyruvate, the corresponding keto acid to alanine; it is principally as alanine and glutamine that NH_2 groups are transported from the periphery to the liver and kidney. As well as being a precursor for renal gluconeogenesis, glutamine also helps to buffer excess acid secretion. Alanine is the major precursor of hepatic gluconeogenesis.

The urea cycle

Urea synthesis takes place in the liver via a cyclic pathway. The key compound is ornithine, on which the urea molecule is 'built'; intermediates in the process include citrulline and arginine. Ammonia is released from amino acids, largely glutamine and alanine (as described earlier), and incorporated, along with carbon dioxide and ATP, into carbamoyl phosphate in the mitochondrion of the hepatocyte. Urea synthesis and its 'release' take place in the cytosol. The whole process is stimulated by glucagon, which is also important in regulating the uptake of amino acids by the liver.

Gluconeogenesis

In times of nutrient shortage, such as simple starvation and the undernutrition that usually complicates sepsis and trauma, the body maintains its glucose requirements by synthesizing glucose from a number of smaller molecules, mainly glycerol, lactate, and amino acids. Essentially, the process is a reversal of glycolysis except for three irreversible steps in glycolysis; in gluconeogenesis, these are bypassed. Most of the amino acids are deaminated and enter the TCA cycle at a variety of points. Pyruvate, the corresponding oxo acid to alanine, is the main precursor and is, of course, closely related to lactate. It is carboxylated to give oxaloacetate (a constituent of the TCA cycle), and then converted into phosphoenolpyruvate by the enzyme phosphoenolpyruvate carboxykinase (PEPCK). Phosphoenolpyruvate is a constituent of the second part of the glycolytic pathway, which is reversed to form glucose. Stages of glycolysis that are otherwise irreversible – the conversion of fructose-6-phosphate into fructose-1,6-bisphosphate by phosphofructokinase and the formation of glucose from glucose-6-phosphatase – are bypassed by fructose-1,6 bisphosphatase and glucose-6-phosphatase, respectively. Glycerol, the third main precursor, is converted into glycerol-3-phosphate and dihydroxyacetone, which are also constituents of the second part of the glycolytic pathway.

Gluconeogenesis is controlled by the rate of arrival of the precursors at the liver from peripheral tissue, and by the activity of PEPCK, fructose-1,6 bisphosphatase, and glucose-6-phosphatase. The delivery of gluconeogenic precursors to the liver is controlled by events in peripheral tissues such as the production of lactate from muscle during exercise (or shock), glycerol from lipolysis in starvation or after adrenergic stimulation, and amino acids in starvation or injury, brought about by inhibition of insulin release or resistance to its action. Activity of the various enzymes is stimulated principally by glucagon, but cortisol and insulin lack have some effect as well.

Regulation of protein metabolism

In the normal individual who has a stable body mass, protein intake, protein synthesis, and protein degradation are in balance. Insulin normally stimulates protein synthesis and maintains protein balance, although other hormones are important, particularly in skeletal muscle (the largest depot of protein in the body). They include growth hormone, insulin-like growth factor-1 (IGF-1), glucocorticoids, and thyroxine. Insulin secretion is stimulated by amino acids, but protein taken in excess of requirements is not stored so does not lead to an increase in lean body mass. Exogenous stimuli that increase lean body mass include exercise and anabolic steroids, and also growth hormone and IGF-1. In animals, β_2-adrenergic stimulants are anabolic, but such an effect has not yet been convincingly shown in humans. However, during recovery from a wasting illness, such as trauma, sepsis, or malnutrition, the body avidly retains ingested nitrogen by mechanisms that remain unclear.

In trauma and sepsis the balance between protein synthesis and breakdown is disturbed. In relatively mild trauma, such as elective surgery, protein synthesis is depressed but degradation may be normal so the net effect is a loss of lean body mass. In severe sepsis and multiple injury both are elevated; in absolute terms breakdown is elevated more than synthesis, so lean tissue is lost. The situation is also affected by feeding in that an increase in nutrient intake elevates both breakdown and synthesis, but in a complex fashion that depends on the level of feeding.

An increase in gluconeogenesis occurs in starvation and following sepsis and trauma. The use of amino acids as gluconeogenic precursors is of concern because they arise from the breakdown of lean tissue mass. In the normal individual glucose infusion suppresses gluconeogenesis completely, but in the septic or injured patient gluconeogenesis is suppressed by about 50% only. By feeding the severely septic or injured individual the most that can be achieved is to attenuate the rate of loss of lean tissue, not prevent it.

The stimulus to this catabolism of protein in trauma and sepsis is considered to be the counterregulatory hormones – catecholamines, cortisol, glucagon, and growth hormone – but infusion of these substances into normal volunteers does not reproduce a catabolic state of the severity seen after injury or sepsis. Somehow cytokines must be involved also. They are certainly involved centrally in terms of stimulating the counterregulatory hormone output, but the extent to which they affect peripheral protein metabolism either directly or via an effect on hepatic protein metabolism is not known.

WHOLE BODY PROTEIN AND ENERGY METABOLISM

Measurement of energy expenditure

The energy released by the oxidation of carbohydrate, fat, and protein is taken up to produce high-energy phosphate compounds, which are used in various energy-requiring processes. Two methods of measuring energy expenditure consist of either measuring the energy liberated (*direct calorimetry*) or the oxygen consumed (*indirect calorimetry*). The latter technique requires assumptions about the amount of energy liberation that consumption of a given quantity of oxygen denotes.

Heat and energy

The terms heat and energy have so far been used interchangeably; heat, however, is a form of energy. Since the early metabolic measurements in humans were of heat output, the units used in energy metabolism are usually those of heat [the calorie or kilocalorie (kcal)], and the techniques of biologic energy measurement are referred to as *calorimetry*. The calorie is defined as the amount of heat required to raise the temperature of 1 g of water by 1°C. The unit of energy or work is the Joule; this is the work done when a force of 1 Newton moves through a distance of 1m. The two are interrelated by a constant known as the *mechanical equivalent of heat*: 1 calorie = 4.2 Joules.

With the arrival of the SI system of units nearly 40 years ago, it was deemed more correct to report metabolic measurements in Joules, or more conveniently kiloJoules, as this was the true unit of energy, but the kilocalorie is still in common use.

Indirect calorimetry

Direct calorimetry is a tedious and cumbersome technique, and is not discussed here.

The traditional method, and probably still the simplest way of measuring oxygen consumption, is the use of a spirometer, such as the Benedict–Roth's design (Fig. 62.6). It consists of a volume of oxygen in a spirometer bell and a closed circuit through which the subject breathes. Carbon dioxide is absorbed and the rate of decrease of the bell's volume over a given period is calculated from the tracing on the kymograph. Gas volumes in indirect calorimetry are conventionally reported at standard temperature and pressure dry [STPD; i.e. at 32°F (0°C) and 101.3kPa (760mmHg)].

The energy value of oxygen consumed depends on the substrate metabolized. Equations 62.1–62.3 summarize energy values for carbohydrate (62.1), fat (62.2), and amino acid (62.3) oxidation; Equation 62.4 shows the synthesis of fat from carbohydrate. The respiratory quotient (RQ) is the ratio of carbon dioxide produced to oxygen consumed.

Equation 62.1

$$1\ \text{glucose} + 6O_2 \rightarrow 6CO_2 + 6H_2O + 673\text{kcal}\ (2827\text{kJ})$$
$$\text{i.e. } 5.03\text{kcal}\ (21.1\ \text{kJ})/\text{L}\ O_2$$
$$RQ = 1.0$$

Equation 62.2

$$1\ \text{palmitate} + 23O_2 \rightarrow 16CO_2 + 16H_2O + 2398\text{kcal}\ (10{,}072\text{kJ})$$
$$\text{i.e. } 4.68\text{kcal}\ (19.7\text{kJ})/\text{L}\ O_2$$
$$RQ = 0.7$$

Equation 62.3

$$1\ \text{amino acid} + 5.1O_2 \rightarrow 4.1CO_2 + 0.7\ \text{urea} + 28H_2O + 475\text{kcal}\ (1995\text{kJ})$$
$$\text{i.e. } 4.18\text{kcal}\ (17.4\text{kJ})/\text{L}\ O_2$$
$$RQ = 0.8$$

Equation 62.4

$$4.5\ \text{glucose} + 4O_2 \rightarrow 1\ \text{palmitoyl}-[11CO_2 + 11H_2O + 630\text{kcal}\ (2646\text{kJ})]$$
$$\text{i.e. } 7.06\text{kcal}\ (29.7\text{kJ})/\text{L}\ O_2$$
$$RQ = 2.75$$

It can be seen that the relationships between oxygen consumed, carbon dioxide produced, and energy released vary. At STPD, in the oxidation of fat the calorific value of 1L of oxygen is 19.7kJ (4.68kcal) and in the oxidation of carbohydrate it is 21.1kJ (5.03kcal). An RQ in excess of 1.0 denotes net fat synthesis from carbohydrate. The RQ, however, is a biochemical concept and is impossible to measure in the whole body. What can be measured is the pulmonary exchange of oxygen and carbon dioxide, but this is affected by factors other than substrate oxidation. It is more correctly known as the respiratory exchange ratio (RER). For RER to approximate RQ, the subject has to be in a steady state and the measurement has to be made over at least 30 minutes.

The RQ of protein depends on the precise make-up of the protein, and is generally in the region of 0.80–0.85, but protein is not oxidized completely into carbon dioxide and water; a variety of other nitrogen- and energy-containing products of protein metabolism are excreted in the urine. The relationship between protein oxidation and urinary nitrogen is fairly constant; on average, 1g of urinary nitrogen denotes oxidation of 6.3g of protein. The amount of protein used as an energy substrate over a given period can thus be quantified purely from a measure of urinary nitrogen collected over that period, with a correction made as necessary for alterations in the body urea pool (estimated from changes in blood urea). In practice, urinary nitrogen is rarely measured because of technical difficulties; it is more usual to measure urinary urea. Of the urinary nitrogen, 80% is excreted as urea, although this is highly variable (both between and within individuals) and has a range of 60–100%. Also, during starvation more nitrogen is excreted in the form of ammonia. As a technique to assess protein metabolism for research purposes, urea measurement is not really acceptable, but for clinical purposes it is probably adequate.

Excretion of 1g of nitrogen also denotes the consumption of 5.94L of oxygen and the production of 4.76L of carbon dioxide; thus, the gas exchange associated with protein metabolism can be calculated and subtracted from total gas exchange as measured, to give the gas exchange associated with fat and carbohydrate oxidation only. The RQ so calculated and associated with only fat and carbohydrate oxidation is called the

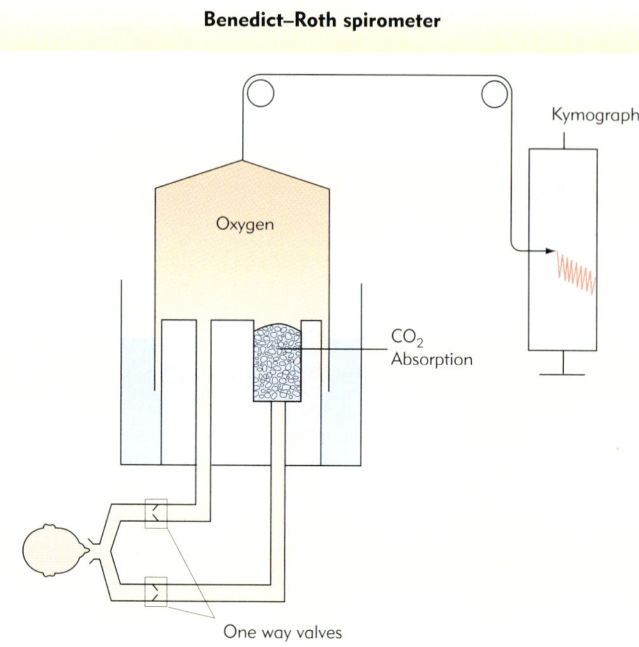

Figure 62.6 The Benedict–Roth spirometer. This simple measurement of oxygen consumption requires only two one-way valves and a motor to turn the kymograph.

nonprotein RQ and, assuming RQ and RER to be equivalent, allows the proportions of energy expenditure derived from fat and carbohydrate oxidation to be calculated. This in combination with the oxygen consumption figure also enables values for total quantities of fat and carbohydrate to be calculated. Equations 62.5 and 62.6 are used to quantify fat and carbohydrate oxidation, in which C and F are carbohydrate and fat oxidation in grams, $\dot{V}O_2$ and $\dot{V}CO_2$ are expressed in liters (at STPD), and N represents urinary nitrogen excretion in grams.

Equation 62.5

$$C = 4.14\dot{V}CO_2 - 2.908\dot{V}O_2 - 2.543N$$

Equation 62.6

$$F = 1.689(\dot{V}O_2 - \dot{V}CO_2) - 1.943N$$

The problem with using the spirometer to measure oxygen consumption is that it has to be 'driven' by the subject who interfaces with the instrument via a mouthpiece and nose clip. This works for a trained volunteer, but seriously ill patients tolerate it poorly.

An alternative technique is to measure inspired ($\dot{V}I$) and expired ($\dot{V}E$) air volumes and the concentrations of oxygen and carbon dioxide in each, either via a mouthpiece and nose clip or face mask, or by drawing a measured volume of air past the subject's face and collecting the mixed expired air for analysis. Equations 62.7 and 62.8 are used, in which FI and FE are the fractional concentrations of oxygen and carbon dioxide in inspired and mixed expired air, respectively. The concentration of carbon dioxide in inspired air is usually ignored.

Equation 62.7

$$\dot{V}O_2 = (\dot{V}I \times FIO_2) - (\dot{V}E \times FEO_2)$$

Equation 62.8

$$\dot{V}CO_2 = \dot{V}E \times FECO_2$$

Inspired and expired volume are measured separately as they are usually unequal – less carbon dioxide is normally expired than oxygen is consumed since the RQ is usually in the range 0.7–1.0. To measure both inspired and expired volumes is complex and probably introduces more errors than would exist if the difference between the two volumes were ignored completely. The conventional procedure is for one of these two volumes to be measured and the other calculated using the inspired and expired nitrogen concentrations, as in Equation 62.9, in which NI and NE are the concentrations of nitrogen in the inspired and mixed expired air, respectively.

Equation 62.9

$$\dot{V}E = \dot{V}I \times \frac{NI}{NE}$$

This is known as the Haldane transformation and assumes that the net ventilatory exchange of nitrogen is zero (i.e. the subject is in a steady state). Nitrogen is not normally measured, but is taken to be the nonoxygen, noncarbon dioxide gas in the inspired and expired gas volumes.

This works well when the subject breathes air and the nitrogen concentration in the system is high, but in the presence of a high FIO_2, as in ventilated patients, the concentration of nitrogen is diminished; with an inspired oxygen concentration of 100%, no nitrogen is in the system, so the Haldane transformation is not applicable. In practice, with most indirect calorimeters that use the Haldane transformation, the system ceases to function at an FIO_2 of about 0.7.

There are essentially two ways around the problem; one is to measure the inspired and expired volumes separately, but this is complex and demands a very high degree of accuracy from the volume measuring devices. The other is to calculate $\dot{V}CO_2$ from measurement of $\dot{V}I$ and the mixed expired carbon dioxide concentration alone, then assume RQ and calculate $\dot{V}O_2$ and energy expenditure accordingly. This can introduce an error of up to about 15%, but for clinical purposes is not unreasonable. In a critically ill patient in multiple organ failure it is certainly better than not to make the measurement at all.

Factors that affect respiratory exchange ratio

Factors other than substrate oxidation also affect RER, and include hyperventilation (or hypoventilation), which produces a transient rise (or fall) in RER until a new steady state is achieved, and metabolic acidosis (or alkalosis) in which carbon dioxide is excreted (or retained) to compensate. As a result of the different solubilities of the two gases in the body, a change in body temperature produces a differential retention of carbon dioxide should temperature fall, or a rise in carbon dioxide excretion should temperature go up. All of these limitations need to be borne in mind when interpreting measurements of RER as an indicator of substrate oxidation.

Energy expenditure in humans

The principal components of energy expenditure in humans are basal energy expenditure, dietary-induced thermogenesis, activity, nonshivering thermogenesis, and hormonal control of metabolic rate.

Basal energy expenditure

Basal energy expenditure is the energy expended when the body is totally at rest in such processes as the maintenance of cell membrane potentials, ventilation, and the action of the heart. It is the largest single component of 24 hour energy expenditure and is conventionally measured at rest, after an overnight fast and with the subject thermoneutral (i.e. neither hot enough to stimulate heat loss nor cold enough to stimulate heat generation).

Although ideally basal metabolism is measured, it is possible to predict it using a number of formulae. One such is the Harris–Benedict formula, in which B is 24 hour basal energy expenditure (kcal), W is body weight (kg), H is height (cm), and A is age (years). Equation 62.10 is for men, and Equation 62.11 is for women.

Equation 62.10

$$B = 66.47 + 13.75W + 5.003H - 6.750A$$

Equation 62.11

$$B = 655.1 + 9.563W + 1.850H - 4.676A$$

The more recent Schofield analysis gives a series of equations of the form $y = mx + c$ (x is weight) for various age groups. The factors common to these formulae and to others of the same type are *body size* (i.e. height and/or weight), *age* (metabolic rate decreases steadily from the age of 6 months, with a minor rise at puberty), and *gender* (women generally have more body fat than men; this is metabolically less active than lean tissue and is a better insulator).

Dietary-induced thermogenesis

Dietary-induced thermogenesis, formerly called specific dynamic action, is the rise in metabolic rate associated with the ingestion of food and is said to represent the energy cost of digestion and assimilation. The argument for this centered around whether the rise in expenditure is related only to the size and timing of a discrete meal or whether it is related more to the general 'level of nutrition', that is whether a means exists for the human to oxidize food eaten in excess of requirements, perhaps by mechanisms such as nonshivering thermogenesis. Certainly, starvation is associated with a decrease in basal metabolism, but the conventional view is that a mechanism to metabolize energy eaten in excess of requirements probably does not exist.

Activity

Energy expenditure rises with activity. In hospital practice the addition of 10–30% to basal expenditure (measured or calculated) is usually enough to take activity into account. For a very active individual such as a manual laborer or a professional sportsman a figure closer to 100% is more appropriate.

Nonshivering thermogenesis

Nonshivering thermogenesis is a mechanism of heat production that occurs in hibernating animals and, in humans, in the first 6 months of life, whereby neonates thermoregulate and hibernating animals warm themselves up after winter. It is associated with a special type of fat called *brown adipose tissue*. In rodents this is found in depots in the back (between the scapulae), and in human neonates in the supra renal fat, in axillary fat, and around the great vessels of the heart and vertebral arteries. The tissue appears brown because of large numbers of mitochondria, which can be uncoupled; that is instead of ATP being generated when foodstuffs are metabolized to carbon dioxide and water, free energy is released to serve as a direct heat source. This is associated with the presence of a specific *uncoupling protein* in the walls of the mitochondria, which has been named thermogenin. The protons that pass down the electrochemical gradient and across the inner membrane of the mitochondrion release free energy instead of generating ATP. The process is under the control of the sympathetic nervous system and brown adipose tissue is richly innervated with sympathetic nerve endings.

This is the principal means available for varying heat production that does not involve muscle contraction. It has been unclear whether the mechanism exists in adult humans as a means of body weight control, as referred to earlier, or to raise body temperature and heat output in response to a pyrogen. The consensus at the moment is that it probably does not.

Hormonal control of metabolic rate

Overall control of metabolic rate in the body is via the thyroid hormones. Thyrotoxicosis is associated with a high metabolic rate and myxedema with a reduced one. The catecholamines also increase metabolism, certainly when given in pharmacologic doses and probably also in response to stimulation of endogenous catecholamine output, possibly secondary to a stimulation of glycolysis, lipolysis, an increase in myocardial contractility, and an increase in muscle tone.

The measurement of 24 hour energy expenditure

Indirect calorimetry

The classic method to assess an individual's 24 hour energy expenditure is to keep a record of the individual's activity and measure the energy cost of each type of activity using indirect calorimetry.

Heart rate is also a useful index of energy expenditure, and is monitored by telemetry or a portable monitor and energy expenditure is measured simultaneously by indirect calorimetry and at various levels of expenditure for discrete periods. A regression line is then constructed for an individual that relates heart rate to energy expenditure. If heart rate is measured over 24 hours, expenditure over that period can be predicted from the regression line. This technique is also reasonably accurate for the population, but individual errors are large.

Doubly labeled water is now the standard method of measuring energy expenditure in the free-living individual. A mixture of two isotopes of water (^2H_2O and $H_2{}^{18}O$) is drunk; ^2H_2O equilibrates with the body water pool and $H_2{}^{18}O$ with both the body water and the bicarbonate pools. The (logarithmic) rate of decline of ^2H_2O in the body is a function of whole body water turnover, and the rate of decline of $H_2{}^{18}O$ is a function of both body water and carbon dioxide turnover, so the difference between the two is a function of carbon dioxide output. A value can be assumed for RQ and energy expenditure calculated, or a dietary record can be kept and RQ derived from the food intake.

The application of this technique is limited by the length of time it takes for isotope enrichment in the body to decline such that a reasonable assessment of carbon dioxide production over that period can be made. This is usually 10–15 days, but obviously varies with the intensity of the activity. Also, only an average measure of energy expenditure is obtained for the period of measurement; if energy expenditure varies widely from day to day, this variability is not identified. Obviously, the longer the period of measurement the smaller the errors. Other limitations are the expense of the isotopes and the specialized nature of the analysis (mass spectrometry).

Rates of decline in isotope enrichment are measured by monitoring body water in blood, urine, or saliva. These can be measured every day for accuracy, but one assessment 10–15 days after administration and mathematic assumptions about the rate of isotope excretion are most convenient.

ENERGY AND NUTRIENT INTAKE

Foodstuffs in the body are metabolized to give carbon dioxide and water, or in the case of protein to give carbon dioxide, water, and urea, creatinine, uric acid, and ammonia. With fat and carbohydrate there is no difference in terms of waste products and energy released when these substrates are oxidized via the numerous biochemical pathways described earlier, or if they are merely burnt (the energy content of fat and carbohydrate can be determined by doing just that in a *bomb calorimeter*). The substance under investigation, in this case food, is dried (either freeze dried or dried in an oven) and ground into a fine powder. A weighed quantity is burnt in oxygen under pressure, which ensures its complete combustion (oxidation). Heat output is measured either in absolute quantities by absorption into a water jacket of known thermal capacity or, in a simpler type of instrument that measures relative heat production, the heat emitted is absorbed by a steel jacket that surrounds the sample. The temperature of this jacket rises transiently to a value that is a function of the total amount of heat emitted, which is compared with the heat emitted by combustion of a known quantity of a standard substance, such as glucose.

The heat energy released from foodstuffs by combustion is the 'gross energy' (GE). For carbohydrate and fat this is the same as the 'metabolizable energy' (ME; i.e. the energy available to the body for metabolic purposes). Equation 62.12 can be used to calculate ME from GE.

Equation 62.8

$$ME = 0.95GE - 0.075\%N$$

Equation 62.12 assumes 95% absorption of all foodstuffs – an average value for a standard, mixed western diet (this is somewhat nearer 90% for a high roughage or high fiber diet) – and allows for excretion of the products of protein metabolism. A sample has to be analyzed for its nitrogen content.

Assessment of nutrient intake

Methods to assess an individual's energy and nitrogen intake include:

- collecting a duplicate sample of everything the individual eats over a period and subjecting it to the bombing and nitrogen analysis procedures described above;
- collecting a duplicate sample and analyzing it for carbohydrate, fat, and protein content; standard factors are used to convert the figures obtained into energy [carbohydrate, 16.8kJ/g (4kcal/g); fat, 37.8kJ/g (9kcal/g), and protein, 15.5kJ/g (3.7kcal/g); these nutrient conversion factors are average figures – the precise values depend on the particular carbohydrate, fat, or protein being eaten].
- in clininical practice the patient keeps a record of what they eat, either weighing their food or describing portion size or, food intake may be assessed by interview, usually with a dietician. Nutrient analysis is then performed using food composition tables (see Holland et al for further reading) Many of the these are now computerised.

Key References

Frayn KN. Metabolic regulation. A human perspective. Portland Press, London. 1996.

Frayn KN. Calculation of substrate oxidation rates in vivo from gaseous exchange. J Appl Physiol. 1989;55:628–34.

Hinkle PL, McCarty RE. How cells make ATP. Sci Am. 1978;238:104–23.

Pilkus SJ, El-Maghrahi MR. Hormonal regulation of hepatic gluconeogenesis and glycolysis. Ann Rev Biochem. 1988;57:755–83.

Schofield WN. Predicting basal metabolic rate, new standards and review of previous work. Hum Nutr Clin Nutr. 1985; 39(suppl 1):5–41.

Further Reading

Bender DA. Introduction to nutrition and metabolism. London: UCL Press; 1993.

Burzstein S, Elwyn DH, Askanazi J, Kinney JM. Energy metabolism, indirect calorimetry and nutrition. London: Williams and Wilkins; 1989.

Girardier L, Stock MJ. Mammalian thermogenesis. London: Chapman and Hall; 1983.

Holland B, Welch AA, Unwin ID, Buss DH, Paul AA, Southgate DAT. McCance and Widdowson's the composition of foods, 5th edn. Royal Society of Chemistry and Ministry of Agriculture, Fisheries and Food. 1991.

Kinney JM, ed. Assessment of energy metabolism in health and disease. Columbus: Ross Laboratories; 1981.

Kleiber M. The fire of life; an introduction to animal energetics. Huntington: Robert Kreiger Publishing Company; 1975.

Matthews HR, Freedland RA, Miesfield RL. Biochemistry. A short course. New York: Wiley–Liss; 1997.

Stryer L. Biochemistry, 4th edn. San Francisco: Freeman and Co; 1995.

Wilmore DW. The metabolic management of the critically ill. New York: Plenum Medical Book Company; 1977.

Acknowledgement The author is grateful for the comments of Dr Keith Frayn.

Chapter 63 Endocrinology

H Michael Marsh and David C Leach

Topics covered in this chapter

This chapter outlines the major endocrine syndromes encountered in anesthesiology, emphasizing the theoretic essentials underlying perioperative care. Hormones can be defined as chemical, non-nutrient, intercellular messengers that are effective at micromolar concentrations or less (Chapter 3); their study is endocrinology. Hormones are structurally extremely diverse (Fig. 63.1), ranging in humans from peptides and proteins (the most common), to modified amino acids (tyrosine-based catecholamines and thyroid hormones, tryptophan-based serotonin and indoleacetic acid, and histidine-based histamine) and lipids (steroids, prostaglandins, platelet-activating factor). Hormones can be differentiated into two classes with broadly different properties: hydrophilic or hydrophobic types.

Hydrophilic hormones such as peptides, catecholamines, and amino acids cannot cross cell membranes easily. Therefore, these compounds can be contained within membrane vesicles and stored there after synthesis for quantal release. Typically, they interact with receptors at the target cell surface and require second messengers within the target cell to achieve their effect and to amplify their signal. They are transported free in serum and usually have short half-lives (minutes) for action.

By contrast, *hydrophobic hormones* do not dissolve readily in plasma or intercellular fluid and require transport within hydrophobic pockets of serum transport proteins. This protects these compounds from destructive enzymes and partially serves to prolong their half-lives (hours to days). Their hydrophobicity also allows them to cross cell membranes to intracellular receptors, where they have usually a direct effect without amplification through second messengers. Their receptors are cytoplasmic or nuclear proteins, and their actions may include effects on gene transcription and, consequently, on protein synthesis by the affected target cell.

Hormones coordinate metabolism, growth, and reproduction within the organism. Metabolism includes all processes that handle or alter materials within the organism (e.g. mineral, water, and energy metabolism; see Chapter 62), and growth is defined as enlargement of tissues or organs or retention by the organism of material that results in net enlargement. Hormones also coordinate inflammatory responses (Chapter 52). The local signs of inflammation, calor, rubor, dolor, and tumor, may be accompanied by systemic changes. The mechanisms underlying these changes include release of cytokines. Chemokines, a subset of the cytokines, precisely control the movement and activities of leukocytes. Cytokines affect calorigenesis and overall metabolism and set in train events that may lead to multiple organ dysfunction by creating widespread effects known as the sepsis-related syndrome.

Hormones may also control cell death in tissues. Cell death induced in individual cells is an orderly process known as apoptosis (programmed cell death); the process of cell disintegration and tissue destruction induced by more noxious stimuli is known as tissue necrosis. Apoptosis-signaling mechanisms may also be regarded as hormonal signals, initially determining organ remodeling during development and later controlling the apoptotic engines in cells, allowing healthy cells to proliferate while encouraging damaged cells to kill themselves. Disorder of this apoptotic engine occurs in cancerous cells, permitting unregulated proliferation of cells in some tumors, and is the cause of some cancers. One signaling ligand for apoptotic receptors on cells is Apo2L or tumor necrosis factor-related apoptosis-inducing ligand (TRAIL). Thus apoptosis of tissue cells may be induced, along with inflammation of that tissue.

Neurotransmitters can also be regarded as hormones. Many molecules can function as either neurotransmitters or hormones, for example catecholamines and several of the gastrointestinal hormones. The neural crest is a common site of embryologic origin for cells producing both hormones (e.g. adrenal catecholamines) and neurotransmitters (e.g. sympathetic ganglion neurons). In the hierarchic system that controls the hypothalamic–pituitary–adrenal (HPA) axis, which is the feedback control mechanism for many of the classical hormonal systems, the distinction between the neural and endocrine elements is blurred and this should be considered as a neuroendocrine system. Further, the very close links between the proinflammatory mediator system embodied in the immune mechanism activated by infection or invasion and the anti-inflammatory mediator system, driven by the classical HPA responses set in train by stress, suggest that this whole mechanism should be considered as a neuro-immuno-endocrine system, with much broader relevance to pathogenesis of disease.

Major vertebrate hormones and their characteristics

Hormones	Structure	Mechanism	Source	Target	Action
Calcium metabolism					
Parathormone (PTH)	Peptide	cAMP	Parathyroid gland	Bone, kidney	Bone resorption; renal Ca^{2+} resorption
Calcitonin (CT)	Peptide	cAMP	C cells (thyroid gland)	Bone	Inhibits bone resorption
1,25-Dihydroxycholecalciferol (1,25-DHCC)	Steroid derivative	DNA binding	Skin, liver, kidney	Intestine	Intestinal Ca^{2+} absorption
Tropic hormones					
Adrenocorticotropic hormone (ACTH)	Peptide	cAMP	Adenohypophysis	Adrenal cortex	Stimulates glucocorticoid synthesis and secretion
Luteinizing hormone (LH)/human chorionic gonadotropin (hCG)	Protein	cAMP	Adenohypophysis/ placenta	Gonads	Stimulates progesterone (♀) and testosterone (♂) synthesis and secretion
Follicle-stimulating hormone (FSH)	Protein	cAMP	Adenohypophysis	Gonads	Stimulates estrogen synthesis and secretion (♀) and gamete development
Thyroid-stimulating hormone (TSH)	Protein	cAMP	Adenohypophysis	Thyroid	Stimulates thyroid hormone synthesis and secretion
Melanocyte-stimulating hormone (MSH)	Peptide	cAMP	Hypophysis	Melanocyte	Skin darkening
Sodium and water metabolism					
Antidiuretic hormone (ADH)/ Vasopressinn (VP)	Peptide	cAMP, Ca^{2+}	Neurohypophysis	Kidney, liver	Renal water resorption and glycogenolysis
Aldosterone	Steroid	DNA binding	Adrenal cortex	Kidney	Renal Na^{+} and water resorption
Growth factors					
Insulin-like growth factors	Peptides	Tyrosine kinase	Liver	Multiple	Cellular and body growth
Neurotransmitters					
Norepinephrine (NE)	Tyrosine derivative	cAMP, Ca^{2+}	Central and sympathetic nervous system	Multiple	'Fight-or-flight' response
Dopamine	Tyrosine derivative	cAMP, Ca^{2+}	Hypothalamus, etc.	Adenohypo-physis, etc.	Inhibitor of PRL secretion
Acetylcholine (ACh)	Amine	Na^{+}, Ca^{2+}, cAMP, NO, cGMP	Central and parasympa-thetic nervous system	Muscles, etc.	Maintenance of involuntary activity and muscle contraction/relaxation
γ-Aminobutyric acid (GABA)	Glutamate derivative	Cl^-	CNS	CNS	Inhibitory transmitter
Glycine	Amino acid	Cl^-	Spinal cord	Spinal cord	Inhibitory transmitter
Parahormones					
Prostaglandins	Arachidonic acid derivative	cAMP (some)	Multiple	Multiple	Smooth muscle contraction, inflammation
Thromboxanes	Arachidonic acid derivative	cAMP, Ca^{2+}	Platelets, neutrophils, brain, lung	Smooth muscle, platelets	Smooth muscle contraction, platelet aggregation
Leukotrienes	Arachidonic acid derivative	Ca^{2+}	Platelets, neutrophils, mast cells lung	Multiple	Smooth muscle contraction, inflammation
Opioid peptides	Peptides	K^{+},Ca^{2+}, cAMP	CNS, pituitary, adrenal medulla	CNS	Analgesia, euphoria, sedation
Reproductive hormones					
Estrogens	Steroids	DNA binding	Ovary, placenta	Reproductive tract, etc.	Sexual characteristics
Androgens	Steroids	DNA binding	Testis, adrenal cortex	Reproductive tract, etc.	Sexual characteristics, spermatogenesis
Progesterone	Steroid	DNA binding	Ovary, placenta	Reproductive tract, etc.	Pregnancy maintenance
Prolactin (PRL)	Peptide	Unknown	Adenohypophysis	Mammary gland	Lactation
Oxytocin (OT)	Peptide	Ca^{2+}	Neurohypophysis	Mammary gland, uterus	Milk ejection, parturition
Inhibin/activin	Peptides	Unknown	Gonads	Hypopthalamo-pituitary axis	Inhibition/stimulation of FSH
Energy metabolism					
Growth hormone (GH)/somatotrophin	Peptide	Unknown	Adenohypophysis	Multiple	Lipolysis, glucose sparing, general body growth
Glucocorticoids	Steroids	DNA binding	Adrenal cortex	Muscle, liver	Gluconeogenesis
Thyroid hormones (T_3, T_4)	Tyrosine derivative	DNA binding	Thyroid gland	Multiple	Lipolysis, glycogenolysis
Glucagon	Peptide	cAMP	α Cells (pancreas)	Liver	Glucogenolysis, gluconeogenesis
Epinephrine (E)	Tyrosine derivative	cAMP, Ca^{2+}	Adrenal medulla	Fat, muscle	Lipolysis, glycogenolysis
Insulin	Peptide	Tyrosine kinase, oligo-saccharides	β Cells (pancreas)	Multiple	Lipid, protein, and glycogen synthesis

Figure 63.1 Major vertebrate hormones and their characteristics.

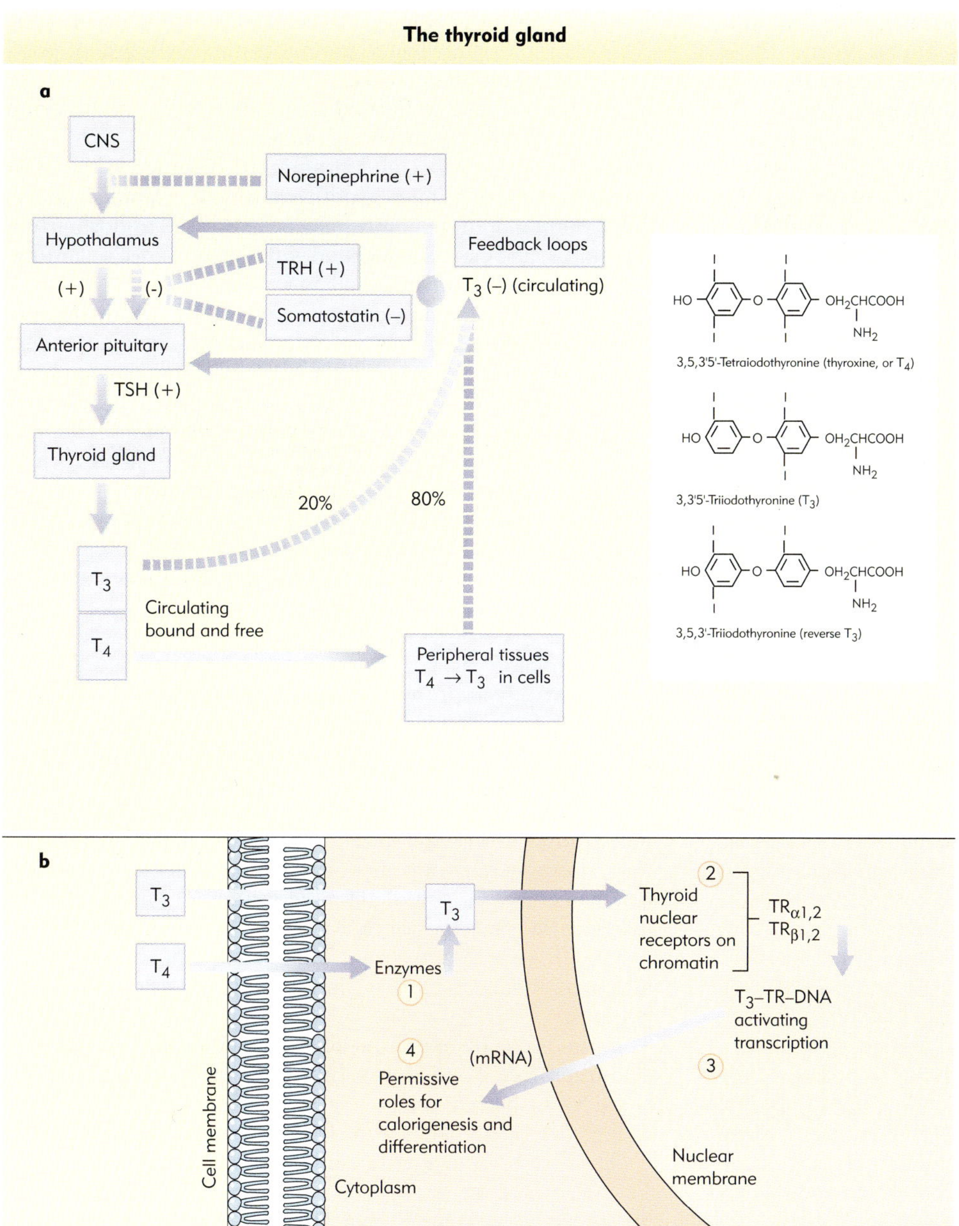

Figure 63.2 The thyroid gland. (a) The hypothalamic–pituitary–thyroid axis: factors controlling release of hormones. (b) Cellular effects of thyroid hormones in four steps. (1) T4 conversion to T3, (2) T3 binds to receptor, (3) transcription now occurs, (4) mRNA yields proteins which have permissive roles.

THYROID

Normal physiology

The normal thyroid gland is situated in the midline of the neck anterior to the trachea and the thyroid cartilage; it is bilobar and H-shaped, with the two lobes joined by an isthmus. It weighs about 25–30g and consists of follicles containing iodothyroglobulin, a 19S, ~660kDa glycoprotein dimer made up of two 330kDa polypeptide monomers. The uniodinated polypeptide chains are synthesized and secreted by follicular cells, which surround the follicular lumen. Each molecule of thyroglobulin contains about 115 tyrosine residues, of which only two to five are usually converted to thyroxine (T_4). Inorganic iodide from the diet is taken up by follicular cells by active transport against a gradient. Of about 50mg of total iodine in the body, 10–15mg is in the thyroid. Thyroglobulin is iodinated in the follicular lumen after it has been secreted by the follicular cell. The follicular cells are surrounded by a sheath of loose connective tissue; this also contains parafollicular C cells, which synthesize and secrete calcitonin. These C cells are involved in medullary thyroid cancers, which may be familial and can be part of the *multiple endocrine neoplasia* (MEN) syndromes.

Secretion of thyroid hormones into the blood is under the control of the hypothalamic–pituitary–thyroid axis (Fig. 63.2). Euthyroidism is maintained by a negative feedback system. Thyrotropin-releasing hormone (TRH) and somatostatin stimulate or inhibit, respectively, release of thyroid-stimulating hormone (TSH) or thyrotropin from the pituitary. Formation of T_4 occurs exclusively in the thyroid gland, whereas triiodothyronine (T_3) is formed in both the thyroid (20%) and in peripheral tissues (80%), which convert T_4 to T_3. TSH stimulates follicular cells to take up iodinated thyroglobulin, hydrolyze it, and secrete T_4 and T_3; mono- and diiodotyrosine are retained for reuse. After secretion into the plasma, T_4 is mostly bound (99.95%) to the transport proteins thyroid-binding globulin (TBG) and transthyretin [also called thyroid-binding prealbumin, (TBPA)], in part covalently; T_3 (99.5% bound) binds only to TBG. Since the bound forms are physiologically inert, T_3 is 10-fold more available than T_4. The elimination half-lives are also affected by the protein binding: T_4 is eliminated slowly with a half-life of 6 to 7 days while T_3, which is less avidly bound, has a half-life of about 1 day. The normal daily secretion of T_4 and T_3 is 70–90 and 15–30mg, respectively. About 40% of T_4 is converted to T_3; 40% is converted to the inactive reverse T_3, and 20% is metabolized in other ways.

Feedback control by thyroid hormones at the pituitary level is remarkably precise. Serum concentrations of TSH are inversely log-linearly related to those of free T_4 in such a manner that minor changes in free T_4 produce marked changes in serum TSH in the opposite direction. This amplification effect on TSH makes it a very sensitive and accurate indicator of thyroid dysfunction. The development in the 1990s of third-generation TSH radioimmunoassay techniques, including use of chemiluminescence for detection, allows TSH determination to sensitivities of 0.01mU/L.

The two major areas of thyroid hormone action on tissues are calorigenesis and growth and development (Fig. 63.2), where it has a critical role particularly in postpartum growth and the development of the brain. Cretinism is a particularly devastating syndrome evident in infants deprived of thyroid hormone throughout the first few months and years of life. Thyroid hormones also directly and indirectly influence cardiac function and interact with the sympathetic nervous system. These effects are mediated through hormone binding to receptors within the cell nucleus. Thyroid hormone receptors belong to the steroid hormone receptor superfamily. The thyroid hormone receptors are 408 amino acid residues in length with a variable N-terminal domain, a DNA-binding domain of about 88 residues, and a 225–285 residue domain for binding to the thyroid hormones. The preferred form for binding appears to be T_3. The thyroid hormone receptor binds to promoter/regulator regions of specific genes. It is bound to its DNA response elements in the absence of hormone and functions as a transcription suppressor. In the presence of T_3 or T_4, the receptor–hormone–DNA response element complex dissociates and activates transcription.

Thyroid dysfunction

The distinction between euthyroid, hyperthyroid, and hypothyroid states depends on testing initiated on the basis of an adequate history and physical examamination. *Thyroid function testing* includes free T_4 or a free T_4 index (FTI) and serum TSH using the newer assays.

Hypothyroidism

Hypothyroidism may present in a variety of ways and is known as a great mimicker. Four patterns of hypothyroidism are seen of which all but the first are disease states:

- subclinical hypothyroidism (free T_4 normal, serum TSH elevated);
- primary thyroid failure (free T_4 low, serum TSH elevated); this is responsible for 95% of cases and is either permanent (as in postablative or primary atrophic states) or reversible (as in iodine deficiency or in the hypothyroid phase of subacute thyroiditis);
- secondary/tertiary failure or central hypothyroidism (free T_4 low, serum TSH low); this is responsible for 5% of cases, as seen in organic hypothalamic–pituitary disease or postpartum pituitary necrosis;
- tissue resistance to thyroid hormone (free T_4 high, serum TSH high); this is rarely encountered.

Hashimoto's thyroiditis, an autoimmune disorder, is the most common cause of primary hypothyroidism. It is familial, affects older women predominantly, may be expressed as postpartum thyroiditis, and can be associated with the presence of antithyroglobulin and antimicrosomal antibodies.

Synthetic T_4 is the drug of choice for treating hypothyroidism. Replacement doses are of the order of 1.5μg/kg body weight, and maintenance doses are of the order of 0.1mg/day. It can be given orally as a once daily medication because of its long half-life. It may also be used to reduce goiter size. Goiter, defined as the presence of an enlarged thyroid gland in the neck, may be present in hypothyroid, euthyroid, and hyperthyroid states. It may be caused by goitrogens or by iodine deficiency (so-called simple goiter), by Hashimoto's thyroiditis, Graves' disease, lymphoma, and Riedel's thyroiditis. Mild hypothyroidism does not contraindicate anesthesia or surgery.

Hyperthyroidism

Hyperthyroidism presents classically with hypermetabolism, low-grade fever, moderate tachycardia, and easy fatiguability, or it can present atypically. Atypically it may have various presentations: cardiac (dysrhythmias, congestive failure or systolic hypertension, high output syndrome), gastrointestinal (hyperdefecation, chronic diarrhea, or mild liver enzyme abnormalities), reproductive (oligomenorrhea or amenorrhea in women or gynecomastia in males), neurologic (myopathy or hypokalemic periodic paralysis), and/or osteoporosis.

Free T_4 or FTI and serum TSH are the most useful tests, although serum T_3 assays may be needed for 10–20% of patients:

- normal free T_4 and serum TSH exclude hyperthyroidism;
- normal free T_4 and low serum TSH may indicate subclinical hyperthyroidism;
- high free T_4 and low serum TSH indicate euthyroid sick syndrome or thyrotoxicosis of any type except that induced by a TSH-producing tumor;
- low free T_4 and low serum TSH indicate the need for a T_3 assay, where high T_3 indicates T_3 toxicosis (seen in about 10–20% of patients) while low T_3 indicates euthyroid sick syndrome or hypothalamic–pituitary disease;
- high free T_4 and serum TSH point to a TSH-producing tumor or to peripheral hormonal resistance, depending on the clinical picture.

Uptake of $^{131}I^-$ is indicated for the differential diagnosis of thyrotoxicosis with diffuse goiter (Graves' disease has a high uptake while silent thyroiditis has a low uptake). The diagnosis of exogenous or ectopic hyperthyroidism (low thyroid gland uptake) and follow-up of differentiated thyroid malignancies may also require [$^{131}I^-$]-uptake scans.

Hyperthyroidism may be treated using drugs or surgery. The useful drugs fall into four categories:

- antithyroid drugs, such as propylthiouracil and methimazole (thiamazole), which directly inhibit thyroid hormone synthesis;
- ionic inhibitors, such as thiocyanate, perchlorate, or lithium, which block iodide transport;
- high concentration of iodine itself, which blocks hormone

release from the gland and decreases synthesis;

- radioactive iodine in doses sufficient to induce radiation damage to the gland and decrease its function.

Adjuvant drugs, such as the β blockers and calcium channel blockers, may be useful to control peripheral manifestations of thyrotoxicosis.

Thyroidectomy may be indicated for the treatment of hyperthyroidism refractory to $^{131}I^-$, for the excision of an enlarged gland causing airway compression or cosmetic discomfort, or for malignancy. Kocher (1841–1917), a surgeon in Switzerland where endemic goiter was prevalent, was the modern pioneer of thyroid surgery, for which he was awarded the Nobel prize in 1909. Kocher observed a high incidence of postoperative hypothyroidism and little tetany, while Billroth of Vienna saw little hypothyroidism but did observe tetany. Halsted from Baltimore saw both of these surgeons operate and commented: 'the explanation probably lies in the operative methods of the two'. Kocher was slow and meticulous, removing all of the thyroid but doing no damage outside its sheath to the parathyroids. Billroth was quicker and left small amounts of thyroid, enough to provide some hormone, while potentially damaging the parathyroids by straying outside the sheath and also damaging their blood supply.

Anesthetic implications

In preparing a patient with thyroid disease for surgery, a euthyroid state is ideal. However, mild or moderate hypothyroidism poses no direct threat, and surgery can usually be performed without fear of major complication. Subclinical hypothyroidism is seen in 8–10% of women and 1–2% of men in the USA. By contrast, hypothyroidism in pregnancy does necessitate treatment, even for this subclinical state, since there is an increased risk for fetal abnormalities in offspring from the hypothyroid parturient. Myxedema or severe overt hypothyroidism, seen in 0.5–1.5% of women and 0.05–0.15% of men, necessitates treatment preoperatively, but the risk of cardiovascular disease exacerbation must be kept in mind. Secondary adrenal insufficiency may also be unmasked.

Hyperthyroidism requires preoperative treatment to avoid potential complications. There are about 400,000 new cases of hyperthyroidism detected in the USA each year, and 5% of pregnant females develop this condition; the prevalence is 1/1000 females and 1/3000 males. In preparing patients with medullary thyroid cancer for surgery, the association with MEN 2 syndromes and the possibility for undiagnosed pheochromocytoma must be considered.

The complications most commonly seen in patients undergoing thyroid surgery include thyroid storm, tetany, recurrent laryngeal nerve damage, postoperative hypoparathyroidism, and cardiac complications, including accelerated coronary artery disease in hypothyroidism and cardiac dysrhythmias or decompensation in hyperthyroidism. Because of the long half-life of T_4, it is not likely that anesthetic agents acutely affect thyroid function. The mechanical effects from thyroid enlargement in proximity to the trachea, with possible tracheomalacia, and the surgical complications of bullous edema or bleeding in the neck with airway narrowing must also be considered.

HYPOTHALAMIC–PITUITARY AXIS

Normal physiology

The diencephalon, the most rostral part of the brainstem, comprises four parts: the epithalamus and pineal, the thalamus, the hypothalamus, and the subthalamus. The hypothalamus lies in the walls and floor of the third ventricle and contains a number of nuclei, which communicate, either directly or indirectly, with the hypophysis or pituitary. Direct communication occurs in the posterior pituitary (neurohypophysis) where axons from the supraoptic and paraventricular nuclei release two nonapeptides, arginine-vasopressin [known simply as vasopressin, as AVP, or as antidiuretic hormone (ADH)] and oxytocin, in this part of the gland. Indirect communication occurs in the anterior pituitary (adenohypophysis) where axons secrete releasing or inhibiting factors into the blood of the hypothalamic–adenohypophyseal portal venous system (Fig. 63.3). These factors are then carried to the gland proper, the anterior pituitary, to act on cells that produce the pituitary hormones.

The pituitary gland is a 0.5–0.7g reddish gray structure attached to the floor of the third ventricle by an infundibular stalk lying just behind the optic chiasm. The pituitary is really two glands fused together, which have different embryonic origin, secrete different classes of hormone, and are regulated very differently. The *anterior pituitary* comprises the anterior lobe, the pars intermedia, and the pars tuberalis; the *posterior pituitary* comprises the supraoptic and paraventricular nuclei of the hypothalamus, their axons, the pituitary stalk, and the posterior lobe of the pituitary gland. Neurohypophyseal functions are discussed in Chapter 55.

The anterior pituitary secretes 10 peptide hormones, contains three stain-distinguishable cell types, and responds to six well-characterized releasing or inhibiting factors that are hormones from the hypothalamus (Fig. 63.1). The hormones of the adenohyphysis can be classified as somatotrophs (growth hormone and prolactin) secreted by acidophils and as glycoprotein hormones [TSH, luteinizing hormone (LH) and follicle-stimulating hormone (FSH)] and the products derived from proopiomelanocortin (POMC) [adrenocorticotropic hormone (ACTH), melanocyte-stimulating hormone (α- and β-MSH), and lipotropic pituitary hormone (β- and γ-LPH)] secreted by basophils. The third cell type, the chromophobe cell, does not secrete known hormones.

Growth hormone (GH) stimulates release of insulin-like growth factors (IGF-1 and IGF-BP3) from liver and other tissues; both GH and the IGF are required for cell differentiation and growth. GH is secreted in bursts under neural control, is entrained during sleep, and is subject to feedback control by IGF-1 and amino and fatty acids. GH-releasing hormone is the dominant hypothalamic control, while somatostatin is an inhibitor of GH secretion. Insulin-induced hypoglycemia induces release of counter-regulatory hormones, including GH. This is the basis for provocative tests sometimes used in children suspected of hypopituitarism. The lack of suppression of GH release from the pituitary by glucose infusion is also useful in diagnosis of acromegaly.

Prolactin (PRL) is a mammotroph and stimulates lactogenesis. It is also under neural control and is sleep entrained. Dopamine is the principal hypothalamic controlling factor and is inhibitory. Prolactin levels increase with pregnancy, stress, estrogens, and suckling.

TSH, LH, and FSH are glycoprotein hormones released under neural control from the hypothalamus when releasing factors (releasing hormones, RH) LH/FSH-RH or TSH-RH are secreted into the portal venous system feeding the anterior pituitary. The tight feedback control for TSH has been described

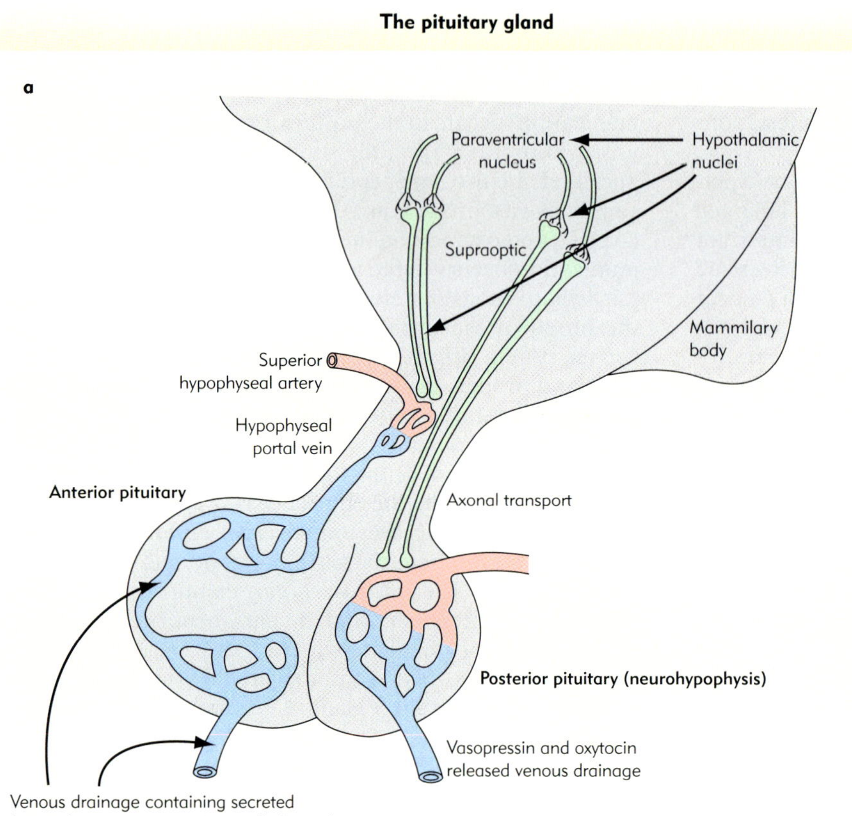

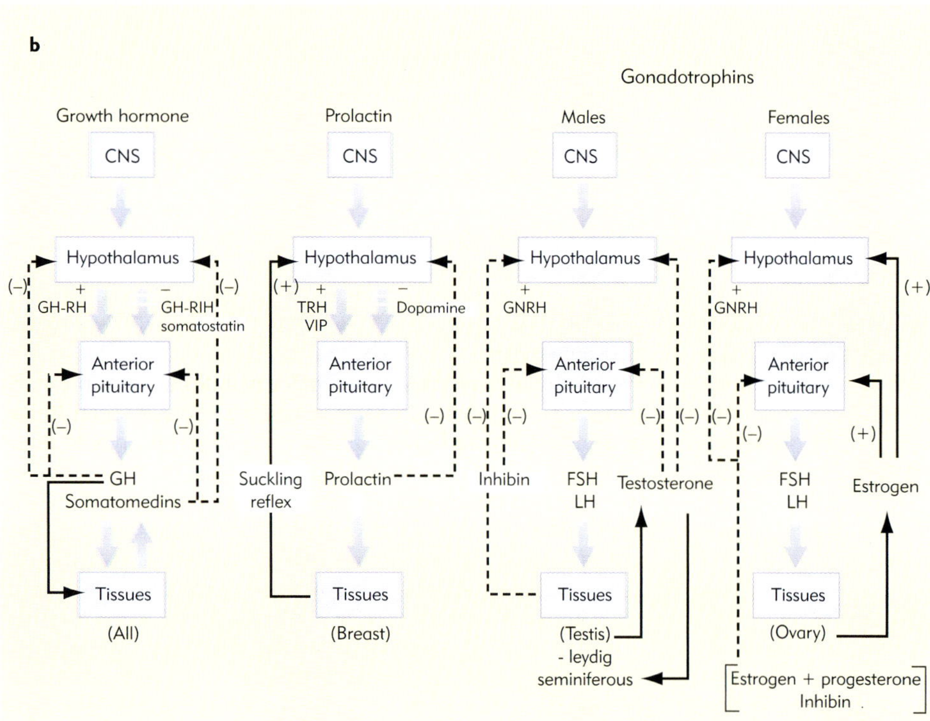

Figure 63.3 The pituitary gland. (a) The hypothalamic–pituitary axis, showing the hypophyseal portal venous system for delivery of releasing factors, and (b) the hypothalamic–pituitary hormone axes.

above (see Fig. 63.2). LH and FSH are gonadotropins responsible for estrogen and androgen secretion from their target organs; they are also subject to feedback effects.

POMC-derived products include ACTH, MSH, and LPH. ACTH will be further discussed below (Fig. 63.4).

Dysfunctional syndromes

Hypothalamic dysfunction

Hypothalamic dysfunction may occur as a result of diseases that disrupt the brain tissue surrounding the third ventricle (e.g. craniopharyngioma, germinoma, metastatic carcinomas);

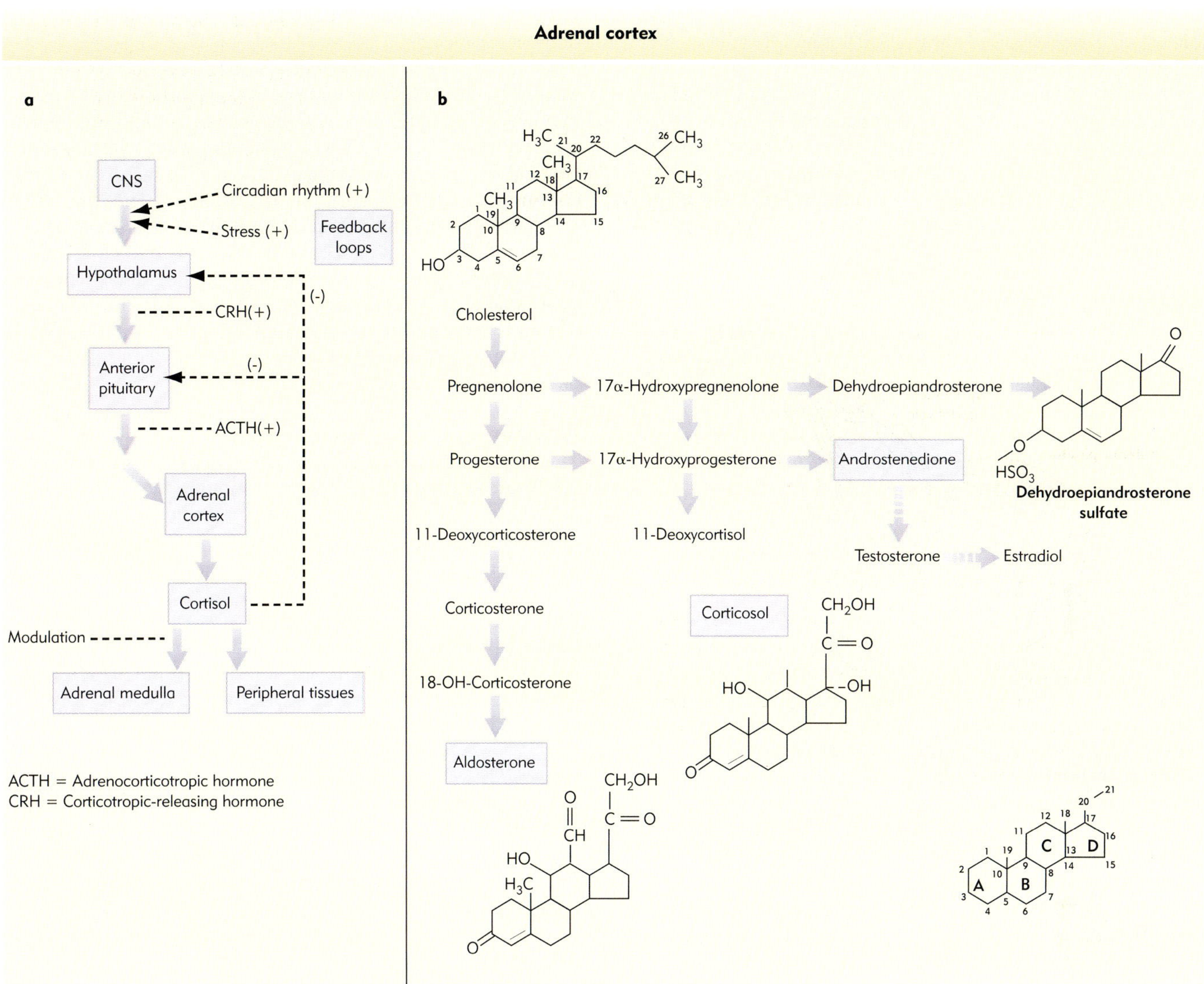

Figure 63.4 The adrenal cortex. (a) Hypothalamic–pituitary–adrenal axis: factors controlling release of hormones. (b) Principal pathways for human adrenal steroid hormone synthesis.

these often present with obstructive hydrocephalus and/or the optic chiasmal syndrome. Dysfunction of the hypothalamus causes vegetative changes, such as thirst, appetite, and temperature dysregulation, and endocrine disorders involving both the anterior and posterior pituitary. Diabetes insipidus, syndrome of inappropriate vasopressin secretion (SIADH), and hypo- or hyperpituitarism may be seen.

Hypopituitarism

Hypopituitarism may manifest as a failure of production of one, more than one, or all of the hormones produced by the pituitary. Failure can occur in any sequence. While usually slow in onset, hypopituitarism can present acutely as acute adrenocortical insufficiency with hypoglycemia and hyponatremia or as sedative or anesthetic sensitivity. Causes of hypopituitarism include primary pituitary disease from trauma, neurosurgery, or radiotherapy; from vascular disease with ischemia or apoplexy; or from neoplasia. Hypopituitarism may also be secondary to hypothalamic disease or associated with extrasellar tumors, cysts, or aneurysms, which destroy the gland or interfere with its blood supply or drainage.

Hyperpituitarism

Hyperpituitarism is most frequently a manifestation of pituitary tumors. These tumors are microadenomas if smaller than 10mm or macroadenomas if over 10mm in diameter; they may be functioning or nonfunctioning. Macroadenomas may be sellar or sellar/extrasellar in extent. They produce prolactin 50% of the time, GH 15%, ACTH 15%, LH/FSH 5%, and αTSH 5%. The remaining 10% of tumors are nonfunctional and may lead to hypopituitarism as they enlarge. Mixed production of two or more hormones is also seen. These tumors may be part of MEN syndrome type 1 (see below).

Diagnosis

Levels of all of the hormones produced by the pituitary (GH, prolactin, LH/FSH, ACTH, and TSH) can be assayed. However, this is not the best strategy for diagnosis under usual circumstances. It is more common to test target organ function (cortisol, T_4 and FTI, testosterone or estradiol) first and then add tests of pituitary function and anatomy (imaging and visual fields) where indicated. Pituitary tumors occur at a rate of 0.2–2.8/100,000 population per year, with a prevalence of 8.9/100,000, and show a 2:1 female preponderance. Releasing-factor analogs (Lupron), inhibitory-factor analogs (octreotide, bromocriptine), replacement therapy (hGH), or replacement of end-target organ functional hormone (cortisol, T_4, estradiol or testosterone) are all viable treatment options. Trans-sphenoidal resection of pituitary tumors is the preferred surgical approach for small tumors. Craniotomy may be preferred for larger tumors but carries a greater risk for optic chiasmal damage.

Anesthetic implications

The major concerns associated with pituitary surgery arise in replacing the hormonal elements that have vegetative function (cortisol and T_4). Diabetes insipidus should be treated with fluid replacement and vasopressin. Corticosteroid replacement or supplementation may also be required for intercurrent surgery where pituitary reserves are compromised. Longer-term thyroid supplements may also be necessary. The mass effect of tumors in this region should also be anticipated. Cerebrospinal fluid rhinorrhea may be seen postoperatively.

ADRENAL

The adrenal glands are situated bilaterally at the upper poles of the kidneys and weigh 5–6g each (3cm × 5cm × <1cm) when healthy. They consist of a cortex and a medulla, each with different embryologic origins. The cortex develops from the mesothelium of the abdominal cavity and envelops the medulla, which originates from the neural crest. During fetal development, each portion of the combined gland has its own blood supply.

Adrenal cortex

Normal physiology

The cortex is divided into three layers: the zona glomerulosa, just under the capsule, from whence arterial blood flows to the cortex; the zona fasciculata, the middle layer; and the zona reticularis, a net-like patterned area innermost, with reticular veins draining into medullary capillaries. This exposes the medulla to high concentrations of adrenocortical steroid hormones; consequently these hormones modulate medullary function, in part regulating epinephrine (adrenaline) synthesis. The zona glomerulosa makes the mineralocorticoid aldosterone exclusively, its cells lacking 17α-hydrolase. The zonae fasciculata and reticularis produce glucocorticoids and androgens (Fig. 63.4). The hydroxylases are P450 enzymes, akin to the hepatic P450 enzymes (Chapter 7), which degrade the hormones produced by the adrenal.

The three major regulatory influences affecting the hypothalamic secretion of corticotropin-releasing hormone (CRH or ACTH-RH), and thus ACTH from the pituitary, are circadian diurnal rhythms, stress, and feedback from free cortisol levels in blood and body fluids (Fig. 63.4). ACTH stimulates the cortex to release its hormonal products. Cortisol, the major free circulating adrenocortical hormone, is a hydrophobic hormone, being a steroid, and, therefore, circulates bound to protein. The bound form accounts for about 98% of circulating cortisol. Only the free form is biologically active. Glucocorticoids play a critical permissive role in intermediary metabolism, are counter-regulatory in relation to insulin, modulate inflammatory and immune responses, and optimize cardiovascular and central nervous system function, while mineralocorticoids allow the kidney to reatain Na^+ and water.

Adrenocortical dysfunction

Adrenal insufficiency

The major clinical features of adrenal insufficiency include weakness, fatiguability, poor appetite, orthostatic hypotension, hypoglycemia, hyponatremia, hyperkalemia, and skin hyperpigmentation. About 25% of patients present with adrenocortical crisis. Autoimmune Addison's disease is the most common cause of adrenal insufficiency in the USA (~1/100,000 population), and about 40% of patients have a history of associated endocrinopathies. Secondary failure is most commonly associated with long-standing steroid therapy, with exogenous suppression of the adrenal. Adrenogenital syndrome is responsible for a small proportion of patients with borderline adrenocortical function who may require attention during surgical stress.

Glucocorticoid excess: Cushing's syndrome

The major clinical features of glucocorticoid excess (Cushing's syndrome) include obesity with cushingoid features such as a 'buffalo' hump; evidence of protein wasting and muscle loss; diabetes mellitus; hypertension, with or without hypokalemia; hyperandrogenicity; psychiatric symptoms; growth failure in children; and a pituitary, ectopic, or adrenal mass lesion. In 90% of patients presenting with Cushing's syndrome, the cause is pituitary tumors (Cushing's disease~7500 cases per year in the USA) and in 10% it is adrenal hyperplasia. However iatrogenic Cushing's syndrome is the most frequent cause of this clinical picture.

Hyperaldosteronism

Hyperaldosteronism, Conn's syndrome (primary hyperaldosteronism) and secondary hyperaldosteronism, lead to hypokalemia, and sodium ion conservation with increased intravascular and extracellular volume and hypertension (Chapter 56).

Treatment

For adrenal dysfunction, ACTH and natural and synthetic steroids are used for replacement therapy; inhibitors of steroid biosynthesis (mitotane, aminoglutethimide, ketoconazole, trilostane, and metyrapone) and antagonists active at the glucocorticoid receptor (mifepristone or RU486) are used for suppression. Cushing's disease and Conn's syndrome are preferentially treated by trans-sphenoidal resection of the pituitary, with a >80% cure rate. Bilateral adrenalectomy may be required.

Anesthetic implications

Surgical stress increases plasma cortisol levels five- to sixfold at 6 hours postoperatively, with return to normal at 24 hours unless stress continues. Patients who have received corticosteroids equivalent to 30mg/day cortisol for longer than 3 weeks may have impairment in this stress response, and steroid supplementation should be considered. All patients with Cushing's syndrome require steroid supplementation postoperatively. Adrenocortical insufficiency is life threatening and necessitates urgent treatment.

Adrenal medulla

The adrenal medulla is a derivative of the neural crest and the sympathetic portion of the autonomic nervous system. The hormones produced by the medulla [epinephrine, dopamine, and norepinephrine (noradrenaline)] are also produced by the central nervous system and their actions are supplemented by sympathetic system effects.

Adrenal medulla dysfunction

Pheochromocytoma is a rare tumor of the chromaffin tissue that involves the adrenal medulla 90% of the time, the remaining 10% being extra-adrenal. Extra-adrenal tumors usually occur in the abdomen but can be in the chest or neck. Most (90%) pheochromocytomas are sporadic, nonfamilial, adrenal, unilateral, and benign.

Familial pheochromocytomas are often part of the *MEN syndrome* type 2A or 2B but may be seen in von Hippel–Lindau disease or with neurofibromatosis (Fig. 63.5). The MEN syndromes have been divided into two major types, 1 and 2. Type 1 is an autosomal dominant disorder affecting the parathyroid glands, endocrine pancreas, and pituitary; it may include carcinoid tumors, adrenal adenomas, and thyroid gland disease plus subcutaneous lipomas. A locus on chromosome 11 for MEN 1 has been identified. Type 2A involves medullary carcinoma of the thyroid gland in 80% of instances, pheochromocytoma in 38%, and hyperparathyroidism in 25%. Type 2B involves medullary carcinoma of the thyroid and pheochromocytoma, together with mucosal neuromas, a marfanoid habitus, and ganglioneuromatosis of the bowel; there are no parathyroid effects. Genetic linkage studies have identified a locus on chromosome 10 that is closely linked to, or identical with, the *ret* proto-oncogene. The gene product Ret is a transmembrane receptor that has a tyrosine kinase domain. Its ligand and function are as yet undefined, but it is likely a growth promoter. The MEN 2 syndromes are also autosomal dominant. Their incidence is of the order 3–30/100,000 population per year.

Diagnosis

Metabolism of the catecholamines (see Fig. 63.5) results in urinary excretion of both free catecholamines and their metabolites, metanephrines and vanillylmandelic acid (VMA). Plasma catecholamine assays are conducted under controlled circumstances, as adjuncts to urinary studies, or as part of a suppression (clonidine) or provocation (glucagon or histamine) test with α-adrenergic blockade.

Anesthetic implications

With pheochromocytoma, medical treatment to reduce perioperative risk is prudent. α-adrenoceptor blockade is the cornerstone of therapy. Blockade of β-adrenoceptors may be necessary to reduce tachydysrhythmia but should only be instituted once satisfactory α-blockade is established to avoid unapposed α-adrenergic effects. Surgical excision of the tumor is usually curative.

PARATHYROIDS: CALCIUM REGULATION

Normal physiology

Calcium homeostasis for the whole organism is regulated in a simple, closed system involving three hormones: *parathormone* from the parathyroid glands, *calcitonin* from theparathyroid oxyphil cells and interfollicular C cells of the thyroid gland, and the active form of vitamin D [*1,25-dihydroxycholecalciferol* (1,25-dihydroxyvitamin D)] produced in the kidneys (Fig. 63.6). These hormones act on three target organs: bones, gut, and kidneys. This system maintains constant free Ca^{2+} levels in blood because of the critical need for this ion by excitable tissues such as nerves and muscle, including cardiac muscle.

The concentration of Ca^{2+} in blood is kept at 8.8–10.4mg/dL (2.2–2.6mmol/L)in three forms: bound, complexed, and free. About 30% of Ca^{2+} is bound to serum albumin, ~10% is complexed with various chelators such as citrate, and ~60% is in the free form ('ionized'). Hypercalcemia depresses electrical activity in tissues, causing muscle weakness, bradycardia, lethargy, and confusion, progressing in severe instances to coma. Hypercalcemia can also lead to ectopic calcification. Hypocalcemia, by contrast, leads to hyperexcitability, producing muscular spasms (tetany), cardiac irritability, psychosis, and seizures.

Bone is the major reservoir for Ca^{2+} in the body (99%), with an additional ~0.9% being bound in intracellular stores in mitochondria and the sarcoplasmic reticulum. Consequently, only approximately 0.1% of total body Ca^{2+} is circulating in blood and distributed in the intercellular fluid. The concentration of free Ca^{2+} in the cytoplasm inside the cell is maintained at a very low level, approximately 100nmol/L. Bone contains Ca^{2+} as an hydroxyapatite salt bound to osteoid, the primary component of which is collagen.

The parathyroid glands, of which there are usually four attached to the posterior surface of the thyroid in the neck and upper anterior mediastinum, are small (3mm × 6mm × 2mm) and richly vascularized. They contain two cell types: chief cells, which have clear cytoplasm and secrete parathormone, and oxyphil cells, which contain oxyphil granules and secrete calcitonin. Parathormone elevates Ca^{2+} levels by promoting the dissolution of the salts in bone, activating osteoclasts, and promoting phosphate and bicarbonate excretion by the kidney while blocking the excretion of Ca^{2+}. The second messenger cAMP acts in this process. Calcitonin is an antagonist of parathormone; it is nonessential and the system can regulate Ca^{2+} quite effectively in its absence.

The kidneys produce 1,25-dihydroxyvitamin D, which acts on the gut inducing a Ca^{2+}-binding protein that is essential for Ca^{2+} absorption and promotes phosphate absorption. The Ca^{2+}-binding protein is a member of the calmodulin family.

These three compounds, parathormone, calcitonin, and 1,25-dihydroxyvitamin D, act through feedback control to maintain constant Ca^{2+} levels in the blood. Low serum Ca^{2+} stimulates parathormone release and inhibits calcitonin. Parathormone releases Ca^{2+} from bone and acts on the kidney to reduce its excretion. The inactive 24,25-dihydroxy derivative of vitamin D is converted to 1,25-dihydroxyvitamin D by 1α-hydroxylase, an enzyme activated by parathormone and hypocalcemia. High serum Ca^{2+} levels create a reverse effect, lowering parathormone levels, releasing calcitonin, and activating a 24-hydroxylase, which inactivates vitamin D. In the gut, Ca^{2+} in the lumen stimulates the release of members of the gastrin family, which stimulate secretion of calcitonin to turn metabolism from bone resorption to gut absorption. This serves to conserve bone.

Calcium is essential for the normal functioning of cells in all body tissues, acting as a regulator for a variety of enzymatic, contractile, secretory, and signaling functions (see Fig. 63.6). It exerts complex, discrete effects on microenvironments within the cell through very localized changes in concentration. Intracellular Ca^{2+} concentrations are tightly regulated by uptake and release from intracellular stores in the endoplasmic reticulum and mitochondria, by operation of cell membrane pumps (Ca^{2+} ATPase), transporters (Na^+/Ca^{2+}

Figure 63.5 The adrenal medulla. (a) Metabolic pathways for catecholamines and (b) disease patterns in multiple endocrine neoplasiae.

Adrenal medulla

a

Phenylalanine → **Tyrosine** (HO–C_6H_4–$CH_2CH(NH_2)$-COOH)

Tyrosine hydroxylase → **Dopa** (HO, HO – $CH_2CH(NH_2)$-COOH)

Aromatic amino acid decarboxylase → **Dopamine** (HO, HO – $CH_2CH_2NH_2$)

Dopamine → Catecholamine O-methyl transferase (COMT) → **Homovanillic acid (HVA)** (CH_3O, HO – CH_2COOH)

Dopamine β-hydroxylase → **Norepinephrine** (HO, HO – $CH(OH)CH_2NH_2$)

Norepinephrine → *N*-Methyl transferase → **Epinephrine** (HO, HO – $CH(OH)$-CH_2NHCH_3)

Norepinephrine → COMT → **Normetanephrine** (CH_3O, HO – $CH(OH)CH_2NH_2$)

Norepinephrine → Monoamine oxidase (MAO) → **3,4-Dihydroxymandelic acid** (HO, HO – $CH(OH)COOH$)

Epinephrine → MAO → **3,4-Dihydroxymandelic acid**

Epinephrine → COMT → **Metanephrine** (HO, HO – $CH(OH)NHCH_3$)

Normetanephrine → MAO; 3,4-Dihydroxymandelic acid → COMT; Metanephrine → MAO → **Vanillylmandelic acid (VMA)** (CH_3O, HO – C(OH)-COOH)

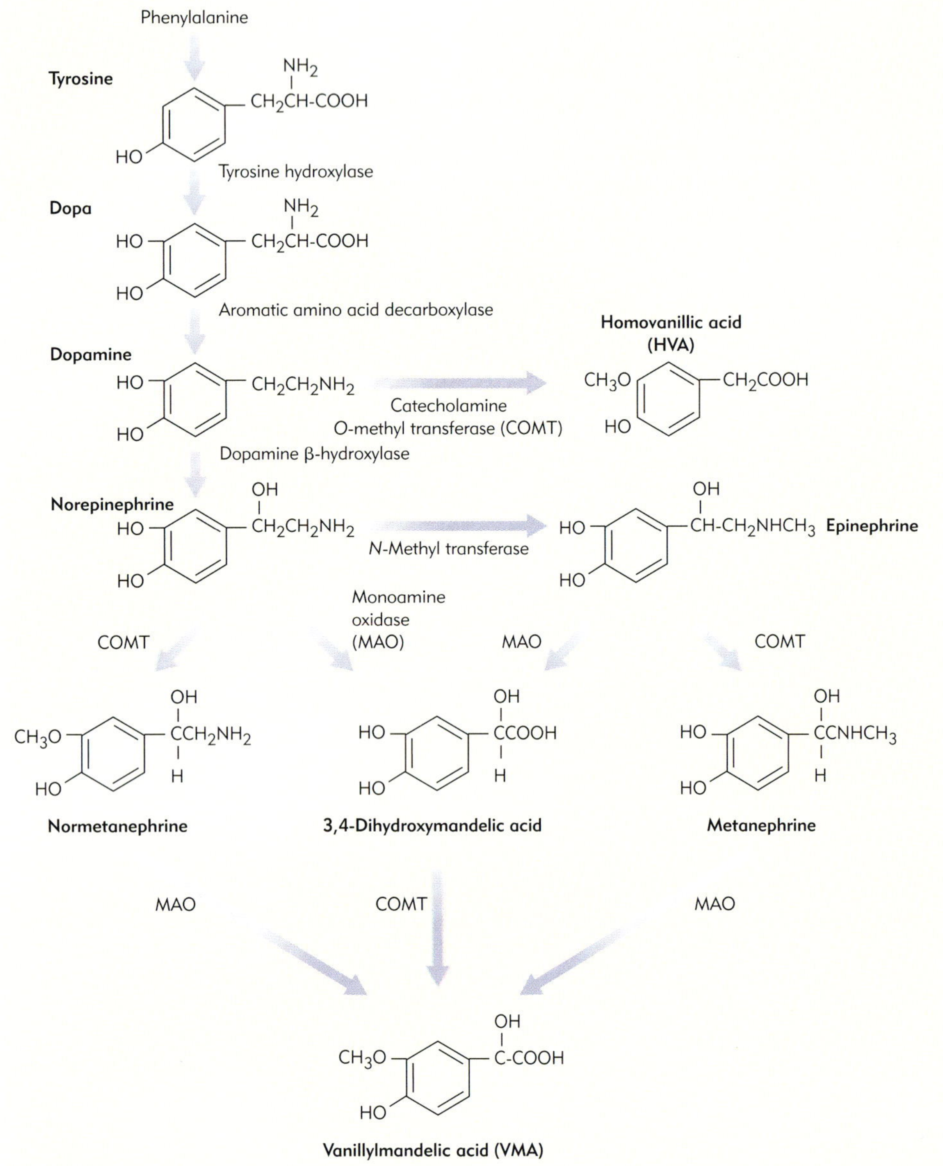

b

MEN type 1 (Wermer's)	MEN type 2	Mixed syndromes
Autosomal dominant Parathyroid (hyperplasia or adenoma) Pancreatic islet cell (hyperplasia, adenomas, or carcinoma) Pituitary (hyperplasia or adenoma) Rare: carcinoid, pheochromocytoma, lipomas	**2A (Sipple's)** Parathyroid (hyperplasia, adenoma) Thyroid medullary carcinoma (MTC) Pheochromocytoma (Occasionally cutaneous lichen amyloidosis) **Familial MTC** **2B (Mucosal neuroma syndrome)** MTC Pheochromocytoma Mucosal and gastrointestinal neuromas Marfanoid habitus	Familial pheochromocytoma or islet cell tumors Von Hippel–Lindau Neurofibromatosis and MEN 1 or 2 features Myoxoma, pigmentation, and generalized endocrine overactivity in one family

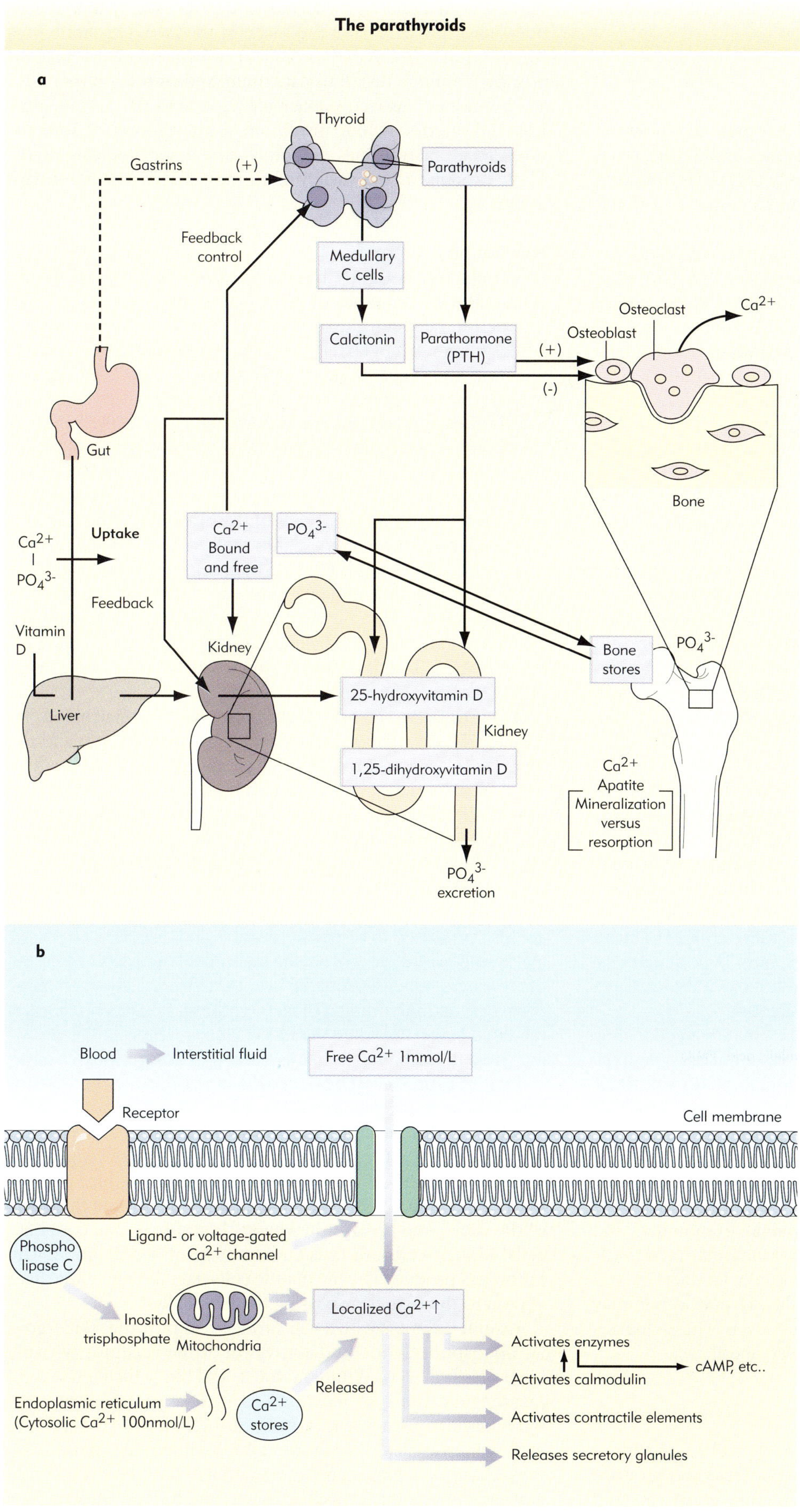

Figure 63.6 The parathyroids. (a) Calcium control mechanisms and (b) the role of calcium in the cell.

exchanger), and ligand- [*N*-methyl-D-asparate (NMDA) receptor] or voltage-gated Ca^{2+} channels.

Dysfunctional states

Hypercalcemia

Hypercalcemia may be asymptomatic or may present as polyuria and polydipsia or with renal problems (stones, renal colic, renal failure). Neuropsychiatric symptoms may also occur, ranging from fatigue, weakness, and confusion to coma. Anorexia, nausea, vomiting, peptic ulceration, and pancreatitis also occur, as does metastatic calcification with band keratopathy, and cardiovascular effects including hypertension, short Q–T interval on the electrocardiogram, and dysrhythmias. Causes can be parathyroid dependent (e.g. hyperparathyroidism, familial benign hypercalciuric hypercalcemia, and drug-induced hypercalcemia with thiazides and lithium) or parathyroid independent (e.g. malignancy, other endocrine disorders as in hyperthyroidism and Addison's disease, immobilization with Paget's disease, hypervitaminosis D, and milk-alkali syndrome).

Specific treatment of the cause is the mainstay of therapy; for example, resection of parathyroid adenomas or control of thyrotoxicosis. Glucocorticoids may be useful for those conditions with excess vitamin D (malignancy, granulomatous disease such as sarcoid, exogenous vitamin D). Nonspecific therapy to decrease bone resorption and to increase Ca^{2+} excretion may also be needed. Rehydration and furosemide (frusemide)-induced diuresis, calcitonin, bisphosphonates [e.g. pamidronate, plicamycin (mithramycin), gallium nitrate] to inhibit osteoclastic activity, and intravenously administered phosphate buffer all lower serum Ca^{2+} levels. Dialysis is reserved for patients with renal failure.

Hypocalcemia

Hypocalcemia may present acutely with profound symptoms at modest levels of deficit or it may be asymptomatic. The cardinal sign is tetany (positive Chvostek's and Trousseau's signs), with possible carpopedal spasms, laryngeal stridor, convulsions, a prolonged Q–T interval, and cardiac dysrhythmias. Causes include hypoparathyroidism, pseudohypoparathyroidism (an inherited disorder with end-organ resistance to PTH action caused by PTH receptor mutations), vitamin D deficiency or resistance, phosphate excess, increased bone avidity for Ca^{2+} (osteoblastic metastases), or acute pancreatitis.

In acute hypocalcemia, intravenous Ca^{2+} may be needed. For chronic therapy, Ca^{2+} taken orally and vitamin D supplementation is needed. Osteoporosis and osteomalacia do not affect Ca^{2+} homeostasis.

Anesthetic implications

The primary risk in anesthetizing patients with either hypo- or hypercalcemia is cardiac dysrhythmias. Hypercalcemia decreases the refractory period, increases ventricular excitability, and enhances digitalis action. Maternal hypercalcemia may profoundly affect fetal and newborn Ca^{2+} levels, usually leading to fetal hypocalcemia and increased fetal mortality. Hypocalcemia may also be accompanied by alteration in Mg^{2+} levels. These changes should be corrected before proceeding with anesthesia.

PANCREAS: DIABETES MELLITUS

The endocrine pancreas comprises the islets of Langerhans. Pancreatic islet cells make up 1% of the pancreas and produce several peptide hormones including insulin, glucagon, and somatostatin. Pancreatic islet cells are part of the system of peptide-secreting cells from the foregut, the APUD (amine precursor uptake and decarboxylation) cell system, which take up precursor amines, decarboxylate them, and secrete polypeptides and hormones [vasoactive intestinal peptide (VIP), gastrin, etc.]. Islet cell tumors include insulinomas, glucagonomas, somatostatinomas, gastrinomas, VIPomas, and associated carcinoids. These produce a wide variety of hormones each associated with unique syndromes.

Normal physiology

Blood glucose is tightly regulated normally between 70 and 100mg/dL (4.0–5.5mmol/L) in the postabsorptive state through interaction between the liver (which stores and then releases glucose from glycogen), the glucose-utilizing tissues (including brain, muscle, and other active tissue), and fat cells (which convert excess glucose to fat for storage). Hepatocyte surface membranes appear to be freely permeable to glucose, whereas cells from extrahepatic tissues are relatively impermeable to glucose and depend on insulin to stimulate uptake. Insulin stimulates the movement of glucose-transport proteins (GLUT) across cell membranes and cells of the blood–brain barrier; this increases transport of glucose into the cerebral spinal fluid and brain extracellular fluid. The rate of uptake or output of glucose by the liver is mainly dependent on the activity of rate-limiting enzymes such as the hexokinase isozymes, while in nonhepatic cells, it is controlled by membrane permeability and regulation of GLUT activity. Insulin also leads to increased activity of hepatic glycogen synthase.

Three states are relevant to the hormonal control of blood glucose levels: the postabsorptive state, the fasted state, and the immediate response to a glucose meal. In the postabsorptive state, blood glucose is maintained by the opposing actions of insulin and glucagon, insulin being secreted when glucose rises and glucagon when it falls. Other counter-regulatory hormones are produced by the pituitary (ACTH and GH) and the adrenal cortex (cortisol) and medulla (epinephrine and norepinephrine). These counter-regulatory hormones show circadian rhythms and are also produced in response to stress and exercise. After fasting, glucagon is released from the mantle cells and acts to increase the release of glucose from the liver by activating glycogen phosphorylase and inhibiting glycogen synthase. Glucagon release is inhibited by insulin when the blood glucose levels in the inflowing blood to the pancreas rise as a result of absorption of a meal.

Insulin is produced by beta cells in the core of the islets of Langerhans in the pancreas (Fig. 63.7). These cells constitute 60–80% of all cells in the islets. The other three cell types are the alpha cells, which produce glucagon, the delta cells, which produce somatostatin, and the F cells, which produce pancreatic polypeptide. These cells lie in the mantle around the edges of the islets, and receive the venous blood from the core beta cells. Mantle cells are thus bathed by insulin-rich blood. The hormones produced by the mantle cells pass directly to the liver and on to the tissues, bypassing the beta cells.

Insulin interacts with a cell surface receptor that undergoes autophosphorylation and activation of the receptor tyrosine kinase (Chapter 3). Within minutes, and likely through second messengers, there is activation of hexose metabolism, with upregulation of glucose transport through exocytosis of GLUT-containing vesicles, alterations in intracellular enzymatic activities, changes in gene expression, and activation of hexokinase and glycogen synthase. Insulin, IGF-1, and IGF-BP3 also induce

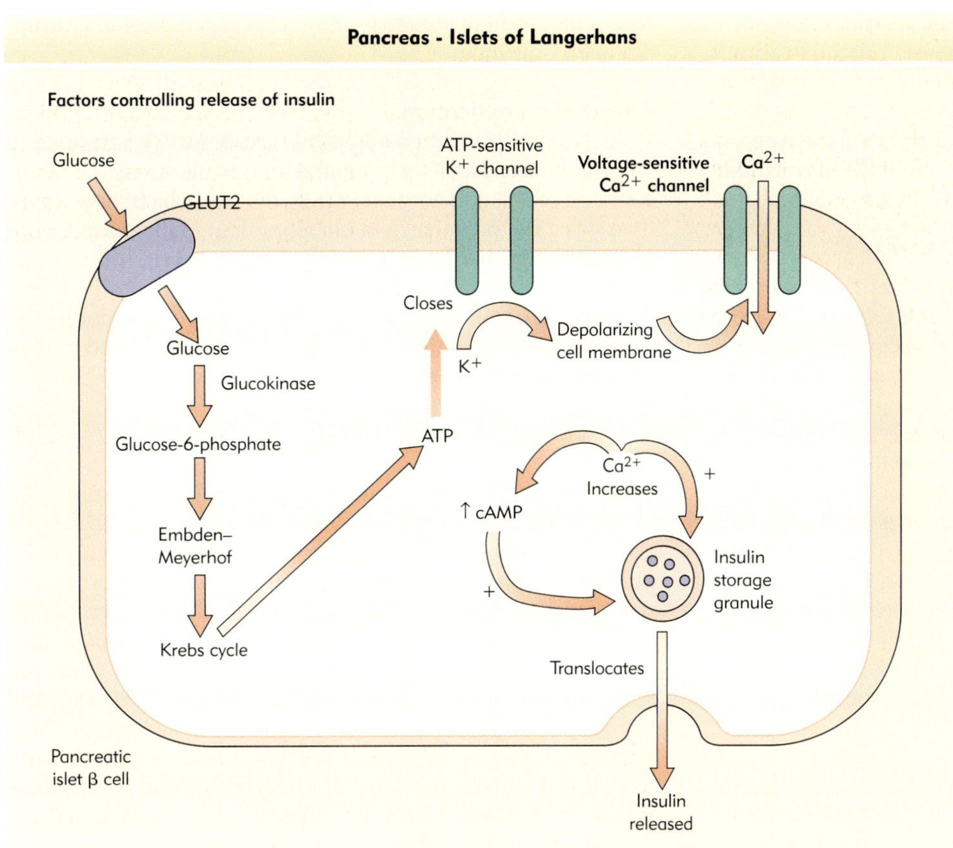

Figure 63.7 Factors controlling the release of insulin from pancreatic islet cells.

cell growth, with induction of DNA, RNA, protein, and lipid synthesis. Finally, insulin-induced downregulation and internalization of insulin receptors occurs.

Dysfunctional states

Hyperglycemic states

Diabetes mellitus is a common disease, afflicting about 6% of the population of the USA, with half of these being undiagnosed. Age, gender, and race affect the prevalence and incidence: 11% of the population aged 65–74 years are affected; the gender ratio (female/male) is 55/45, and 50% of Pima Indians from Arizona are afflicted. The incidence in the USA is about 240/100,000 per annum, or just over 500,000 new cases each year. In addition, there are about 22 million of that population who have prediabetes, as revealed through impaired glucose tolerance. Diabetes mellitus is a set of syndromes characterized by hyperglycemia and caused by disease states involving the glucose regulatory and counter-regulatory mechanisms. Diabetes mellitus is usually defined as a metabolic disease characterized by an absolute or relative lack of insulin from the pancreas. There are two major types of diabetes mellitus, type I and II.

Type I diabetes, also called ketotic, juvenile, or insulin-dependent diabetes mellitus (IDDM), is characterized by absolute insulin deficiency caused by islet cell destruction. It usually has an abrupt onset, occurs at age less than 20 years, shows a 50% concordance in twins, and is responsible for 10–20% of diabetes. The risk for developing type I diabetes is roughly 1/500. The pathogenesis of type I diabetes is partly genetic, with links to HLA determinants on chromosome 6, partly environmental, being initiated by viral or inflammatory triggers, and partly autoimmune, with concomitant antibodies directed at beta cell components.

Type II diabetes, so-called nonketotic, adult-onset, or non-insulin-dependent diabetes mellitus (NIDDM), is characterized by insulin resistance occurring usually at a postreceptor site, particularly in activation of glycogen synthase. This type has a slow insidious onset passing through three phases: hyperinsulinemic normal glucose tolerance, hyperinsulinemic impaired glucose tolerance, and frank diabetes. The hyperinsulinemic state is a condition in which the mitogenic activity of insulin may induce microvascular changes, with deterioration of organ function in target sites such as the eye, kidney, and heart. Syndrome X is seen with insulin resistance, dyslipidemia, hypertension, central obesity, and accelerated atherosclerosis. Coronary artery disease is responsible for about 55% of deaths in diabetics, with diabetes mellitus being the sixth leading cause of death in the USA.

Secondary diabetes is seen with certain endocrine syndromes, stress, pregnancy, and some infections. Destructive surgery or pancreatic disease may also cause secondary disease.

Diagnosis

A diagnosis of diabetes mellitus is made if fasting blood glucose values are greater than 126mg/dL (7mmol/L) on two separate occasions. The main value of an oral glucose tolerance test is to confirm the presence of diabetes when the fasting values are borderline [115–126mg/dL (6.4–7.0mmol/L)]. Blood glucose values over 200mg/dL (11mmol/L) at 2 hours postingestion with one other value between 30 and 60 minutes also exceeding this value are diagnostic. A 2-hour value less than 126mg/dL effectively rules out the diagnosis.

Replacement therapy with insulin is the treatment of choice for IDDM, which usually has an abrupt onset related to abrupt severe insulin deficiency. NIDDM usually has an insidious onset, with episodes of recurrent infection, or evidence of chronic diabetic complications. Restoration of euglycemia should be the goal of therapy, which for NIDDM may include diet, exercise, oral sulfonylureas, biguanides, or insulin.

Diabetic control

The extent to which metabolism in a patient varies from that in a normal healthy subject is assessed by measurement of glucose levels in the blood or urine at defined times, by estimation of ketones in blood or urine, and by estimation of glycated proteins in the patient (e.g. hemoglobin A_{1c} or fructosamine assays). Glycated hemoglobins measure integrated glycemic control over the preceding 2–3 months, with extra weighting toward the immediately preceding month. There are a number of hemoglobins formed by post-translational modification of globin chains, with slow nonenzymatic glycosylation of amino acid residues in the affected chain. Hemoglobin A_{1c} is the largest component (60–80%). Serum proteins are also glycosylated and these are measured using the fructosamine assay. This assay represents glycemic control over a period of 2–3 weeks. Ketones indicate acute insulin deficiency with potential for ketoacidosis.

Hypoglycemic states

Hypoglycemia may arise from a number of causes; these can be classified as either postprandial, caused by excessive insulin secretion following prandial plasma glucose increases (rapid gastric emptying), or reactive, occurring as fasting hypoglycemia. Fasting hypoglycemia may be caused by insulinoma, exogenous insulin, hypopituitarism, cortisol deficiency, alcohol, other drugs or poisons (β blockers, salicylate overdose, hepatotoxins), or hepatic disease.

Measurement of an elevated C-peptide level with elevated insulin levels may confirm the presence of an insulinoma, or recent ingestion of sulfonylureas. Surgery is indicated if insulinoma is confirmed.

Anesthetic implications

Diabetes mellitus is considered a risk factor for surgery and anesthesia because of the potential for complications. The most common problem is coronary artery disease, which shows more than twice the prevalence in diabetics than in the normal population. Congestive heart failure is also prevalent in the diabetic population (males show twice and females five times the risk in the general population). Oculopathy, kidney dysfunction, diabetic neuropathy, both peripheral and autonomic, and gastroparesis with aspiration potential may also occur.

INFLAMMATION AND THE STRESS RESPONSE

Trauma and stress induce diffuse changes in limbic function, expressed in alterations in autonomic nervous system activity and in hormonal secretions controlled by the hypothalamic–pituitary axis. The exact sequence and extent of release of inflammatory mediators in response to tissue damage or infection is being clarified; however, the part these factors play as hormonal determinants of organ function in response to the stress of trauma and infection remains poorly defined. The local expression of inflammation in response to tissue disruption or invasion and the systemic response to trauma and stress is controlled by complex feedback interactions. These interactions include those between neural elements (the locus coeruleus and neurons releasing norepinephrine and CRH), endocrine elements (HPA axis), and immune-mediated inflammatory elements, particularly expressed through the circulating defense system humoral mediators (tumor necrosis factor α and the interleukins). They affect energy metabolism and biochemical homeostasis, electrolyte and fluid metabolism, vascular permeability, and cardiopulmonary function. These responses are discussed in detail in Chapter 69.

Key References

Brown EM. Extracellular Ca^{2+} sensing, regulation of parathyroid cell function, and role of Ca^{2+} and other ions as extracellular first messengers. Physiol Rev. 1991;71:371–411.

Chrousos GP. The hypothalamic–pituitary–adrenal axis and immune-mediated inflammation. N Engl J Med. 1995;332:1351–62.

Edelman SV. Type II diabetes mellitus. Adv Int Med. 1998;43:449–500.

Gifford RW, Manger WM, Bravo EL. Pheochromocytoma. Endocrinol Metab Clin North Am. 1994;23:387–404.

Lazar MA. Thyroid hormone receptors: multiple forms, multiple possibilities. Endocrinol Rev 1993;14:184–93.

Reichlin S. Neuroendocrine–immune interactions. N Engl J Med. 1993;329:1246–53.

Further Reading

Kahn CR. New concepts in the pathogenesis of diabetes mellitus. Adv Int Med. 1996;41:285–321.

Luster A.D.Chemokines – chemotactic cytokines that mediate inflammation. N Engl J Med. 1998;338:436–45.

Oelkers W. Adrenal insufficiency. N Engl J Med. 1996;335:1206–12.

Orth DN. Cushing's syndrome. N Engl J Med. 1995;332:791–803.

Petti GHJ. Hyperparathyroidism. Otolaryngol Clin North Am. 1990;23:339–55.

Vance ML. Hypopituitarism. N Engl J Med. 1994;330:1651–62.

Chapter 64 Thermoregulation

Steven M Frank

Topics covered in this chapter

Thermoregulation
Heat balance
Measurement of body temperature
Effects of anesthetics on thermoregulation
Benefits of hypothermia
Consequences of hypothermia
Hyperthermia

Normally, body temperature is maintained within a very narrow range by an integrated thermoregulatory system that is centered in the hypothalamus. This system is impaired by virtually all anesthetics, which creates a state of poikilothermia wherein body temperature tends to equilibrate with ambient temperature. At typical operating room temperatures [16–21°C (60.8–69.8°F)], hypothermia occurs in >50% of patients when no measures are taken to maintain body temperature. In contrast, malignant hyperthermia (MH) is a rare syndrome triggered by specific anesthetic drugs, and may lead to fatal outcomes in the absence of prompt diagnosis and treatment. Thus, alterations in body temperature at either end of the spectrum (hypo- or hyperthermia) are associated with morbid outcomes. Consequently, body temperature must be routinely monitored and controlled. In this chapter the mechanisms of thermoregulatory control, the effects of anesthetics on thermoregulation, and the consequences and treatment of alterations in body temperature are examined.

THERMOREGULATION

The three general components of the thermoregulatory system are (Fig. 64.1):

- afferent input of thermal information;
- central processing of this information; and
- efferent responses that control heat loss and production.

Thermoreceptors are found in the hypothalamus, other parts of the brain and spinal cord, deep visceral tissues, and the skin surface. The relative contribution of information to the central thermoregulatory system is 80% from the core and deep body tissues and 20% from the skin surface. In the preoptic area of the anterior hypothalamus, this information is integrated and compared with an internal set-point temperature analogous to the setting on a thermostat. When body temperature is above or below this set point, the first response to correct body temperature is a behavioral one that involves changing the ambient temperature to which the person is exposed, or altering clothing to

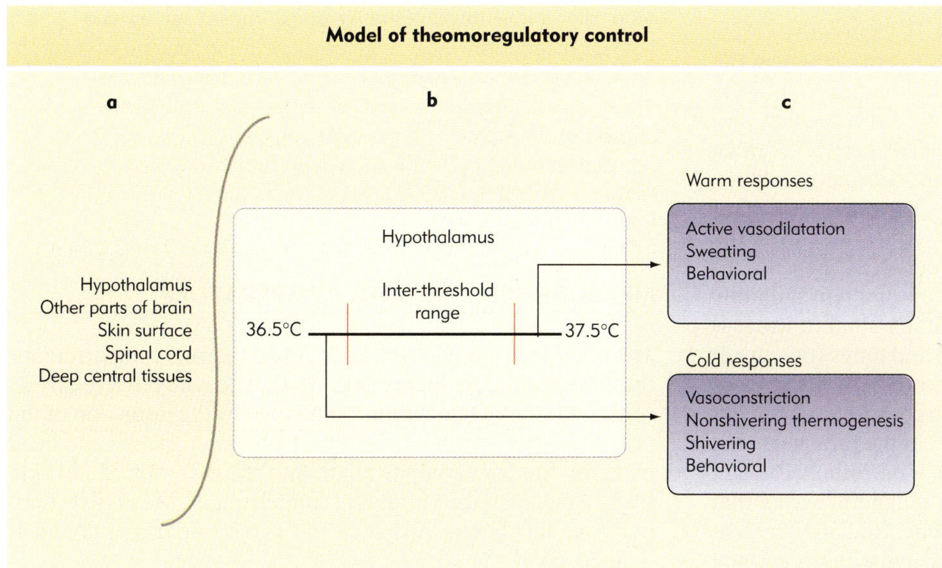

Figure 64.1 A model of thermoregulatory control. The three components of the thermoregulatory system are (a) afferent temperature input, (b) central processing of this information, and (c) the efferent responses that control heat balance. Afferent thermal information is derived from tissues throughout the body, including the brain, skin surface, spinal cord, and deep tissues. Central processing occurs in the preoptic area of the hypothalamus. A mean body temperature below or above the set point initiates the efferent cold or warm responses respectively. (Modified with permission from Sessler DI. Temperature monitoring. In: Miller RD, ed. Anesthesia, 3rd edn. New York: Churchill Livingstone; 1990:315–37.)

optimize heat balance. When behavioral thermoregulation is inadequate, and temperature exceeds the set point, vasodilatation and sweating are triggered to release heat. When temperature is below the set point, vasoconstriction is triggered to conserve heat, and shivering and nonshivering thermogenesis are triggered to produce heat. Nonshivering thermogenesis is not thought to occur in adult humans, but contributes significantly to heat production in neonates.

Efferent thermoregulatory responses are characterized by three concepts – threshold, gain, and maximum intensity. Threshold is the core temperature at which the response is triggered. The interthreshold range is the range of core temperatures over which no thermoregulatory responses occur. The difference between sweating and vasoconstriction thresholds is normally about 0.2°C (0.36°F) in adult humans. Gain is the change in response intensity for a given change in body temperature. Maximum intensity of a response is the highest value that occurs under maximal thermal stress.

HEAT BALANCE

Basal metabolic energy appears as heat at the rate of 1kcal/kg per hour. If all this heat were to be retained, body temperature would increase at the rate of 1°C/h (1.8°F/h). The liver, heart, and skeletal muscle are major heat generators, whereas skin and respiratory mucosal surfaces provide opportunities for heat dissipation. Muscle tension (tone) alone, in the absence of shivering, generates additional heat.

Approximately 12,600kJ (3000kcal) of heat are lost per day by the average adult male, most of which is dissipated through the skin and respiratory mucosa. Cutaneous blood flow is specifically regulated by the opening and closing of arteriovenous (AV) shunts to serve as a heat exchanger (Fig. 64.2). In some areas, blood flow through AV shunts can be altered 10,000 fold by changes in vasomotor tone. Regulation of flow is determined by peripheral sympathetic nerve activity and norepinephrine (noradrenaline)-mediated vasoconstriction. Thermoregulatory vasoconstriction is mediated by α_1-adrenergic receptors and can be blocked by α_1-antagonists. α_1-Antagonists, however, have no effect on shivering or metabolic heat production in response to cold challenge.

The four mechanisms of heat loss are convection, conduction, evaporation, and radiation (Fig. 64.3). Convective transfer, which accounts for 15% of total heat loss, occurs by the moving air. Heat loss is proportional to the square root of the air velocity. Conductive heat loss occurs by direct contact with a cooler material, such as the cold mattress of a stretcher or by intravenous (IV) infusion of cold solutions. Normally, only 3% of total heat loss is through conduction. Conversion of 1ml of water from a liquid into a vapor state (evaporation) from the skin or respiratory tract permits dissipation of 2.4kJ (0.58kcal) of energy. Evaporation is facilitated by low ambient humidity and hindered in humid atmospheres. Nearly 30ml of water is lost each hour from the skin (two thirds) and lungs (one third) at room temperature, which accounts for 67.2kJ (16kcal) of energy. Radiation of heat through the skin constitutes the major mechanism of heat loss, and reaches 60% of the total heat loss, or about 210kPa (50kcal/h) when a person is unclothed. Radiant heat transfer occurs by infrared electromagnetic waves that travel from a warmer object to a cooler one. Radiant heat loss increases with the temperature differential and with the amount of exposed surface.

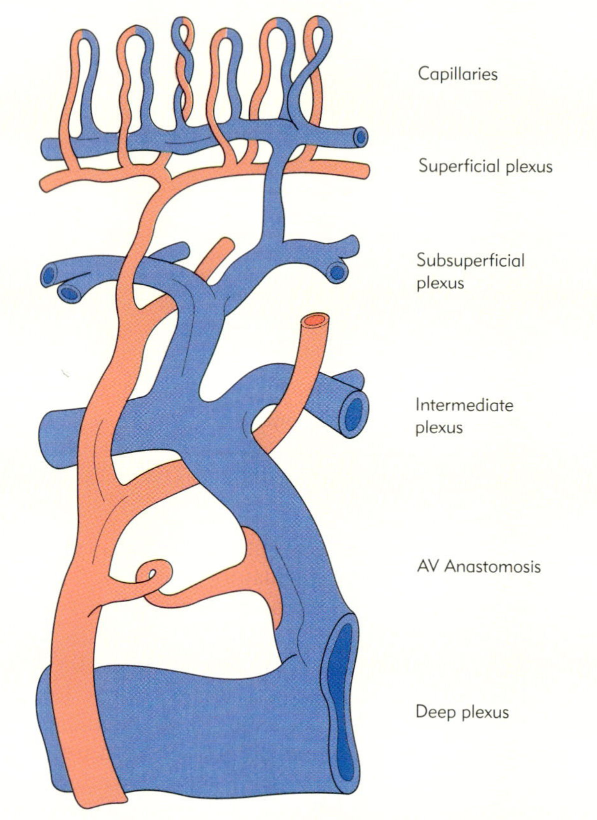

Figure 64.2 Anatomy of the cutaneous circulation. A special feature of the cutaneous vasculature is the presence of AV anastomoses, which are most numerous in the palmar surfaces of the hands and feet, but are also present in the nose and ears. The AV anastomoses are coiled vessels with thick, muscular, highly innervated walls that connect the arterioles and venules in the dermis. Under steady-state conditions, most heat exchange occurs in the terminal capillary loops that are closest to the external environment and have the greatest surface-to-volume ratio. Blood flow through the AV anastomoses serves as a backup mechanism when capillary flow is inadequate to control heat exchange. Although their surface area is small, AV anastomoses can dramatically alter flow and thus heat exchange. (Adapted with permission from Conrad MC. Functional anatomy of the circulation to the lower extremities. Chicago: Year Book; 1971).

MEASUREMENT OF BODY TEMPERATURE

The body can be modeled simply as two thermal compartments, the core and the periphery (Fig. 64.4). The core has a relatively constant internal temperature protected by the insulation of the peripheral compartment. The chest, abdomen, pelvis, and head make up the core compartment, and the extremities and skin surface make up the peripheral compartment. Mean body temperature lies between that of the two compartments and is defined as:

$$(0.66 \times \text{CT}) + (0.34 \times \text{mean skin surface temperature}).$$

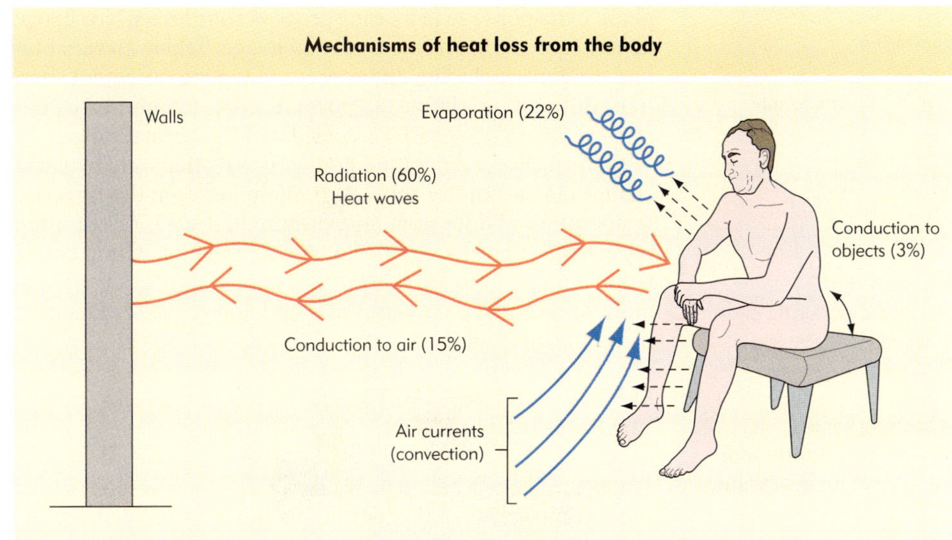

Figure 64.3 Mechanisms of heat loss from the body. The majority of heat is lost by radiation in the form of infrared heat waves, which occurs when the surrounding ambient temperature is less than the body temperature. Heat loss by evaporation occurs from the skin, lungs, and (in the surgical patient) open wounds. Convection is merely radiation heat loss that is increased by air currents. Conduction through physical contact with objects results in little heat loss. (Adapted with permission from Guyton AC. Metabolism and temperature regulation. In: Textbook of physiology, 9th edn. Philadelphia: WB Saunders; 1991:849–60).

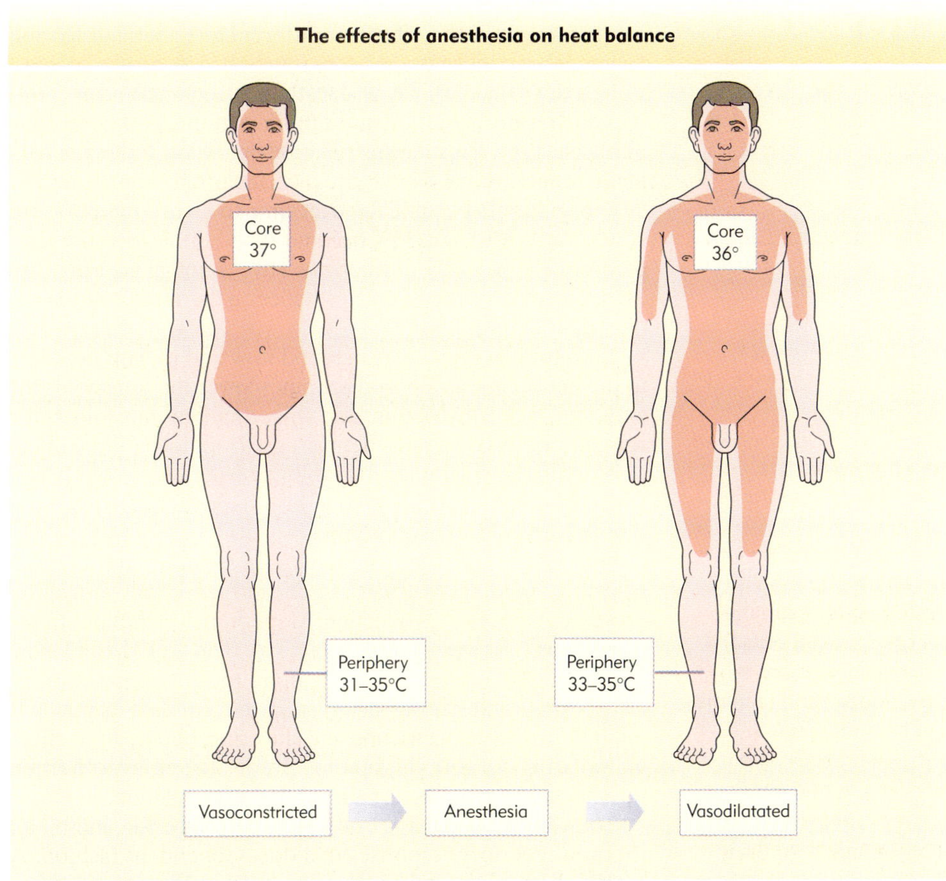

Figure 64.4 The effects of anesthesia on heat balance. In a simplified model, the human body is composed of two compartments, the core and the periphery. Under baseline conditions, the core is considerably warmer than the periphery. By decreasing vasomotor tone, both regional and general anesthesia decrease core temperature by redistribution of heat, whereby heat flows from the core to the peripheral thermal compartment. This effect decreases core temperature by about 1°C (1.8°F) in the first 30–60 minutes following induction of anesthesia. This redistribution predisposes to further hypothermia, since an increased temperature gradient results between the skin surface and the surrounding environment.

The best sites for monitoring temperature during anesthesia and surgery are those that are closest to blood temperature, which is considered the 'true' core temperature (Fig. 64.5).

When body temperature changes (i.e. during anesthesia and surgery), bladder and rectal temperatures are the slowest to change, and are likely to underestimate the magnitude of alteration in body temperature. In some clinical situations (i.e. cardiac surgery) these sites are deliberately monitored since the 'slow-to-change' characteristic helps to assess the 'completeness' of cooling and warming on cardiopulmonary bypass. The skin surface temperature is usually 2–3°C (3.6–5.4°F) lower than core temperature, but the core-to-skin temperature gradient depends on ambient temperature and vasomotor tone. For this reason, monitoring of skin-surface temperature can be misleading in the perioperative period. The relative changes in body temperature from various monitoring sites during

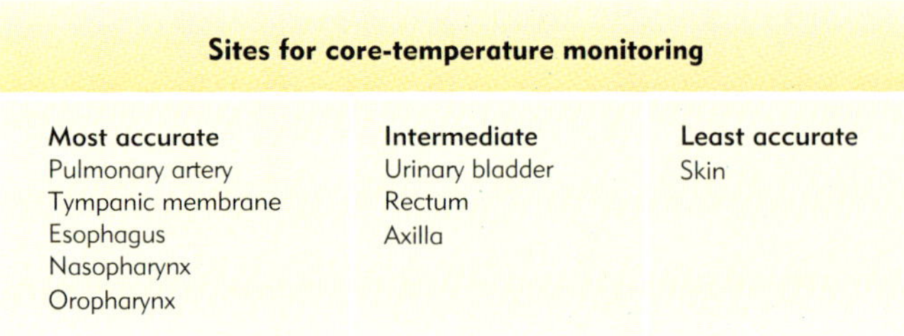

Sites for core-temperature monitoring

Most accurate	Intermediate	Least accurate
Pulmonary artery	Urinary bladder	Skin
Tympanic membrane	Rectum	
Esophagus	Axilla	
Nasopharynx		
Oropharynx		

Figure 64.5. Core temperature monitoring sites and correlation with blood temperature. Most to least accurate sites for correlation with blood temperature are listed.

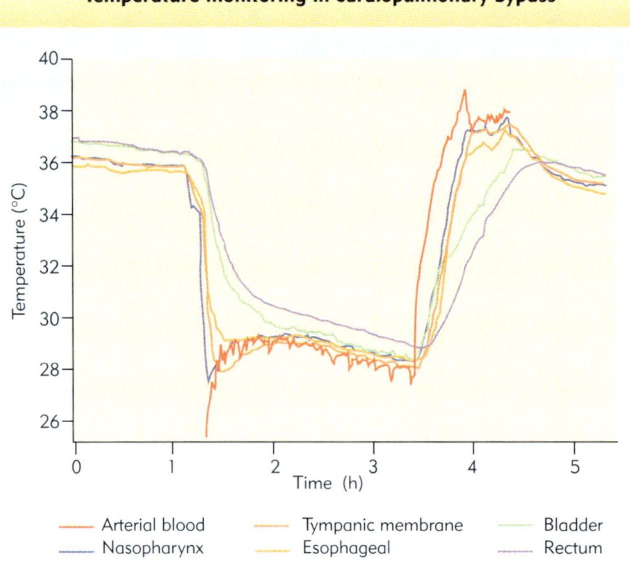

Figure 64.6 Temperature monitoring in a patient on cardiopulmonary bypass. The relative ability of each monitoring site to reflect core temperature is shown, including the temperature of arterial blood passing from the bypass pump into the ascending aorta, and various sites that are used to monitor 'core' temperature. The sites that show the fastest temperature change during cooling and warming (other than arterial blood) are those measured at the nasopharynx, tympanic membrane, and esophagus. Temperatures in the urinary bladder and rectum are slower to change and are considered to be 'intermediate' temperatures rather than core temperatures. These sites help to assess the completeness of cooling and warming during cardiac surgery. Although skin-surface temperature is not shown, changes in skin temperature occur even more slowly than those measured in the rectum or urinary bladder.

cooling and rewarming on cardiopulmonary bypass are shown in Figure 64.6.

The definition of normal core temperature varies, since a circadian variation of about 1°C occurs with a nadir in the morning and a peak in the afternoon. Also, a monthly variation occurs in menstruating women, with a sudden increase in core temperature [about 0.5°C (0.9°F)] at the onset of the luteal phase in response to increasing progesterone levels. No change in basal core temperature is related to age. Taking all variables into account, including differences among measurement sites, it is difficult to define a 'normal' core temperature, but 36.5–37.5°C (97.7–99.5°F) is considered the normal range.

Skin-surface temperature gradients are often used to assess changes in vasomotor tone. A gradient between the fingertip temperature and forearm temperature of 4°C (7.2°F) or more represents clinically significant vasoconstriction. Good correlation is found between skin-surface temperature gradients and more sophisticated measures of blood flow (i.e. laser Doppler, plethysmography).

EFFECTS OF ANESTHETICS ON THERMOREGULATION

Drugs can modify heat balance by altering one or more of the three components of the thermoregulatory system – the afferent pathway, central control mechanism, or efferent responses. General anesthetics impair all three components while regional anesthetics (major conduction blockade) impair the afferent and efferent components. Over the past decade numerous studies characterized the effects of different anesthetic drugs and techniques on thermoregulatory function. The results of these studies show that virtually all anesthetics (regional and general) impair thermoregulation and render patients poikilothermic during surgery. Considering the cold operating-room environment, unintentional hypothermia occurs often. Approximately 50% of patients become hypothermic to a core temperature <36°C (<96.8°F), and 33% become hypothermic to a core temperature <35°C (<95°F) when no active warming measures are used. The overall effects of anesthetics on thermoregulation are illustrated in Figure 64.7.

Barbiturates increase skin blood flow and radiant heat loss to the environment. Benzodiazepines lower the thresholds for sweating, vasoconstriction, and shivering, but only minimally compared with other anesthetic drugs. Propofol has little effect on sweating, but significantly inhibits responses to cold (vasoconstriction and shivering) in a dose-dependent fashion, and thus predisposes to hypothermia.

Systemic opioids in high doses cause hypothermia. This is a centrally mediated effect since intracerebral morphine decreases body-heat production. Meperidine (pethidine) treats postoperative shivering more effectively than fentanyl and morphine, an effect related to its κ-opioid receptor agonist properties. Alfentanil (a μ-agonist) causes a linear dose-dependent inhibition of vasoconstriction and shivering, but has little effect on sweating. In general, opioids predispose to hypothermia through significant impairment of thermoregulation.

The volatile anesthetics, as well as nitrous oxide, inhibit all thermoregulatory responses in a dose-dependent fashion. A sudden redistribution of heat occurs within the body after induction of general anesthesia, characterized by a 1°C (1.8°F) decrease in core temperature over the first 30–60 minutes. This represents heat flow from the core to the peripheral thermal compartment because of vasodilatation. At typical doses of volatile anesthetics, the interthreshold range is expanded 10-fold and vasoconstriction is not triggered until core temperature is near 34°C (93.2°F). Thus, core temperature continues to decrease over the first 2–3 hours of general anesthesia, whereupon the core temperature often plateaus because of vasoconstriction. Active vasoconstriction and shivering are fre-

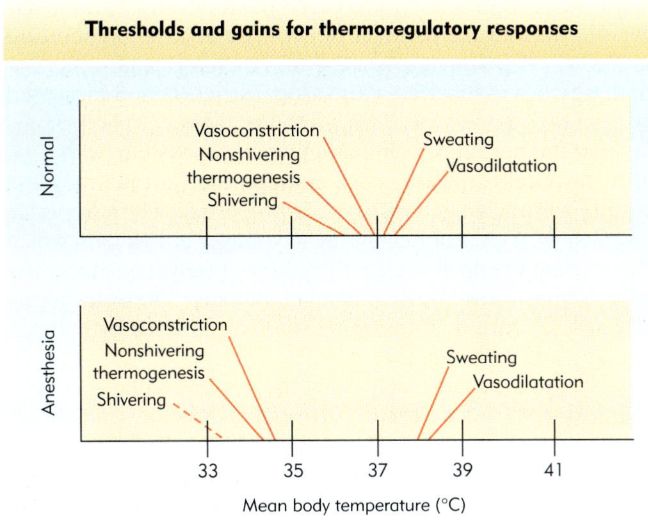

Figure 64.7 Thresholds and gains for thermoregulatory responses in awake and anesthetized humans. For each individual thermoregulatory response, the threshold is indicated by the intersection with the x-axis and the gain is represented by the slope of the intersecting line. The interthreshold range is shown as the range of temperatures that do not trigger a response. This range (between sweating and vasoconstriction) is expanded by approximately 10-fold in the anesthetized patient. This effect of anesthetic renders patients 'poikilothermic', and body temperature drifts towards environmental temperature. (Adapted with permission from Sessler DI. Temperature monitoring. In: Miller RD, ed. Anesthesia, 3rd edition. New York: Churchill Livingstone; 1990:1227–42).

quently observed as the anesthetic is discontinued in the hypothermic patient (Fig. 64.8).

In contrast to general anesthesia, epidural or spinal anesthetics do not modify central thermoregulatory activity. However, major conduction blockade is associated with approximately the same magnitude of hypothermia as occurs during general anesthesia, when all other factors are the same (see Fig. 64.8). The effects of regional anesthesia on afferent thermal signals are such that the hypothalamus is fooled by apparent warm signals from the lower body as the dominant cold signals are blocked. The efferent responses are also blocked, as vasoconstriction and shivering cannot occur below the level of the block and heat loss continues without the plateau phase, as with general anesthesia. Some evidence suggests that higher block levels predispose to more hypothermia. Shivering occurs, but results in less heat production since only the upper body contributes.

BENEFITS OF HYPOTHERMIA

Neuroprotection

The benefits of hypothermia during surgical procedures that put the brain or spinal cord at risk of ischemic injury are well recognized (Chapter 20). These procedures include cerebral aneurysm clipping, carotid endarterectomy, cardiac surgery, or aortic surgery with high cross clamps. Hypothermia reduces oxygen consumption by 5–7% for each 1°C (1.8°F) of cooling and this reduction is linear. At a typical hypothermic cardiopulmonary bypass temperature [28°C (82.4°F)], brain metabolism is reduced by about 50% (Chapter 41). Several animal studies suggest that even mild hypothermia [(34°C (93.2°F)] provides significant cerebral protection, perhaps not only by reducing brain oxygen consumption but also by decreasing the release of excitatory amino acids. Conversely, mild hyperthermia [39°C (102.2°F)] increases injury during ischemia. In addition to brain protection, mild hypothermia protects the spinal cord during ischemia. Paraplegia is a well-recognized complication of aortic surgical procedures, especially when aortic cross clamps are placed high on the aorta. Certainly, many variables contribute to spinal cord injury, but mild-to-moderate hypothermia [30–34°C (86.0–102.2°F)] is protective. Animal studies show a two-fold prolongation in the duration of aortic cross-clamp required to produce paraplegia at 35°C (95.0°F) versus 37°C (98.6°F).

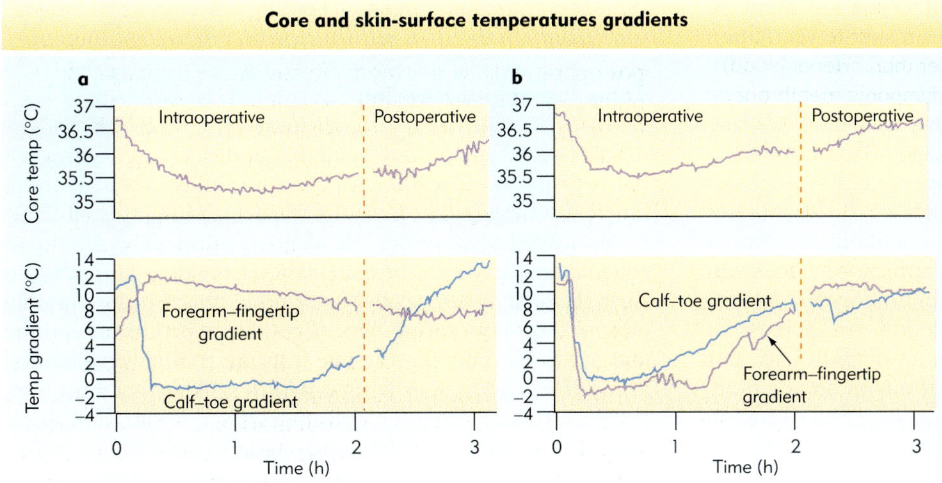

Figure 64.8 Core temperature and skin-surface temperature gradients during epidural and general anesthesia. The typical temperature pattern is shown for two patients who underwent open prostatectomy. (a) Epidural anesthetic with bupivacaine to a T4 level. (b) General anesthetic included thiopental (thiopentone), morphine, and isoflurane. The core temperature patterns were somewhat similar. The skin surface gradients illustrate vasodilatation in the lower extremities with both general and epidural anesthesia. The upper extremities showed vasodilatation with general anesthesia, but a compensatory vasoconstriction with epidural anesthesia. These vasomotor changes return to baseline in the early postoperative period. Regional anesthesia is associated with a similar degree of core hypothermia compared with general anesthesia.

CONSEQUENCES OF HYPOTHERMIA

Shivering and metabolism

One of the most commonly recognized effects of hypothermia is postoperative shivering. Despite earlier suggestions that inhalational anesthetics cause shivering by disassociation of spinal reflexes from cortical centers in the brain, it is now believed that virtually all perioperative shivering (with general or regional anesthesia) is thermoregulatory in origin. Based on older studies with very small numbers of patients and questionable methods, the myth has been perpetuated that postoperative shivering increases total body oxygen consumption by about four-fold above baseline. Although these earlier studies included single patients that reportedly increased their metabolic rates by 400%, the average increase with shivering was about 100%. Recent, more carefully conducted studies, show that postoperative shivering increases oxygen consumption, but the average increase is about 40%, with a maximum increase by about two-fold above baseline. Although shivering is uncomfortable for most patients, it is unlikely that this relatively small increase in total body oxygen consumption in the average shivering patient is associated with perioperative morbidity.

Although all opioids reduce shivering, meperidine is the most effective because of the agonist effect at the κ-opioid receptor. Other drugs that treat shivering effectively include clonidine, neostigmine, and ketanserin (a serotonin antagonist). Thermal comfort is significantly improved and shivering can be virtually eliminated by cutaneous warming using forced air during or following surgery. For every 1°C (1.8°F) of core hypothermia, approximately 4°C (7.2°F) of skin-surface warming is required to attenuate the shivering response.

Respiratory

Whole-body carbon dioxide production decreases with hypothermia. The magnitude of this decrease reflects the behavior of most enzyme-controlled biologic phenomena [i.e. a halving of activity with a fall in temperature of 10°C (18°F)]. This halving is formally expressed as a Q_{10}, or quotient of measured activities at two temperatures 10°C (18°F) apart. Decreases in both tidal volume and respiratory rate contribute to decreased minute ventilation in hypothermic patients. Body carbon dioxide content remains constant at hypothermia. It might be expected that the magnitude of decrease in minute ventilation would parallel that of carbon dioxide production. However, ventilatory dead space increases with hypothermia, and thus blunts the decrease in minute ventilation.

Hypothermia blunts the ventilatory response to carbon dioxide. The slope of the carbon dioxide response curve decreases from 0.38L/min per mmHg at 37°C (98.6°F) to 0.10L/min per mmHg at 28°C (82.4°F). The respiratory quotient, or ratio of carbon dioxide production to oxygen utilization, does not change with hypothermia. Thus, oxygen utilization decreases at the same rate as carbon dioxide production. An increase of oxygen solubility in blood compounds an overall 7.5% per degree centigrade increase in oxygen affinity of hemoglobin. Thus, the arterial partial pressure of oxygen decreases with cooling. Even mild hypothermia induces pulmonary vasoconstriction, which interferes with hypoxic pulmonary vasoconstriction.

Cardiovascular

A significant adrenergic occurs in response to hypothermia. Although this is not manifested during anesthesia, norepinephrine is significantly increased postoperatively in mildly hypothermic awake patients. A decrease in core temperature to 35.0°C (95.0°F) triggers a 2–7 fold increase in norepinephrine, which is associated with vasoconstriction and increased arterial blood pressure. This response appears to be primarily from the peripheral sympathetic nervous system, with little or no adrenal response, since epinephrine (adrenaline) and cortisol are unchanged with core hypothermia. The adrenergic response is of greater magnitude in younger individuals, which may explain the decreased ability of the elderly to protect their core temperature during cold challenge. The adrenergic response to core hypothermia can be attenuated by increasing skin-surface temperature.

Cold stress can adversely affect the cardiovascular system by triggering myocardial ischemia. A seasonal variation in death rate from myocardial infarction has been recognized, with increased mortality during winter months. The classic model of cold stress used to precipitate myocardial ischemia is the cold pressor test. The stimulus triggers a significant increase in both norepinephrine and epinephrine, along with α-adrenergically mediated coronary vasoconstriction. In high-risk patients (e.g. those who undergo vascular surgery), a core temperature <35°C (<95°F) is associated with a 2 to 3-fold increase in the incidence of early postoperative myocardial ischemia. This 'cold-induced' myocardial ischemia is independent of anesthetic technique (regional or general). In a recently completed randomized trial in high-risk noncardiac surgery patients, the relative risk for early postoperative cardiac morbidity was reduced by 55% in patients who were aggressively warmed during surgery. The incidences of postoperative ventricular tachycardia and morbid cardiac events were reduced in the normothermic group [36.7°C (98.0°F)] compared with the hypothermic group [35.4°C (95.7°F)], while cardiac outcomes occurred with similar frequency in the two groups intraoperatively. This suggests that cold-induced perioperative cardiovascular morbidity is adrenergically mediated, since the effect of temperature on outcome is significant in the postoperative period after emergence, not during anesthesia (when the adrenergic response to hypothermia is attenuated). Atrial fibrillation is common when core temperature approaches 30°C (86°F), especially when the atrium is traumatized by cannulation for cardiopulmonary bypass. Between 24°C (75.2°F) and 28°C (82.4°F), ventricular fibrillation develops. Hypothermia-induced ventricular fibrillation is refractory to pharmacologic therapy.

Coagulation and bleeding

The coagulation system is significantly influenced by hypothermia caused by impaired platelet function, decreased activity of the coagulation cascade, and increased fibrinolysis. Platelet function is impaired by hypothermia because of reduced levels of thromboxane B_2 at the site of tissue injury. The activity of coagulation factors in the coagulation cascade is also reduced since the activity of enzymes involved in the cascade, as for all enzymes, is temperature dependent. Since prothrombin time and partial thromboplastin time tests are routinely performed at 37°C (98.6°F) in most laboratories, it is likely that most temperature-related coagulopathies are missed in the clinical setting. Fibrinolysis is enhanced with hypothermia, which destabilizes clot and predisposes to increased bleeding. Patients who undergo total hip arthroplasty show a significant reduction in blood loss and decreased requirements for allogeneic blood transfusion when maintained normothermic compared with those who have mild hypothermia [35.0°C (95.0°F)].

Wound healing and infection

Wound healing is impaired and patients are more susceptible to wound infection when hypothermia [core <35°C (<95.°F)] occurs during surgery. Mild hypothermia [34.7°C (94.5°F)] increases the incidence of wound infection more than three-fold (19% versus 6%) compared with normothermia [36.6°C (97.9°F)] in patients who undergo colon surgery. This effect is thought to be related to impaired macrophage function and reduced tissue oxygen tension secondary to thermoregulatory vasoconstriction. Collagen deposition in the wound is also impaired with hypothermia. Increased susceptibility to infection with hypothermia at the time of inoculation of bacteria into the skin has been shown in animal models. The 'window of opportunity' for infection to become established is reportedly in the first 3 hours following inoculation. If hypothermia occurs at this critical time, infection occurs more frequently.

Pharmacodynamics and pharmacokinetics

The minimal anesthetic concentration (MAC) for volatile anesthetics is reduced by about 5% for each 1°C (1.8°F) reduction in body temperature. In addition, the blood/gas solubility ratio for volatile anesthetics is increased with hypothermia. In combination, these effects contribute to the slow emergence from general anesthesia in hypothermic patients, which suggests that substantial cost savings may be achieved by maintaining normothermia and expediting recovery from general anesthesia.

Mild hypothermia increases the duration of action of nondepolarizing neuromuscular blockers. At 34°C (93.2°F) the duration of action of vecuronium is doubled, an effect thought to be pharmacokinetic rather than pharmacodynamic. The duration of action of atracurium is also prolonged, but somewhat less – a 60% increase in duration occurs at 34°C (93.2°F). When added to the changes in MAC and solubility for inhaled anesthetics, this prolongation of neuromuscular blockade can delay or prevent emergence from general anesthesia, especially in the elderly who already have a reduced MAC and are especially susceptible to hypothermia.

Methods of controlling body temperature

Modern operating rooms are maintained at cool temperatures [16–20°C (61–68°F)], primarily for the comfort of the staff, which predisposes patients to hypothermia. This is exacerbated by the high rate of air exchange, which creates a 'wind-chill' effect. When ambient temperature is >23°C (>73.5°F), unintentional hypothermia occurs less frequently during surgery, but this warm environment is not well tolerated by the surgical staff.

Active heating and humidification of inspired gases have little or no effect on core temperature, except in neonates for whom this may help maintain normothermia. In adult patients, <10% of the total heat loss during surgery occurs from the respiratory tract, but this fraction increases in small children. Passive humidification with heat-moisture exchangers increases humidity in the airway, but has no effect on the core temperature.

Fluid warming can reduce the magnitude of hypothermia during surgery, but cannot be used to warm patients since fluids cannot be delivered at temperatures significantly >37°C (>98.5°F). When transfusion is likely, a fluid–blood warmer should be used, since blood is stored at 4°C (39.2°F). When a unit of cold blood or liter of room temperature crystalloid is given to a patient, mean body temperature is reduced by about 0.25°C (0.45°F). Adding this to the ongoing heat loss from the skin surface compounds the problem of unwarmed fluids. When fluid warmers are used, two factors must be considered in determining the temperature at which the fluid is delivered to the patient – flow rate and length of IV tubing. At low flow rates, after it leaves the warmer the fluid returns to ambient room temperature before it reaches the patient. At high flows, fluids pass through the warmer so quickly that they cannot be warmed sufficiently.

A layer of passive insulation reduces heat loss from the skin surface by 30%. The type of insulator is relatively unimportant as there is little difference between materials (plastic, cotton, paper, or reflective 'space blankets'). The layer of air between the insulation cover and the patient's skin provides the insulation, independent of the material itself. Prewarmed cotton blankets are commonly used in the operating room. Patients feel immediate warmth and comfort, but actual heat flux through the skin is virtually identical with both warmed and unwarmed cotton blankets.

Although passive insulation and IV fluid warming can reduce heat loss, they cannot be used to transfer heat into the patient. Therefore, active warming is required to maintain normothermia during the intraoperative period. Of the available warming systems, the most effective is forced air. This was initially used to warm hypothermic patients actively in the postoperative period, but it quickly became recognized that intraoperative prevention was more desirable than postoperative treatment. The forced-air system consists of two components – the forced-air generator and the blanket. The blankets may cover the upper body, lower body, or full body, and the appropriate design is chosen based on the location of the surgical field. Heat transfer with these systems is between 60 and 100W, which makes this therapy more efficient than other warming systems.

Circulating water mattresses are placed beneath the patient and connected to a warm water source that circulates flow through the mattress. Heat transfer with these devices is limited, since cutaneous blood flow to the back is limited because of pressure on the capillary beds from the body's weight. Heat flux through the skin surface over the back is 7W compared with the 3W of the standard foam mattress used on operating room tables. Water mattresses most effectively transfer heat when used over the ventral surface of the patient, but this is impractical during surgery.

Radiant heat is another type of active warming system. Radiant heaters should be used with a skin-surface thermistor that provides thermostatic feedback to the warmer and reduces the risk of burning. As it warms the skin surface, shivering is immediately attenuated with radiant warming.

HYPERTHERMIA

Environmental and disease induced

During anesthesia, iatrogenic hyperthermia can result from active warming of patients by application of warming blankets or unintentional overuse of heated airway humidifiers. Hyperthermia, usually mild, can also occur during long procedures in which the patient is covered with impermeable drapes and the operative area is small. Before temperature control of the operating room and air conditioning, heat stroke during anesthesia was not uncommon.

Thyrotoxicosis and thyroid storm can cause intraoperative hyperthermia. Thyroid storm presents with hypertension, hyperthermia, and tachycardia. Unlike with MH, muscle rigidity does not occur and acidosis is unusual. Elevated body temperature also complicates the Riley–Day syndrome, in which dopamine β-hydroxylase is deficient. People who have this syndrome exhibit pronounced instability of the autonomic nervous system, with wide variation in blood pressure, heart rate, and temperature, apparently unrelated to external stimuli. Hyperthermia can occur during anesthesia in patients who have osteogenesis imperfecta, a metabolic bone disease characterized by easy and frequent bone fractures and blue sclerae. Although a few episodes of true MH have been reported with osteogenesis imperfecta, in many cases clinical and laboratory tests reveal that MH was diagnosed mistakenly. Sepsis, bacteremia, and hyperthermia may be induced by surgical manipulation, which leads to postoperative hyperthermia. Surgical procedures that involve the oral cavity or gastrointestinal tract are associated with bacteremia and fever.

Cytokines, such as interleukin-1 (Chapter 52), that are released by pyrogens (e.g. bacterial lipopolysaccharide) stimulate prostaglandin E_2 (PGE_2) synthesis in the hypothalamus, which activates the thermoregulatory center and increases the set point to cause fever. The PGE_2 involved in the febrile response is probably synthesized by cyclo-oxygenase-2 in nonneuronal cells (Chapter 27).

Drug induced

Two syndromes of hyperthermia related to drug administration are MH and the neuroleptic malignant syndrome (NMS). The former occurs in genetically predisposed persons treated with volatile anesthetic agents or succinylcholine (Chapter 30). Transmission is thought to be autosomal dominant, and the incidence of MH is about 1 in 50,000 anesthetics. The syndrome occurs most frequently in younger individuals, more often males, and in those who undergo head-and-neck or orthopedic surgical procedures. The incidence depends on the gene pool for MH (the prevalence of genetic susceptibility is about 1:10,000) as well as on the frequency of use of triggering agents. The elderly appear to be more resistant to MH triggers.

The precise cause of MH is unknown. Increased intracellular Ca^{2+} concentration in skeletal muscle cells clearly constitutes part of the mechanism, since early recognition and treatment with dantrolene, which blocks the release of Ca^{2+} from intracellular stores, is an effective therapy (see below). The occurrence of MH requires both a susceptible patient and exposure to specific drugs. The 'trigger' drugs include all the volatile anesthetic agents and the depolarizing neuromuscular blocker succinylcholine. Local anesthetics, both amides and esters, do not trigger MH, nor do IV induction agents, including propofol, barbiturates, and benzodiazepines. Mild hypothermia protects against the development of MH. Although MH may occur in pigs during physical or emotional stress in the absence of drug intervention, in humans no direct evidence indicates that full-blown MH occurs in the absence of triggering drugs. The clinical consequences of MH include hyperkalemia, myoglobinemia, and disseminated intravascular coagulation.

The other drug-induced syndrome is NMS, which is characterized by hyperthermia, muscle rigidity, rhabdomyolysis, arrhythmia, acidosis, and death. It is precipitated by dopamine antagonist (e.g. antipsychotics). Despite its clinical similarity to MH, the cause of NMS is probably different. Most investigators believe that NMS results from blockade of dopamine receptors in the central nervous system – the dopamine agonist bromocriptine is one of the drugs that effectively treats NMS. Whether patients who have experienced NMS are at risk for MH is unclear. Succinylcholine, if preceded by barbiturate (as may occur for electroconvulsive therapy), does not precipitate MH syndrome in the patient who has NMS. There is little experience, however, with general anesthesia in patients who have experienced NMS.

Diagnosis and treatment of malignant hyperthermia

The signs and symptoms of MH are individually nonspecific and include tachycardia, tachypnea, and diaphoresis, but unexplained elevation in end-tidal carbon dioxide is the earliest and most sensitive sign. Temperature elevation is a later sign that follows the increase in oxygen consumption. Other signs of MH include muscle destruction with increased levels of creatine kinase (CK), myoglobinuria, myoglobinemia, and hyperkalemia. Respiratory and metabolic acidosis frequently accompany MH.

At the present time, the most popular diagnostic test for MH is the halothane–caffeine contracture test, which uses skeletal muscle from a biopsy to test the contracture response to halothane and caffeine separately. The sensitivity and specificity of the tests are high and no patient who had a negative biopsy has subsequently developed MH, even when challenged. Serum CK levels are not an appropriate screening test for MH.

Dantrolene, a hydantoin derivative, inhibits the release of Ca^{2+} from sarcoplasmic reticulum and may also enhance reuptake of Ca^{2+} into the sarcoplasmic reticulum. The use of dantrolene was first described in 1975 and has contributed to the reduction in mortality from MH. Other therapeutic measures include stopping the administration of trigger drugs, cold IV saline, surface cooling, hyperventilation with 100% oxygen, and treatment of the secondary effects of MH (acidosis, hyperkalemia, arrhythmias, coagulopathy). Importantly, in the treatment of arrhythmias the combination of Ca^{2+} channel blockers and dantrolene causes profound myocardial depression. The urine must be alkalinized and a diuresis established in an attempt to prevent myoglobin-induced nephropathy.

Key References

Frank SM, Raja SN, Fleisher LA, Beattie C, Higgins MS, Breslow MJ. Adrenergic and cardiovascular manifestations of cold stress. In: Zeisberger E, Schonbaum E, Lomax P, eds. Thermal balance in health and disease: recent basic research and clinical progress. Basel: Birkhauser Verlag; 1994:325–31.

Frank SM. Body temperature monitoring. In: Levitt RC, ed. Anesthesiology clinics of North America. Philadelphia: W. Saunders and Co; 1994:387–407.

Hopkins PM, Ellis FR, eds. Hyperthermic and hypermetabolic disorders. Cambridge: Cambridge University Press; 1996.

Sessler DI. Perianesthetic thermoregulation and heat balance in humans. FASEB J. 1993;7:638–44.

Sessler DI. Consequences and treatment of perioperative hypothermia. In: Levitt RC, ed. Temperature regulation during anesthesia. Philadelphia: Saunders; 1994:425–56.

Further Reading

Busto R, Dietrich WD, Globus MY, et al. Small differences in intraischemic brain temperature critically determine the extent of ischemic neuronal injury. J Cereb Blood Flow Metab. 1987;7:729–38.

Frank SM, Fleisher LA, Breslow MJ, et al. Perioperative maintenance of normothermia reduces the incidence of morbid cardiac events: A randomized trial. JAMA. 1997;277:1127–34.

Frank SM, Higgins M, Breslow M, et al. The catecholamine, cortisol, and hemodynamic responses to mild perioperative hypothermia: a randomized clinical trial. Anesthesiology. 1995;82:83–93.

Frank SM, Gorman RB, Higgins MS, Breslow MJ, Fleisher LA, Sitzman JV. Multivariate determinates of early postoperative oxygen consumption: The effects of body temperature, shivering, and gender. Anesthesiology. 1995;83:241–9.

Frank SM, El-Gamal N, Raja SN, Wu PK, Afifi O. Role of alpha-adrenoceptors in the maintenance of core temperature in humans. Clin Sci. 1995;89:219–25.

Frank SM, Higgins MS, Fleisher LA, et al. Core hypothermia and skin-surface temperature gradients: Epidural vs. general anesthesia and the effects of age. Anesthesiology. 1994;80:502–8.

Frank SM, Shir Y, Raja SN, et al. The adrenergic, respiratory, and cardiovascular effects of core cooling in humans. Am J Physiol. 1997;272:R557–62.

Kurz A, Sessler DI, Lenhardt R, et al. Perioperative normothermia to reduce the incidence of surgical-wound infection and shorten hospitalization. N Engl J Med. 1996;334:1209–15.

MacIntyre PE, Pavlin EG, Dwersteg JF. Effect of meperidine on oxygen consumption, carbon dioxide production, and respiratory gas exchange in postanesthetic shivering. Anesthesiol Analg. 1987;66:751–5.

Sessler DI. Mild perioperative hypothermia. N Engl J Med. 1997;336:1730–7.

Vacanti FX, Ames AA. Mild hypothermia and Mg2+ protect against irreversible damage during CNS ischemia. Stroke. 1983;15:695–8.

Chapter 65 Pregnancy

Norman L Herman

Topics covered in this chapter

Maternal physiology
Uterine blood flow
Drugs in pregnancy
Preeclampsia, eclampsia, and HELLP syndrome
Pregnancy and local anesthetic action and toxicity
Epidural and spinal anesthesia: effect on labor
Non-obstetric surgery during pregnancy
Complications

MATERNAL PHYSIOLOGY

Pregnancy induces many physiologic changes within the body of a woman that have important anesthetic implications. A good working knowledge of these alterations is important for the safe and appropriate anesthetic care of the pregnant (gravid) patient.

Cardiovascular system

With pregnancy several notable changes occur in blood volume, pressure, and resistance. The gravid patient rapidly expands her blood volume by 25 to 40% during the first half of pregnancy. However, an imbalance exists between the increases in plasma volume (50%) and red cell mass (15%), which peaks at about 25 weeks of pregnancy (Fig. 65.1). The resultant hemodilution causes the physiologic anemia of pregnancy. The increase in plasma volume dilutes protein concentrations, which can markedly alter the bound:free ratio of protein-bound agents and reduce the concentrations of circulating enzymes (e.g. plasma cholinesterase).

Cardiac output increases by 30–40% by the 20th week of pregnancy, and remains stable until labor. With the initiation of uterine contractions, cardiac output increases by an additional 30% during contraction in active labor and 45% during the second stage of labor. The greatest increase occurs after autotransfusion of as much as 800mL of blood from the contracting uterus following delivery, which elevates cardiac output by 80% above prelabor values.

Despite the increases in both blood volume and cardiac output, maternal blood pressure is lowest during the first half of pregnancy, but increases toward normal prepregnancy values by term. This results from a 35% reduction in systemic vascular resistance, which is thought to result from the low-resistance intervillous circulation in the placenta and the vasodilator properties of circulating progesterone, prostacyclin, and estrogen. Blood pressures greater than prepregnancy values usually signify a pathophysiologic entity of pregnancy (e.g. preeclampsia).

The weight of a gravid uterus can markedly affect the cardiovascular system in the pregnant patient. By term, almost 90% of parturients completely obstruct their inferior vena cava when supine. However, only 15% exhibit symptoms of supine hypotensive syndrome, which results from a reduction in venous return. The remaining women have an efficient alternative pathway via the lumbrosacral venous plexus (including the epidural vessels), which return blood to the heart via the azygous vein (Fig. 65.2). This engorgement of the epidural vessels can alter the response to regional anesthetics in pregnancy (see below).

Changes in maternal blood volume during pregnancy

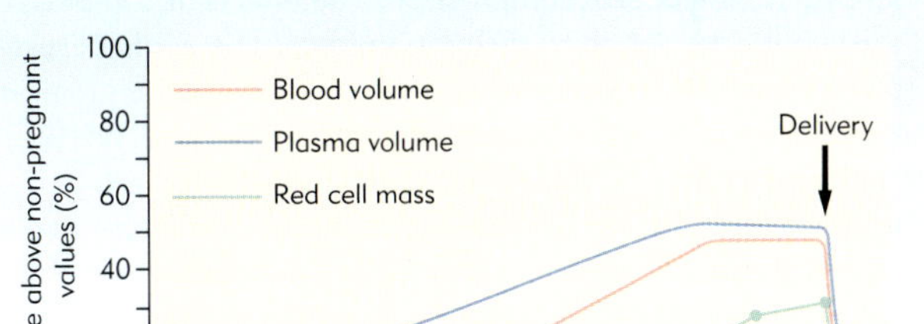

Figure 65.1 Changes in maternal blood volume during pregnancy. A plot depicting the increases in blood volume and its constituent components during pregnancy. (Adapted with permission from Chamberlain G. The changing body during pregnancy. Br Med J. 1991;302:719–22.)

Respiratory system

Minute ventilation increases by up to 45%, beginning very early in pregnancy primarily because of an increased tidal volume. This results from progesterone-induced changes in carbon dioxide sensitivity and the increased metabolic rate and oxygen demands of pregnancy. Renal excretion of bicarbonate partially compensates for the resultant respiratory alkalosis.

As the gravid uterus expands into the abdomen, the lower ribs flare and the diaphragm elevates. This induces a decrease in both the expiratory and residual volumes, and thereby lowers the functional residual capacity (Fig. 65.3). This decrease, along with the profound increase in oxygen consumption seen with

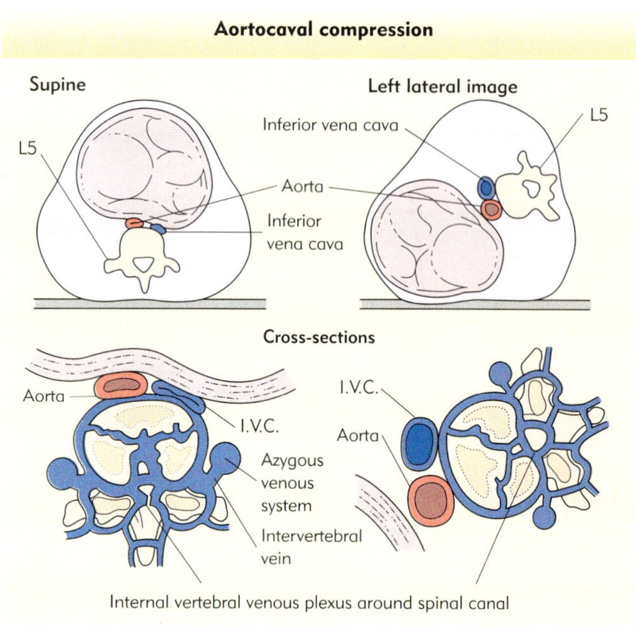

Figure 65.2 Aortocaval compression. The effects of compression of the central circulation by the gravid uterus. The epidural vessels become engorged as venous blood takes an alternative route when the inferior vena cava is compressed in the supine position. IVC, inferior vena cava; L5, 5th lumbar vertebra. (Adapted with permission from Bonica JJ. Obstetric analgesia and anesthesia. Amsterdam: World Federation of Societies of Anaesthesia; 1980.)

pregnancy, explains the precipitous drop in arterial oxygen saturation after short periods of apnea (e.g. rapid sequence induction and intubation). Otherwise, vital capacity is unaltered.

The increases in maternal blood volume cause an engorgement of the capillaries of the nasal passages and upper airway, which bleed easily and briskly. These changes can markedly alter the view of and ability to intubate the trachea of the parturient. In conjunction with weight gain, these changes explain the increased risk of failed intubation in the pregnant patient undergoing anesthesia.

Central nervous system

Pregnancy induces a 25–40% decrease in the minimum alveolar concentration (MAC) for inhalational anesthetics. The sedating effects of progesterone and elevated levels of endogenous opioids are two of the factors believed to contribute to this reduction. Intravenous anesthetics are apparently affected as well (e.g. the dose of thiopental required for induction is 18% less in the pregnant patient). Changes in the spread and sensitivity to local anesthetics during pregnancy are described below.

Gastrointestinal system

Gastric volume and acidity increase early in pregnancy because of the release of placental gastrin. Gastric emptying is affected by the mechanical restrictions on stomach mobility induced by the gravid uterus. In addition, progesterone has a relaxing effect on the entire gastrointestinal tract and may delay gastric emptying throughout pregnancy. Although this seems true during labor, most clinical evidence indicates no difference in stomach emptying between pregnant and nonpregnant patients.

Renal system

Concomitant with the increase in cardiac output is an increase in glomerular filtration rate. Tubular reabsorption also increases, so no net change in fluid or electrolyte excretion occurs. The 40% decline in plasma creatinine and blood urea nitrogen reflect this increase in renal filtration, which may accelerate the excretion of agents cleared by the kidney.

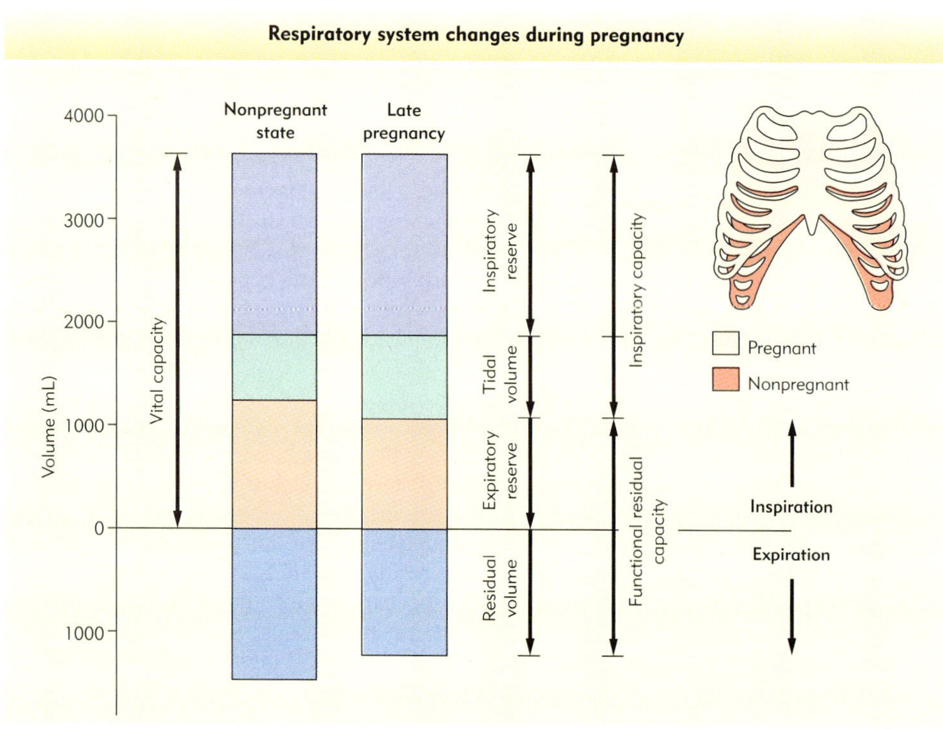

Figure 65.3 Respiratory system changes during pregnancy. The inset shows changes in the chest cavity with pregnancy. The changes in inspiratory and expiratory volumes lead to significant reductions in functional residual capacity during pregnancy. (Adapted with permission from Chamberlain G. The changing body during pregnancy. Br Med J. 1991;302:719–22.)

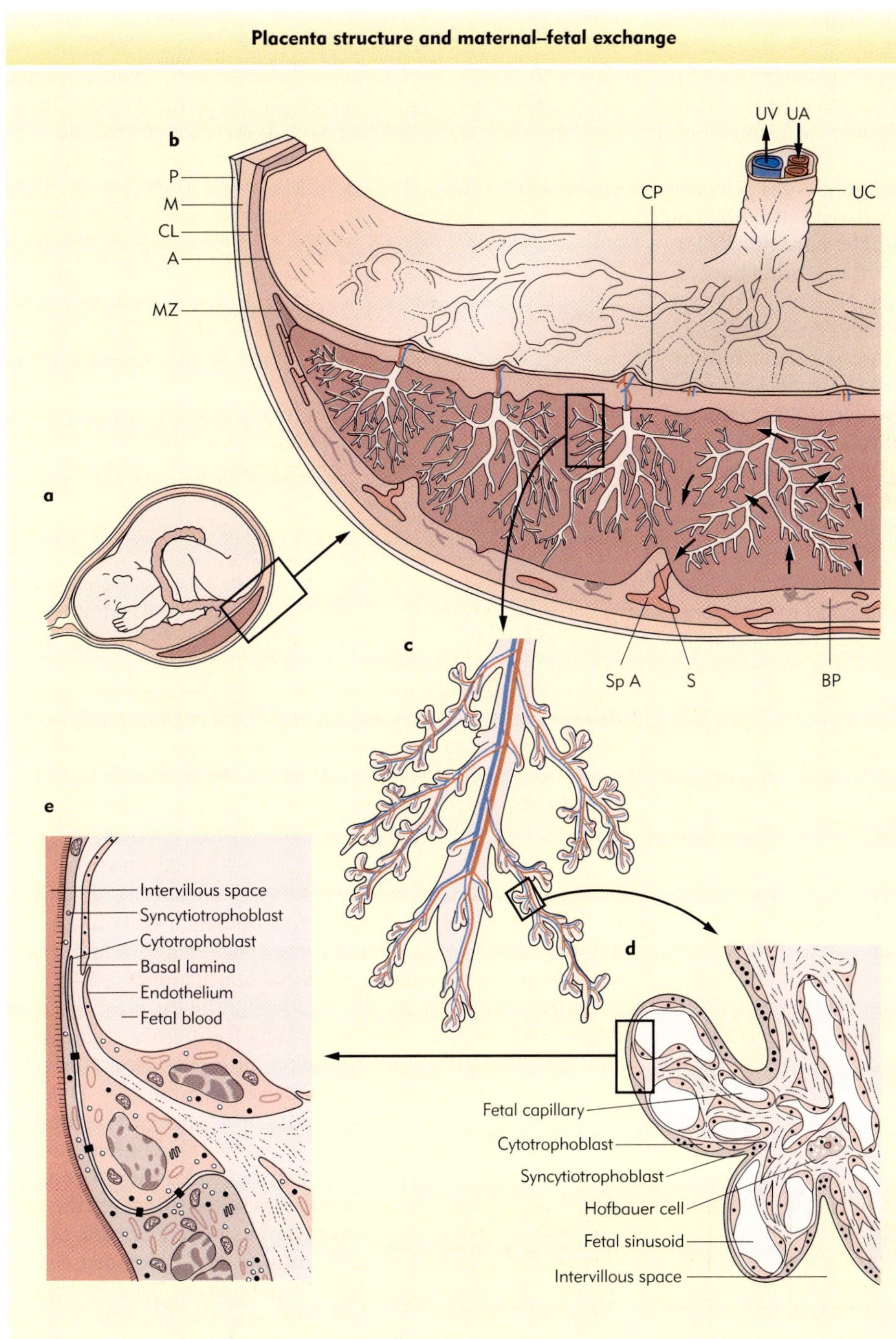

Figure 65.4 Basic structure of the placenta and the site of maternal–fetal exchange. (a) The fetus and placenta *in utero*. (b) The placenta is a complex structure that brings the maternal and fetal circulations into close apposition for exchange. The arrows illustrate the flow characteristics of maternal blood around the villous trees that contain the fetal vessels. A, amnion; BP, basal plate; CP, chorionic plate; CL, chorionic laeve; M, myometrium; MZ, marginal zone; P, perimetrium; S, septum; SpA, spiral artery; UA, umbilical artery; UC, umbilical cord; UV, umbilical vein. (c) The villi branch into multiple generations (the terminal branchings are shown). (d) Light microscope view through a terminal villous showing the fetal sinusoids, which are enlarged fetal capillaries that serve to increase surface area for transfer. (e) Simplified electron micrograph of the 'placental barrier' in which maternal–fetal interchange takes place. (Adapted with permission from both Kaufmann P, Schaffen I. Placental development. In: Polin RA, Fox WW, eds. Fetal and neonatal physiology. Philadelphia: WB Saunders; 1998:59–66; and Kaufmann P. Basic morphology of the fetal and maternal circuits in the human placenta. Contrib Gynecol Obstetr. 1985;13:5–17.)

UTERINE BLOOD FLOW

The flow of blood to the uterus undergoes a dramatic increase throughout pregnancy, rising from 50–100mL/min to more than 700mL/min at term, or nearly 20% of cardiac output. Nearly 90% of blood flow to the gravid uterus is directed to the placental intervillous spaces for transplacental exchange with the fetus (Fig. 65.4).

The 200 or so spiral arteries that underlie the developing placenta undergo changes from the invasion of trophoblastic cells. These cells erode the elastic and muscle components of the vessels and replace it with fibrous tissue, thereby exposing the arteries to systemic pressures that dilate them into funnel-shaped sacs. In addition, the arteries become less sensitive to the effects of vasoconstrictors of all types (α-adrenergic agonists, angiotensin II, and endothelial-derived factors). These alterations result in a low-resistance pathway that shunts blood into the intervillous space to ensure adequate placental perfusion. Therefore, to ensure continued fetal well-being, an adequate maternal systemic pressure must be delivered to the uterus to maintain uteroplacental circulation.

DRUGS IN PREGNANCY

Historically, the placenta was believed to be a barrier to protect the fetus from agents given to the mother. It is now clear that no such barrier exists. Most drugs given to a pregnant woman are shared with the fetus to some extent, particularly low molecular weight compounds like anesthetics. Drug permeability through the placenta and pharmacokinetic properties are the important factors in determining fetal exposure. Simple diffusion from maternal blood in the intervillous space to fetal blood within the fetal sinusoids of the villous trees of the placenta is the primary transfer mechanism for anesthetic agents, with the concentration gradient determining their rates (Fig. 65.4). The same properties that allow anesthetics to rapidly cross the blood–brain barrier allow their equally rapid transfer across the placenta. With the notable exception of the muscle relaxants and glycopyrrolate, which are quaternary amines and therefore poorly diffusible across placenta, the majority of drugs used in anesthesia easily transfer across the placenta to rapidly achieve fetal–maternal concentration ratios >0.5. This is essential information for the anesthesiologist and is necessary to understand how much of an agent given to the mother reaches the fetus such that postdelivery neonatal depression can be avoided or minimized.

An important question is whether or not anesthetic agents are safe for the developing fetus if administered for surgery during pregnancy or for anesthesia or analgesia for delivery. Adverse effects of drugs on the fetus can be divided into early and late effects. Early effects center around the potential for teratogenicity (inducing changes in morphology or function through alterations in development). Many drugs have demonstrated teratogenic effects in animal models of gestation, but only a small number of agents have been shown to cause fetal abnormalities or toxicity in humans. In 1980, the US Food and Drug Administration (FDA) published guidelines for drug companies to use to classify agents into risk categories so that practitioners could make rational decisions as to whether a therapeutic intervention was safe for the fetus (Fig. 65.5). With the exceptions of nitrous oxide, which has not been given an FDA classification, and the benzodiazepines, which have been given a category D rating, the anesthetics currently used belong to either category B or C. It is possible that any drug administered in the right amount at the right time could be a teratogen. However, this does not mean that the drug causes defects when given once during pregnancy at its normal therapeutic dose.

Adverse effects of anesthetics later in pregnancy involve the potential for reductions in maternal oxygenation that lead to hypoxemia or blood pressure changes that result in uterine hypoperfusion, either of which can induce fetal asphyxia. A number of anesthetic complications include high or complete spinal blockade and unintended deep inhalation or intravenous anesthesia, which can result in fetal asphyxia. Although a demarcation is made between the injurious effects of drugs in early versus late gestation, drugs can be directly toxic to a fetus after organogenesis (from 2–8 weeks of gestation), and hypotension and hypoxia can be harmful to an embryo.

US Food and Drug Administration guidelines for therapeutic intervention that is safe for the fetus	
Category A	Controlled studies have shown no risk to the fetus during the first trimester, and later trimesters as well. Risk is remote (e.g., water).
Category B	Animal studies have demonstrated no fetal risk, but no controlled studies have been performed in humans or animal studies have shown adverse fetal effects but these results were not confirmed in controlled human studies. No risk is evident after the first trimester.
Category C	Either studies have shown fetal risk in animals (teratogenic or embryocidal) but no controlled human studies have been performed or there are no available data in humans and animals for an agent. Drugs of this class should only be given if benefits outweigh the risks.
Category D	Confirmed evidence exists for human fetal risk, but benefits are acceptable despite known risk, i.e., life-or-limb situations or serious disease for which no safer drugs exist (e.g., diazepam).
Category X	Agents of this class are contraindicated in pregnant patients for any reason because animal or human studies have displayed teratogenicity or there is evidence of fetal risk from prior human experience. Fetal risk clearly outweighs any clinical benefit of its use in pregnancy (e.g., thalidomide).

Figure 65.5 US Food and Drug Administration guidelines for therapeutic intervention that is safe for the fetus. (Adapted with permission from the Food and Drug Administration. Labeling and prescription drug advertising; content and format for labeling for human prescription drugs. Fed Register. 1979;44:37434–67.)

Drugs affecting uterine activity

Analgesics and anesthetics are administered to laboring and delivering parturients to diminish (and in most cases eliminate) pain. Some reports indicate that anesthesia can affect uterus activity, either by impeding the progress of labor (dystocia) or by affecting the postdelivery hemostasis brought about via uterine contraction.

Local anesthetics and opioids do not appear to have a negative effect upon normal uterine activity, and therefore direct uterine effects do not cause the extended first and second stages of labor with epidural analgesia. Measurements of intrauterine pressure in laboring parturients before and after epidural analgesia suggest no differences in uterine force or coordination. With intrathecal opioid analgesia, the opposite concern has emerged. Spinal opioids can produce transient episodes of fetal bradycardia 5–15 minutes after intrathecal injection, particularly in the presence of an infusion of oxytocin or if the contraction pattern is accelerated. The bradycardia is usually associated with hypertonic uterine contraction, with a reduction of uteroplacental blood flow.

Recent data on the effects of intrathecal analgesia on the rate of cervical dilatation may help explain this phenomenon. With epidural analgesia using local anesthetic, the rate of cervical dilatation is about 1.9cm/h, while with spinal sufentanil the rate is 4–5cm/h, apparently as a result of its rapid analgesic effect. Circulating epinephrine (adrenaline) levels plummet within minutes of sufentanil administration, as opposed to a more extended fall with epidural local anesthetics. The natural tocolytic effect of epinephrine most likely balances the constrictor effects of circulating oxytocin released during labor. The sudden reduction in circulating epinephrine leaves oxytocin temporarily unopposed, which results in increased frequency and strength of uterine contraction. The Fergusen reflex resets oxytocin levels to compensate, but the increased rate of cervical dilatation suggests that compensation is not complete. Loss of epinephrine-related β-adrenergic agonism and the subsequent unopposed oxytocic effects can result in tetanic uterine contraction and fetal bradycardia. Uterine relaxants (terbutaline or nitroglycerin) have been effectively utilized to abolish this hypertonic contraction and restore uterine blood flow.

Potent inhalational anesthetics have been both hailed and condemned for their dose-dependent uterine-relaxing effects. Effective uterine relaxation requires significant concentrations of any of the volatile agents, generally in excess of one MAC, which can only be accomplished after securing the airway with an endotracheal tube accompanied by close hemodynamic monitoring, particularly in the face of bleeding. There is insufficient evidence that low concentrations of volatile agents (<0.5 MAC) significantly increase bleeding after cesarean delivery.

Drugs with direct inhibitory affects on uterine activity are intentionally given by obstetricians to parturients in premature labor to reduce or abolish contractions. These tocolytic agents, as they are known, may have implications upon the subsequent administration of anesthesia.

The β-adrenergic agents terbutaline and ritodrine are the first-line tocolytic agents in most obstetric units. The β-adrenoceptor activation by these drugs causes an increase in cyclic adenosine monophosphate (cAMP) within uterine smooth muscle cells, which decreases available intracellular Ca^{2+} for actin and myosin filament interaction and therefore results in uterine relaxation. However, both of these agents also possess β_1-adrenergic agonism, which can cause tachycardia and elevated cardiac output. In addition, β_2-adrenoceptor activation in vascular smooth muscle can induce significant vasodilation and hypotension, which leads to further elevations in inotropic and chronotropic drive via the baroreceptor reflex. Palpitations, chest tightness, and overt chest pain are not uncommon in parturients treated with these drugs. There are reports of patients with supraventricular tachycardia and myocardial ischemia that resulted from β-adrenergic tocolytic therapy.

Another important side effect seen occasionally with ritodrine or terbutaline therapy is pulmonary edema and hypoxemia. An association exists between β-adrenergic-induced pulmonary edema and plasma volume expansion, either by intravenous hydration or through the antidiuretic effect of β-adrenergic stimulation. Whether the pulmonary edema results from decreased diastolic filling time and/or increased pulmonary capillary permeability is unclear. Use of ritodrine and terbutaline for preterm labor can also cause hyperglycemia and hypokalemia.

Concern has been expressed regarding the induction of anesthesia soon after the use of β-adrenergic agents (e.g. if the tocolysis fails and the fetus is about to deliver). Hypotension, ventricular arrhythmia, pulmonary edema, and sinus tachycardia have been reported when general anesthesia is administered soon after ritodrine or terbutaline. Whenever possible, general anesthesia should be delayed at least 15 minutes after discontinuation of a β-agonist. Halothane should be avoided in parturients treated with ritodrine or terbutaline as it sensitizes the myocardium to catecholamine-induced arrhythmias. Epidural analgesia and anesthesia might worsen ritodrine-induced hypotension. Evidence in the gravid ewe suggests that the elevated cardiac output caused by these agents maintains stable hemodynamics during epidural anesthesia. It is advisable, however, to judiciously administer intravenous hydration prior to regional anesthetic in light of the potential for fluid retention and subsequent pulmonary edema.

Magnesium sulfate ($MgSO_4$) reduces uterine contractions by direct competition with Ca^{2+} for uptake and binding and by its action to increase intracellular cAMP, thereby making it an effective tocolytic agent. Both of these actions decrease intracellular Ca^{2+} concentration and decrease actin–myosin interaction. In a dose-related fashion, $MgSO_4$ affects neuromuscular function by decreasing acetylcholine release, desensitizing the motor end-plate, and altering muscle membrane excitability. Patients given long-term therapy with $MgSO_4$ are profoundly sensitive to nondepolarizing neuromuscular blocking agents and their response to succinylcholine is variable. Blockade should be closely monitored and doses of nondepolarizing agents given after recovery from succinylcholine should be decreased. $MgSO_4$ affects vascular smooth muscle activity and can lead to transient reductions in blood pressure. When establishing epidural analgesia in a patient treated with $MgSO_4$, induction should be slow with careful blood pressure monitoring, particularly since the response to vasopressors (e.g. ephedrine, phenylephrine) used to treat hypotension also may be altered.

PREECLAMPSIA, ECLAMPSIA, AND HELLP SYNDROME

Preeclampsia is a complex, multisystem hypertensive disorder of pregnancy that affects up to 10% of parturients. The process affects the heart, blood vessels, kidneys, liver, brain, and platelets and resolves spontaneously after the delivery of the placenta. When neurologic involvement causes convulsions in the absence of a pre-existing seizure disorder, it is classified as *eclampsia*. A severe subtype of preeclampsia or eclampsia that results from profound liver involvement is known as *HELLP syndrome* (hemolysis, elevated liver enzymes, and low platelet count).

For reasons that are unclear, the process by which the trophoblastic cells normally invade and erode the tunica media of high-resistance uterine spiral arteries, replacing it with fibrin matrix and fibroblasts to produce the low-resistance conduits for maternal blood to the placenta, is incomplete in preeclamptic patients (Fig. 65.6). Genetic and immunologic etiologies have been invoked to explain this placental dysfunction. The resultant narrow, constrictable spiral arteries provide inadequate perfusion to the intervillous space, especially as the placenta enlarges, leading to placental ischemia. The varying clinical presentation may reflect the degree to which trophoblastic cells fail to alter spiral arterial integrity.

Peripheral vascular resistance is markedly elevated in preeclamptic patients and results in elevated blood pressures, decreased vascular capacitance, and (consequently) relative hypovolemia. The pathophysiologic process for this increased resistance is unclear. Animal models suggest that an imbalance in endothelial-derived factors that vasodilate and vasoconstrict vascular smooth muscle is involved. The exaggerated responses to vasoconstrictors (e.g. angiotensin II), increased capillary permeability, and other evidence of endothelial dysfunction (e.g. reduced prostacyclin production, elevated levels of von Willebrand factor and fibronectin, increased neutrophil activation) suggest that factors released by the ischemic placenta lead to maternal endothelial injury and induce a cascade of pathophysiologic processes.

The mechanism by which placental ischemia induces endothelial damage in preeclampsia is unclear. Current evidence suggests an increased turnover of trophoblast cells within the placenta as the source of endothelial toxic compounds. Under conditions of hypoxia, toxic oxygen radicals are produced by the metabolism by the enzyme xanthine oxidase of increased levels of purines produced by trophoblast cell death. These radicals may cause an increase in lipid peroxidation in the relatively hyperlipidemic maternal plasma. The products of lipid peroxidation are toxic to endothelial cells. It has been suggested that fragments of trophoblastic cells within the maternal blood may also directly alter endothelial cell function. The multisystem disruption of preeclampsia results from endothelial damage in the various affected organs. Recent studies of human sympathetic nerve activity suggest that the increased vascular resistance in preeclampsia may

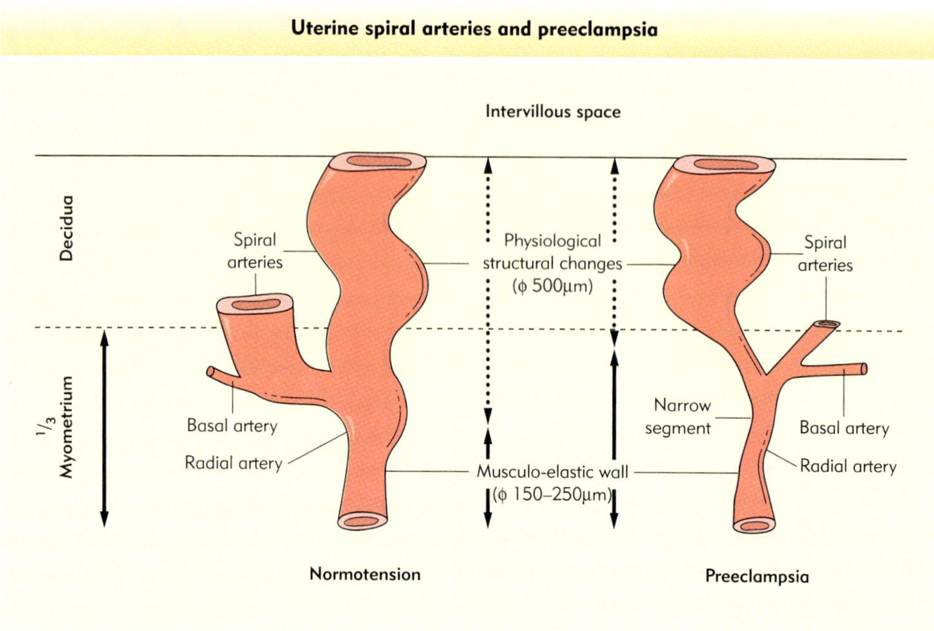

Figure 65.6 Differences in uterine spiral arteries in normal and preeclamptic patients. The failure of complete trophoblastic erosion of the tunica media of the spiral arteries beyond the deciduomyometrial junction causes arterial narrowing, diminished uteroplacental blood flow, and ultimately placental ischemia in preeclampsia. (Adapted from Bronsens IA. Morphological changes in the utero-placental bed in pregnancy hypertension. Clin Obstet Gynaecol. 1977;4:573–93.)

result in part from elevated efferent nerve traffic (almost a three times greater burst rate than in nonpreeclamptic parturients).

PREGNANCY AND LOCAL ANESTHETIC ACTION AND TOXICITY

Physiologic changes of pregnancy increase the sensitivity of parturients to the effects of local anesthetics. The decreased physical capacities of the epidural and intrathecal spaces produced by the engorgement of epidural vessels increase the spread of a sensory blockade to comparable doses of local anesthetic in pregnant versus nonpregnant women (Fig. 65.7). Data that compare median nerve blockade with lidocaine (lignocaine) in pregnant and nonpregnant women suggest that pregnancy may increase the sensitivity of nervous tissue to local anesthetics as well. However, recent data from dorsal root nerve axons in pregnant rats suggest a decrease in sensitivity to local anesthetics, which suggests that the increased sensitivity observed *in vivo* resides outside the nerve cell itself, and possibly results from alterations in pharmacokinetics (e.g. higher maternal pH may increase the proportion of un-ionized local anesthetic) or from increased concentrations of endorphins during pregnancy. The elevated cardiac output and dilution of plasma protein concentrations during pregnancy may influence the distribution and elimination (pharmacokinetics) of local anesthetic agents.

Systemic toxicity of local anesthetics occurs primarily by accidental injection into the circulation, although high systemic levels can also follow absorption from the site of injection (Chapter 28). The first symptoms of increasing plasma concentrations of local anesthetics result from the effects of these agents on the CNS. As brain concentrations rise, local anesthetics selectively block inhibitory pathways, which leads to unopposed CNS stimulation that manifests initially as perioral numbness, metallic taste, tinnitus, etc., and ultimately as seizures. Coma and respiratory arrest follow as even higher levels inhibit excitatory pathways and brainstem centers. The CNS toxicity of individual local anesthetic agents is related to local anesthetic potency. The relative toxicity of agents commonly used in obstetrics is 2-chloroprocaine < lidocaine < ropivacaine < tetracaine < bupivacaine. Factors such as speed of injection and metabolic or respiratory acidosis can lower the cumulative dose necessary for seizures.

As plasma lidocaine concentrations rise, even highly resistant myocardial tissues manifest signs of depression. Cardiac arrest is rare and preventable by supporting respiratory and hemodynamic function. Plasma levels at which severe cardiovascular toxicity symptoms occur are almost double those that cause seizures. This margin of safety is not seen with bupivacaine. In many cases of bupivacaine-induced cardiac arrest, seizures occur concurrently, if at all. Bupivacaine induces refractory ventricular arrhythmia (ventricular tachycardia or fibrillation). This difference between bupivacaine and lidocaine may be the result of the slow dissociation of bupivacaine from cardiac Na^+ channels. The greater lipid solubility of bupivacaine may lead to rapidly increasing brainstem concentrations that may also produce bradycardia, hypotension, and arrhythmia. The sensitivity to the cardiotoxic effects of bupivacaine increases with pregnancy; this is not so with lidocaine. The higher protein-binding ability of bupivacaine may lead to greater free concentrations with comparable doses because of the dilution of plasma protein during pregnancy. In addition, animal studies demonstrate an increase in cardiotoxic and arrhythymogenic potential of bupivacaine after progesterone and β-estradiol treatment. These properties are unique to bupivacaine in pregnancy.

Ropivacaine was introduced into clinical practice recently. The substitution of a propyl group on the piperidine nitrogen, instead of a methyl group as in mepivacaine or a butyl group as in bupivacaine (see Chapter 28), confers a side-effect profile for ropivacaine that is intermediate between the profiles of these agents. Unlike bupivacaine, which is a racemic mixture, ropivacaine is prepared as a pure *S*-enantiomer – the *S*-enantiomer is the more potent local anesthetic, while the *R*-enantiomer is more cardiotoxic. Using the same technology, a pure *S*-enantiomer of bupivacaine (levobupivacaine) has been formulated recently and possesses the same reduced cardiotoxicity.

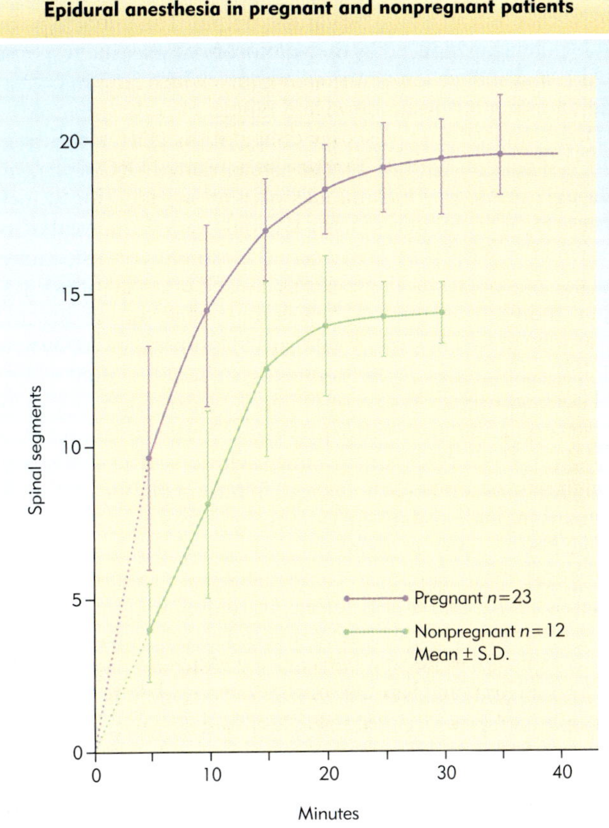

Figure 65.7 Differences in the spread of epidural anesthesia in pregnant versus nonpregnant patients. Pregnancy alters the rate and extent of spread of epidural analgesia as shown by a study that compared nonpregnant and pregnant women in their first trimester given comparable doses of local anesthetic. (Adapted with permission from Fagraeus L, Urban BJ, Bromage PR. Spread of epidural analgesia in early pregnancy. Anesthesiology. 1983;58:184–7. Philadelphia: Lippincott–Raven. Copyright, American Society of Anesthesiologists.)

EPIDURAL AND SPINAL ANESTHESIA: EFFECT ON LABOR

Studies have demonstrated as much as a 20-times greater incidence of fetal malrotations that require intervention in parturients with epidural analgesia versus those without, reflected in a doubling of forceps delivery rate. Other studies report no such differences, and one study showed an increase in forceps delivery rate when epidural analgesia was discontinued. These examples illustrate the uncertainties of the relationship between epidural analgesia and dystocia.

Studies on the effects of epidural analgesia on the progress of labor suffer from design flaws and selection biases. Deciding whether the assisted delivery was indicated or simply convenient because anesthesia was present is difficult. As Chestnut (1997) succinctly comments:

> '... women at increased risk of operative delivery are more likely to request and receive epidural anesthesia during labor than are women with rapid uncomplicated labor ...'

That is patients with pre-existing dystocia have more pain and are over-represented in epidural groups. Conducting blind randomized trials to compare epidural and parenteral analgesia is difficult (and possibly unethical). Such problems hinder the interpretation of the results of these studies.

The mechanism of dystocia related to epidural analgesia is believed to involve motor blockade of the pelvic diaphragm by local anesthetics. The pelvic diaphragm in normal labor acts as a fixed outlet, forcing the fetus to rotate to pass beyond and enter the pelvic outlet in the correct position for delivery. With the loss of pelvic floor tone because of motor blockade induced by local anesthetic in epidural anesthesia, the fetus can enter the pelvis malrotated, which increase the chances of dystocia.

NON-OBSTETRIC SURGERY DURING PREGNANCY

Each year about 50,000 pregnant patients in the US undergo nonobstetric surgical procedures; about 2.2% of all parturients require surgery during pregnancy. This is likely an underestimate, since surgery may take place before a woman knows she is pregnant. Although it is recommended that elective surgery be delayed until after completion of pregnancy, a number of nonobstetric conditions require surgical intervention during pregnancy (e.g. trauma, appendicitis, perforated gall bladder, bleeding cerebral aneurysm, and refractory decompensating valvular or ischemic heart disease).

Surgery during pregnancy is not benign. The fetus is exposed to risks such as exposure to numerous pharmacologic agents (including anesthetics), potential disruption of uteroplacental blood flow by surgical manipulation of the uterus, and the potential for spontaneous abortion or preterm delivery of the fetus. The greatest risk for loss occurs during the first trimester and when the surgical field is near the uterus. Whether the increased risk of abortion or fetal loss is the result of the anesthetic or the surgery has not been established. This indicates the need for continued close monitoring of uterine activity perioperatively and the aggressive use of tocolytic therapy if uterine activity is associated with cervical changes.

Monitoring maternal parameters during surgery in the parturient is no different than monitoring those in a nonpregnant patient. The difficulty involves assessing the effects of the anesthetic and surgery on the fetus. As described above, uteroplacental circulation represents a low-resistance circuit that requires a narrow range of perfusion pressure to maintain adequate circulation and provide adequate oxygen to the fetus. Disruptions in the supply of oxygen to the infant are reflected in changes in baseline fetal heart rate (FHR). An abrupt hypoxic event generally results in fetal bradycardia (<120 beats/minute), as has been noted at the onset of cardiopulmonary bypass in gravid patients. The bradycardia is a reflex response to chemoreceptor activation mediated by the parasympathetic nervous system. If hypoxia is prolonged, the fetus develops acidemia, which has a direct depressant effect on contractility and heart rate. If, however, the onset of hypoxemia is slower, the initial fetal response is a transient fetal tachycardia (>160 beats/minute) and hypertension. Hypoxemia induces epinephrine release from the fetal adrenal medulla. The insidious onset of the hypoxemia may depress the parasympathetic response and may explain the difference in response with abrupt ischemia. Recovery is rapid upon restoration of fetal oxygenation (by increasing uterine blood flow, maternal oxygen saturation, or oxygen-carrying capacity).

Rebound tachycardia may initially follow the episode and reflects the stress on the fetus (e.g. adrenal stimulation).

Around the 25th to 27th week of gestation, FHR begins to fluctuate between 6 and 8 beats/minute. This beat-to-beat variability, as it is known, reflects changes in sympathetic and parasympathetic nerve activity from the fetal medulla and as such is an indicator of fetal well-being. The most reliable method of assessing this variability is with a fetal scalp electrode, which records well-defined electrocardiographic R-wave potentials for the cardiotachograph to integrate and plot. A fetal scalp electrode is not practical in the vast majority of surgical procedures in parturients and therefore an external or vaginal Doppler probe is used to monitor FHR. The signal-to-noise ratio of a Doppler transducer is poor when compared with that of a fetal scalp electrode and is not as useful in assessing subtle changes in FHR variability. However, gross changes in FHR variability, such as complete loss of beat-to-beat variability, are reliable indications of changes in fetal well-being. If fetal tachycardia or bradycardia develops during surgery, the anesthesiologist must search for maternal hypoxemia, hypotension, hypovolemia, or other causes of altered oxygen exchange within the placenta. Minimally, FHR should be assessed before and after induction of anesthesia and again at the end of surgery.

Most obstetric anesthesiologists prefer a regional anesthetic whenever possible to reduce the risk of maternal aspiration and fetal drug exposure, and possibly of spontaneous abortion when compared with a general anesthetic. This does not mean that general anesthetics cannot be delivered safely when the surgical site or patient preference excludes the option of a regional technique. If a general anesthetic is used, the patient should be carefully preoxygenated and should undergo a rapid-sequence induction–tracheal intubation.

COMPLICATIONS

Amniotic fluid embolism

Amniotic fluid embolism (AFE) represents one of the most devastating and unpreventable, although thankfully rare (incidence from 1:8000 to 1:80,000 pregnancies), events of the peripartum period. Amniotic fluid enters the maternal circulation, which results in sudden respiratory distress, cyanosis, cardiovascular collapse, and coma. These patients can exhibit severe bleeding secondary to uterine atony as well as coagulopathy. Mortality is very high (up to 86%), and accounts for 7–13% of all maternal deaths in the US. Even with aggressive care, the outcome is dismal.

The complication of AFE has occurred under many circumstances during pregnancy, from first trimester abortions to the postpartum period. It requires a route of entry (i.e. amniotomy, endocervical laceration, or uterine vessels) and an intense pressure gradient to force fluid against venous or arterial pressure. A strong association is found between AFE and placental abruption (in 50% of cases and fetal death in up to 40% of patients with AFE before symptoms).

The pathophysiology of AFE was initially believed to result solely from pulmonary hypertension and subsequent cor pulmonale, as observed in some animal models. This may be true in the first hour of the episode, but since over half of the patients die within this time, hemodynamic data in the initial period are sparse. The vast majority of patients who survive this early insult do not exhibit symptoms of right heart failure. In fact, the major defects seen in parturients who enter the second phase of AFE are left heart failure and noncardiogenic pulmonary edema, which require aggressive inotropic support and afterload reduction to maintain an adequate cardiac output. The initial hypoxia and hypotension induced by the pulmonary vasospastic response to AFE may induce left ventricular injury, which later manifests as left ventricular dysfunction and failure.

Disseminated intravascular coagulation (DIC) occurs in >50% of patients with AFE. The mechanism of DIC is unclear, although amniotic fluid induces platelet aggregation, which causes release of platelet factor III, and has a thromboplastin-like effect. Aggravating DIC-related bleeding is uterine atony, which leaves open spiral arteries that bleed into the former placental bed. With as much as 20% of the cardiac output directed toward the gravid uterus, bleeding can be brisk. The atony may result from a uterine relaxation factor in amniotic fluid.

The diagnosis of AFE is often made by exclusion. It may be diagnosed definitively by the presence of fetal squamous cells and hair in smaller pulmonary vessels. However, the almost uniform finding of fetal squamous cells in the circulation of normal pregnant individuals has thrown this into doubt.

The best therapy for these patients is supportive, directed at correcting the three major derangements – cardiorespiratory instability, DIC, and uterine atony. Cardiopulmonary resuscitation is necessary to restore circulation and blood component therapy to replace circulating volume and to treat coagulopathy. Intubation and ventilation with 100% oxygen is essential. Inotropic therapy with dopamine has proved effective, and hydrocortisone administration may improve survival. Restoration of blood pressure is imperative to treat uterine atony when intractable to oxytocins. If the patient is to survive this cataclysmic event, resuscitation efforts must be rapid and aggressive.

Aspiration

Anesthesia is the third and fifth leading cause of direct maternal mortality in the UK and the US, respectively. Aspiration of stomach contents remains one of the greatest risks of general anesthesia during pregnancy, accounting for up to 25–50% of anesthesia-related deaths. The mortality from aspiration varies widely in reports, from 3 to 60%, which most likely reflects the differences in degree and type of aspirate, diagnostic criteria, and therapy.

The physiologic changes in gastrointestinal function during pregnancy (see above) enhance the risks of aspiration during induction and intubation. Modern obstetric anesthesia practice has relegated general endotracheal anesthesia primarily to emergent situations when, unfortunately, the risk of failed intubation and aspiration are even higher.

Three factors play a major role in the morbidity and mortality of aspiration – the pH of the aspirate, whether it is particulate or nonparticulate, and the total volume. Classic teaching suggested that greatest morbidity and mortality in nonparticulate aspiration occurred if the was pH <2.5 and the volume >25mL. However, recent reports suggest that the required volume for aspiration pneumonitis may be higher (>50mL), although the threshold pH may be higher as well (<3.5). Acid within the alveoli induces edema, fibrin, and cellular debris (red and white blood cells). The loss of normal surfactant function causes a decreased compliance, further alveolar edema, loss of lung volume, and shunting of pulmonary blood flow. These pathophysiologic responses lead to hypoxemia, which is the universal presenting symptom. The damage and the subsequent cascade of response to injury by attracted neutrophils and macrophages lead to oxygen radical formation and may result in adult respiratory distress syndrome (see Chapters 49 and 50). When aspiration includes large particulate matter, obstruction of bronchi or bronchioles and distal atelectasis occur.

Clinical response depends upon the character and volume of the aspirate. Bronchospasm is common, hypoxemia can be immediate or delayed, and hypotension in combination with increased cardiac filling pressures can accompany severe hypoxemia.

Therapy for aspiration is directed at treating hypoxemia, supporting hemodynamics, and removing obstruction if aspiration is particulate. Continuous positive airway pressure (CPAP) or positive end expiratory pressure (PEEP) therapy is administered to spontaneously breathing or ventilated patients, respectively, although the efficacy of either is questionable. These therapeutic measures allow for a decrease in fractional inspired oxygen concentration (FIO_2). However, CPAP and PEEP can reduce left ventricular filling, and thereby decrease cardiac output, and can alter regional pulmonary blood flow, both of which may ultimately decrease oxygen delivery. FIO_2 should be reduced to <50% to maintain arterial oxygen saturation at least in the 90–95% range. Bronchoscopy may be necessary to remove large particles. The response to corticosteroids and prophylactic antibiotics is unclear and their use lacks objective evidence of efficacy.

The best treatment for aspiration is prevention. Prophylactic therapy includes:

- ingestion of a nonparticulate antacid (e.g. 0.3mol/L sodium citrate) before induction to raise stomach pH;
- H_2-receptor antagonists (e.g. cimetidine, ranitidine, or famotidine) either orally or intravenously to reduce acid secretion; and
- metoclopramide to lower stomach volume.

Induction and intubation should be in rapid sequence with cricoid pressure using Sellick's maneuver to reduce the chances of passive aspiration of stomach contents.

Hemorrhage

Blood loss following vaginal delivery can routinely be 250–700mL. Maternal blood volume increases during pregnancy not only to provide the increase in blood flow for the increased demands of pregnancy, but also to buffer the parturient from detrimental effects of postdelivery bleeding. However, bleeding either before or following delivery can be profound and life threatening. Hemorrhage is still a major cause of maternal mortality worldwide.

Placenta previa

Placenta previa represents the cause of about one-third of vaginal bleeding in the late second and third trimester (incidence from 0.1 to 1% of pregnancies). However, since the bleeding it produces can be so profuse, all vaginal bleeding in the third trimester is considered placenta previa until proved otherwise. Placenta previa literally means 'placenta going ahead'. It involves implantation of the placenta near or over the internal os of the cervix, with potential for maternal hemorrhage as the placenta is torn off the uterine wall (Fig. 65.8). The blood that is lost is maternal (with the rare exception of vasa previa in which the blood loss is fetal). Since the placenta is implanted in the lower segment of the uterus, an area with sparse smooth muscle contribution, the normal mechanisms of contraction of the uterine wall around open spiral arteries works poorly. It appears to be more prevalent in patients who are multiparous and in those with a history of previous cesarean section; each of these risk factors is consistent with the understanding that

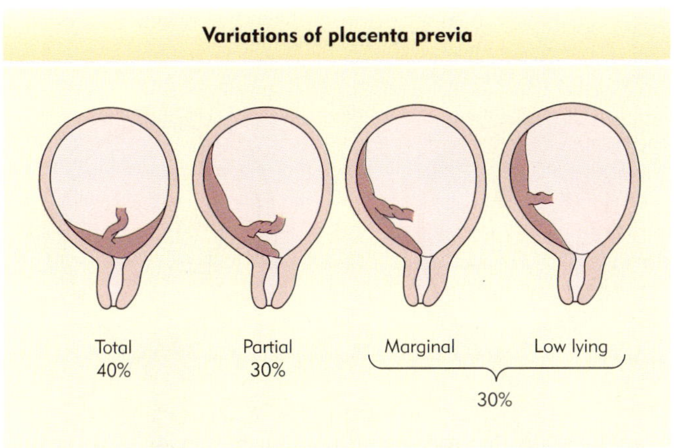

Figure 65.8 Variations of placenta previa. If the placenta covers the cervical os, it is said to be complete or total. Other variations of placenta previa are classified by the proximity to the placenta and the degree to which it overlies the cervix. (Adapted with permission from Suresh MS, Belfort MA. Antepartum hemorrhage. In: Datta S, ed. Anesthetic and obstetric management of high-risk pregnancy. St Louis: Mosby; 1996:76–109.)

endometrial damage causes the lower implantation site. The sentinel bleeding episode generally occurs well into the second trimester, when the uterus undergoes its greatest increase in size and in so doing disrupts spiral arteries as the placenta undergoes a tug-of-war from all sides of the cervix.

Placental abruption

Abruptio placentae represents the premature separation of the placenta from the basalis membrane of the uterus with resultant bleeding from the exposed spiral arteries (incidence of 0.2–2.4% of pregnancies). This separation, which occurs most commonly within the final 10 weeks of pregnancy, can be complete or partial. The abruption causes a disruption of the spiral arteries in the region of the separation and the formation of a decidual hematoma, which pushes the placenta further away from its basal attachments and results in a vicious cycle of more disruption (Fig. 65.9). As the abruption expands, more placental function is lost. If the disruption extends to the placental margin, blood can either escape into the amniotic cavity to mix with amniotic fluid ('port wine' fluid) or track out to escape through the cervix. Even when the hemorrhage is revealed in this fashion, a true estimation of blood loss can be difficult to make. Extensive amounts of hemorrhage can be concealed behind the placenta, which may lead to misdiagnosis of the problem and then to profound maternal hypovolemia. Blood tracking below the decidua induces contraction of the uterus. As the pressure within the uterus rises, tissue thromboplastins and/or amniotic fluid may be pushed into the maternal circulation, which results in DIC and possibly AFE (see above).

Placenta accreta, percreta, or increta

When the placenta implants deep into the uterus, beyond the basalis membrane, it becomes unusually adherent and may result in incomplete separation of the placenta or tearing of the uterus with severe maternal bleeding. These abnormal implantations are categorized according to the degree of penetration into or beyond the uterine myometrium (Fig. 65.10). In *placenta accreta*, the syncytiotrophoblasts anchor the placenta onto the myometrium. Placental penetration and adherence into the myometrium is

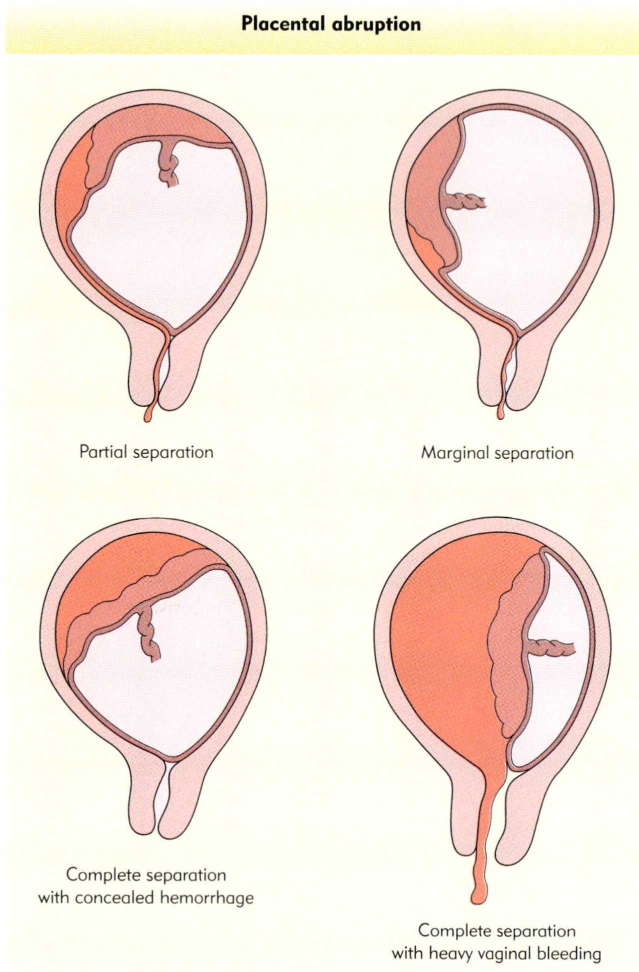

Figure 65.9 Placental abruption is classified by the degree of placental separation from the uterus. Bleeding is generally overt, but sometimes it is concealed and can be extensive. (Adapted with permission from Suresh MS, Belfort MA. Antepartum hemorrhage. In: Datta S, ed. Anesthetic and obstetric management of high-risk pregnancy. St Louis: Mosby; 1996:76–109.)

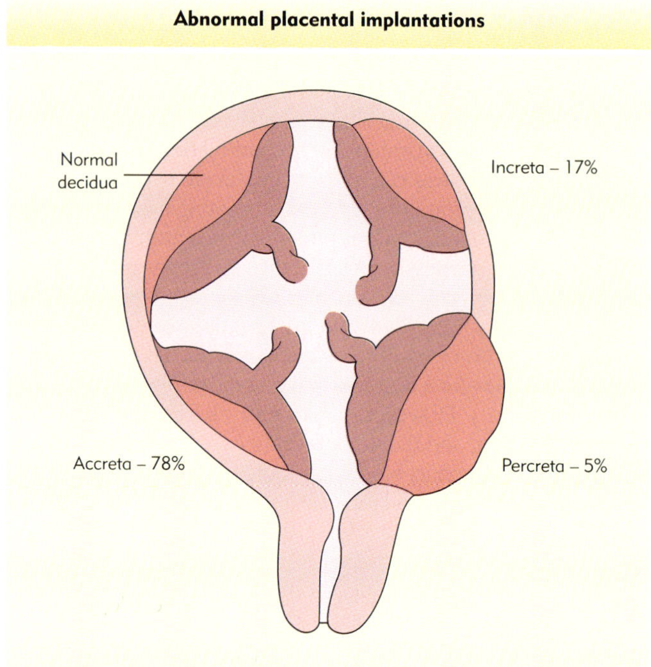

Figure 65.10 Unusual placental adherence can signal abnormal placentation. The classification placenta accreta, increta, and percreta refers to the extent to which the placenta anchors into or through the uterine myometrium. (Adapted with permission from Suresh MS, Belfort MA. Antepartum hemorrhage. In: Datta S, ed. Anesthetic and obstetric management of high-risk pregnancy. St Louis: Mosby; 1996:76–109.)

called *placenta increta*. There is an association between placenta accreta and increta and placenta previa, particularly when a prior cesarean section has occurred. With open uterine spinal arteries, either because the surrounding myometrium has been avulsed away during placental removal (thereby preventing hemostasis by contraction) or because retained placental attachments with the arteries essentially act as stents, bleeding can be catastrophic. Blood loss in excess of 4L is not uncommon. Over 20% of patients with placenta accreta and increta develop coagulopathies as a result of the aggressive resuscitation of shock and as many as 70% require cesarean hysterectomy.

The most dangerous subtype of placenta accreta is *placenta percreta*, in which placental villi completely penetrate the myometrium and in rare instances actually implant onto abdominal organs (e.g. bladder, colon, and small bowel). Attempts to remove the placenta in this situation lead not only to observable uterine bleeding, but also to intra-abdominal hemorrhage from the uterus and other organs. Mortality can be high (>60%) without immediate cesarean hysterectomy and prompt fluid and blood product resuscitation.

Uterine rupture

Another rare but dangerous complication of pregnancy and delivery is a rupture of the uterus (incidence 0.1–0.2% of deliveries). The etiologies of uterine rupture include trauma, dehiscence of a prior uterine scar (cesarean or myomectomy), and spontaneous. It has been associated with use of oxytocin, multigravidity, podalic version (internal and external), and cephalopelvic disproportion. Mortality in traumatic and spontaneous uterine rupture is as high as 56%, which accounts for nearly one half of all deaths from uterine hemorrhage and for 5% of total maternal mortality. Fetal mortality is up to 80%.

Key References

Chestnut DH. Epidural analgesia and the incidence of cesarean section: time for another close look. Anesthesiology. 1997;87:472–6.
Clark SL. Amniotic fluid embolism. Crit Care Clin. 1991;7:877–82.
Herman NL. The placenta: anatomy, physiology, and transfer of drug. In: Chestnut DH, ed. Obstetric anesthesia: principles and practice. St Louis: Mosby; 1999:57–74.
Herman NL. Surgery during pregnancy. In: Norris MC, ed. Obstetric anesthesia. Philadelphia: JB Lippincott; 1999:161–85.
Williams DJ, de Swiet M. The pathophysiology of pre-eclampsia. Intensive Care Med. 1997;23:620–9.

Further Reading

Clark SL, Hankins GD, Dudley DA, Dildy GA, Porter TF. Amniotic fluid embolism: analysis of the national registry. Am J Obstet Gynecol. 1995;172:1158–67.
Dewan DM, Cohen SE. Epidural analgesia and the incidence of cesarean section. Time for a closer look. Anesthesiology. 1994;80:1189–92.
Guyton TS, Gibbs CP. Aspiration: risk, prophylaxis, and treatment. In: Chestnut DH, ed. Obstetric anesthesia: principles and practice. St Louis: Mosby; 1999:578–89.
Schobel HP, Fischer T, Heuszer K, Geiger H, Schmieder RE. Preeclampsia – a state of sympathetic overactivity. N Engl J Med. 1996;335:1480–5.
Suresh MS, Belfort MA. Antepartum hemorrhage. In: Datta S, ed. Anesthetic and obstetric management of high-risk pregnancy. St Louis: Mosby; 1996:76–109.

Chapter 66 Geriatrics

Jeffrey H Silverstein and
Michael Zaugg

Topics covered in this chapter

Theories of aging
Neurologic system
Cardiovascular system
Respiratory system
Drug disposition

In 1927, an age of 50 years was considered a relative contraindication to surgical repair of an inguinal hernia. By 1994, 31,000 patients over the age of 65 years were discharged from US hospitals following inguinal hernia repair while another 114,000 had the same procedure done on an ambulatory surgery basis. Two parallel phenomena underlie this change. Anesthesia developed from an infant adjunct of surgery into a complicated, and much safer, medical specialty. Simultaneously, the 20th century has witnessed the greatest increase in longevity in recorded history (Fig. 66.1) In 1995, the estimated life expectancy at birth was 75.8 years. Improvements in public health have been primarily responsible for the increase in life expectancy. As a result of increased longevity, the population of older individuals continues to grow. It is projected that there will be 35.3 million persons over the age of 65 years in the USA by the year 2000. Today, patients over 65 years of age represent an important proportion of most anesthetic practices. Roughly 50% of people over age 65 years will have at least one operation before death.

Aging might be described as the composite of all changes that occur in an organism with the passage of time, incorporating the findings that functional impairment and the likelihood of death increase with aging. Aging has also been characterized as a progressive deterioration of those physiologic processes necessary to maintain homeostasis, death being the ultimate failure of these mechanisms. Senescence may be defined as the progressive loss of physiologic functions with aging. Longevity, then, is the summation of forces that prevent or retard senescence. Aging clearly progresses at different rates in different individuals; physiologic age of older patients is more important than chronologic age. Physiologically, all 20-year-old humans are more similar than all 75-year-old humans. This variability represents a key modulating concept in aging; the balance between senescence and longevity provides the basis for this variability. An important distinction is between normal aging, that which would be identified in an aging cohort thought to be relatively free of disease, and 'successful aging', which is the process by which individuals reach advanced age with relatively

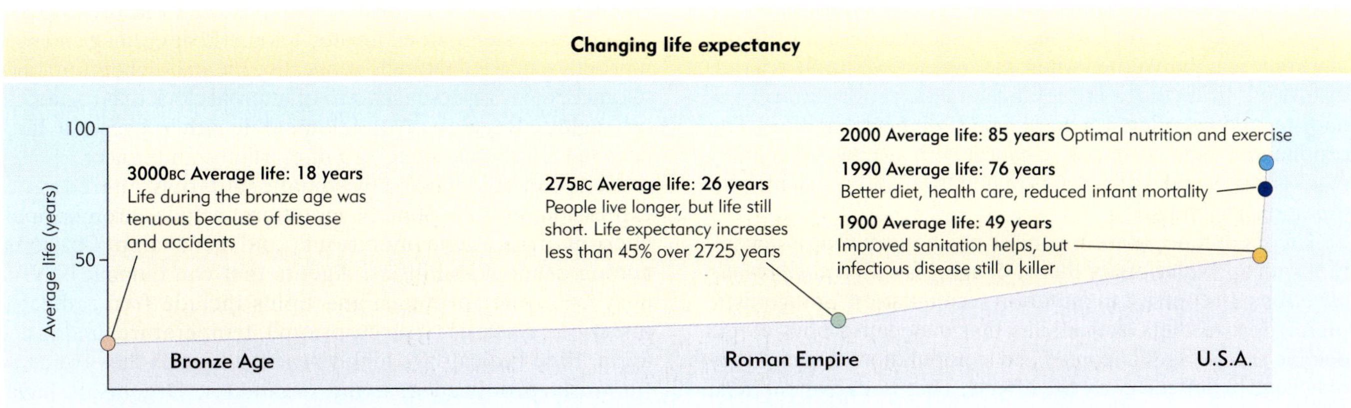

Figure 66.1 Changing life expectancy. The 20th century has seen the greatest increase in life expectancy in recorded history, primarily through improvements in public health and an associated decrease in infant mortality. (With permission from American Federation of Aging Research, 1995.)

minimal impairment. A balance in favor of longevity over senescence defines successful aging. This concept also highlights a singularly difficult aspect of aging research, that of defining the population to be included in any study of aging phenomena. Modern gerontology eschews the previous assumption that, in the absence of disease, other age-related alterations such as modest cognitive deterioration or changes in blood glucose metabolism were normal. Successful aging includes low probability of disease and related disability, high physical and cognitive function, and active engagement with life.

Research into the aging process and its implications has been extensive since the 1960s. This chapter provides a foundation for the science underlying anesthetic care of the geriatric patient; a few areas have been selected for more extensive treatment as examples of the depth and breadth of knowledge. Multiple concomitant diseases are the rule in geriatric patients, and are associated with increased risk of perioperative complications.

THEORIES OF AGING

Many theories of aging have been proposed. Each theory must explain three basic observations: why organisms undergo physiologic decline in later life; why there is variation in life span within and between species; and why certain experimental paradigms such as dietary restriction and selection for delayed reproduction delay the onset of aging and extend the life span of animals.

Gerontology as a science is but three to four decades old. Consequently, much of the theoretic basis of this scientific endeavor is still developing. Most theories refer to aging as if it were a single process, but gerontologists now suggest that a single unitary theory of aging is unlikely and unnecessary.

Two population genetic mechanisms have been invoked in the development of the evolutionary theory of aging. The first, *mutation accumulation*, posits that alleles with neutral early effects will not be eliminated by natural selection despite deleterious effects in later life. The frequency of the allele will be determined by genetic drift and, therefore, it will not be present in high frequency in large populations. Continuous damage occurs to DNA but is rapidly eliminated by a number of repair enzymes. In mutation accumulation, DNA mutations would be expected to correlate with life span. In addition, genetic diseases in which higher levels of DNA damage or a marked deficiency in DNA repair are present should also manifest premature aging. Genetic defects in enzymes called helicases, which unwind the DNA double helix, are responsible for the Bloom syndrome and the Werner syndrome. Werner syndrome is a rare disorder that includes bilateral cataracts, progeria, hypogonadism, and a tendency toward type II diabetes mellitus. The exponential increase in risk of cancer with age, which in many cases is associated with a series of mutations, is consistent with mutation accumulation.

The second population genetic mechanism that is consistent with an evolutionary theory of aging is called *antagonistic pleiotropy*. In contrast to mutation accumulation, antagonistic pleiotropy predicts that alleles that may cause physiologic decline at later ages become fixed in populations because they may have beneficial early life effects. That is, early beneficial effects lead to selection and accumulation, even though the subsequent effect is deleterious to the organism. This mechanism suggests that there is a means to determine time in life, a biologic clock of sorts. This 'clock' has yet to be detected. There are a very few disease entities that are consistent with antagonistic pleiotropy, that is genetic disorders that have late-life onset such as Huntington's chorea and idiopathic hemochromatosis. Both mechanisms and their associated predictions have been supported by experimentation in animal models including *Drosophilia* (fruit fly) and *Caenorhabditis elegans* (round worm).

In spite of any success that evolutionary theory may have had in unifying concepts of aging, many theories of aging remain capable of explaining certain aspects. Theories of aging are divided into physiologic, cellular, and molecular categories (Fig. 66.2). Wear and tear theory proposes that death is the result of cumulative damage to vital body parts. While originally conceived in terms of organs or organisms, at the level of DNA the question once again becomes one of the balance between damage and repair capacity. The active agent of senescence could then be the accumulated detritus or the damaged DNA itself. At the physiologic level, senescence can be correlated with metabolic rate, the higher the metabolic rate per unit of body mass the shorter the life span. Thermal manipulation of metabolic rate was utilized in the original experiments examining this concept. Manipulation by persistent exercise has shown no effect on life span. In certain species, reproductive exhaustion can be seen to have dramatic effects. For example, the life span of a salmon, which spawns and then dies, can be dramatically extended by castration. Hormonal dysregulation, particularly of glucocorticoids, have been implicated, particularly in neuronal aging. The idea that cells possess a limited capacity to divide was initially developed by Hayflick working with human fibroblasts. There are a limited number of 'passages' in cultured cells, which are related to the life span of the source of the cells (i.e. a cell can only divide a limited number of times). The broader concept of the Hayflick limit is sometimes used to represent the theoretic upper limit of survivability of a given species.

A potential underlying mechanism of limited cell division is telomere shortening. Telomeres are repeated sequences of DNA at the ends of each chromosome that maintain the integrity of the chromosome. They protect chormosomes from degradation or fusion with other chromosomes. Telomere length is shortened each time a cell divides, and a mutation in yeast that shortens telomeres causes early senescence. Once the telomeres reach a critically short length, the cell stops dividing. Telomerase, an enzyme that replaces telomeric DNA, has recently been expressed in mortal human cells. The presence of this enzyme essentially eliminated telomeric shortening and significantly extended the cells' replicative life span. Therefore, the telomeres may represent a form of internal clock that regulates cell aging. Regulation of telomere length suggests a link between telomeres, aging, cell immortality, and cancer.

Cells can be damaged by somatic mutation, altered gene expression, or both. Somatic mutations include chromosomal abnormalities, gene mutations, and gene amplifications among other possibilities. Agents that can damage DNA, enzymes, other proteins, and lipids include free radicals, infectious diseases (viruses, prions), temperature, and radiation. Free radicals are highly reactive species that are continuously produced in living organisms. Organisms have developed extensive antioxidant defense systems such as the enzymes superoxide dismutase, catalase, and glutathione peroxidase. The administration of antioxidants has been reported to increase life span, but alterations in other aspects of metabolism cannot be excluded in interpreting these experiments.

Some theories of aging		
Physiologic effects	**Cellular effects**	**Molecular effects**
Wear and tear	Limited cellular replication	Somatic mutation
Infectious disease	Pathogies of metabolism	Autoimmune failure
Depletion of resources	Differentiation	Vertebrate oncogenes
Reproductive exhaustion	Telomere shortening	RNA: error/catastrophe
Rate of living		Free radicals
Hormonal controls		Collagen cross-linkage DNA methylation

Figure 66.2 Some theories of aging. (Reprinted from Graves JL Jr, General theories of aging: unification and synthesis. In: Dani SU, Hori A, Walter GF, eds. Principles for neural aging. Copyright 1997, p.37, with kind permission of Elsevier Science–NL, Sara Burgerhartstraat 25, 1055 KV Amsterdam, The Netherlands.)

Proponents of these theories suggest that persistent minor damage accumulates over time, resulting in the changes observed as aging (i.e. mutation accumulation). Support for this theory includes the observations that overexpression of antioxidant enzymes can extend the the life span of *Drosophilia* spp.; variation in the rates of mitochondrial superoxide anion is inversely correlated with longevity, and caloric restriction is associated with a decrease in oxidative stress.

Theoretic considerations have generally followed extensive descriptive evaluation of the aged and aging. Folkow and Svanbourg focused on four general manifestations of aging: a slow progressive reduction of both peripheral and central neuronal networks; slow decline in muscle cell number, strength, and speed of contraction; slow decline in tissue compliance or distensibility; and modest decline in basal metabolic rate and oxygen consumption per unit body weight.

Within aging studies, it is possible to study different cohorts of individuals, for example a young group of college students compared with an elderly cohort. A number of difficulties are associated with this approach. First, many physiologic variables peak between the ages of 20 and 30 years and then decline. A second issue is that the elderly individuals included in a study are those that survived, while the 'control' group of young individuals includes those who have potentially higher and earlier mortality. Finally, utilization of a general linear statistical model is substantially limited by the use of only two age points. Many of these drawbacks are avoided by the use of longitudinal study designs, in which a single group or multiple age groups are followed over a prolonged period of time. However, this design strategy incurs significant logistical difficulties.

NEUROLOGIC SYSTEM

Central neurologic changes are some of the most profound changes associated with aging and account for approximately 50% of disability after age 65 years. Neuronal loss was long thought to be a hallmark of aging, although the mechanism of neuronal attrition is not understood. Extensive neuroanatomic studies discerned, for example, a 48% decrease in neuronal density in the visual cortex from the third to the ninth decade of life. Similar losses were reported to occur in the cortex, hippocampus, anterior thalamus, and the locus ceruleus. This well-accepted concept was brought into question by recent evidence in which advanced screening methods were used to eliminate patients who had signs of Alzheimer's disease. One important study found age-related decrements in brain weight, cortical thickness in the midfrontal and superior temporal areas, large neurons in all three areas, and the neuron:glia ratio in the midfrontal and inferior parietal areas. However, the total number of neurons, percentage of cell area, and neuronal density were all unchanged. The number of small neurons in the midfrontal cortex and glia in the midfrontal and superior temporal areas increased with age.

Evaluation at the ultrastructural level provides similar, highly specific findings that defy a simplistic view of brain aging. For example, both the perforant path and *N*-methyl-D-aspartate (NMDA) receptors are important in memory formation. A 30.6% decrease in the ratio of NMDA receptor type 1 immunofluorescence intensity in the distal dendrites relative to proximal dendrites of rat dentate gyrus granule cells without a similar alteration of non-NMDA receptors occurred with aging. These findings suggest a circuit-specific alteration in the intradendritic concentration of NMDA type 1 receptors without concomitant gross structural changes in dendritic morphology or a significant change in the total synaptic density. Extensive evaluation of other receptors has produced a catalog of contradictory age-related alterations that currently defies elucidation of a clear pattern.

Age-related alterations of γ-aminobutyric acid (GABA) receptors are relevant to anesthesia (see Chapters 6 & 22). Early studies were fairly consistent in describing a 20–30% decrease in benzodiazepine-binding sites in cerebral cortex, hippocampus, and cerebellum. However, more recent work has found changes only in specific regions, but these observations are inconsistent between different studies. A series of reports concerning subunit densities in the inferior colliculus (associated with hearing) have found alterations in messenger ribonucleic acid (mRNA) of specific subunits of the $GABA_A$ receptor. This is interesting given the correlation between auditory evoked mid-latency potentials and anesthetic potency. Preliminary findings suggest a correlation between altered $GABA_A$ receptors and age-related alterations of anesthetic potency.

The change in perception of patterns of neuronal loss and reactive gliosis in the brain has yet to be evaluated to the same extent in the spinal cord. Reports of loss of small neurons in the intermediate zone of the ventral horn associated with preservation of larger neurons in the medial and lateral nuclei suggest a lack of generalized neuron loss. Conduction velocities of spinal nerves decrease to a clinically insignificant extent. The clinical result is not necessarily apparent from these alterations. In a series of experiments evaluating the effects of aging on spinal opioid-induced antinociception, aging animals responded more rapidly to painful stimuli and required higher doses of intrathecal opioid agonists to produce significant increases in tail-flick latency (time to pain response) in aged rats.

The routine mental state examination in the elderly should be normal. While complaints of subjective memory loss and cognitive deficits are common and neuropsychologic evaluation does show slowing of central processing time, acquisition of new information, and a decline in 'fluid intelligence', these changes are below the threshold of detectability of most clinical mental state examinations. Clear abnormalities in mental state should not be attributed to aging but should lead to consideration of a differential diagnosis. Aging does appear to be a significant risk factor for cognitive dysfunction following anesthesia. A recent study of 1218 patients over 60 years of age found a 9.8% incidence of cognitive dysfunction following general anesthesia at 3 months following operation. Age was significantly correlated with this effect.

CARDIOVASCULAR SYSTEM

Hypertension and atherosclerosis are the most common disorders of the elderly, and more than 50% have significant coronary artery disease, often without symptoms. The chemical and ultrastructural changes of the aging myocardium have been studied quite extensively. Two major areas of research are of particular interest in anesthesiology: age-related alterations in β-adrenergic function and structural alterations of the heart and vessels. Both areas have expanded our understanding of cardiovascular function in the elderly.

In healthy humans in the absence of coronary artery disease, hypertension, or severe deconditioning, resting cardiovascular performance is not significantly altered (Fig. 66.3). However, during significant exercise there is less of an increase in heart rate while stroke volume is maintained or increased. This pattern is similar to that in younger individuals who undergo exercise in the presence of β-adrenergic blockade. This is particularly intriguing given that circulating levels of norepinephrine (noradrenaline), but not epinephrine (adrenaline), increase progressively with aging. Extensive studies of myocardium as well as other tissues have failed to identify a decrease in β-adrenoceptor density. The β-adrenoceptors are G-protein linked and exist in at least two states, described as high- and low-affinity states (see Chapter 29). Beta-adrenergic agonist binding affinity is significantly decreased with aging in rat myocardium; this observation is associated primarily with a decrease in the proportion of receptors in the high-affinity state. Affinity for β-adrenergic antagonists, however, is not altered with age. Other aspects of the β-adrenergic cascade including G-protein activity and the adenylyl cyclase catalytic subunit have also been shown to decrease with aging but somewhat less consistently than the relative affinity alterations of the β-adrenoceptor. Phosphorylation mediated by β-adrenoceptors, but not dephosphorylation of troponin I, is decreased in aging myocytes. Therefore, alterations in the function of the β-adrenergic system in aging myocardium are not the result of a single specific alteration but rather of multiple changes that occur at different levels of the β-adrenergic signaling cascade. It is not known whether alterations in other segments of the cascade [e.g. β-adrenoceptor kinase (β-ARK) and β-arrestin] occur with normal aging. In contrast to β-adrenergic system function, α_1-adrenergic functions appear to be preserved during aging while α_2-adrenergic responses appear to be decreased. Vagal cholinergic tone increases in aging rats. Finally, there is a suggestion that thyroid hormone can compensate for age-related alterations in adrenergic tone.

Structural changes in the heart and major vessels contribute greatly to the altered physiology of the aging cardiovascular system. Some of the hemodynamic alterations seen in aging are explained in part by physical alterations in the vessels and myocardium. Aging is associated with a decrease in connective tissue compliance and distensibility, primarily as a result of increased cross-bridging between elastin and collagen filaments. One result is the well-known elongation, stiffening, and widening of the aorta. Stiffening of the aorta results in a higher peak systolic pressure, which considerably increases afterload. In addition to systemic vascular resistance, pulse-wave reflection from the periphery is integrated into the overall pressure characteristics that constitute the afterload of the left ventricle. When the ventricle contracts, a pulse wave is transmitted and at least partially reflected back into the great vessels. Pulse-wave velocity increases two- to threefold with aging. In the cardiovascular systems of the young, the reflected pulse wave tends to arrive following systole, but in the elderly this component is appended to the end-systolic afterload. Standard measurement of blood pressure by sphygmomanometry fails to discern this aspect of pressure as the reflected wave is not retransmitted significantly down the arterial tree.

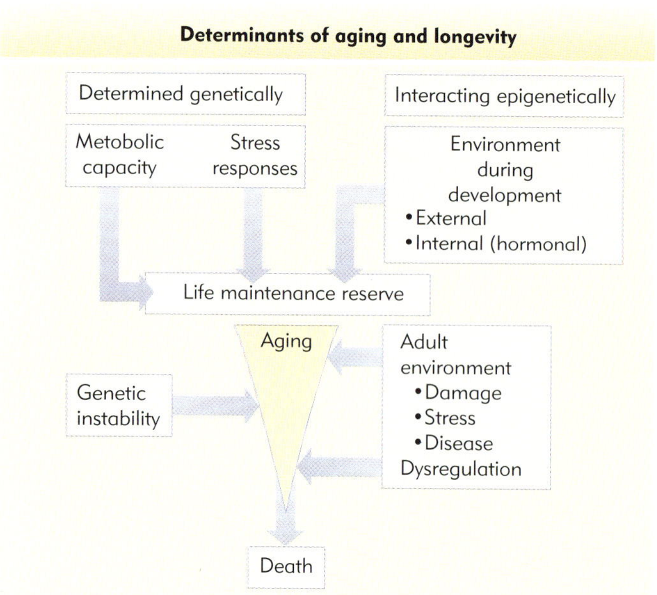

Figure 66.3 Determinants of aging and longevity. Rather than molecular mechanisms, physiologic mechanisms of aging are described. Environment, metabolic capacity, and stress responses all contribute to the life maintenance reserve. Genetic instability is influenced by environmental factors. The essential concept is that aging functions at all levels of biological organization; itis not possible to seperate cellular changes from organismal aging. (With permission from Jazwinski SM. Longevity, Genes, and Aging. Science:1996;273:57.)

Age-related alteration in aortic-arterial stiffness is one of the most serious normal changes that affect the aging human cardiovascular system. Figure 66.4 depicts the essential alterations of the aging heart as a response to increased afterload. The heart is unusual in that it does not decrease in size with age whereas that of most other organs does increase. While fewer myocytes are present, there is a general hypertrophy of the cells and a marked increase in connective tissue. Cardiac structural alterations in the human are not well represented by rat models but are well described. The two primary alterations that are noted in elderly hearts in the absence of disease states and severe deconditioning are concentric left ventricular hypertrophy and a substantial decline in diastolic compliance. Left ventricular wall thickness increases with age secondary to myocardial hypertrophy and there are increases in connective tissue components, including fibrous tissue, lipids, and collagen. Echocardiographic measurements describe a 30% increase in left ventricular wall thickness, with intraventricular septal thickness increasing to the greatest extent.

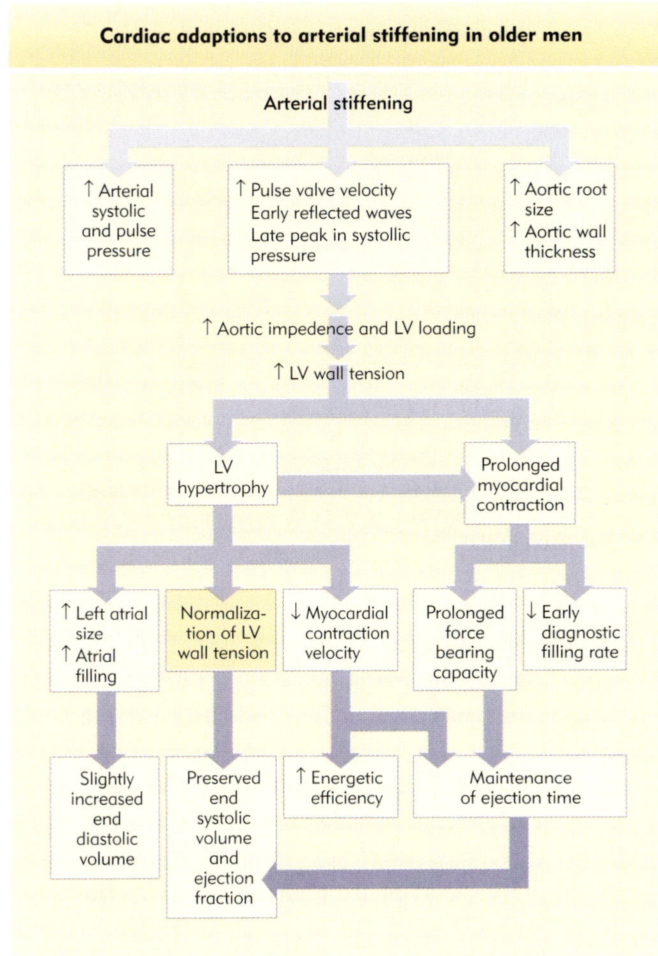

Figure 66.4 Cardiac adaptations to arterial stiffening in older men. Most of the changes in the aging heart can be seen to be the result of alterations in stiffness of the aorta. (LV, left ventricular.) (With permission from Lakkata E. In: Abrams WB,. Beer MH, Berkow R, eds. The Merck manual of geriatrics, 2nd edn. Copyright 1995 by Merck & Co., Inc., Whitehouse Station: NJ.)

Alterations in diastolic compliance are seen primarily in humans and not in elderly rats. Calcium ions are removed from the myocardial cytoplasm to the sarcoplasmic reticulum during diastole, a process requiring substantial energy (see Chapter 34). Relaxation is dependent on this process, which is substantially impaired during aging. There is also a suggestion of decreased oxygen utilization by mitochondria. Finally, a prolonged action potential and isovolemic relaxation time in senescent hearts delays diastolic filling. The result is a 50% decline in early diastolic ventricular filling in the aged. The importance of atrial contraction to ventricular filling increases from 10% in young adults to 30% in elderly subjects. Recently, a decrease in early diastolic filling was described in a group of older male athletes. From a comparison of these conditioned individuals with a sedentary cohort, it was concluded that diastolic dysfunction is intrinsic to aging rather than the result of a reduction in aerobic capacity.

Left ventricular end-diastolic pressure is increased, both at rest and during exercise, secondary to altered diastolic relaxation. Higher pressure is needed to achieve the same stroke volume. The upper limit of pressure at which hydrostatic forces are overcome is not altered with age. Therefore, the aged heart can be exquisitely sensitive to alterations in ventricular preload, particularly loss of the atrial systole. Cardiac output, despite multiple reports of progressive decline with age, is essentially maintained in subjects who are carefully screened to exclude occult disease.

The response to exercise by the elderly as an index of organ reserve has long been of interest to anesthesiologists. While cardiac performance at rest may not be altered, major limitations occur during strenuous exercise. Maximum aerobic capacity decreases with age. Conditioning and the presence of even occult coronary artery disease play an important limiting role. While maximum oxygen consumption declines with age, this is not entirely a consequence of alterations in the central circulation. It is possible that an age-related difference in muscle mass, oxidation capacity per unit muscle, and/or inability to shunt blood to exercising muscles could also contribute.

The nature of the physiologic changes of the aging heart predicts the clinical implications. Diastolic-based cardiac dysfunction has been distinguished from systolic dysfunction as a cause of heart failure (see Chapter 39). A number of studies indicate a significant and increasing prevalence of coronary artery disease in elderly patients. Therefore, although pure age-related alterations in the cardiovascular system have been well delineated, it is the unusual patient who has a cardiovascular system altered solely by the processes of normal aging, particularly in Western civilizations.

RESPIRATORY SYSTEM

The loss of respiratory function with aging varies widely between individuals of the same chronologic age. In general, the elderly have a greater predisposition to pulmonary dysfunction during the perioperative period. The primary age-related alterations are progressive (20–30%) loss of alveolar surface area, a reduction of the elastic recoil of lung tissue combined with stiffening of the chest wall, decreased strength of the respiratory muscles, and impaired nervous control of ventilation.

Chronic oxidative damage to lung tissue by environmental factors, including oxygen free radicals, is thought to be responsible for the tissue alterations typically found in the aged lung. Antioxidant consumption (e.g. vitamins C and E) can improve lung function in elderly patients. Microscopically, senile respiratory bronchioles and alveolar ducts are dilated and the pores of Kohn become larger and more numerous. Whole alveolar septa may be eliminated by this process, which is called interalveolar fenestration or ductectasia. In contrast to emphysematous lung tissue, no signs of destruction or inflammation can be demonstrated in this process. However, marked fibrosis is frequently present. The direct consequences of the reduced alveolar surface area are a slightly increased alveolar deadspace and a decreased oxygen diffusing capacity. From youth to age 80 years, maximal diffusing capacity can decrease by up to 50%.

The elastic properties of lung tissue and thoracic wall gradually change with aging. The chest wall becomes stiffer (calcification of the ribs, arthritic changes in rib and vertebral joints) and less compliant, while the lung parenchyma loses elastic recoil and becomes more compliant secondary to modified protein cross-linking, rearrangement of collagen fibrils and elastin, and an altered surfactant composition. Clinically, this results in a more barrel-shaped chest with a flattened diaphragm. The new equilibrium of the opposing thoracic and pulmonary forces increases the interpleural pressure by 2–4cmH_2O and has a significant impact on the static and dynamic lung volumes, as well as on the respiratory mechanics (Fig. 66.5; see Chapter 42). Residual volume (RV) increases with age by 5–10% per decade and the functional residual capacity (FRC) by 1–3% per decade. Expiratory and inspiratory reserve volumes (ERV, IRV) and, therefore, vital capacity (VC = ERV + IRV) decrease. Specific (height-adapted) total lung capacity (TLC) does not change with aging. The small increase in FRC with aging is disputed but is not clinically relevant since it is overcome by a 20% reduction in FRC following induction of anesthesia. Forced expiratory volume in 1 second (FEV_1) can be significantly reduced in old people (by 6–8% per decade), and FEV_1/VC may even fall below 70% in apparently healthy individuals. The loss of elastic recoil results in a narrowing of small airways (diameter less than 1mm) and increases the closing volume (CV). The closing capacity (RV + CV) may even be larger than FRC, thus closing the small airways during normal tidal breathing. This may significantly impair pulmonary gas exchange.

Application of Laplace's law to diaphragmatic contraction demonstrates that the flattened diaphragm of old people must generate more power to attain necessary transpulmonary pressure. The diaphragmatic efficacy is additionally impaired by a significant age-related loss of motor neurons, particularly fast twitch fibers II. While the work of breathing at rest is unchanged with age, vigorous exercise may elevate the work of breathing by 30%.

Arterial oxygen tension falls approximately 5mmHg per decade from 20 years of age. This is primarily a result of increased ventilation/perfusion maldistribution rather than decreased diffusing capacity. Alterations in hypoxic pulmonary vasoconstriction and hypocapnic bronchoconstriction may also contribute to age-related ventilation/perfusion maldistribution. The magnitude of shunting can be markedly increased by atelectasis following induction of anesthesia. Unfortunately, positive end-expiratory pressure has a limited impact on atelectasis since the elastic recoil curves of atelectatic and nonatelectactic lung units can be quite different (zones of different time constants). Finally, an increased tendency for upper airway collapse, decreased tonic activity of upper airway muscles (pharyngeal collapse), and decreased ventilatory response to both hypercapnia and hypoxia are present in the elderly. Consequently, a dangerous predisposition to hypoxemia exists in the perioperative period. The loss of protective reflexes also increases the risk of aspiration. Finally, both hypercapnic and hypoxemic respiratory drive are decreased to a greater degree in older people by both sedative drugs and analgesic medications.

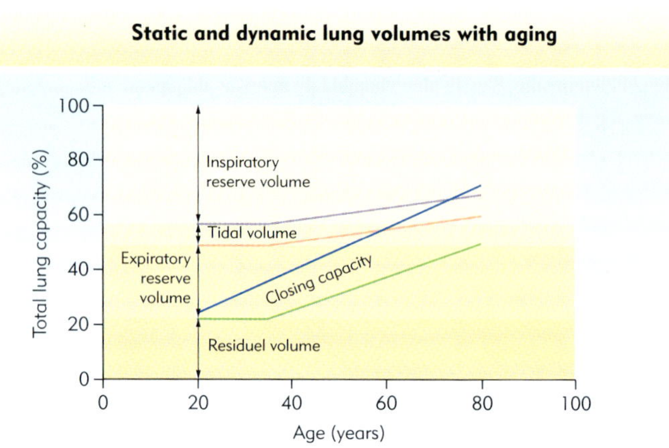

Figure 66.5 Static and dynamic lung volumes with aging. Changes in lung volumes and the consequences for anesthesia are discussed in the text.

DRUG DISPOSITION

Essentially all clinically relevant data on drug disposition in the elderly can be summarized by stating that elderly patients require smaller doses of intravenous anesthetics. A number of age-related physiologic changes affect the pharmacokinetics of many anesthetic agents, including reduced total body water, blood volume, and skeletal muscle mass, altered protein binding, and increased body fat. Pharmacodynamic changes result in increased sensitivity to opioids, benzodiazepines, and volatile anesthetics [minimum alveolar concentration (MAC) decreases about 4% per decade after age 40 years]. Animal models have limited applicability in determining age-related alterations in humans to drug action, and each drug must be considered individually. Renal mass, renal blood flow, glomerular blood flow, and number of glomeruli (cortical more than medullary) decrease with age. Glomerular filtration rate decreases approximately 1mL/min each year after age 40 years. Because there is a decline in muscle mass and creatinine production, serum creatinine concentration is not a useful indicator of glomerular filtration in the elderly. Creatinine clearance (C_{cr}) can be estimated from the serum creatinine (S_{cr}) by the following formula:

$$C_{cr}\ (\text{ml/min}) = \frac{[140 - \text{age(years)}] \times \text{weight(kg)}}{72 \times S_{cr}\ (\text{mg/dL})}$$

Apart from clearance issues, changes in body composition of the elderly prove important in the alterations seen and expected in the elderly patient's response to pharmaceutic agents. Aging humans manifest a decrease in total body water and lean body mass while total body fat increases. While this may be expected to increase the volume of distribution at steady state for lipophilic drugs, the volume of the central compartment is reduced, which increases initial blood concentrates. For example, the principle drug-binding proteins, albumin and α_1-acid glycoprotein are affected differently by the aging process. Albumin decreases while α_1-acid glycoprotein levels typically increase. Alterations in free fraction and thus the clearance and volume of distribution of a given drug will depend on which protein provides the principle binding site for a drug.

Figure 66.6 summarizes the observed alterations for various drugs in aged patients and Figure 66.7 summarizes a recent examination of the pharmacokinetics and pharmacodynamics of the narcotic remifentanil as an example. This study showed that the necessary initial bolus dose in an 80-year-old patient is 50% that of a 20 year old, and the infusion rate is about two thirds less.

OTHER EFFECTS

Loss of hearing with age affects over 30% of adults between the ages of 65 and 74 and about 50% of individuals between the ages of 75 and 80. Presbycusis is the bilaterally symmetric, sensiorineural hearing loss that is associated with aging. Hearing loss is 2.5–5 times more frequent in men than women and likely to be more severe. Presbycusis can be divided into sensory, neural, metabolic, and cochlear conductive defects. High frequencies are much more affected than lower frequencies. Acute sensorineural hearing loss can occur following general anesthesia (not ear surgery) or spinal anesthesia. This

Age-related pharmacologic changes of anesthetics and drugs in anesthesia practice			
Anesthetic/drug	**Pharmacodynamics**	**Pharmacokinetics**	**Anesthetic management**
Inhalational anesthetics	Sensistivity of the brain ↑ (cerebral metabolic rate ↓)	Ventilation/perfusion mismatch with slow rise of alveolar/inspired ratio of inhaled gases; maximal cardiac output ↓; volume of distribution ↑	Minimum alveolar concentration down 30%; slower induction and emergence; delayed but more profound onset of anesthesia
Hypnotics			
Thiopental	No changes	Central volume of distribution ↓; intercompartmental clearance ↑	Induction dose reduced by 15% (20-year-old patient: 2.5–5.0mg/kg i.v.; 80-year-old patient: 2.1mg/kg i.v.). Maintenance dose: same maintenance dose requirements 60 minutes after starting a continuous infusion. Emergence: slightly faster
Propofol	No changes	Central volume of distribution ↓; intercompartmental clearance ↑	Induction dose reduced by 20% (slower induction requires lower doses) (20-year-old: 2.0–3.0mg/kg/ i.v.; 80-year-old: 1.7mg/kg i.v.). Maintenance dose: same maintenance dose requirements 120 minutes after starting a continuous infusion. Emergence: slightly faster (?)
Midazolam	Sensitivity of the brain ↑	Clearance ↓	Sedation/induction dose reduced by 50% (20-year-old: 0.07–0.15mg/kg i.v.; 80-year-old: 0.02–0.03mg/kg i.v.). Maintenance dose reduced by 25%. Recovery: delayed (hours)
Etomidate	No changes	Central clearance ↓; volume of distribution ↓	Induction dose reduced by 20% (20-year-old: 0.3mg/kg i.v.; 80-year-old: 0.2mg/kg i.v.). Emergence: slightly faster (?)
Ketamine	?	?	Use with caution: hallucinations, seizures, mental disturbance, release of catecholamines: avoid in combination with levodopa (tachycardia, arterial hypertension)
Opioids			
Fentanyl, afentanil, sufentanil	Sensitivity of the brain ↑	No changes	Induction dose reduced by 50%. Maintenance dose rduced by 30–50%. Emergence: may be delayed
Remifentanil	Sensitivity of the brain ↑	Central volume of distribution ↓; intercompartmental clearance ↓	Induction dose reduced by 50%. Maintenance dose reduced by 70%. Emergence: may be delayed
Muscle relaxants			
Mivacurium	No changes	Plasma cholinesterase ↓; muscle blood flow ↓; cardiac output ↓; intercompartmental clearance ↓	Onset time ↑. Maintenance dose requirements↓. Duration of action ↑
Succinylcholine			Clinically indistinguishable from mivacurium. Differences: no changes in initial dose, prolonged block with metoclopramide
Pancuronium, doxacuronium, pipecuronium, vecuronium, rocuronium	No changes	Plasma cholinesterase ↓; muscle blood flow ↓; cardiac output ↓; intercompar-mental clearance ↓ Clearance ↓; (volume of distribution ↓)	Onset time ↑. Maintenance dose requirements ↓. Duration of action ↑. Recommended dose reduced by 20%
Atracurium	No changes	No changes	No changes
Reversal agents			
Neostigmine, pyridostigmine	No changes	Clearance ↓	Duration of action ↑↑; since muscle relaxants have a markedly prolonged duration of action, larger doses of reversal agents are needed in elderly patients
Edrophonium	No changes	No changes	No change
Local anesthetics	Sensitivity of the nervous tissue ↑ (?)	Hepatic microsomal metabolism of amide local anesthetics [lidocaine (lignocaine), bupivacaine]; plasma protein binding ↓; cephalad spread ↑	Epidural (and spinal) dose requirements ↓. Duration of spinal and epidural anesthesia seems clinically independent of age, toxicity ↑ (percent free drug ↑)

Figure 66.6 Age-related pharmacologic changes of anesthetics and drugs in anesthesia practice.

10–20dB hearing loss appears to be more common in the elderly and is generally transient; the cause is still unknown. Postoperative hearing deficits can exacerbate postoperative confusion or simply impair communication.

Elderly patients are more prone to hypothermia as a result of reduced basal metabolic rate (about 1% per year) causing decreased heat production and a lower threshold for cold-induced peripheral vasoconstriction.

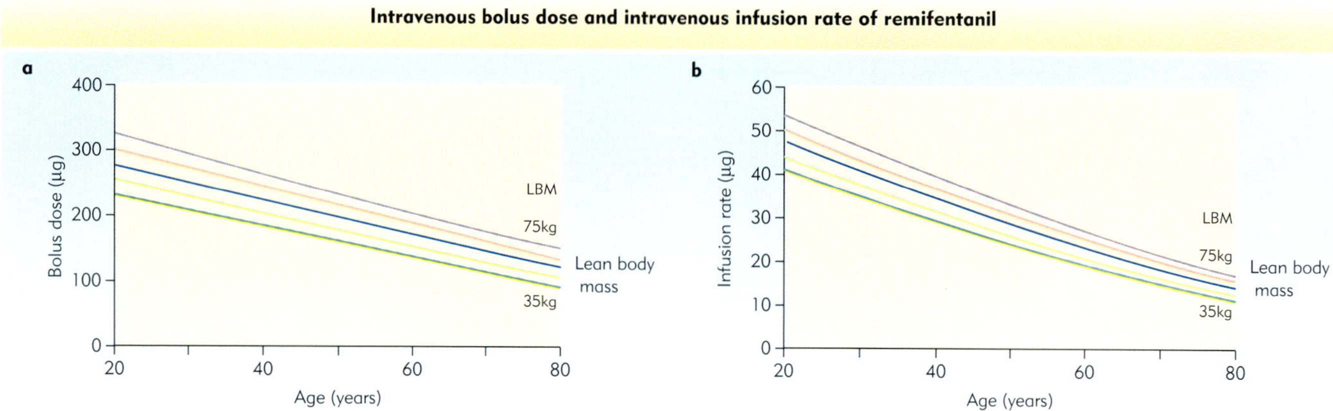

Figure 66.7 Nomogram for calculating intravenous bolus dose (a) and intravenous infusion rate (b) of remifentanil required to cause 50% of the maximum effect as a function of age and lean body mass (LBM). Note that the principal effect of age is altered significantly by the relative lean body mass. This highlights some of the multiple factors to consider when choosing drug dosages for elderly patients. (With permission from Minto et al., 1997.)

Key References

American Federation for Aging Research. Putting aging on hold. Official Report to the 1995 White House Conference on Aging. New York: American Federation of Aging Research and the Alliance for Aging Research; 1995.

Dani SU, Hori A, Walter GF, eds. Principles of neural aging. Amsterdam: Elsevier; 1997.

Folkow B, Svanborg A. Physiology of cardiovascular aging. Physiol Rev. 1993;73:725–64.

Graves JL, Jr. General theories of aging: unification and synthesis. In: Dani SU, Hori A, Walter GF, eds. Principle for neural aging. Amsterdam: Elsevier; 1997:35–55.

Jazwinski SM. Longevity, genes, and aging. Science. 1996;273:54–9.

Lakkata E. In: Abrams WB, Beer MH, Berkow R, eds. Normal changes of aging. In: The Merck manual of geriatrics, 2nd edn. Whitehouse Station, NJ: Merck; 1995:425-41.

Minto CF, Schnider TW, Shafer SL. Pharmacokinetics and pharmacodynamics of remifentanil. II. Model application. Anesthesiology. 1997;86:24–33.

Rowe JW, Kahn RL. Successful aging. Gerontologist. 1997;7:433–40.

Shafer SL. Pharmacokinetics and pharmacodynamics of the elderly. In: McLeskey CH, ed. Geriatric anesthesiology. Baltimore, MD: Williams & Wilkins; 1997:123–42.

Xiao RP, Lakatta EG. Deterioration of beta-adrenergic modulation of cardiovascular function with aging. Ann N Y Acad Sci. 1992;673:293–310.

Further Reading

Evan KE, Tavill MA, Goldberg AN, Silverstein H. Sudden sensorineural hearing loss after general anesthesia for nonotologic surgery. Laryngoscope. 1997;107:747–52.

Fleg JL, Schulman SP, O'Connor FC, et al. Cardiovascular responses to exhaustive upright cycle exercise in highly trained older men. J Appl Physiol. 1994;77:1500–6.

Geokas MC, Lakatta EG, Makinodan T, Timiras PS. The aging process. Ann Intern Med. 1990;113:455–66.

Moller JT, Cluitsman P, Ramussen LS, et al. Long term postoperative cognitive dysfunction in the elderly. Lancet 1998;135:857-61.

Muravchick S. Geroanesthesia. Principles for Management of the Elderly Patient. St Louis, PA: Mosby; 1997.

Ruano D, Araujo F, Bentareha R, Victoria J. Age-related modification on the GABAA receptor binding properties from Wistar rat prefrontal cortex. Brain Res. 1996;738:103–8.

Sapolsky RM, Krey LC, McEwen BS. The neuroendocrinology of stress and aging: the glucocorticoid cascade hypothesis. Endocr Rev. 1986;7:284–301.

Schneider EL, Rowe JW, eds. Handbook of the biology of aging, 4th edn. San Diego, CA: Academic Press; 1996.

Sohal RS, Weindruch R. Oxidative stress, caloric restriction and aging. Science. 1996;273:59–63.

Wei JY. Age and the cardiovascular system. N Engl J Med. 1992;327:1735–9.

Chapter 67 Neonatology

Ian G Wilson

Topics covered in this chapter

The neonatal period is defined as the first 28 days of life following delivery. For a baby born at term (that is 40 weeks postconception), many of the immature physiologic systems will have begun their progress to maturity by the end of this period. Advances in neonatal and reproductive medicine have resulted in the survival of babies born after 24 or 25 weeks gestation, a time at which many systems are extremely immature, and in these babies the neonatal period should be considered to last until 44 weeks postconception. Thus, the concept of postconceptional age in weeks is important to grasp for anyone involved in the management of these patients. Anyone who witnesses the delivery of an infant surely cannot fail to marvel at the resilience and adaptability required to complete the transition to extrauterine life. A reduction in the time allowed to prepare for this transition is bound to result in increased morbidity and mortality. In this chapter important differences in basic physiology that are relevant to the practice of neonatal anesthesia are highlighted.

RESPIRATORY PHYSIOLOGY

The function of respiration is provided for the fetus by the placenta, which allows gas exchange. However, the fetus does engage in irregular breathing movements that may be essential to the normal development of the lungs. When fetal breathing is abolished by section of the phrenic nerve in lambs they are born with hypoplastic lungs. These movements occur during rapid eye movement (REM) sleep and are suppressed by maternal smoking and alcohol ingestion, and are abolished by hypoxemia. It is likely that these effects on fetal breathing are central, and result from a reduction in REM sleep. This is an indication of the differing response of the fetus and premature infant to hypoxemia, which is discussed with the control of breathing below.

Lung development

Lung development begins in the first few weeks with a groove in the foregut. The bronchial tree develops apace by budding and is complete by the seventeenth week. At this point the airways are blind tubules lined with nonrespiratory epithelium. Capillaries begin to grow adjacent to these bronchioles and the blood–gas barrier forms and thins. Disturbance or restriction of development at this stage (such as the presence of gut in the chest with a diaphragmatic hernia) results in hypoplasia of all lung tissue. Alveoli are not present at this stage, but are initiated as terminal saccules at 24 weeks that do not start to develop until 34 weeks; the majority are formed after birth in the first 18 months of life. Some species, like the rat, have no alveoli at term. The Type II alveolar epithelial cells or pneumocytes, which are the sole site of surfactant synthesis, begin to differentiate at 24 weeks and this process is complete by 32 weeks. The Laplace formula indicates that the pressure within a sphere required to prevent collapse because of surface tension is inversely proportional to the radius (Chapter 42). Thus if spheres are connected, as in the lungs, the pressure within the smallest ones would be higher and they would tend to empty their contents into the larger ones. This creates instability and areas of collapse as seen in respiratory distress syndrome (RDS). The likelihood of RDS in a fetus can be predicted by an examination of the various surface-active components of the amniotic fluid e.g. levels of surfactant protein A or the ratio of the phospholipids lecithin (phosphatidylcholine) and sphingomyelin.

The ability of the very preterm infant to perform gas exchange in the lungs depends on all these various processes maturing together.

Control of breathing

Breathing starts before birth; the rate in a 30-week fetus is around 58 breaths/minute, dropping to 47 breaths/minute near term. Neural and chemical control of breathing is similar to that in adults, but the neural system is relatively immature at birth and there are important differences in the responses to changes in oxygen and carbon dioxide partial pressures (P_{O_2} and P_{CO_2}, respectively).

Premature and full-term neonates show a biphasic response to hypoxemia. A transient increase in ventilation is followed by prolonged depression of ventilation. If the environment is cold even the transient stimulation is abolished in a preterm neonate. This effect seems to last longer after birth in preterm infants, but the normal adult response to hypoxemia, that is sustained hyperventilation, is usually in place by 3 weeks.

The control of breathing in infants has been of great interest to investigators of sudden infant death syndrome (SIDS). The cause of this tragic syndrome remains uncertain, although disturbances of respiratory control, thermal regulation, and sleeping position are the most promising candidates.

Anecdotal reports of two cases of SIDS after long-haul air travel led to a recent investigation into the effects of 15% oxygen on breathing patterns and oxygenation in infants. Aircraft cabins are pressurized to the equivalent of about 2500m above sea level. This reduces arterial Po_2 (Pao_2) to 56mmHg (7.5kPa) and the arterial oxygen saturation (Sao_2) to about 89% in healthy adults. The study examined 34 infants aged between 1 and 6 months and found a 3.5-fold increase in the time spent in periodic apnea and a significant fall in Sao_2 (from 97.6 to 92.8%) during the exposure to 15% oxygen. It may be that the adult response of respiratory stimulation in the face of hypoxia takes a little longer to be established. Some evidence also suggests that respiratory tract infections can cause infants, especially those born prematurely, to revert to a neonatal immature pattern of apnea in response to hypoxia.

Gas transport

As Po_2 in fetal blood is much lower than that in the mother, the fetus has developed a mechanism to improve oxygen carriage. Fetal hemoglobin (HbF) reacts poorly with 2,3-diphosphoglycerate, which binds to deoxyhemoglobin and not oxyhemoglobin. This increases the affinity of HbF for oxygen. The oxygen–hemoglobin dissociation curve is shifted to the left and thus Po_250 (the Po_2 at which oxygen saturation is 50%) is reduced. Adult Po_250 is 27mmHg (3.6kPa), whereas the neonate value is 20mmHg (2.7kPa; Fig. 67.1). This increases to beyond the adult value by 3 months, when Po_250 is about 30mmHg (4.0kPa), and declines during the first decade.

Although the fetus can carry more oxygen at low Po_2 values, oxygen delivery at the tissues should be impaired. However, carbon dioxide shifts the curve to the right and the slope of the dissociation curve is so steep at this point that oxygen delivery is assured. The newborn can suffer severe tissue hypoxia with falls in Pao_2 caused by the poor oxygen unloading of HbF.

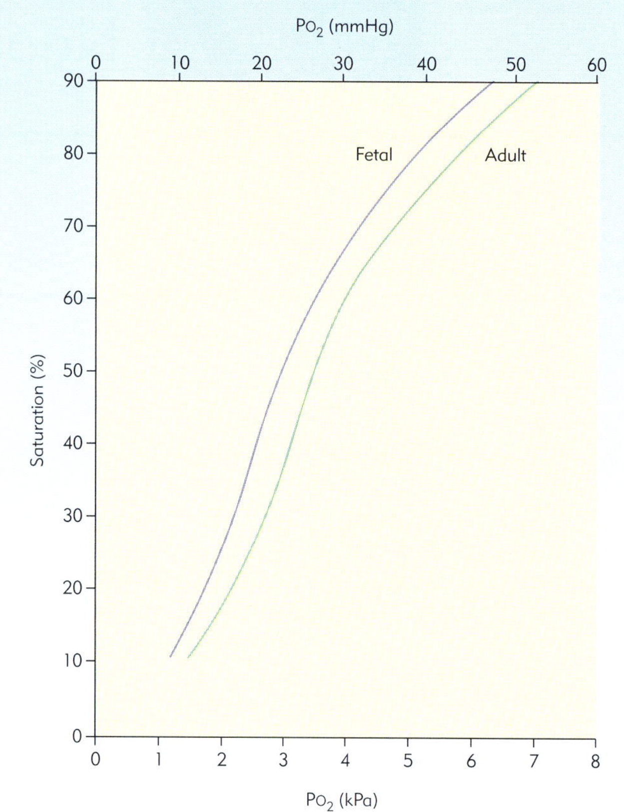

Figure 67.1 Oxygen–hemoglobin dissociation curves for fetal and adult blood. (Reproduced with permission from Darling *et al.* J Clin Invest. 1941;20;739–47.)

CARDIOVASCULAR PHYSIOLOGY

While the lungs take a back seat to the placenta, the fetal heart must function from an early stage to ensure survival. As the lungs only require enough of the cardiac output to supply nutrition, the fetus must have shunts to minimize the pulmonary flow and maximize the supply of oxygen to the brain and heart. These shunts are the foramen ovale, the ductus arteriosus, and the ductus venosus.

As every fetal organ receives a mix of blood from the right and left ventricles, fetal circulation is often referred to as a parallel circulation. That of the adult is of course in series, as blood must follow a path around the left and then the right side of the circulation.

Fetal circulation

Oxygenated blood from the placenta, with a Po_2 of 35mmHg (4.7pKa) flows via the umbilical vein to the fetus; 50% bypasses the liver in the ductus venosus. The crista terminalis, which is the superior border of the foramen ovale, directs the majority of this flow through the foramen ovale and into the left atrium. This ensures that the blood perfusing the cerebral and coronary arteries has the highest oxygen content.

That portion of blood that enters the right atrium and stays on the right side of the circulation joins blood from the superior vena cava and is ejected into the pulmonary artery, where 90% is shunted across the huge ductus arteriosus into the descending aorta (Fig. 67.2).

The transition to extrauterine life

The changes required at birth are dramatic and deserve to be considered separately. Some occur almost instantaneously, but others take much longer. Thus the neonate has what is referred to as a transitional circulation for some time after birth.

The first breath and clamping of the umbilical cord reduce right atrial pressure. Pulmonary blood flow increases as a result of decreased pulmonary vascular resistance (PVR), so that left atrial pressure rises. This reversal of the pressure difference closes the foramen ovale. Decreases in PVR result from the direct effects of increased oxygenation and local mediators such as bradykinin.

The initiation of breathing is complex. During a vaginal delivery, fluid within the lungs is squeezed out as a result of pressure on the thorax; when this pressure is released air enters the airways passively. Removal of the placental circulation decreases prostaglandin E_2 (PGE_2) levels, which inhibit respiration, and rising values of Po_2 stimulate breathing. The first few breaths rapidly establish a residual capacity (Fig. 67.3). Surprisingly high

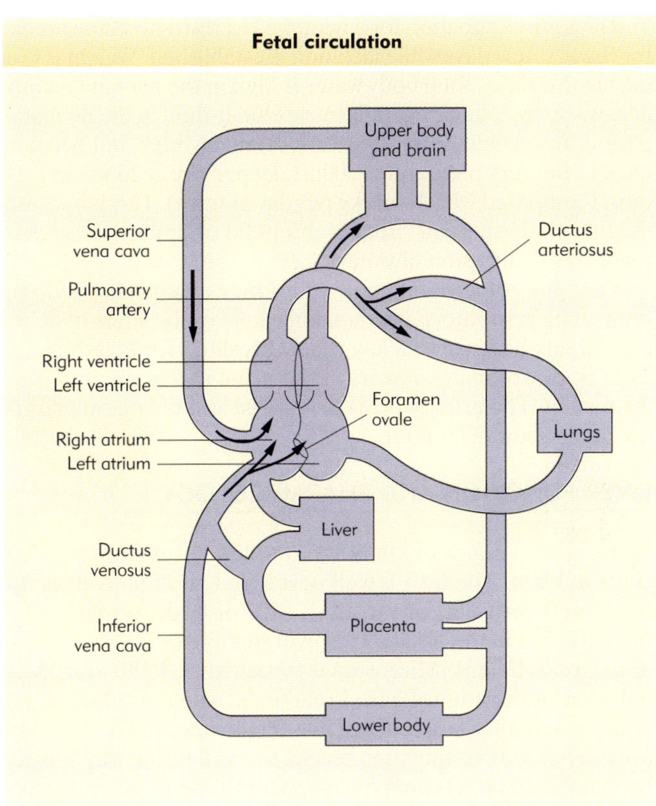

Figure 67.2 The fetal circulation. The wide arrows show the preferential flow through the fetal shunts to avoid the lungs. Also shown is the diversion of deoxygenated blood from the superior vena cava via the right ventricle to avoid the brain.

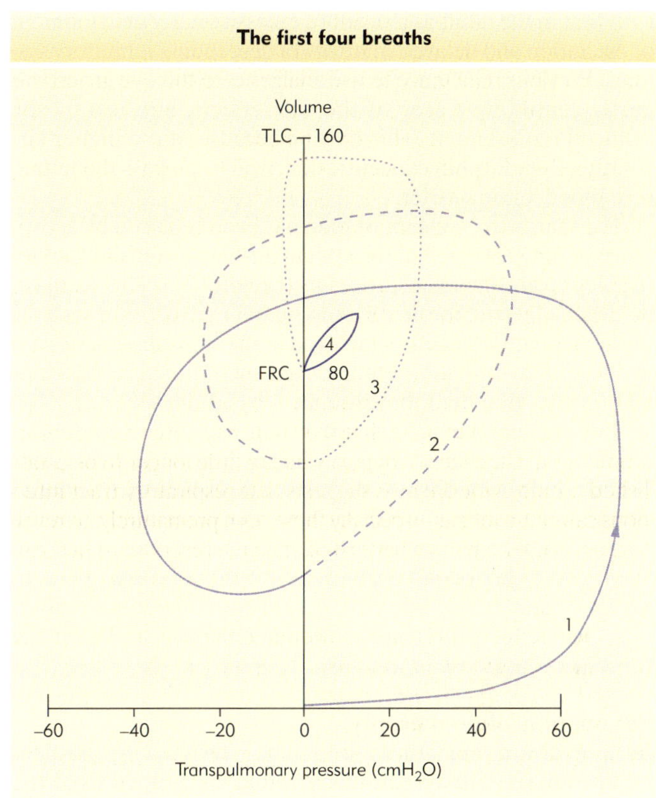

Figure 67.3 The first four breaths. Each successive breath requires less pressure and increases the functional residual capacity (FRC). TLC, total lung capacity. (With permission from Hatch D, Sumner E, Hellmann J. Hatch D, Sumner E, Hellmann J, eds. The surgical neonate: anaesthesia and intensive care. London: Edward Arnold; 1995.)

inspiratory pressures are required at first to overcome viscous forces, but these pressures decrease over the first four or five breaths. The hypercarbia is reduced within 5 minutes and acidemia resolves over the first day of life.

The ductus arteriosus also begins to close in response to increasing Pao_2 and decreasing prostaglandins. The spiral smooth muscle constricts and cushions of mucoid protrude into the lumen. This initial physiologic closure occurs in the first 12 hours. Permanent closure takes 2–4 weeks in term infants and longer in premature infants.

As these shunts do not close anatomically at first, they can open in response to physiologic challenges, most importantly hypoxia, hypercarbia, and acidemia. This is the danger of the transitional circulation, and neonatal anesthetists must be prepared for this to happen. Obviously, the patency of the ductus is vital to the fetus. Hypoxia and PGE_1 and PGE_2 maintain patency and can continue to do so after birth. The constrictor response to rises in Pao_2 increases with age, so premature infants are more likely to keep their ductus open.

The main pathophysiologic change that may reopen fetal channels and produce a transitional circulation is increased PVR. The state in which PVR rises to systemic levels and opens the ductus is referred to as persistent pulmonary hypertension of the neonate (PPHN). In addition to the dangerous triad of hypoxia, hypercarbia, and acidosis, PPHN may result from excessive muscularization of the pulmonary arterioles; an overall reduction in cross-sectional area of pulmonary vessels because of hypoplastic lungs; or reduced flow from a hyperviscosity or congenital abnormality. This scenario is not unusual in neonates that present to the anesthetist. Manipulations of PVR involve adjustments to mechanical ventilation to produce alkalosis and hyperoxia (temporarily), vasodilators, and inhaled nitric oxide.

THE NERVOUS SYSTEM

The brain has a different rate of growth from other body systems. There are two spurts – neuronal cells multiply at 15–20 weeks gestation and glial cells from 25 weeks to 2 years. Myelination is incomplete at birth and continues until the third year of life. The brain is relatively large at birth, representing a tenth of total body weight, and it has about a quarter of the number of brain cells as the adult. Poor nutrition during these rapid growth spurts severely impairs brain development.

Immature reflexes (such as the Moro reflex) depend on cutaneous stimuli and owe their presence to immature myelination. Neurologic development and gestational age can be estimated by examining these reflexes.

The apparently low pain sensitivity that preterm babies exhibit is also caused by incomplete myelination and anatomic immaturity. However, even preterm babies respond to a painful stimulus by withdrawal, autonomic stimulation, and stress hormone release. Indeed some workers argue that the transmission of pain in the spinal cord of the young is exaggerated compared with that in the adult as a result of excessive early development of excitation and delayed maturity of descending inhibitory systems. Previous reluctance to use analgesics in this age group was partly caused by a fear of the side effects, but also by the reduced requirement. This may be because of the higher circulating β-endorphin concentration, which can pass the immature blood–brain barrier.

The 'hardwire' concept of pain has been replaced by acceptance of the 'plasticity' of the system through astonishing adaptive neural and chemical processes (Chapter 21). This seems to be especially true in the developing pain-perception systems of the neonate. Receptors involved in the transmission of pain at the spinal cord subunits undergo such dramatic developmental alteration that they disappear by adulthood.

Pain experience in this age group can alter subsequent responses of the patient. Babies who are given serial heel pricks become more responsive over time, and babies who undergo circumcision without anesthetic have an exaggerated response to inoculations when compared with controls. Concern has also arisen as to the longer-term effects of opioid drugs given to neonates undergoing intensive care. These exogenous opioids may change the proportion of opioid receptors and alter the subsequent response to opioids.

Retinopathy of prematurity

Retinopathy of prematurity used to be referred to as retrolental fibroplasia. The vessels in the retina are formed from the nasal side to the temporal side by 44 weeks of gestation. Exposure to high oxygen concentrations during the process, especially early on, causes vascular spasm. The retinal tissue necroses and heals with fibrosis. New vessels proliferate in the fibrosed area and can cause retinal detachment. Those babies most at risk are the premature, those on high inspired oxygen, and those who receive adult blood (the dissociation curve is shifted to the right). Keeping the Pao_2 at 45–60mmHg (6–8kPa) is the best preventative measure.

RENAL PHYSIOLOGY

Despite the fact that the fetus maintains metabolic homeostasis through the placenta, the kidney is remarkably well developed by 34 weeks of gestation. At this stage all the nephrons have formed, but growth continues well into childhood, particularly tubule length. Nevertheless the fetal kidney has an important role in maintaining amniotic fluid volume. Neonates with renal agenesis develop fetal compression or Potter's syndrome and exhibit facial deformity, low-set ears, pulmonary hypoplasia, and skeletal deformities.

Although the neonatal kidney is pressed into action straight from birth the demands required of it differ from those made of the adult's kidney, as it uses around 50% of the nitrogen intake.

Physiological differences are, of course, present. Glomerular filtration rate is only 15–30% that of the adult in the first few days, but reaches 50% by the tenth day. Renal blood flow increases from around 5% of cardiac output at birth, rapidly at first, to the adult value of 20% by 24 months. This limits the ability to excrete Na^+ and water loads (and drugs). Concentrating ability (to a maximum of 800osmol/L) is reduced by fewer and shorter loops of Henle, but also by the low urea production because of growth. The concentrating gradient caused by urea in the medulla is therefore less. The ability to dilute urine is better.

The normal situation for a neonate is a restricted fluid intake for the first few days while lactation is established. Weight is lost during this time. Total body water is high in the neonate mainly because extracellular exceeds intracellular fluid in the neonatal period. Insensible water losses are relatively high, but become huge in the very premature (200mL/kg per day at 26 weeks gestation compared with 10mL/kg per day at term). This is because the thin epidermis and virtually absent fat offer much less resistance to the diffusion of water.

The 'physiologic acidemia' of infancy extends beyond the immediate respiratory and metabolic load of the stress of delivery, largely because of a low renal threshold for bicarbonate. That is, bicarbonate appears in the urine at a low serum concentration. The urinary pH is 6 or above and the plasma bicarbonate is about 20mmol/L.

LIVER FUNCTION AND PHARMACOLOGY

Once again a major organ is asked to take over from the placenta at birth. The liver is well developed and relatively large compared with that of the adult (4% of body weight in the neonate, 2% in the adult). However, many of the enzyme systems are deficient. Microsomal cytochrome P450 activity is half that of the adult. Phase I reactions, which produce more polar metabolites, are reduced in effectiveness, but less so than are the phase II conjugation reactions. As a result, physiologic neonatal jaundice is common; it appears by 48 hours and peaks on the fourth day. Reabsorption of bilirubin from the gut, rapid red-cell breakdown, and hematomas from trauma at delivery overload the immature liver. The danger is the formation of bilirubin–membrane complexes in the basal ganglia and brainstem, which cause serious damage. This process, known as kernicterus, is more likely to occur in sick premature infants. The problem is avoided by phototherapy – blue light (425–475nm) converts bilirubin into biliverdin, which is excreted more easily.

Hepatic enzyme systems develop quickly, reaching adult levels by 3 months in both premature and term infants. Both quantitative plasma protein concentrations and qualitative plasma protein binding are reduced, which results in an apparent larger volume of distribution for many drugs. This protects the fetus from placental transfer of drugs to a certain extent, as the fetal protein binding is less than the maternal. However, all drugs can cross the placenta.

Low carbohydrate reserves and immature liver function place the neonate, especially preterm, at risk of hypoglycemia. Blood glucose levels drop rapidly after birth because of high circulating catecholamines,.

It is often held that the blood–brain barrier is poorly developed in the neonate. In practice, that drugs seem to pass this barrier with relative ease is the net result of a number of factors:

- less fat deposits in the lipid interface between blood vessels and the extracellular fluid;
- higher total and extracellular water;
- greater cerebral blood flow as a proportion of cardiac output; and
- increased sensitivity of receptors.

The gastric pH is high in neonates and after oral administration, basic drugs such as penicillins have high bioavailability, and acidic drugs such as phenobarbital and phenytoin show reduced absorption.

Increased surface area, skin water content, and less keratin all predispose the neonate to greater percutaneous drug absorption. This has caused problems with methemoglobinemia following the use of Emla® [the eutectic mixture of lidocaine (lignocaine) and prilocaine] in neonates. The use of Emla® in infants is not recommended.

The end result of the complex interactions of hepatic, renal, and other physiologic variables is that the loading dose of many drugs is increased in the neonate to account for the higher volume of distribution, while the longer elimination half-lives require less frequent doses.

THERMOREGULATION

Humans are homeothermic, which means they can maintain a stable core temperature in the face of changes in ambient temperature. Neonates, however, are especially prone to heat loss. Radiation is the major source of loss, as newborns have a larger ratio of surface area to volume, although convection and evaporation are also very important (Chapter 64).

To maintain body temperature in cold environments, the homeotherm must be able to produce heat. Three mechanisms are available – voluntary muscle activity, involuntary muscle activity (shivering), and nonshivering thermogenesis.

Shivering is poorly developed in the neonate and voluntary activity is inadequate. Thus nonshivering thermogenesis is vital for the neonate. While heat production can occur in muscle, liver, and brain, the metabolism of brown fat is by far the most important mechanism. Brown fat, which differentiates between 26 and 30 weeks gestation, comprises around 11% of the total body fat of the neonate. It is found between the scapulae, in the axillae and mediastinum, around major blood vessels in the neck, and around the kidneys. It is well vascularized and well innervated by the sympathetic nervous system. The many mitochondria in brown fat cells are packed with cristae. The stress of cold stimulates release of norepinephrine (noradrenaline), which metabolizes brown fat to free fatty acids and glycerol. This mechanism of thermogenesis can be inhibited by surgical or pharmacologic sympathetic block.

The range over which a neonate can thermoregulate is considerably more limited than that in an adult. The lower limit in adults is 0°C (32°F) whereas that of the neonate is 22°C (71.6°F).

However, a more useful concept is that of the neutral thermal environment, which is the range of temperatures at which body temperature can be maintained at minimum oxygen expenditure. In the first few days of life this range is narrow and the temperature surprisingly high (Fig. 67.4). The importance of maintaining body temperature cannot be stressed enough. The metabolism required to increase temperature rapidly results in hypoxia and hypoglycemia.

EVALUATION AND RESUSCITATION OF THE NEWBORN

In 1953 Dr Virginia Apgar formulated a scoring system to evaluate the physiologic status of the neonate (Fig. 67.5). This system is in universal use and has been employed to compare numerous variables in perinatal care and their outcomes.

Preparation for neonatal resuscitation is all important. Those areas in which delivery can be expected should be well equipped. More importantly, if antenatal events indicate a risk for neonatal resuscitation (Fig. 67.6), the necessary personnel must be made available.

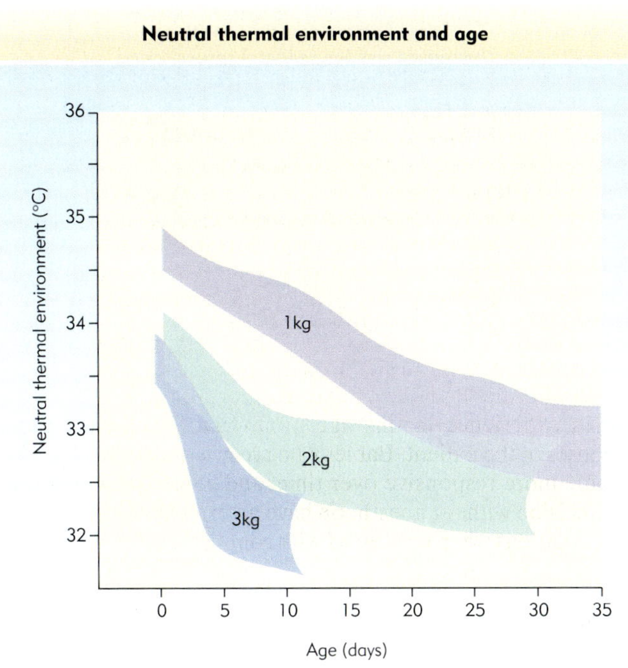

Figure 67.4 Neutral thermal environment for babies of various birth weight in the first month of life. (With permission from Hey EN, Katz G. Arch Dis Child. 1970:45;328–34.)

The Apgar Score

Sign	Score		
	0	1	2
Heart Rate per min	Absent	Less than 100	More than100
Respirations	Absent	Slow and irregular	Good crying
Muscle tone	Limp	Some flexion	Active motion
Reflex irritability (catheter in nostril)	No response	Grimace	Cough or sneeze
Color	Blue or pale	Pink body, blue extremities	Completely pink

Figure 67.5 The Apgar score.

Of course, most babies do not require aggressive resuscitation. In cases of hypoxia and inadequate perfusion in the fetus that become severe during birth, the asphyxiated baby follows a pattern of primary and secondary apnea. Mild hypoxia occurs with each contraction during labor and the fetus has protective responses to this. Blood is diverted to vital organs and the diving reflex results in bradycardia and raised mean arterial pressure. The pattern of heart-rate response to uterine contractions is used to interpret the degree of fetal distress. Once the severely asphyxiated fetus is delivered, an initial phase of tachypnea, tachycardia, and hypertension occurs. Rapidly this progresses to bradycardia and primary apnea. Gasping intercedes briefly, fading away to secondary or terminal apnea. Spontaneous recovery usually occurs if the baby is stimulated before secondary apnea. However, once secondary apnea is

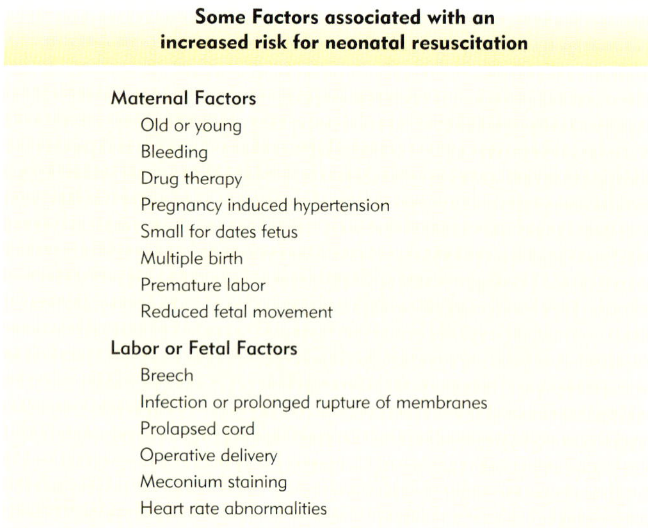

Some Factors associated with an increased risk for neonatal resuscitation

Maternal Factors
- Old or young
- Bleeding
- Drug therapy
- Pregnancy induced hypertension
- Small for dates fetus
- Multiple birth
- Premature labor
- Reduced fetal movement

Labor or Fetal Factors
- Breech
- Infection or prolonged rupture of membranes
- Prolapsed cord
- Operative delivery
- Meconium staining
- Heart rate abnormalities

Figure 67.6 Some factors associated with an increased risk for neonatal resuscitation.

apparent the baby succumbs without active intervention. As it may be difficult to distinguish primary from secondary apnea, every apneic neonate must be treated aggressively.

The familiar sequence of airway, breathing, and circulation (ABC) is appropriate, with the addition of the simple maneuvers of drying, warming, suctioning, and stimulating being performed in all babies. Temperature control must be at the front of the anesthetist's mind. Hypothermia exacerbates the effects of acidosis, impairs myocardial function, and reduces the production of surfactant. The mild stimulation of drying, warming, and suctioning helps to initiate breathing in the majority of newborns. Flicking the soles of the feet can be tried in addition, but more vigorous stimulation should be avoided. These actions should be achieved virtually simultaneously and before any assessment of breathing is made. After 10 seconds of stimulation, breathing is assessed. If adequate, oxygen is administered while heart rate is checked. If inadequate (i.e. slow, shallow, or gasping), positive pressure ventilation is started immediately with 100% oxygen.

Heart rate can be checked at the base of the umbilical cord or by stethoscope. If >100 beats/minute, assessment can continue. If <80 beats/minute, chest compressions should be commenced at 120 compressions/minute. The method of choice may well be that of encircling the babies' chest with the hands. The thumbs press over the lower sternum while the fingers support the back. This is certainly the most comfortable technique and allows accurate application of 1–2cm of compression. Full cardiopulmonary resuscitation is now under way and the ratio of compressions to ventilations should be 3:1.

Drug therapy

If, despite adequate ventilation with 100% oxygen and external cardiac massage, the heart rate remains below 80 beats/minute, drug treatment is indicated. Epinephrine (adrenaline) 0.01mg/kg is given intravenously. The site of choice for infusion is the umbilical vein, which is usually readily identified as it is larger than the two arteries, and the arteries are in spasm by this time. The dose is repeated if necessary, and doses of 0.1mg/kg may be required. Bicarbonate should be reserved for documented acidosis or prolonged resuscitation. Consideration must always be given to the possible diagnoses of hypovolemia, pneumothorax, or severe malformations.

Meconium

If a term (>37 week) fetus is subjected to hypoxia, the gut vessels constrict, peristalsis increases, and the sphincters relax. This results in the passage of meconium into the amniotic fluid. During the hypoxic period the shallow, rapid fetal breathing ceases, but if hypoxia continues deep gasping intervenes and amniotic fluid together with meconium is aspirated into the respiratory tract. Whether before or after delivery, meconium aspiration causes respiratory distress by airway obstruction or chemical pneumonitis.

If meconium is visible before delivery, the mouth and pharynx should be suctioned as the head is delivered. Subsequently, the larynx is inspected by laryngoscopy and any meconium aspirated from the trachea directly via a tracheal tube before the baby is stimulated to breath or positive pressure breaths are given.

ANESTHETIC CONSIDERATIONS

By their nature, neonates who require surgery and therefore anesthesia usually have a major problem. Operations in this age group are normally required to correct a congenital malformation or a disease process related to prematurity such as necrotizing enterocolitis or inguinal hernia. This is at a time when the infant is undergoing dramatic changes in physiology, particularly cardiovascular, to adapt to extrauterine life. An appreciation of the scientific principles involved in these changes is vital to the safe delivery of anesthetic care to these babies.

Ventilation

The foregoing description of respiratory development demands that tracheal intubation and controlled ventilation be employed for virtually all anesthetics for neonates. Careful monitoring of inspired oxygen concentration and of oxygenation is required to avoid the pitfalls of the altered ventilatory response to hypoxemia and retinopathy. Reduced functional residual capacity (FRC) and collapse associated with RDS dictate the use of continuous positive airway pressure (CPAP) or of positive end-expiratory pressure. Infants actually apply their own CPAP, not only by nasal breathing but also by expiratory braking with a partially closed glottis. These problems are exacerbated by the use of nitrous oxide, so this agent is avoided. Air should be the carrier gas, and the lowest inspired oxygen concentration that provides satisfactory oxygenation is used. On anesthetic machines that deliver a minimum flow of oxygen it can be difficult to achieve inspired concentrations below 25%.

Temperature regulation

The neonate is vulnerable to changes in temperature, particularly hypothermia. Ambient and body temperature should be monitored throughout the perioperative period. Conductive and radiant warming devices should be used and all fluids and gases that come into contact with the baby should be warmed.

Clinical pharmacology

Inhalation agents

Neonates are particularly susceptible to cardiorespiratory depression from inhaled agents. The uptake and time to equilibration is more rapid in infants (Chapter 8). because alveolar ventilation is greater in relation to FRC, blood gas solubilities are lower, and the distribution of cardiac output to brain and heart is greater.

Baroreceptor responses are depressed by volatile agents to a greater degree in neonates. These effects combine to reduce the therapeutic ratio between satisfactory anesthesia and myocardial depression.

Minimal alveolar concentration for all agents is low at birth and increases to a maximum at around 6 months before gradually declining throughout life. Many theories have been put forward to explain this, including reduced response to pain, increased permeability of the blood–brain barrier, and low blood-gas solubility.

Muscle relaxants

Larger doses of succinylcholine per kilogram are required in neonates, because of a combination of an increased volume of distribution and immature receptors. Infants have lower plasma cholinesterase activity. As extracellular fluid and surface area have a constant relationship throughout life, doses calculated on this basis are more constant. The duration of action is similarly reduced.

Neonates have long been held to be sensitive to nondepolarizing agents and this is certainly true of tubocurarine. Now that newer agents are available the evidence is unclear. Vecuronium seems to be required in lower dosage, whereas atracurium is generally less effective and seems to have a shorter duration of action. The message is that these drugs are unpredictable in this age group and great care should be taken.

Fluid management

Fluid management is more important in this patient group than in any other; the margins for error are small, and every drug and flush has to be taken into account.

The physiologic approach of considering that neonates require 420kJ/kg per day (100kcal/kg per day), and that 100mL of fluid is used for every 420kJ (100kcal) metabolized is well established. However, the individual situation must also be considered. Not only maintenance fluid, but also fluid-deficit 'third space losses' as well as blood and gastrointestinal losses have to be taken into account. Urine volume and osmolality, together with clinical assessment of circulation, form the basis of minute-by-minute assessment of fluid requirements.

Key References

Apgar V. A proposal for a new method of evaluation of the newborn infant. Curr Res Anesth Analg. 1953;32:253–67.

Anand KJS, Brown MJ, Causon RC, Christofides ND, Bloom SR, Aynsley-Green A. Can the human neonate mount an endocrine and metabolic response to surgery? J Pediatr Surg. 1985;20:41–8.

Han VKM. Neonatal anatomy, physiology and development. Curr Opinion Pediatr. 1990;2:275–81.

Hatch D, Sumner E, Hellmann J. Perinatal physiology and medicine. In: Hatch D, Sumner E, Hellmann J, eds. The surgical neonate: anaesthesia and intensive care. London: Edward Arnold; 1995:1–97.

Krishna G, Emhardt JD. Anesthesia for the newborn and ex-preterm infant. Semin Pediatr Surg. 1992;1:32–44.

Motoyama EK, Davis PJ. Basic principles in pediatric anesthesia. In: Motoyama EK, Davis PJ, eds. Smith's anesthesia for infants and children. St Louis: Mosby; 1996:1–212.

Further Reading

Anas N, Boettrich C, Hall CB, Brooks JG. The association of apnea and respiratory syncytial virus in infants. J Pediatr. 1982;101:65–8.

Aynsley-Green A, Ward Platt MP, Lloyd-Thomas AR. Clinical paediatrics: stress and pain in infancy and childhood. London: Baillière Tindall; 1995.

Levine MI, Tudehope D, Thearle MJ. Essentials of neonatal medicine. Oxford: Blackwell Science; 1993.

Milner AD. Effects of 15% oxygen on breathing patterns and oxygenation in infants. Br Med J. 1998;316:873–4.

Parkin KJ, Poets CF, O'Brien LM, Stebbings VA, Southall DP. Effects of exposure to 15% oxygen on breathing patterns and oxygen saturation in infants: interventional study. Br Med J. 1998;316:887–94.

Taddio A, Goldbach M, Ipp M, Stevens B, Koren G. Effect of neonatal circumcision on pain responses during vaccination in boys. Lancet. 1995;345:291–2.

Chapter 68 Obesity

Paul G Murphy

Topics covered in this chapter

Epidemiology
Obesity and the heart
Obesity and the respiratory system
Obesity and other medical conditions
Altered drug handling in obesity
Postoperative outcomes in morbidly obese patients

It has been known since ancient times that obesity is associated with increased morbidity and premature death. Hippocrates wrote: 'Those naturally fat are more liable to sudden death than the thin'. Contemporary actuarial data supports the view that obesity is the most common nutritional disorder of the Western world and its prevalence continues to increase. Much of our current knowledge of the pathophysiology of obesity comes from studies on morbidly obese patients undergoing bariatric (weight reduction) surgery and justifiably centers on the cardiovascular, respiratory, and metabolic consequences of the condition. It should be understood that this is a selected group of (younger) patients who represent the fittest examples of their type, and that (older) individuals presenting with other medical or surgical conditions may provide attending physicians with far greater challenges than those faced by anesthesiologists involved in anesthesia for surgical correction of severe obesity.

Definitions

Obesity is a condition of excessive body fat (from the Latin *obesus*: fattened by eating). What is a 'normal' body fat content varies with the affluence and the age distribution of the population studied and does not necessarily equate with the content that is optimal for health. Examples of body fat contents in adults from affluent westernized societies are:

- average female 20–30%;
- average male 18–25%;
- professional soccer player 10–12%; and
- marathon runner 7%.

Most measures of obesity involve an evaluation of weight for a given height, which is then compared with an ideal, rather than on estimates of body fat itself. The concept of *ideal body weight* (IBW) originates from life insurance studies, such as those presented by the Metropolitan Life Insurance Company in 1959 and 1979, which describe the weight associated with the lowest mortality rate for a given height and gender (and in some studies body frame size). Although such study populations are highly selective (North American individuals holding life insurance policies), the population size is impressive (>4 million), and the findings have been confirmed in more robust population studies, particularly when the sample size has been sufficient, the follow-up period has been long enough, and other influences such as tobacco usage have been eliminated (e.g. that of the American Cancer Society, published in 1979). For most day-to-day clinical purposes, IBW can be estimated from the following:

- adult males: IBW(kg) = height(cm) – 100; and
- adult females: IBW(kg) = height(cm) – 105.

The *body mass index* (BMI) is a more robust assessment of weight for height and has gained widespread use in most clinical and epidemiologic studies of obesity. The BMI (weight/height^2 in kg/m^2) correlates reasonably well with measures of body fat content (r >0.5). Definitions of obesity in terms of the IBW and BMI are listed in Figure 68.1.

Definitions of obesity

Definition	Weight related to ideal body weight (IBW)	Body mass index
Normal		15–25
Overweight	110–119% IBW	27
Obesity	120–199% IBW	30
Morbid obesity	>200% IBW or IBW + 100lb (45.5kg)	35
Super-morbid obesity	IBW + 200lb (90kg)	50

Figure 68.1 Definitions of obesity.

EPIDEMIOLOGY

Most epidemiologic studies use a BMI of 30kg/m^2 to define obesity, since mortality risk rises sharply at this level. Using such a definition, many studies have detailed a worldwide increase in the prevalence of obesity, which has been attributed largely to the widespread adoption of Western lifestyles and dietary habits in the developing world. For example, the prevalence of obesity in the UK has increased from 6% in men and 8% in women to 13% in men and 15% in women from 1980 to 1991. The prevalence also increases with age. For example, the prevalence in men of 3% in those aged 16–24 years increases to 9% in those aged 50–64 years; in women the increase is from 6 to 18%.

Mortality

A wealth of epidemiologic and actuarial studies have linked obesity to increased mortality. While there is little evidence that a modest excess of body fat (actual body weight of 110–120% IBW) is harmful, mortality risk in young adults begins to rise when BMI exceeds 30kg/m^2 (Fig. 68.2). Morbid obesity (BMI >35kg/m^2) is associated with a twofold increase in overall mortality, a 13-fold increase in sudden unexplained female deaths, and a severalfold increase in mortality from diabetes, respiratory, cerebrovascular, and cardiovascular diseases, and certain forms of cancer. In the Framingham study, being overweight was associated with a mortality rate nearly four times that of the normal weight group.

The risks of obesity are proportional to the duration of obesity, that is, young adults who are obese are far more at risk than older individuals, in whom the acceptable weight for height is higher. Continued weight gain in obese individuals is associated with a higher risk than that for obese individuals whose weight is constant, and weight loss reduces the risks of previous obesity. For a given degree of obesity, males are more at risk than females.

Visceral obesity

There is increasing evidence that the risks of obesity are determined as much by the distribution of body fat as by the extent of its excess. Two different types of obesity are recognized. In the central or *android* type, which is more common in males, the distribution is predominantly upper body and it may also be associated with increased proportions of intra-abdominal or visceral fat. In the peripheral or *gynecoid* type, fat is located predominantly around the hips, buttocks, and thighs.

Coronary artery disease and noninsulin-dependent diabetes mellitus are more common in obese individuals who have a higher proportion of visceral or intra-abdominal fat. The basis for such increased risks is unclear, although one widely quoted hypothesis proposes that the breakdown of visceral adipose tissue results in the delivery of excessive quantities of lipid breakdown products directly into the portal circulation. This, in turn, establishes secondary metabolic imbalances [e.g. dyslipidemia, glucose intolerance and hyperinsulinemia, elevated plasma triglycerides, low plasma high-density lipoprotein (HDL) levels], which might account for such increased morbidities.

OBESITY AND THE HEART

Cardiovascular disease figures prominently among the causes of morbidity and mortality in obesity. Specifically, obesity is considered to be a significant risk factor for hypertension, ischemic heart disease, and a form of ventricular impairment unique to severe obesity, so-called obesity cardiomyopathy. Right-sided heart failure may result from coexisting respiratory disease and add to the cardiovascular problems.

Hypertension

The link between obesity and hypertension has been well established in several large epidemiologic studies. The Framingham study showed that a 10% gain in body fat was associated with a 6mmHg rise in systolic and a 4mmHg rise in diastolic blood pressure. The proportion of individuals requiring antihypertensive therapy increases steadily with body weight. In individuals who have a BMI of 30kg/m^2 or more, 60% will be hypertensive and the hypertension will be severe in one in six. Under such circumstances, hypertension leads to concentric left ventricular (LV) hypertrophy and a progressively noncompliant LV.

Mortality risk charged with body mass index, and the effects of smoking

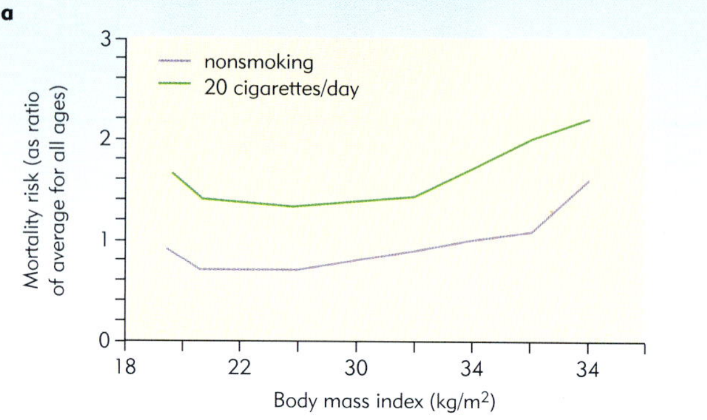

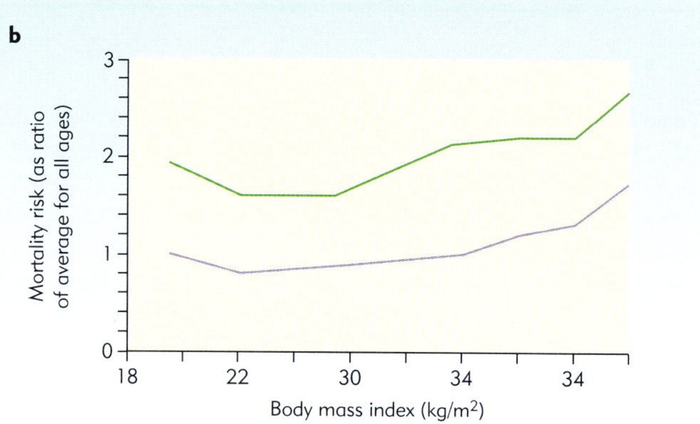

Figure 68.2 Relationship between body mass index and mortality risk in men (a) and women (b), and the effects of coincident cigarette smoking

Ischemic heart disease

Epidemiologic studies have demonstrated a clear association between obesity and sudden death, acute myocardial infarction, and coronary insufficiency. Although previously controversial, it is now generally accepted that this increased risk is independent of confounding influences such as hypertension, hypercholesterolemia, reduced HDL levels, diabetes mellitus, and other diseases, all of which are more common in the obese. Ischemic heart disease is particularly common in individuals who have a central or visceral distribution of excess body fat: for any given degree of obesity, a visceral distribution approximately doubles cardiac risk.

Obesity cardiomyopathy

In 1933, Smith and Willius reported a systematic autopsy study of heart morphology in 135 severely obese individuals. They demonstrated a more or less linear relationship between heart weight and body weight up to 105kg, beyond which the heart continued to increase in weight but in a decreasing manner. In contrast to early ideas, founded on the Victorian belief in the 'fatty heart' (*cor adiposum*), this and later studies demonstrated that the increased heart weight was largely a consequence of dilatation and eccentric hypertrophy of the LV and, to a lesser extent, right ventricle (RV). Although increases in epicardial fat were often noted, fatty infiltration of the myocardium (previously believed to account for sudden death by causing

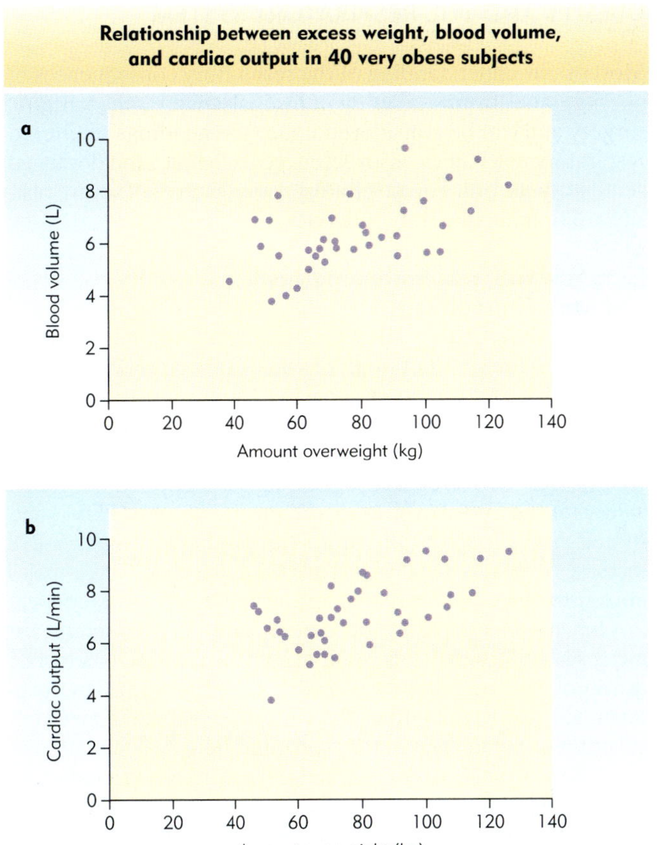

Figure 68.3 Changes in blood volume (a) and cardiac output (b) in obesity. Relationships between excess weight, blood volume, and cardiac output in 40 very obese subjects.

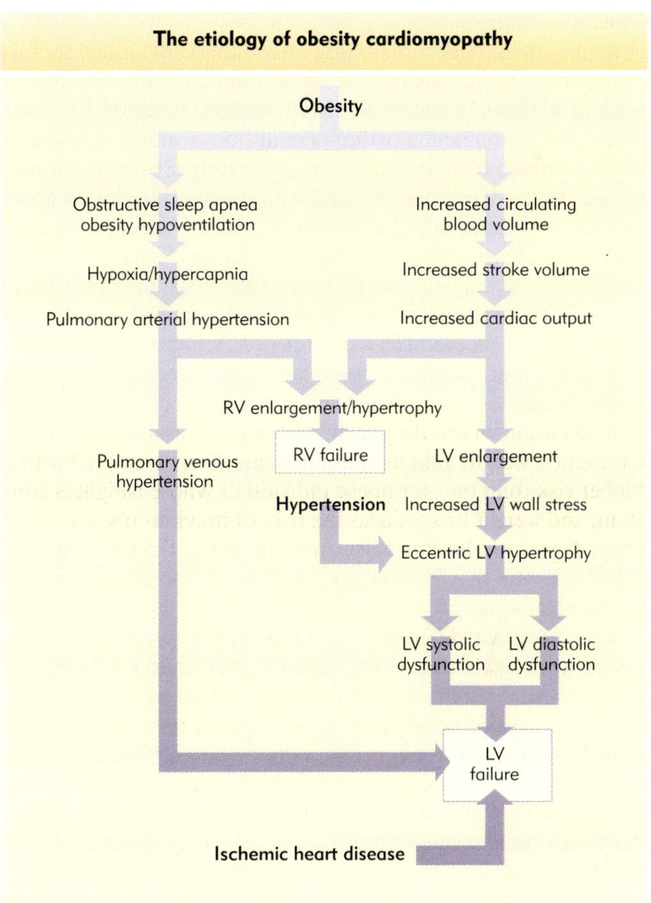

Figure 68.4 The etiology of obesity cardiomyopathy, and its interaction with hypertension, ischemic heart disease, and respiratory impairment.

arrhythmias) was uncommon and restricted to the RV. Although many of the patients studied in these reports appeared both clinically and *post mortem* to have suffered a cardiac death (most notably congestive cardiac failure), the nature of the underlying cause remained unclear.

Functional studies have added considerable clarity to our understanding of the cardiovascular consequences of obesity, specifically by identifying a form of cardiomyopathy specific to severe obesity and by showing its interaction with systemic hypertension. In the 1960s, Alexander described a striking relationship between the degree of obesity and both circulating blood volume and resting cardiac output (Fig. 68.3), which in an 170kg individual are approximately double those found in a subject weighing 70kg. These increases are mostly attributable to an increased blood flow to the (enlarged) fat organ (which requires 2–3mL/min per 100g tissue at rest). Radionucleide and echocardiographic studies in normotensive morbidly obese individuals undergoing weight-reduction surgery have elaborated our understanding of the hemodynamic response to obesity.

The increased cardiac output is achieved largely through an increase in stroke volume resulting from an increase in LV cavity size. As predicted by LaPlace's law, LV wall stress increases as the cavity dilates, and the ventricular wall hypertrophies as a result. Such *eccentric* hypertrophy (as opposed to the *concentric* pattern seen in nonobese hypertensive individuals in which increased LV wall thickness is associated with a reduction in cavity size) serves to reduce LV wall stress. Eccentric hypertrophy is associated with diastolic LV dysfunction, with higher LV end-diastolic pressures at rest, during exercise, or in response to increased venous return; pulmonary edema may, therefore, develop under such circumstances. The capacity of the dilated ventricle to hypertrophy is limited, whereupon systolic dysfunction ensues. Superimposed systemic hypertension compounds these problems. The adverse changes in LV cavity size, wall thickness, and stress and adverse changes in function in both systole and diastole worsen with increasing duration of obesity and improve with weight loss. Morbidly obese individuals tolerate exercise badly. Consequently, they exhibit a lower than anticipated increase in cardiac output in response to graded work. In these individuals, increase in cardiac output is achieved solely by an increase in heart rate, without an increase in stroke volume or ejection fraction and often at the expense of rises in filling pressures; this may cause pulmonary edema. The obstructive sleep apnea/obesity hypoventilation syndrome occurs in 5% of morbidly obese individuals. Recurrent hypoxemia and hypercapnia lead to chronic pulmonary hypertension and eventually to RV failure. It is invariably the case in such patients that the LV is also impaired, heart failure then being biventricular.

The etiology of obesity cardiomyopathy and its interaction with hypertension, ischemic heart disease, and respiratory impairment is illustrated in Figure 68.4.

Clinical features

Patients who have severe obesity often have very limited mobility and may, therefore, appear asymptomatic in the face of significant ventricular impairment. The earliest symptoms include exertional dyspnea and orthopnea, although many individuals sleep sitting in a chair and, therefore, rarely if ever lie supine. Symptoms may be episodic and initially associated with good systolic but reduced diastolic function. Accelerated weight gain may indicate decompensating ventricular function before peripheral edema becomes clinically obvious; it may be precipitated by the onset of the sleep apnea/obesity hypoventilation syndrome, or accelerated hypertension. Clinical examination may be difficult, although the signs of congestive cardiac failure (added heart sounds, pulmonary crepitations, elevated jugular venous pressure, hepatomegaly, ascites, and peripheral edema) have the usual significance. Placing the patient in the supine position and observing the effect on cardiorespiratory function should be a routine part of clinical examination; acute decompensation and cardiac arrest have been reported. Systemic blood pressure may be overestimated if a standard-sized, rather than large, blood pressure cuff is employed.

The electrocardiogram is frequently of low voltage and significantly underestimates the severity of RV and LV hypertrophy. Axis deviation and atrial tachyarrhythmias are relatively common. Cardiomegaly may be seen by chest X-ray examination, although it is often normal. Echocardiography can be very informative: eccentric LV hypertrophy suggests significant obesity-induced changes even if LV function appears good. Although such examinations may be difficult in inexperienced hands, studies can be improved if nonstandard echocardiographic windows are used in recognition of the distorted architecture of the intrathoracic contents.

Anesthetic implications

The severity of ventricular impairment is often underestimated by standard clinical evaluation; in experienced hands, transthoracic echocardiography adds considerably to the preoperative assessment. Ventricular impairment is inevitable in patients who have coexisting respiratory failure, and such patients should be considered as extremely high risk. Sudden weight gain may indicate fluid retention and biventricular failure. Intraoperative ventricular failure may develop for several reasons: increased venous return associated with rapid intravenous fluid administration or the supine or Trendelenburg positions; negative inotropic effects of anesthetic agents; or pulmonary hypertension caused by hypoxemia and hypercapnia. It is good practice to have a range of inotropes and vasodilators immediately to hand so as to be able to respond quickly in the event of difficulties.

A cuff of large size will be required for noninvasive measurement of arterial pressure; however, this can often be disturbed by external compression of the cuff by arm supports or members of the surgical team. Invasive arterial pressure monitoring is recommended because it avoids these problems and allows regular estimation of blood gas and acid–base status. Central venous pressure monitoring is more debatable, although it does provide secure venous access in patients who might otherwise present difficulties and also allows cardiovascular support to be instituted if necessary. Placement of right internal jugular lines does not usually present undue difficulty. Patients who have clinical evidence of heart failure who are undergoing major surgery may benefit from the use of a pulmonary artery flotation catheter. Monitoring should be extended into the postoperative period.

OBESITY AND THE RESPIRATORY SYSTEM

Most of our understanding of the respiratory consequences of obesity comes from studies on individuals undergoing bariatric surgery and can be considered under the headings of altered respiratory mechanics, disordered gas exchange, and deranged ventilatory control. The respiratory consequences of severe obesity are summarized in Figure 68.5.

Lung volumes, respiratory mechanics, and work of breathing

Morbid obesity is associated with reductions in the expiratory reserve volume, functional residual capacity (FRC) (see Chapter 42), and total lung capacity. These changes appear to be caused by splinting of the diaphragm during tidal ventilation and can be reversed by weight loss. In contrast, the residual volume may be increased, suggesting gas trapping. Although values for the forced expiratory volume in 1 second (FEV_1) and forced vital capacity fall within the predicted range, 6–7% increases following weight loss have been reported. Obese males appear to be at greater risk of airflow limitation than females.

Oxygen consumption and carbon dioxide production are increased in the obese, as a result of both the increased metabolic activity of the fat organ and the increased work performed by skeletal muscle. At the same time, there is evidence that the mechanical efficiency of the respiratory apparatus falls. Accumulation of fat in the chest wall, diaphragm, and abdomen leads to a reduction in both pulmonary and chest wall compliance; as a result, the respiratory pattern typically becomes shallow and rapid. This reduction in compliance, along with increased intra-abdominal pressure, increases the pulmonary work load and limits the maximum ventilatory capacity. On occasions, this capacity may fall short of the metabolic requirements, and relative hypoventilation results. Such derangements are at their most extreme in patients who have carbon dioxide retention, when compliance can fall to 35% and work of breathing can rise to 400% of predicted values.

Gas exchange defects and the interaction with anesthesia

Hedenstierna and Santesson have detailed the perioperative changes in oxygenation in patients undergoing bariatric surgery (Fig. 68.6). Preoperatively, these patients exhibit a modest defect in gas exchange, as shown by a reduced arterial oxygen partial pressure, increased alveolar to arterial oxygen difference, and increased shunt fraction. All these indices deteriorate dramatically on the induction of anesthesia, necessitating the use of high inspired oxygen fractions to maintain a satisfactory arterial oxygen tension. Furthermore, although positive end-expiratory pressure (PEEP) helps to correct the deterioration in gas exchange, this is at the expense of cardiac output and oxygen delivery.

Defects in gas exchange are explained on the basis of the effect of obesity on FRC and its relationship to the closing volume (Fig. 68.7). Functional residual capacity is reduced by 25% in awake morbidly obese subjects awaiting bariatric surgery. Further reductions can be anticipated on the assumption of the supine position and with induction of anesthesia, thereby causing the tidal excursion to encroach upon the closing volume of the lung (i.e. the lung volume at which airways begin to collapse). This, in turn, leads to increased ventilation/perfusion mismatching and hypoxemia. The use of PEEP may improve gas exchange by restoring the FRC to preanesthetic levels, thereby avoiding such encroachment and preventing airway closure.

Pulmonary abnormalities in severe obesity	
Lung functions	**Abnormalities**
Lung volumes	Reduced expiratory reserve volume, reduced functional residual capacity, reduced total lung capacity, increased residual volume
Lung mechanics	Reduced lung compliance, reduced chest wall compliance, increased airway resistance, increased work of breathing, reduced respiratory muscle efficiency
Gas exchange	Increased O_2 consumption; increased CO_2 production; increased ventilation/perfusion abnormalities, particularly during anaesthesia; limited maximum lung capacity (inability to increase ventilation in response to increased demand); increased sensitivity to respiratory depressant drugs
Respiratory control	Obstructive sleep apnea, obesity hypoventilation syndrome, high risk of airway and intubation difficulties at induction of anesthesia

Figure 68.5 Pulmonary abnormalities in severe obesity.

The reduced FRC also impairs the capacity of obese individuals to tolerate apnea. Obese individuals lose arterial oxygen (desaturate) rapidly following induction of anesthesia, even if they have had preoxygenation. In patients who have a normal BMI, at least 450 seconds of apnea can elapse before arterial saturation drops below 90% after a standard period of preoxygenation, compared with 300 seconds in the morbidly obese. This may be a result of obese individuals having a lower FRC and, therefore, a smaller reservoir of oxygen that can be used during periods of apnea.

Ventilatory control

Severe obesity is associated with two disorders of ventilatory control: obstructive sleep apnea (OSA) and obesity hypoventilation syndrome. Since the two often coexist, they can be considered together.

The occurrence of OSA is a common and potentially serious medical problem characterized by frequent episodes of apnea and/or hypopnea during sleep. Its consequences include repeated arousal from sleep, along with recurrent episodes of hypoxemia and hypercapnia. It occurs because during sleep the pharyngeal muscles relax, promoting upper airway collapse under the influence of the subatmospheric intrathoracic pressure generated during inspiration. Total occlusion becomes more likely when the pharyngeal soft tissues are expanded, if the airway morphology is abnormally narrowed, or if pharyngeal muscle tone is further reduced by drugs, alcohol, etc. The airway only reopens when the pharyngeal muscle tone is restored; this occurs when the individual is aroused from sleep in response to the hypoxemia/hypercapnia. An obstructive apneic episode is defined arbitrarily as a total cessation of airflow for 10 seconds or more despite continued respiratory efforts against an obstructed pharyngeal airway, while hypopnea is defined as a 50% reduction in airflow or a reduction sufficient to lead to 4% or greater reduction in arterial oxygen saturation. The precise definition of significant OSA is disputed and relies as much on the incidence of clinical sequelae as the precise number of apneic/hypopneic episodes, although a frequency of five or more episodes per hour of sleep, or more than 30 episodes per night is often quoted. In extreme cases, there may be 300–400 obstructive episodes per night.

Severe obesity and the male gender combine to be significant risk factors for significant OSA (≥ 30 apneic episodes per night). The coexistence of other risk factors (e.g. evening alcohol or sedative ingestion) may compound the problems. There are a number of typical clinical and laboratory features of OSA; the definitive diagnosis of OSA requires polysomnography in a sleep laboratory.

Snoring

Snoring occurs that is typically *crescendo* snoring, which gets louder as the airway obstruction worsens, followed by silence when airflow ceases altogether, and finally gasping or choking as the patient is aroused and airway patency is restored. The patient himself may be completely unaware of his snoring until complaints are made by a partner or even the neighbours!

Daytime somnolence

Frequent arousals each night severely fragment sleep and cause marked daytime sleepiness. This is associated with memory problems, poor attention and concentration skills, personality changes, and a high incidence of accidents (sufferers are 10 times more likely to be involved in road traffic accidents than normal individuals).

Perioperative changes in oxygenation, and the influence of the peak end-expiratory pressure (PEEP)

Ventilation conditions	Pa_{O_2} (kPa)	Pa_{CO_2} (kPa)	$PA_{O_2} - Pa_{O_2}$ (kPa)	Cardiac output (QT) (L/min)	Shunt fraction (QS/QT) (%)	Oxygen delivery (D_{O_2}) (mL/min)
Preoperative, air	10.9 ± 1.1	4.6 ± 0.3	3.5 ± 1.1	7.3 ± 1.1	10 ± 4	1346 ± 222
Intermittent positive-pressure ventilation [fraction inspired O_2 = 0.5] at peak end-expiratory pressures of:						
0	14.0 ± 2.7	4.5 ± 0.5	28.4 ± 2.6	5.5 ± 1.1	21 ± 5	1039 ± 239
10cmH_2O	15.8 ± 3.0	4.5 ± 0.3	26.7 ± 3.0	5.2 ± 0.9	17 ± 3	996 ± 210
15cmH_2O	21.5 ± 7.2	4.5 ± 0.3	21.2 ± 7.1	4.4 ± 0.6	13 ± 4	862 ± 170

Figure 68.6 Perioperative changes in oxygenation, and the influence of the peak end-expiratory pressure (PEEP). A modest defect in gas exchange and increased shunt fraction deteriorates dramatically following induction of anesthesia despite intubation and ventilation (zero PEEP) and requires an increase in the inspired oxygen fraction. (Pa_{O_2}, arterial partial pressure of oxygen; PA_{O_2}, alveolar partial pressure of oxygen.)

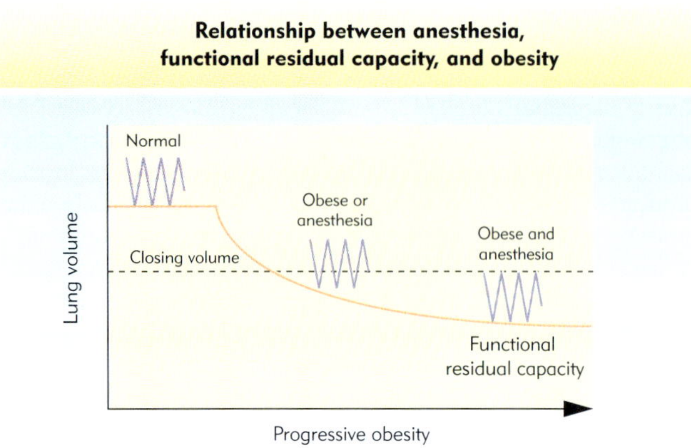

Figure 68.7 Relationship between anesthesia, functional residual capacity (FRC), and closing volume in obese patients. Obesity is associated with a progressive fall in the FRC, so that tidal ventilation increasingly encroaches on the lung closing volume. Anesthesia also results in a fall in FRC, adding to the intrapulmonary shunt suffered by patients who have severe obesity.

Physiologic responses

The physiologic responses to recurrent apnea include hypoxemia and hypercapnia as well as pulmonary and systemic vasoconstriction. Repeated episodes of hypoxemia leads to secondary polycythemia, while recurrent pulmonary vasoconstriction leads to right ventricular impairment.

Obesity hypoventilation syndrome

A further response to long-term severe OSA is a progressive alteration in the central control of breathing. These changes are limited initially to sleep and are manifested by a reduction in respiratory drive leading to central apneic events (i.e. apnea without respiratory effort) and are accompanied by altered chemoreceptor sensitivity to carbon dioxide. Eventually, however, there is loss of normal respiratory control during the day, and daytime respiratory failure develops: the so-called obesity hypoventilation syndrome.

Other features

Features that help to identify significant OSA include BMI over 30kg/m^2, hypertension, observed apneic episodes during sleep, collar size greater than 16.5, polycythemia, hypoxemia/hypercapnia, and right ventricular strain/impairment on electrocardiography and echocardiography. Overnight oximetry is also a practical assessment in many institutions.

Anesthetic implications

Preoperative assessment should include lung function tests, arterial blood gases, overnight pulse oximetry, and full blood count (to exclude polycythemia). Patients who have symptoms of significant OSA may benefit from polysomnography and even from preoperative treatment of such airway problems.

Induction of anesthesia is a particularly hazardous time, for a number of reasons. Although BMI *per se* is a poor predictor of perioperative airway difficulties, the same factors that promote OSA in obese patients (fatty infiltration of the soft tissues of the neck) make airway maintenance and intubation more difficult. All patients who have OSA are at risk of airway obstruction on induction of anesthesia and should be considered to be a potentially difficult intubation.

Obese patients tolerate periods of apnea badly, even if an adequate period of preoxygenation has been used. Bag/mask ventilation is likely to be very difficult because of upper airway obstruction and the low chest compliance. The increased risk of regurgitation and inspiration of stomach contents will be increased by gastric insufflation during ineffective mask ventilation.

Awake fiberoptic intubation should be considered in patients likely to present airway/intubation difficulties. Otherwise a rapid sequence induction technique with succinylcholine (suxamethonium) following a period of preoxygenation will provide the best conditions in which to intubate the trachea as quickly and safely as possible. It is particularly important under these circumstances to have skilled and physically strong anesthetic assistance, along with a comprehensive range of aids for a difficult intubation.

Episodes of hypoxemia and hypercapnia may increase pulmonary vascular resistance and precipitate right-sided heart failure. Hypoventilation is likely to occur if obese patients are allowed to breathe spontaneously under anesthesia. The lithotomy or Trendelenburg positions may further impair respiratory function. Intubation and mechanical ventilation with high inspired oxygen fractions should be employed in all but the briefest of cases, and PEEP may be required to maintain adequate oxygenation. Care must be taken to ensure that a sufficiently powerful and sophisticated mechanical ventilator is available. End-tidal capnography may significantly underestimate arterial carbon dioxide levels because of an increased alveolar to arterial carbon dioxide difference and it is, therefore, a poor guide to ventilation. Adequacy of minute ventilation is best assessed by frequent arterial blood gas measurements, particularly in those patients at risk of pulmonary hypertension and right-sided heart failure.

The postoperative period is often the time of greatest danger. Whether or not a period of postoperative ventilation is employed, such patients should be monitored closely. Patients may be very sensitive to the effects of sedatives, opioids, and anesthetic drugs, all of which may further worsen upper airway control and ventilatory drive. Postoperative ventilation may be indicated in such circumstances in order to allow the safe elimination of residual sedative agents; regional anesthetic techniques should be used if at all possible.

Anesthesia abolishes rapid eye movement (REM) sleep in the first two or three postoperative nights, which leads to a compensatory increase in REM sleep in subsequent nights (Chapter 13). Since OSA episodes are worse during REM sleep, obstructive airway problems may be worse on the third to fifth postoperative nights. High-risk patients may, therefore, require appropriate monitoring (e.g. continuous pulse oximetry) for longer periods of time than might otherwise be anticipated from the surgery alone.

OBESITY AND OTHER MEDICAL CONDITIONS

The diverse medical consequences of obesity are listed in Figure 68.8. The increased incidence of surgical pathologies such as neoplasia, osteoarthritis, gallstones, incontinence, and infertility means that obese individuals present for anesthesia more frequently than their lean peers. The medical consequences of obesity make this group of patients more difficult to manage in

Medical and surgical conditions associated with obesity

Cardiovascular
- Sudden (cardiac) death
- Obesity cardiomyopathy
- Hypertension
- Ischemic heart disease
- Hyperlipidemia
- Cor pulmonale
- Cerebrovascular disease
- Peripheral vascular disease
- Varicose veins
- Deep vein thrombosis and pulmonary embolism

Respiratory
- Restrictive lung disease
- Obstructive sleep apnea
- Obesity hypoventilation syndrome

Endocrine
- Diabetes mellitus
- Cushing's disease
- Hypothyroidism
- Infertility

Gastrointestinal
- Hiatus hernia
- Gallstones
- Inguinal hernia

Genitourinary
- Menstrual abnormalities
- Female urinary incontinence
- Renal calculi

Musculoskeletal
- Osteoarthritis of weight-bearing joints
- Back pain

Malignancy
- Breast
- Prostate
- Colorectal
- Cervical and endometrial

Figure 68.8 Medical and surgical conditions associated with obesity.

the perioperative period. While most of the conditions listed in Figure 68.8 require no specific consideration, a number merit some attention.

Hiatus hernia and gastroesophageal reflux

Obese individuals are more at risk of aspiration of gastric contents during anesthesia, for several reasons. First, there is an increased incidence of esophageal reflux and hiatus hernia; this may be exacerbated by the raised intra-abdominal pressure associated with obesity and the supine lithotomy and Trendelenburg positions. Second, 75% of obese patients have a resting volume of gastric contents that is greater than 25mL, with a low pH (<2.5). Third, gastric emptying may be delayed (although this is disputed). Finally, there is a higher incidence of difficult intubation. Precautions against acid aspiration at induction and reduction of anesthesia should always be taken. Approaches include reduction in the volume and acidity of gastric contents with histamine H_2 antagonists, antacids, and prokinetic agents such as metoclopramide or cisapride; rapid sequence induction with cricoid pressure; and extubation with the patient fully awake.

Diabetes mellitus

In one perioperative series, more than 10% of patients undergoing bariatric surgery had an abnormal glucose tolerance test. There is a clear causal relationship between obesity and type II or maturity-onset diabetes mellitus, so much so that it is now considered to be a surgically correctable disease in the morbidly obese population. The catabolic response to (surgical) trauma or sepsis may worsen glucose intolerance to the extent that insulin becomes necessary to control blood sugar perioperatively. The preoperative workup of morbidly obese individuals should include a random blood sugar and, if necessary, a glucose tolerance test.

Thromboembolic disease

The incidence of deep vein thrombosis following nonmalignant abdominal surgery in obese individuals, as revealed by iodine-labeled fibrinogen uptake scans, is twice that of lean patients (48 versus 23%), and there is a similar increased risk of pulmonary embolus in patients weighing more than 91kg. Furthermore, it is the most serious nonsurgical complication of bariatric surgery, with an incidence as high as 4.5%. The higher incidence of thromboembolic disease in obese patients is likely to be multifactorial in origin, including venous stasis owing to reduced mobility, increased pressure on deep venous channels of lower limb, and global reductions in cardiac output because of ventricular impairment; the occurrence of prolonged surgery; increased blood viscosity resulting from polycythemia; and reduced fibrinolysis.

There is no general agreement as to how to reduce the risk of perioperative thromboembolism. Approaches include the use of anticoagulant regimens such as subcutaneous heparin (including low-molecular-weight preparations such as enoxaparin), elasticated stockings, intermittent calf compression devices, axial sympathetic blockade to increase lower limb blood flow, and prompt postoperative mobilization.

ALTERED DRUG HANDLING IN OBESITY

Obesity is associated with alterations in the distribution, binding, and elimination of many drugs; the resulting pharmacokinetic consequences may be of considerable importance to the anesthesiologist. The implications for the use of specific anesthetic drugs are summarized in Figure 68.9.

Volume of distribution

Factors that influence volume of distribution of a drug in obesity include increased size of the fat organ, increased lean body mass, increased blood volume and cardiac output, reduced total body water, and alterations in blood concentrations of species that alter protein binding, such as free fatty acids and α_1-acid glycoprotein.

The consequences of these changes on the clinical effectiveness of a drug will depend upon its lipid solubility, its route of administration, and upon whether the effect is achieved at bolus or steady-state concentrations. Any increase in the volume of distribution will reduce the elimination half-life unless the clearance is increased. The altered kinetics of thiopental (thiopentone) illustrate these effects. Because of an increased blood volume, cardiac output, and muscle mass, there is an increase in its central volume of distribution; therefore, the absolute dose should be increased: up to 1g may be required, although on a weight per weight basis (mg/kg) the dose required is less than in nonobese patients. As with other highly lipid-soluble drugs, the terminal disposition and steady-state volumes of distribution for thiopental are three to four times greater than normal; as a result, the elimination of thiopental can be expected to be delayed. This is of particular clinical importance following the administration of benzodiazepines, when the effects may persist for some days after discontinuation.

Drug	Altered pharmacokinetics	Clinical implications
Hypnotics		
Thiopental	Increased central volume of distribution, prolonged elimination half-life	Increased absolute dose, reduced dose/unit body weight, prolonged duration of action
Propofol	Little known	Increased absolute dose, reduced dose/unit body weight
Midazolam, diazepam	Central volume of distribution increases in line with body weight, prolonged elimination half-life	Increased absolute dose, same dose/unit body weight, prolonged duration of action, particularly after infusion
Muscle relaxants		
Succinylcholine	Plasma cholinesterase activity increases in proportion to body weight	Increased absolute dose, reduced dose/unit body weight, doses of 120–140mg appear satisfactory
Atracurium	No change in absolute clearance, absolute volume of distribution and absolute elimination half-life	Unchanged dose/unit body weight
Vecuronium	Impaired hepatic clearance and increased volume of distribution lead to delayed recovery time	Give according to estimated lean body weight
Pancuronium, tubocurarine chloride (d-tubocurarine)	Low lipid solubility, elimination half-life increases in proportion with the degree of obesity	Unchanged dose/unit body weight, give according to estimated lean body weight
Opioids		
Fentanyl	No change in elimination following 10μg/kg	Dose per unit body weight unchanged
Alfentanil	Elimination may be prolonged	Adjust dose to lean body weight
Morphine	No information available	–
Local anesthetics		
Lidocaine (lignocaine)	Increased absolute volume of distribution, unchanged if adjusted for body weight; increased epidural fat content and epidural venous engorgement	Intravenous dose unchanged as dose/unit body weight, extradural dose is 75% of dose calculated according to total body weight
Bupivacaine	No information available	–
Inhalational anesthetics		
Nitrous oxide	Little information	Increases fraction of inspred O_2, which limits practical usefulness; intestinal distension may contribute to perioperative difficulties
Halothane	Considerable deposition in adipose tissue, increased risk of reductive hepatic metabolism	Possible increased risk of halothane hepatitis
Enflurane	Blood:gas partition coefficient falls with increasing obesity, inorganic fluoride levels rise twice as fast in obese individuals	Possibly lower minimum alveolar concentration (MAC)
Sevoflurane	No difference in fluoride levels between obese and nonobese patients	Increased risk of fluoride nephrotoxicity following prolonged administration

Figure 68.9 Influence of obesity on the pharmacokinetics of anesthetic drugs. (Adapted from Shenkman et al., 1993.)

Drug clearance

Renal clearance increases in obesity because of the increased renal blood flow and glomerular filtration rate. The effects of obesity on liver metabolism are more unpredictable, although reduction in liver blood flow in patients who have congestive cardiac failure may slow the elimination of drugs with a rapid hepatic elimination such as lidocaine (lignocaine) and midazolam.

Inhalational anesthetics

It has been traditionally held that the slow emergence from anesthesia often experienced by obese patients results from the delayed release of the highly lipid-soluble volatile agents from the excessive amount of adipose tissue. This is probably not the case because reductions in fat blood flow may limit the delivery of volatile agents to such fat stores, and the slow emergence is more likely to result from increased central sensitivity to anesthetic drugs.

Obese patients may be more at risk from ill-effects as a consequence of changed hepatic metabolism of volatile agents (see Chapter 24). For example, plasma bromide levels – a marker of both oxidative and reductive metabolism of halothane – are higher in obese patients. Increased reductive metabolism of halothane is considered to be an important factor in the etiology of liver injury following halothane exposure and may be more likely in obese individuals at risk of hypoxemia and reduced hepatic blood flow. The hepatic metabolism of the halogenated volatile agents may also result in increased plasma concentrations of inorganic free fluoride ions, which are potentially nephrotoxic if levels exceed 95mg/dL (50mmol/L). Plasma fluoride levels following methoxyflurane, halothane, and enflurane are all higher in obese patients, although this does not appears to occur with sevoflurane. The increased levels following enflurane may be of practical importance, fluoride concentrations being up to 60% higher in obese patients.

POSTOPERATIVE OUTCOMES IN MORBIDLY OBESE PATIENTS

It is traditionally held that severe obesity is associated with higher rates of postoperative morbidity and mortality, although the data are conflicting. For instance, while obesity does not influence mortality after hysterectomy or open cholecystectomy, in a survey of more than 2000 patients undergoing duodenal ulcer surgery the mortality rate was 6.6% in obese patients and 2.7% in the nonobese. Mortality rates following renal transplantation are considerably higher in obese patients. Furthermore, life insurance statistics have associated obesity with a two- to threefold increase in mortality from appendicitis and cholelithiasis. The most common causes of death following surgery for severe obesity are pulmonary embolism and anastamotic breakdown.

Logistic regression analysis of more than 3000 patients undergoing surgery for severe obesity suggests that postoperative complications are related to age, preoperative BMI, and the male gender. Respiratory problems are the most common postoperative complication in obese patients. The reduced lung volumes observed during anesthesia persist for some days postoperatively, particularly following abdominal surgery, and correlate with hypoxemia. In one series of obese individuals undergoing bariatric surgery, there was a 22% incidence of postoperative lung collapse. Wound infections are also more common and presumably result from longer incisions, extended operative times, difficulty in obliterating tissue deadspace, and the inability of adipose tissue to resist infection. The morbidly obese parturient represents a particularly high-risk group. In comparison with nonobese parturients, they carry a higher risk of premature labor, emergency cesarean section (with longer operative times), and failed epidural analgesia. There may also be a higher incidence of accidental dural puncture.

Key References

Alpert MA, Hashimi MW. Obesity and the heart. 1993;306:117–23.

Millman RP, Meyer TJ, Eveloff SE. Sleep apnea in the morbidly obese. Rhode Island Med. 1992;75:483–6.

Shenkman Z, Shir Y, Brodsky JB. Perioperative management of the obese patient. Anesthesiology. 1993;70:349–59.

Further Reading

Caterson ID, ed. Ballière's clinical endocrinology and metabolism, Vol. 8, Obesity. London: Ballière-Tindall; 1994. Several articles of interest, including Hodge AM, Zimmet PZ. The epidemiology of obesity. pp. 577–600; Grunstein RR, Wilcox I. Sleep-disordered breathing and obesity. pp. 601–28; Després J-P. Dyslipidemia and obesity. pp. 629–60.

Chapter 69 Physiologic responses to surgery and trauma

Joan P Desborough

Topics covered in this chapter

Surgery and trauma evoke a range of physiologic responses, which are part of a widespread systemic inflammatory reaction to injury. These responses include endocrinologic, immunologic, and hematologic changes and the release of inflammatory mediators such as cytokines (Fig. 69.1). This so-called 'stress response' is seen after all major systemic disturbances, including traumatic injury, burns, and major infection, as well as surgery. The aim of the response is to restore homeostasis by activating defense mechanisms, mobilizing substrates, and promoting healing and repair.

The hormonal and metabolic changes are initiated by activation of the hypothalamic–pituitary–adrenal (HPA) axis, which leads to increased secretion of pituitary hormones and cortisol. As a result, catabolism of stored body fuels occurs, with an increase in metabolic rate and oxygen consumption. In addition to alterations in endocrine secretion, other characteristic changes occur that are known as the 'acute-phase response' (Fig. 69.2).

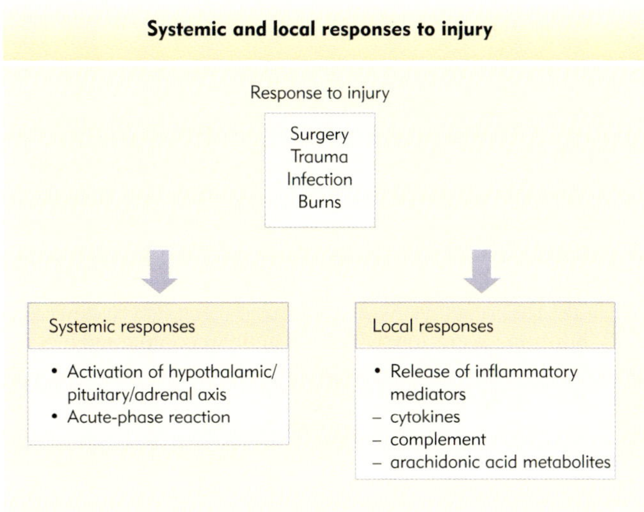

Figure 69.1 Systemic and local responses to injury.

Acute-phase responses to surgery and trauma

- Acute-phase protein production in the liver (e.g. C-reactive protein, fibrinogen)
- Decreased hepatic synthesis of albumin and transferrin
- Decreased circulating concentrations of divalent cations
- Neutrophil leukocytosis
- Lymphocyte proliferation and differentiation
- Increased body temperature

Figure 69.2 Acute-phase responses to surgery and trauma.

HORMONAL AND METABOLIC RESPONSES TO SURGERY

Afferent neuronal impulses from the site of the operation activate the sympathetic nervous system and stimulate hormonal secretion from the hypothalamus and pituitary gland. Both autonomic and somatic nerve pathways are involved. In addition to neural activation, many substances are released from cells as a result of tissue injury. These mediators, which include cytokines, augment the acute-phase reaction and have both local and systemic effects.

The magnitude and duration of the hormonal and metabolic response to surgery depends largely on the severity of the surgical stimulus. As discussed below, the responses can be modified by local and general anesthesia. The principal hormonal and metabolic sequelae are shown in Figure 69.3.

AUTONOMIC SYSTEM

The sympathetic nervous system is activated and epinephrine (adrenaline) is released from the adrenal medulla. Norepinephrine is released at adrenergic nerve terminals and may spill over into the circulation. Therefore, the concentrations of circulating catecholamines become elevated, which leads to tachycardia, hypertension, and increased systemic vascular resistance, although these effects are often obtunded by general or local anesthesia.

Pituitary hormones

The hypothalamus is stimulated to produce releasing factors that increase anterior pituitary hormone secretion. β-Endorphin,

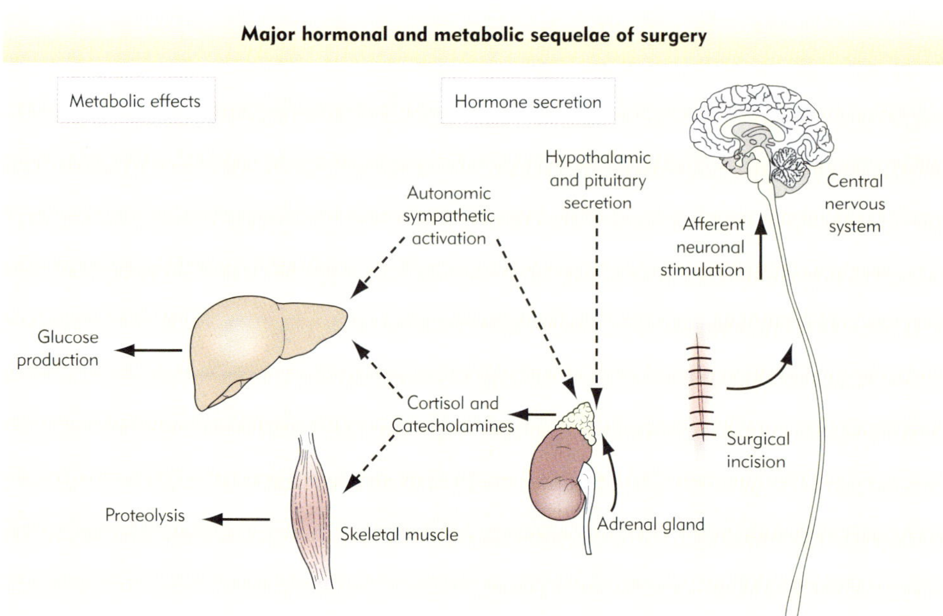

Figure 69.3 Major hormonal and metabolic sequelae of surgery.

prolactin, adrenocorticotropic hormone (ACTH), and growth hormone (GH) are secreted, of which ACTH and GH have significant hormonal and metabolic effects. Much of the research on hormonal responses to surgery is centered on changes in catecholamines, cortisol production, and the glycemic responses. Changes in thyroid hormone and gonadotropin secretion also occur, but have received less attention. Overall, the endocrine response is characterized by an increase in catabolic hormone secretion, which is usually accompanied by suppression of the release of the anabolic hormones testosterone and insulin (Fig. 69.4).

Increased amounts of arginine vasopressin are secreted from the posterior pituitary, with a resultant conservation of salt and water by the kidney.

Insulin and glucagon

Insulin is secreted from the β cells of the islets of Langerhans in the pancreas in response to increases in blood glucose (Chapter 63). Insulin is an anabolic hormone; it promotes the uptake of glucose and its storage as glycogen, and it inhibits the mobilization of fat and muscle protein. After the onset of surgery, circulating concentrations of insulin may increase or decrease, but occasionally do not change. However, insulin secretion fails to increase appropriately for the hyperglycemia that is provoked by surgery.

The exact mechanism(s) for the relative lack of insulin remains unclear. It is possible that secretion may be inhibited by anesthesia, either directly or through decreased blood flow. It is widely assumed that sympathetic stimulation and circulating epinephrine inhibit insulin secretion through α-adrenoceptors. In addition to the relative hyposecretion of insulin in the perioperative period, insulin appears to be less effective metabolically; this is known as insulin resistance.

Glucagon is released from the α cells of the pancreas. This hormone increases blood glucose concentrations by glycogenolysis in the liver and gluconeogenesis. It stimulates lipolysis and ketone body formation. Secretion of glucagon changes little after surgical stimulation.

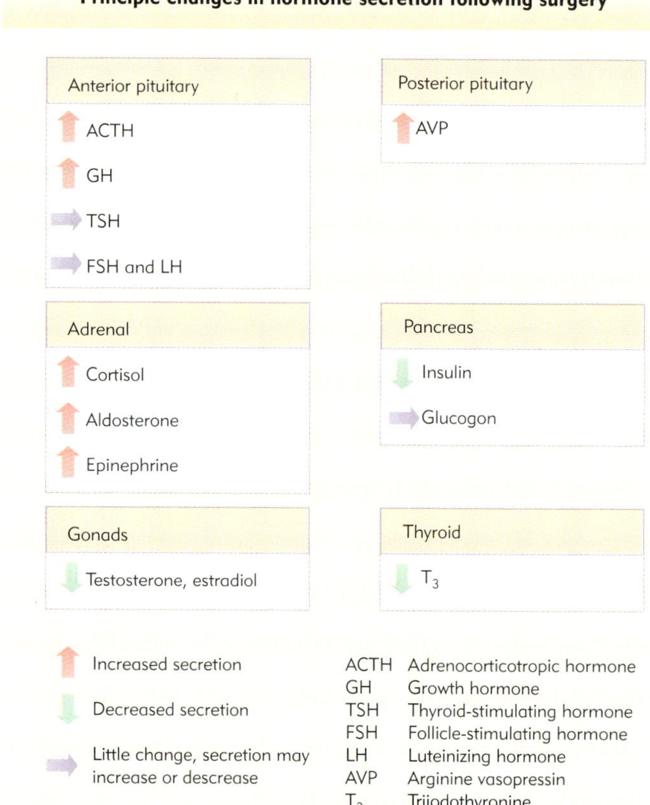

Figure 69.4 Principal changes in hormone secretion following surgery.

Thyroid hormones

The influence of surgery on thyroid hormone concentrations is well defined. For example, in one study of abdominal surgery, total and free triiodothyronine (T_3) values decreased markedly during surgery, returning to normal after about 7 days. Free thyroxine (T_4) concentrations increased during surgery itself and remained constant during the postoperative period despite a slight postoperative decrease in total T_4. Thyroid-stimulating hormone (TSH) values showed a profound decrease during the first 24 hours postoperatively and returned to preoperative levels. Such changes, the cause of which remains unclear, suggest that TSH and T_3 production is suppressed in the early postoperative period. A relationship between thyroid hormones, cortisol, and catecholamines after surgery and other trauma has been suggested. Thus, hyperadrenocortisolism may suppress T_3. An alternative theory is that since thyroid hormones have a stimulatory effect on metabolism, suppression of these hormones guards against excessive catabolism in the presence of high concentrations of catecholamines.

Gonadotropins

Pituitary secretion of leutenizing hormone increases during surgery, returning close to preoperative values by the first postoperative day. Serum values of follicle-stimulating hormone show no significant changes in the perioperative period. Circulating concentrations of testosterone and estradiol are decreased following surgery, reaching minimum values around the fourth and fifth postoperative days.

METABOLIC SEQUELAE

The effect of catabolic hormone secretion is substrate mobilization. In evolutionary terms, this probably represents a survival mechanism that allows injured animals to sustain themselves using their own stored body fuel. Hyperglycemia occurs during surgery as a result of increased hepatic glycogenolysis and gluconeogenesis. This is facilitated by catecholamines and cortisol, together with a relative suppression of insulin secretion. Protein catabolism releases amino acids, which are used in the synthesis of acute-phase proteins by the liver, and in gluconeogenesis. Production of free fatty acids from triglyceride breakdown is stimulated by catecholamines.

The glycemic response

Blood glucose values vary with the intensity of surgical stimulation. For example, concentrations of blood glucose may reach up to 180mg/dL (10mmol/L) in cardiac surgery, but are much lower after cataract surgery. The changes are closely associated with increases in catecholamine secretion, which suggests that catecholamines have a key role in the glycemic response. Interestingly, the feedback mechanisms that usually restore normoglycemia are ineffective after surgery so that hyperglycemia continues unabated until the stimulus subsides.

Evidence that prolonged hyperglycemia may be harmful is increasing, particularly in diabetic patients. In diabetic subjects, poor glycemic control is associated with an increased incidence of diabetic complications. Potential risks of perioperative hyperglycemia include impaired wound healing and wound infection. In addition, ischemic damage to the myocardium and nervous system is worsened by the presence of hyperglycemia.

Protein catabolism

Following major surgery, muscle protein is catabolized. Considerable weight loss up to 0.5kg of lean body mass per day can occur after major surgery or trauma. The amino acids mobilized are used in gluconeogenesis and the formation of new acute-phase proteins in the liver. The stimulus for protein breakdown is likely to be a combination of factors, which include catabolic hormone secretion, low insulin concentrations, and cytokines.

Fat metabolism

The effects of surgical trauma on fat metabolism have received much less attention than the glycemic changes – there are few changes, unless starvation is an important feature. In cardiac surgery, heparinization leads to marked increases in circulating nonesterified fatty acids (NEFAs) values. Heparin activates lipoprotein lipase which acts on triglycerides, ultimately releasing NEFAs.

Renal effects

The neuroendocrine control of the kidney, and the regulation of blood volume and electrolyte concentrations are described in Chapter 54. In response to surgery, a number of hormonal changes occur that influence salt and water metabolism and allow the preservation of an adequate circulating blood volume. The release of vasopressin from the posterior pituitary leads to water retention and the production of concentrated urine by a direct action on the kidney. Increased vasopressin release may last for 3–5 days, depending on the severity of surgery and the development of complications such as sepsis. Renin secretion is increased partly as a result of sympathetic stimulation of the juxtaglomerular cells of the kidney, which promotes the production of angiotensin II. This has a number of important effects, including stimulation of the release of aldosterone from the adrenal cortex, which promotes Na^+ and water reabsorption from the distal tubules in the kidney.

CYTOKINES

Cytokines are low molecular weight (up to 80kDa) proteins produced from activated white blood cells, in particular monocytes, and from activated fibroblasts and endothelial cells. These proteins together with other inflammatory mediators are released as an early cellular response to tissue injury. The cytokines act on surface receptors of many different target cells and their effects ultimately result from an influence on protein synthesis within these target cells. Cytokines play a major role in the inflammatory responses to trauma and infection, but they also have longer term effects on cells as regulators of cell growth and differentiation.

The main cytokine produced after major surgery is interleukin-6 (IL-6). Other cytokines released after surgical stimuli are tumor necrosis factor-α and IL-1. Under normal circumstances in healthy individuals, circulating values of cytokines are low, if at all detectable. Increased circulating values of IL-6 are found within 30–60 minutes of the start of surgery, with significant increases after 2–4 hours. The response reflects the degree of tissue trauma, so that cytokine production is lowest with minimally invasive and laparoscopic procedures. The largest increases in IL-6 concentrations are found after surgery such as joint arthroplasty, vascular reconstruction, and colorectal surgery. Following these operations, cytokine values are elevated for further 48–72 hours. Peak values occur at about 24 hours. If complications such as sepsis arise in the postoperative period, concentrations of cytokines remain elevated until the stimulus subsides.

It is now recognized that acute-phase responses that cannot be explained by activation of the HPA axis are stimulated by cytokines. Although IL-1 was thought initially to be responsible for inducing the fever that follows surgery, IL-6 is likely to be involved in this response. One of the principal effects of IL-6 is to stimulate the manufacture in the liver of acute-phase proteins (one of the early names for IL-6 was hepatocyte-stimulating factor). The acute-phase proteins act as inflammatory mediators in scavenging and in tissue repair. They include C-reactive protein (CRP), fibrinogen, and α_2-macroglobulin and other antiproteinases. The changes in circulating CRP values lag behind the changes in IL-6, and CRP acts as a nonspecific opsonin to augment the phagocytosis of bacteria.

Another key action of cytokines is their effect on the immune system. The production and maturation of B and T lymphocytes and the maturation of hemopoietic stem cells are stimulated by IL-6. The cytokines also interact with the neuroendocrine system (e.g. IL-6 stimulates pituitary hormone secretion). Conversely, glucocorticoids have anti-inflammatory actions, and in large doses have inhibitory actions on cytokine production and the subsequent synthesis of acute-phase proteins.

EFFECT OF ANESTHESIA ON THE ENDOCRINE RESPONSE

Nerve blockade

A complete afferent and efferent nerve blockade prevents the hormonal responses to surgery. Such total blockade is possible if there is a specific nerve supply to the operative site (e.g. the optic nerve). Thus, the hormonal responses to cataract surgery can be abolished with retrobulbar or peribulbar block of the optic nerve.

Regional analgesia

Extradural analgesia with local anesthetic agents effectively inhibits the hormonal and metabolic consequences of surgery in the pelvis or lower limbs. The blockade must be extensive, from dermatomal levels T4 to S5. Afferent impulses from the operative site to the brain and efferent autonomic pathways to the liver and adrenal gland are blocked. Thus, the cortisol and glycemic responses to surgery are abolished. Less extensive blockade does not completely prevent the hormonal and metabolic changes.

For surgery in the upper abdomen and the chest, extensive blockade with local anesthetic modifies the glycemic responses. In a classic study, Bromage showed that, despite extensive block (up to the C6 dermatomal level in some cases), the hypercortisolemia of surgery was unaffected. Bromage suggested that afferent impulses were able to pass through the vagus nerve. Thus, the hypothalamus and pituitary were stimulated with subsequent release of ACTH and cortisol. The glycemic response was inhibited because the extradural block effectively inhibited the efferent sympathetic supply to the liver and adrenal gland. Other investigators suggest that, in upper abdominal and thoracic surgery, afferent impulses might also pass via diaphragmatic or peritoneal innervation. The failure of regional anesthesia to prevent endocrine responses in this type of surgery is caused by inadequate neural blockade.

Opioids

Opioids suppress hypothalamic and pituitary hormone secretion. It was demonstrated many years ago that morphine inhibited ACTH release from the pituitary gland, with subsequent suppression of cortisol secretion by an effect at hypothalamic level. High-dose opioids have been used to suppress the endocrine changes that occur during surgery. Although these techniques are valuable in elucidating hormonal responses, they are of limited use in clinical practice because of the associated ventilatory depression.

Fentanyl (50μg/kg) abolishes the endocrine and metabolic changes found during pelvic surgery, but larger doses are needed to inhibit responses to surgery in the upper abdomen. In a study using a dose of 100μg/kg fentanyl, the hormonal responses to cholecystectomy (by laparotomy) were suppressed, but postoperative ventilation of the lungs was required.

Morphine (4mg/kg) and fentanyl (50–100μg/kg) suppress the hormonal responses to cardiac surgery until the onset of cardiopulmonary bypass (CPB). At the beginning of CPB, intense afferent stimulation results from sudden and profound hemodilution, hypothermia, and the perturbations associated with flow through the bypass circuit. The consequent hormonal changes cannot be suppressed by high-dose opioids.

Intravenous and inhalational agents

Etomidate directly inhibits corticosteroid production in the adrenal gland by inhibition of the enzyme 11β-hydroxylase – the synthesis of both cortisol and aldosterone are blocked. Following a single dose of etomidate, production of these two hormones is inhibited for 6–12 hours. In healthy patients undergoing routine, elective surgery, no deleterious effects seem to result from this adrenal suppression. However, in the early 1980s an audit of the use of etomidate in the sedation of critically ill patients found the drug to be associated with increased mortality. As a result, it is no longer licensed to be used in long-term sedation.

Benzodiazepines inhibit hormone production from adrenocortical cells *in vitro*. In clinical studies, midazolam decreased the cortisol response in both minor surgery and cholecystectomy. In one of these studies, cortisol secretion was enhanced by the administration of exogenous ACTH, which demonstrates that the effect is at the level of the hypothalamus and pituitary, although a direct effect on the adrenal cortex may occur.

The volatile anesthetic agents have little influence on hormonal and metabolic responses to surgery. In high inspired concentrations, these agents may obtund the responses to minor surface operations, but were found to be ineffective in inhibiting the hormonal changes associated with pelvic surgery.

Multimodal therapy

Although regional techniques with local anesthetics and opioids provide excellent analgesia, they are ineffective in suppressing the hormonal responses to abdominal surgery. Combinations of other drugs, including analgesics, have been used with regional analgesia in an attempt to enhance hormone suppression after surgery. The addition of a nonsteroidal anti-inflammatory drug to a regimen of extradural bupivacaine and morphine gave very good postoperative analgesia following conventional cholecystectomy. However, it was no more effective in hormonal blockade than the extradural analgesia alone.

The addition of high-dose corticosteroid (methylprednisolone 30mg/kg) to the combined regimen was associated with a small decrease in the acute-phase and IL-6 responses.

Influence of inhibition of hormonal responses on surgical outcome

Much diligent research has been carried out in an attempt to determine anesthetic and analgesic regimens that inhibit the endocrine responses to surgery. Little evidence, apart from a few occasional reports, indicates that suppression of the hormonal and metabolic changes associated with surgery leads to improved patient outcome. Two reviews examined a large number of studies, and the most recent of these suggested that further work was required to establish a direct association between stress responses and patient outcome.

PHYSIOLOGIC RESPONSES TO HEMORRHAGE AND ANEMIA

Immediate changes

Loss of circulating volume by hemorrhage decreases cardiac filling and cardiac output falls, which activates numerous compensatory mechanisms (Fig. 69.5). Arterial baroreceptors are situated in the carotid sinus and aortic arch; cardiopulmonary baroreceptors are located in the pulmonary circulation and left ventricle. The rate of afferent discharge from these receptors depends on the degree of stretch to which the baroreceptor tissue is subjected. As circulating volume decreases, afferent nerve discharge decreases, and sympathetic activity increases, stimulating the cardiovascular system. The sympathetic reflexes are activated within 30 seconds of the onset of hemorrhage. Tachycardia helps maintain cardiac output and intense vasoconstriction maintains arterial pressure by an increase in total peripheral resistance.

Vasoconstriction is most intense in the skin (causing pallor), viscera, and kidneys. Reflex venoconstriction also helps maintain cardiac filling pressure. Blood is shifted out of venous reservoirs in the skin, and from the pulmonary veins and the visceral circulation into the systemic circulation. Contraction of the spleen also mobilizes a small volume of blood. Vasoconstriction spares the coronary and cerebral circulations, but not the kidneys. In the brain and heart, local autoregulation allows maintenance of blood flow at near-normal levels, provided mean arterial pressure is >70mmHg (9.3kPa). Both afferent and efferent arterioles of the kidney are constricted, the efferent vessels to a greater degree. Glomerular filtration is decreased and blood is shunted away from the cortical glomeruli. Urine output is decreased, which conserves circulating blood volume.

The decrease in cardiac output and vasoconstriction decreases tissue perfusion, with consequent anaerobic cell metabolism and increased production of lactic acid. Blood lactate levels may increase markedly from the normal value of about 1mmol/L. The metabolic acidosis can cause myocardial depression. Fluid is redistributed from the interstitial spaces into the intravascular compartment, which helps to maintain circulating blood volume. The pressure in the capillary beds is decreased because arterioles are constricted and the venous pressure is decreased by reduced blood volume. According to Starling forces that govern fluid transfer across capillary membranes, fluid moves into the capillaries from the interstitial spaces. Subsequently, the interstitial fluid volume is decreased and fluid moves out of cells.

Hemorrhage stimulates the release of catecholamines through increased sympathetic activity. Adrenal medullary secretion of epinephrine increases and circulating values of norepinephrine also increase as a result of release from sympathetic noradrenergic nerve terminals. The circulating catecholamines make a small contribution to the stimulus for vasoconstriction.

Other hormones are also secreted as a result of hemorrhage. Increased secretion of angiotensin II results from increased renin activity – angiotensin II is a very powerful vasoconstrictor and its release contributes to the maintenance of blood pressure. Arginine vasopressin, released from the posterior pituitary, also has an important role in maintaining blood pressure, as well as in promoting the preservation of water at the kidneys. Anterior pituitary hormone secretion increases in response to the stress of hemorrhage. Together with angiotensin, ACTH increases the release of aldosterone from the adrenal cortex. Aldosterone and vasopressin act on the kidney to conserve salt and water, which helps to maintain circulating blood volume. This mechanism takes at least 30 minutes to have an effect; the immediate decrease in urine output and Na^+ excretion is caused by the hemodynamic changes in the kidney.

During hemorrhage, anemia and stagnant hypoxia stimulate the chemoreceptors in the carotid and aortic bodies. Metabolic acidosis may also stimulate the chemoreceptors. Increased afferent nerve activity stimulates respiration, and also adds to the stimulus for vasoconstriction.

The osmoreceptors in the hypothalamus of the brain are sensitive to changes in osmolarity of the extracellular fluid and decreases in extracellular fluid volume. Increased afferent neural activity leads to the sensation of thirst in conscious patients.

Immediate physiologic responses to hemorrhage

Cause	Effect
Decreased cardiac filling	Decreased cardiac output
Decreased baroreceptor activity	Increased sympathetic stimulation Tachycardia, hypotension, peripheral vasoconstriction
Fluid redistribution	Venoconstriction, decreased ECF volume
Increased pituitary and adrenal hormone secretion	Increased circluating catecholamines Oliguria
Increased chemoreceptor stimulation	Tachypnea

Figure 69.5 Immediate physiologic responses to hemorrhage. ECF, extracellular fluid.

EFFECTS OF BLOOD LOSS

Circulatory shock is the term used when inadequate blood flow results in damage to body tissues. Provided that sympathetic reflexes are intact, about 10% of the blood volume can be lost with little change in either arterial pressure or cardiac output. At this stage, shock is reversible. With larger amounts of blood loss, cardiac output starts to decrease, followed by arterial pressure. The reflex compensatory mechanisms allow systemic arterial pressure to be maintained at an adequate level with blood volume losses of up to about 30–35%. Without intervention, losses >35–45% are not likely to be compatible with survival. In such circumstances, cardiac output declines progressively. Coronary blood flow decreases, which damages the myocardium and further decreases cardiac output. Blood flow to the vasomotor area of the brain falls so that the center becomes inactive and sympathetic output fails. Tissue hypoxia ensues as the circulation to the capillary beds becomes inadequate for cell survival.

Longer term compensatory mechanisms

In the longer term, changes occur to restore body fluid volume and blood components that have been lost. Most of the fluid that moves into the intravascular compartment is protein free.

Albumin moves into capillaries from stores in the skin and other sites. Plasma protein production in the liver is increased to replace the losses over a period of 3–4 days. Secretion of erythropoietin increases, which stimulates the formation of new red blood cells. The reticulocyte count increases and peaks at about 10 days after the hemorrhagic event. The red cell mass is restored to normal in 4–8 weeks.

Fluid therapy

The basis of fluid replacement is to maintain circulating fluid volume and ensure blood flow to the vital organs. Obviously, blood is required to replace losses, but whole blood is used rarely in current clinical practice. A combination of concentrated blood cells and plasma or plasma substitutes must be infused to replace lost blood and maintain intravascular volume. Plasma substitutes are colloidal solutions that contain particles of such a molecular size that they stay in the intravascular space for a useful period of time. Thus they provide more rapid and effective circulatory support than do crystalloid solutions. When crystalloid solutions are infused, the water is distributed throughout the extracellular fluid space; if used alone, large volumes are required. However, some crystalloid solutions are needed to replace fluid that has been lost from the intracellular and interstitial fluid spaces. An ideal regimen would be an infusion of 1500mL colloid to restore intravascular volume, followed by a 2:1 crystalloid:colloid mixture together with red cells to maintain hematocrit at 30%.

BURNS

Burn injury is associated with a widespread systemic disturbance that involves endocrinologic, metabolic, physiologic, and immunologic changes.

Burn injury results in significant fluid losses because of local and systemic increases in capillary permeability. Edema occurs in the burn wound and also in unburned tissue. The loss of fluid into the tissues decreases the extracellular and circulating volume, which leads to a decline in cardiac output. Hypovolemic shock follows unless fluid resuscitation is prompt.

In addition to the gross systemic disturbance, many local changes occur. Inflammatory mediators are released at the burn site and contribute to the increased vascular permeability and a hypermetabolic state, with the potential for wound infection, sepsis, and multiorgan failure. Increased plasma concentrations of the cytokines IL-1β and IL-6 are found in many patients following burn injury. Although these mediators are beneficial, very high cytokine concentrations may exacerbate tissue damage. Prostaglandins and leukotrienes are vasoactive products of arachidonic acid metabolites that are released at the burn site with a variety of effects. They increase permeability in the microvascular circulation, and prostaglandin E_2 allows the accumulation of neutrophils at the burn site, but not all of the mediators contribute to tissue repair and healing. For example, some of the thromboxanes cause local tissue ischemia and can lead to decreased perfusion of the gut and the kidneys. Sepsis and multiorgan failure may develop, even if the initial fluid resuscitation is adequate.

Resuscitative measures and fluid therapy

The mainstay of the initial management of burn injury is adequate fluid resuscitation. Most regimens are derived from retrospective data of fluid requirements and are based on the size of the burn. Many formulae now use similar volumes of fluid and no single regimen has been shown to be superior to any other. One example is a crystalloid infusion of 4mL/kg multiplied by the percentage of body size affected by the burn during the first 24 hours. Other regimens differ in the type of fluid that is given. The use of colloid decreases the total volume required, although its use has declined because controlled trials have shown it to provide no advantage. In adults, an hourly urine output >0.5mL/kg is a useful guide to adequate tissue perfusion.

The use of hypertonic fluid, such as crystalloid that contains sodium 250mmol/L, can decrease the total fluid volume requirements. This may theoretically be beneficial in patients who have poor cardiopulmonary function, as the risks of volume overload are lessened. However, the safety of hypertonic saline is unclear so very careful patient monitoring is required. One study reported that the use of hypertonic saline in burns increased the incidence of renal failure and death.

Hypermetabolism

Increased circulating concentrations of cortisol, catecholamines, and glucagon occur after burn injury. Patients become hypermetabolic with proteolysis, lipolysis, and gluconeogenesis. Massive protein catabolism may occur, with severe weight loss and muscle wasting. The release of inflammatory mediators, including cytokines, from the injured tissue contributes to the hypermetabolic state. The metabolic rate is also increased because of the fluid and heat losses from burned skin.

In addition to essential treatment with fluid volume resuscitation, many strategies have been suggested to ameliorate the catabolic changes that occur after burns. Early closure of burn wounds and raised environmental temperature have been used to decrease fluid losses and metabolic rate in thermally injured rats, although clinical studies of large burns show that early wound closure alone does not suppress the metabolic response.

The administration of GH to ameliorate the protein catabolic effects of burns and other injury received much interest in the past. However, GH alone may not be the ideal anabolic hormone in this situation as it has diabetogenic properties. Insulin-like growth factors (IGFs), such as IGF-1, have protein anabolic effects, but do not have the hyperglycemic effects of GH. A combination of GH and IGF-1 may be most suitable, to maximize protein anabolism and decrease the incidence of hyperglycemia.

Key References

Bruttig SP, Calgani DE. Hemorrhage and its treatment. Curr Opin Anaesthesiol. 1997;10:124–9.

Hall GM, Desborough JP. Endocrine and metabolic responses to surgery and injury – effects of anaesthesia. In: Prys-Roberts C, Brown BJ Jr, eds. International practice of anaesthesia, Vol. 1. Oxford: Butterworth Heinneman; 1996:Ch 79,1–11.

Monafo WW. Initial management of burns. N Engl J Med. 1996;335:1581–6.

Nguyen TT, Gilpin DA, Meyer NA, Herndon DN. Current treatment of severely burned patients. Ann Surg. 1996;223:14–25.

Ramsey G. Intravenous volume replacement: indications and choices. Br Med J. 1988;196:1422–3.

Further Reading

Kehlet H. Multimodal approach to control postoperative pathophysiology and rehabilitation. Br J Anaesth. 1997;78:606–17.

Liu S, Carpenter RL, Neal JM. Epidural anesthesia and analgesia. Their role in postoperative outcome. Anesthesiology. 1995;82:1474–506.

Scott NB, Kehlet H. Regional anaesthesia and surgical morbidity. Br J Surg. 1988;75:299–304.

Sheeran P, Hall GM. Cytokines in anaesthesia. Br J Anaesth. 1997;78:201–19.

Chapter 70 Sepsis

Nigel R Webster and Helen F Galley

Topics covered in this chapter

Definitions
Pathophysiology
Cytokines
Process of the inflammatory response
Multiorgan failure
Treatment
Genetic studies

Sepsis and septic shock are the most common causes of death in the intensive care unit (ICU). An estimated 400,000–500,000 patients develop sepsis each year in both European and American ICUs and some 50% of these demonstrate signs of shock. Sepsis often leads to multiorgan dysfunction and failure, with an associated high mortality rate. Of those patients developing septic shock, some 50–60% will die despite the best of currently available treatment. The incidence of sepsis in the ICU is increasing. This is most likely a consequence of our ability to sustain life through better organ support techniques and because of the more widespread use of invasive procedures in patients, more of whom are now immunocompromised.

DEFINITIONS

Definitions of sepsis and shock have been agreed at a recent consensus meeting of the American Thoracic Society and the American Society of Critical Care Medicine.

- *Infection* is an inflammatory response to the presence of microorganisms or the invasion of normally sterile host tissue by those organisms.
- *Bacteremia* is the presence of viable bacteria in the blood.
- *Septicemia is* a clinical term, the use of which is now discouraged.
- *Sepsis* is the systemic response to infection, manifested by two or more of the following conditions as a result of infection: temperature >100.4°F (>38°C) or <96.8°F (<36°C); heart rate >90 beat/min; respiratory rate >20 breaths/min or a requirement for artificial ventilation; and white blood cell count $>12{,}000/mm^3$ or $<4{,}000/mm^3$ ($>12 \times 10^9$ cells/L or $<4 \times 10^9$ cells/L).
- *Severe sepsis* is sepsis associated with organ dysfunction, hypoperfusion, or hypotension.
- *Septic shock* is sepsis-induced hypotension (systolic blood pressure <90mmHg) or a requirement for vasoconstrictors, despite adequate fluid resuscitation.
- *Multiple organ dysfunction syndrome* (MODS) is the presence of altered organ function such that homeostasis cannot be maintained without intervention.

In addition, it is now appreciated that no source of infection is found in many patients demonstrating all the signs of classical sepsis. This condition is referred to as the *systemic inflammatory response syndrome* (SIRS). It is thought that this condition results when inflammatory mediators (probably identical to those found in bacteremic patients) are released from ischemic and infarcted tissue.

Other terms have recently been added to this list to reflect the growing understanding of the relationship of the two counter systems that regulate the inflammatory response: namely the proinflammatory and anti-inflammatory processes. It is now thought that there is a carefully maintained balance between these two processes with *compensatory anti-inflammatory response syndrome* (CARS) and *mixed anti-inflammatory response syndrome* (MARS) suggested as suitable titles to describe this. These phases of the inflammatory response occur at differing time intervals from the initial insult, as depicted in Figure 70.1.

PATHOPHYSIOLOGY

Much evidence supports the hypothesis that molecules released from bacteria [called either *exotoxins* (secreted from live bacteria) or *endotoxins* (present in the cell wall of bacteria and usually released on bacterial death)] are responsible for the altered physiology seen in sepsis. These molecules are complexes of polysaccharide and fatty acids, with endotoxin commonly being called lipopolysaccharide (LPS). Examples of exotoxins include tetanus and botulinus toxins and the toxins seen in toxic shock syndrome. All of the signs and symptoms of sepsis can be reproduced by the injection of endotoxin into human volunteers. These subjects display an increased heart rate and cardiac output with a fall in blood pressure owing to vasodilatation and a decreased systemic vascular resistance. Respiratory rate increases, with a decreased arterial carbon dioxide partial pressure; while arterial oxygenation is maintained initially, it eventually falls because of an increased alveolar to arterial oxygen gradient caused by ventilation/perfusion mismatch. In addition, there is an accumulation of edema fluid because of increased capillary permeability. The endotoxin also causes changes in white blood cell and capillary endothelial function. A cascade of inflammatory mediators is released that will activate and recruit white cells to the affected region. It is against this inflammatory mediator cascade that most of the current research to improve treatment is directed.

Mediator release in sepsis

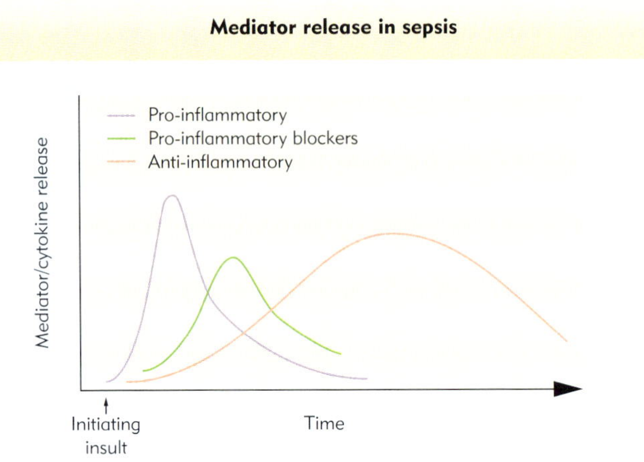

Figure 70.1 The time course of mediator release in sepsis. An early proinflammatory response is mounted (e.g. TNF-α and IL-1β), followed by a later release of proinflammatory blockers (e.g. IL-1 receptor antagonist) and anti-inflammatory cytokines (e.g. IL-10).

Outcome from sepsis is determined not only by the infection but also by the intensity of the immunoinflammatory response. This response is essential for the resolution of infection but may occur in an uncontrolled manner, causing damage to the host. The pronounced synergy and interaction of the components of the immune system dictate that modulation may result in either immunostimulation or immunosuppression. Co-ordination is, therefore, vital for an optimum response. Mediators of immunity and inflammation (families of protein and lipid molecules) are part of an intricate intercellular signaling system that enables cells, tissues, and organs to produce a response to an insult. This response may be modified if previous exposure to the insult has occurred.

The body possesses a range of barriers to prevent microorganisms from entering, including the skin, mucous secretion, ciliary action, and gastric acid. If these barriers are crossed, microorganisms are destroyed by soluble factors such as lysozyme and by phagocytosis with intracellular digestion (termed innate immunity). The complement system is a multicomponent triggered enzyme cascade that attracts phagocytes to microorganisms, increasing capillary permeability and neutrophil chemotaxis and adhesion. Specific acquired immunity in the form of antibodies inactivates microorganisms that are not destroyed by the innate immune system. Microorganisms evading the innate system either fail to activate the complement pathway or prevent activation of phagocytes. Acquired immune defense against specific microorganisms (antigen) forms the second component of the immune response. Antibodies activate the complement system, stimulate phagocytic cells, and specifically inactivate microorganisms (Chapter 52).

CYTOKINES

Cytokines are low-molecular-weight proteins produced by a variety of cells; they regulate the amplitude and duration of the inflammatory response (described in detail in Chapter 52). Cytokines have multiple effects on growth and differentiation in a variety of cell types, with considerable overlap and redundancy between different cytokines, partially accounted for by their shared ability to induce the synthesis of several proteins. Cytokines are transiently active and tightly regulated; they interact with specific high-affinity cell surface receptors to regulate gene expression. Interactions between cytokines may occur in a variety of ways: a cascade system in which one cytokine induces another; modulation of the receptor of another cytokine; synergism or antagonism between two cytokines acting on the same cell; release of receptor antagonists; and release of soluble receptors that bind cytokine without causing biologic actions.

Metabolic responses to tumor necrosis factor implicated in septic shock syndrome

System	Effects
Cardiovascular	Hypotension, myocardial suppression, decreased peripheral vascular resistance, capillary leakage syndrome
Pulmonary	Adult respiratory distress syndrome, capillary leakage with edema, leukocyte margination, respiratory arrest
Renal	Acute renal tubular necrosis
Gastrointestinal	Hemorrhagic necrosis, decreased motility, absorption
Hematologic	Neutrophilia or neutropenia, increased procoagulant activity, diffuse intravascular coagulopathy, endothelial activation
Central nervous	Fever, increased sympathetic outflow, anorexia, altered hypothalamic–pituitary outflow
Metabolic	Lactic acidosis, catabolic stress hormone release (catecholamines, glucagon, adrenocorticotropic hormone, cortisol), hyperglycemia followed by hypoglycemia, hyperaminoacidemia
Musculoskeletal	Myalgia, decreased resting membrane potential in skeletal muscle, increased skeletal muscle amino acid release

Figure 70.2 Metabolic responses to tumor necrosis factor is implicated in septic shock syndrome. (With permission from Tracey and Cerami, 1992.)

The local balance of cytokine effects is an important determinant of immune responses. Specific induction of each subset of T helper cells causes the production of a distant and specific range of cytokines and inflammatory mediators, which may have important implications for outcome in patients who have sepsis.

Not all of the effects of the inflammatory response are deleterious; indeed, the inflammatory response is a normal host defense mechanism. Nitric oxide and oxygen-derived free radicals are released by activated white cells and form peroxynitrite and prevent patients progressing to a systemic inflammatory response.

Several studies have shown that infusion of endotoxin or tumor necrosis factor-α (TNF-α) in animal models effectively mimics severe sepsis syndrome with ensuing organ dysfunction and leads to the appearance of other proinflammatory cytokines (Fig 70.2). Elevated circulating TNF-α concentrations are not found in all patients who have sepsis but are higher than in nonseptic critically ill patients (and highest levels are associated with the development of shock and lung injury).

Several studies of patients who have severe sepsis have shown that peak TNF-α concentrations are higher in those patients who die than in those who survive; they also fail to decrease in patients who die. However, other studies have found no association with outcome. It is possible that tissue or local concentrations of mediators are important for their actions rather than circulating levels, which may be too low to be measured in the peripheral circulation (Fig. 70.3).

Interleukin (IL)-6 concentrations are also increased in patients who have sepsis and are associated with the onset of shock. High levels have been linked to increased mortality in some studies, although again other studies have not found such a correlation. Levels of IL-1β are raised in some patients who have sepsis and are reported to be higher in nonsurvivors, although this difference is not found in all studies. In addition, a combined cytokine score encompassing endotoxin, TNF-α, Il-1β, and IL-6 concentrations was also found to correlate with mortality. Therapeutic administration of antibodies to TNF-α has been successful in increasing survival in primate models of sepsis, but human studies showed no effect on mortality, although TNF-α and IL-6 levels were attenuated and cardiac function improved. Concentrations of the anti-inflammatory cytokine IL-10 are also elevated in sepsis and are highest in those patients who have shock. Elevated IL-10 correlated with the subsequent development of sepsis in trauma patients and was highest in those septic patients who did not survive. Although there are no human studies, administration of IL-10 after caecal ligation and puncture in mice blunted the rise in TNF-α and improved survival.

Biologic activities of cytokines are regulated by specific cellular receptors. Soluble receptors released either as unique proteins or from shedding of cell surface expressed receptors, compete with membrane-bound receptors and appear in response to stimuli as part of a naturally occurring independent regulatory process to limit deleterious effects of the cytokine. Soluble receptors for TNF-α are elevated in patients who have severe sepsis, particularly in nonsurvivors. Circulating concentrations of the endogenous antagonist to the IL-1 receptor (IL-1RA) are elevated in patients who have sepsis but the relationship with outcome is unclear.

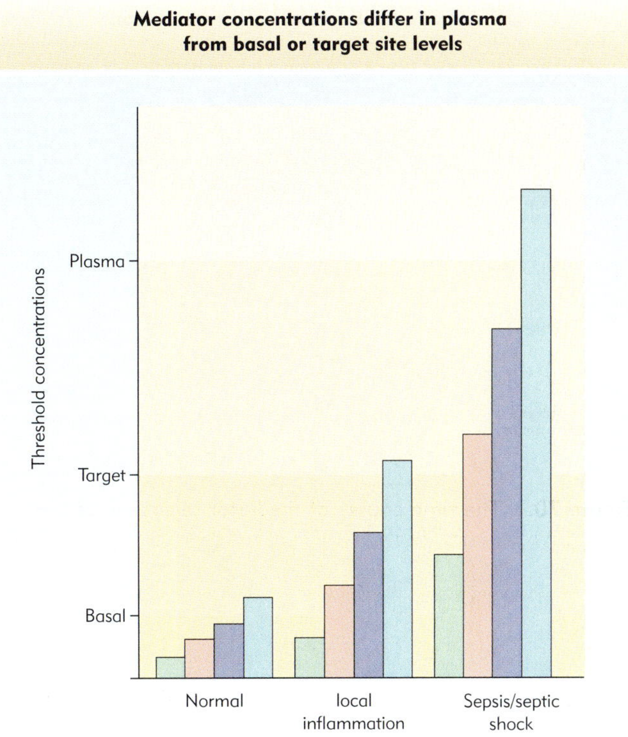

Figure 70.3 The difference between mediator concentrations basally, at target cell site, and in plasma. Different bars represent different mediators or tissue sites during sepsis, in local inflammation, and normally. Plasma concentrations may, therefore, not represent either target cell or tissue levels and may have little bearing on outcome from sepsis.

PROCESS OF THE INFLAMMATORY RESPONSE

Severe infection leads to the appearance of LPS in the bloodstream, which triggers innate immune responses such as activation of phagocytic cells and the complement cascade and leads to the production of the primary proinflammatory mediators TNF and IL-1. Secondary mediators, including other cytokines, prostaglandins, and platelet-activating factor (PAF), are then released, with further activation of complement, the initiation of the acute-phase response, expression of adhesion molecules, T-cell selection, antibody production, and release of oxygen-derived free radicals. Other toxins and cellular debris must also trigger such a systemic inflammatory response since this process can occur in the absence of LPS release.

Prolonged systemic exposure to high concentrations of cytokines and other components of the immunoinflammatory cascade may contribute to the development of MODS. Damage and activation of the endothelium, which plays a pivotal role in the regulation of hemostasis, vascular tone, and fibrinolysis, has profound consequences. The endothelium produces several substances that regulate inflammation and regional perfusion, including nitric oxide, vasoactive arachidonic acid metabolites, and cytokines. Changes in the balance of concentrations of these substances may contribute to the pathogenesis of the inflammatory response during sepsis and injury. Phagocytic cells are in constant contact with the endothelium, and disturbance of the relationship between these two cell types may result in direct tissue damage through local production of oxygen-derived free radicals, hypochlorous acid, and proteolytic enzymes.

Nitric oxide

Nitric oxide has many potential roles in the inflammatory process. Besides its vasodilatory effects (see Chapter 33), it reduces platelet aggregation, prevents monocyte chemotaxis, and inhibits leukocyte adhesion to the endothelium. Trials are currently ongoing using nitric oxide synthase (NOS) inhibitors to increase blood pressure in sepsis (Fig. 70.4). However, nitric oxide also reduces cytokine-induced expression of a number of effector molecules important in sepsis. Nitric oxide donors inhibit cytokine-induced vascular cell adhesion molecule (VCAM) expression and monocyte adhesion. This effect is more interesting since it appears that it is not caused by the usual activation of guanylyl cyclase but is most likely caused by inhibition of the transcription factor nuclear factor-kappa B (NF-κB) (Fig. 70.5). This transcription factor regulates the expression of adhesion molecules and various inflammatory cytokines such as IL-6 and IL-8. Since activation of NF-κB by TNFα is thought to occur via reactive oxygen species, nitric oxide may inhibit NF-κB by scavenging and inactivating superoxide anion. Nitric oxide has also been found to stabilize the inhibitory subunit of NF-κB (IκB).

In alveolar cells grown in culture, nitric oxide has been shown to modulate the cytotoxic effects of superoxide anion. Basal rates

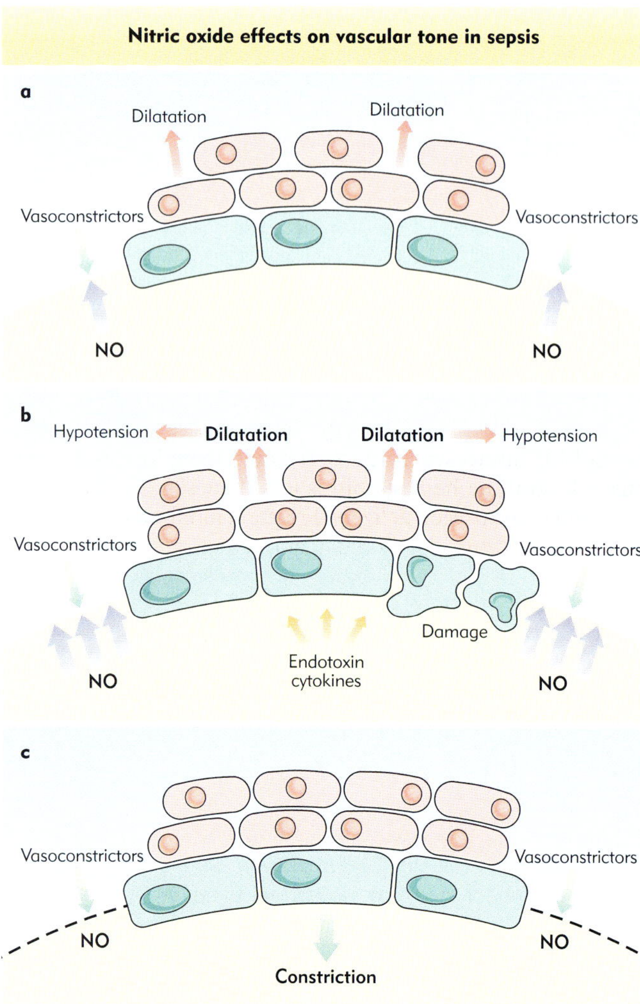

Figure 70.4 Nitric oxide effects on vascular tone in sepsis. Constitutively produced nitric oxide usually maintains a state of constant vasodilatation (a). During septic shock, large quantities of nitric oxide are produced in response to endotoxin and cytokines, resulting in excessive vasodilatation and hypotension (b). Inhibition of nitric oxide synthase in septic shock blocks the production of nitric oxide and results in vasoconstriction and reversal of shock (c).

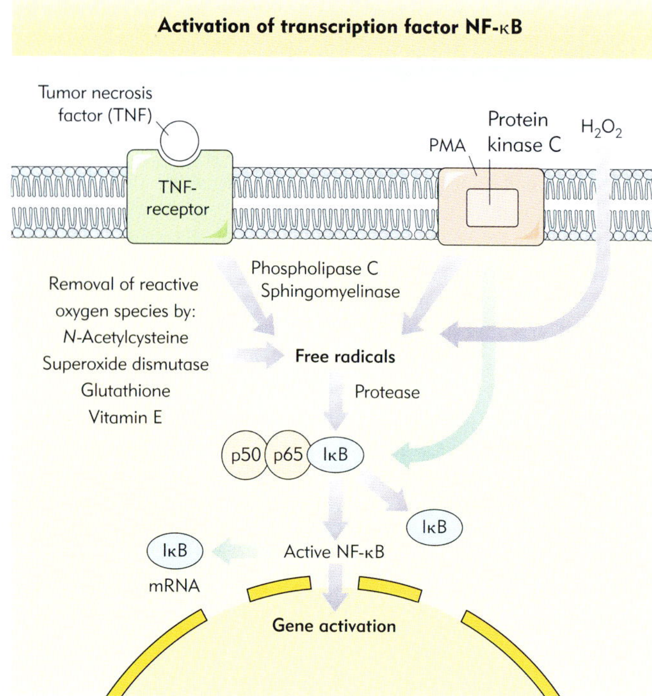

Figure 70.5 Schematic representation of the activation of the transcription factor nuclear factor-kappa B (NF-κB). Activation of NF-κB occurs by a common route involving free radicals and leading to removal of the inhibitory subunit IκB. The active NF-κB, consisting of the two subunits p50 and p65, then moves into the cell nucleus and binds to target DNA, leading to gene activation and transcription of mRNA for adhesion molecules, cytokines, NOS, and other inflammatory proteins. Antioxidants such as *N*-acetylcysteine block NF-κB activation by removal of reactive oxygen species.

of cytolysis and superoxide-dependent oxidative damage to the cells was attenuated by either enhanced rates of endogenous nitric oxide production following cytokine stimulation or by exogenous nitric oxide administration using either nitric oxide itself or the potentially more biologically important nitrosothiol compounds. In this model, nitric oxide alone was not cytotoxic. When control and cytokine-stimulated cells were treated with L-*N*-monomethylarginine (L-NMMA), a competitive inhibitor of NOS, cell injury was significantly increased, suggesting a protective role for endogenously produced nitric oxide.

MULTIORGAN FAILURE

Once the inflammatory response has been activated, many organ systems can be adversely affected. Of prime importance are the effects on the cardiovascular system that characterize severe sepsis. There is a marked fall in systemic vascular resistance resulting from arterial and venous dilatation; this is accompanied by leakage of plasma into the extravascular space, leading to relative hypovolemia. With adequate fluid resuscitation, the cardiac output is usually elevated. Despite this, myocardial performance is below normal, possibly because of the occurrence of circulating factors with myocardial depressant properties. Myocardial contractility is decreased and the left ventricular ejection fraction reduced, with high cardiac output being maintained by an increase in heart rate. The microcirculation is adversely affected, with maldistribution of blood flow (Fig. 70.6). Measurements of arteriovenous oxygen content difference and mixed venous saturations suggest that oxygen is neither reaching nor being effectively extracted by the cells. The reason for this is not fully understood but may be related to arteriovenous shunting or abnormalities in cellular metabolism. It has recently been demonstrated that nitric oxide can irreversibly inhibit enzymes involved in the electron transport chain of oxidative phosphorylation. Most patients have a raised blood lactate level and are acidotic.

Pulmonary manifestations of sepsis are common, ranging from mild hypoxemia to adult respiratory distress syndrome (ARDS). Hyperventilation occurs at first, probably because of the fall in arterial oxygen partial pressure, which is a consequence

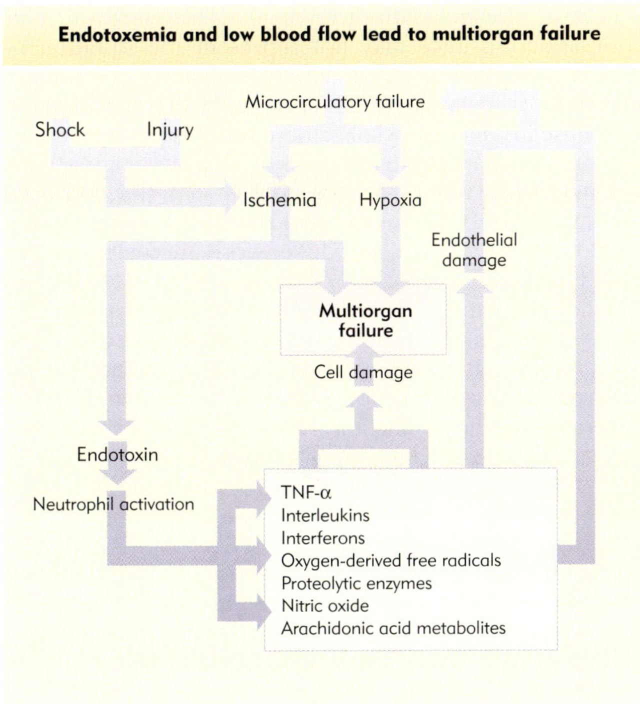

Figure 70.6 Endotoxemia and low blood flow in critically ill patients, resulting in multiorgan dysfunction syndrome.

of ventilation/perfusion mismatch. This progresses to acute lung injury with severe abnormalities in pulmonary gas exchange and the appearance of pulmonary edema that can be seen by chest X-ray. The edema results from margination of activated polymorphonuclear leukocytes within the pulmonary vascular bed and the release of mediators that increase vascular leakage.

Coagulation abnormalities are common, ranging from mild derangement of clotting times to disseminated intravascular coagulation (DIC) and thrombocytopenia. Decreased synthesis by the liver is one possible explanation. However, the vascular endothelium has an important role in the synthesis and release of antithrombotic and antiplatelet agents, and these are altered by the presence of inflammatory mediators.

Blood flow is altered to other organ systems in the presence of sepsis; this is particularly noticeable in the CNS, the kidneys, and the gastrointestinal system. Despite increased total hepatosplanchnic perfusion in sepsis and an accompanying rise in oxygen extraction across the gut wall, oxygen demand frequently outstrips supply, leading to inadequate oxygenation of the splanchnic bed.

TREATMENT

Recognition of sepsis often requires a high index of suspicion: while some cases will be obvious with fever and an identifiable source of sepsis, others will be much more subtle, particularly in the elderly and immunocompromised. A full microbiologic screen is imperative. Further investigations including sophisticated imaging techniques to identify possible sources of infection can be guided by the findings on initial clinical assessment. Because bacteriologic confirmation of the responsible organism is not usually immediately available, two or more antibiotics are often administered empirically. These should provide coverage against a broad spectrum of organisms but can often be 'targeted' at likely organisms based on the site of infection and the local patterns of sensitivity of common organisms. Vigorous steps should be taken to eradicate any source of infection; collections of pus must be drained (either surgically or using radiologically guided drain insertion) and nonviable tissue excised. Resuscitative measures are then instituted.

Oxygen is administered and many patients may require ventilatory support. Fluid resuscitation is commenced in an attempt to reverse the hypotension and tissue hypoperfusion. Septic patients often require large amounts of fluids to attain a reasonable cardiac preload. The choice of fluid used is a matter of some controversy, and the type may be of little significance, but it must be remembered that almost three times as much crystalloid as colloid will be required to achieve an equal expansion of the intravascular space. It would seem logical to transfuse blood if the hemoglobin is less than 10g/dL in order to facilitate tissue oxygen delivery. Frequent monitoring of the cardiovascular status is required. Central venous pressure rarely gives an accurate assessment of left ventricular preload in sepsis because of myocardial dysfunction, and pulmonary artery catheterization is currently recommended. Fluids are given to optimize both cardiac output and blood pressure and a Frank–Starling curve can readily be estimated by measuring cardiac output as fluid resuscitation continues. Inotropes and vasoconstrictors, including dopamine, dobutamine, epinephrine (adrenaline), phenylephrine, and norepinephrine (noradrenaline), are given to elevate cardiac output and systemic vascular resistance as appropriate (Chapters 36–38).

Immunotherapy

Steroids are well known immunomodulators and have been shown to alter the production of TNF by a specific effect on TNF messenger ribonucleic acid (mRNA). However, clinical studies have not shown that the use of steroids is beneficial. Similarly, pentoxyphylline (oxpentifylline) alters TNF production but has not been proven to be useful clinically. Both soluble receptors and monoclonal antibodies directed against receptors can be used to block the interaction of a cytokine with its receptor. This prevents transduction of the relevant biologic signal in the target cell. Use of a recombinant soluble receptor might also prevent the deleterious effect of excessive cytokine production. Administration of a recombinant form of the human IL-1RA to a heterogeneous group of patients who had sepsis was unsuccessful in reducing mortality. In addition to soluble receptors, monoclonal antibodies that block cellular cytokine receptors can be used as anticytokine therapy. However, it has been shown that cytokine complexed to such binding proteins is still available for receptor binding and will act as an agonist. Another approach to minimize the deleterious effects of the uncontrolled inflammatory process is to blunt the final common pathways of damage (i.e. using either agents that decrease free radical production or antioxidants that inactivate free radicals as they are produced). Monoclonal antibodies to TNF-α have been used both in clinical and animal studies. The use of soluble TNF receptors has also been evaluated in sepsis. The naturally occurring IL-1RA has been studied in two large clinical trials. Specific chemical antagonists, for example against PAF, have also been evaluated in patients who have sepsis.

Blockade of any single inflammatory mediator or a combination of mediators may not be successful for a number of reasons. First, the immunoinflammatory process is a normal response to infection and is essential not only for the resolution of infection but also for the initiation of other adaptive stress responses required for host survival (e.g. acute-phase and heat-shock responses). Second, the profound redundancy of action of many cytokines means that there are many overlapping pathways for cellular activation and further mediator release. Third, the synergism of actions and effects of many cytokines suggests that balance in the process of the immune response may be adversely affected by inhibition of a single agent. Fourth, exogenously administered anticytokine therapy may have hitherto unrecognized effects because of its interaction with other immunomodulators or their receptors. Finally, the timing of any potential anticytokine therapy is clearly crucial. Strategies designed to predict the activation of specific components of the inflammatory response may, therefore, be useful. It is also possible that specific cellular targeting of such therapy may be more beneficial than global inhibition. Preliminary animal studies suggest that the therapeutic use of anti-inflammatory cytokines such as IL-10 and IL-13 may be beneficial in sepsis, although as yet there have been no confirmatory clinical studies.

GENETICS STUDIES

Polymorphisms are variations in genes which occur in a population. They can be either single nucleotide base substitutions – point mutations – or repeated units of two nucleotides called dinucleotide repeats. Polymorphisms may be functional, such that the occurence of a specific allele may lead to, for example, greater protein expression or increased disease susceptibility.

Polymorphisms have been identified for genes for several cytokines and their receptors. In postsurgical patients who have sepsis, homozygotes for the TNFB2– allele had higher TNF-α levels than heterozygotes and were more likely to die from sepsis, strongly suggesting that regulatory polymorphisms of the gene for TNF-α can affect outcome from severe infection. An allele of polymorphism in the gene for the IL-1RA is associated with raised IL-1RA concentrations in patients who have sepsis. The gene for the anti-inflammatory cytokine IL-10 has been assigned to chromosome 1q31, and a functional dinucleotide repeat polymorphism has been identified in the promoter region. The relationship with levels of IL-10 in sepsis is not known. Low-frequency polymorphisms for the IL-6 receptor (IL-6R) gene have been reported in a small group of healthy subjects but there have been no studies of the genetics of these mediators in sepsis. The soluble form of IL-6R, which binds IL-6 and mediates IL-6 signaling through interaction with gp130, may modulate biologic activities of IL-6 in a range of pathologic conditions. Outcome in sepsis has been linked to levels of IL-6, IL-10 and IL-1RA, but there have been no studies investigating the role of these polymorphisms in the outcome from sepsis.

Studies of mice that have been rendered genetically deficient in TNF receptors (TNFRs) or in intercellular cell adhesion molecule 1 (ICAM-1) have revealed the critical role of these molecules in septic shock. These and other experiments suggest that there are differences in the molecular and cellular mechanisms underlying shock induced by endotoxins and exotoxins. Results from these experiments are however, occasionally different from those generated in experiments that use blocking antibodies against the same inflammatory mediators. Also mice are relatively resistant to bacterial toxins, and septic shock in mice may not represent the situation in humans. Nevertheless, a high dose of toxin in mice (the 'high-dose endotoxin' model) might correlate with a substantially lower dose in human shock, Furthermore, it is possible to sensitize mice dramatically to low doses of toxin by impairing their liver metabolism with D-galactosamine (D-Gal) (the 'low-dose endotoxin' model). This model could be relevant to the human situation when recurrent episodes of sepsis are combined with organ failure.

Deficiency of the gene encoding ICAM-1 renders mice resistant to the lethal effects of high-dose LPS. Because levels of TNF and IL-1 after LPS injection are similar to those in the wild-type mice, the protection appears to be distal to the event triggering cytokine production. $TNFR_1$-deficient mice are not protected against lethality, which suggests the involvement of other TNF–TNFR signaling pathways (the same is true of $TNFR_2$-deficient mice). Mice incapable of making IL-1 are markedly protected in the high-dose LPS model.

The increased susceptibility of rodents to TNF-induced lethality after pretreatment with D-Gal was shown to be largely a consequence of a relative and selective liver failure. D-Gal acts as a specific transcriptional inhibitor in hepatocytes. This sensitizes the hepatocyte to the cytotoxic action of TNF and induces death by apoptosis. Transcriptionally arrested primary hepatocytes from $TNFR_1$-deficient mice were found to be protected from TNF-induced apoptosis and these mice showed no signs of liver failure in *in vivo* experiments. Mice deficient in ICAM-1 and IL-1 mice are not resistant to low doses of LPS after D-Gal pretreatment, and ICAM deficiency does not decrease macrophage activation as reflected by normal TNF production. These experiments underlie the importance of TNF in this process.

Future immunogenetic therapy

Because cytokines are potent bioactive molecules, it is not surprising that their production is tightly regulated at several steps. Cytokines exert their effects by binding to their membrane receptors and activating intracellular signal transduction pathways, leading to alterations in targeted cells. Each of these steps may be a target for therapeutic manipulation. In addition, there are soluble receptors and receptor antagonists that modulate cytokine effects. Future therapeutic options for modulating the inflammatory response include neutralizing antibodies to block cytokine inducers, proinflammatory cytokines, and their cell-surface receptors; blocking the interaction between cytokines and cell-surface receptors with naturally expressed molecules; enhancing protective activities in target cells; and the intracellular blockade of cytokine-induced responses.

Gene therapy is a therapeutic approach by which a recombinant gene is introduced into the cells of patients. These genes can then synthesize a novel or missing/defective gene product *in vivo*. The use of genes as drugs, or in combination with drug therapy, to enhance anti-inflammatory responses has tremendous potential in critical care. The first step in the use of gene therapy is to introduce the gene of interest into the target cell. Two general categories of gene transfer vectors have been developed: viral and nonviral. In viral vectors, adenovirus or retrovirus DNA is modified to incorporate the therapeutic gene. The virus then acts as a shuttle for the gene; since the virus can self-replicate, this can be a very efficient mode of transfection. Nonviral vectors include liposomes and molecular conjugates, which exploit endogenous transport systems to permit efficient delivery of the therapeutic gene into the cell. Examples of gene transfers tested in sepsis models include IL-10, soluble TNFR, the antioxidant enzymes superoxide dismutase and catalase, the antiprotease α_1-antitrypsin, and heat-shock proteins (particularly HSP72).

Identification and targeting of those patients likely to benefit from modulation of the inflammatory response may be possible through analysis of polymorphisms of genes of relevant mediators, cytokines, receptors, and antagonists. The future may present a scenario of full genetic screening on admission to the ICU in order to determine the most appropriate therapeutic strategy.

Key References

Bone RC, Balk RA, Cerra FB, et al. American College of Chest Physicians/Society of Critical Care Medicine Consensus Conference: definitions for sepsis and organ failure and guidelines for the use of innovative therapies in sepsis. Crit Care Med. 1992;20:864–74.

Galley HF, Webster NR. The immuno-inflammatory cascade. Br J Anaesth. 1996;77:11–16.

Goode HF, Webster NR. Free radicals and antioxidants in sepsis. Crit Care Med. 1993;21:1770–6.

Lamy M, Thijs LG, eds. Mediators of sepsis. Berlin: Springer-Verlag; 1992:124–35.

Liu M, Slutsky AS. Anti-inflammatory therapies: application of molecular biology techniques in intensive care medicine. Int Care Med. 1997;23:718–31.

Parillo JE. Pathogenic mechanisms of septic shock. N Engl J Med. 1993;328:1471–7.

Tracey KJ, Cerami A. Tumor necrosis factor and regulation of metabolism in infection: role of systemic versus tissue levels. Proc Soc Exp Biol Med. 1992;200:233–9.

Further Reading

Tracey KJ, Cerami A. Tumor necrosis factor: a pleiotropic cytokine and therapeutic target. Annu Rev Med. 1994;45:491–503.

van der Poll T, Lowry SF. Tumor necrosis factor in sepsis; mediator of multiple organ failure or essential part of host defense? Shock. 1995;3:1–12.

Finding Medical Resources on the Internet

Keith J Ruskin

The Internet can be used to gather or distribute information about clinical, scientific, and academic issues. It is used by anesthesiologists around the world to exchange information, between institutions and across time zones and international boundaries. Physicians go online to discuss patient care, to improve medical care in developing nations, and to exchange information about new technology and pharmaceuticals and regulatory issues. Moreover, physicians who share a problem or a similar interest can exchange ideas, and even build a 'virtual community'. The Internet also makes it possible to use resources (e.g., literature searches) from the operating room, from home, or even from an airplane.

Electronic publications play an increasingly important role in medical education, research, and clinical practice. The quality of pictures, sound, and video produced by new, multimedia-equipped computers is rapidly improving, and low cost, wide availability, and ease of use make this technology a potentially valuable tool for clinicians and researchers. The Internet offers a unique opportunity to create a truly global specialty. Moreover, the Internet is growing at a rapid rate, and new resources, which offer new ways to learn and to communicate, are added almost daily. Electronic publication is rapidly maturing, and will probably become the predominant method of communication among medical professionals. The ultimate acceptance of electronic publication depends upon the creation of high-quality, secure resources with clearly identified authors, publishers, and references. The most pressing concern for consumers of electronic medical literature is, therefore, the accuracy and timeliness of the information.

Internet resources are accessed using a variety of computer programs referred to collectively as *Internet services*. Internet services can be divided into two broad classifications. *Basic services* are primarily text-based, and were the first applications to be developed for the Internet; they include a terminal program (telnet), the file transfer protocol (FTP), and electronic mail (email). *Advanced services* include the World Wide Web (WWW) and teleconferencing, and take advantage of the graphical user interface provided by Microsoft Windows, the Apple Macintosh, and other computer operating systems. Even more sophisticated services, such as interactive documents, teleconferencing, and video on demand, are being introduced at a rapid pace. New resources are being added to the Internet each day, while other resources are moved to a new location or removed entirely. This can make finding information on nearly any topic difficult.

Many Internet 'search engines' offer assistance with finding information on a particular topic. Because each of these uses a different strategy for searching for and cataloging information, and because each search engine has a slightly different interface, the information that is returned depends largely on the specific keywords used and on the person who is using the engine. Moreover, some search engines now offer to place web sites higher in the list of sites returned for a particular key word for a fee. Alta Vista (http://www.altavista.com) attempts to find web sites that contain the specific key words typed in by the user. Higher weighting is given to keywords that are contained as 'meta' tags and also to words contained in titles or headings. Excite (http://www.excite.com) attempts to determine the concept that a user is searching for, and returns sites that match a concept, rather than a specific word (e.g., searching for 'hyperpyrexia' might return a page about malignant hyperthermia). Yahoo (http://www.yahoo.com) offers lists of links that represent particularly good starting points on a given subject. Search sites such as Metacrawler (http://www.metacrawler.com) offer an interesting solution to the problems listed above: Metacrawler submits a search phrase to a variety of search engines, compiles the results, and ranks results according to consistent high rankings from the other searches.

One potential solution to the problem of finding high-quality medical sites is external rating. WWW sites are rated according to specific criteria by an external organization. Most rating sites, such as LookSmart (http://www.looksmart.com) and BioMedNet (http://www.biomednet.com), award a single 'medallion' to sites that they have selected. This medallion is then displayed on the site, and a link to reviewed sites is provided from the rating service. Users can then choose to visit only health-related resources that have been rated highly by a well-known organization. Health rating services that evaluate resources and provide some indication of relative value by awarding stars or medals are being developed. However, current external rating systems have problems. In one recent study, popular rating services failed to publish the criteria that they use to rate sites, and the ratings themselves tend to be based on subjective evaluation.

The Health on the Net Foundation (http://www.hon.ch/) is an organization that promotes and evaluates health-related Internet resources. This organization offers a voluntary code of conduct (HONcode) that specifically describes how medical resources should be created and maintained. It also undertakes other initiatives such as monitoring medical use of the Internet, creation of specialized search engines, and hosting WWW sites for other related organizations. About.com (http://www.about.com/) offers a unique solution to the problem of searching for anything on the Internet. Instead of employing text mining software to determine the content of a Web site, About.com employs subject experts who create a web site that contains lists of links, preferred resources, and a chat area.

Medical Internet resources now number in the thousands. Independent organizations, academic medical centers, individuals, publishers, and corporations have all created WWW sites for the medical profession. Some of these resources have been developed especially for electronic media while others have been adapted from printed materials. Because of the rapidly changing structure of the WWW, it is impossible to offer a comprehensive listing of medical Internet resources. Some resources, however, have demonstrated longevity, and are good starting points or demonstrate the unique advantages of electronic publication.

World-Wide Web Resources

ACCRI (Anesthesia and Critical Care Resources on the Internet; http://www.eur.nl/fgg/anest/wright/) is a comprehensive database of nearly every anesthesiology or critical care resource on the Internet. It is maintained by A. J. Wright, a librarian at the University of Alabama at Birmingham, who updates the database almost daily.

The American Society of Anesthesiologists Web site (http://www.asahq.org/) contains information about the Society, including programs and abstracts of the Annual Meeting, information about anesthesiology for lay persons, ASA press releases, and more. It also contains links to Component Societies and anesthesiology resources on the Internet. *Anesthesiology* (http://www.anesthesiology.org/), the scientific journal of the American Society of Anesthesiologists, has a web site with tables of contents of both past and future issues, abstracts of journal articles, and information for authors.

GASNet (http://gasnet.med.yale.edu) is an anesthesia resource created by the author. It contains an on-line journal of anesthesia, pre-published abstracts of journal articles, digests of several discussion groups, a video library, links to anesthesia resources on the Internet, and more.

The Web site of the Malignant Hyperthermia Association of the United States (http://www.mhaus.org/) offers information about MH addressed both to lay people and physicians, including their MH emergency management poster, MH brochures, and information about the MH consultants group.

The National Library of Medicine (http://www.nlm.nih.gov/) now provides free access to MEDLINE via the WWW (http://www.ncbi.nlm.nih.gov/pubmed/).

The Physicians Desk Reference (http://www.pdr.net/) is available free of charge to any physician. Registration is required, and users should note that their email address will be shared with third parties unless they specifically request that their information not be distributed.

The Virtual Anaesthetia Textbook is the project of a team of anesthesiologists (http://www.usyd.edu.au/su/anaes/VAT/), led by Chris Thompson, to categorize and review medical information on the Internet. Individual Web sites are organized into 'chapters' on a given topic.

Mailing Lists

The *GASNet* Anesthesiology Discussion Group is one example of a mailing list designed specifically for anesthesiology professionals. It currently has 2,800 subscribers; its members are located in countries around the world. Topics of discussion range from political developments to questions about patient care or research. Information about the Anesthesiology Discussion Group, as well as digests of all messages since 1993, is available at http://gasnet.med.yale.edu/discussion/anesthesiology.

CCM-L is a moderated mailing list that is used by anesthesiologists and intensivists to discuss clinical care, research, politics, and other subjects. Regular features of the list include the Case of the Week, Ethical Dilemmas, and a Journal Club. The list is moderated by David W Crippen, MD at the University of Pittsburgh. To subscribe to the list, send the command *subscribe ccm-l* to majordomo@list.pitt.edu.

Of the several pediatric anesthesia mailing lists, one on pediatric anesthesia and one on pediatric pain management are particularly helpful to clinicians and researchers. The Pediatric Pain mailing list is maintained by Allen Finley, and has an archive of messages available to subscribers. To subscribe to this list, send the command *sub pediatric-pain* to mailserv@ac.dal.ca. To subscribe to the Pediatric Anesthesia mailing list, which is maintained by Jim Tibbals at the Hospital for Sick Children in Toronto, Canada, send the command subscribe pac to majordomo@anaes.sickkids.on.ca.

TRAUMA-L is a mailing list maintained by Ernest Block for the discussion of all aspects of trauma, including surgery, anesthesiology, and critical care. To subscribe, send the command subscribe *trauma-l [your name]* to listserv@listserv.lsumc.edu.

Index

Page numbers suffixed by 'i' refer to illustrations

A

B

C

D

E

F

G

H

I

M

Q

R

S

T